Handbook of

Geriatric Drug Therapy

Springhouse Corporation
Springhouse, Pennsylvania

Staff

Senior Publisher
Donna O. Carpenter

Editorial Director
William J. Kelly

Clinical Director
Ann M. Barrow, RN, MSN, CCRN

Design Director
John Hubbard

Art Director
Elaine Kasmer Ezrow

Drug Information Editor
Lisa Truong, RPh, PharmD

Associate Editor
Stacey Ann Follin

Clinical Project Editor
Eileen Cassin Gallen, RN, BSN

Editors
Laura Ninger, Joanne Poeggel

Clinical Editors
Theresa P. Fulginiti, RN, BSN, CEN; Pamela S. Messer, RN, MSN; Lori Musolf Neri, RN, MSN, CCRN; Kimberly A. Zalewski, RN, MSN, CEN

Copy Editors
Karen C. Comerford (manager), Colleen Coady, Leslie Dworkin, Karen Stover

Designers
Arlene Putterman (associate design director), Joseph John Clark, Jacalyn Facciolo, Donald G. Knauss, Mary Ludwicki

Typographers
Diane Paluba (manager), Joyce Rossi Biletz

Manufacturing
Deborah Meiris (director), Patricia K. Dorshaw (manager), Otto Mezei (book production manager)

Editorial Assistants
Arlene P. Claffee, Carol A. Caputo

Dr., Danvers, MA 01923. For those organizations that have been granted a photocopy license by CCC, a separate system of payment has been arranged. The fee code for users of the Transactional Reporting Service is 0874349982/00 $00.00 + $.75. Printed in the United States of America.

A member of the Reed Elsevier plc group

Visit our Web site at www.eDrugInfo.com

HGDT–D   N   O   S   A   J   J   M   A   M
03 02 01 00 10 9 8 7 6 5 4 3 2 1
ISBN 0-87434-998-2

Library of Congress Cataloging-in-Publication Data

Handbook of geriatric drug therapy.
   p. cm.
   Includes index.
   1. Geriatric pharmacology–Handbooks,
   manuals, etc.
RC953.7.H36 2000
615.5'8'0846–dc21   99-058888
ISBN 0-87434-998-2 (lexotone,
3-color cover, flex case)   CIP

Contents

Contributors

Christine Arenson, MD
Clinical Assistant Professor of Family
Medicine and Assistant Director of
Geriatric Fellowship
Jefferson Medical College,
Philadelphia, Pa.

Rebecca E. Boehne, RN, PhD
Patient & Family Education Coordinator
Portland VA Medical Center,
Portland, Ore.

Melvin L. Butler, MD, FACP
Staff Physician/Medical Coordinator
Baylor Senior Health Care, Bedford, Tex.

James M. Camamo, PharmD
Clinical Specialist for Medication
Information and Policy Development
University Medical Center, Tucson, Ariz.

Lawrence Carey, PharmD
Clinical Pharmacist Supervisor
Jefferson Home Infusion Service
Philadelphia, Pa.

Toni M. Cutson, MD, MHS
Assistant Clinical Professor
Duke University Medical Center &
GRECC Durham VA Medical Center
Durham, N.C.

Jennifer L. Defilippi, PharmD
Clinical Psychiatric Specialist
Central Texas Veterans Health Care
System, Waco, Tex.

David M. DiPersio, BS, PharmD, BCPS
Clinical Pharmacist, Critical Care
Vanderbilt University Medical Center
Nashville, Tenn.
Assistant Clinical Professor
University of Tennessee

Beverly Sigl Felten, RN,CS, MS, ARNP
President
Gero-Psych Nursing, S.C., Lannon, Wis.

Geriann B. Gallagher, APRN, ND
Gerontological Nurse Practitioner
Rehabilitation Hospital of Connecticut/
St. Francis Care, Hartford, Conn.

Cynthia A. Gobin, PharmD
Clinical Assistant Professor
Temple University School of Pharmacy,
Philadelphia, Pa.

Mildred D. Gottwald, PharmD
Assistant Clinical Professor
Department of Clinical Pharmacy
University of California, San Francisco

Ronald L. Greenberg, RPh, PharmD, BCPS
Clinical Pharmacy Coordinator
Fairview Ridges Hospital,
Burnsville, Minn.

Tatyana Gurvich, PharmD
Clinical Pharmacologist
Glendale Adventist Family Practice
Residency Program, Glendale, Calif.

Barbara S. Kannewurf, BS Pharm, PharmD
Clinical Fellow, Virginia Commonwealth
University Medical College of Virginia
Campus, Richmond, Va.

Thomas E. Lackner, PharmD, CGP, FASCP
Professor of Geriatrics
College of Pharmacy, University of
Minnesota, Minneapolis, Minn.
Director of Clinical Services
Institute of Geriatric Pharmacotherapy,
University of Minnesota

Lawrence A. Lemchen, RPh, FASCP
General Manager
PharMerica, Kent, Wash.

Ellen J. Mangin, MSN, CRNP, CS
Director of Resident Services
Rydal Park, Rydal, Pa.

Rein Tideiksaar, PhD, PA-C
Clinical Program Director
Southwest Medical Associates,
Las Vegas, Nev.

Candy Tsourounis, PharmD
Assistant Clinical Professor
University of California
School of Pharmacy, San Francisco

Grace E. Wert, RN,CS, MSN
Gerontological Clinical Nurse Specialist
Abington Memorial Hospital,
Abington, Pa.

Peter S. Yoon, PharmD, CGP
Consultant Pharmacist Supervisor
PharMerica, San Marino, Calif.

Foreword

I vividly recall my terror as a student nurse in 1970 when I prepared drugs for a geriatric patient for the first time, while my instructor looked over my shoulder. Quickly shuffling 15 3" x 5" handwritten drug cards, I attempted to answer my instructor's rapid-fire questions about each drug's mechanism of action and adverse effects. After this intense grilling, I faced a bigger hurdle: administering 15 oral drugs to an 80-year-old patient on fluid restriction.

Some 12 years later, I completed a geriatric nurse practitioner (GNP) program and found myself responsible not only for administering drugs but also for prescribing them. Though drug management was a critical element of the GNP program and the risks associated with polypharmacy in geriatric patients were well explained, few references dedicated to geriatric pharmacology were available.

How I wish that in both of these circumstances I could have turned to the book you now hold in your hands, the *Handbook of Geriatric Drug Therapy*.

The introductory chapters provide a solid foundation in geriatric pharmacology. They take an in-depth look at the physiologic changes associated with aging and the impact these changes have on drug absorption, distribution, metabolism, and excretion. These chapters also look at the issues that affect patient compliance with drug therapy—and offer practical steps for improving compliance.

Comprehensive profiles of the drugs most commonly prescribed for geriatric patients are arranged alphabetically, making it quicker and easier for you to evaluate your patient's current drug regimen as well as his drug history. The text within each profile is current, concise, and well organized, providing dosage adjustments, patient-teaching points, and key age-specific information to help you better meet the special needs of your geriatric patient.

The full-color photoguide of actual-sized tablets and capsules and the appendices, which gather in one place some of the most relevant geriatric reference information available, complete the book—making *Handbook of Geriatric Drug Therapy* a "must have" for all health care professionals working with geriatric patients. With this invaluable resource, you too can spend less time reviewing drugs and more time teaching your patient about them.

Kathleen Fletcher, RN, CS, MSN, GNP
Director Geriatric Services
University of Virginia Health System
Charlottesville, Va.

How to use this book

The *Handbook of Geriatric Drug Therapy* provides exhaustively reviewed, completely updated, detailed information on drugs commonly prescribed for geriatric patients. It covers all aspects of drug information from fundamental pharmacology to specific management of adverse and toxic reactions. It also includes several features—a comprehensive listing of indications that includes clinically approved but unlabeled uses and specific dosing recommendations for geriatric patients.

GENERIC DRUG ENTRIES

Drug entries are arranged alphabetically by generic name and are complete, eliminating the need for cross-referencing to other sections of the book. A guide word at the top of each page identifies the generic drug presented on that page.

In each drug entry, the generic name (with alternate generic names following in parentheses) precedes an alphabetically arranged list of current trade names. (An asterisk signals products available only in Canada.)

Next come pharmacologic and therapeutic classifications. Listing both classifications helps the reader grasp the multiple, varying, and sometimes overlapping uses of drugs within a single pharmacologic class and among different classes. When appropriate, the next line identifies drugs regulated under the jurisdiction of the Controlled Substances Act of 1970. These drugs are divided into the following groups, or schedules:

- Schedule I (C-I): High abuse potential and no accepted medical use—for example, heroin, marijuana, and LSD.
- Schedule II (C-II): High abuse potential with severe dependence liability—for example, narcotics, amphetamines, and some barbiturates. Emergency telephone orders for limited quantities of these drugs are authorized but the prescriber must provide a written signed prescription order to the pharmacy within 72 hours.

- Schedule III (C-III): Less abuse potential than schedule II drugs and moderate dependence liability—for example, nonbarbiturate sedatives, nonamphetamine stimulants, anabolic steroids, and limited amounts of certain narcotics. Telephone orders are permitted for these drugs.
- Schedule IV (C-IV): Less abuse potential than schedule III drugs and limited dependence liability—for example, some sedatives, anxiolytics, and nonnarcotic analgesics. Telephone orders are permitted for these drugs.
- Schedule V (C-V): Limited abuse potential. Primarily small amounts of narcotics, such as codeine, used as antitussives or antidiarrheals. Under federal law, limited quantities of certain C-V drugs may be purchased without a prescription directly from a pharmacist if allowed under specific state statutes. The purchaser must be at least age 18 and must furnish suitable identification. The dispensing pharmacist must record all such transactions.

The next line lists the preparations available for each drug (for example, tablets, capsules, solution, or injection), specifying available dosage forms and strengths.

Indications & dosage presents all accepted indications for use with general dosage recommendations for adults and geriatric patients; dosage adjustments for specific patient groups, such as patients with renal or hepatic impairment, are included when appropriate. Note that specific usage and dosing guidelines for geriatric patients haven't been established for most drugs. For individual application, dosage must be considered in light of the patient's condition and clinical status. Because age-related changes can affect drug therapy, dosages for geriatric patients should begin low in comparison to those for adult patients, and adjustments should be made slowly and gradually, based on the patient's response. An open diamond signals a clinically accepted but unlabeled use. Dosage instructions reflect current trends in therapeutics and shouldn't be considered as absolute, standard recommendations.

Pharmacodynamics explains the mechanism and effects of the drug's physiologic action.

Pharmacokinetics describes absorption, distribution, metabolism, and excretion of the drug, along with the kinetic changes of the drug as a result of age-related physiologic changes in the geriatric patient; it specifies onset and duration of action, peak levels, and half-life as appropriate.

Contraindications & precautions lists conditions associated with special risks in patients who receive the drug.

Interactions specifies significant additive, synergistic, or antagonistic effects that result from combined use of the drug with other drugs, foods, and lifestyle (such as smoking or alcohol use), along with specific suggestions or actions to take to manage the interaction. The interacting agent is italicized.

Adverse reactions lists the undesirable effects that may follow use of the drug; these effects are arranged by body systems (CNS, CV, EENT, GI, GU, Hematologic, Hepatic, Metabolic, Musculoskeletal, Respiratory, Skin, and Other). Local effects occur at the site of drug administration (by application, infusion, or injection); adverse reactions not specific to a single body system (for example, the effects of hypersensitivity) are listed under Other. Throughout, the most common adverse reactions (those experienced by at least 10% of people taking the drug in clinical trials) are in *italic* type; less common reactions are in roman type; life-threatening reactions are in **bold italic** type; and reactions that are both common and life-threatening are in BOLD CAPITAL letters. At the end of this section, Note signals a list of severe and hazardous reactions that mandate discontinuation of the drug.

Key considerations offers detailed recommendations specific to the drug for the geriatric patient along with drug preparation and administration; patient education about drug therapy; and pertinent information for drug overdose or significant interference with a diagnostic test. This section includes geriatric-specific recommendations for monitoring the effects of drug therapy, for preventing and treating adverse reactions or drug overdose, for promoting patient comfort, and for storing the drug.

PHOTOGUIDE

This extensive section provides full-color photographs of more than 300 of the most commonly prescribed tablets and capsules in the United States. Shown in actual size, the tablets and capsules are organized alphabetically for quick reference.

APPENDICES

Appendices offer information on adverse effects commonly misinterpreted as age-related changes, components of analgesic combination products, age-related changes in laboratory values, and methods for calculating creatinine clearance. They also include guidelines for using antipsychotics, anxiolytics, sedatives, and other drugs in long-term care facilities and resources for geriatric care.

INDEX

The index lists both the generic and trade names, diseases, and pharmacologic classes. Generic drugs and pharmacologic classes appear alphabetically within the main text.

A guide to abbreviations

ACE	angiotensin-converting enzyme	IU	international unit
ADH	antidiuretic hormone	I.V.	intravenous
AIDS	acquired immunodeficiency syndrome	kg	kilogram
		LD	lactate dehydrogenase
ALT	alanine aminotransferase	M	molar
APTT	activated partial thromboplastin time	m^2	square meter
AST	aspartate aminotransferase	MAO	monoamine oxidase
AV	atrioventricular	mcg	microgram
b.i.d.	twice daily	mEq	millequivalent
BPH	benign prostatic hyperplasia	mg	milligram
BUN	blood urea nitrogen	MI	myocardial infarction
cAMP	cyclic 38, 58 adenosine monophosphate	ml	milliliter
		mm^3	cubic millimeter
CBC	complete blood count	msec	millisecond
CK	creatine kinase	Na	sodium
CMV	cytomegalovirus	NaCl	sodium chloride
CNS	central nervous system	NG	nasogastric
COPD	chronic obstructive pulmonary disease	NSAID	nonsteroidal anti-inflammatory drug
		OTC	over the counter
CSF	cerebrospinal fluid	PABA	para-aminobenzoic acid
CV	cardiovascular	PCA	patient-controlled analgesia
CVA	cerebrovascular accident	P.O.	by mouth
D_5W	dextrose 5% in water	P.R.	by rectum
DIC	disseminated intravascular coagulation	p.r.n.	as needed
		PT	prothrombin time
DNA	deoxyribonucleic acid	PTT	partial thromboplastin time
ECG	electrocardiogram	PVC	premature ventricular contraction
EEG	electroencephalogram		
EENT	eyes, ears, nose, throat	q	every
FDA	Food and Drug Administration	q.d.	every day
g	gram	q.i.d.	four times daily
G	gauge	RBC	red blood cell
GFR	glomerular filtration rate	RDA	recommended daily allowance
GGT	gamma-glutamyltransferase	REM	rapid eye movement
GI	gastrointestinal	RNA	ribonucleic acid
gtt	drops	RSV	respiratory syncytial virus
GU	genitourinary	SA	sinoatrial
G6PD	glucose-6-phosphate dehydrogenase	S.C.	subcutaneous
H_1	histamine₁	SIADH	syndrome of inappropriate antidiuretic hormone
H_2	histamine₂		
HIV	human immunodeficiency virus	S.L.	sublingual
hr	hour	T_3	triiodothyronine
h.s.	at bedtime	T_4	thyroxine
ICU	intensive care unit	t.i.d.	three times daily
I.D.	intradermal	U	units
I.M.	intramuscular	USP	United States Pharmacopeia
IND	investigational new drug	UTI	urinary tract infection
INR	international normalized ratio	WBC	white blood cell
IPPB	intermittent positive-pressure breathing		

Geriatric patients require more drugs than patients in other age-groups. With four of five patients older than age 65 having at least one chronic disorder, geriatric patients receive 30% to 40% of all prescriptions issued. That's about 400 million prescriptions a year.

Although drug therapy can extend and enhance a patient's quality of life, many factors can complicate it, including diminished physiological function, chronic disorders and, consequently, altered pharmacokinetics. To ensure that drug therapy is safe and effective, dosages should be adjusted as needed and patients closely monitored.

This chapter defines *aging,* describes changes in the body that affect drug therapy, and explains the way advancing age affects how the body absorbs, distributes, metabolizes, and excretes drugs.

Aging

Aging can be described chronologically, physiologically, and functionally.

Chronological age measures a person's age by the number of years lived. The most commonly used objective method for identifying and measuring age, it also establishes eligibility for such activities as driving, employment, and collection of retirement benefits. Age 65 is the accepted age for attaining senior citizen status in the United States, and according to the Social Security Act and Medicare, age 62 is the minimum age of eligibility for retirement benefits and age 65 is the standard age of eligibility for full retirement benefits. Yet, old age can be further divided into chronological categories—young-old (ages 65 to 74), middle-old (ages 75 to 84), and old-old (ages 85 and older).

Physiological age measures a person's age according to body function. Mental capacity, sensory perception, and organ and body system function provide the basis for this measurement. However, age-related physiological changes affect different patients at different times, and you can't reliably determine a patient's chronological age from his physiological age.

Functional age measures a person's age by his ability to contribute to society and benefit others and himself. It's based on the premise that chronological age doesn't dictate the level of function. Some people remain physically fit, mentally active, productive members of society beyond age 80 or 90. Others decline physically and functionally much earlier. The fastest growing segment of the geriatric population is ages 75 and older. About 25% of those ages 75 to 84 and about 50% of those ages 85 and older who aren't institutionalized need help with daily activities, including overcoming physical barriers to drug therapy.

Drug therapy in the aging body

Older bodies tend to work less efficiently than younger ones, but illness doesn't inevitably accompany old age. Although aging shouldn't be equated with the unavoidable breakdown of body systems, the gradual changes in body function that normally occur with aging should be considered when initiating and adjusting drug therapy. (See *How age affects drug action,* on page 2.)

Central nervous system changes

Aging affects the CNS in many ways. After age 50, brain cells decrease by about 1% per year, but effects usually aren't noticeable until the patient is older. About 20% of the neurons in the cerebral cortex are lost. Neurons of the central and peripheral nervous systems deteriorate. Nerve transmission slows, causing prolonged reaction time to external stimuli. Homeostasis becomes harder to maintain, causing decreased or inadequate recovery from stress. Short-term memory changes diminish the patient's capacity to process and retain new information, such as new drug regimens.

How age affects drug action

As the body ages, body structures and systems change, affecting how the body responds to drugs. Here are some changes that commonly and significantly affect drug therapy.

Body composition
As a person grows older, total body and lean body mass tend to decrease, whereas body fat tends to increase. Total body water decreases, and the amount of plasma albumin available for binding with drugs diminishes. These factors affect the relationship between drug level and solubility in the body.

Digestive system
Decreases in gastric acid secretion and GI motility can significantly reduce the body's ability to absorb many drugs well. This can cause problems with certain drugs, such as digoxin, that have a narrow therapeutic range closely tied to absorption.

Hepatic system
Advancing age almost always reduces the blood supply to the liver, and certain liver enzymes become less active. As a result, the liver loses some of its ability to metabolize drugs. With reduced liver function, higher drug levels remain in circulation, causing more intense drug effects and increasing the risk of drug toxicity.

Renal system
Kidney function also diminishes with age as a result of decreased cardiac output. This alone may impair drug elimination by 50% or more. In many cases, decreased kidney function leads to increased blood levels of certain drugs.

As a result of these changes, CNS drugs sometimes act unpredictably in geriatric patients. And drugs with adverse CNS effects commonly aggravate existing conditions, causing additional signs or symptoms.

Visual changes
With age, the eyes undergo several changes. The cornea loses its luster and flattens. The iris fades or develops irregular pigmentation. The sphincter muscles may undergo sclerosis because of increased connective tissue. The pupil becomes smaller, decreasing the amount of light that reaches the retina. The lens enlarges and loses transparency and elasticity. The cones in the retina deteriorate.

As a result, many geriatric patients have impaired color vision, especially with blues and greens. Furthermore,

changes in visual acuity and color perception may make it difficult for them to self-administer drugs. If they're unable to read their drug labels, they may misidentify drugs of similar size and color, they may be unable to see syringe markings, and they may administer the drugs inaccurately.

Aural changes
Because aging causes degenerative structural changes throughout the auditory system, many geriatric patients suffer from an irreversible, bilateral, sensorineural hearing loss called presbycusis, or senile deafness. Affecting more men than women, this problem usually starts during middle age and slowly worsens. The most common cause is atrophy of the organ of Corti and the auditory nerve. The accompanying hearing loss mostly af-

fects high-pitched sounds. By age 60, most patients have difficulty hearing above 4,000 Hz. (The normal range for speech recognition is 500 to 2,000 Hz.)

Respiratory changes

Pulmonary function decreases with age. Respiratory muscles deteriorate and atrophy. The diffusing capacity of the lungs declines. Vital capacity diminishes because inspiratory and expiratory muscles weaken. Lung tissue deteriorates, decreasing elastic recoil and resulting in an elevated residual volume. Because some airways close, basal areas are poorly ventilated, resulting in decreased surface area for gas exchange and reduced partial pressure of oxygen. So partial pressure of oxygen in arterial blood decreases to 70 to 85 mm Hg, and oxygen saturation decreases by 5%.

Furthermore, the lungs become more rigid, and the number and size of alveoli decline. Respiratory fluids are reduced by 30%, which increases the risk of pulmonary infection and mucus plugs. Thus, maximum breathing capacity, forced vital capacity, vital capacity, and inspiratory reserve volume diminish with age, leaving the geriatric patient less tolerant of oxygen debt.

Cardiovascular changes

As the myocardium of the aging heart becomes more irritable, extra systoles, sinus arrhythmias, and sinus bradycardia occur. More fibrous tissue infiltrates the sinoatrial node and internodal atrial tracts, which may cause atrial fibrillation and flutter. The veins also dilate and stretch with age, and coronary artery blood flow decreases 35% between ages 20 and 60. The aorta becomes more rigid, causing systolic blood pressure to increase disproportionately more than diastolic pressure, resulting in a widened pulse pressure. ECG changes include decreased amplitude of the QRS complex, a leftward shift of the QRS axis, and increased PR, QRS, and QT intervals.

The heart's ability to respond to physical and emotional stress also decreases markedly with age. Aging contributes to arterial and venous insufficiency as the strength and elasticity of blood vessels decrease. Additionally, baroreceptors in the carotid sinus and aortic notch progressively and significantly become less sensitive, increasing the frequency of drug-related orthostatic hypotension among geriatric patients.

Gastrointestinal changes

The physiological changes that accompany aging usually prove less debilitating in the GI system than in most other body systems. Normal changes include diminished mucosal elasticity and reduced GI secretions; as a result, digestion and absorption are altered. GI tract motility, bowel wall and anal sphincter tone, and abdominal muscle strength also may decrease with age. These changes may cause the geriatric patient to lose his appetite, become constipated, or experience other adverse effects.

Because diminished gag reflex and decreased saliva production are common in geriatric patients, it may be more difficult for them to swallow pills.

Normal physiological changes in the liver include decreased liver weight, reduced regenerative capacity, and decreased blood flow to the liver. Because levels of liver enzymes involved in oxidation and reduction markedly decline with age, the liver metabolizes and detoxifies drugs less efficiently.

Genitourinary changes

After age 40, renal function may diminish; in a 90-year-old patient, renal function may decrease by as much as 50%. This change is reflected by a decline in glomerular filtration rate, caused by age-related changes in renal vasculature that disturb glomerular hemodynamics. Renal blood flow decreases by 53% because of reduced cardiac output and age-related atherosclerotic changes. Tubular reabsorption and renal concentrating ability also decline because the size and number of functioning nephrons decrease.

Pharmacokinetics

Age changes the physical influence of drug pharmacokinetics—that is, how the

What alters drug action in geriatric patients

Differences in the way geriatric patients absorb, distribute, metabolize, and eliminate drugs can alter drug effects. The age-related differences are listed below.

Absorption
- Change in quality and quantity of digestive enzymes
- Increased gastric pH
- Decreased number of absorbing cells
- Decreased GI motility
- Decreased intestinal blood flow
- Decreased GI emptying time

Distribution
- Decreased cardiac output and reserve
- Decreased blood flow to target tissues, liver, and kidneys
- Decreased distribution space and area
- Decreased lean body mass
- Increased adipose stores
- Decreased plasma protein levels (decreased protein-binding drugs)
- Decreased total body water

Metabolism
- Decreased microsomal metabolism of drugs
- Decreased hepatic biotransformation

Elimination
- Decreased renal excretion of drugs
- Decreased respiratory and vital capacity with increased carbon dioxide retention
- Decreased number of receptors
- Variability in receptor sensitivity

drug is absorbed, distributed, metabolized, and eliminated from the body. Acute and chronic disorders exacerbate normal physiological changes in the geriatric patient. Together, these factors can increase the risk of toxic and adverse reactions and poor compliance. (See *What alters drug action in geriatric patients.*)

Absorption

Drug absorption depends on *rate of absorption,* which determines the onset of action, and *extent of absorption,* which determines the amount of drug that passes through the absorbing surface. In geriatric patients, several factors can slow drug absorption: mucosal atrophy, decreased gastric emptying, decreased gastric acid secretion, increased pH, reduced splanchnic blood flow, duodenal diverticula, and decreased GI motility. However, because absorption is slowed, oral drugs remain in the system longer, and complete absorption is still possible.

Drugs given I.M. and S.C. may have delayed absorption because of reduced blood flow and altered capillary wall permeability. However, because muscle mass generally decreases with age, a geriatric patient may absorb an I.M. injection faster than a patient in another age-group.

Distribution

Because geriatric patients have more fat and less water in their body, the distribution patterns for most drugs are different than in other patients. Therefore, a highly fat-soluble drug such as diazepam has an increased volume of distribution and a prolonged distribution phase, which prolong the half-life and duration of action. In contrast, a highly water-soluble drug such as gentamicin has a decreased volume of distribution, so more drug remains in the bloodstream, which increases the risk of toxic reaction.

Aging also reduces plasma levels of albumin, which binds and transports many drugs. As a result, more unbound drug may circulate in the bloodstream. This increases the pharmacological action of protein-bound drugs, heightening the risk of adverse and toxic drug effects. If the patient takes multiple drugs, these drugs may compete for protein-binding sites and some drugs may be displaced, resulting in increased free serum levels of the drugs.

Other factors that can alter drug distribution include declining cardiac output, dehydration, electrolyte and mineral imbalances, extremes of body weight, inactivity, poor nutrition, prolonged bed rest, and physical size. Because geriatric patients are typically smaller than younger patients, a drug dose may result in higher blood levels in a geriatric patient because he has a lower volume of fluid.

Metabolism

Drug metabolism by the liver depends primarily on blood flow and metabolic enzyme action. Because aging reduces blood flow to the liver, less drug is delivered there, and consequently, less drug is metabolized into inactive compounds. Liver enzymes metabolize drugs in two major pathways or phases, which operate less efficiently with the diminished liver mass and altered nutritional status that accompany aging. Phase I reactions (oxidation, reduction, and hydrolysis of the drug molecules) are affected more than phase II reactions (coupling of the drug or its metabolite with an acid to produce an inactive compound). Thus, drug effects differ in geriatric patients, depending on whether a drug is metabolized in phase I, phase II, or both.

Excretion

Most drugs are excreted through the kidneys. With aging, glomerular filtration and tubular secretion decline progressively. Dehydration and cardiovascular and renal diseases also impair renal function. Remember, a geriatric patient has a smaller renal reserve than a younger patient, even if BUN and serum creatinine levels are normal. In a geriatric patient with impaired drug metabolism, expect to see signs and symptoms of toxic reaction from delayed drug clearance and excretion.

Pharmacodynamics

In geriatric patients, the aging body and its role in drug-receptor or drug-organ interactions cause many of the changes in drug effect. Drugs bind to these receptors and either activate a cascade of cellular events leading to an anticipated effect or bind to receptors and block the effects of other chemicals that could potentially act on that site. Consequently, drug pharmacodynamics—the action of the drug in the body and its interaction with body tissues, organs, and cells—can be significantly different in geriatric patients.

Aging causes many receptors to function less efficiently and reduces the density of beta receptors. As a result, geriatric patients are more likely to have a toxic reaction from such beta blockers as propranolol and a diminished response to such drugs as isoproterenol. A dose of isoproterenol needed to elicit an increased heart rate of 25 beats/minute in a geriatric patient is up to six times higher than that needed in a younger patient. Aging produces a decline in parasympathetic control, which enhances the effects of anticholinergics. Receptor changes may contribute to adverse neurological effects, including such extrapyramidal adverse effects as dystonia, akathisia, and tardive dyskinesia. To compensate for pharmacodynamic changes, geriatric patients commonly need lower drug dosages.

Noncompliance with a drug regimen can inhibit therapeutic response and lead to unsuccessful treatment. Because cognitive and physical impairments prevent many geriatric patients from complying with their drug regimens, a patient should understand why a drug is important to his regimen as well as how he should take it. Also, supervision and teaching should be individualized to fit each patient's needs.

Evaluating the patient

Determine your patient's ability to comply with his drug regimen, and then intervene to prevent noncompliance. Learn about your patient's health and drug history, and determine his success with previous treatment plans. Ask him which prescription and nonprescription drugs he takes now and which he has taken in the past. If possible, ask to see samples. Have him name each drug and tell you why, when, and how often he takes it. Find out if more than one health care provider prescribes drugs for him. Also, ask if he's taking a drug originally prescribed for another person. Remember, geriatric patients typically are taking several drugs. Such multidrug therapy (called polypharmacy) can trigger synergistic, potentiated, or antagonistic effects.

Evaluate the patient's cognitive skills. Can he remember where he stores his drugs as well as when and how to take them? Assess his beliefs about drug use. For example, he may believe that long-term drug therapy implies sickness or weakness and thus may take drugs erratically. Also, evaluate his physical skills. Can he read drug labels and directions? Can he open drug containers easily?

Finally, assess his lifestyle for things that could interact with the drugs he's taking or prevent him from complying with his drug regimen. Does he consume alcohol, caffeine, or dairy products? Is he regularly exposed to the sun? Does he live alone or does he live with a debilitated spouse, family, or friends?

Monitoring drug administration

Administering drugs to a geriatric patient requires additional precautions. Use these guidelines to modify your approach:
- To maximize drug absorption, encourage a patient who must take a drug before meals to take it on an empty stomach. (Remember, geriatric patients produce less gastric acid, so they take longer to digest food.) Encourage a drug schedule that interferes little with the patient's normal activities. For example, tell him to take his diuretic early in the day so that he won't have to urinate at night.
- To prevent adverse drug interactions, advise the patient to contact his health care provider before taking nonprescription drugs. Regularly monitor serum drug levels to prevent toxic reaction.
- To avoid improper storage and possible drug deterioration, advise the patient to keep drugs in their original containers, out of direct sunlight, and in cool, dry areas (not in the bathroom medicine cabinet or near the kitchen sink). Keep in mind that some drugs deteriorate on contact with other drugs, so advise the patient to consult his pharmacist before storing drugs together. Also, the patient shouldn't store drugs on his bedside table because he may accidentally take an extra dose before he's fully awake and alert.
- To assess a patient's ability to follow a new drug regimen and to monitor his response to therapy, schedule a visiting nurse to provide follow-up care after discharge.
- To ensure the patient doesn't mistakenly continue taking a drug that has been removed from his drug regimen, instruct him to discard the drug.

Teaching the patient

Tailor your patient teaching to account for the patient's learning, motivational, and social differences. Also, keep in mind that aging affects a patient's mental capacity, sensory perception, and psychomotor function.

Changes in mental capacity

Maximize your patient's learning ability by asking him what he already knows about the drugs he's taking. Then, use concrete examples he can understand and relate to (for example, say "2 tablespoons" rather than "30 cc"). Divide instructions into short, discrete steps; wait for your patient to respond to or repeat each one; and provide written material to reinforce your oral instructions. To prevent confusion, label each drug container.

Remember that the geriatric patient may confuse words or symbols. For example, in a discussion about blood glucose levels, he might confuse the terms *hyperglycemia* and *hypoglycemia*. Wait for a response before introducing a new concept or definition, and whenever possible, use appropriate, common lay terms, such as *high blood sugar* and *low blood sugar*.

Because short-term memory decreases with age, give the patient more time to comprehend what you say, and repeat your demonstrations. Also, devise clues to help him remember information, such as colors or shapes of tablets linked to times. Repeat information if the patient seems hesitant.

Changes in sensory perception

When teaching a patient about his drug regimen, make sure he has eyeglasses, contact lenses, or other vision enhancers, such as a magnifying glass, if he needs them. Use large-print, color teaching aids; however, remember to select colors with sufficient contrast so the patient can differentiate between printed text and background. Make sure that reading lights are properly placed and supply bright but diffused light.

Also, if the patient has difficulty hearing, make sure he uses a hearing aid if he needs one. Face him when you talk. Speak slowly and clearly and in a normal tone; don't raise your voice. Remember he may nod his head and agree with what you say, even if he can't hear you.

Changes in psychomotor function

Because patients lose flexibility and fine motor skills as they age, make sure your patient is capable of opening and closing his drug containers. Make this return demonstration a requirement before discharge from a facility or on admission to a home care agency. If he can't open and close the containers and if no children live in the house, tell him to ask his pharmacist for non–child-proof drug containers.

Motivating the patient

Keep patient-teaching sessions brief. Find out about the patient's activities and lifestyle and then present your information in a way that makes it important to him. To avoid frustrating him with too much information, include just a few points in each session.

Teach the patient about his drug regimen when he is alert and ready to learn. Make sure he hasn't recently taken a drug that will impair his concentration or finished a strenuous activity that has depleted his energy. Find out his immediate concerns, and address them. Keep in mind that positive reinforcement increases a patient's confidence in his ability to comply with his prescribed drug regimen, so be supportive.

Explain how your teaching points will help your patient stay well. Some geriatric patients adapt to their conditions so well that they don't consider them problems and don't want to learn about them. To gain his confidence, ask about his sleeping, eating, and other health habits. Ask him what he knows about a technique or health care tip before you explain it. And ask about his health beliefs. Because a patient's beliefs can either reinforce or hinder your teaching, discuss the beliefs with him before you teach something new.

With the patient's permission, include family members or other caregivers in teaching sessions, and enlist their support. However, explain how important it is for the patient to participate in his own care. This might prevent family members from needlessly taking over the responsibility of administering the patient's drugs.

Other obstacles, such as a lack of resources, can sabotage your patient's motivation. If you can detect these problems, you might be able to reduce or overcome them. For example, if he can't afford the prescribed drug, help him find out if relatives or a social service agency can help. If he doesn't have transportation to the pharmacy or the health care provider's office, find out if a friend, family member, or transportation service can help.

Preventing complications

Compile a list of the patient's drugs, potential interactions, possible adverse effects, and suggested ways he can handle any adverse effects. Then, review the findings with the patient and give him the list. If he knows what to expect, he'll be more likely to comply with treatment. Advise him about specific drug-food interactions, and provide a list of foods and beverages to avoid. As your patient receives a drug—regardless of whether it's new or familiar—name it, explain its intended effect, and describe its possible adverse effects.

Encourage the patient to purchase drugs from only one pharmacy, preferably one that maintains a drug profile for each customer. Advise him to consult the pharmacist, who can warn him about potentially harmful drug-drug, drug-food, or drug-lifestyle interactions before they occur.

If the patient's forgetfulness interferes with compliance, devise a system for helping him remember to take his drugs properly. Suggest that he purchase or make a scheduling aid, such as a calendar, checklist, alarm wristwatch, or a drug container with compartments for the different times of the day and the different days of the week.

If he simply can't remember to take his drugs on time and in the right amounts or can't remember where he stored them, see if his family is able to help. If he lives alone or with a debilitated spouse, he may need continuing support from a visiting nurse or another caregiver. Refer him to appropriate community resources for supervision to avoid drug misuse.

To correct problems related to dosage form and administration, help the patient find easier ways to take the drug. For example, if he can't swallow tablets or capsules, see about switching to a liquid or powdered form of the drug or suggest that he slide the tablet down with soft foods such as applesauce. Keep in mind that some drug forms—for example, enteric-coated tablets, timed-release capsules, or sublingual or buccal tablets—shouldn't be crushed. Doing so may affect absorption and effectiveness. Also, some crushed drugs taste bitter or can stain teeth or irritate oral mucosa.

To alter eating habits that lead to noncompliance, emphasize which drugs the patient must take with food and which he must take on an empty stomach. Explain that taking some drugs on an empty stomach may cause nausea, whereas taking some drugs on a full stomach may interfere with absorption. Also, find out whether the patient eats regularly or skips meals. If he skips meals, he may be skipping doses, too. As needed, help him coordinate his drug administration schedule with his eating habits.

If mobility or transportation prevents compliance, help find a pharmacy that delivers or suggest using a mail-order prescription company. If financial considerations prevent compliance, help the patient explore new ways to manage. He may be trying to save money by not having prescriptions filled or refilled or by taking fewer doses than ordered to make the drug last longer. Also, explore ways that family members can help, or refer the patient to the social service department and appropriate community agencies. Many states have programs to help low-income, older people buy needed drugs.

abacavir sulfate
Ziagen

Nucleoside analogue reverse transcriptase inhibitor (NRTI), antiviral

Available by prescription only
Tablets: 300 mg
Oral solution: 20 mg/ml

INDICATIONS & DOSAGE
Treatment of HIV, type 1 infection
Adults: 300 mg P.O. twice daily in combination with other antiretrovirals.

PHARMACODYNAMICS
Antiviral activity: Abacavir is converted intracellularly to the active metabolite carbovir triphosphate, which inhibits the activity of HIV-1 reverse transcriptase by competing with the natural substrate deoxyguanosine triphosphate and by incorporating itself into viral DNA. Because no 3'-OH group exists in the incorporated nucleoside analogue, the 5' to 3' phosphodiester linkage essential for DNA chain elongation is prevented from forming; therefore, viral DNA growth is terminated.

PHARMACOKINETICS
Absorption: Abacavir is rapidly and extensively absorbed after oral administration; the mean absolute bioavailability of the tablet is 83%. Because food doesn't alter absorption of the drug, it can be administered without regard to meals, and because systemic exposure is comparable with both the oral solution and the tablets, they may be used interchangeably.
Distribution: About 50% of the drug binds to plasma proteins, independent of drug level. Total blood and plasma drug-related radioactivity levels are identical, demonstrating that drug readily distributes into erythrocytes.
Metabolism: Cytochrome P-450 enzymes don't metabolize the drug in any significant way. Alcohol dehydrogenase and glucuronyl transferase metabolize it

to form two metabolites that have no antiviral activity.
Excretion: Its elimination half-life in single-dose studies has been 1 to 2 hours.

CONTRAINDICATIONS & PRECAUTIONS
Contraindicated in patients with hypersensitivity to abacavir or its components. Use cautiously in patients with known risk factors for liver disease.

INTERACTIONS
Drug-lifestyle. *Alcohol* decreases elimination of abacavir, increasing overall exposure to drug. Monitor alcohol consumption. Use together cautiously.

ADVERSE REACTIONS
CNS: insomnia and sleep disorders, headache.
GI: *nausea, vomiting,* diarrhea, loss of appetite, anorexia.
Hepatic: elevated triglyceride levels.
Skin: rash.
Other: *hypersensitivity reaction,* fever.

▣ KEY CONSIDERATIONS
● Dosage selection for geriatric patients should be cautious because many of them have decreased hepatic, renal, and cardiac function or concomitant disease or are undergoing other drug therapy.
● Drug should always be used with other antiretrovirals, never alone.
● Drug therapy has caused fatal hypersensitivity reactions. Patients who develop signs or symptoms of these reactions—such as fever, skin rash, fatigue, and GI signs and symptoms such as nausea, vomiting, diarrhea, or abdominal pain—should discontinue the drug as soon as a hypersensitivity reaction is suspected and seek medical attention immediately.
● Don't restart drug therapy following a hypersensitivity reaction because within hours the patient will experience more severe signs and symptoms, possibly including life-threatening hypotension and death. Although signs and symptoms

usually appear within the first 6 weeks of treatment, they can appear anytime.

• An abacavir hypersensitivity registry makes it easy to report hypersensitivity reactions and collect information on each case. Register patients by calling 1-800-270-0425.

• Nucleoside analogues alone or in combination, including abacavir and other antiretrovirals, can cause fatal cases of lactic acidosis or severe hepatomegaly with steatosis.

• Suspend treatment in any patient who develops signs or symptoms of lactic acidosis or pronounced hepatotoxicity (which may include hepatomegaly and steatosis even if the patient doesn't have elevated transaminase levels).

• Provide patient with written information about the drug along with the warning card, which lists the signs and symptoms of a hypersensitivity reaction.

Patient education
• Tell patient if he develops signs or symptoms of hypersensitivity—such as fever; skin rash; severe tiredness; GI signs and symptoms such as nausea, vomiting, diarrhea, or stomach pain; achiness; or a generally ill feeling—to stop taking the drug and call the doctor immediately.

• Instruct patient to always carry the warning card, which summarizes the signs and symptoms of a hypersensitivity reaction.

• Explain that this drug isn't a cure for HIV infection: A patient may continue to experience HIV-related illnesses, including opportunistic infections.

• Advise patient that drug won't reduce his risk of transmitting HIV to others through sexual contact or blood contamination.

• Inform patient to remain under a doctor's care throughout drug therapy.

• Inform patient that the long-term effects of this drug are unknown at this time.

• Advise patient to take drug exactly as prescribed.

• Tell patient he may take drug without regard to meals.

acarbose
Precose

Alpha-glucosidase inhibitor, antidiabetic

Available by prescription only
Tablets: 50 mg, 100 mg

INDICATIONS & DOSAGE
Adjunct to diet to lower blood glucose levels in patients with type 2 diabetes mellitus whose hyperglycemia can't be managed by diet alone or by diet and a sulfonylurea
Adults: Initially, 25 mg P.O. t.i.d. with the first bite of each main meal. Subsequent dosage adjustment made at 4- to 8-week intervals based on 1-hour postprandial glucose levels and tolerance. Maintenance dosage is 50 to 100 mg P.O. t.i.d., depending on patient's weight. Maximum dosage for patients weighing 60 kg (132 lb) or less is 50 mg P.O. t.i.d.; for patients weighing more than 132 lb, maximum dosage is 100 mg P.O. t.i.d.

PHARMACODYNAMICS
Antidiabetic action: The ability of acarbose to the lower blood glucose level results from a competitive, reversible inhibition of pancreatic alpha-amylase and membrane-bound intestinal alpha-glucoside hydrolase enzymes. In diabetic patients, this enzyme inhibition results in delayed glucose absorption and a lowering of postprandial hyperglycemia.

PHARMACOKINETICS
Absorption: Acarbose is minimally absorbed.
Distribution: Drug acts locally in the GI tract.
Metabolism: Drug is metabolized exclusively in the GI tract, principally by intestinal bacteria and partially by digestive enzymes.
Excretion: Within 96 hours, 51% of dose is excreted in feces as unabsorbed drug. The kidneys excrete most of the absorbed drug. Plasma elimination half-life of drug is about 2 hours. Because drug is dosed orally three times daily, it doesn't accumulate in the body.

Reactions may be *common*, uncommon, *life-threatening*, or COMMON AND LIFE-THREATENING.

CONTRAINDICATIONS & PRECAUTIONS

Contraindicated in patients with hypersensitivity to acarbose, diabetic ketoacidosis, cirrhosis, inflammatory bowel disease, colonic ulceration, or partial intestinal obstruction and in those predisposed to intestinal obstruction. Also contraindicated in patients with chronic intestinal diseases from digestive or absorptive disorders, conditions that may deteriorate because of increased gas formation in the intestine, or serum creatinine levels exceeding 2 mg/dl. Use cautiously in patients with mild to moderate renal impairment.

INTERACTIONS

Drug-drug: *Calcium channel blockers, corticosteroids, estrogens, isoniazid, nicotinic acid, oral contraceptives, phenothiazines, phenytoin, sympathomimetics, thiazides and other diuretics,* and *thyroid products* may cause hyperglycemia or hypoglycemia when withdrawn. When acarbose is used with a *sulfonylurea* or *insulin,* it may increase the hypoglycemic potential of these drugs. Monitor patient's blood glucose level.

Intestinal adsorbents such as *activated charcoal* and *digestive enzyme preparations containing carbohydrate-splitting enzymes* such as *amylase* and *pancreatin* may reduce the effect of acarbose. Don't administer concomitantly.

ADVERSE REACTIONS

GI: *abdominal pain, diarrhea, flatulence.*
Hepatic: elevated serum transaminase levels particularly in dosages exceeding 50 mg t.i.d.

▣ KEY CONSIDERATIONS

● When given alone, acarbose doesn't cause hypoglycemia. However, when given with a sulfonylurea or insulin, it may increase the hypoglycemic potential of the sulfonylurea. Monitor patient receiving both drugs closely. If hypoglycemia occurs, treat only with oral glucose (dextrose) because the body absorbs it more readily than sucrose (table sugar) when given concomitantly with acarbose. Severe hypoglycemia may require I.V. glucose infusion or glucagon

administration. To prevent further episodes of hypoglycemia, dosages of acarbose and sulfonylurea may need to be adjusted.
● During periods of increased stress—such as infection, fever, surgery, or trauma—patient may require insulin therapy. During these periods, monitor patient closely for hyperglycemia.
● To determine therapeutic effectiveness of acarbose and to identify appropriate dosage, monitor patient's 1-hour postprandial plasma glucose level. Thereafter, his glycosylated hemoglobin level should be measured every 3 months. Treatment goals include decreasing both postprandial plasma glucose and glycosylated hemoglobin levels to normal or near normal by using the lowest effective dosage of acarbose, either as monotherapy or in combination with a sulfonylurea.
● Monitor serum transaminase level every 3 months during 1st year of therapy and then periodically thereafter in patients receiving more than 50 mg t.i.d. Abnormal findings may require dosage adjustment or withdrawal of drug.

Patient education
● Tell patient to take acarbose with the first bite of each of three main meals daily.
● Make sure patient understands that drug relieves symptoms but doesn't cure disease.
● Stress the importance of adhering to the prescribed diet, reducing weight, exercising, and following personal hygiene programs. Explain how and when patient should check his blood glucose level and how to recognize and treat hyperglycemia.
● If patient takes a sulfonylurea, teach him how to recognize and treat hypoglycemia—that is, with something containing oral glucose, or dextrose, rather than sucrose, or table sugar.
● Advise patient to carry medical identification to alert others that he has diabetes.

acebutolol
Sectral

Beta blocker, antihypertensive, antiarrhythmic

Available by prescription only
Capsules: 200 mg, 400 mg

INDICATIONS & DOSAGE
Hypertension
Adults: 400 mg P.O. either as a single daily dose or divided b.i.d. Patients may receive as much as 1,200 mg divided b.i.d.
Ventricular arrhythmias
Adults: 200 mg P.O. b.i.d. daily. Increase dosage to provide an adequate response. Usual daily dosage is 600 to 1,200 mg.
◇**Angina**
Adults: Initially, 200 mg b.i.d. Increase up to 800 mg daily until angina is controlled. Patients with severe angina may require higher doses.
✦ **Dosage adjustment.** Reduce dosage in geriatric patients and avoid doses over 800 mg/day. In patients with impaired renal function, if creatinine clearance is 25 to 49 ml/minute, decrease dose by 50%. If it's less than 25 ml/minute, decrease dose by 75%.

PHARMACODYNAMICS
Antihypertensive action: Exact mechanism of action is unknown. Acebutolol has cardioselective beta-blocking properties and mild intrinsic sympathomimetic activity.
Antiarrhythmic action: Drug decreases heart rate, myocardial contractility, cardiac output, and SA and AV nodal conduction velocity and prevents exercise-induced increases in heart rate.

PHARMACOKINETICS
Absorption: Acebutolol is well absorbed after oral administration. Plasma levels peak at about 2½ hours.
Distribution: Drug is about 26% protein-bound; minimal quantities are detected in CSF.
Metabolism: Drug undergoes extensive first-pass metabolism in the liver; levels of its major active metabolite, diacetolol, peak within about 3½ hours.
Excretion: Between 30% and 40% of a given dose is excreted in urine; the rest is excreted in feces and bile. Half-life of acebutolol is 3 to 4 hours; half-life of diacetolol, 8 to 13 hours.

CONTRAINDICATIONS & PRECAUTIONS
Contraindicated in patients with persistent severe bradycardia, second- and third-degree heart block, overt cardiac failure, and cardiogenic shock. Use cautiously in patients at risk for heart failure and in patients with bronchospastic disease, diabetes, hyperthyroidism, or peripheral vascular disease.

INTERACTIONS
Drug-drug. Acebutolol may potentiate hypotensive effects of other *antihypertensives*; it also may alter *insulin* or *oral antidiabetic* dosage requirements in patients whose diabetes is stable. Hypotensive effects of drug may be antagonized by *indomethacin, NSAIDs,* and *alpha-adrenergic stimulants* such as those contained in OTC cold remedies.

ADVERSE REACTIONS
CNS: depression, dizziness, fatigue, headache, hyperesthesia, hypoesthesia, impotence, insomnia.
CV: bradycardia, chest pain, edema, *heart failure,* hypotension.
GI: abdominal pain, constipation, diarrhea, dyspepsia, flatulence, nausea, vomiting.
Musculoskeletal: arthralgia, myalgia.
Respiratory: *bronchospasm,* cough, dyspnea.
Skin: rash.

🔳 KEY CONSIDERATIONS
Besides the recommendations relevant to all beta blockers, consider the following:
● Don't discontinue drug abruptly.
● Drug may cause positive antinuclear antibody titers.

Patient education
● Advise patient to report wheezing promptly.

Overdose & treatment
• Signs and symptoms of overdose include severe hypotension, bradycardia, heart failure, and bronchospasm.
• After acute ingestion, empty stomach by inducing vomiting or performing gastric lavage and reduce absorption by administering activated charcoal. Then provide symptomatic and supportive treatment.

acetaminophen
Acephen, Anacin-3, Bromo-Seltzer, Feverall, Panadol, Tempra, Tylenol

Para-aminophenol derivative, nonnarcotic analgesic, antipyretic

Available without a prescription
Tablets: 160 mg, 325 mg, 500 mg, 650 mg
Tablets (chewable): 80 mg, 160 mg
Capsules: 325 mg, 500 mg
Suppositories: 80 mg, 120 mg, 125 mg, 300 mg, 325 mg, 650 mg
Solution: 48 mg/ml, 80 mg/ml*, 100 mg/ml, 80 mg/5 ml, 120 mg/5 ml, 160 mg/5 ml, 167 mg/5 ml, 500 mg/15 ml
Suspension: 48 mg/ml, 80 mg/ml*, 80 mg/5 ml*, 100 mg/ml, 160 mg/5 ml
Sprinkle capsules: 80 mg, 160 mg
Caplets: 160 mg, 500 mg, 650 mg
Syrup: 16 mg/ml

INDICATIONS & DOSAGE
Mild pain; fever
Adults: 325 to 650 mg P.O. or P.R. q 4 to 6 hours, p.r.n. Maximum dose shouldn't exceed 4 g daily. Maximum dosage for long-term therapy is 2.6 g daily.

PHARMACODYNAMICS
Mechanism of action and site of action are unclear. Acetaminophen may inhibit prostaglandin synthesis in the CNS.
Analgesic action: Drug may exert its analgesic effect by elevating the pain threshold.
Antipyretic action: Drug is believed to exert its antipyretic effect by directly acting on the temperature-regulating center of the hypothalamus to block the effects of endogenous pyrogen, causing more heat to dissipate through sweating and vasodilation.

PHARMACOKINETICS
Absorption: Acetaminophen is absorbed rapidly and completely via the GI tract. Plasma levels peak in 1½ to 2 hours; they peak slightly faster for liquid preparations.
Distribution: Drug is 25% protein-bound. Plasma levels don't correlate well with analgesic effect, but they do correlate with toxicity.
Metabolism: Some 90% to 95% of drug is metabolized in the liver.
Excretion: Drug is excreted in urine. Average elimination half-life ranges from 1 to 4 hours. In acute overdose, toxic effects occur because elimination half-life is prolonged. Half-life exceeding 4 hours is associated with hepatic necrosis; exceeding 12 hours, coma.

CONTRAINDICATIONS & PRECAUTIONS
No known contraindications exist. Use acetaminophen cautiously in patients with history of chronic alcohol abuse because hepatotoxicity has occurred after therapeutic doses. Also use cautiously in patients with hepatic or CV disease, impaired renal function, or viral infection.

INTERACTIONS
Drug-drug. *Antacids* delay and decrease the absorption of acetaminophen; don't give together. Acetaminophen may potentiate the effects of *anticoagulants* and *thrombolytics,* but this effect appears to be insignificant. Use with *anticonvulsants* or *isoniazid* may increase the risk of hepatotoxicity. Use in large doses with *phenothiazines* may result in hypothermia. Use cautiously together.
Drug-food. Use with *caffeine* may enhance the therapeutic effect of acetaminophen, so use cautiously together. Because *food* delays and decreases the absorption of acetaminophen, drug should be taken on an empty stomach.
Drug-lifestyle. Use with *alcohol* increases the risk of hepatic damage. Don't use together.

ADVERSE REACTIONS
Hematologic: hemolytic anemia, *neutropenia, leukopenia, pancytopenia*.
Hepatic: jaundice, *severe liver damage*.
Metabolic: hypoglycemia.
Skin: rash, urticaria.

▣ KEY CONSIDERATIONS
● Geriatric patients are more sensitive to acetaminophen. Use with caution.
● Drug doesn't have a significant anti-inflammatory effect. Even so, studies have shown substantial benefit in patients with osteoarthritis of the knee. Therapeutic benefits may stem from the analgesic effects of drug.
● Many OTC products contain acetaminophen. Be aware of this when calculating total daily dosage.
● Monitor PT and INR in patients receiving warfarin and high dosages of acetaminophen (3 to 4 g/day).
● Patients unable to tolerate aspirin may be able to tolerate acetaminophen.
● Monitor vital signs, especially temperature, to evaluate effectiveness of the drug.
● Assess patient's level of pain and response before and after drug administration.
● Store rectal acetaminophen suppositories in refrigerator.
● Drug may cause a false-positive test result for urine 5-hydroxyindoleacetic acid.

Patient education
● Instruct patient how to properly administer prescribed form of drug.
● For a patient on long-term high-dose acetaminophen therapy, arrange for monitoring of laboratory values, especially BUN and serum creatinine levels, liver function tests, and CBC.
● Warn patient with current or past rectal bleeding to avoid using rectal acetaminophen suppositories. If they are used, they must be retained in the rectum for at least 1 hour.
● Warn patient that high doses or unsupervised long-term use of drug can cause liver damage. Use with alcohol increases the risk of liver toxicity.
● Tell patient not to self-medicate with drug for a fever above 103° F (39° C), a fever persisting longer than 3 days, or a recurrent fever.
● Tell patient not to take acetaminophen with an NSAID on a regular basis.
● Warn patient to avoid taking tetracycline antibiotics within 1 hour after taking buffered acetaminophen effervescent granules.
● Tell patient not to take drug for arthritic or rheumatic conditions without medical approval.
● Tell patient not to take drug for more than 10 days without medical approval.
● Tell patient on high-dose or long-term therapy that regular follow-up visits are essential.

Overdose & treatment
● In acute overdose, plasma levels of 300 µg/ml 4 hours after ingestion or 50 µg/ml 12 hours after ingestion are associated with hepatotoxicity. Signs and symptoms of overdose include cyanosis, anemia, jaundice, skin eruptions, fever, vomiting, CNS stimulation, delirium, methemoglobinemia progressing to depression, coma, vascular collapse, seizures, and death. Acetaminophen poisoning develops in stages.
● After a toxic overdose of acetaminophen, empty stomach immediately by inducing vomiting with ipecac syrup if patient is conscious or by performing gastric lavage. Administer activated charcoal via an NG tube. Then, administer oral acetylcysteine (Mucomyst), which is an antidote for acetaminophen poisoning. Although acetylcysteine is most effective if started within 10 to 12 hours after ingestion, it can help if started within 24 hours after ingestion. Administer a loading dosage of 140 mg/kg P.O., followed by a maintenance dosage of 70 mg/kg P.O. every 4 hours for an additional 17 doses. If patient vomits within 1 hour of administration, dose must be repeated. Because charcoal may interfere with absorption of this antidote, charcoal administration should stop before acetylcysteine administration begins.
● Hemodialysis may help remove acetaminophen from the body. Monitor laboratory values and vital signs closely. Provide symptomatic and supportive mea-

---

Reactions may be *common*, uncommon, *life-threatening*, or COMMON AND LIFE-THREATENING.

sures (respiratory support, correction of fluid and electrolyte imbalances). Determine plasma acetaminophen levels at least 4 hours after overdose. If plasma acetaminophen levels indicate hepatotoxicity, perform liver function tests every 24 hours for at least 96 hours.

acetazolamide
Dazamide, Diamox, Diamox Sequels

acetazolamide sodium
Diamox

Carbonic anhydrase inhibitor, antiglaucoma drug, anticonvulsant, diuretic, altitude sickness drug (prevention and treatment)

Available by prescription only
Tablets: 125 mg, 250 mg
Capsules (extended-release): 500 mg
Injection: 500 mg

INDICATIONS & DOSAGE
Preoperative management of acute angle-closure glaucoma
Adults: 250 mg P.O. q 4 hours; 250 mg P.O. b.i.d.; or 500 mg (extended-release) P.O. b.i.d. For short-term rapid-relief therapy, 500 mg I.V., which may be repeated in 2 to 4 hours, if necessary, followed by 125 to 250 mg P.O. q 4 hours.
Open-angle glaucoma, secondary glaucoma
Adults: 250 mg to 1 g P.O. or I.V. q.i.d. or 500 mg (extended-release) P.O. b.i.d.
Myoclonic seizures, refractory generalized tonic-clonic or absence seizures, mixed seizures
Adults: 375 mg P.O. or I.V. every day up to 250 mg q.i.d. Initial dosage when used with other anticonvulsants usually is 250 mg/day.
Edema in heart failure, drug-induced edema
Adults: 250 to 375 mg P.O. as single daily morning dose for 1 to 2 days alternating with 1 drug-free day.
Prevention or amelioration of acute mountain sickness
Adults: 500 to 1,000 mg P.O. in divided doses taken preferably 48 hours before

ascent and continued for at least 48 hours after arrival at the high altitude.
◇ *Periodic paralysis*
Adults: 250 mg P.O. b.i.d. or t.i.d. Maximum dosage, 1.5 g/day.

PHARMACODYNAMICS
Antiglaucoma action: Acetazolamide and acetazolamide sodium decrease formation of aqueous humor, lowering intraocular pressure.
Anticonvulsant action: Acetazolamide and acetazolamide sodium inhibit carbonic anhydrase in the CNS, which appears to slow down abnormal paroxysmal discharge from the neurons.
Diuretic action: Acetazolamide and acetazolamide sodium inhibit the enzyme carbonic anhydrase, which is responsible for forming hydrogen and bicarbonate ions from carbon dioxide and water. Noncompetitive and reversible, this inhibition results in decreased hydrogen levels in the renal tubules, which promotes excretion of bicarbonate, sodium, potassium, and water; because carbon dioxide isn't eliminated as rapidly, systemic acidosis may occur.
Altitude sickness action: Acetazolamide shortens the period of high-altitude acclimatization; by inhibiting conversion of carbon dioxide to bicarbonate, drug may increase carbon dioxide tension in tissues and decrease it in the lungs. The resultant metabolic acidosis may also increase oxygenation during hypoxia.

PHARMACOKINETICS
Absorption: Acetazolamide is well absorbed from the GI tract after oral administration.
Distribution: Drug is distributed throughout body tissues.
Metabolism: None.
Excretion: Drug is excreted primarily in urine via tubular secretion and passive reabsorption.

CONTRAINDICATIONS & PRECAUTIONS
Contraindicated in patients with hypersensitivity to acetazolamide, hyponatremia or hypokalemia, renal or hepatic disease or dysfunction, adrenal gland failure, or hyperchloremic acidosis and in those receiving long-term therapy for

chronic noncongestive angle-closure glaucoma. Use cautiously in patients with respiratory acidosis, emphysema, diabetes, or COPD and in those receiving other diuretics.

INTERACTIONS
Drug-drug. Acetazolamide alkalinizes urine and thus may decrease excretion of *amphetamines, flecainide, procainamide,* and *quinidine;* monitor for toxicity. Acetazolamide may increase excretion of *lithium, phenobarbital,* and *salicylates*, lowering plasma levels of these drugs and possibly necessitating dosage adjustments.

ADVERSE REACTIONS
CNS: confusion, drowsiness, paresthesia, *seizures*.
EENT: hearing dysfunction, transient myopia, tinnitus.
GI: anorexia, altered taste, diarrhea, nausea, vomiting.
GU: hematuria, polyuria.
Hematologic: *aplastic anemia*, hemolytic anemia, *leukopenia.*
Metabolic: hyperuricemia with no signs or symptoms, hyperchloremic acidosis, hypokalemia.
Skin: rash.

▣ KEY CONSIDERATIONS
● Observe geriatric patients closely because they're more susceptible to drug-induced diuresis. Excessive diuresis promotes rapid dehydration—leading to hypovolemia, hypokalemia, and hyponatremia—and may cause circulatory collapse. Reduced dosages may be indicated for these patients.
● Suspensions containing 250 mg/5 ml of syrup are the most palatable and can be made by a pharmacist. These suspensions remain stable for about 1 week. Tablets won't dissolve in fruit juice.
● Reconstitute powder by adding at least 5 ml sterile water for injection.
● Direct I.V. administration is preferred if drug must be given parenterally.
● Because acetazolamide alkalinizes urine it may cause false-positive proteinuria in Albustix or Albutest. Drug may also decrease thyroid iodine uptake.

Patient education
● Warn patient to use caution while driving or performing tasks that require alertness, coordination, or dexterity because drug may cause drowsiness.

acetylcholine chloride
Miochol

Cholinergic agonist, miotic

Available by prescription only
Ophthalmic solution: 1%

INDICATIONS & DOSAGE
To produce miosis during surgery
Adults: 0.5 to 2 ml of 1% solution instilled gently in anterior chamber of eye. Drug is used during ophthalmic surgery to cause rapid, complete miosis.

PHARMACODYNAMICS
Miotic action: The cholinergic activity of acetylcholine causes contraction of the sphincter muscles of the iris, resulting in miosis and contraction of the ciliary muscle, leading to accommodation. It also deepens the anterior chamber and vasodilates conjunctival vessels of the outflow tract.

PHARMACOKINETICS
Absorption: Action begins within seconds.
Distribution: Unknown.
Metabolism: Probably local, by cholinesterases.
Excretion: Duration of activity is 10 to 20 minutes.

CONTRAINDICATIONS & PRECAUTIONS
Contraindicated in patients with hypersensitivity to acetylcholine or its components.

INTERACTIONS
None reported.

ADVERSE REACTIONS
CV: bradycardia, hypotension, diaphoresis, flushing.
EENT: corneal edema, clouding, decompensation.
Respiratory: breathing difficulties.

▣ KEY CONSIDERATIONS
• Because acetylcholine chloride solution is unstable, prepare it immediately before use. Discard unused solution and solution that isn't clear and colorless.
• If the center rubber plug seal doesn't go down or is already down when reconstituting, don't use the vial.
• Don't gas-sterilize the vial. Ethylene oxide may produce formic acid.

Overdose & treatment
• Overdose may cause miosis, flushing, vomiting, bradycardia, bronchospasm, increased bronchial secretion, sweating, tearing, involuntary urination, hypotension, and seizures.
• Flush eyes with normal saline solution or sterile water. If drug was accidentally swallowed, vomiting should be spontaneous; if not, induce vomiting with activated charcoal or a cathartic. Treat accidental dermal exposure by washing the area twice with water. Epinephrine may be used to treat adverse CV reactions.

acetylcysteine
Mucomyst, Mucosil, Parvolex*

Amino acid (L-cysteine) derivative, mucolytic, acetaminophen antidote

Available by prescription only
Solution: 10%, 20%
Injection*: 200 mg/ml

INDICATIONS & DOSAGE
Acute and chronic bronchopulmonary disease, tracheostomy care, pulmonary complications of surgery, diagnostic bronchial studies
Administer by nebulization, direct application, or intratracheal instillation.
Adults: 1 to 2 ml of 10% or 20% solution via direct instillation into trachea hourly; or 3 to 5 ml of 20% solution or 6 to 10 ml of 10% solution via nebulization q 2 to 3 hours. For instillation through a percutaneous intratracheal catheter, 1 to 2 ml of 20% solution or 2 to 4 ml of 10% solution every 1 to 4 hours via a syringe attached to the catheter. For instillation through a tracheal catheter to treat a specific bron-

chopulmonary tree segment, administer 2 to 5 ml of 20% solution. For diagnostic bronchial studies (administered before procedure), administer 1 to 2 ml of 20% solution or 2 to 4 ml of 10% solution for two or three doses.
Acetaminophen toxicity
Adults: Initially, 140 mg/kg P.O., followed by 70 mg/kg q 4 hours for 17 doses (a total of 1,330 mg/kg) or until acetaminophen assay reveals a nontoxic level.
Alternatively, 150 mg/kg I.V. in 200 ml D_5W over 15 minutes as a loading dose, followed by 50 mg/kg I.V. in 500 ml D_5W over 4 hours, followed by 100 mg/kg I.V. in 1,000 ml D_5W over 16 hours.

PHARMACODYNAMICS
Mucolytic action: Acetylcysteine splits the disulfide bonds of mucoprotein, the substance responsible for increased viscosity of mucus secretions in the lungs; thus, pulmonary secretions become less viscous and more liquid.
Acetaminophen antidote: Mechanism of action isn't fully understood; however, acetylcysteine may restore hepatic stores of glutathione or inactivate the toxic metabolite of acetaminophen via a chemical interaction, thereby preventing hepatic damage.

PHARMACOKINETICS
Absorption: Most inhaled acetylcysteine acts directly on the mucus in the lungs; the remainder is absorbed by pulmonary epithelium. Action begins within 1 minute after inhalation and immediately upon direct intratracheal instillation; peak effect occurs in 5 to 10 minutes. After oral administration, drug is absorbed from the GI tract.
Distribution: Unknown.
Metabolism: Drug is metabolized in the liver.
Excretion: Unknown.

CONTRAINDICATIONS & PRECAUTIONS
Contraindicated in patients hypersensitive to acetylcysteine. Use cautiously in geriatric patients, especially those with severe respiratory insufficiency.

INTERACTIONS
Drug-drug. *Activated charcoal* adsorbs orally administered acetylcysteine, preventing its absorption.

ADVERSE REACTIONS
CV: hypotension, hypertension, tachycardia.
EENT: *rhinorrhea.*
GI: *nausea, stomatitis, vomiting.*
Respiratory: *bronchospasm* (especially in asthmatic patients).
Other: clamminess, chest tightness, fever.

🔲 KEY CONSIDERATIONS
• Geriatric patients may have inadequate cough and be unable to clear airway completely of mucus. Keep suction equipment available and monitor patient closely.
• Acetylcysteine solutions release hydrogen sulfide and discolor on contact with rubber and some metals (especially iron, nickel, and copper); drug tarnishes silver (this doesn't affect drug potency).
• Solution may turn light purple; this discoloration doesn't affect safety or efficacy of the drug. Use plastic, stainless steel, or other inert metal when administering drug via a nebulizer. Don't use handheld bulb nebulizers; output is too small and particle size too large.
• After opening, store in refrigerator or use within 96 hours.
• Monitor cough type and frequency; for maximum effect, instruct patient to clear airway by coughing before aerosol administration. Many doctors treat with bronchodilators before administering acetylcysteine. Keep suction equipment available; if patient has insufficient cough to clear increased secretions, suction will be needed to maintain open airway.
• When used orally for acetaminophen overdose, dilute with cola, fruit juice, or water to a 5% concentration and administer within 1 hour.
• Don't place acetylcysteine solutions directly in the chamber of a heated (hot pot) nebulizer.

Patient education
• Warn patient of unpleasant odor (rotten egg odor of hydrogen sulfide), and explain that increased amounts of liquefied bronchial secretion plus unpleasant odor may cause nausea and vomiting; have patient rinse mouth with water after nebulizer treatment.

activated charcoal
Actidose-Aqua, Charcoaid, CharcoCaps

Adsorbent, antidote, antidiarrheal, antiflatulent

Available without a prescription
Tablets: 325 mg, 650 mg
Tablets with 40 mg simethicone: 200 mg
Tablets (delayed-release) with 80 mg simethicone: 250 mg
Capsules: 260 mg
Powder: 30 g, 50 g
Suspension: 0.625 g/5 ml, 0.7 g/5 ml (50 g), 1 g/5 ml, 1.25 g/5 ml

INDICATIONS & DOSAGE
Poisoning
Adults: Five to ten times the estimated weight of drug or chemical ingested. (Larger dosages are necessary if food is in the stomach.) Dosage is 30 to 100 g in 250 ml water to make a slurry, given orally, preferably within 30 minutes of the drug or chemical ingested.

Activated charcoal is used as an adjunct in treating poisoning from or overdose of acetaminophen, amphetamines, antimony, arsenic, aspirin, atropine, barbiturates, camphor, cardiac glycosides, cocaine, glutethimide, ipecac, malathion, morphine, opium, oxalic acid, parathion, phenol, phenothiazines, phenytoin, poisonous mushrooms, potassium permanganate, propoxyphene, quinine, strychnine, sulfonamides, or tricyclic antidepressants. To enhance removal of a drug from the bloodstream and promote gastric dialysis, activated charcoal may be given 20 to 60 g q 4 to 12 hours. Monitor serum drug level.
◊ *To relieve GI disturbances—such as halitosis, anorexia, nausea, or vomiting—in uremic patients*
Adults: 20 to 50 g daily.

Flatulence or dyspepsia
Adults: 600 mg to 5 g P.O. as a single dose, or 975 mg to 3.9 g t.i.d. after meals.

PHARMACODYNAMICS

Antidote action: Activated charcoal adsorbs ingested toxins, thereby inhibiting GI absorption.
Antidiarrheal action: Drug adsorbs toxic and nontoxic irritants that cause diarrhea or GI discomfort.
Antiflatulent action: Drug adsorbs intestinal gas to relieve discomfort.

PHARMACOKINETICS

Absorption: Activated charcoal isn't absorbed from the GI tract.
Distribution: None.
Metabolism: None.
Excretion: Drug is excreted in feces.

CONTRAINDICATIONS & PRECAUTIONS

No known contraindications exist.

INTERACTIONS

Drug-drug. Activated charcoal inactivates *syrup of ipecac* and also adsorbs and inactivates *many oral drugs* when used concomitantly, including orally administered *acetylcysteine.* Gastric lavage should be used to remove the charcoal before acetylcysteine is administered. If administering activated charcoal for indications other than poisoning, give other drugs 1 hour before or 2 hours after it.
Drug-food. *Dairy products* decrease the effectiveness of activated charcoal. Don't give it in ice cream or milk.

ADVERSE REACTIONS

GI: black stools, constipation, nausea.

▣ KEY CONSIDERATIONS

• Don't give activated charcoal by mouth to a semiconscious or unconscious patient; instead, administer drug through an NG tube.
• Because drug adsorbs and inactivates syrup of ipecac, give only after patient stops vomiting.
• Drug is most effective when used within 30 minutes of toxin ingestion; a cathartic is commonly administered with or after activated charcoal to speed removal of the toxin-charcoal complex.

• Powder form is most effective. Mix with tap water to form consistency of thick syrup. A small amount of fruit juice or flavoring may be added to make mixture more palatable.
• Dose may need to be repeated if patient vomits shortly after administration.
• Prolonged use (more than 72 hours) may impair patient's nutritional status.
• Drug may be used orally to decrease colostomy odor.

Patient education

• Tell patient to call poison information center or hospital emergency department before taking activated charcoal as an antidote.
• If patient is using drug as an antidiarrheal or antiflatulent, instruct him to take other drugs 1 hour before or 2 hours after activated charcoal. Advise him to report diarrhea that persists after 2 days of therapy, fever, or flatulence that persists after 7 days.
• Warn patient that activated charcoal turns stools black.
• Advise patient not to mix drug with dairy products, which may lessen its effectiveness.

---

acyclovir (acycloguanosine)

acyclovir sodium
Zovirax

Synthetic purine nucleoside, antiviral

Available by prescription only
Tablets: 400 mg, 800 mg
Capsules: 200 mg
Oral suspension: 200 mg/5 ml
Injection: 500 mg/vial, 1 g/vial
Ointment: 5%

INDICATIONS & DOSAGE

Initial and recurrent mucocutaneous herpes simplex virus (HSV type 1 and HSV type 2) or severe initial genital herpes or herpes simplex in immuno-compromised patient
Adults: 5 mg/kg, given at a constant rate over 1 hour by I.V. infusion q 8 hours for 7 days (5 days for genital herpes).

◇ *Treatment of disseminated herpes zoster*
Adults: 5 to 10 mg/kg I.V. q 8 hours for 7 to 10 days. Infuse over at least 1 hour.
Treatment of initial genital herpes
Adults: 200 mg P.O. q 4 hours while awake (a total of five capsules daily). Treatment should continue for 10 days.
Treatment of acute herpes zoster infections
Adults: 800 mg P.O. five times daily for 7 to 10 days. Initiate therapy within 48 hours of rash onset.
Intermittent therapy for recurrent genital herpes
Adults: 200 mg P.O. q 4 hours while awake (a total of five capsules daily). Treatment should continue for 5 days. Initiate therapy at first sign of recurrence.
Long-term suppressive therapy for recurrent genital herpes
Adults: 400 mg P.O. b.i.d. for up to 1 year, followed by reevaluation.
Genital herpes; non-life-threatening herpes simplex infection in immunocompromised patients
Adults: Apply sufficient quantity of ointment to adequately cover all lesions q 3 hours, six times daily for 7 days.
Treatment of acute varicella (chickenpox) infections
Adults weighing more than 40 kg (88 lb): 800 mg P.O. q.i.d. for 5 days.
Adults weighing less than 88 lb: 20 mg/kg P.O. q.i.d. for 5 days.
Immunocompromised patient
Adults: 10 mg/kg I.V. over 1 hour q 8 hours for 7 days.
Herpes simplex encephalitis
Adults: 10 mg/kg I.V. over 1 hour q 8 hours for 10 days; usual daily dose is 30 mg/kg.
✦ *Dosage adjustment.* In patients with renal failure, adjust normal oral dosage (200 to 400 mg) to 200 mg q 12 hours if creatinine clearance drops below 10 ml/minute/1.73 m². For normal dosages exceeding 400 mg, refer to package insert.

In patients with renal failure, give 100% of the I.V. dose q 8 hours if creatinine clearance exceeds 50 ml/minute/1.73 m²; 100% of the dose q 12 hours if it ranges between 25 and 50 ml/minute/1.73 m²; 100% of the dose q 24 hours if it ranges between 10 and 25 ml/minute/1.73 m²; and 50% of the dose q 24 hours if it falls below 10 ml/minute/1.73 m².

PHARMACODYNAMICS
Antiviral action: Acyclovir, which the viral cell converts into triphosphate (its active form), inhibits viral DNA polymerase.

In vitro, acyclovir is active against HSV type 1, HSV type 2, varicella-zoster virus, Epstein-Barr virus, and cytomegalovirus. In vivo, acyclovir may reduce the duration of acute infection and speed lesion healing in initial genital herpes episodes. Oral acyclovir may be prescribed to prevent recurrences in patients with frequent herpes infections (more than six episodes a year) or to reduce the frequency of these infections.

PHARMACOKINETICS
Absorption: With oral administration, acyclovir is absorbed slowly and incompletely (15% to 30%). Levels peak in 1½ to 2 hours. Food doesn't affect absorption. With topical administration, absorption is minimal.
Distribution: Drug is distributed widely to organ tissues and body fluids. CSF levels equal about 50% of serum levels. About 9% to 33% of a dose binds to plasma proteins.
Metabolism: Drug is metabolized inside the viral cell to its active form. About 10% of dose is metabolized extracellularly.
Excretion: Up to 92% of systemically absorbed acyclovir is excreted as unchanged drug from the kidneys through glomerular filtration and tubular secretion. In patients with normal renal function, half-life is 2 to 3½ hours. Renal failure may extend half-life to 19 hours.

CONTRAINDICATIONS & PRECAUTIONS
Contraindicated in patients with hypersensitivity to acyclovir. Use cautiously in patients with underlying neurologic problems, renal disease, or dehydration and in those receiving nephrotoxic drugs.

Reactions may be *common*, uncommon, *life-threatening*, or COMMON AND LIFE-THREATENING.

INTERACTIONS

Drug-drug. Use with *probenecid* may result in reduced renal tubular secretion of acyclovir, leading to increased drug half-life, reduced elimination rate, and decreased urine excretion. This reduced clearance causes more sustained serum drug levels. Use with *zidovudine* may result in increased levels of acyclovir, causing toxicity.

ADVERSE REACTIONS

CNS: *encephalopathic changes (lethargy, obtundation, tremor, confusion, hallucinations, agitation, **seizures, coma**), headache, malaise.*
GI: diarrhea, nausea, vomiting.
GU: hematuria, *transient elevations of serum creatinine levels,* **acute renal failure.**
Hematologic: bone marrow hypoplasia, **leukopenia,** megaloblastic hematopoiesis, thrombocytosis, **thrombocytopenia.**
Skin: itching, rash, transient burning and stinging, pruritus, urticaria, vulvitis.
Other: *inflammation, phlebitis (at injection site).*

▣ KEY CONSIDERATIONS

• Administer acyclovir cautiously to geriatric patients because they may suffer from renal dysfunction or dehydration.
• Drug shouldn't be administered S.C., I.M., by I.V. bolus, or ophthalmically.
• I.V. dose should be infused over at least 1 hour to prevent renal tubular damage.
• Solubility of acyclovir in urine is low. To prevent nephrotoxicity, make sure that the patient taking the systemic form of drug is well hydrated.
• Monitor serum creatinine level. If level doesn't return to normal within a few days after therapy begins, increase hydration, adjust dosage, or discontinue drug.
• Encephalopathic signs are more likely in patients who have experienced neurologic reactions to cytotoxic drugs.
• Serum creatinine and BUN levels may increase.

Patient education

• Warn patient that although drug helps manage the disease, it doesn't cure it or prevent it from spreading to others.
• For best results, tell patient to begin taking drug when early infection symptoms (such as tingling, itching, or pain) occur.
• Instruct patient who's taking ointment to use a finger cot or rubber glove and to apply about a ½" ribbon of ointment for every 4 square inches of area to be covered. Ointment should thoroughly cover each lesion. Warn patient to avoid getting ointment in the eye.
• Instruct patient to avoid sexual intercourse during active genital infection.

Overdose & treatment

• Overdose has followed I.V. bolus administration in patients with unmonitored fluid status or in patients receiving inappropriately high parenteral dosages. Acute toxicity hasn't been reported after high oral dosage.
• Hemodialysis decreases plasma drug levels by 60%.
• Signs and symptoms of overdose include signs of nephrotoxicity, including elevated serum creatinine and BUN levels, progressing to renal failure.

albuterol sulfate
Proventil, Proventil HFA, Proventil Repetabs, Proventil Syrup, Ventolin, Ventolin Syrup, Volmax

Adrenergic, bronchodilator

Available by prescription only
Tablets: 2 mg, 4 mg
Tablets (sustained-release): 4 mg, 8 mg
Syrup: 2 mg/5 ml
Aerosol inhaler: 90 mcg/metered-spray
Solution for nebulization: 0.083%, 0.5%
Capsules for inhalation: 200 mcg microfine

INDICATIONS & DOSAGE

To prevent and treat bronchospasm in patients with reversible obstructive airway disease
Adults: 2 to 4 mg (immediate-release tablets) P.O. t.i.d. or q.i.d.; maximum dosage, 8 mg q.i.d. Alternatively, use

sustained-release tablets. Usual starting dosage is 4 mg q 12 hours. Increase to 8 mg q 12 hours if patient fails to respond. Cautiously increase stepwise as needed and tolerated to 16 mg q 12 hours.

Aerosol inhalation: 1 or 2 inhalations q 4 to 6 hours. More frequent administration or a greater number of inhalations isn't usually recommended. However, because deposition of inhaled drugs is variable, higher doses are occasionally used, especially in patients with acute bronchospasm.

Solution for inhalation: 2.5 mg t.i.d. or q.i.d. by nebulizer.

Capsules for inhalation: 200 mcg inhaled q 4 to 6 hours using a Rotahaler inhalation device.

Geriatric patients: 2 mg (tablets) P.O. t.i.d. or q.i.d.

To prevent exercise-induced bronchospasm

Adults: Two inhalations 15 minutes before exercise.

PHARMACODYNAMICS

Bronchodilator action: Albuterol selectively stimulates beta receptors of the lungs, uterus, and vascular smooth muscle. Bronchodilation results from relaxation of bronchial smooth muscles, which relieves bronchospasm and reduces airway resistance.

PHARMACOKINETICS

Absorption: After oral inhalation, albuterol appears to be absorbed gradually (over several hours) from the respiratory tract; however, dose is mostly swallowed and absorbed through the GI tract. Onset of action occurs within 5 to 15 minutes, peaks in ½ to 2 hours, and lasts 3 to 6 hours. After oral administration, albuterol is well absorbed through the GI tract. Onset of action occurs within 30 minutes and peaks in 2 to 3 hours. Drug effect lasts 4 to 6 hours with immediate-release tablets and 12 hours with extended-release tablets.

Distribution: Drug doesn't cross the blood-brain barrier.

Metabolism: Drug is extensively metabolized in the liver to inactive compounds.

Excretion: Drug is rapidly excreted in urine and feces. After oral inhalation, 70% of a dose is excreted in urine unchanged and as metabolites within 24 hours; 10% is excreted in feces. Elimination half-life is about 4 hours. After oral administration, 75% of a dose is excreted in urine within 72 hours as metabolites; 4% is excreted in feces.

CONTRAINDICATIONS & PRECAUTIONS

Contraindicated in patients with hypersensitivity to albuterol or any component of its formulation. Use cautiously in patients with CV disorders, including coronary insufficiency and hypertension; in patients with hyperthyroidism or diabetes mellitus; and in those who are unusually responsive to adrenergics.

INTERACTIONS

Drug-drug. Use of orally inhaled albuterol with *epinephrine* and *other orally inhaled sympathomimetic amines* may increase sympathomimetic effects and risk of toxicity. Serious CV effects may follow use with *MAO inhibitors* and *tricyclic antidepressants*. *Propranolol* and *other beta blockers* may antagonize the effects of albuterol.

ADVERSE REACTIONS

CNS: *tremor, nervousness,* dizziness, insomnia, *headache, hyperactivity,* weakness, CNS stimulation, malaise.

CV: *tachycardia, palpitations,* hypertension.

EENT: dry and irritated nose and throat (with inhaled form), nasal congestion, epistaxis, hoarseness, taste perversion.

GI: heartburn, *nausea, vomiting,* anorexia, increased appetite.

Metabolic: hypokalemia.

Musculoskeletal: muscle cramps.

Respiratory: *bronchospasm,* cough, wheezing, dyspnea, bronchitis, increased sputum.

Other: hypersensitivity reactions.

▣ KEY CONSIDERATIONS

Besides the recommendations relevant to all adrenergics, consider the following:
• Geriatric patients may be more sensitive to sympathomimetic amines and require a lower dosage.

• Small, transient increases in blood glucose levels may occur after oral inhalation.

• Although serum potassium levels may decrease after the drug is administered I.V. or via inhalation, potassium supplementation is usually unnecessary.

• Effectiveness of treatment is measured by periodic monitoring of patient's pulmonary function.

Patient education

• Instruct patient on how to properly use the inhaler and tell him to read the directions before use. Alert him that he may experience dryness in his mouth and throat and that rinsing with water after each dose may help.

Administration by metered-dose nebulizer: Shake canister thoroughly to activate; place mouthpiece well into mouth, aimed at back of throat. Close lips and teeth around mouthpiece. Exhale through nose as completely as possible; then inhale through mouth slowly and deeply while actuating the nebulizer to release dose. Hold breath 10 seconds (count "1-100, 2-100, 3-100," until "10-100" is reached), remove mouthpiece, and then exhale slowly.

Administration by metered-powder inhaler: Instruct patient to breathe with normal force and depth, not to force a deep breath. Observe him closely for exaggerated systemic drug action.

Administration by oxygen aerosolization: Administer over 15- to 20-minute period, with oxygen flow rate adjusted to 4 L/minute. Turn on oxygen supply before patient places nebulizer in mouth. Lips need not be closed tightly around nebulizer opening. Placement of Y tube in rubber tubing permits patient to control administration. Advise patient to rinse mouth immediately after inhalation therapy to help prevent dryness and throat irritation. To prevent clogging, rinse mouthpiece thoroughly with warm running water at least once daily. (It isn't dishwasher-safe.) After cleaning, wait until mouthpiece is completely dry before storing. Don't place near heat (for example in a dishwasher or an oven). Replace reservoir bag every 2 to 3 weeks

or as needed; replace mouthpiece every 6 to 9 months or as needed.

Note: Replacement of bags or mouthpieces may require a prescription.

• Tell patient that if he experiences paradoxical bronchospasm from repeated use, he should discontinue the drug and call his health care provider.

• Tell patient to call his health care provider if troubled breathing persists 1 hour after using drug, if symptoms return within 4 hours, if condition worsens, or if new (refill) canister is needed within 2 weeks.

• Tell patient to wait 15 minutes after using inhaled albuterol before using an adrenocorticoid, such as beclomethasone, dexamethasone, flunisolide, or triamcinolone.

• Warn patient to use the drug only as directed and not to use more than prescribed amount or more often than prescribed.

Overdose & treatment

• Signs and symptoms of overdose include exaggeration of common adverse reactions, particularly angina, hypertension, hypokalemia, and seizures.

• To treat, use selective beta blockers (such as metoprolol) with extreme caution; they may induce an asthma attack. Dialysis is inappropriate. Monitor vital signs and electrolyte levels closely.

alclometasone dipropionate
Aclovate

Topical adrenocorticoid, anti-inflammatory

Available by prescription only
Cream, ointment: 0.05%

INDICATIONS & DOSAGE
Inflammation of corticosteroid-responsive dermatoses
Adults: Apply a thin film to affected areas b.i.d. or t.i.d. Gently massage until the drug disappears, or apply a thick layer and cover with an occlusive dressing and tape and leave in place overnight or at least 6 hours. Course of treatment may

last 2 to 6 weeks. Use occlusive dressing for severe or resistant dermatoses.

PHARMACODYNAMICS

Anti-inflammatory action: Alclometasone stimulates the synthesis of enzymes needed to decrease the inflammatory response. It's a group VI nonfluorinated topical glucocorticoid with less anti-inflammatory activity than hydrocortisone 0.2% or greater. Its potency is similar to desonide 0.05% and fluocinolone acetonide 0.01%. Applied topically, it may be used for refractory lesions of psoriasis and other deep-seated dermatoses such as localized neurodermatitis.

PHARMACOKINETICS

Absorption: Amount of alclometasone absorbed depends on amount of drug applied and the skin at the application site. It ranges from about 1% in areas with thick stratum corneum (such as the palms, soles, elbows, and knees) to as high as 36% in areas of the thinnest stratum corneum (such as the face, eyelids, and genitals). Absorption increases in areas of skin damage, inflammation, or occlusion. Some systemic absorption of topical steroids may occur, especially through the oral mucosa.
Distribution: After topical application, drug is distributed throughout the local skin. If drug is absorbed into the circulation, it's rapidly removed from the blood and distributed into muscle, liver, skin, intestines, and kidneys.
Metabolism: After topical administration, drug is metabolized primarily in the skin. The small amount that's absorbed into systemic circulation is metabolized primarily in the liver to inactive compounds.
Excretion: The kidneys excrete inactive metabolites, primarily as glucuronides and sulfates, but also as unconjugated products. Small amounts of the metabolites are also excreted in feces.

CONTRAINDICATIONS & PRECAUTIONS

Contraindicated in patients hypersensitive to corticosteroids.

INTERACTIONS

None reported.

ADVERSE REACTIONS

EENT: cataracts, glaucoma (if used around eyes for a prolonged period).
GU: glycosuria.
Metabolic: hyperglycemia.
Skin: burning, pruritus, irritation, dryness, erythema, folliculitis, acneiform eruptions, perioral dermatitis, hypopigmentation, hypertrichosis, allergic contact dermatitis; secondary infection, maceration, atrophy, striae, miliaria (with occlusive dressings).
Other: hypothalamic-pituitary-adrenal axis suppression, Cushing's syndrome.

▣ KEY CONSIDERATIONS

• Systemic absorption of topical corticosteroids can produce reversible hypothalamic-pituitary-adrenal axis suppression with the potential for glucocorticosteroid insufficiency after discontinuing therapy.
• Systemic absorption may also cause symptoms of Cushing's syndrome, hyperglycemia, and glycosuria in some patients.
• Periodically evaluate patients applying topical steroid to a large surface area or to areas occluded for hypothalamic-pituitary-adrenal axis suppression.

Patient education

• Tell patient to use it only as directed—and to use it only to treat the disorder for which it was prescribed.
• Inform patient that he shouldn't bandage or otherwise occlude the affected area, unless instructed to do so.
• Advise patient to notify doctor if he experiences localized adverse reactions or if he doesn't see improvement within 2 weeks.

alendronate sodium
Fosamax

Osteoclast-mediated bone resorption inhibitor, antiosteoporotic

Available by prescription only
Tablets: 5 mg, 10 mg, 40 mg

INDICATIONS & DOSAGE
Osteoporosis in postmenopausal women
Adults: 10 mg P.O. daily taken with water at least 30 minutes before first food, beverage, or drug of the day.
Prevention of osteoporosis in post-menopausal women
Adults: 5 mg P.O. daily taken with water at least 30 minutes before first food, beverage, or drug of the day.
Paget's disease of bone
Adults: 40 mg P.O. daily for 6 months taken with water at least 30 minutes before first food, beverage, or drug of the day.

PHARMACODYNAMICS
Antiosteoporotic action: At the cellular level, alendronate suppresses osteoclast activity on newly formed resorption surfaces, which reduces bone turnover. Bone formation exceeds bone resorption at bone remodeling sites and thus leads to progressive gains in bone mass.

PHARMACOKINETICS
Absorption: Alendronate is absorbed from the GI tract. Food or beverages can decrease bioavailability significantly.
Distribution: Drug is distributed to soft tissues but is then rapidly redistributed to bone or excreted in urine. About 78% binds to proteins.
Metabolism: None.
Excretion: Drug is excreted in urine.

CONTRAINDICATIONS & PRECAUTIONS
Contraindicated in patients with hypersensitivity to any component of alendronate, hypocalcemia, or severe renal insufficiency (creatinine clearance below 35 ml/minute).

Use cautiously in patients with active upper GI problems—such as dysphagia, symptomatic esophageal diseases, gastritis, duodenitis, or ulcers—and in patients with mild to moderate renal insufficiency (creatinine clearance between 35 and 60 ml/minute).

INTERACTIONS
Drug-drug. *Antacids* and *calcium supplements* impair absorption of alendronate. Instruct patient to wait at least 30 minutes after taking alendronate before consuming other drugs. *Aspirin* and *NSAIDs* increase risk of upper GI adverse reactions with alendronate dosages above 10 mg daily. Monitor patient closely. *Hormone replacement therapy* shouldn't be used concomitantly to treat osteoporosis because of the lack of sufficient evidence regarding effectiveness.
Drug-food. *Food* decreases absorption of drug. Administer with a full glass of water 30 minutes before eating or drinking.

ADVERSE REACTIONS
CNS: headache.
GI: abdominal pain, nausea, dyspepsia, constipation, diarrhea, flatulence, acid regurgitation, esophageal ulcer, vomiting, dysphagia, abdominal distention, gastritis, taste perversion.
Musculoskeletal: musculoskeletal pain.

▣ KEY CONSIDERATIONS
• Some geriatric patients may be sensitive to the drug, so use cautiously.
• Hypocalcemia must be corrected before drug therapy begins. Other disturbances of mineral metabolism (such as vitamin D deficiency) should also be corrected before initiating therapy.
• When drug is used to treat osteoporosis in postmenopausal women, disease is confirmed by low bone mass findings on diagnostic studies or history of an osteoporotic fracture.
• Drug is indicated for patients with Paget's disease who have alkaline phosphatase levels at least twice the upper limit for normal, who are symptomatic, or who are at risk for future complications from the disease.
• Monitor patient's serum calcium and phosphate levels throughout therapy.

Patient education
• Stress importance of taking each tablet with a glass of plain water (not mineral water or other beverages) first thing in the morning, at least 30 minutes before ingesting food, beverages, or other drugs. Tell patient that waiting more than 30 minutes improves absorption of drug.

---

*Canada only   ◇ Unlabeled clinical use

- To facilitate delivery to stomach and to reduce the potential for esophageal irritation, warn patient not to lie down for at least 30 minutes after taking drug.
- Tell patient to take supplemental calcium and vitamin D if daily dietary intake is inadequate.
- Inform patient that weight-bearing exercises increase bone mass, and stress the importance of modifying excessive cigarette smoking and alcohol consumption, if these factors are part of patient's lifestyle.

Overdose & treatment

- Signs and symptoms of oral overdose include hypocalcemia, hypophosphatemia, and upper GI adverse effects, such as upset stomach, heartburn, esophagitis, gastritis, and ulcer.
- Although specific information is lacking regarding the treatment of an overdose, consider administering milk or antacids (to bind alendronate). Dialysis isn't beneficial in removing drug from circulation.

allopurinol
Purinol*, Zyloprim

Xanthine oxidase inhibitor, antigout drug

Available by prescription only
Tablets (scored): 100 mg, 300 mg

INDICATIONS & DOSAGE
Gout, primary or secondary hyperuricemia
Gout may be secondary to diseases such as acute or chronic leukemia, polycythemia vera, multiple myeloma, or psoriasis or after administration of chemotherapeutic drugs. Dosage varies with severity of disease; can be given as single dose or divided, but doses larger than 300 mg should be divided.
Adults: Mild gout, 200 to 300 mg P.O. daily; severe gout with large tophi, 400 to 600 mg P.O. daily. Same dose is applicable for maintenance in secondary hyperuricemia.

To prevent acute gouty attacks
Adults: 100 mg P.O. daily; increase at weekly intervals by 100 mg without exceeding maximum dose (800 mg), until serum uric acid level falls to 6 mg/100 ml or less.
To prevent uric acid nephropathy during cancer chemotherapy
Adults: 600 to 800 mg P.O. daily for 2 to 3 days, with high fluid intake.
Recurrent calcium oxalate calculi
Adults: 200 to 300 mg P.O. daily in single dose or divided doses.
✦ *Dosage adjustment.* In adults with creatinine clearance up to 9 ml/minute, give 100 mg q 3 days; 10 to 19 ml/minute, give 100 mg every other day; 20 to 39 ml/minute, 100 mg/day; 40 to 59 ml/minute, 150 mg/day; 60 to 79 ml/minute, 200 mg/day; and if it is 80 ml/minute, give 250 mg/day.
◊ *Stomatitis from fluorouracil*
Adults: Allopurinol mouthwash, 600 mg/day.

PHARMACODYNAMICS
Antigout action: Allopurinol inhibits xanthine oxidase, the enzyme catalyzing the conversion of hypoxanthine to xanthine, and the conversion of xanthine to uric acid. By blocking this enzyme, allopurinol and its metabolite, oxypurinol, prevent the conversion of oxypurines (xanthine and hypoxanthine) to uric acid, thus decreasing serum and urine levels of uric acid. Drug has no analgesic, antiinflammatory, or uricosuric action.

PHARMACOKINETICS
Absorption: After oral administration, 80% to 90% of a dose is absorbed. Allopurinol levels peak 2 to 6 hours after a usual dose.
Distribution: Drug is distributed widely throughout the body except in the brain, where drug levels are 50% of those found in the rest of the body. Allopurinol and oxypurinol don't bind to plasma proteins.
Metabolism: Drug is metabolized to oxypurinol by xanthine oxidase. Half-life of allopurinol is 1 to 2 hours; oxypurinol, about 15 hours.

Reactions may be *common*, uncommon, *life-threatening*, or COMMON AND LIFE-THREATENING.

Excretion: Within 6 hours of ingestion, 5% to 7% of an allopurinol dose is excreted in urine unchanged. After this, the kidneys excrete the drug as oxypurinol, allopurinol, and oxypurinol ribonucleosides. Within 48 to 72 hours, about 70% of the administered daily dose is excreted in urine as oxypurinol and an additional 2% appears in feces as unchanged drug.

CONTRAINDICATIONS & PRECAUTIONS
Contraindicated in patients with hypersensitivity to allopurinol and in those with idiopathic hemochromatosis.

INTERACTIONS
Drug-drug. Use with *ampicillin* or *amoxicillin* may increase the likelihood of rash, so use cautiously together. Use with *azathioprine* and *mercaptopurine* may increase the toxic effects of these drugs, particularly bone marrow depression, and requires reduction of initial doses of *azathioprine* or *mercaptopurine* to 25% to 33% of the usual dose, with subsequent doses adjusted according to patient response and toxic effects.

Because allopurinol or its metabolites may compete with *chlorpropamide* for renal tubular secretion, patients who receive both drugs should be observed for excessive hypoglycemia.

Use with *co-trimoxazole* may cause thrombocytopenia. Use with *cyclophosphamide* may increase the incidence of bone marrow depression through an unknown mechanism. Allopurinol inhibits hepatic microsomal metabolism of *dicumarol,* thus increasing the half-life of dicumarol; patients receiving both drugs should be observed for increased anticoagulant effects. In patients with decreased renal function, use with a *thiazide diuretic* may increase the risk of allopurinol-induced hypersensitivity reactions. Use cautiously together.

Use with large doses of allopurinol (600 mg/day) can decrease *theophylline* clearance, leading to increased plasma theophylline levels; monitor closely.

ADVERSE REACTIONS
CNS: drowsiness, headache, paresthesia, peripheral neuropathy, neuritis.

CV: hypersensitivity vasculitis, necrotizing angiitis.
EENT: epistaxis, taste loss or perversion.
GI: nausea, vomiting, diarrhea, abdominal pain, gastritis, dyspepsia.
GU: *renal failure,* uremia.
Hematologic: *agranulocytosis,* anemia, *aplastic anemia, thrombocytopenia, leukopenia,* leukocytosis, eosinophilia.
Hepatic: altered liver function studies, hepatitis, hepatic necrosis, hepatomegaly, cholestatic jaundice.
Musculoskeletal: arthralgia, myopathy.
Skin: alopecia; ecchymoses; *rash (usually maculopapular);* exfoliative, urticarial, and purpuric lesions; *Stevens-Johnson syndrome (erythema multiforme);* severe furunculosis of nose; ichthyosis; *toxic epidermal necrolysis.*
Other: fever, chills.

▣ KEY CONSIDERATIONS
- Rash occurs mostly in patients taking diuretics and in those with renal disorders.
- Monitor patient's intake and output. Daily urine output of at least 2 L and maintenance of neutral or slightly alkaline urine is desirable.
- If renal insufficiency occurs during treatment, reduce allopurinol dosage.
- Monitor CBC, serum uric acid levels, and hepatic and renal function at start of therapy and periodically thereafter.
- Acute gout attacks may occur in first 6 weeks of therapy. To prevent these attacks, allopurinol may be used concomitantly with colchicine or another anti-inflammatory.
- Minimize GI adverse reactions by administering drug with meals or immediately after. Tablets may be crushed and administered with fluid or food.
- Allopurinol may predispose a patient who is concomitantly taking ampicillin to an ampicillin-induced rash.
- Allopurinol-induced rash may occur weeks after discontinuation of drug.
- Increased alkaline phosphatase, AST, and ALT levels have been reported in patients taking allopurinol.

Patient education

• Encourage patient to drink plenty of fluids (10 to 12 8-oz [240-ml] glasses daily) while taking drug unless otherwise contraindicated.

• When treating recurrent calcium oxalate stones, advise patient to reduce dietary intake of animal protein, sodium, refined sugars, vitamin C, oxalate-rich foods, and calcium.

• Advise patient to avoid hazardous activities requiring alertness until CNS response to drug is known because drowsiness may occur.

• Advise patient to avoid alcohol because it decreases effectiveness of allopurinol.

• Tell patient to report all adverse reactions immediately.

• Advise patient to take a missed dose as soon as he remembers it, unless it's time for the next scheduled dose, in which case he shouldn't double-dose.

• Inform patient to discontinue drug and call immediately at first sign of rash or other signs that may indicate an allergic reaction.

• Tell patient to take drug with food or milk.

---

alprazolam
Alprazolam Intensol, Apo-Alpraz*, Novo-Alprazol*, Xanax

Benzodiazepine, anxiolytic
Controlled substance schedule IV

Available by prescription only
Tablets: 0.25 mg, 0.5 mg, 1 mg, 2 mg
Oral solution: 0.1 mg/ml, 1 mg/ml

INDICATIONS & DOSAGE
Anxiety
Adults: Usual starting dose is 0.25 to 0.5 mg P.O. t.i.d. Increase dose, p.r.n., q 3 to 4 days. Maximum total daily dosage is 4 mg in divided doses.
Geriatric patients: 0.25 mg P.O. b.i.d. or t.i.d.
✦ *Dosage adjustment.* In debilitated patients or in those with hepatic impairment, initial dose is 0.25 mg P.O. b.i.d. or t.i.d.

Panic disorder
Adults: Initially, 0.5 mg P.O. t.i.d. Increase as needed and tolerated at intervals of 3 to 4 days in increments of 1 mg daily. Most patients require more than 4 mg daily; however, dosages from 1 to 10 mg daily have been reported.
◊ *Agoraphobia with social phobia*
Adults: 2 to 8 mg/day P.O.
◊ *Depression*
Adults: 0.25 mg P.O. t.i.d.

PHARMACODYNAMICS
Anxiolytic action: Alprazolam depresses the CNS at the limbic and subcortical levels of the brain. It reduces anxiety by enhancing the effect of the neurotransmitter gamma-aminobutyric acid on its receptor in the ascending reticular activating system, which increases inhibition and blocks both cortical and limbic arousal.

PHARMACOKINETICS
Absorption: When administered orally, alprazolam is well absorbed. Onset of action occurs within 15 to 30 minutes, with peak action in 1 to 2 hours.
Distribution: Drug is distributed widely throughout the body. About 80% to 90% of an administered dose binds to plasma protein.
Metabolism: Drug is metabolized in the liver equally to alpha-hydroxyalprazolam and inactive metabolites.
Excretion: Alpha-hydroxyalprazolam and other metabolites are excreted in urine. The half-life of alprazolam is 12 to 15 hours. The mean half-life of alprazolam in healthy geriatric patients in clinical studies was 16.3 hours, compared with 11 hours in healthy younger adult patients.

CONTRAINDICATIONS & PRECAUTIONS
Contraindicated in patients with hypersensitivity to alprazolam or other benzodiazepines or acute angle-closure glaucoma. Use cautiously in patients with hepatic, renal, or pulmonary disease.

INTERACTIONS
Drug-drug. Alprazolam potentiates the CNS depressant effects of *antidepressants, antihistamines, barbiturates, gen-*

Reactions may be *common*, uncommon, *life-threatening*, or COMMON AND LIFE-THREATENING.

eral anesthetics, *MAO inhibitors, narcotics, and phenothiazines.* Use with *cimetidine* or *disulfiram* may diminish hepatic metabolism of alprazolam, increasing its plasma level. Use with *digoxin* may increase plasma digoxin levels. Use with *rifampin* may decrease effects of alprazolam. And use with *theophylline* may increase the sedative effects of alprazolam. Use together cautiously.

Drug-lifestyle. Alprazolam potentiates the CNS depressant effects of *alcohol. Heavy smoking* accelerates alprazolam metabolism, thus lowering the effectiveness of the drug. Use together cautiously.

ADVERSE REACTIONS

CNS: *drowsiness, light-headedness,* headache, confusion, tremor, dizziness, syncope, *depression,* insomnia, nervousness.
CV: hypotension, tachycardia.
EENT: blurred vision, nasal congestion.
GI: *dry mouth,* nausea, vomiting, *diarrhea, constipation.*
Metabolic: weight gain or loss.
Musculoskeletal: muscle rigidity.
Skin: dermatitis.

▣ KEY CONSIDERATIONS

Besides the recommendations relevant to all benzodiazepines, consider the following:
• Lower dosages are usually effective in geriatric patients because of altered pharmacokinetics and in patients with renal or hepatic dysfunction.
• During initiation of therapy and after an increase in dosage, geriatric patients should be supervised when walking and performing activities of daily living.
• To prevent withdrawal symptoms, patients receiving long-term high-dose therapy should be weaned from the drug gradually, perhaps over 2 to 3 months.
• Anxiety associated with depression is also responsive to alprazolam but may require more frequent dosing.
• Store drug in a cool, dry place away from direct light.
• Alprazolam may elevate liver function test results. Minor changes in EEG patterns—usually low-voltage, fast activity—may occur during and after alprazolam therapy.

Patient education

• Make sure patient understands potential for physical and psychological dependence with long-term use of alprazolam.
• Instruct patient not to alter drug regimen.
• Warn patient that sudden position changes can cause dizziness. To prevent falls and injury, advise him to dangle his legs for a few minutes before getting out of bed.

Overdose & treatment

• Signs and symptoms of overdose include somnolence, confusion, coma, hypoactive reflexes, dyspnea, labored breathing, hypotension, bradycardia, slurred speech, unsteady gait, and impaired coordination.
• Support blood pressure and respiration until drug effects subside, and monitor vital signs. Flumazenil, a specific benzodiazepine antagonist, may be useful. To maintain a patent airway and support adequate oxygenation, mechanical ventilatory assistance via endotracheal tube may be required. To treat hypotension, use I.V. fluids and vasopressors, such as dopamine and phenylephrine, as needed. If the patient is conscious, induce vomiting. Perform gastric lavage if ingestion was recent, but only if an endotracheal tube is in place to prevent aspiration. After patient vomits or receives gastric lavage, administer activated charcoal with a cathartic as a single dose. Dialysis is of limited value. Because barbiturates may exacerbate excitation or CNS depression, avoid using them in patients who experience excitation.

alprostadil
Caverject, Muse

Prostaglandin, corrective drug for impotence

Available by prescription only
Sterile powder for injection: 6.15-mcg vial, 11.9-mcg vial, 23.2-mcg vial
Urethral suppository pellet: 125 mcg, 250 mcg, 500 mcg, 1,000 mcg

INDICATIONS & DOSAGE

Erectile dysfunction of vasculogenic, psychogenic, or mixed origin

Adults: Dosages are highly individualized. *For injection:* initial dose is 2.5 mcg intracavernously. If partial response occurs, increase second dose by 2.5 to 5 mcg, and then increase dose further in increments of 5 to 10 mcg until patient achieves an erection (suitable for intercourse but not lasting for more than 1 hour). If initial dose is ineffective, increase second dose to 7.5 mcg within 1 hour; then increase dose further in 5- to 10-mcg increments until patient achieves an erection. Patient must remain in health care provider's office until complete detumescence occurs. If patient responds, don't repeat procedure for 24 hours. *For pellet:* start initially with lower dosages (125 mcg or 250 mcg). Increase or decrease dosage gradually on separate occasions until patient achieves an erection that's sufficient for sexual intercourse.

Erectile dysfunction of pure neurologic origin (spinal cord injury)

Adults: Dosages are highly individualized. Initial dosage is 1.25 mcg intracavernously. If partial response occurs, give second dosage of 1.25 mcg and then a third dosage of 2.5 mcg; increase dosage further in 5-mcg increments until patient achieves an erection (suitable for intercourse but not lasting for more than 1 hour). If initial dosage is ineffective, increase second dosage to 2.5 mcg within 1 hour; then increase further in 5-mcg increments until patient achieves an erection. Patient must remain in health care provider's office until complete detumescence occurs. If patient responds, don't repeat procedure for 24 hours.

PHARMACODYNAMICS

Corrective action of impotence: Alprostadil is a prostaglandin derivative that induces erection by relaxing trabecular smooth muscle and dilating cavernosal arteries. As a result, lacunar spaces expand and blood is trapped by compressing the venules against the tunica albuginea. This process is referred to as the corporal veno-occlusive mechanism.

PHARMACOKINETICS

Absorption: The absolute bioavailability of alprostadil hasn't been determined.
Distribution: Drug is bound in plasma protein primarily to albumin (81%).
Metabolism: Drug is rapidly converted to compounds that are further metabolized before excretion.
Excretion: Most metabolites are excreted in urine; the rest are excreted in feces.

CONTRAINDICATIONS & PRECAUTIONS

Contraindicated in patients with hypersensitivity to alprostadil, conditions associated with priapism (sickle cell anemia or trait, multiple myeloma, or leukemia), or penile deformation (angulation, cavernosal fibrosis, or Peyronie's disease). Don't give to men who have penile implants or in whom sexual activity is contraindicated.

INTERACTIONS

Drug-drug. *Anticoagulants* increase the risk of bleeding from intracavernosal injection site. Alprostadil may decrease serum *cyclosporine* levels. Monitor patient closely.

ADVERSE REACTIONS

CNS: headache, dizziness, fainting.
CV: hypertension, hypotension, swelling of leg veins.
GU: *penile pain,* prolonged erection, penile fibrosis, penis disorder, penile rash, penile edema, prostatic disorder, testicular and perineal aching, minor urethral burning.
Musculoskeletal: back pain.
Respiratory: upper respiratory tract infection, flulike syndrome, sinusitis, nasal congestion, cough.
Other: hematoma, ecchymosis (at injection site); localized trauma; localized pain.

▣ KEY CONSIDERATIONS

• Patient must have underlying treatable medical causes of erectile dysfunction diagnosed and treated before therapy begins.
• Regular follow-up with careful examination of the penis is strongly recommended to detect penile fibrosis. Dis-

---

continue drug in patients in whom penile angulation, cavernosal fibrosis, or Peyronie's disease develops.
• Monitor a patient using Muse for hypotension; titrate drug to the lowest effective dosage.
• Female partners of patients who use Muse may experience vaginal itching and burning.

Patient education
• To ensure safe and effective use, thoroughly instruct patient how to prepare and administer alprostadil before beginning intracavernosal treatment at home. Stress the importance of following instructions carefully.
• Tell patient to discard vials with precipitate or discoloration. A reconstituted vial should only be used once and should be discarded once the proper volume of solution has been withdrawn.
• Instruct patient not to shake the contents of a reconstituted vial.
• Stress the importance of not reusing or sharing needles or syringes and not sharing the drug.
• Make sure patient has the manufacturer's instructions for administration that are included in each package of alprostadil to refer to at home.
• Tell patient that he shouldn't change the dosage that the health care provider established without approval.
• Inform patient that he can expect an erection within 5 to 20 minutes after drug administration and that the goal is to produce an erection that doesn't last for more than 1 hour.
• Instruct patient to seek medical attention immediately if he develops an erection that lasts for more than 6 hours after alprostadil injection.
• Tell patient that drug shouldn't be used more than three times weekly, with at least 24 hours between each use. Muse shouldn't be administered more than twice within a 24-hour period.
• Review possible adverse reactions with patient. Instruct patient to immediately report penile pain that wasn't present before or increases in intensity and penile nodules or hard tissue.
• Instruct patient to inspect penis daily for redness, swelling, tenderness, or cur-vature of the erect penis, which might suggest infection. Tell him to call the doctor if these signs or symptoms occur.
• Remind patient regular follow-up visits are necessary to evaluate effectiveness and safety of therapy.
• Inform patient that drug doesn't protect against transmission of sexually transmitted diseases and that he must continue to take protective measures.
• Warn patient that slight bleeding may occur at the injection site, which may increase the risk of transmitting blood-borne diseases, if present, to his sexual partner.
• To prevent potential vaginal burning and itching in female partner, a patient using Muse should use a condom when having sexual intercourse.

alteplase (recombinant alteplase, tissue plasminogen activator)
Activase

Thrombolytic enzyme

Available by prescription only
Injection: 20-mg (11.6 million IU), 50-mg (29 million IU), 100-mg (58 million IU) vials

INDICATIONS & DOSAGE
Lysis of thrombi obstructing coronary arteries in management of an acute MI (3-hour infusion)
Adults weighing more than 65 kg (143 lb): 60 mg in 1st hour, with 6 to 10 mg I.V. bolus over first 1 to 2 minutes; then 20 mg/hour for an additional 2 hours. Total dose, 100 mg.
Adults weighing 143 lb or less:
1.25 mg/kg I.V. given over 3 hours as described above.
Lysis of thrombi obstructing coronary arteries in management of an acute MI (accelerated infusion)
Adults weighing more than 67 kg (148 lb): 15 mg I.V. push, 50 mg over 30 minutes, then 35 mg over 60 minutes.
Adults weighing 148 lb or less: 15 mg I.V. push, 0.75 mg/kg over 30 minutes

(not to exceed 50 mg), then 0.50 mg/kg over 60 minutes (not to exceed 35 mg).

Pulmonary embolism

Adults: 100 mg by I.V. infusion over 2 hours. Heparin therapy should be initiated at the end of the infusion.

Acute ischemic stroke

Adults: 0.9 mg/kg (maximum dose, 90 mg). Administer 10% of dose as an I.V. bolus over 1 minute; remaining 90%, over 1 hour.

PHARMACODYNAMICS

Thrombolytic action: Alteplase is an enzyme that catalyzes the conversion of tissue plasminogen to plasmin in the presence of fibrin. This fibrin specificity produces local fibrinolysis in the area of recent clot formation, with limited systemic proteolysis. In patients with an acute MI, this allows for reperfusion of ischemic cardiac muscle and improved left ventricular function with a decreased incidence of heart failure after an MI.

PHARMACOKINETICS

Absorption: Alteplase must be given I.V.

Distribution: Drug is rapidly cleared from the plasma by the liver; 80% of a dose is cleared within 10 minutes after infusion is discontinued.

Metabolism: Drug is metabolized primarily in the liver.

Excretion: More than 85% of drug is excreted in urine; 5%, in feces. Plasma half-life is less than 10 minutes.

CONTRAINDICATIONS & PRECAUTIONS

Contraindicated in patients with history or evidence of intracranial hemorrhage, suspected subarachnoid hemorrhage, seizure at the onset of stroke, active internal bleeding, intracranial neoplasm, arteriovenous malformation, aneurysm, and severe uncontrolled hypertension (more than 185 mm Hg systolic or 110 mm Hg diastolic). Also contraindicated in patients with a history of CVA, recent (within 2 months) intraspinal or intracranial trauma or surgery, or known bleeding diathesis (see package insert).

Use cautiously in patients with recent (within 10 days) major surgery; organ biopsy; trauma (including cardiopulmonary resuscitation); GI or GU bleed-

ing; cerebrovascular disease; hypertension; likelihood of left-sided heart thrombus; hemostatic defects, including those secondary to severe hepatic or renal disease; hepatic dysfunction; occluded AV cannula; severe neurologic deficit (NIH Stroke Scale over 22); signs of major early infarct on a computed tomographic (CT) scan; mitral stenosis; atrial fibrillation; acute pericarditis or subacute bacterial endocarditis; septic thrombophlebitis; or diabetic hemorrhagic retinopathy or other hemorrhagic ophthalmic conditions. Also use cautiously in patients receiving anticoagulants and in patients ages 75 and older.

INTERACTIONS

Drug-drug. Use of alteplase with *drugs that antagonize platelet function*—such as *abciximab, aspirin,* and *dipyridamole*—may increase risk of bleeding if administered before, during, or after alteplase therapy. Use cautiously together.

ADVERSE REACTIONS

CNS: *cerebral hemorrhage,* fever.

CV: hypotension, *arrhythmias,* edema.

GI: nausea, vomiting.

Hematologic: *severe, spontaneous bleeding (cerebral, retroperitoneal, GU, GI).*

Other: bleeding at puncture sites, *hypersensitivity reactions (anaphylaxis).*

▣ KEY CONSIDERATIONS

• Expect to begin alteplase infusions as soon as possible after onset of MI signs and symptoms (angina that lasts for more than 30 minutes, angina that's unresponsive to nitroglycerin, or ECG evidence of an MI).

• Administer drug within 3 hours after onset of stroke symptoms once a CT scan or another diagnostic imaging method capable of detecting hemorrhage has ruled out intracranial hemorrhage. Treatment should only be performed in facilities that can appropriately evaluate and manage intracranial hemorrhage.

• Heparin is usually administered during or after alteplase as part of the treatment regimen for an acute MI or pulmonary embolism. When alteplase is used to treat acute ischemic stroke, 24-hour anti-

---

Reactions may be *common,* uncommon, *life-threatening,* or COMMON AND LIFE-THREATENING.

coagulant or antiplatelet therapy is contraindicated.

• If pretreatment PT exceeds 15 seconds or an elevated APTT is identified in a patient who hasn't recently received an oral anticoagulant or heparin, drug therapy for acute ischemic stroke should be discontinued.

• After coronary thrombolysis, monitor ECG for transient arrhythmias (sinus bradycardia, ventricular tachycardia, accelerated idioventricular rhythm, premature ventricular depolarization) caused by reperfusion. Have antiarrhythmics available.

• Avoid I.M. injections, venipuncture, and arterial puncture during therapy. Use pressure dressings or ice packs on recent puncture sites to prevent bleeding. If arterial puncture is necessary, select a site on the arm and apply pressure for 30 minutes afterward.

• Prepare solution using supplied sterile water for injection. Don't use bacteriostatic water for injection.

• Don't mix other drugs with alteplase. Use an 18G needle for preparing solution. Aim water stream at the lyophilized cake, which will foam slightly. Don't use if you don't have a vacuum.

• To yield a concentration of 0.5 mg/ml, drug may be further diluted with normal saline solution injection or D_5W. Reconstituted or diluted solutions are stable for up to 8 hours at room temperature.

• Altered results may be expected in coagulation and fibrinolytic tests. The use of aprotinin (150 to 200 U/ml) in the blood sample may attenuate this interference.

Patient education
• Teach patient signs and symptoms of internal bleeding and tell him to report these immediately.

• To prevent excessive gum trauma, advise patient about proper dental care.

aluminum carbonate
Basaljel

Inorganic aluminum salt, antacid, hypophosphatemic

Available without a prescription
Tablets or capsules: aluminum hydroxide equivalent 500 mg
Suspension: aluminum hydroxide equivalent 400 mg/5 ml

INDICATIONS & DOSAGE
Antacid
Adults: 10 ml suspension P.O. q 2 hours p.r.n. or 1 or 2 tablets or capsules q 2 hours p.r.n.
Treatment of hyperphosphatemia and prevention of renal calculi (with low-phosphate diet)
Adults: 1 g P.O. t.i.d. or q.i.d.; adjust to lowest possible dosage after therapy begins, monitoring diet and serum levels.

PHARMACODYNAMICS
Antacid action: Aluminum carbonate neutralizes gastric acid, which increases pH and thus decreases pepsin activity.
Hypophosphatemic action: Drug reduces serum phosphate levels by combining with phosphate in the gut. This results in the formation of insoluble, nonabsorbable aluminum phosphate, which is then excreted in feces. Calcium absorption increases secondary to reduced phosphate absorption.

PHARMACOKINETICS
Absorption: Aluminum carbonate is largely unabsorbed; a small amount may be absorbed systemically.
Distribution: None.
Metabolism: None.
Excretion: Drug is excreted in feces.

CONTRAINDICATIONS & PRECAUTIONS
No known contraindications. Use cautiously in patients with chronic renal disease.

INTERACTIONS
Drug-drug. Aluminum carbonate may decrease absorption of many drugs—including *antimuscarinics, chenodiol,*

◊ Unlabeled clinical use

chlordiazepoxide, coumarin anticoagulants, diazepam, digoxin, indomethacin, iron salts, isoniazid, phenothiazines (especially chlorpromazine), quinolones, sodium or potassium phosphate, tetracycline, and *vitamin A*—thereby making them less effective. Administer at least 2 hours apart. Use with *enteric-coated drugs* causes premature drug release. Administer drugs at least 1 hour apart.

ADVERSE REACTIONS
CNS: encephalopathy.
GI: *constipation,* intestinal obstruction.
Metabolic: hypophosphatemia.
Musculoskeletal: osteomalacia.

▣ KEY CONSIDERATIONS
● Because geriatric patients commonly have decreased GI motility, they may become constipated more easily from aluminum carbonate.
● Manage constipation with stool softeners or bulk laxatives, or alternate drug with magnesium-containing antacids (unless patient has renal disease).
● When administering a suspension, shake well and give with a small amount of water or fruit juice.
● After administering drug through an NG tube, flush tube with water to prevent obstruction.
● When administering drug as an antiurolithic, encourage increased fluid intake to enhance drug effectiveness.
● Monitor serum calcium and phosphate levels periodically; reduced serum phosphate levels may lead to increased serum calcium levels.
● Long-term aluminum carbonate use can lead to calcium resorption and subsequent bone demineralization.
● Aluminum carbonate may interfere with imaging techniques using sodium pertechnetate technetium 99m (^{99m}Tc), thus impairing evaluation of Meckel's diverticulum, and reticuloendothelial imaging of liver, spleen, or bone marrow using technetium ^{99m}Tc sulfur colloid. Drug may also antagonize the effect of pentagastrin during gastric acid secretion tests.
● Aluminum carbonate may increase serum gastrin levels and decrease serum phosphate levels.

Patient education
● Advise patient to take drug only as directed and not to take more than 24 capsules or tablets or more than 120 ml (24 tsp) of regular suspension per day. Instruct patient to shake suspension well.
● As needed, advise patient to restrict sodium intake, drink plenty of fluids, and follow a low-phosphate diet.
● Advise patient not to switch antacids without his doctor's approval.

aluminum hydroxide
Alterna-GEL, Alu-Cap, Alu-Tab, Amphojel, Dialume, Nephrox

Aluminum salt, antacid, hypophosphatemic

Available without a prescription
Tablets: 300 mg, 500 mg, 600 mg
Capsules: 475 mg, 500 mg
Suspension: 320 mg/5 ml, 450 mg/5 ml, 675 mg/5 ml
Liquid: 600 mg/5 ml

INDICATIONS & DOSAGE
Antacid; treatment of hyperphosphatemia
Adults: 500 to 1,500 mg P.O. (tablet or capsule) 1 hour after meals and h.s.; or 5 to 30 ml of suspension, p.r.n., 1 hour after meals and h.s.

PHARMACODYNAMICS
Antacid action: Aluminum hydroxide neutralizes gastric acid, reducing the direct acid irritant effect. This increases pH, thereby decreasing pepsin activity.
Antihyperphosphatemic action: Drug reduces serum phosphate levels by combining with phosphate in the gut, which results in insoluble, nonabsorbable aluminum phosphate, which is then excreted in feces. Calcium absorption increases secondary to decreased phosphate absorption.

PHARMACOKINETICS
Absorption: Aluminum hydroxide is largely unabsorbed; a small amount may be absorbed systemically.
Distribution: None.
Metabolism: None.

Excretion: Drug is excreted in feces.

CONTRAINDICATIONS & PRECAUTIONS
No known contraindications. Use cautiously in patients with renal disease.

INTERACTIONS
Drug-drug. Aluminum hydroxide may decrease absorption of many drugs—including *antimuscarinics, chenodiol, chlordiazepoxide, coumarin anticoagulants, diazepam, digoxin, indomethacin, iron salts, isoniazid, phenothiazines (especially chlorpromazine), quinolones, sodium or potassium phosphate, tetracycline,* and *vitamin A*—thereby decreasing their effectiveness. Administer drugs at least 2 hours apart. Use with *enteric-coated drugs* causes premature drug release. Administer drugs at least 1 hour apart.

ADVERSE REACTIONS
CNS: encephalopathy.
GI: *constipation,* intestinal obstruction.
Metabolic: hypophosphatemia.
Musculoskeletal: osteomalacia.

▣ KEY CONSIDERATIONS
• Because geriatric patients commonly have decreased GI motility, they may become constipated more easily from aluminum hydroxide than younger patients.
• Manage constipation with stool softeners or bulk laxatives, and alternate aluminum hydroxide with magnesium-containing antacids (unless patient has renal disease).
• Shake suspension well (especially extra-strength suspension), and give with a small amount of water or fruit juice.
• After administering drug through an NG tube, flush tube with water to prevent obstruction.
• When administering drug as an antiurolithic, encourage increased fluid intake to enhance drug effectiveness.
• Periodically monitor serum calcium and phosphate levels; decreased serum phosphate levels may lead to increased serum calcium levels. Observe patient for symptoms of hypophosphatemia, such as anorexia, muscle weakness, and malaise.

• Drug therapy may interfere with imaging techniques using sodium pertechnetate technetium 99m (^{99m}Tc), thus impairing evaluation of Meckel's diverticulum, and reticuloendothelial imaging of liver, spleen, and bone marrow using technetium ^{99m}Tc sulfur colloid. It may also antagonize the effect of pentagastrin during gastric acid secretion tests. Drug may elevate serum gastrin levels and reduce serum phosphate levels.

Patient education
• Caution patient to take drug only as directed, to shake suspension well or chew tablets thoroughly, and to follow with sips of water or juice.
• As indicated, instruct patient to restrict sodium intake, drink plenty of fluids, or follow a low-phosphate diet.
• Advise patient not to switch to another antacid without the doctor's approval.

---

amantadine hydrochloride
Symmetrel

Synthetic cyclic primary amine, antiviral, antiparkinsonian

Available by prescription only
Tablets: 100 mg
Capsules: 100 mg
Syrup: 50 mg/5 ml

INDICATIONS & DOSAGE
Prophylaxis or symptomatic treatment of influenza type A virus, respiratory tract illnesses in geriatric patients
Adults ages 64 and younger: 200 mg P.O. daily in a single dose or divided b.i.d.
Geriatric patients: 100 mg P.O. once daily.

Treatment should continue for 24 to 48 hours after symptoms disappear. Prophylaxis should start as soon as possible after initial exposure and continue for at least 10 days after exposure. Prophylaxis may be continued up to 90 days for repeated or suspected exposures if influenza virus vaccine is unavailable. If used with influenza virus vaccine, continue dose for 2 to 4 weeks until protection from vaccine develops.

Treatment of drug-induced extrapyramidal reactions
Adults: 100 to 300 mg/day P.O. in divided doses.

Treatment of idiopathic parkinsonism, parkinsonian syndrome
Adults: 100 mg P.O. b.i.d.; in patients who are seriously ill or receiving other antiparkinsonians, 100 mg/day for at least 1 week, then 100 mg b.i.d., p.r.n. Patient may benefit from as much as 400 mg/day, but dosages over 200 mg must be closely supervised.

✦ ***Dosage adjustment.*** In patients with renal dysfunction, base maintenance dosage on creatinine clearance value, as follows:

If creatinine clearance is between 30 and 50 ml/minute/1.73 m^2, give 200 mg the first day and then 100 mg daily; if it's between 15 and 29 ml/minute/1.73 m^2, 200 mg on the first day and 100 mg q alternating day; and if it's below 15 ml/minute/1.73 m^2, 200 mg q 7 days.

Note: Patients receiving long-term hemodialysis therapy should receive 200 mg q 7 days.

PHARMACODYNAMICS
Antiviral action: Amantadine interferes with viral uncoating of the RNA in lysosomes. In vitro, amantadine is active only against influenza type A virus. (However, spontaneous resistance commonly occurs.) In vivo, amantadine may protect against influenza type A virus in 70% to 90% of patients; when administered within 24 to 48 hours of onset of illness, it reduces duration of fever and other systemic symptoms.

Antiparkinsonian action: Amantadine is thought to cause the release of dopamine in the substantia nigra.

PHARMACOKINETICS
Absorption: With oral administration, amantadine is well absorbed from the GI tract. Serum levels peak in 1 to 8 hours; usual serum level is 0.2 to 0.9 µg/ml. (Neurotoxicity may occur at levels exceeding 1.5 µg/ml.)

Distribution: Drug is distributed widely throughout body and crosses the blood-brain barrier.

Metabolism: About 10% of dose is metabolized.

Excretion: About 90% of dose is excreted unchanged in urine, primarily by tubular secretion. Excretion rate depends on urine pH (acidic pH enhances excretion). Elimination half-life in patients with normal renal function is about 24 hours; in those with renal dysfunction, about 10 days.

CONTRAINDICATIONS & PRECAUTIONS
Contraindicated in patients with hypersensitivity to amantadine. Use cautiously in geriatric patients, especially those with seizure disorders, heart failure, peripheral edema, hepatic disease, mental illness, eczematoid rash, renal impairment, orthostatic hypotension, and CV disease.

INTERACTIONS
Drug-drug. Use with *benztropine* or *trihexyphenidyl* may potentiate the anticholinergic adverse effects of these drugs when they're given in high doses, possibly causing confusion and hallucinations. Use with a *combination of hydrochlorothiazide and triamterene* may decrease urinary amantadine excretion, resulting in increased serum amantadine levels and possible toxicity. Use with *CNS stimulants* may cause additive stimulation. Use cautiously together.

Drug-lifestyle. Use with *alcohol* may result in light-headedness, confusion, fainting, and hypotension. Avoid using together.

ADVERSE REACTIONS
CNS: depression, fatigue, confusion, *dizziness,* hallucinations, anxiety, *irritability,* ataxia, *insomnia,* headache, *light-headedness.*

CV: peripheral edema, orthostatic hypotension, **heart failure.**

GI: anorexia, *nausea,* constipation, vomiting, dry mouth.

Skin: *livedo reticularis (with prolonged use).*

▣ KEY CONSIDERATIONS
• Geriatric patients are more susceptible to adverse neurologic effects; dividing

daily dose into two doses may reduce risk.

• To prevent orthostatic hypotension, instruct patient to move slowly when changing position (especially when rising to standing position).

• If patient experiences insomnia, administer dose several hours before bedtime.

• Prophylactic drug use is recommended for selected high-risk patients who can't receive influenza virus vaccine. Manufacturer recommends prophylactic therapy lasting up to 90 days with possible repeated or unknown exposure.

Patient education

• Warn patient that drug may impair mental alertness.

• Advise patient to take drug after meals to ensure best absorption.

• Caution patient to avoid abrupt position changes because these may cause light-headedness or dizziness.

• If drug is being taken to treat parkinsonism, warn patient not to discontinue it abruptly because doing so could precipitate a parkinsonian crisis.

• Warn patient to avoid alcohol while taking drug.

• Instruct patient to report adverse effects promptly, especially dizziness, depression, anxiety, nausea, and urine retention.

Overdose & treatment

• Signs and symptoms of overdose include nausea, vomiting, anorexia, hyperexcitability, tremors, slurred speech, blurred vision, lethargy, anticholinergic symptoms, seizures, and possible ventricular arrhythmias, including torsades de pointes and ventricular fibrillation. CNS effects result from increased levels of dopamine in the brain.

• Treatment includes immediately performing gastric lavage or inducing vomiting along with providing supportive measures, forcing fluids and, if necessary, administering fluids I.V. Urine acidification may be used to increase drug excretion. Physostigmine may be given (1 to 2 mg by slow I.V. infusion at 1- to 2-hour intervals) to counteract CNS toxicity. Seizures or arrhythmias may be treated with conventional therapy. Patient should be monitored closely.

amifostine
Ethyol

Organic thiophosphate, cytoprotective drug

Available by prescription only
Injection: 500 mg anhydrous basis and 500 mg mannitol/10-ml vial

INDICATIONS & DOSAGE
Reduction of cumulative renal toxicity caused by repeated administration of cisplatin in patients with advanced ovarian cancer
Adults: 910 mg/m^2 daily as a 15-minute I.V. infusion, starting within 30 minutes before chemotherapy. If hypotension occurs and blood pressure doesn't return to normal within 5 minutes of treatment, subsequent cycles should use 740 mg/m^2.

PHARMACODYNAMICS
Cytoprotective action: Amifostine is dephosphorylated by alkaline phosphatase in tissues to a pharmacologically active free thiol metabolite. The higher levels of free thiol in normal tissues is available to bind to—and thereby detoxify—reactive metabolites of cisplatin, which can reduce the toxic effects of cisplatin on renal tissue. Free thiol can also scavenge for free radicals that may be generated in tissues exposed to cisplatin.

PHARMACOKINETICS
Absorption: Not applicable because amifostine is administered I.V.
Distribution: Drug is rapidly cleared from the plasma with a distribution half-life of less than 1 minute. It has been found in bone marrow cells 5 to 8 minutes following administration.
Metabolism: Drug is rapidly metabolized to an active free thiol metabolite. A disulfide metabolite is produced subsequently and is less active than the free thiol.

Excretion: Amifostine and the two metabolites are minimally excreted in the urine.

CONTRAINDICATIONS & PRECAUTIONS

Contraindicated in patients hypersensitive to aminothiol compounds or mannitol. Amifostine shouldn't be used in patients receiving chemotherapy for malignancies that are potentially curable (certain malignancies of germ cell origin), except in clinical studies. Also contraindicated in hypotensive or dehydrated patients and in those receiving antihypertensives that can't be stopped for 24 hours preceding amifostine administration.

Use cautiously in geriatric patients, especially those with ischemic heart disease, arrhythmias, heart failure, or history of stroke or transient ischemic attacks. Also use cautiously in patients in whom the common adverse effects of nausea, vomiting, and hypotension are likely to have serious consequences.

INTERACTIONS

Drug-drug. Use with *antihypertensives* or *other drugs that could potentiate hypotension* requires special consideration because of the increased risk of hypotension.

ADVERSE REACTIONS

CNS: loss of consciousness, dizziness, somnolence.
CV: *hypotension.*
GI: *nausea, vomiting.*
Metabolic: hypocalcemia.
Other: flushing or feeling of warmth, chills or feeling of coldness, hiccups, sneezing, allergic reactions ranging from rash to rigors.

▣ KEY CONSIDERATIONS

• Amifostine should be used cautiously in patients older than age 70 because experience with use in patients from this age-group is limited.
• Reconstitute each single-dose vial with 9.5 ml of sterile normal saline injection, normal saline solution. Reconstituting the drug with other solutions isn't recommended. Reconstituted solution (500 mg amifostine/10 ml) is chemically stable for up to 5 hours at room temperature (about 77° F [25° C]) or up to 24 hours if refrigerated (35° to 46° F [2° to 8° C]).
• Drug can be prepared in polyvinyl chloride bags at concentrations of 5 to 40 mg/ml and has the same stability as when it's reconstituted in the single-use vial.
• Inspect vial for particulate matter and discoloration before administration whenever solution and container permit. Don't use vials that are cloudy or contain precipitate.
• If possible, stop antihypertensive therapy 24 hours before administering amifostine. If antihypertensive therapy can't be stopped, don't use drug because of the risk of severe hypotension.
• Patients receiving amifostine should be adequately hydrated before drug is administered and be kept in a supine position during the infusion.
• Monitor blood pressure every 5 minutes during infusion. If hypotension occurs, requiring interruption of therapy, place patient in Trendelenburg's position and give an infusion of normal saline solution using a separate I.V. line. If blood pressure returns to normal within 5 minutes and patient is asymptomatic, infusion may be restarted so that the full dose of drug can be given. If full dose of amifostine can't be administered, drug dosage for subsequent cycles should be 740 mg/m^2.
• Don't infuse for more than 15 minutes because a longer infusion time has been linked to a higher incidence of adverse reactions.
• Administer an antiemetic, including 20 mg of I.V. dexamethasone and a serotonin 5HT receptor antagonist, before and together with amifostine. Additional antiemetics may be required, based on the chemotherapy drugs administered.
• When amifostine is used with highly emetogenic chemotherapy, monitor fluid balance of patient.
• Monitor serum calcium level in patients at risk for hypocalcemia, such as those with nephrotic syndrome. If necessary, administer a calcium supplement.

Reactions may be *common,* uncommon, *life-threatening,* or COMMON AND LIFE-THREATENING.

Patient education
• Instruct patient to remain in a supine position during infusion.

amikacin sulfate
Amikin

Aminoglycoside, antibiotic

Available by prescription only
Injection: 50 mg/ml, 250 mg/ml

INDICATIONS & DOSAGE
Serious infections caused by susceptible organisms
Adults: 15 mg/kg/day divided q 8 to 12 hours I.M. or I.V. (in 100 to 200 ml D_5W or normal saline solution administered over 30 to 60 minutes). Don't exceed 1.5 g/day.
◊*Adults:* 4 to 20 mg given intrathecally or intraventricularly as a single dose in conjunction with I.M. or I.V. administration.
Uncomplicated urinary tract infections
Adults: 250 mg I.M. or I.V. b.i.d.
✦ *Dosage adjustment.* In a patient with renal failure, initially, 7.5 mg/kg. Subsequent doses and frequency determined by blood amikacin levels and renal function studies. One method is to administer additional 7.5 mg/kg doses and alter dosing interval based on steady-state serum creatinine level:

$$\frac{\text{creatinine}}{\text{(mg/dl)}} \times 9 = \frac{\text{dosing interval}}{\text{(hours)}}$$

Keep peak serum levels between 15 and 30 µg/ml; trough serum levels shouldn't exceed 5 to 10 µg/ml.

PHARMACODYNAMICS
Antibiotic action: Amikacin is bactericidal; it binds directly to the 30S ribosomal subunit, thus inhibiting bacterial protein synthesis. Its spectrum of activity includes many aerobic gram-negative organisms (including most strains of *Pseudomonas aeruginosa*) and some aerobic gram-positive organisms. Amikacin may act against some organisms resistant to other aminoglycosides, such as *Proteus, Pseudomonas,* and *Serratia;* some strains of these may be resis-

tant to amikacin. The drug is ineffective against anaerobes.

PHARMACOKINETICS
Absorption: Amikacin is poorly absorbed after oral administration and is given parenterally; after I.M. administration, serum levels peak in 45 to 120 minutes.
Distribution: Drug is distributed widely after parenteral administration; intraocular penetration is poor. Factors that increase volume of distribution (such as burns or peritonitis) may increase dosage requirements. CSF penetration is low, even in patients with inflamed meninges. Intraventricular administration produces high levels throughout the CNS. Protein binding is minimal.
Metabolism: None.
Excretion: Drug is excreted primarily in urine through glomerular filtration; a small amount may be excreted in bile. Elimination half-life in adults is 2 to 3 hours. In patients with severe renal damage, half-life may extend to 30 to 86 hours. Over time, amikacin accumulates in inner ear and kidneys; urine levels approach 800 µg/ml 6 hours after a 500-mg I.M. dose.

CONTRAINDICATIONS & PRECAUTIONS
Contraindicated in patients with hypersensitivity to amikacin or other aminoglycosides. Use cautiously in geriatric patients, especially those with impaired renal function or neuromuscular disorders.

INTERACTIONS
Drug-drug. Use with *amphotericin B, capreomycin, cephalosporins, cisplatin, loop diuretics, methoxyflurane, polymyxin B, vancomycin,* or *other aminoglycosides* may increase the risk of nephrotoxicity, ototoxicity, and neurotoxicity. Use with *bumetanide, ethacrynic acid, furosemide, mannitol,* or *urea* may increase the risk of ototoxicity. Use with *dimenhydrinate* or *other antiemetics and antivertigo drugs* may mask amikacin-induced ototoxicity. Amikacin may potentiate neuromuscular blockade from *general anesthetics* or *neuromuscular*

blockers such as *succinylcholine* and *tubocurarine.* Use cautiously together.

Use with *penicillin* results in a synergistic bactericidal effect against *Citrobacter, Enterobacter, Escherichia coli, Klebsiella, Proteus mirabilis, Pseudomonas aeruginosa,* and *Serratia.* However, the drugs are physically and chemically incompatible and are inactivated when mixed or given together. In vivo inactivation has also been reported when aminoglycosides and penicillins are used concomitantly.

ADVERSE REACTIONS
CNS: *neuromuscular blockade.*
EENT: *ototoxicity.*
GU: *nephrotoxicity, azotemia.*
Musculoskeletal: arthralgia, acute muscular paralysis.

▣ KEY CONSIDERATIONS
Besides the recommendations relevant to all aminoglycosides, consider the following:
• Because geriatric patients may have impaired renal function, which may not be evident in routine screening tests such as BUN and serum creatinine levels, a creatinine clearance may be more useful.
• Because drug is dialyzable, patients undergoing hemodialysis need dosage adjustments.
• Recommendations for care and teaching of patients during therapy are the same as for all aminoglycosides.
• Drug-induced nephrotoxicity may elevate patient's BUN, nonprotein nitrogen, or serum creatinine level and increase urinary excretion of casts.
• Review renal function studies and hearing evaluation before initiating therapy.
• Peak blood levels above 35 µg/ml and trough levels above 10 µg/ml may increase the risk of toxicity.

Patient education
• Instruct patient to report adverse reactions promptly.
• Encourage adequate fluid intake.

Overdose & treatment
• Signs and symptoms of overdose include ototoxicity, nephrotoxicity, and neuromuscular toxicity.
• To reverse neuromuscular blockade, treat with calcium salts or anticholinesterases. Drug can be removed through hemodialysis or peritoneal dialysis.

amiloride hydrochloride
Midamor

Potassium sparing diuretic, antihypertensive

Available by prescription only
Tablets: 5 mg

INDICATIONS & DOSAGE
Hypertension; edema caused by heart failure, usually in patients who are also taking thiazide or another potassium wasting diuretic
Adults: Usually 5 mg P.O. daily. Dosage may be increased to 10 mg daily, if necessary. Don't exceed 20 mg daily.
◊ ***Lithium-induced polyuria***
Adults: 5 to 10 mg b.i.d.
◊ ***Cystic fibrosis***
Adults: Aerosolized amiloride dissolved in 0.3% NaCl solution.

PHARMACODYNAMICS
Diuretic action: Amiloride acts directly on the distal renal tubule to inhibit sodium reabsorption and potassium excretion, thereby reducing potassium loss.
Antihypertensive action: Drug is commonly used in combination with more effective diuretics to manage edema that results from heart failure, hepatic cirrhosis, and hyperaldosteronism. Mechanism of action is unknown.

PHARMACOKINETICS
Absorption: About 50% of an amiloride dose is absorbed from the GI tract. Food decreases absorption to 30%. Diuresis usually begins in 2 hours and peaks in 6 to 10 hours.
Distribution: Drug has wide extravascular distribution.
Metabolism: Insignificant.

Excretion: Most of the amiloride dose is excreted in urine; half-life is 6 to 9 hours in patients with normal renal function.

CONTRAINDICATIONS & PRECAUTIONS

Contraindicated in patients with elevated serum potassium level (over 5.5 mEq/L). Don't administer to patients receiving another potassium sparing diuretic, such as spironolactone or triamterene. Also contraindicated in patients with anuria, acute or chronic renal insufficiency, diabetic nephropathy, and hypersensitivity to drug.

Use with extreme caution in patients with diabetes mellitus.

INTERACTIONS

Drug-drug. Use with *ACE inhibitors, potassium-containing drugs (parenteral penicillin G), potassium sparing diuretics,* or *potassium supplements* increases the risk of hyperkalemia. Use cautiously together. Use with *digoxin* may decrease renal clearance of digoxin, along with the inotropic effect. Amiloride may reduce renal clearance of *lithium* and increase lithium blood levels. *NSAIDs, such as ibuprofen or indomethacin,* may alter renal function and thus affect potassium excretion. Use cautiously together.

Amiloride may potentiate hypotensive effects of other *antihypertensives;* this may be used to therapeutic advantage.
Drug-food. Use with *salt substitutes* or *food high in potassium* increases the risk of hyperkalemia. Avoid use.

ADVERSE REACTIONS

CNS: fatigue, *headache,* weakness, dizziness, encephalopathy.
CV: orthostatic hypotension.
GI: *nausea, anorexia, diarrhea, vomiting,* abdominal pain, constipation, appetite changes.
GU: impotence.
Hematologic: *aplastic anemia, neutropenia.*
Metabolic: hyperkalemia.
Musculoskeletal: muscle cramps.
Respiratory: dyspnea.

▣ KEY CONSIDERATIONS

Besides the recommendations relevant to all potassium sparing diuretics, consider the following:
• Geriatric patients require close observation because they're more susceptible to drug-induced diuresis and hyperkalemia. Reduced dosages may be indicated.
• Transient abnormal renal and hepatic function tests have been noted. Amiloride therapy causes severe hyperkalemia in diabetic patients following I.V. glucose tolerance testing; discontinue amiloride at least 3 days before testing.

Patient education

• Tell patient to take drug with food because it may cause stomach upset.
• Tell patient to call the doctor if signs of dehydration are present.
• Advise patient not to consume large quantities of high-potassium foods, such as oranges and bananas.

Overdose & treatment

• Signs and symptoms of overdose are consistent with those for dehydration and electrolyte disturbance.
• Treatment is supportive and symptomatic. In acute ingestion, empty stomach by inducing vomiting or performing gastric lavage. In severe hyperkalemia (6.5 mEq/L or more), reduce serum potassium levels with I.V. sodium bicarbonate or glucose with insulin. A cation exchange resin, sodium polystyrene sulfonate (Kayexalate), given orally or as a retention enema, may also reduce serum potassium levels.

aminophylline
Phyllocontin, Truphylline

Xanthine derivative, bronchodilator

Available by prescription only
Tablets: 100 mg, 200 mg
Tablets (controlled-release): 225 mg
Liquid: 105 mg/5 ml
Injection: 250-mg and 500-mg vials and ampules
Rectal suppositories: 250 mg, 500 mg

INDICATIONS & DOSAGE
Symptomatic relief of acute broncho-spasm
Patients not receiving theophylline:
Loading dosage is 6 mg/kg (equivalent to 4.7 mg/kg anhydrous theophylline) I.V. slowly (25 mg/minute or less), then maintenance infusion.
Patients receiving theophylline: Aminophylline loading infusions of 0.63 mg/kg (0.5 mg/kg anhydrous theophylline) will increase plasma levels of theophylline by 1 mcg/ml, after serum levels have been evaluated. Some doctors recommend a loading dose of 3.1 mg/kg I.V. (2.5 mg/kg anhydrous theophylline) if no obvious signs of theophylline toxicity are present, then maintenance infusion.
Otherwise healthy, adult nonsmokers:
0.7 mg/kg/hour I.V. for 12 hours, then 0.5 mg/kg/hour I.V.; or 3 mg/kg P.O. q 6 hours for two doses, then 3 mg/kg q 8 hours.
Otherwise healthy, adult smokers:
1 mg/kg/hour I.V. for 12 hours, then 0.8 mg/kg/hour I.V.; or 3 mg/kg P.O. q 4 hours for three doses, then 3 mg/kg q 6 hours.
Geriatric patients and adults with cor pulmonale: 0.6 mg/kg/hour I.V. for 12 hours, then 0.3 mg/kg/hour I.V.; or 2 mg/kg P.O. q 6 hours for two doses, then 2 mg/kg q 8 hours.
Adults with heart failure or liver disease: 0.5 mg/kg/hour I.V. for 12 hours, then 0.1 to 0.2 mg/kg/hour I.V.; or 2 mg/kg P.O. q 8 hours for two doses, then 1 to 2 mg/kg q 12 hours.
Chronic bronchial asthma
Adults: 400 mg P.O. t.i.d. or q.i.d.
Monitor serum theophylline levels to ensure that they range from 10 to 20 µg/ml.
◊ *Periodic apnea associated with Cheyne-Stokes respirations; left-sided heart failure*
Adults: 200 to 400 mg I.V. bolus.

PHARMACODYNAMICS
Bronchodilating action: Aminophylline acts at the cellular level after it is converted to theophylline. (Aminophylline [theophylline ethylenediamine] is 79% theophylline.) Theophylline acts by either inhibiting phosphodiesterase or blocking adenosine receptors in the bronchi, thus relaxing the smooth muscle. Drug also stimulates the respiratory center in the medulla and prevents diaphragmatic fatigue.

PHARMACOKINETICS
Absorption: Most dosage forms are absorbed well; absorption of the suppository, however, is unreliable and slow. Rate and onset of action also depend on the dosage form selected. Food may alter the rate, but not the extent of absorption, of oral doses.
Distribution: Distributed in all tissues and extracellular fluids except fatty tissue.
Metabolism: Drug is converted to theophylline and then metabolized to inactive compounds.
Excretion: Excreted in urine as theophylline (10%).

CONTRAINDICATIONS & PRECAUTIONS
Contraindicated in patients with hypersensitivity to xanthine compounds (caffeine, theobromine) and ethylenediamine and in patients with active peptic ulcer disease and seizure disorders (unless adequate anticonvulsant therapy is given). Rectal suppositories are also contraindicated in patients who have an irritation or infection of the rectum or lower colon.

Use cautiously in geriatric patients with heart failure, CV disorders, COPD, cor pulmonale, renal or hepatic disease, hyperthyroidism, diabetes mellitus, peptic ulcer, severe hypoxemia, or hypertension.

INTERACTIONS
Drug-drug. Use with *alkali-sensitive drugs* reduces activity of aminophylline. Don't add these drugs to I.V. fluids containing aminophylline.

Use with *allopurinol* (high dose), *cimetidine, erythromycin, propranolol, quinolones,* or *troleandomycin* may increase serum aminophylline level by decreasing hepatic clearance. Use with *aminoglutethimide, carbamazepine, phenobarbital, phenytoin,* or *rifampin* decreases effects of aminophylline. Aminophylline increases the excretion of *lithium*. Monitor closely.

Drug-lifestyle. Use with *marijuana* or *tobacco* decreases effects of aminophylline. Avoid using together.

ADVERSE REACTIONS

CNS: *nervousness, restlessness,* headache, *insomnia,* **seizures,** muscle twitching, irritability.

CV: *palpitations, sinus tachycardia,* extrasystoles, flushing, marked hypotension, **arrhythmias.**

GI: *nausea, vomiting,* diarrhea, epigastric pain, hematemesis.

Metabolic: hyperglycemia.

Respiratory: tachypnea, *respiratory arrest.*

Skin: urticaria.

Other: irritation (with rectal suppositories), fever.

▣ KEY CONSIDERATIONS

• Use in patients older than age 55 usually requires reduced dosage and close monitoring because of reduced clearance of drug, which commonly results in higher and potentially toxic serum levels.

• Before giving loading dose, check that patient hasn't received theophylline recently.

• Don't combine in the following fluids for I.V. infusion: ascorbic acid, chlorpromazine, codeine phosphate, dimenhydrinate, dobutamine, epinephrine, erythromycin gluceptate, hydralazine, insulin, levorphanol tartrate, meperidine, methadone, methicillin, morphine sulfate, norepinephrine bitartrate, oxytetracycline, penicillin g potassium, phenobarbital, phenytoin, prochlorperazine, promazine, promethazine, tetracycline, vancomycin, or vitamin B complex with C.

• Don't crush controlled-release tablets.

• I.V. drug administration includes I.V. push at a very slow rate or preferably an infusion with 100 to 200 ml of D_5W or normal saline solution.

• Although taking the drug while food is in stomach delays absorption, adverse GI reactions may be relieved by taking oral drug with full glass of water at meals. Enteric-coated tablets may also delay absorption. No evidence that antacids reduce adverse GI reactions exists.

• Suppositories are slowly and erratically absorbed; retention enemas may be absorbed more rapidly. Rectal preparations can be administered when patient can't take drug orally. To increase the likelihood of retention, schedule administration after evacuation, if possible, and before a meal. Advise patient to remain recumbent 15 to 20 minutes after insertion.

• Patients metabolize xanthines at different rates. Adjust dose by monitoring response, tolerance, pulmonary function, and blood theophylline levels. Therapeutic level is 10 to 20 µg/ml, but some patients may respond at lower levels; toxicity occurs at levels exceeding 20 µg/ml.

• Plasma clearance may be decreased in patients with heart failure, hepatic dysfunction, or pulmonary edema. Smokers show accelerated clearance. Dosage adjustments are necessary.

• Aminophylline may alter the assay for uric acid, depending on method used, and increases plasma-free fatty acid and urinary catecholamine levels. Theophylline levels may be falsely elevated if patient has taken in furosemide, phenylbutazone, probenecid, theobromine, caffeine, tea, chocolate, cola beverages, or acetaminophen, depending on type of assay used.

Patient education

• Teach patient rationale for therapy and importance of compliance with prescribed regimen; if a dose is missed, patient should take it as soon as possible but shouldn't double-dose. Advise patient to avoid taking extra "breathing pills."

• Warn patients of dizziness, a common adverse reaction at start of therapy.

• Advise patient of adverse effects and possible signs of toxicity.

• Tell patient not to eat or drink a large quantity of xanthine-containing foods and beverages.

• Warn patient that OTC remedies may combine ephedrine with theophylline salts; excessive CNS stimulation may result. Tell patient to seek medical approval before taking other drugs.

Overdose & treatment

• Signs and symptoms of overdose include nausea, vomiting, insomnia, irritability, tachycardia, extrasystoles, tachypnea, and tonic-clonic seizures. Onset of toxicity may be sudden and severe; arrhythmias and seizures are the first signs.

• Induce vomiting, except in patients with seizures, then use activated charcoal and a cathartic. Charcoal hemoperfusion may be beneficial. Treat arrhythmias with lidocaine and seizures with I.V. benzodiazepine; support respiratory and CV systems.

---

amiodarone hydrochloride
Cordarone

Benzofuran derivative, ventricular and supraventricular antiarrhythmic

---

Available by prescription only
Tablets: 100 mg*, 200 mg
Injection: 50 mg/ml

INDICATIONS & DOSAGE

Recurrent ventricular fibrillation and unstable ventricular tachycardia; ◇ *supraventricular arrhythmias;* ◇ *atrial fibrillation;* ◇ *angina;* ◇ *hypertrophic cardiomyopathy*
Adults: Loading dosage of 800 to 1,600 mg P.O. daily for 1 to 3 weeks until initial therapeutic response occurs. Maintenance dosage is 200 to 600 mg P.O. daily. Alternatively, for first 24 hours 150 mg I.V. over 10 minutes (mixed in 100 ml D₅W); then 360 mg I.V. over 6 hours (mix 900 mg in 500 ml D₅W); then maintenance of 540 mg I.V. over 18 hours at a rate of 0.5 mg/minute. After first 24 hours, continue a maintenance infusion of 0.5 mg/minute in a 1 to 6 mg/ml concentration. For infusions lasting than 1 hour, concentrations shouldn't exceed 2 mg/ml unless a central venous catheter is used. Don't use for more than 3 weeks.

Conversion from I.V. to P.O.
Adults: Daily dosage of 720 mg (rate 0.5 mg/minute): for 1 week, 800 to 1,600 mg daily; 1 to 3 weeks, 600 to 800 mg daily; more than 3 weeks, 400 mg daily.

PHARMACODYNAMICS
Ventricular antiarrhythmic action: Although amiodarone has mixed class Ic and III antiarrhythmic effects, it's generally considered a class III drug. It widens the action potential duration (repolarization inhibition). With prolonged therapy, the effective refractory period increases in the atria, ventricles, AV node, His-Purkinje system, and bypass tracts, and conduction slows in the atria, AV node, His-Purkinje system, and ventricles; sinus node automaticity decreases. Amiodarone also noncompetitively blocks beta receptors. It has little, if any, negative inotropic effect. Coronary and peripheral vasodilator effects may occur with long-term therapy. Amiodarone is among the most effective antiarrhythmics, but its therapeutic applications are somewhat limited by its severe adverse reactions.

PHARMACOKINETICS
Absorption: Amiodarone has slow, variable absorption. Bioavailability is 22% to 86%. Plasma levels peak 3 to 7 hours after oral administration; however, onset of action may be delayed from 2 to 3 days to 2 to 3 months—even with loading doses.
Distribution: Drug is distributed widely because it accumulates in adipose tissue and in organs—such as the lungs, liver, and spleen—with marked perfusion. It's also highly protein-bound (96%). The therapeutic serum level isn't well defined but may range from 1 to 2.5 µg/ml.
Metabolism: Drug is metabolized extensively in the liver to a pharmacologic active metabolite, desethyl amiodarone.
Excretion: Drug is excreted mainly by the liver, through the biliary tree (with enterohepatic recirculation). Because none of the drug is excreted by the kidneys, patients with impaired renal function don't require dosage reduction. Terminal elimination half-life—25 to 110 days—is the longest of any antiarrhyth-

---

Reactions may be *common*, uncommon, *life-threatening*, or COMMON AND LIFE-THREATENING.

mic; in most patients, half-life ranges from 40 to 50 days.

CONTRAINDICATIONS & PRECAUTIONS

Contraindicated in patients with hypersensitivity to amiodarone and in those with severe SA node disease resulting in preexisting bradycardia. Unless an artificial pacemaker is present, drug is also contraindicated in patients with second- or third-degree AV block or bradycardia-induced syncope. Use with caution in patients already receiving antiarrhythmics, beta blockers, or calcium channel blockers.

INTERACTIONS

Drug-drug. Use with *beta blockers* or *calcium channel blockers* may cause sinus bradycardia, sinus arrest, or AV block. Use with *disopyramide, phenothiazines, quinidine,* or *tricyclic antidepressants* may cause additive effects that lead to a prolonged QT interval, possibly resulting in torsades de pointes ventricular tachycardia. Don't use together.

Use with *cholestyramine* increases elimination of amiodarone. Use with *cimetidine* increases amiodarone levels. Use with *cyclosporine, digoxin, flecainide, lidocaine, phenytoin, procainamide, quinidine,* or *theophylline* may lead to increased serum levels of these drugs, resulting in enhanced effects. Use with *phenytoin* decreases amiodarone levels. Use with *warfarin* may prolong PT, as a result of enhanced drug displacement from protein-binding sites. Monitor closely.

Drug-lifestyle. Exposure to *sunlight* may cause photosensitivity reactions. Take precautions.

ADVERSE REACTIONS

CNS: peripheral neuropathy, ataxia, paresthesia, tremor, insomnia, sleep disturbances, headache, *malaise, fatigue.*
CV: bradycardia, hypotension, ***arrhythmias, heart failure, heart block, sinus arrest,*** edema.
EENT: *corneal microdeposits,* visual disturbances.
GI: *nausea, vomiting,* constipation, abdominal pain.

Hematologic: coagulation abnormalities.
Hepatic: *altered liver enzyme levels,* hepatic dysfunction, ***hepatic failure.***
Metabolic: hypothyroidism, hyperthyroidism.
Respiratory: SEVERE PULMONARY TOXICITY (PNEUMONITIS, ALVEOLITIS).
Skin: *photosensitivity,* blue-gray skin pigmentation, solar dermatitis.

▣ KEY CONSIDERATIONS

• Relatively high dosages of amiodarone should be used cautiously because geriatric patients may be more susceptible to the bradycardia and conduction disturbances that this drug causes.
• Amiodarone can alter thyroid function test results, increasing serum T_4 levels and decreasing serum T_3 levels, particularly in geriatric patients, especially those with thyroid dysfunction. Thyroid function tests should be performed before initiating therapy and about every 3 to 6 months thereafter.
• Drug is effective in treating arrhythmias resistant to other drug therapy. However, its high frequency of adverse effects limits its use.
• To minimize GI intolerance, divide loading dosage into three equal doses, and give with meals. Maintenance dosage may be given once daily but may be divided into two doses and taken with meals if GI intolerance occurs.
• Monitor blood pressure and heart rate and rhythm frequently for significant changes.
• Periodically monitor hepatic and thyroid function tests. To assess corneal microdeposits, perform periodic ophthalmologic evaluations.
• Monitor for signs and symptoms of pneumonitis, such as exertional dyspnea, nonproductive cough, and pleuritic chest pain. Also, check pulmonary function tests and chest X-ray. (Pulmonary toxicity is more common with daily dosages exceeding 600 mg.) If patient develops pulmonary complications, amiodarone will need to be discontinued and patient may need to be treated with corticosteroids.
• To avoid toxicity, digoxin, quinidine, phenytoin, and procainamide dosages

should be decreased during amiodarone therapy.

• Adverse effects are more prevalent with high doses but usually resolve within about 4 months of stopping drug therapy.

• I.V. amiodarone infusions lasting more than 2 hours must be administered in glass or polyolefin bottles containing D_5W.

• Tell patient to notify doctor for episodes of chest pain or aggravation of cardiovascular disease because amiodarone-induced hyperthyroidism may be present.

Patient education

• Advise patient to use sunscreen to prevent photosensitivity, which may result in sunburn and blistering from ultraviolet light or sunlight.

• Although corneal microdeposits typically appear 1 to 4 months after therapy begins, only 2% to 3% of patients have actual visual disturbances. To minimize this complication, recommend frequent instillation of methylcellulose ophthalmic solution.

Overdose & treatment

• Signs and symptoms of overdose include bradyarrhythmias.

• Treatment to restore an acceptable heart rate may include beta agonists (such as isoproterenol) and artificial pacing. Treatment for hypotension may include positive inotropic drugs (such as dopamine and dobutamine) and vasopressors (such as epinephrine and norepinephrine). General supportive measures should be used, as necessary. Drug can't be removed through dialysis.

---

amitriptyline hydrochloride
Amitriptyline, Elavil, Levate*, Novotriptyn*

Tricyclic antidepressant

Available by prescription only
Tablets: 10 mg, 25 mg, 50 mg, 75 mg, 100 mg, 150 mg
Injection: 10 mg/ml

INDICATIONS & DOSAGE
Depression; anorexia or bulimia associated with depression; adjunctive treatment of neurogenic pain
Adults: Initial outpatient, 75 to 150 mg/day P.O. in divided doses or 50 to 150 mg h.s.; inpatient, 100 to 300 mg/day. I.M. dosage is 20 to 30 mg q.i.d., which should be changed to oral route as soon as possible. Maintenance dosage is 50 to 100 mg/day.
Geriatric patients: 10 mg P.O. t.i.d. and 20 mg h.s.

PHARMACODYNAMICS
Antidepressant action: Amitriptyline inhibits reuptake of norepinephrine and serotonin in CNS nerve terminals (presynaptic neurons), resulting in increased levels and enhanced activity of these neurotransmitters in the synaptic cleft. Amitriptyline more actively inhibits reuptake of serotonin than norepinephrine; it increases the risk of undesirable sedation, but tolerance to this effect usually develops within a few weeks.

PHARMACOKINETICS
Absorption: Amitriptyline is absorbed rapidly from the GI tract after oral administration and from muscle tissue after I.M. administration.
Distribution: Drug is distributed widely into the body, including the CNS; 96% is protein-bound. Peak effect occurs 2 to 12 hours after a given dose, and steady state is achieved in 4 to 10 days; full therapeutic effect usually occurs in 2 to 4 weeks.
Metabolism: Drug is metabolized in the liver to the active metabolite nortriptyline; a significant first-pass effect may explain why serum levels vary in different patients taking the same dosage.
Excretion: Drug is excreted mostly in urine.

CONTRAINDICATIONS & PRECAUTIONS
Contraindicated in patients who are in the acute recovery phase of an MI, in those with hypersensitivity, and in patients who have received an MAO inhibitor within the past 14 days.

Use cautiously in patients with recent history of an MI and in those with unsta-

---

Reactions may be *common*, uncommon, *life-threatening*, or COMMON AND LIFE-THREATENING.

ble heart disease or renal or hepatic impairment.

INTERACTIONS

Drug-drug. Use with *antiarrhythmics—such as quinidine, disopyramide,* or *procainamide—pimozide, or thyroid hormones* may increase incidence of arrhythmias and conduction defects. Use with *atropine* or *other anticholinergics—including antihistamines, antiparkinsonians, meperidine, and phenothiazines—*increases sedation, paralytic ileus, and hyperthermia. Use with *disulfiram* or *ethchlorvynol* may cause delirium and tachycardia. Use cautiously.

Use with *barbiturates* induces amitriptyline metabolism, increases sedation, and decreases therapeutic efficacy. Use with *beta blockers, cimetidine, methylphenidate, oral contraceptives, propoxyphene,* or *selective serotonin reuptake inhibitors (such as Prozac)* may inhibit amitriptyline metabolism, increasing plasma levels and toxicity.

Amitriptyline may decrease the hypotensive effects of *centrally acting hypertensives, such as clonidine, guanethidine, guanabenz, guanadrel, methyldopa,* and *reserpine.* Use with *CNS depressants—including analgesics, anesthetics, narcotics,* and *tranquilizers—*may increase the likelihood of additive effects. Use with *ephedrine, phenylephrine, phenylpropanolamine,* or *sympathomimetics—including epinephrine (found in many nasal sprays)—*may increase blood pressure. Use with *metrizamide* increases risk of seizures. Use with *phenothiazines* or *haloperidol* decreases metabolism and increases blood levels of amitriptyline. Use with *warfarin* may increase PT and INR and cause bleeding. Monitor closely.
Drug-lifestyle. Use with *alcohol* increases the risk of additive effects. *Heavy smoking* induces amitriptyline metabolism and decreases therapeutic efficacy. Don't use together.

ADVERSE REACTIONS

CNS: *coma, seizures,* hallucinations, delusions, disorientation, ataxia, tremor, peripheral neuropathy, anxiety, insomnia, restlessness, drowsiness, dizziness, weakness, fatigue, headache, extrapyramidal reactions.
CV: *MI, stroke, arrhythmias,* heart block, *orthostatic hypotension, tachycardia, ECG changes,* hypertension, edema.
EENT: *blurred vision,* tinnitus, mydriasis, increased intraocular pressure.
GI: *dry mouth,* nausea, vomiting, anorexia, epigastric distress, diarrhea, constipation, paralytic ileus.
GU: urine retention.
Hematologic: *agranulocytosis, thrombocytopenia, leukopenia,* eosinophilia.
Skin: rash, urticaria, photosensitivity.
Other: *diaphoresis, hypersensitivity reaction.*
After abrupt withdrawal of long-term therapy: nausea, headache, malaise (doesn't indicate addiction).

🔲 KEY CONSIDERATIONS

Besides the recommendations relevant to all tricyclic antidepressants, consider the following:

● Geriatric patients may be at greater risk for adverse cardiac effects.

● Amitriptyline also may be used to prevent migraine and cluster headaches, intractable hiccups, and posttherapeutic neuralgia.

● Drug produces sedative effects in many patients. Although tolerance to these effects usually develops over several weeks, some patients never become tolerant.

● The full dose may be given at bedtime to help offset daytime sedation.

● Drug should be switched from parenteral to oral administration as soon as possible.

● I.M. administration may result in a more rapid onset of action than oral administration.

● Don't withdraw drug abruptly.

● Discontinue drug at least 48 hours before surgical procedures.

● Sugarless chewing gum or hard candy or ice may alleviate dry mouth. Stress the importance of regular dental hygiene because dry mouth can increase the risk of dental caries.

● Depressed patients, particularly those with known manic depressive illness, may experience a shift to mania or hypomania.

• Amitriptyline may prolong conduction time (elongation of QT and PR intervals, flattened T waves on ECG); it also may elevate liver function test results, decrease WBC counts, and decrease or increase serum glucose levels.

Patient education
• Tell patient to take drug exactly as prescribed and not to double-dose if he misses a dose.
• Advise patient that a full dose may be taken at bedtime to alleviate daytime sedation. Alternatively, it may be taken in the early evening to avoid morning "hangover."
• Explain that full effects of drug may not become apparent for up to 4 weeks after initiation of therapy.
• Warn patient that drug may cause drowsiness or dizziness. Tell him to avoid hazardous activities that require alertness until full effects of drug are known.
• Warn patient not to drink alcoholic beverages while taking drug.
• Suggest taking drug with food or milk if it causes stomach upset and using sugarless gum or candy to relieve dry mouth.
• After initial doses, advise patient to lie down for about 30 minutes and raise to upright position slowly to prevent dizziness or fainting.
• Warn patient not to stop taking drug suddenly.
• Encourage patient to report troublesome or unusual effects, especially confusion, movement disorders, rapid heartbeat, dizziness, fainting, or difficulty urinating.
• Tell patient to store drug safely away from children.

Overdose & treatment
• The first 12 hours after acute ingestion make up the stimulatory phase, which is characterized by excessive anticholinergic activity (agitation, irritation, confusion, hallucinations, hyperthermia, parkinsonian symptoms, seizure, urine retention, dry mucous membranes, pupillary dilation, constipation, and ileus). CNS depressant effects—including hypothermia, decreased or absent reflexes, sedation, hypotension, cyanosis, and cardiac irregularities, including tachycardia, conduction disturbances, and quinidine-like effects on the ECG—follow this phase.
• Severity of overdose is best indicated by widening of the QRS complex and usually represents a serum level in excess of 1,000 mg/ml; metabolic acidosis may follow hypotension, hypoventilation, and seizures. Delayed cardiac anomalies and death may occur.
• Treatment is symptomatic and supportive, including maintaining airway, a stable body temperature, and fluid and electrolyte balance. Induce vomiting with ipecac if gag reflex is intact; follow with gastric lavage and activated charcoal to prevent further absorption. Dialysis is of little use. Physostigmine may be cautiously used to reverse the symptoms of tricyclic antidepressant poisoning in life-threatening situations. Treatment of seizures may include parenteral diazepam or phenytoin; treatment of arrhythmias, parenteral phenytoin or lidocaine; and treatment of acidosis, sodium bicarbonate. Because barbiturates may enhance CNS and respiratory depressant effects, they shouldn't be administered.

---

amlodipine besylate
Norvasc

Dihydropyridine calcium channel blocker, antianginal, antihypertensive

Available by prescription only
Tablets: 2.5 mg, 5 mg, 10 mg

INDICATIONS & DOSAGE
Chronic stable angina, vasospastic angina (Prinzmetal's or variant angina)
Adults: Initially, 5 to 10 mg P.O. daily.
Hypertension
Adults: Initially, 5 mg P.O. daily. Adjust dosage based on patient response and tolerance. Maximum daily dose, 10 mg.
Geriatric patients: 2.5 mg P.O. daily.
✦ **Dosage adjustment.** In small, frail patients; patients receiving other antihypertensives; or patients with hepatic insufficiency, give 2.5 mg P.O. daily.

PHARMACODYNAMICS
Antianginal and antihypertensive actions: Contractility of cardiac muscle and vascular smooth muscle depends on movement of extracellular calcium ions into cardiac and smooth-muscle cells through specific ion channels. Amlodipine inhibits the transmembrane influx of calcium ions into vascular smooth muscle and cardiac muscle, thus decreasing myocardial contractility and oxygen demand. As a peripheral arterial vasodilator, the drug acts directly on vascular smooth muscle to reduce peripheral vascular resistance and blood pressure. It also dilates coronary arteries and arterioles.

PHARMACOKINETICS
Absorption: After oral administration of therapeutic dosages of amlodipine, plasma levels peak within 6 to 12 hours. Estimated absolute bioavailability is between 64% and 90%.
Distribution: About 93% of the circulating drug binds to plasma proteins in hypertensive patients.
Metabolism: Drug is extensively metabolized in the liver, with about 90% converted to inactive metabolites.
Excretion: Drug is excreted primarily in urine.

CONTRAINDICATIONS & PRECAUTIONS
Contraindicated in patients with hypersensitivity to amlodipine. Use cautiously in patients receiving other peripheral dilators and in those with aortic stenosis, heart failure, or severe hepatic disease.

INTERACTIONS
None reported.

ADVERSE REACTIONS
CNS: *headache,* somnolence, fatigue, dizziness, light-headedness, paresthesia.
CV: *edema,* flushing, palpitations.
GI: nausea, abdominal pain.
Musculoskeletal: muscle pain.
Respiratory: dyspnea.
Skin: rash, pruritus.

◎ KEY CONSIDERATIONS
• Some patients, especially those with severe obstructive coronary artery disease, have developed increased frequency, duration, or severity of angina or even an acute MI after initiation of calcium channel blocker therapy or at time of dosage increase. Monitor patient carefully.
• Because the vasodilation induced by amlodipine is gradual in onset, acute hypotension has rarely been reported after oral administration of amlodipine. However, the drug should be administered cautiously, particularly in patients with severe aortic stenosis.

Patient education
• Tell patient to take nitroglycerin S.L. as needed for acute angina. If patient continues nitrate therapy during adjustment of amlodipine dosage, stress the importance of continued compliance.
• Caution patient to continue taking amlodipine even when he feels better.
• Tell patient to notify doctor about signs and symptoms of heart failure, such as swelling of hands and feet or shortness of breath.

Overdose & treatment
• Signs and symptoms of overdose include nausea, weakness, dizziness, drowsiness, confusion, and slurred speech. Overdose also can cause excessive peripheral vasodilation with marked hypotension and bradycardia, both of which may reduce cardiac output. Junctional rhythms and second- or third-degree AV block also can occur. Massive overdose warrants active cardiac and respiratory monitoring and frequent blood pressure measurements.
• Treatment of hypotension consists of CV support, including elevation of the extremities and judicious administration of fluids. If hypotension remains unresponsive to these conservative measures, administration of vasopressors (such as phenylephrine) should be considered, with attention to circulating volume and urine output. I.V. calcium gluconate may help reverse the effects of calcium entry blockade. Because amlodipine is highly protein-bound, hemodialysis isn't likely to benefit the patient.

amobarbital

amobarbital sodium
Amytal

Barbiturate, sedative-hypnotic, anticonvulsant
Controlled substance schedule II

Available by prescription only
Tablets: 30 mg
Capsules: 200 mg
Powder for injection: 250-mg vial, 500-mg vial

INDICATIONS & DOSAGE
Sedation
Adults: Usually 30 to 50 mg P.O. b.i.d. or t.i.d. but may range from 15 to 120 mg b.i.d. to q.i.d.
Insomnia
Adults: 65 to 200 mg P.O. or deep I.M. h.s.; I.M. injection not to exceed 5 ml in any one site. Maximum dosage is 500 mg.
Preanesthetic sedation
Adults: 200 mg P.O. 1 to 2 hours before surgery.
Anticonvulsant
Adults: 65 to 500 mg by slow I.V. injection (rate not exceeding 100 mg/minute). Maximum dose is 1 g.

PHARMACODYNAMICS
Sedative-hypnotic action: Amobarbital acts throughout the CNS as a nonselective depressant with an intermediate onset and duration of action. The mesencephalic reticular activating system, which controls CNS arousal, is particularly sensitive to this drug. Amobarbital decreases both presynaptic and postsynaptic membrane excitability by facilitating the action of gamma-aminobutyric acid (GABA).
Anticonvulsant action: The exact cellular site and mechanism of action are unknown. By enhancing the effect of GABA, parenteral amobarbital suppresses the spread of seizure activity from the epileptogenic foci in the cortex, thalamus, and limbic systems. Both presynaptic and postsynaptic excitability are decreased.

PHARMACOKINETICS
Absorption: Amobarbital is well absorbed after oral administration. Absorption after I.M. administration is 100%. Onset of action is 45 to 60 minutes.
Distribution: Drug is well distributed throughout body tissues and fluids.
Metabolism: Drug is metabolized in the liver through oxidation to a tertiary alcohol.
Excretion: Less than 1% of a dose is excreted unchanged in the urine; the rest is excreted as metabolites. The half-life is biphasic, with a first phase half-life of about 40 minutes and a second phase of about 20 hours. Duration of action is 6 to 8 hours.

CONTRAINDICATIONS & PRECAUTIONS
Contraindicated in patients with bronchopneumonia or other severe pulmonary insufficiency or hypersensitivity to barbiturates or porphyria.
Use cautiously in patients with suicidal tendencies, acute or chronic pain, history of drug abuse, hepatic or renal impairment, or pulmonary or CV disease.

INTERACTIONS
Drug-drug. Amobarbital may add to or potentiate CNS and respiratory depressant effects of *antidepressants, antihistamines, MAO inhibitors, narcotics, sedative-hypnotics,* and *tranquilizers.* Amobarbital enhances hepatic metabolism of *corticosteroids, digitoxin, doxycycline, oral contraceptives and other estrogens,* and *theophylline and other xanthines.* Amobarbital may cause unpredictable fluctuations in serum *phenytoin* levels. Use with *rifampin* may decrease amobarbital levels by increasing metabolism. Amobarbital enhances the enzymatic degradation of *warfarin and other oral anticoagulants;* patients may require increased dosages of the anticoagulants. Monitor closely.
Use with *disulfiram, MAO inhibitors,* or *valproic acid* decreases the metabolism of amobarbital and can increase its toxicity. Amobarbital impairs the effectiveness of *griseofulvin* by decreasing absorption from the GI tract. Don't use together.

Reactions may be *common*, uncommon, *life-threatening*, or COMMON AND LIFE-THREATENING.

Drug-lifestyle. Amobarbital may add to or potentiate CNS and respiratory depressant effects of *alcohol.* Don't use together.

ADVERSE REACTIONS

CNS: *drowsiness, lethargy, hangover,* paradoxical excitement, somnolence.
CV: bradycardia, hypotension, syncope.
GI: nausea, vomiting.
Hematologic: exacerbation of porphyria.
Respiratory: *respiratory depression, apnea.*
Skin: rash; urticaria; *Stevens-Johnson syndrome;* pain, irritation, sterile abscess at injection site.
Other: *angioedema,* physical and psychological dependence.

▣ KEY CONSIDERATIONS

Besides the recommendations relevant to all barbiturates, consider the following:
• Geriatric patients usually require lower dosages of amobarbital. Confusion, disorientation, and excitability may occur in geriatric patients. Use with caution.
• Drug isn't commonly used as a sedative or an aid to sleeping; barbiturates have been replaced by safer benzodiazepines for such use.
• Administer drug orally before meals or on an empty stomach to enhance rate of absorption.
• Reconstitute powder for injection with sterile water for injection. Roll vial between palms; don't shake. Use 2.5 ml or 5 ml (for 250 mg or 500 mg of amobarbital) to make 10% solution. For I.M. use, prepare 20% solution by using 1.25 ml or 2.5 ml of sterile water for injection.
• Administer reconstituted parenteral solution within 30 minutes after opening the vial.
• Don't administer amobarbital solution that's cloudy or forms a precipitate after 5 minutes of reconstitution.
• To prevent possible hypotension and respiratory depression, administer I.V. dose at a rate no greater than 100 mg/minute in adults. Have emergency resuscitative equipment available.
• Administer I.M. dose deep into large muscle mass, giving no more than 5 ml in any one injection site. Sterile abscess or tissue damage may result from inadvertent superficial I.M. or S.C. injection.
• Administering a full loading dosage over a short period of time to treat status epilepticus may require ventilatory support in adults.
• Assess cardiopulmonary status frequently for possible alterations. Monitor blood counts for potential adverse reactions.
• To ensure adequate drug removal, assess renal and hepatic laboratory studies.
• Amobarbital may cause a false-positive phentolamine test. It may also impair absorption of cyanocobalamin ^{57}Co, decrease serum bilirubin levels in patients with a seizure disorder or congenital nonhemolytic unconjugated hyperbilirubinemia, and alter EEG patterns, with a change in low-voltage, fast-activity. Changes in EEG patterns persist for a time after therapy has been discontinued.
• Monitor PT and INR carefully when patient taking amobarbital starts or ends anticoagulant therapy. Anticoagulant dosage may need to be adjusted.

Patient education
• Warn patient of possible physical or psychological dependence with prolonged use.
• Tell patient to avoid alcohol while taking drug.

Overdose & treatment
• Signs and symptoms of overdose include unsteady gait, slurred speech, sustained nystagmus, somnolence, confusion, respiratory depression, pulmonary edema, areflexia, and coma. Oliguria, jaundice, hypothermia, fever, and shock with tachycardia and hypotension may occur.
• Treatment aims to maintain and support ventilation and pulmonary function as necessary; support cardiac function and circulation with vasopressors and I.V. fluids as needed. If patient is conscious with a functioning gag reflex and ingestion is recent, then induce vomiting by administering ipecac syrup. To prevent aspiration when vomiting is inappropriate, you may perform gastric lavage if a cuffed endotracheal tube is in

place. Then, administer activated charcoal or sodium chloride cathartic. Measure fluid intake and output, vital signs, and laboratory parameters. Maintain body temperature. Maintain and support ventilation as necessary; support circulation with vasopressors and I.V. fluids as needed. Alkalinization of urine may be helpful in removing amobarbital from the body; hemodialysis may be useful in severe overdose.

amoxapine
Asendin

Dibenzoxazepine, tricyclic antidepressant

Available by prescription only
Tablets: 25 mg, 50 mg, 100 mg, 150 mg

INDICATIONS & DOSAGE
Depression
Adults: Initial dosage is 50 mg P.O. b.i.d. or t.i.d; may increase to 100 mg b.i.d. or t.i.d. by end of first week. Increases above 300 mg daily should be made only if this dosage has been ineffective during a trial period of at least 2 weeks. When effective dosage is established, entire dosage (not exceeding 300 mg) may be given h.s. Maximum dosage in hospitalized patients is 600 mg.
Geriatric patients: Recommended starting dosage is 25 mg P.O. b.i.d. or t.i.d.
   Note: Don't give more than 300 mg in a single dose.

PHARMACODYNAMICS
Antidepressant action: Amoxapine inhibits reuptake of norepinephrine and serotonin in CNS nerve terminals (presynaptic neurons), which results in increased levels and enhanced activity of these neurotransmitters in the synaptic cleft. Amoxapine has a greater inhibitory effect on norepinephrine reuptake than on serotonin. Drug also blocks CNS dopamine receptors, which may account for the increasing number of movement disorders during therapy.

PHARMACOKINETICS
Absorption: Amoxapine is absorbed rapidly and completely from the GI tract after oral administration.
Distribution: Drug is distributed widely into the body, including the CNS, and is 92% protein-bound. Drug effect peaks in 8 to 10 hours; steady state, within 2 to 7 days. Proposed therapeutic plasma levels (parent drug and metabolite) range from 200 to 500 ng/ml.
Metabolism: Drug is metabolized in the liver to the active metabolite 8-hydroxyamoxapine; a significant first-pass effect may explain why serum levels vary in different patients taking the same dosage.
Excretion: Drug is excreted in urine and feces (7% to 18%); about 60% of a given dose is excreted as the conjugated form within 6 days.

CONTRAINDICATIONS & PRECAUTIONS
Contraindicated in patients who are hypersensitive, are in the acute recovery phase of an MI, or have received an MAO inhibitor within the past 14 days.
   Use cautiously in patients with history of urine retention, CV disease, angle-closure glaucoma, or increased intraocular pressure. Also, use with extreme caution in patients with a history of seizures.

INTERACTIONS
Drug-drug. Use with *antiarrhythmics* (such as *disopyramide, procainamide,* and *quinidine), pimozide,* or *thyroid drugs* may increase the incidence of arrhythmias and conduction defects. Use with *atropine* or *other anticholinergics* (including *antihistamines, antiparkinsonians, meperidine,* and *phenothiazines)* increases sedation, hyperthermia, and paralytic ileus. Use with *disulfiram* or *ethchlorvynol* may cause delirium and tachycardia. Use cautiously.
   Use with *barbiturates* increases sedation and increases metabolism of amoxapine, possibly decreasing its therapeutic effect. Amoxapine may decrease the hypotensive effects of *centrally acting antihypertensives* such as *clonidine, guanabenz, guanadrel, guanethidine, methyldopa,* and *reserpine.* Use with

---

CNS depressants (including *analgesics, anesthetics, narcotics,* and *tranquilizers)* may increase the likelihood of adverse effects. Use with *beta blockers, cimetidine, methylphenidate, oral contraceptives,* or *propoxyphene* may inhibit amoxapine metabolism, increasing plasma levels and toxicity. Use with *haloperidol* or *phenothiazines* decreases metabolism and increases bloods levels of amoxapine. Use with *metrizamide* increases the risk of seizures.

Use with *sympathomimetics—including ephedrine (found in many nasal sprays), epinephrine, phenylephrine, and phenylpropanolamine—*may increase blood pressure. Use with *warfarin* may increase PT and INR and cause bleeding. Monitor closely.

Drug-lifestyle. Use with alcohol increases CNS effects. *Heavy smoking* induces metabolism of amoxapine and decreases its therapeutic effect. Avoid concomitant use.

ADVERSE REACTIONS

CNS: *drowsiness, dizziness,* excitation, tremor, weakness, confusion, anxiety, insomnia, restlessness, nightmares, ataxia, fatigue, headache, nervousness, *tardive dyskinesia, EEG changes, **seizures, neuroleptic malignant syndrome (high fever, tachycardia, tachypnea, profuse diaphoresis).***
CV: *orthostatic hypotension, tachycardia,* hypertension, palpitations.
EENT: *blurred vision.*
GI: *dry mouth, constipation,* nausea, excessive appetite.
GU: *urine retention, acute renal failure.*
Skin: rash, edema.
Other: *diaphoresis.*
After abrupt withdrawal of long-term therapy: nausea, headache, malaise.

◻ KEY CONSIDERATIONS

Besides the recommendations relevant to all tricyclic antidepressants, consider the following:
● Geriatric patients are more sensitive to the therapeutic and adverse effects (especially tardive dyskinesia and extrapyramidal symptoms) of drug and require a lower dosage.

● Amoxapine has been known to cause seizures in many patients.
● Antidepressants can cause manic episodes during the depressed phase in patients with bipolar disorder.
● The full dose may be given at bedtime to help reduce daytime sedation.
● The full dose shouldn't be withdrawn abruptly.
● Tolerance to sedative effects usually develops over the first few weeks of therapy.
● Drug should be discontinued at least 48 hours before surgical procedures.
● Sugarless chewing gum or hard candy or ice may alleviate dry mouth.
● Tardive dyskinesia and other extrapyramidal effects may occur because of the dopamine-blocking activity of amoxapine. Geriatric patients appear to be more susceptible to these effects.
● Watch for gynecomastia in males and females because amoxapine may increase cellular division in breast tissue.
● Amoxapine may prolong conduction time (elongation of QT and PR intervals, flattened T waves on ECG); it also may elevate liver function test results, decrease WBC counts, and decrease or increase serum glucose levels.

Patient education
● Explain that full effects of drug may not become apparent for at least 2 weeks or more after therapy begins, perhaps not for 4 to 6 weeks.
● Tell patient to take drug exactly as prescribed; however, full dose may be taken at bedtime to alleviate daytime sedation. Patient shouldn't double-dose if he misses one.
● Warn patient that because drug may cause drowsiness or dizziness, hazardous activities that require alertness should be avoided until drug's full effects are known.
● Tell patient not to drink alcoholic beverages while taking drug.
● Suggest that patient takes drug with food or milk if it causes stomach upset; dry mouth can be relieved with sugarless gum or hard candy.
● After initial doses, tell patient to lie down for about 30 minutes and rise slowly to prevent dizziness.

• Warn patient not to discontinue drug suddenly.

• Encourage patient to report unusual or troublesome reactions immediately, especially confusion, movement disorders, rapid heartbeat, dizziness, fainting, or difficulty urinating.

• Warn patient of risks of tardive dyskinesia and explain its symptoms.

• Inform patient that exposure to sunlight, sunlamps, or tanning beds may burn the skin or cause abnormal pigmentary changes.

Overdose & treatment

• The first 12 hours after acute ingestion are a stimulatory phase characterized by excessive anticholinergic activity (agitation, irritation, confusion, hallucinations, hyperthermia, parkinsonian symptoms, seizures, urine retention, dry mucous membranes, pupillary dilation, constipation, and ileus). This initial period is then followed by CNS depressant effects, including hypothermia, decreased or absent reflexes, sedation, hypotension, cyanosis, and cardiac irregularities, including tachycardia, conduction disturbances, and quinidine-like effects on the ECG.

• Amoxapine overdose causes CNS toxicity in more patients than other antidepressants. Acute deterioration of renal function (evidenced by myoglobin in urine) occurs in 5% of patients who overdosed; this is most likely to occur in patients with repeated seizures after the overdose. Seizures may progress to status epilepticus within 12 hours.

• Severity of overdose is best indicated by widening of the QRS complex, which generally represents a serum level in excess of 1,000 ng/ml; serum levels aren't usually helpful. Metabolic acidosis may follow hypotension, hypoventilation, and seizures.

• Treatment is symptomatic and supportive, including maintaining airway, a stable body temperature, and fluid and electrolyte balance; monitor renal status because of the risk of renal failure. Induce vomiting with ipecac if patient is conscious; follow with gastric lavage and activated charcoal to prevent further absorption. Dialysis is of little use. Treat seizures with parenteral diazepam or phenytoin (the value of physostigmine is less certain); arrhythmias, with parenteral phenytoin or lidocaine; and acidosis, with sodium bicarbonate. Don't give barbiturates; these may enhance CNS and respiratory depressant effects.

---

amoxicillin/clavulanate potassium
Augmentin, Clavulin*

Aminopenicillin and beta-lactamase inhibitor, antibiotic

Available by prescription only
Tablets (chewable): 125 mg of amoxicillin trihydrate, 31.25 mg of clavulanic acid; 200 mg of amoxicillin trihydrate, 31.25 mg of clavulanic acid; 250 mg of amoxicillin trihydrate, 62.5 mg of clavulanic acid; 400 mg of amoxicillin trihydrate, 62.5 mg of clavulanic acid
Tablets (film-coated): 250 mg of amoxicillin trihydrate, 125 mg of clavulanic acid; 500 mg of amoxicillin trihydrate, 125 mg of clavulanic acid; 875 mg of amoxicillin trihydrate, 125 mg of clavulanic acid
Oral suspension: 125 mg of amoxicillin trihydrate and 31.25 mg of clavulanic acid/5 ml (after reconstitution), 200 mg of amoxicillin trihydrate and 28.5 mg of clavulanic acid/5 ml (after reconstitution); 250 mg of amoxicillin trihydrate and 62.5 mg of clavulanic acid/5 ml (after reconstitution); 400 mg of amoxicillin trihydrate and 57 mg of clavulanic acid/5 ml (after reconstitution)

INDICATIONS & DOSAGE
Lower respiratory tract infections, otitis media, sinusitis, skin and skin-structure infections, and urinary tract infections caused by susceptible organisms
Adults weighing more than 40 kg (88 lb): 250 mg (based on amoxicillin component) P.O. q 8 hours or one 500-mg tablet q 12 hours. For more severe infections, 500 mg q 8 hours or 875 mg q 12 hours.
Adults weighing less than 88 lb: 20 to 40 mg/kg/day P.O. (based on amoxicillin component) given in divided doses q 8 hours.

Reactions may be *common,* uncommon, *life-threatening,* or COMMON AND LIFE-THREATENING.

PHARMACODYNAMICS

Antibiotic action: Amoxicillin is bactericidal; it adheres to bacterial penicillin-binding proteins, thus inhibiting bacterial cell wall synthesis.

Clavulanate has only weak antibacterial activity and doesn't affect the mechanism of action of amoxicillin. However, clavulanic acid has a beta-lactam ring and is structurally similar to penicillin and cephalosporins; it binds irreversibly with certain beta-lactamases and prevents them from inactivating amoxicillin, thus enhancing its bactericidal activity.

This combination acts against penicillinase- and non-penicillinase-producing gram-positive bacteria, *Neisseria gonorrhoeae, N. meningitidis, Haemophilus influenzae, Escherichia coli, Proteus mirabilis, Citrobacter diversus, Klebsiella pneumoniae, P. vulgaris, Salmonella,* and *Shigella.*

PHARMACOKINETICS

Absorption: Amoxicillin and clavulanate potassium are well absorbed after oral administration; peak serum levels occur at 1 to 2½ hours.
Distribution: Both amoxicillin and clavulanate potassium are distributed into pleural fluid, lungs, and peritoneal fluid; high urine levels are attained. Amoxicillin also is distributed into synovial fluid, liver, prostate, muscle, and gallbladder and penetrates into middle ear effusions, maxillary sinus secretions, tonsils, sputum, and bronchial secretions. Amoxicillin and clavulanate potassium have minimal protein-binding of 17% to 20% and 22% to 30%, respectively.
Metabolism: Amoxicillin is metabolized only partially. The metabolic fate of clavulanate potassium isn't completely identified, but it appears to undergo extensive metabolism.
Excretion: Amoxicillin is excreted principally in urine through renal tubular secretion and glomerular filtration. Clavulanate potassium is excreted through glomerular filtration. In adults, elimination half-life of amoxicillin is 1 to 1½ hours; in patients with severe renal impairment, 7½ hours. In adults, half-life of clavulanate is 1 to 1½ hours; in patients with severe renal impairment, 4½ hours.

Both drugs are removed readily through hemodialysis and minimally through peritoneal dialysis.

CONTRAINDICATIONS & PRECAUTIONS

Contraindicated in patients with hypersensitivity to drug or other penicillins and in those with a previous history of amoxicillin-associated cholestatic jaundice or hepatic dysfunction. An oral penicillin shouldn't be used in patients with severe pneumonia, empyema, bacteremia, pericarditis, meningitis, and purulent or septic arthritis. Use with caution in patients with mononucleosis.

INTERACTIONS

Drug-drug. Use with *allopurinol* appears to increase incidence of rash from both drugs. Large doses of penicillins may interfere with renal tubular secretion of *methotrexate,* thus delaying elimination and prolonging elevated serum methotrexate levels. Use with *probenecid* blocks tubular secretion of amoxicillin, raising its serum levels, but has no effect on clavulanate. Monitor closely.

ADVERSE REACTIONS

CNS: agitation, anxiety, insomnia, confusion, behavioral changes, dizziness.
GI: *nausea,* vomiting, *diarrhea,* indigestion, gastritis, stomatitis, glossitis, black "hairy" tongue, enterocolitis, pseudomembranous colitis.
GU: vaginitis.
Hematologic: anemia, ***thrombocytopenia***, thrombocytopenic purpura, eosinophilia, *leukopenia, agranulocytosis.*
Other: hypersensitivity reactions (erythematous maculopapular rash, urticaria, *anaphylaxis*), overgrowth of nonsusceptible organisms.

▣ KEY CONSIDERATIONS

Besides the recommendations relevant to all penicillins, consider the following:
● In geriatric patients, diminished renal tubular secretion may prolong half-life of amoxicillin.

- Oral dosage is best absorbed from an empty stomach, but food doesn't cause significant impairment of absorption.
- Suspension is stable for 10 days in refrigerator after reconstitution.
- When using film-coated tablets, be aware that both dosages contain different amounts of amoxicillin, but the same amount of clavulanate; therefore two "250-mg" tablets aren't the equivalent of one "500-mg" tablet.
- Because amoxicillin/clavulanate potassium is dialyzable, patients undergoing hemodialysis may need dosage adjustments.
- Amoxicillin/clavulanate potassium can alter results of urine glucose tests that use cupric sulfate (Benedict's reagent or Clinitest). Make urine glucose determinations with glucose oxidase methods (Chemstrip uG or Diastix or glucose enzymatic test strip). Positive Coombs' tests have been reported with other clavulanate combinations. Amoxicillin/clavulanate potassium may produce a positive direct antiglobulin test.

Patient education
- Tell patient to chew chewable tablets thoroughly or crush before swallowing and wash down with liquid to ensure adequate absorption of drug; capsule may be emptied and contents swallowed with water.
- Instruct patient to report diarrhea promptly.
- Inform patient to complete full course of drug therapy.

Overdose & treatment
- Signs of overdose include neuromuscular sensitivity and seizures.
- After recent ingestion (4 hours or less), empty the stomach by inducing vomiting or performing gastric lavage; to reduce absorption, follow with activated charcoal. Amoxicillin/clavulanate potassium can be removed by hemodialysis.

amoxicillin trihydrate
Amoxil, Polymox, Trimox, Wymox

Aminopenicillin, antibiotic

Available by prescription only
Tablets (chewable): 125 mg, 250 mg
Capsules: 250 mg, 500 mg
Suspension: 125 mg/5 ml, 250 mg/5 ml

INDICATIONS & DOSAGE
Systemic infections, acute and chronic urinary or respiratory tract infections caused by susceptible organisms, uncomplicated urinary tract infections caused by susceptible organisms
Adults: 250 mg P.O. q 8 hours. In adults who have severe infections or those caused by susceptible organisms, 500 mg q 8 hours may be needed.
Uncomplicated gonorrhea
Adults: 3 g P.O. as a single dose.
✦ *Dosage adjustment.* In patients with renal failure who require repeated doses, dosing interval may need to be adjusted. If creatinine clearance is 10 to 30 ml/minute, increase interval to q 12 hours; if creatinine clearance is less than 10 ml/minute, administer q 24 hours. Supplemental doses should be given both during and after hemodialysis.
Oral prophylaxis of bacterial endocarditis
Consult current American Heart Association recommendations before administering drug.
Adults: 2 g P.O. 1 hour before procedure.

PHARMACODYNAMICS
Antibacterial action: Amoxicillin is bactericidal; it adheres to bacterial penicillin-binding proteins, thus inhibiting bacterial cell wall synthesis.

Drug is effective against non-penicillinase-producing gram-positive bacteria, *Streptococcus* group B, *Neisseria gonorrhoeae, Proteus mirabilis, Salmonella,* and *Haemophilus influenzae.* It's also effective against non-penicillinase-producing *Staphylococcus aureus, S. pyogenes, Streptococcus bovis, S. pneumoniae, S. viridans, N. meningitidis, Escherichia coli, Salmo-*

Reactions may be *common,* uncommon, *life-threatening,* or COMMON AND LIFE-THREATENING.

nella typhi, Bordetella pertussis, Peptococcus, and *Peptostreptococcus.*

PHARMACOKINETICS

Absorption: About 80% of amoxicillin is absorbed after oral administration; serum levels peak at 1 to 2½ hours after an oral dose.

Distribution: Drug distributes into pleural peritoneal and synovial fluids and into the lungs, prostate, muscle, liver, and gallbladder; it also penetrates middle ear, maxillary sinus and bronchial secretions, tonsils, and sputum. Between 17% and 20% binds to proteins.

Metabolism: Drug is only partially metabolized.

Excretion: Drug is excreted principally in urine through renal tubular secretion and glomerular filtration. Elimination half-life in adults is 1 to 1½ hours; severe renal impairment increases half-life to 7½ hours.

CONTRAINDICATIONS & PRECAUTIONS

Contraindicated in patients with hypersensitivity to amoxicillin or other penicillins. Use with caution in patients with mononucleosis.

INTERACTIONS

Drug-drug. Use with *allopurinol* appears to increase the incidence of rash from both drugs. Use with *clavulanate potassium* enhances the effect of amoxicillin against certain beta-lactamase-producing bacteria. Large doses of penicillins may interfere with renal tubular secretion of *methotrexate,* thus delaying elimination and prolonging elevated serum methotrexate levels. Use with *probenecid* blocks renal tubular secretion of amoxicillin, raising its serum levels. Monitor closely.

ADVERSE REACTIONS

CNS: lethargy, hallucinations, *seizures,* anxiety, confusion, agitation, depression, dizziness, fatigue.

GI: *nausea,* vomiting, *diarrhea,* glossitis, stomatitis, gastritis, abdominal pain, enterocolitis, pseudomembranous colitis, black "hairy" tongue.

GU: interstitial nephritis, nephropathy, vaginitis.

Hematologic: anemia, *thrombocytopenia,* thrombocytopenic purpura, eosinophilia, *leukopenia,* hemolytic anemia, *agranulocytosis.*

Other: hypersensitivity reactions (erythematous maculopapular rash, urticaria, *anaphylaxis*), overgrowth of nonsusceptible organisms.

▣ KEY CONSIDERATIONS

Besides the recommendations relevant to all penicillins, consider the following:

• Because of diminished renal tubular secretion, half-life may be prolonged in geriatric patients.

• Oral dosage is maximally absorbed from an empty stomach, but food doesn't cause significant loss of potency.

• Suspension and drops are stable for 14 days in refrigerator after reconstitution.

• Amoxicillin is less likely to cause diarrhea than ampicillin.

• Amoxicillin may alter results of urine glucose tests that use cupric sulfate (Benedict's reagent or Clinitest). Make urine glucose determinations with glucose oxidase methods (Chemstrip uG, Diastix, or glucose enzymatic test strip).

• Amoxicillin may falsely decrease serum aminoglycoside levels.

Patient education

• Tell patient to chew tablets thoroughly or crush before swallowing and wash down with liquid to ensure adequate absorption of drug; capsule may be emptied and contents swallowed with water.

• Tell patient to report diarrhea promptly.

• Instruct patient to complete full course of drug therapy.

Overdose & treatment

• Signs and symptoms of overdose include neuromuscular sensitivity or seizures.

• After recent ingestion (4 hours or less), empty the stomach by inducing vomiting or performing gastric lavage; follow with activated charcoal to reduce absorption. Drug can be removed through hemodialysis.

---

*Canada only   ◊ Unlabeled clinical use

amphotericin B
Abelcet, AmBisome, Fungizone

Polyene macrolide, antifungal

Available by prescription only
Injection: 50-mg lyophilized cake, 50-mg vial, 100-mg/20-ml vial (Abelcet)
Oral suspension: 100 mg/ml
Suspension for injection: 5 mg/ml
Cream: 3%
Lotion: 3%
Ointment: 3%

INDICATIONS & DOSAGE
Systemic (potentially fatal) fungal infections, caused by susceptible organisms; ◇fungal endocarditis; fungal septicemia
Adults: Some health care providers recommend an initial dose of 1 mg I.V. in 20 ml D_5W infused over 20 minutes. If test dose is tolerated, then give daily dosages of 0.25 to 0.30 mg/kg, gradually increasing by 5 to 10 mg/day until daily dosage is 1 mg/kg/day or 1.5 mg/kg q alternate day. Duration of therapy depends on the severity and nature of the infection.
Abelcet (only): 5 mg/kg given as a single infusion, administered 2.5 mg/kg/hour. If infusion lasts longer than 2 hours, mix bag q 2 hours by shaking.
Sporotrichosis: 0.4 to 0.5 mg/kg amphotericin B daily I.V. for up to 9 months. Total I.V. dosage over 9 months is 2.5 g.
Aspergillosis: 0.5 to 0.6 mg/kg I.V. daily. Higher dosages (1 to 1.5 mg/kg daily) may be necessary in neutropenic patients or in the treatment of rapidly progressing, potentially fatal infections. Total dosages of 1.5 to 4 g have been given over an 11-month period.
◇Fungal meningitis
Adults: Intrathecal injection of 25 mcg/0.1 ml diluted with 10 to 20 ml of CSF and administered by barbotage two or three times weekly. Initial dosage shouldn't exceed 50 mcg.
◇Candidal cystitis
Adults: Bladder irrigations in concentrations of 5 to 50 mcg/ml instilled periodically or continuously for 5 to 7 days.

Oropharyngeal candidiasis
Adults: 100 mg/ml oral suspension q.i.d. swished and swallowed.
Topical fungal infections (3% cream, lotion, ointment)
Adults: Apply liberally and rub well into affected area b.i.d. to q.i.d.
Cutaneous or mucocutaneous candidal infections
Adults: Apply topical product b.i.d., t.i.d., or q.i.d. for 1 to 3 weeks; apply up to several months for interdigital or paronychial lesions.
◇Histoplasmal pulmonary and intrapleural effusion
Adults: 15 to 20 mg with 25 mg hydrocortisone sodium succinate.
◇Pulmonary coccidioidomycosis
Adults: Via intermittent positive pressure breathing device, 5 to 10 mg q.i.d.
◇Ophthalmic candidal infection
Adults: 0.1 to 1 mg/ml drop suspension q 30 minutes.

PHARMACODYNAMICS
Antifungal action: Amphotericin B is fungistatic or fungicidal, depending on the concentrations available in body fluids and on the susceptibility of the fungus. It binds to sterols in the fungal cell membrane, increasing membrane permeability of fungal cells, causing subsequent leakage of intracellular components; it also may interfere with some human cell membranes that contain sterols.

Spectrum of activity includes *Histoplasma capsulatum, Coccidioides immitis, Blastomyces dermatitidis, Cryptococcus neoformans, Candida* species, *Aspergillus fumigatus, Mucor* species, *Rhizopus* species, *Absidia* species, *Entomophthora* species, *Basidiobolus* species, *Paracoccidioides brasiliensis, Sporothrix schenckii,* and *Rhodotorula* species.

PHARMACOKINETICS
Absorption: Amphotericin B is absorbed poorly from the GI tract.
Distribution: Drug distributes well into inflamed pleural cavities and joints and in low levels into aqueous humor, bronchial secretions, pancreas, bone, muscle, and parotids. CSF levels reach

---

Reactions may be *common,* uncommon, *life-threatening,* or COMMON AND LIFE-THREATENING.

about 3% of serum levels. Some 90% to 95% of drug binds to plasma proteins.
Metabolism: Not well defined.
Excretion: Elimination of amphotericin B is biphasic: Initial serum half-life of 24 hours, followed by a second phase half-life of about 15 days. Two to five percent of drug is excreted unchanged in urine. Drug isn't readily removed through hemodialysis.

CONTRAINDICATIONS & PRECAUTIONS

Contraindicated in patients with hypersensitivity to amphotericin B. Use cautiously in patients with renal impairment.

INTERACTIONS

Drug-drug. Use with *aminoglycosides, cisplatin,* or *other nephrotoxic drugs* increases the risk of added nephrotoxic effects. If possible, don't use together.

Use with *corticosteroids* causes added potassium depletion. Carefully monitor serum electrolyte levels and cardiac function.

Because amphotericin B induces hypokalemia and hypomagnesemia, concomitant use with *digoxin* increases the risk of digitalis toxicity.

Amphotericin potentiates the effects of *flucytosine* and *other antibiotics,* presumably by increasing cell membrane permeability.

Amphotericin B–induced hypokalemia may enhance effects of *skeletal muscle relaxants.* Monitor closely.

ADVERSE REACTIONS

CNS: *malaise, generalized pain, headache,* peripheral neuropathy, **seizures** (with systemic form).
CV: *phlebitis, thrombophlebitis,* hypotension, **arrhythmias, asystole,** hypertension (with systemic form).
EENT: hearing loss, tinnitus, transient vertigo, blurred vision, diplopia (with systemic form).
GI: *anorexia, weight loss, nausea, vomiting, dyspepsia, diarrhea, epigastric pain, cramping,* melena, **hemorrhagic gastroenteritis** (with systemic form).
GU: *abnormal renal function with hypokalemia, azotemia, hyposthenuria, renal tubular acidosis, nephrocalcinosis;* with large doses, **permanent renal im-** **pairment,** anuria, oliguria (with systemic form).
Hematologic: *normochromic, normocytic anemia,* **thrombocytopenia, leukopenia, agranulocytosis,** eosinophilia, leukocytosis (with systemic form).
Hepatic: hepatitis, jaundice, **acute liver failure** (with systemic form).
Musculoskeletal: arthralgia, myalgia.
Respiratory: dyspnea, tachypnea, **bronchospasm,** wheezing (with systemic form).
Skin: tissue damage with extravasation, maculopapular rash, pruritus without rash (with systemic form); possible dryness, contact sensitivity, erythema, burning, pruritus (with topical administration).
Other: *pain at injection site, fever, chills,* flushing, **anaphylactoid reactions** (with topical administration).

▣ KEY CONSIDERATIONS

● In patient who isn't immunocompromised, cultures and histologic sensitivity testing must be completed and diagnosis confirmed before therapy begins.
● Prepare infusion as manufacturer directs, with strict aseptic technique, using only 10 ml of sterile water to reconstitute. To avoid precipitation, don't mix with solutions containing normal saline, other electrolytes, or bacteriostatic agents such as benzyl alcohol.
● Lyophilized cake contains no preservatives. Don't use if solution contains a precipitate or other foreign particles. Store cake at 35.6° to 46.4° F (2° to 8° C). Protect drug from light, and check the expiration date.
● When mixed with D_5W, liposomal amphotericin B (AmBisome) is stable for 6 hours after dilution.
● Liposomal amphotericin B shouldn't be mixed with other I.V. solutions.
● Note dosage difference between conventional amphotericin and lipid products. Don't interchange. Total daily dosage of conventional amphotericin B shouldn't exceed 1.5 mg/kg/day.
● For I.V. infusion, use an in-line membrane with a mean pore diameter larger than 1 micron. Abelcet shouldn't be used with a filter.

• Infuse slowly; rapid infusion may cause CV collapse.

• Don't mix or piggyback antibiotics with amphotericin B infusion; the I.V. solution appears compatible with a small amount of heparin sodium, hydrocortisone sodium succinate, and methylprednisolone sodium succinate.

• Administer into distal veins, and monitor site for discomfort or thrombosis; if thrombosis occurs, consider alternate-day therapy.

• Vital signs should be checked every 30 minutes for at least 4 hours after start of I.V. infusion; fever may appear in 1 to 2 hours but should subside within 4 hours of discontinuing drug.

• Monitor intake and output and check for changes in urine appearance or volume; renal damage may be reversible if drug is stopped at earliest sign of dysfunction.

• Monitor potassium and magnesium levels closely; monitor calcium and magnesium levels twice weekly; perform liver and renal function studies and CBCs weekly.

• Reduce the severity of some adverse reactions by premedicating the patient with aspirin or acetaminophen, antihistamines, antiemetics, meperidine, or a small dosage of corticosteroids; by adding a phosphate buffer to the solution; or by dosing the drug on alternate days. If reactions are severe, drug may have to be discontinued for varying periods.

• Use topical products for folds of groin, neck, or armpit; avoid occlusive dressing with ointment, and discontinue if patient develops signs of hypersensitivity.

• Topical products may stain skin or clothes.

• Store at room temperature. Solution is stable at room temperature and in indoor light for 24 hours or in the refrigerator for 1 week.

• Amphotericin B may increase BUN, serum creatinine, alkaline phosphatase, and bilirubin levels.

• Amphotericin B may cause hypokalemia and hypomagnesemia and may decrease WBC, RBC, and platelet counts.

Patient education

• Teach patient signs and symptoms of hypersensitivity and other adverse reactions, especially those associated with I.V. therapy. Warn that fever and chills are likely to occur and can be quite severe when therapy is initiated but that they usually subside with repeated doses. Encourage patient feedback during infusion.

• Warn patient that therapy may take several months; teach personal hygiene and other measures to prevent spread and recurrence of lesions.

• Urge patient to adhere to regimen and to return, as instructed, for follow-up.

• Tell patient that topical products may stain skin and clothing; cream or lotion may be removed from clothing with soap and water.

amphotericin B cholesteryl sulfate complex
Amphotec

Polyene macrolide, antifungal

Available by prescription only
Injection: 50 mg/20 ml, 100 mg/50 ml

INDICATIONS & DOSAGE
Invasive aspergillosis in patients in whom renal impairment or unacceptable toxicity precludes use of amphotericin B deoxycholate in effective dosages and in those with invasive aspergillosis in whom amphotericin B deoxycholate therapy has failed in the past; ◊ **Candida *and* Cryptococcus *infections in patients who failed to respond or couldn't tolerate conventional amphotericin B therapy***
Adults: 3 to 4 mg/kg/day I.V.; may increase to 6 mg/kg/day if no improvement occurs or if fungal infection has progressed. Administer by continuous infusion at 1 mg/kg/hour.

PHARMACODYNAMICS
Fungistatic or fungicidal action: Depends on level of drug and susceptibility of fungus. Drug binds to sterols in cell membranes of sensitive fungi, resulting in leakage of intracellular contents and

---

Reactions may be *common*, uncommon, *life-threatening*, or COMMON AND LIFE-THREATENING.

causing cell death due to changes in membrane permeability. Also binds to sterols in mammalian cell membranes, which is believed to account for human toxicity. Spectrum of activity includes *Aspergillus fumigatus, Candida albicans, Coccidioides immitis,* and *Cryptococcus neoformans.*

PHARMACOKINETICS

Absorption: For an infusion rate of 1 mg/kg/hour and dosage ranges from 3 to 6 mg/kg/day, maximum plasma level at end of an infusion ranges from 2.6 to 3.4 µg/ml.

Distribution: Multicompartmental; steady-state volume increases with higher dosages, possibly from uptake by tissues.

Metabolism: Unknown.

Excretion: Unclear; elimination half-life, 27 to 29 hours; increasing dosages increase the elimination half-life. Drug may not be removed through dialysis.

CONTRAINDICATIONS & PRECAUTIONS

Contraindicated in patients with hypersensitivity to any component of drug unless the benefits outweigh the risk of hypersensitivity.

INTERACTIONS

Drug-drug. Use with *aminoglycosides, cisplatin,* or *other nephrotoxic drugs* increases the risk of added nephrotoxic effects. Avoid using together, when possible.

Use with *corticosteroids* causes added potassium depletion. Carefully monitor serum electrolyte levels and cardiac function.

Because amphotericin B induces hypokalemia and hypomagnesemia, concomitant use with *digoxin* increases the risk of digitalis toxicity.

Use potentiates the effects of *flucytosine* and *other antibiotics,* probably by increasing cell membrane permeability.

Amphotericin B-induced hypokalemia may enhance effects of *skeletal muscle relaxants.* Monitor closely.

ADVERSE REACTIONS

CNS: asthenia, abnormal thoughts, anxiety, agitation, confusion, depression, dizziness, hallucinations, headache, hypertonia, neuropathy, paresthesia, *seizures,* somnolence, stupor.

CV: edema; *arrhythmias, atrial fibrillation, bradycardia, **cardiac arrest, heart failure, hemorrhage,*** hypertension, hypotension, phlebitis, syncope, orthostatic hypotension, *shock, supraventricular tachycardia,* tachycardia, *ventricular extrasystoles.*

EENT: eye hemorrhage, tinnitus.

GI: anorexia, GI disorder, GI hemorrhage, hematemesis, melena, *nausea,* stomatitis, *vomiting.*

GU: abnormal renal function, hematuria, *renal failure.*

Hematologic: anemia, *agranulocytosis,* coagulation disorders, hypochromic anemia, increased PT and INR, sepsis, leukocytosis, *leukopenia, thrombocytopenia.*

Hepatic: jaundice, abnormal liver function test results, *hepatic failure.*

Metabolic: *hypokalemia;* hypocalcemia; hyperglycemia; hypervolemia; hypophosphatemia; hyponatremia; hyperkalemia; *increased creatinine, bilirubinemia,* hypomagnesemia, alkaline phosphatase, BUN, AST, ALT, and LD levels.

Musculoskeletal: arthralgia, myalgia.

Respiratory: *apnea,* asthma, dyspnea, epistaxis, hemoptysis, hyperventilation, hypoxia, increased cough, lung or respiratory disorders, *pulmonary edema.*

Skin: pruritus, rash, sweating, skin disorders.

Other: *allergic reaction; anaphylaxis; chills; fever;* abdominal, chest, or back pain; peripheral or facial edema; infection, mucous membrane disorder; pain or reaction at injection site.

▣ KEY CONSIDERATIONS

• Pretreating with antihistamines and corticosteroids or reducing the rate of infusion (or both) may reduce the risk of acute infusion-related reactions.

• Dilute in D_5W and administer by continuous infusion at 1 mg/kg/hour. Perform a test dose before starting a new course of treatment; infuse a small amount of drug (10 ml of final preparation containing 1.6 to 8.3 mg of amphotericin B) over 15 to 30 minutes and monitor patient for the next 30 minutes. Can shorten infusion time to 2 hours or lengthen infusion time based on patient tolerance.

• Drug is incompatible with normal saline and electrolyte solutions and bacteriostatic agents.

• Infuse drug over at least 2 hours.

• Don't mix with other drugs. If administered through an existing I.V. line, flush line with D_5W before infusion or use a separate line.

• Store vials at room temperature. Reconstitute 50-mg vial with rapid addition of 10 ml of sterile water for injection, and 100-mg vial with rapid addition of 20 ml sterile water with a sterile syringe and 20G needle. Shake vial gently. Don't use diluent other than sterile water for injection.

• Reconstituted drug is clear or opalescent liquid and is stable for 24 hours refrigerated. Discard partially used vials.

• Don't administer undiluted drug.

• Don't filter or use an in-line filter and don't freeze.

• Monitor vital signs every 30 minutes during initial therapy. Acute infusion-related reactions (fever, chills, hypotension, nausea, tachycardia) usually occur 1 to 3 hours after starting I.V. infusion. These reactions are usually more severe after initial doses and usually diminish with subsequent doses. If severe respiratory distress occurs, stop infusion immediately and don't treat further with drug.

• Monitor intake and output; report changes in urine appearance or volume.

• Monitor renal and hepatic function tests, serum electrolyte levels (especially potassium, magnesium, and calcium), CBCs, and PT and INR.

Patient education

• Instruct patient to report symptoms of hypersensitivity immediately.

• Warn patient of possible discomfort at I.V. site.

• Advise patient of potential adverse effects, such as fever, chills, nausea, and vomiting. Tell him that these can be severe with initial treatment but usually subside with repeated doses.

Overdose & treatment

• Amphotericin B deoxycholate overdose may result in cardiorespiratory arrest.

• If overdose is suspected, discontinue therapy, monitor clinical status, and administer supportive therapy. Drug isn't dialyzable.

ampicillin
Apo-Ampi*, Novo-Ampicillin*, Omnipen, Penbritin*

ampicillin sodium
Ampicin*, Omnipen-N, Penbritin*

ampicillin trihydrate
Omnipen, Principen, Totacillin

Aminopenicillin, antibiotic

Available by prescription only
Capsules: 250 mg, 500 mg
Suspension: 125 mg/5 ml, 250 mg/5 ml, 500 mg/5 ml (after reconstitution)
Parenteral: 125 mg, 250 mg, 500 mg, 1 g, 2 g
Infusion: 500 mg, 1 g, 2 g

INDICATIONS & DOSAGE
Systemic infections, acute and chronic urinary tract infections caused by susceptible organisms
Adults: 250 to 500 mg P.O. q 6 hours.
Meningitis
Adults: 8 to 14 g I.V. divided q 3 to 4 hours for 3 days; then may give I.M. if desired.
Uncomplicated gonorrhea
Adults: 3.5 g P.O. with 1 g probenecid given as a single dose.
✦ *Dosage adjustment.* Dosing interval should be increased to q 12 hours in patients with severe renal impairment (creatinine clearance of 10 ml/minute or less).
Prophylaxis for salmonella in patients infected with HIV
Adults: 50 to 100 mg P.O. q.i.d. for several months.

Prophylaxis for bacterial endocarditis before dental or minor respiratory procedures
Adults: 2 g (I.V. or I.M.) 30 minutes before procedure.

PHARMACODYNAMICS

Antibiotic action: Ampicillin is bactericidal; it adheres to bacterial penicillin-binding proteins, thus inhibiting bacterial cell wall synthesis.

Spectrum of action includes nonpenicillinase-producing gram-positive bacteria. It's also effective against many gram-negative organisms, including *Neisseria gonorrhoeae, N. meningitidis, Haemophilus influenzae, Escherichia coli, Proteus mirabilis, Salmonella,* and *Shigella.* Ampicillin should be used in gram-negative systemic infections only when organism sensitivity is known.

PHARMACOKINETICS

Absorption: About 42% of ampicillin is absorbed after an oral dose; serum levels peak in 1 to 2 hours. After I.M. administration, serum levels peak in 1 hour.
Distribution: Drug distributes into pleural, peritoneal and synovial fluids, lungs, prostate, liver, and gallbladder; it also penetrates middle ear effusions, maxillary sinus and bronchial secretions, tonsils, and sputum. Drug is minimally protein-bound (15% to 25%).
Metabolism: Drug is only partially metabolized.
Excretion: Drug is excreted in urine through renal tubular secretion and glomerular filtration. Elimination half-life is 1 to 1½ hours; in patients with extensive renal impairment, half-life is 10 to 24 hours.

CONTRAINDICATIONS & PRECAUTIONS

Contraindicated in patients with hypersensitivity to ampicillin or other penicillins. Use with caution in patients with mononucleosis.

INTERACTIONS

Drug-drug. Use with *allopurinol* appears to increase incidence of rash from both drugs. Large doses of penicillins may interfere with renal tubular secretion of *methotrexate,* thus delaying elim-

ination and elevating serum methotrexate levels. Use with *probenecid* inhibits renal tubular secretion of ampicillin, raising its serum levels. Monitor closely.

Use with *aminoglycosides* causes a synergistic bactericidal effect against some strains of enterococci and group B streptococci; however, the drugs are physically and chemically incompatible and are inactivated if mixed or given together.

Use with *clavulanate* results in increased bactericidal effects because clavulanic acid is a beta-lactamase inhibitor. Concomitant use is suggested.

ADVERSE REACTIONS

CNS: lethargy, hallucinations, *seizures,* anxiety, confusion, agitation, depression, dizziness, fatigue.
CV: vein irritation, thrombophlebitis.
GI: *nausea,* vomiting, *diarrhea,* glossitis, stomatitis, gastritis, abdominal pain, enterocolitis, pseudomembranous colitis, black "hairy" tongue.
GU: interstitial nephritis, nephropathy, vaginitis.
Hematologic: anemia, ***thrombocytopenia,*** thrombocytopenic purpura, eosinophilia, *leukopenia,* hemolytic anemia, *agranulocytosis.*
Other: hypersensitivity reactions (erythematous maculopapular rash, urticaria, *anaphylaxis,* overgrowth of nonsusceptible organisms, pain at injection site).

▣ KEY CONSIDERATIONS

Besides the recommendations relevant to all penicillins, consider the following:
● Because of diminished renal tubular secretion in geriatric patients, half-life of drug may be prolonged.
● Administer I.M. or I.V. only when patient is too ill to take oral drug.
● Ampicillin can alter results of urine glucose tests that use cupric sulfate (Benedict's reagent or Clinitest). Make urine glucose determinations with glucose oxidase methods (Chemstrip uG, Diastix, or glucose enzymatic test strip).
● Ampicillin may falsely decrease serum aminoglycoside levels.

Patient education
• Encourage patient to report diarrhea promptly.
• Instruct patient to finish taking all of the prescribed drug.

Overdose & treatment
• Signs and symptoms of overdose include neuromuscular sensitivity or seizures.
• After recent ingestion (within 4 hours), empty the stomach by inducing vomiting or performing gastric lavage; follow with activated charcoal to reduce absorption. Drug can be removed through hemodialysis.

ampicillin sodium/sulbactam sodium
Unasyn

Aminopenicillin/beta-lactamase inhibitor combination, antibiotic

Available by prescription only
Injection: Vials and piggyback vials containing 1.5 g (1 g ampicillin sodium with 500 mg sulbactam sodium) and 3 g (2 g ampicillin sodium with 1 g sulbactam sodium)

INDICATIONS & DOSAGE
Skin and skin-structure infections, intra-abdominal and gynecologic infections caused by susceptible beta-lactamase–producing strains of **Staphylococcus aureus, Escherichia coli, Klebsiella** *(including* **K. pneumoniae***),* **Proteus mirabilis, Bacteroides** *(including* **B. fragilis***),* **Enterobacter,** *and* **Acinetobacter calcoaceticus**
Adults: 1.5 to 3 g I.M. or I.V. q 6 hours. Don't exceed 4 g/day sulbactam sodium.
✦ *Dosage adjustment.*

Creatinine clearance (ml/min/ 1.73 m²)	Half-life (hr)	Recommended dosage
≥ 30	1	1.5-3 g q 6-8 hr
15-29	5	1.5-3 g q 12 hr
5-14	9	1.5-3 g q 24 hr

PHARMACODYNAMICS
Antibiotic action: Ampicillin is bactericidal; it adheres to bacterial penicillin-binding proteins, thus inhibiting bacterial cell wall synthesis. Sulbactam inhibits beta-lactamase, an enzyme produced by ampicillin-resistant bacteria that degrades ampicillin.

PHARMACOKINETICS
Absorption: Peak plasma levels occur immediately after I.V. infusion and within 1 hour after I.M. injection.
Distribution: Both drugs distribute into pleural, peritoneal and synovial fluids, lungs, prostate, liver, and gallbladder; they also penetrate middle ear effusions, maxillary sinus and bronchial secretions, tonsils, and sputum. Ampicillin is minimally protein-bound at 15% to 25%; sulbactam is about 38% bound.
Metabolism: Both drugs are metabolized only partially; only 15% to 25% of both drugs are metabolized.
Excretion: Both ampicillin and sulbactam are excreted in the urine by renal tubular secretion and glomerular filtration. Elimination half-life is 1 to 1½ hours; in patients with extensive renal impairment, half-life may be 10 to 24 hours.

CONTRAINDICATIONS & PRECAUTIONS
Contraindicated in patients with hypersensitivity to drug or other penicillins. Use cautiously in patients with maculopapular rash.

INTERACTIONS
Drug-drug. Use with *allopurinol* may lead to an increased incidence of rash. Large doses of I.V. penicillins can increase bleeding risks of *anticoagulants* because of a prolongation of bleeding times. Use with *probenecid* decreases excretion of both ampicillin and sulbactam. Monitor closely.

The ampicillin component may cause in vitro inactivation of *aminoglycosides* if these antibiotics are mixed in the same infusion container. Don't mix in same container.

Reactions may be *common*, uncommon, **life-threatening**, or COMMON AND LIFE-THREATENING.

ADVERSE REACTIONS

GI: *nausea,* vomiting, *diarrhea,* glossitis, stomatitis, gastritis, black "hairy" tongue, enterocolitis, pseudomembranous colitis.

Hematologic: anemia, ***thrombocytopenia,*** thrombocytopenic purpura, eosinophilia, ***leukopenia, agranulocytosis.***

Other: hypersensitivity reactions (erythematous maculopapular rash, urticaria, ***anaphylaxis***), ***overgrowth of nonsusceptible organisms,*** pain at injection site, vein irritation, thrombophlebitis.

▣ KEY CONSIDERATIONS

• Because of diminished renal tubular secretion in geriatric patients, half-life of drug may be prolonged.

• I.V. administration should be given by slow injection over at least 10 to 15 minutes or infused in greater dilutions with 50 to 100 ml of a compatible diluent over 15 to 30 minutes.

• For I.V. use, reconstitute powder in piggyback units to desired concentrations with sterile water for injection, normal saline injection, D_5W injection, lactated Ringer's injection, 1/6 M sodium lactate injection, dextrose 5% in half-normal saline solution, or 10% invert sugar.

• If piggyback bottles are unavailable, reconstitute standard vials of sterile powder with sterile water for injection to yield solutions of 375 mg/ml (250 mg ampicillin/125 mg sulbactam). Then immediately dilute an appropriate volume with a suitable diluent to yield solutions of 3 to 45 mg/ml (2 to 30 mg ampicillin/1 to 15 mg sulbactam/ml).

• For I.M. injection, reconstitute with sterile water for injection, or 0.5% or 2% lidocaine hydrochloride injection. To obtain 375 mg/ml solutions (250 mg ampicillin/125 mg sulbactam/ml), add contents of the 1.5-g vial to 3.2 ml of diluent to produce 4 ml withdrawal volume; add 3-g vial to 6.4 ml of diluent to produce 8 ml withdrawal volume.

• Reconstituted solutions are stable for varying periods (from 2 hours to 72 hours) depending on diluent used. Check with pharmacist. For patients on sodium restriction, note that a 1.5-g dose of ampicillin sodium/sulbactam sodium yields 5 mEq of sodium.

• Ampicillin can alter results of urine glucose tests that use cupric sulfate (Benedict's reagent or Clinitest). Make urine glucose determinations with glucose oxidase methods (Chemstrip uG, Diastix, or glucose enzymatic test strip).

Patient education

• Advise patient to report a rash, fever, or chills. A rash is the most common allergic reaction.

Overdose & treatment

• Neurologic adverse reactions, including seizures, are likely with an overdose.

• Treatment is supportive. Although confirming data are lacking, ampicillin and sulbactam are likely to be removed by hemodialysis.

---

amrinone lactate
Inocor

Bipyridine derivative, inotropic, vasodilator

Available by prescription only
Injection: 5 mg/ml

INDICATIONS & DOSAGE

Short-term management of heart failure

Adults: Initially, 0.75 mg/kg I.V. bolus over 2 to 3 minutes; then, begin maintenance infusion of 5 to 10 mcg/kg/minute. Additional bolus of 0.75 mg/kg may be given 30 minutes after therapy starts. Maximum daily dose is 10 mg/kg.

PHARMACODYNAMICS

Inotropic action: The mechanism of action responsible for the apparent inotropic effect isn't fully understood; however, it may be associated with inhibition of phosphodiesterase activity, resulting in increased cellular levels of adenosine 3',5'-cyclic phosphate; this, in turn, may alter intracellular and extracellular calcium levels. The role of calcium homeostasis hasn't been determined. Effects include increased cardiac output mediated by reduced afterload and, possibly, inotropism.

Vasodilative action: The primary vasodilating effect of amrinone seems to stem from a direct effect on peripheral vessels.

PHARMACOKINETICS

Absorption: With I.V. administration, onset of action occurs in 2 to 5 minutes, with peak effects in about 10 minutes. CV effects may persist for 1 to 2 hours.
Distribution: Distribution volume is 1.2 L/kg. Distribution sites are unknown. Protein-binding ranges from 10% to 49%. Therapeutic steady-state serum levels range from 0.5 to 7 µg/ml (ideal level is 3 µg/ml).
Metabolism: Drug is metabolized in the liver to several metabolites of unknown activity.
Excretion: Normally, amrinone is excreted in the urine, with a terminal elimination half-life of about 4 hours. Half-life may be prolonged slightly in patients with heart failure.

CONTRAINDICATIONS & PRECAUTIONS

Contraindicated in patients with hypersensitivity to amrinone or bisulfites. It shouldn't be used in patients with severe aortic or pulmonic valvular disease in place of surgical intervention or during an acute phase of an MI.

INTERACTIONS

Drug-drug. Use with *disopyramide* may cause severe hypotension. Monitor closely.

ADVERSE REACTIONS

CV: *arrhythmias,* hypotension, chest pain.
GI: nausea, vomiting, anorexia, abdominal pain.
Hematologic: *thrombocytopenia (based on dose and duration of therapy).*
Hepatic: elevated enzyme levels, *hepatotoxicity (rare).*
Other: burning at injection site, *hypersensitivity reactions (pericarditis, ascites, myositis vasculitis, pleuritis),* fever.

▣ KEY CONSIDERATIONS

● Administer drug as supplied or dilute in normal or half-normal saline solution to concentration of 1 to 3 mg/ml. Don't dilute drug with solutions containing dextrose because a slow chemical reaction occurs over 24 hours. However, amrinone can be injected into running dextrose infusions through Y-connector or directly into tubing. Use diluted solution within 24 hours.
● Don't administer furosemide in I.V. lines containing amrinone because a chemical reaction occurs immediately.
● Monitor blood pressure and heart rate throughout infusion. Infusion should be slowed or stopped if patient's blood pressure decreases or if arrhythmias (ventricular or supraventricular) occur. Dosage may need to be reduced.
● Monitor platelet counts. A count below 150,000/mm³ usually necessitates dosage reduction. Thrombocytopenia usually occurs after long-term treatment.
● Monitor electrolyte levels (especially potassium) because drug increases cardiac output, which may cause diuresis.
● Hemodynamic monitoring may be useful in guiding therapy.
● Monitor liver function tests to detect hepatic damage (rare).
● Observe for adverse GI effects (such as nausea, vomiting, and diarrhea); reduce dosage or discontinue drug.
● Amrinone is prescribed primarily for patients who haven't responded to therapy with cardiac glycosides, diuretics, and vasodilators.
● The physiological effects of amrinone may decrease serum potassium levels or increase serum hepatic enzyme levels.

Overdose & treatment

● Signs and symptoms of overdose include severe hypotension.
● Treatment may include administration of a potent vasopressor, such as norepinephrine, and other general supportive measures, such as cautious fluid volume replacement.

anagrelide hydrochloride
Agrylin

Platelet-reducing drug

Available by prescription only
Capsules: 0.5 mg, 1 mg

Reactions may be *common,* uncommon, *life-threatening,* or COMMON AND LIFE-THREATENING.

INDICATIONS & DOSAGE

Essential thrombocythemia to reduce the elevated platelet count, risk of thrombosis and to ameliorate associated symptoms

Adults: 0.5 mg P.O. q.i.d. or 1 mg b.i.d. for at least 1 week; then adjust dosage to lowest effective dose required to maintain platelet count below 600,000/mm^3, and ideally to the normal range. Don't increase dosage to more than 0.5 mg/day in any 1 week; don't exceed 10 mg/day or 2.5 mg in a single dose.

PHARMACODYNAMICS

Platelet-reducing action: Mechanism of action is still under investigation; reduction in platelet production is thought to result from a decrease in megakaryocyte hypermaturation. Drug inhibits cAMP phosphodiesterase and adenosine diphosphate- and collagen-induced platelet aggregation.

PHARMACOKINETICS

Absorption: After oral administration of 1 mg in healthy individuals, plasma levels peak in about 1 hour. Plasma levels decline to less than 10% of peak levels in 24 hours.

Distribution: Plasma half-life at fasting and at 0.5 mg dosages is 1.3 hours. Drug doesn't accumulate in plasma after repeated administration and bioavailability is modestly reduced by food.

Metabolism: Drug is extensively metabolized.

Excretion: Drug is eliminated in urine; less than 1% is recovered unchanged in urine.

CONTRAINDICATIONS & PRECAUTIONS

Use with caution in patients with CV disease because anagrelide may cause vasodilation, tachycardia, palpitations, and heart failure. Use cautiously in patients with creatinine clearance over 2 mg/dl and in those with liver function tests exceeding 1.5 times the upper normal limits. Interruption of drug use will cause platelet counts to rise within 4 days of discontinuation.

INTERACTIONS

Drug-drug. Use with *sucralfate* may interfere with anagrelide absorption.

Drug-lifestyle. Exposure to *sunlight* may cause a photosensitivity reaction.

ADVERSE REACTIONS

CNS: malaise, amnesia, *asthenia,* confusion, *CVA,* depression, *dizziness, headache,* insomnia, migraine, nervousness, pain, paresthesia, somnolence.

CV: *arrhythmias, angina pectoris, chest pain,* CV disease, *heart failure, hemorrhage,* hypertension, palpitations, orthostatic hypotension, vasodilatation, *edema,* syncope, *tachycardia.*

EENT: abnormal vision, amblyopia, diplopia, tinnitus, visual field abnormality.

GI: anorexia, *abdominal pain,* aphthous stomatitis, constipation, *diarrhea,* dyspepsia, eructation, *flatulence,* GI distress, GI hemorrhage, gastritis, melena, *nausea,* vomiting.

GU: dysuria, hematuria.

Hematologic: anemia, ecchymosis, lymphadenoma, *thrombocytopenia.*

Metabolic: dehydration.

Musculoskeletal: arthralgia, back pain, leg cramps, myalgia, neck pain.

Respiratory: *dyspnea,* rhinitis, epistaxis, respiratory disease, sinusitis, pneumonia, bronchitis, asthma.

Skin: alopecia, pruritus, rash, skin disorder, urticaria, photosensitivity.

Other: chills, fever, flulike syndrome.

▣ KEY CONSIDERATIONS

• Evaluate use of drug carefully in patients with renal, liver, or CV disease.

• During the first 2 weeks of treatment, monitor blood counts and liver and renal function tests.

• Perform platelet counts every 2 days during 1st week then weekly until maintenance dosage reached.

Patient education

• Tell patient to use drug only as prescribed.

• Inform patient that drug can be taken without regard to meals.

• Instruct patient to report increased bleeding, bruising, or cardiac symptoms.

- Advise patient to take precautions in the sun because photosensitivity reactions may occur.

anastrozole
Arimidex

Nonsteroidal aromatase inhibitor, antineoplastic

Available by prescription only
Tablets: 1 mg

INDICATIONS & DOSAGE
Treatment of advanced breast cancer in postmenopausal women with disease progression after tamoxifen therapy
Adults: 1 mg P.O. daily.

PHARMACODYNAMICS
Antineoplastic action: A potent and selective nonsteroidal aromatase inhibitor, anastrozole significantly lowers serum estradiol levels. (The principal estrogen circulating in postmenopausal women, estradiol can stimulate breast cancer cell growth.)

PHARMACOKINETICS
Absorption: Anastrozole is absorbed from the GI tract; food affects the extent of absorption.
Distribution: Drug is 40% bound to plasma proteins in the therapeutic range.
Metabolism: Drug is metabolized in the liver.
Excretion: About 11% of drug is excreted in urine as parent drug and about 60% is excreted in urine as metabolites. Half-life is about 50 hours.

CONTRAINDICATIONS & PRECAUTIONS
None known.

INTERACTIONS
None reported.

ADVERSE REACTIONS
CNS: *asthenia, headache,* dizziness, depression, paresthesia.
CV: chest pain, edema, thromboembolic disease.
GI: increased appetite, dry mouth, *nausea,* vomiting, diarrhea, constipation, abdominal pain, anorexia.
GU: vaginal hemorrhage, vaginal dryness.
Metabolic: weight gain.
Musculoskeletal: pelvic pain, *back pain,* bone pain.
Respiratory: dyspnea, increased cough, pharyngitis.
Skin: *hot flashes,* rash, sweating.
Other: *pain,* peripheral edema.

▣ KEY CONSIDERATIONS
- Patients treated with this drug don't require glucocorticoid or mineralocorticoid therapy.
- Drug should be administered under supervision of qualified staff experienced in the use of anticancer drugs.

Patient education
- Instruct patient to report adverse reactions.
- Stress importance of follow-up care.

Overdose & treatment
- A single dose of anastrozole isn't known to cause life-threatening symptoms. Single oral doses that exceed 100 mg/kg may cause severe stomach irritation (necrosis, gastritis, ulceration, and hemorrhage).
- Because no specific antidote to overdosage exists, treatment must be symptomatic. Vomiting may be induced if the patient is alert. Dialysis may be helpful. General supportive care, including frequent monitoring of vital signs and close observation of the patient, is indicated.

anistreplase (anisoylated plasminogen-streptokinase activator complex, APSAC)
Eminase

Thrombolytic enzyme

Available by prescription only
Injection: 30 U/single-dose vial

Reactions may be *common,* uncommon, *life-threatening,* or COMMON AND LIFE-THREATENING.

INDICATIONS & DOSAGE
Treatment of acute coronary arterial thrombosis
Adults: 30 U by direct I.V. injection over 2 to 5 minutes.

PHARMACODYNAMICS
Enzymatic action: Anistreplase is derived from Lys-plasminogen and streptokinase. It activates the endogenous fibrinolytic system to produce plasmin, which degrades fibrin clots, fibrinogen, and other plasma proteins, including procoagulant factors V and VIII.

PHARMACOKINETICS
Absorption: Anistreplase is administered I.V.
Distribution: Unknown.
Metabolism: Immediately after injection, drug is deacylated by a nonenzymatic process to form the active streptokinase-plasminogen complex. The half-life of acylated and deacylated anistreplase is 88 to 112 minutes.
Excretion: Unknown. Duration of fibrinolytic activity is 4 to 6 hours and is limited by the deacylation of the anistreplase.

CONTRAINDICATIONS & PRECAUTIONS
Contraindicated in patients with history of severe allergic reaction to anistreplase or streptokinase; active internal bleeding, CVA, recent (within the past 2 months) intraspinal or intracranial surgery or trauma, aneurysm, arteriovenous malformation, intracranial neoplasm, uncontrolled hypertension, or known bleeding diathesis.

Use cautiously in patients with recent (within 10 days) major surgery, trauma (including cardiopulmonary resuscitation), GI or GU bleeding, cerebrovascular disease, hypertension, mitral stenosis, atrial fibrillation, acute pericarditis, subacute bacterial endocarditis, septic thrombophlebitis, and diabetic hemorrhagic retinopathy; in patients receiving anticoagulants; and in patients older than age 75.

INTERACTIONS
Drug-drug. Use with *adrenocorticoids, cefamandole, cefoperazone, cefotetan, glucocorticoids, long-term corticotropin or ethacrynic acid therapy, plicamycin,* or *valproic acid* may increase the risk of severe hemorrhage. Use with *antihypertensives* may increase risk of severe hypotension. Use with *heparin, oral anticoagulants, drugs that alter platelet function (including aspirin and dipyridamole), NSAIDs,* or *sulfinpyrazone* may increase the risk of bleeding. Don't use together.

ADVERSE REACTIONS
CNS: *intracranial hemorrhage.*
CV: ARRHYTHMIAS, *conduction disorders, hypotension.*
EENT: hemoptysis, gum or mouth hemorrhage.
GI: hemorrhage.
GU: hematuria.
Hematologic: *bleeding tendency,* eosinophilia.
Musculoskeletal: arthralgia.
Skin: hematoma, urticaria, pruritus, flushing, delayed purpuric rash (2 weeks after therapy).
Other: bleeding at puncture sites, *anaphylaxis or anaphylactoid reactions (rare).*

▣ KEY CONSIDERATIONS
• No age-specific problems have been reported to date. Risk-benefit must be assessed in patients ages 75 and older because preexisting conditions increase the risk of hemorrhagic complications.
• The following tests may be needed before and after drug administration: activated partial thromboplastin time (APTT), PT and INR, thrombin time, hemoglobin level, hematocrit, fibrinogen determination, platelet count, and fibrin-fibrinogen degradation products.
• Anistreplase prolongs APTT, PT and INR, and thrombin time. The drug remains active in vitro and can cause degradation of fibrinogen in blood samples drawn for analysis. It also decreases the activity of alpha$_2$-antiplasmin, factor V, factor VIII, fibrinogen, and plasminogen; moderately reduces hemoglobin level and hematocrit; and increases levels of fibrinogen- and fibrin-degradation products.
• Coronary angiography can help monitor drug effectiveness.

• ECG monitoring is recommended to detect arrhythmias associated with an acute MI or reperfusion and may help determine effectiveness of treatment.

• Initiate therapy as soon as possible after signs and symptoms of an acute MI begin.

• Monitor vital signs, mental status, and neurologic status.

• Anistreplase is derived from human plasma. No cases of hepatitis or HIV infection have been reported to date.

• Store lyophilized powder in refrigerator.

• Reconstitute by slowly adding 5 ml sterile water for injection. Direct the stream against the side of the vial, not at the drug itself. Gently roll the vial to mix the dry powder and water. To avoid excessive foaming, don't shake vial. Solution should be colorless to pale yellow.

• Don't mix with other drugs or further dilute after reconstitution.

• Discard drug that isn't administered within 30 minutes of reconstituting.

• To decrease risk of rethrombosis, heparin therapy may be initiated after administration.

• Adding a fibrinolysis inhibitor (for example, aprotinin) or aminocaproic acid to blood samples drawn to measure fibrinogen will attenuate the degradation of fibrinogen typically associated with patients treated with a thrombolytic.

• Keep patient on strict bed rest and apply pressure dressings to recently invaded sites. To minimize risk of bleeding, avoid nonessential handling or moving of patient, invasive procedures such as biopsies, and I.M. injections.

Patient education

• Instruct patient to recognize and report signs and symptoms of internal bleeding.

• Instruct patient about importance of strict bed rest.

---

apraclonidine hydrochloride
Iopidine

Alpha-adrenergic agonist, ocular hypotensive

Available by prescription only
Ophthalmic solution: 0.5%, 1%

INDICATIONS & DOSAGE

Prevention or control of intraocular pressure (IOP) elevations after argon laser trabeculoplasty or iridotomy
Adults: Instill 1 gtt (1% solution) in the eye 1 hour before initiation of laser surgery on the anterior segment, followed by 1 gtt immediately on completion of surgery.

Short-term adjunctive therapy in patients on maximally tolerated medical therapy who require IOP reduction
Adults: Instill 1 or 2 gtt (0.5% solution) in the eye t.i.d.

◊ ***Open-angle glaucoma***
Adults: Instill 1 gtt (0.5% solution) in the eye b.i.d. or t.i.d.

PHARMACODYNAMICS

Ocular hypotensive action: Apraclonidine is an alpha-adrenergic agonist that reduces IOP, possibly by decreasing aqueous humor production.

PHARMACOKINETICS

Absorption: Unknown.
Distribution: Onset of action is within 1 hour after instillation, and maximum effect on reducing IOP occurs in 3 to 5 hours.
Metabolism: Unknown.
Excretion: Unknown.

CONTRAINDICATIONS & PRECAUTIONS

Contraindicated in patients who are hypersensitive to apraclonidine or clonidine or who are concomitantly taking an MAO inhibitor. Use cautiously in patients with severe cardiac disease, including hypertension and vasovagal attacks.

INTERACTIONS

Drug-drug. Use with *pilocarpine* or *topical beta blockers* may produce additive lowering of IOP. Monitor closely.

ADVERSE REACTIONS

CNS: insomnia, irritability, dream disturbances, headache, irritability, paresthesia.

CV: *bradycardia,* vasovagal attack, palpitations, hypotension, orthostatic hypotension.

EENT: upper eyelid elevation, conjunctival blanching and microhemorrhage, mydriasis, eye burning or discomfort, foreign body sensation in eye, eye dryness and *itching, hyperemia,* conjunctivitis, blurred vision, nasal burning or dryness or increased pharyngeal secretions.

GI: abdominal pain, discomfort, diarrhea, vomiting, taste disturbances, dry mouth.

Skin: pruritus not associated with rash, sweaty palms.

Other: body heat sensation, decreased libido, extremity pain or numbness, allergic response.

▣ KEY CONSIDERATIONS

● Protect stored drug from light and freezing.

Patient education

● Warn patient about the potential for dizziness and drowsiness.

● Tell patient if using more than one form of eyedrops, to allow a 5-minute interval between doses to prevent the previous dose from washing out.

---

ardeparin sodium
Normiflo

Low-molecular-weight heparin, anticoagulant

Available by prescription only
Injection: 5,000 anti-factor Xa U/0.5 ml, 10,000 anti-factor Xa U/0.5 ml

INDICATIONS & DOSAGE

Prevention of deep venous thrombosis, which may lead to pulmonary embolism after knee replacement surgery
Adults: 50 anti-factor Xa U/kg S.C. q 12 hours for 14 days or until patient is ambulatory, whichever is shorter. Give initial dosage the evening of day of surgery or the following morning.

PHARMACODYNAMICS

Anticoagulant action: Ardeparin is a low-molecular-weight heparin that binds to and accelerates the activity of antithrombin III. This results in an inactivation of factor Xa and thrombin, which prevents the formation of clots. Ardeparin also inhibits thrombin by binding to heparin cofactor II.

PHARMACOKINETICS

Absorption: Mean peak plasma anti-factor Xa and anti-factor IIa activity occurs about 3 hours after S.C. injection. Mean absolute bioavailability based on anti-factor Xa activity is 92%.

Distribution: Steady state volume of distribution based on anti-factor Xa activity is about 99 ml/kg.

Metabolism: Information not available.

Excretion: Elimination half-life based on anti-factor Xa activity is about 3 hours.

CONTRAINDICATIONS & PRECAUTIONS

Contraindicated in patients with known hypersensitivity to ardeparin, active bleeding, or thrombocytopenia associated with antiplatelet antibodies in the presence of drug. Don't use in patients with known hypersensitivity to pork products.

Use with extreme caution in patients with history of heparin-induced thrombocytopenia and in those with a known hypersensitivity to methylparaben, propylparaben, and sulfites. Use cautiously in patients at increased risk for hemorrhage (bacterial endocarditis), in patients concomitantly taking a platelet inhibitor, and in patients with congenital or acquired bleeding disorders; active ulcerative disease; angiodysplastic GI disease; hemorrhagic stroke; recent eye, spinal, or brain surgery or procedures; or severe uncontrolled hypertension. When epidural or spinal anesthesia or spinal puncture is used, patients who are anticoagulated or scheduled to be anticoagulated with low-molecular-weight heparins are at risk for developing epidural or spinal hematomas, which can result in long-term paralysis.

INTERACTIONS
Drug-drug. Use with *anticoagulants* or *antiplatelets (including aspirin and NSAIDs)* increases the risk of bleeding. Use cautiously.

ADVERSE REACTIONS
CNS: dizziness, headache, *CVA,* insomnia.
CV: chest pain, peripheral edema.
GI: nausea, vomiting.
Hematologic: anemia, ecchymosis, *hemorrhage, thrombocytopenia,* hematoma (at injection site).
Musculoskeletal: arthralgia.
Skin: pruritus, rash, local reaction.
Other: fever, pain.

▣ KEY CONSIDERATIONS
• Base dosing on actual body weight.
• Ardeparin can't be used interchangeably (unit for unit) with heparin sodium or other low-molecular-weight heparins.
• Routinely monitor CBC, platelet counts, urinalysis, and occult blood in stools throughout therapy. Routine monitoring of coagulation parameters isn't required.
• Don't mix with other injections or infusions.
• With patient sitting or lying down, administer drug with deep S.C. injection in the abdomen, (avoiding the navel), outer aspect of upper arm, or anterior thigh. Extrude air and excess drug before administration. The full length of the needle should be introduced into the skinfold held between the thumb and forefinger. Hold skinfold throughout the injection. Rotate injection site.
• To avoid hematoma at the injection site, don't give drug I.M.
• Ardeparin may decrease platelet count and increase transaminase and serum triglyceride levels.

Patient education
• Instruct patient to report abnormal bruising, bleeding, or dark stools.
• Instruct patient to observe for hematoma at injection site.
• Tell patient to avoid use of OTC drugs such as aspirin or NSAIDs.

Overdose & treatment
• Bleeding is the principal sign of an ardeparin overdose.
• Most bleeding can be stopped by discontinuing the drug, applying pressure to the site, and replacing hemostatic blood elements if necessary. Protamine sulfate can also be administered. Dose of protamine should be equal to the dose of ardeparin administered (1 mg of protamine neutralizes 100 anti-factor Xa U of ardeparin). If bleeding persists after 2 hours, blood should be drawn and residual anti-factor Xa levels determined. Additional protamine can be administered if bleeding persists or if anti-factor Xa levels remain high. Drug doesn't appear to be dialyzable.

ascorbic acid (vitamin C)
Ascorbicap, Cebid Timecelles, Cecon, Cevalin, Cevi-Bid, Ce-Vi-Sol, Dull-C, Flavorcee

Water-soluble vitamin

Available by prescription only
Injection: 250 mg/ml in 2-ml ampules and 2-ml and 30-ml vials; 500 mg/ml in 2-ml and 5-ml ampules and 50-ml vials; 500 mg/ml (with monothioglycerol) in 1-ml ampules
Available without a prescription
Tablets: 25 mg, 50 mg, 100 mg, 250 mg, 500 mg, 1,000 mg
Tablets (chewable): 100 mg, 250 mg, 500 mg
Tablets (timed-release): 500 mg, 1,000 mg, 1,500 mg
Capsules (timed-release): 500 mg
Lozenges: 60 mg
Crystals: 100 g (4 g/tsp), 1,000 g (4 g/tsp, sugar-free)
Powder: 100 g (4 g/tsp), 500 g (4 g/tsp)
Liquid: 50 ml (35 mg/0.6 ml)
Solution: 50 ml (100 mg/ml)
Syrup: 20 mg/ml in 120 ml and 480 ml; 500 mg/5 ml in 5 ml, 10 ml, 120 ml, and 473 ml

INDICATIONS & DOSAGE
Frank and subclinical scurvy
Adults: 100 to 250 mg, depending on severity, P.O., S.C., I.M., or I.V. daily or

b.i.d., then at least 50 mg/day for maintenance.

Prevention of ascorbic acid deficiency in those with poor nutritional habits or increased requirements
Adults: 45 to 60 mg P.O., S.C., I.M., or I.V. daily.
◊ **Potentiation of methenamine in urine acidification**
Adults: 4 to 12 g daily in divided doses.
◊ **Adjunctive therapy in the treatment of idiopathic methemoglobinemia**
Adults: 300 to 600 mg P.O. daily in divided doses.

PHARMACODYNAMICS
Nutritional action: Ascorbic acid, an essential vitamin, is involved with the biologic oxidations and reductions used in cellular respiration. It's essential for the formation and maintenance of intracellular ground substance and collagen. In the body, ascorbic acid is reversibly oxidized to dehydroascorbic acid and influences tyrosine metabolism, conversion of folic acid to folinic acid, carbohydrate metabolism, resistance to infections, and cellular respiration. Ascorbic acid deficiency causes scurvy, a condition marked by degenerative changes in the capillaries, bone, and connective tissues. Restoring adequate ascorbic acid intake completely reverses symptoms of ascorbic acid deficiency. Data regarding use of ascorbic acid as a urinary acidifier are conflicting.

PHARMACOKINETICS
Absorption: After oral administration, ascorbic acid is readily absorbed. After very large doses, absorption may be limited because absorption is an active process. Absorption also may be reduced in patients with diarrhea or GI diseases. Normal plasma ascorbic acid levels are 10 to 20 µg/ml. Plasma levels below 1.5 µg/ml are associated with scurvy. However, leukocyte counts (although not usually measured) may better reflect ascorbic acid tissue saturation. About 1.5 g of ascorbic acid is stored in the body. Within 3 to 5 months of ascorbic acid deficiency, signs of scurvy become evident.

Distribution: Distributed widely in the body, with significant levels found in the liver, leukocytes, platelets, glandular tissues, and lens of the eye.
Metabolism: Ascorbic acid is metabolized in the liver.
Excretion: Ascorbic acid is reversibly oxidized to dehydroascorbic acid. Some is metabolized to inactive compounds that are excreted in urine. The renal threshold is about 14 µg/ml. When the body is saturated and blood levels exceed the threshold, unchanged ascorbic acid is excreted in urine. Renal excretion is directly proportional to blood levels. Hemodialysis removes ascorbic acid from circulation.

CONTRAINDICATIONS & PRECAUTIONS
No known contraindications. Use cautiously in patients with renal insufficiency.

INTERACTIONS
Drug-drug. Use in large doses (more than 2 g/day) with *acidic drugs* may lower urine pH, causing renal tubular reabsorption of acidic drugs. Use with *basic drugs (such as amphetamines* or *tricyclic antidepressants)* may decrease reabsorption and therapeutic effect. Use with *dicumarol* or *warfarin* influences the intensity and duration of the anticoagulant effect; use with warfarin may inhibit the anticoagulant effect. Use with *ethinyl estradiol* may increase plasma ethinyl estradiol levels. Use with *iron* keeps the iron in the ferrous state and increases iron absorption in the GI tract, but this increase may be insignificant; a combination of 30 mg of iron with 200 mg of ascorbic acid is sometimes recommended. Use with *salicylates* inhibits ascorbic acid uptake by leukocytes and platelets; although salicylates aren't known to precipitate ascorbic acid deficiency, patients receiving high doses of salicylates with ascorbic acid supplements must be observed for symptoms of ascorbic acid deficiency. Use with *sulfonamides* may cause crystallization. Monitor closely.
Drug-lifestyle. Because *smoking* can decrease serum ascorbic acid levels, dosage requirements of this vitamin

should be increased in a patient who smokes.

ADVERSE REACTIONS
CNS: faintness, dizziness (with too-rapid I.V. administration).
GI: diarrhea.
GU: acid urine, oxaluria, renal calculi.
Other: discomfort at injection site.

▣ KEY CONSIDERATIONS
• Administer large doses of ascorbic acid (1,000 mg/day) in divided amounts because the body uses only a limited amount and excretes the rest in urine. Large doses may increase small-intestine pH and impair absorption of vitamin B_{12}. The RDA for ascorbic acid is as follows:
Adults: 60 mg/day
Smokers: 100 mg/day
Patients on long-term hemodialysis: 100 to 200 mg/day.
• Administer oral solutions of ascorbic acid directly into the mouth or mix with food.
• Administer I.V. solution slowly.
• Conditions that elevate the metabolic rate (hyperthyroidism, fever, infection, burns and other severe trauma, postoperative states, neoplastic disease, and chronic alcoholism) significantly increase ascorbic acid requirements.
• Reportedly, patients taking oral contraceptives require ascorbic acid supplements.
• Smokers appear to have increased requirements for ascorbic acid because the vitamin is oxidized and excreted more rapidly than in nonsmokers.
• Use ascorbic acid cautiously in patients with renal insufficiency because the vitamin is normally excreted in urine.
• Patients with diets that are deficient in fruits and vegetables can develop subclinical ascorbic acid deficiency. Observe for such deficiency.
• Signs and symptoms of ascorbic acid deficiency include irritability; emotional disturbances; general debility; pallor; anorexia; sensitivity to touch; limb and joint pain; follicular hyperkeratosis (particularly on thighs and buttocks); easy bruising; petechiae; bloody diarrhea; delayed healing; loosening of teeth; sensitive, swollen, and bleeding gums; and anemia.
• Protect ascorbic acid solutions from light.
• Ascorbic acid is a strong reducing agent; it alters results of tests that are based on oxidation-reduction reactions. Large doses of ascorbic acid (over 500 mg) may cause false-negative glucose determinations using the glucose oxidase method, or false-positive results using the copper reduction method or Benedict's reagent. Ascorbic acid shouldn't be used for 48 to 72 hours before an amine-dependent test for occult blood in the stool is conducted because a false-negative result may occur. Depending on the reagents used, ascorbic acid may also cause interactions with other diagnostic tests.

Patient education
• Teach patient about good dietary sources of ascorbic acid, such as citrus fruits, leafy vegetables, tomatoes, green peppers, and potatoes.
• Inform patient to cover foods and fruit juices tightly and to use them promptly.
• Advise patients with ascorbic acid deficiency to decrease or stop smoking. Replacement ascorbic acid dosages are greater for the smoker.
• Tell patients who are prone to renal calculi, who have diabetes, who are undergoing tests for occult blood in stools, or who are on sodium-restricted diets or anticoagulant therapy to avoid high dosages of ascorbic acid.

Overdose & treatment
• Serious adverse effects or toxicity is uncommon but require discontinuation of therapy. After tissue saturation, the kidneys excrete excessively high dosages of parenteral ascorbic acid, so they rarely accumulate.

---

aspirin
A.S.A., Ascriptin, Aspergum, Bufferin, Ecotrin, Empirin, Halfprin, Novasen*, ZORprin

Salicylate, nonnarcotic analgesic, antipyretic, anti-inflammatory, antiplatelet

Available by prescription only
Tablets (enteric-coated): 975 mg
Tablets (extended-release): 800 mg
Available without a prescription
Tablets: 81 mg, 325 mg (5 grains), 500 mg, 650 mg
Tablets (enteric-coated): 81 mg, 162 mg, 165 mg, 325 mg, 500 mg, 650 mg
Tablets (extended-release): 650 mg
Chewing gum: 227.5 mg
Suppositories: 60 mg, 120 mg, 125 mg, 200 mg, 300 mg, 600 mg

INDICATIONS & DOSAGE
Mild pain or fever
Adults: 325 to 650 mg P.O. or P.R. q 4 hours, p.r.n.
Rheumatic fever
Adults: 4.9 to 7.8 g P.O. daily divided q 4 to 6 hours for 1 to 2 weeks; then decrease to 60 to 70 mg/kg daily for 1 to 6 weeks; then gradually withdraw over 1 to 2 weeks.
Arthritis
Adults: 3.6 to 5.4 g P.O. daily in divided doses.
Transient ischemic attacks and thromboembolic disorders
Adults: 650 mg P.O. b.i.d. or 325 mg q.i.d.
Reduction of the risk of heart attack in patients with a previous MI or unstable angina
Adults: 160 to 325 mg P.O. once daily.
Treatment of Kawasaki (mucocutaneous lymph node) syndrome
Adults: 80 to 100 mg/kg P.O. daily in four divided doses. Some patients may require up to 120 mg/kg daily to maintain acceptable serum salicylate levels (over 200 µg/ml during the febrile phase). After the fever subsides, reduce dosage to 3 to 5 mg/kg once daily. Therapy is usually continued for 6 to 8 weeks.

PHARMACODYNAMICS
Analgesic action: Aspirin produces analgesia by producing an ill-defined effect on the hypothalamus (central action) and by blocking generation of pain impulses (peripheral action). The peripheral action may involve blocking of prostaglandin synthesis via inhibition of cyclo-oxygenase enzyme.
Antipyretic action: Drug relieves fever by acting on the hypothalamic heat-regulating center to produce peripheral vasodilation. This increases peripheral blood supply and promotes sweating, which leads to loss of heat and to cooling by evaporation.
Anti-inflammatory action: Although the exact mechanism is unknown, drug is believed to inhibit prostaglandin synthesis; it may also inhibit the synthesis or action of other mediators of inflammation.
Antiplatelet action: At low dosages, drug appears to impede clotting by blocking prostaglandin synthetase action, which prevents the platelet-aggregating substance thromboxane A_2 from forming. This interference with platelet activity is irreversible and can prolong bleeding time. However, at high dosages, aspirin interferes with prostacyclin production, a potent vasoconstrictor and inhibitor of platelet aggregation, possibly negating its anticlotting properties.

PHARMACOKINETICS
Absorption: Aspirin is absorbed rapidly and completely from the GI tract. Therapeutic blood salicylate levels for analgesia and anti-inflammatory effect are 150 to 300 µg/ml; responses vary with the patient.
Distribution: Drug is distributed widely into most body tissues and fluids. Protein-binding to albumin depends on drug level, ranges from 75% to 90%, and decreases as serum level increases. Severe toxic effects may occur at serum levels greater than 400 µg/ml.
Metabolism: Drug is hydrolyzed partially in the GI tract to salicylic acid with almost complete metabolism in the liver.
Excretion: Drug is excreted in urine as salicylate and its metabolites. Elimina-

tion half-life ranges from 15 to 20 minutes.

CONTRAINDICATIONS & PRECAUTIONS

Contraindicated in patients with hypersensitivity to aspirin, G6PD deficiency, bleeding disorders such as hemophilia, von Willebrand's disease, or telangiectasia. Also contraindicated in patients with NSAID-induced sensitivity reactions.

Use cautiously in patients with GI lesions, impaired renal function, hypoprothrombinemia, vitamin K deficiency, thrombotic thrombocytopenic purpura, or hepatic impairment.

INTERACTIONS

Drug-drug. Use with *ammonium chloride* or *other urine acidifiers* increases blood aspirin levels. Monitor for aspirin toxicity.

Antacids in high dosages and other *urine alkalizers* decrease blood aspirin levels. Monitor for decreased salicylate effect. Use delays and decreases absorption of aspirin.

Use with *anticoagulants* or *thrombolytics* may potentiate the platelet-inhibiting effects of aspirin. Use with *corticosteroids* enhances aspirin elimination. Use with *drugs that are highly protein-bound*—such as *phenytoin, sulfonylureas,* and *warfarin*—may cause displacement of either drug and adverse effects. Aspirin decreases renal clearance of *lithium,* thus increasing serum lithium levels and the risk of adverse effects. Use with *ototoxic drugs*—such as *aminoglycosides, bumetanide, capreomycin, ethacrynic acid, furosemide, cisplatin, vancomycin,* and *erythromycin*—may potentiate ototoxic effects. Aspirin antagonizes the uricosuric effect of *phenylbutazone, probenecid,* and *sulfinpyrazone.* Monitor closely.

Use with *GI irritants*—such as *antibiotics, steroids,* and *other NSAIDs*—may potentiate the adverse GI effects of the aspirin. Use together with caution.
Drug-food. *Food* delays and decreases absorption of aspirin. Don't use together.
Drug-lifestyle. *Alcohol* may potentiate the adverse GI effects of the aspirin. Use together with caution.

ADVERSE REACTIONS

EENT: *tinnitus, hearing loss.*
GI: *nausea, GI distress, occult bleeding, dyspepsia,* **GI bleeding.**
Hematologic: *leukopenia, thrombocytopenia,* prolonged bleeding time.
Hepatic: abnormal liver function test results, hepatitis.
Skin: *rash,* bruising, urticaria, angioedema.
Other: hypersensitivity reactions (***anaphylaxis,*** asthma), *Reye's syndrome.*

☒ KEY CONSIDERATIONS

Besides the recommendations relevant to all salicylates, consider the following:
● Patients older than age 60 may be more susceptible to the toxic effects of aspirin. Use with caution.
● Effects of aspirin on renal prostaglandins may cause fluid retention and edema, a significant drawback for geriatric patients.
● Enteric-coated products are absorbed slowly and aren't suitable for immediate therapy. They are ideal for long-term therapy such as for arthritis.
● Aspirin isn't known to reduce the incidence of transient ischemic attacks in women.
● Avoid giving effervescent aspirin preparations to sodium-restricted patients.
● Stop aspirin therapy 1 week before elective surgery, if possible.
● Moisture may cause aspirin to lose potency. Store in a cool, dry place, and avoid using if tablets smell like vinegar.
● Aspirin will cause an increased bleeding time. Aspirin interferes with urinary glucose analysis performed with Diastix, Chemstrip uG, glucose enzymatic test strip, Clinitest, and Benedict's solution, and with urinary 5-hydroxyindoleacetic acid and vanillylmandelic acid tests. Serum uric acid levels may be falsely increased. Aspirin may interfere with the Gerhardt test for urine acetoacetic acid.

Patient education
● Tell patients to keep aspirin out of children's reach because it's a leading cause of poisoning.

Reactions may be *common,* uncommon, *life-threatening,* or **COMMON AND LIFE-THREATENING.**

- Advise patients receiving high-dose, long-term aspirin therapy to watch for petechiae, bleeding gums, and signs of GI bleeding.
- Instruct patient to avoid use of aspirin if allergic to tartrazine dye.
- Tell patient to take drug with food or after meals to avoid GI upset.

Overdose & treatment

- Signs and symptoms of overdose include GI discomfort, oliguria, acute renal failure, hyperthermia, EEG abnormalities, and restlessness as well as metabolic acidosis with respiratory alkalosis, hyperpnea, and tachypnea because of increased carbon dioxide production and direct stimulation of the respiratory center.
- To treat aspirin overdose, empty the patient's stomach immediately by inducing vomiting with ipecac syrup if patient is conscious or by performing gastric lavage. Administer activated charcoal via an NG tube. Provide symptomatic and supportive measures (respiratory support and correction of fluid and electrolyte imbalances). Closely monitor laboratory parameters and vital signs. Enhance renal excretion by administering sodium bicarbonate to alkalize urine. Use cooling blanket or sponging if patient's rectal temperature is more than 104° F (40° C). Hemodialysis is effective in removing aspirin but is only used in severely poisoned individuals or those at risk for pulmonary edema.

---

atenolol
Tenormin

Beta blocker, antihypertensive, antianginal

Available by prescription only
Tablets: 25 mg, 50 mg, 100 mg
Injection: 5 mg/10 ml

INDICATIONS & DOSAGE

Hypertension
Adults: Initially, 50 mg P.O. as a single daily dosage. May increase dosage to 100 mg/day after 7 to 14 days. Higher dosages are unlikely to produce further benefit.

Chronic stable angina pectoris
Adults: 50 mg P.O. once daily; may be increased to 100 mg/day after 7 days for optimal effect. Maximum daily dosage is 200 mg/day.

To reduce risk of CV mortality in patients with an acute MI
Adults: 5 mg I.V. over 5 minutes, followed by another 5 mg I.V. 10 minutes later. In patients who tolerate the full I.V. dose, initiate oral therapy 10 minutes after the final I.V. dose. Give 50 mg P.O. q 12 hours for 2 doses; then give 100 mg P.O. daily or 50 mg P.O. b.i.d. for 6 to 9 days or until discharged from the hospital.

♦ *Dosage adjustment.* In patients with renal failure, adjust dosage if creatinine clearance is below 35 ml/minute. In patients with creatinine clearance of 15 to 35 ml/minute/1.73 m², give 50 mg/day; in patients with creatinine clearance below 15 ml/minute/1.73 m², give 25 mg/day; in patients undergoing hemodialysis, dosage is 25 to 50 mg after each treatment under close supervision.

PHARMACODYNAMICS

Antihypertensive action: Atenolol may reduce blood pressure by blocking adrenergic receptors, thus decreasing cardiac output by decreasing sympathetic outflow from the CNS and by suppressing renin release. At low dosages, atenolol, like metoprolol, selectively inhibits cardiac beta$_1$ receptors; it has little effect on beta$_2$ receptors in bronchial and vascular smooth muscle.

Antianginal action: Atenolol helps treat chronic stable angina by decreasing myocardial contractility and heart rate (negative inotropic and chronotropic effect), thus reducing myocardial oxygen consumption.

Cardioprotective action: The mechanism whereby atenolol improves survival in patients with an MI is unknown. However, it reduces the frequency of PVCs, chest pain, and elevated enzyme levels.

PHARMACOKINETICS

Absorption: Some 50% to 60% of an atenolol dose is absorbed. Drug usually

affects heart rate within 60 minutes, with peak effect in 2 to 4 hours. Antihypertensive effect persists for about 24 hours.
Distribution: Drug distributes into most tissues and fluids except the brain and CSF; 5% to 15% binds to proteins.
Metabolism: Drug is metabolized only minimally.
Excretion: Some 40% to 50% of a given dose is excreted unchanged in urine; remainder is excreted as unchanged drug and metabolites in feces. In patients with normal renal function, plasma half-life is 6 to 7 hours; half-life increases as renal function decreases.

CONTRAINDICATIONS & PRECAUTIONS
Contraindicated in patients with sinus bradycardia, greater than first-degree heart block, overt cardiac failure, or cardiogenic shock. Use cautiously in patients at risk for heart failure and in those with bronchospastic disease, diabetes, or hyperthyroidism.

INTERACTIONS
Drug-drug. Atenolol may potentiate the antihypertensive effects of *other antihypertensives*. It may also alter a diabetic patient's *insulin* or *oral antidiabetic* dosage requirements. Monitor closely.
   Indomethacin, NSAIDs, and *alpha-adrenergics such as those found in OTC cold remedies* may antagonize the antihypertensive effects of atenolol. Use with caution.

ADVERSE REACTIONS
CNS: *fatigue,* lethargy, vertigo, drowsiness, *dizziness.*
CV: *bradycardia, hypotension, **heart failure,*** intermittent claudication.
GI: nausea, diarrhea.
Respiratory: dyspnea, ***bronchospasm.***
Skin: rash.
Other: fever, leg pain.

▣ KEY CONSIDERATIONS
Besides the recommendations relevant to all beta blockers, consider the following:
● Geriatric patients may require lower maintenance dosages of atenolol because of increased bioavailability or delayed metabolism; they also may experience enhanced adverse effects.

● Give oral single daily dose at same time each day.
● Drug may be taken without food.
● Dosage may need to be reduced in patients with renal insufficiency.
● I.V. atenolol affords a rapid onset of the protective effects of beta blockade against reinfarction.
● Patients who can't tolerate I.V. atenolol after an MI may be candidates for oral atenolol therapy. Gastric absorption of atenolol may be delayed in the early phase of an MI. This may result from the physiological changes that accompany the MI or from the effects of morphine, which is commonly administered to treat chest pain. However, oral therapy alone may still provide benefits. Clinical trials suggest giving 100 mg of atenolol daily P.O. (either as 50 mg b.i.d. or 100 mg once daily) for at least 7 days. In the absence of contraindications, some may continue therapy for 1 to 3 years.
● Although such use is controversial, atenolol has been used as an adjunct in treating alcohol withdrawal.
● Atenolol may increase or decrease serum glucose levels in diabetic patients; it doesn't potentiate insulin-induced hypoglycemia or delay recovery of serum glucose to normal levels.
● Atenolol also may cause changes in exercise tolerance and ECG; it has reportedly elevated platelet count and serum levels of potassium, uric acid, transaminase, alkaline phosphatase, LD, creatinine, and BUN.

Patient education
● Stress importance of not missing doses, but tell patient not to double-dose if one is missed, especially if taking drug once daily.
● Advise patient to seek medical approval before taking OTC cold preparations.

Overdose & treatment
● Signs and symptoms of overdose include severe hypotension, bradycardia, heart failure, and bronchospasm.
● After acute ingestion, empty stomach by inducing vomiting or performing gastric lavage; follow with activated char-

---

Reactions may be *common,* uncommon, *life-threatening,* or COMMON AND LIFE-THREATENING.

coal to reduce absorption. Thereafter, treat symptomatically and supportively.

atorvastatin calcium
Lipitor

3-hydroxy-3-methylglutaryl-coenzyme A (HMG-CoA) reductase inhibitor, antilipemic

Available by prescription only
Tablets: 10 mg, 20 mg, 40 mg

INDICATIONS & DOSAGE
Adjunct to diet to reduce elevated low-density lipoprotein (LDL), total cholesterol, apo B, and triglyceride levels in patients with primary hypercholesterolemia and mixed dyslipidemia
Adults: Initially, 10 mg P.O. once daily. Increase dosage, p.r.n., to maximum of 80 mg daily as single dose. Dosage based on blood lipid levels drawn within 2 to 4 weeks after starting therapy.
Alone or as an adjunct to lipid-lowering treatments such as LDL apheresis in patients with homozygous familial hypercholesterolemia
Adults: 10 to 80 mg P.O. once daily.

PHARMACODYNAMICS
Antilipemic action: Atorvastatin inhibits HMG-CoA reductase, an early (and rate-limiting) step in cholesterol biosynthesis.

PHARMACOKINETICS
Absorption: Atorvastatin is rapidly absorbed. Plasma levels peak within 1 to 2 hours. Therapeutic response can be seen within 2 weeks; maximum response within 4 weeks and maintained during long-term therapy.
Distribution: Mean volume of distribution is about 565 L. Some 98% or more of drug binds to plasma proteins with poor drug penetration into RBCs.
Metabolism: Drug is extensively metabolized to orthohydroxylated and parahydroxylated derivatives and various beta-oxidation products. In vitro inhibition of HMG-CoA reductase by orthohydroxylated and parahydroxylated metabolites is equivalent to that of atorvastatin.

About 70% of circulating inhibitory activity for HMG-CoA reductase is attributed to active metabolites. In vitro studies suggest the importance of atorvastatin metabolism by cytochrome P450 3A4.
Excretion: Drug and its metabolites are eliminated primarily in bile after hepatic or extrahepatic metabolism; however, drug doesn't appear to undergo enterohepatic recirculation. Mean plasma elimination half-life of atorvastatin is about 14 hours, but the half-life of inhibitory activity for HMG-CoA reductase is 20 to 30 hours because of the contribution of active metabolites. Less than 2% of a dose of atorvastatin is recovered in urine after oral administration.

CONTRAINDICATIONS & PRECAUTIONS
Contraindicated in patients who are hypersensitive to atorvastatin or who have active hepatic disease or conditions with unexplained persistent elevations of serum transaminase levels.

Use cautiously in patients with history of hepatic disease or heavy alcohol use.

INTERACTIONS
Drug-drug. Use with *azole antifungals, cyclosporine, erythromycin, fibric acid derivatives,* or *niacin* may increase the risk of rhabdomyolysis. Don't use together.

Use with *digoxin* or *erythromycin* may increase plasma levels of these drugs. Monitor closely.

ADVERSE REACTIONS
CNS: asthenia, *headache.*
GI: abdominal pain, constipation, diarrhea, dyspepsia, flatulence.
Musculoskeletal: arthralgia, back pain, myalgia.
Respiratory: pharyngitis, sinusitis.
Skin: rash.
Other: accidental injury, allergic reaction, flulike syndrome, *infection.*

▣ KEY CONSIDERATIONS
• Safety and efficacy in patients ages 70 and older with drug doses up to 80 mg daily were similar to those of patients younger than age 70.

• Drug should be withheld or discontinued in patients with serious, acute conditions that suggest myopathy and in patients at risk for renal failure secondary to rhabdomyolysis as a result of trauma; major surgery; severe metabolic, endocrine, and electrolyte disorders; severe acute infection; hypotension; or uncontrolled seizures.

• Use drug only after diet and other nonpharmacologic treatments prove ineffective. Patient should follow a standard low-cholesterol diet before and during therapy.

• Before initiating treatment, exclude secondary causes for hypercholesterolemia and perform a baseline lipid profile. Periodic liver function tests and lipid levels should be done before starting treatment, at 6 weeks and 12 weeks after initiation, or after an increase in dosage and periodically thereafter.

• Drug may be given as a single dose at any time of day without regard for food.

• Watch for signs of myositis.

• Drug may increase liver function test results.

Patient education

• Teach patient proper dietary management, weight control, and exercise. Explain the importance of controlling elevated serum lipid levels.

• Warn patient to avoid alcohol.

• Tell patient to report adverse reactions, such as muscle pain, malaise, and fever.

atovaquone
Mepron

Ubiquinone analogue, antiprotozoal

Available by prescription only
Suspension: 750 mg/5 ml

INDICATIONS & DOSAGE
Mild to moderate Pneumocystis carinii pneumonia in patients who can't tolerate trimethoprim-sulfamethoxazole
Adults: 750 mg P.O. b.i.d. for 21 days given with food.

PHARMACODYNAMICS
Antiprotozoal action: The mechanism of action of atovaquone against *P. carinii* is unclear. In *Plasmodium* species, the site of action appears to be the cytochrome bc_1 complex (complex III). Several metabolic enzymes are linked to the mitochondrial electron transport chain via ubiquinone. Inhibition of electron transport by atovaquone results in indirect inhibition of these enzymes. The ultimate metabolic effects of such a blockade may include inhibition of nucleic acid and adenosine triphosphate synthesis.

PHARMACOKINETICS
Absorption: Absorption of atovaquone is limited. However, food increases bioavailability of drug threefold. In particular, fat has been shown to enhance absorption significantly.
Distribution: Drug binds extensively (99.9%) to plasma proteins.
Metabolism: Drug isn't metabolized.
Excretion: Drug undergoes enterohepatic cycling and is primarily excreted in feces. Less than 0.6% is excreted in urine.

CONTRAINDICATIONS & PRECAUTIONS
Contraindicated in patients with hypersensitivity to atovaquone.

INTERACTIONS
Drug-drug. Use with other *highly plasma protein–bound drugs with narrow therapeutic indices* may increase competition for binding sites. (Phenytoin, however, isn't affected.) Use caution when administering together.

Use with *rifampin* can significantly decrease plasma drug levels. Don't use together.

ADVERSE REACTIONS
CNS: *headache, insomnia,* asthenia, anxiety, dizziness.
CV: hypotension.
EENT: *cough,* sinusitis, rhinitis, taste perversion.
GI: *oral candidiasis, nausea, diarrhea,* vomiting, constipation, abdominal pain, anorexia, dyspepsia.
Metabolic: hypoglycemia.

Reactions may be *common,* uncommon, ***life-threatening***, or **COMMON AND LIFE-THREATENING**.

Skin: *rash,* pruritus, *diaphoresis.*
Other: *fever, pain.*

▣ KEY CONSIDERATIONS

• Use cautiously in geriatric patients because they're more likely to have decreased hepatic, renal, and cardiac function.
• Drug hasn't been systematically studied for use in the treatment of more severe episodes of *Pneumocystis carinii* pneumonia, nor has it been evaluated as prophylaxis against *P. carinii* pneumonia. Also, the efficacy of atovaquone in patients who are failing therapy with trimethoprim-sulfamethoxazole hasn't been systematically studied.
• GI disorders may limit absorption of the oral form and prevent the patient from achieving plasma drug levels that indicate he's responding to therapy.
• Drug is ineffective for concurrent pulmonary conditions, such as bacterial, viral, or fungal pneumonia or mycobacterial disease.
• Patients with acute *Pneumocystis carinii* pneumonia should be carefully evaluated for other possible causes of pulmonary disease and treated with additional drugs as appropriate.

Patient education

• Instruct patient to take drug with meals because food enhances absorption significantly.

atropine sulfate

Anticholinergic, belladonna alkaloid, antiarrhythmic, vagolytic

Available by prescription only
Tablets: 0.4 mg
Injection: 0.05 mg/ml, 0.1 mg/ml, 0.3 mg/ml, 0.4 mg/ml, 0.5 mg/ml, 0.8 mg/ml, 1 mg/ml
Ophthalmic ointment: 1%
Ophthalmic solution: 0.5%, 1%, 2%

INDICATIONS & DOSAGE

Symptomatic bradycardia, bradyarrhythmia (junctional or escape rhythm)
Adults: Usually 0.5 to 1 mg by I.V. push; repeat q 3 to 5 minutes, to maximum of 2 mg. Lower dosages (less than 0.5 mg) may cause bradycardia.

Preoperatively for diminishing secretions and blocking cardiac vagal reflexes
Adults: 0.4 mg I.M. or S.C. 30 to 60 minutes before anesthesia.

Antidote for anticholinesterase insecticide poisoning
Adults: 1 to 2 mg I.M. or I.V. repeated q 20 to 30 minutes until muscarinic symptoms disappear.

Hypotonic radiograph of the GI tract
Adults: 1 mg I.M.

Acute iritis, uveitis
Adults: 1 or 2 gtt (0.5% or 1% solution) into the eye q.i.d. or a small amount of ointment in the conjunctival sac t.i.d.

Cycloplegic refraction
Adults: 1 or 2 gtt (1% solution) 1 hour before refraction.

PHARMACODYNAMICS

Antiarrhythmic action: An anticholinergic (parasympatholytic) with many uses, atropine remains the mainstay of pharmacologic treatment for bradyarrhythmias. It blocks the effects of acetylcholine on the SA and AV nodes, thereby increasing SA and AV node conduction velocity. It also increases sinus node discharge rate and decreases the effective refractory period of the AV node. These changes result in increased atrial and ventricular heart rates.

Atropine has variable—and clinically negligible—effects on the His-Purkinje system. Small dosages (below 0.5 mg) and occasionally larger dosages may lead to a paradoxical slowing of the heart rate, which may be followed by a more rapid rate.
Vagolytic action: As an anticholinergic, atropine decreases the action of the parasympathetic nervous system on bronchial, salivary, and sweat glands, resulting in decreased secretions. It also decreases cholinergic effects on the iris, ciliary body, and intestinal and bronchial smooth muscle.

As an antidote for cholinesterase poisoning, atropine blocks the cholinomimetic effects of these pesticides.

PHARMACOKINETICS

Absorption: The I.V. route is the most common route when treating bradyarrhythmia. With endotracheal administration, atropine is well absorbed from the bronchial tree (drug has been used in 1-mg doses in acute bradyarrhythmia when an I.V. line hasn't been established). Effects on heart rate peak within 2 to 4 minutes after I.V. administration. Drug is well absorbed after oral and I.M. administration, and inhibitory effects on salivation peak 30 minutes to 1 hour after either route.

Distribution: Drug is well distributed throughout the body, including the CNS. Only 18% of drug binds with plasma protein (clinically insignificant).

Metabolism: Drug is metabolized in the liver to several metabolites.

Excretion: The kidneys excrete 30% to 50% of a dose as unchanged drug; however, small amounts may be excreted in feces and expired air. Elimination half-life is biphasic, with an initial 2-hour phase followed by a terminal half-life of about 12½ hours.

CONTRAINDICATIONS & PRECAUTIONS

Contraindicated in patients with hypersensitivity to atropine or sodium metabisulfite, acute angle-closure glaucoma, obstructive uropathy, obstructive disease of GI tract, paralytic ileus, toxic megacolon, intestinal atony, unstable CV status in acute hemorrhage, asthma, and myasthenia gravis.

Ophthalmic form is contraindicated in patients with glaucoma or hypersensitivity to drug or belladonna alkaloids and in those who have adhesions between the iris and lens.

Use cautiously in patients with Down syndrome. Ophthalmic form should be used with caution in geriatric patients, especially those with increased intraocular pressure.

INTERACTIONS

Drug-drug. Use with *amantadine* may result in an increase in anticholinergic adverse effects. Use with *other anticholinergics* or *drugs with anticholinergic effects* produces additive effects. Monitor closely.

ADVERSE REACTIONS

CNS: *headache, restlessness,* ataxia, disorientation, hallucinations, delirium, *insomnia, dizziness,* excitement, agitation, confusion, especially in geriatric patients (with systemic or oral form); confusion, somnolence, headache (with ophthalmic form).

CV: palpitations and bradycardia after a low dose of atropine, tachycardia after higher doses (with systemic or oral form); tachycardia (with ophthalmic form).

EENT: photophobia, increased intraocular pressure, *blurred vision, mydriasis,* cycloplegia (with systemic or oral form), ocular congestion with long-term use, conjunctivitis, contact dermatitis of eye, ocular edema, eye dryness, transient stinging and burning, eye irritation, hyperemia (with ophthalmic form).

GI: *dry mouth,* thirst, *constipation,* nausea, vomiting (with systemic or oral form).

GU: urine retention, impotence (with systemic or oral form).

Hematologic: leukocytosis (with systemic or oral form).

Skin: dryness (with ophthalmic form).

Other: severe allergic reactions, including ***anaphylaxis*** and urticaria (with systemic or oral form).

▣ KEY CONSIDERATIONS

• Monitor closely for urine retention in geriatric male patient with benign prostatic hyperplasia.

• Observe for tachycardia if patient has cardiac disorder.

• With I.V. administration, drug may cause paradoxical initial bradycardia, which usually disappears within 2 minutes.

• Monitor patient's fluid intake and output; drug causes urine retention and urinary hesitancy. If possible, patient should void before taking drug.

• High dosages may cause hyperpyrexia, urine retention, and CNS effects, including hallucinations and confusion (anticholinergic delirium).

• Adverse reactions vary considerably with dosage.

Reactions may be *common,* uncommon, *life-threatening,* or COMMON AND LIFE-THREATENING.

attapulgite

Diasorb, Donnagel, Fowler's*, Kaopectate, Kaopectate Advanced Formula, Kaopectate Maximum Strength, K-Pek, Parepectolin, Rheaban, Rheaban Maximum Strength

Hydrated magnesium aluminum silicate, antidiarrheal

Available without a prescription
Tablets: 300 mg, 600 mg*, 630 mg*, 750 mg
Tablets (chewable): 600 mg
Oral suspension: 600 mg/15 ml, 750 mg/5 ml, 750 mg/15 ml*, 900 mg/15 ml*

INDICATIONS & DOSAGE
Acute, nonspecific diarrhea
Adults: 1.2 to 1.5 g (unless using Diasorb, in which case dosage can be as high as 3 g) P.O. after each loose bowel movement; don't exceed 9 g within 24 hours.

PHARMACODYNAMICS
Antidiarrheal action: Although the exact action of attapulgite is unknown, attapulgite is thought to absorb a large number of bacteria and toxins and reduce water loss in the GI tract.

PHARMACOKINETICS
Absorption: Attapulgite isn't absorbed.
Distribution: Not applicable.
Metabolism: Not applicable.
Excretion: Drug is excreted unchanged in feces.

CONTRAINDICATIONS & PRECAUTIONS
Contraindicated in patients with dysentery or suspected bowel obstruction. Use cautiously in dehydrated patients.

INTERACTIONS
Drug-drug. Use with *oral drugs* may impair their absorption. Administer attapulgite not less than 2 hours before or 3 to 4 hours after these drugs, and monitor the patient for decreased effectiveness.

ADVERSE REACTIONS
GI: constipation.

◙ KEY CONSIDERATIONS
• Use cautiously and only under medical supervision.
• To compensate for fluid loss from diarrhea, ensure that patient achieves adequate fluid intake.
• Drug shouldn't be used if fever or blood or mucus in the stool accompanies the diarrhea. Discontinue drug if patient experiences these effects during treatment.

Patient education
• Tell patient to take drug after each loose bowel movement until diarrhea is controlled.
• Instruct patient to call if diarrhea isn't controlled within 48 hours or if fever develops.

auranofin
Ridaura

Gold salt, antarthritic

Available by prescription only
Capsules: 3 mg

INDICATIONS & DOSAGE
Rheumatoid arthritis, ◇ *psoriatic arthritis,* ◇ *active systemic lupus erythematosus,* ◇ *Felty's syndrome*
Adults: 6 mg P.O. daily, administered either as 3 mg b.i.d. or 6 mg once daily. After 4 to 6 months, may be increased to 9 mg daily. If response remains inadequate after 3 months at 9 mg daily, discontinue drug.

PHARMACODYNAMICS
Antarthritic action: Auranofin prevents adult arthritis and synovitis. In patients with active arthritis, drug is thought to reduce inflammation by altering the immune system; it also decreases high serum levels of immunoglobulins and rheumatoid factors. However, the exact mechanism of action is unknown.

PHARMACOKINETICS
Absorption: When administered orally, 25% of the gold in auranofin is absorbed through the GI tract. Plasma levels peak in 1 to 2 hours.

Distribution: Drug is 60% protein-bound and is distributed widely in body tissues. Oral gold from auranofin is bound to a higher degree than gold from the injectable form. Synovial fluid levels are about 50% of blood levels. No correlation between blood-gold level and safety or efficacy has been determined.
Metabolism: The metabolic fate of auranofin is unknown, but it probably isn't broken down into elemental gold.
Excretion: 60% of absorbed auranofin (15% of the administered dosage) is excreted in urine and the remainder in feces. Average plasma half-life is 26 days, compared with about 6 days for gold sodium thiomalate.

CONTRAINDICATIONS & PRECAUTIONS

Contraindicated in patients with history of severe gold toxicity, necrotizing enterocolitis, pulmonary fibrosis, exfoliative dermatitis, bone marrow aplasia, severe hematologic disorders, or history of severe toxicity caused by previous exposure to other heavy metals.

Use cautiously with other drugs that cause blood dyscrasias or in patients with renal, hepatic, or inflammatory bowel disease; rash; or bone marrow depression.

INTERACTIONS

Drug-drug. Use with *drugs that may cause blood dyscrasias* can produce additive hematologic toxicity. Use cautiously.

ADVERSE REACTIONS

CNS: confusion, hallucinations, *seizures.*
EENT: conjunctivitis.
GI: *diarrhea, abdominal pain, nausea, stomatitis,* glossitis, anorexia, metallic taste, dyspepsia, flatulence, constipation, dysgeusia, *ulcerative colitis.*
GU: proteinuria, hematuria, *nephrotic syndrome,* glomerulonephritis, *acute renal failure.*
Hematologic: *thrombocytopenia (with or without purpura), aplastic anemia, agranulocytosis, leukopenia,* eosinophilia, anemia.
Hepatic: jaundice, elevated liver enzyme levels.
Respiratory: interstitial pneumonitis.

Skin: *rash, pruritus, dermatitis,* exfoliative dermatitis, urticaria, erythema, alopecia.

🖵 KEY CONSIDERATIONS

• Discontinue auranofin if platelet count falls below 100,000/mm^3.
• When switching from injectable gold, start auranofin at 6 mg P.O. daily.
• Serum protein-bound iodine test, especially when done by the chloric acid digestion method, gives false readings during and for several weeks after gold therapy.

Patient education

• Emphasize importance of monthly follow-up to monitor patient's platelet count.
• Reassure patient that beneficial drug effect may be delayed for 3 months. However, if response is inadequate after 6 to 9 months, auranofin will probably be discontinued.
• Encourage patient to take drug as prescribed and not to alter the dosage schedule.
• Diarrhea is the most common adverse reaction. Tell patient to continue taking drug if patient experiences mild diarrhea; however, tell him to call immediately if blood occurs in stool.
• Tell patient to continue taking concomitant drug therapy, such as NSAIDs, if prescribed.
• Because dermatitis is a common adverse reaction, advise patient to report rash or other skin problems immediately.
• Tell patient that drug may cause stomatitis, which is commonly preceded by a metallic taste. Advise him to call the health care provider immediately.

Overdose & treatment

• In acute overdose, empty gastric contents by inducing vomiting or performing gastric lavage. When severe reactions to gold occur, corticosteroids, dimercaprol (a chelate), or penicillamine may be given to aid recovery. Administering 40 to 100 mg of prednisone daily in divided doses is recommended to manage severe renal, hematologic, pulmonary, or enterocolitic reactions to gold. Dimercaprol may be used with

---

Reactions may be *common*, uncommon, *life-threatening*, or COMMON AND LIFE-THREATENING.

steroids to help remove the gold when steroid treatment alone is ineffective. Use of chelates is controversial, and caution is recommended. Appropriate supportive therapy is indicated as necessary.

azathioprine
Imuran

azathioprine sodium
Imuran

Purine antagonist, immunosuppressant

Available by prescription only
Tablets: 50 mg
Injection: 100-mg vial

INDICATIONS & DOSAGE
Prevention of the rejection of kidney transplants
Adults: Initially, 3 to 5 mg/kg P.O. daily beginning on day of (or 1 to 3 days before) transplantation. After transplantation, dosage may be administered I.V., until patient is able to tolerate oral dosage. Usual maintenance dosage is 1 to 3 mg/kg daily. Dosage varies with patient response.
Severe, refractory rheumatoid arthritis
Adults: Initially, 1 mg/kg (about 50 to 100 mg) P.O. taken as a single dose or in divided doses. If patient response is unsatisfactory after 6 to 8 weeks, dosage may be increased by 0.5 mg/kg daily (up to a maximum of 2.5 mg/kg daily) at 4-week intervals.

PHARMACODYNAMICS
Immunosuppressant action: The mechanism of immunosuppressive activity is unknown; however, azathioprine may inhibit RNA and DNA synthesis, mitosis, or (in patients undergoing renal transplantation) coenzyme formation and functioning. Azathioprine suppresses cell-mediated hypersensitivity and alters antibody production.

PHARMACOKINETICS
Absorption: Azathioprine is well absorbed orally.

Distribution: Drug and its major metabolite, mercaptopurine, are distributed throughout the body; both are 30% protein-bound.
Metabolism: Azathioprine is metabolized primarily to mercaptopurine.
Excretion: Small amounts of azathioprine and mercaptopurine are excreted in urine intact; most of a given dose is excreted in urine as secondary metabolites.

CONTRAINDICATIONS & PRECAUTIONS
Contraindicated in patients hypersensitive to azathioprine. Use cautiously in patients with impaired renal or hepatic function.

INTERACTIONS
Drug-drug. Use with *tubocurarine* or *pancuronium,* which are nondepolarizing muscle relaxants, may reverse the neuromuscular blockade that these drugs cause. Don't use together.

Allopurinol, which competes for the oxidative enzyme xanthine oxidase, inhibits the major metabolic pathway of azathioprine; concomitant use is potentially hazardous and should be avoided. If concomitant use is unavoidable, dosage should be reduced by one-third to one-fourth the usual dosage.

Use with *ACE inhibitors* may cause anemia and severe leukopenia. Use with *cyclosporine* may decrease plasma cyclosporine levels. Use with *methotrexate* may increase plasma levels of the metabolite 6-MP. Monitor closely.

ADVERSE REACTIONS
GI: *nausea, vomiting, pancreatitis,* steatorrhea, diarrhea, abdominal pain.
Hematologic: LEUKOPENIA, *bone marrow suppression,* anemia, *pancytopenia, thrombocytopenia, immunosuppression (possibly profound).*
Hepatic: *hepatotoxicity,* jaundice.
Musculoskeletal: arthralgia, myalgia
Skin: alopecia, rash.
Other: *infections,* fever, *increased risk of neoplasia.*

▣ KEY CONSIDERATIONS
• Monitor patient for signs and symptoms of hepatic damage: clay-colored

stools, dark urine, jaundice, pruritus, and elevated liver enzyme levels.
• If infection occurs, reduce azathioprine dosage and treat infection.
• If nausea and vomiting occur, divide dose or give with or after meals.
• Monitor for unusual bleeding or bruising, fever, or sore throat.
• If used to treat rheumatoid arthritis, NSAIDs should be continued when azathioprine therapy is initiated.
• Hematologic status should be monitored while patient is receiving azathioprine. CBCs, including platelet counts, should be taken at least weekly during the first month, twice monthly for the second and third months, then monthly.
• Chronic immunosuppression with azathioprine is associated with an increased risk of neoplasia.
• Azathioprine alters CBC and differential blood counts, decreases serum uric acid levels, and elevates liver enzyme levels.

Patient education
• Teach patient about disease and rationale for therapy. Explain possible adverse effects and importance of reporting them, especially unusual bleeding or bruising, fever, sore throat, mouth sores, abdominal pain, pale stools, or dark urine.
• Encourage compliance with therapy and follow-up visits.
• Tell patient with rheumatoid arthritis that a response to drug may not be apparent for up to 12 weeks.
• Suggest taking drug with or after meals or in divided doses to prevent nausea.

Overdose & treatment
• Signs and symptoms of overdose include nausea, vomiting, diarrhea, and extension of hematologic effects.
• Supportive treatment may include blood products if necessary.

azithromycin
Zithromax

Azalide macrolide, antibiotic

Available by prescription only
Tablets: 250 mg

Powder for oral suspension:
100 mg/5 ml, 200 mg/5 ml; 300 mg*, 600 mg*, 900 mg*, 1,000-mg packet
Injection: 500 mg

INDICATIONS & DOSAGE
***Acute bacterial exacerbations of COPD caused by* Haemophilus influenzae, Moraxella (Branhamella) catarrhalis,** *or* **Streptococcus pneumoniae;** *uncomplicated skin and skin-structure infections caused by* **Staphylococcus aureus, Streptococcus pyogenes,** *or* **S. agalactiae;** *and second-line therapy of pharyngitis or tonsillitis caused by* **S. pyogenes**
Adults: Initially, 500 mg P.O. as a single dose on day 1, followed by 250 mg daily on days 2 through 5. Total cumulative dosage is 1.5 g.
***Community-acquired pneumonia caused by* Chlamydia pneumoniae, H. influenzae, Mycoplasma pneumoniae, S. pneumoniae;** *I.V. form can be used for above infections and those caused by* **Legionella pneumophila, M. catarrhalis,** *and* **S. aureus**
Adults: 500 mg P.O. as a single dose on day 1, followed by 250 mg P.O. daily on days 2 to 5. Total dosage is 1.5 g. For those who require initial I.V. therapy, 500 mg I.V. as a single daily dose for 2 days, followed by 500 mg P.O. as a single daily dose to complete a 7- to 10-day course of therapy. Based on patient's response, the health care provider will determine the timing of the change from I.V. to P.O. therapy.
***Nongonococcal urethritis or cervicitis caused by* Chlamydia trachomatis**
Adults: 1 g P.O. as a single dose.
***Pelvic inflammatory disease caused by* C. trachomatis, Neisseria gonorrhoeae,** *or* **Mycoplasma hominis** *in patients requiring initial I.V. therapy*
Adults: 500 mg I.V. as a single daily dose for 1 to 2 days, followed by 250 mg P.O. daily to complete a 7-day course of therapy. Based on patient's response, the health care provider will determine the timing of the change from I.V. to P.O. therapy.
Chancroid
Adults: 1 g P.O. as a single dose.

Reactions may be *common,* uncommon, *life-threatening,* or COMMON AND LIFE-THREATENING.

Disseminated Mycobacterium avium complex (MAC) in patients with advanced infection with HIV
Adults: 1.2 g P.O. once weekly alone or in combination with rifabutin.

PHARMACODYNAMICS

Antibiotic action: Azithromycin, a derivative of erythromycin, binds to the 50S subunit of bacterial ribosomes, blocking protein synthesis. It's bacteriostatic or bactericidal, depending on concentration.

PHARMACOKINETICS

Absorption: Azithromycin is rapidly absorbed from the GI tract; food decreases both maximum plasma levels and amount of drug absorbed.
Distribution: Drug is rapidly distributed throughout the body and readily penetrates cells; it doesn't readily enter the CNS. It concentrates in fibroblasts and phagocytes. Significantly higher levels of drug are reached in the tissues as compared with the plasma. Uptake and release of drug from tissues contributes to the long half-life. With a loading dose, peak and trough blood levels are stable within 48 hours. Without a loading dosage, 5 to 7 days are required before steady state is reached.
Metabolism: Drug isn't metabolized.
Excretion: Drug is excreted mostly in feces after excretion into the bile. Less than 10% is excreted in urine. Terminal elimination half-life is 68 hours.

CONTRAINDICATIONS & PRECAUTIONS

Contraindicated in patients with hypersensitivity to erythromycin or other macrolides. Use cautiously in patients with impaired hepatic function.

INTERACTIONS

Drug-drug. Use with *ergotamine* or *dihydroergotamine* causes acute ergot toxicity. Don't use together.

Administration with *aluminum-* or *magnesium-containing antacids* may lower peak plasma azithromycin levels. Separate administration times by at least 2 hours.

Use with drugs *metabolized by the hepatic cytochrome P-450 system* (such as *barbiturates, carbamazepine, cyclosporine,* and *phenytoin*) may impair metabolism of these drugs and increase the risk of toxicity. Macrolides may increase plasma *theophylline* levels by decreasing theophylline clearance. Use with *triazolam* may decrease clearance of this drug, increasing the risk of toxicity. Monitor closely.

Use with *warfarin* may increase PT and INR. Monitor PT and INR carefully.
Drug-food. *Food* decreases both maximum plasma levels and amount of drug absorbed. Administer on an empty stomach.
Drug-lifestyle. Exposure to *sunlight* may cause a photosensitivity reaction. Take precautions.

ADVERSE REACTIONS

CNS: dizziness, vertigo, headache, fatigue, somnolence.
CV: palpitations, chest pain.
GI: *nausea, vomiting, diarrhea, abdominal pain,* dyspepsia, flatulence, melena, cholestatic jaundice, pseudomembranous colitis.
GU: candidiasis, vaginitis, nephritis.
Skin: rash, photosensitivity.
Other: *angioedema.*

▣ KEY CONSIDERATIONS

• Obtain culture and sensitivity tests before giving first dose. Therapy can begin before results are obtained.
• Azithromycin may cause overgrowth of nonsusceptible bacteria or fungi. Watch for signs and symptoms of superinfection.
• Serologic tests for syphilis and cultures for gonorrhea should be taken from patients diagnosed with sexually transmitted urethritis or cervicitis. Drug shouldn't be used to treat gonorrhea or syphilis.
• Reconstitute 500-mg vial with 4.8 ml of sterile water for injection. Shake well until drug is dissolved (yields a concentration of 100 mg/ml). Dilute solution further in at least 250 ml of normal or half-normal saline solution, D_5W, or lactated Ringer's solution to yield a concentration range of 1 to 2 mg/ml.
• Infuse 500-mg dose of azithromycin I.V. over 1 or more hours. Don't give as a bolus or I.M. injection.

• In clinical trials of patients with normal hepatic and renal function, using the 5-day dosage regimen, no significant pharmacokinetic differences were seen in patients between ages 65 and 85.

Patient education
• Tell patient to take all of drug prescribed, even if he is feeling better.
• Remind patient that drug should always be taken on an empty stomach because food or antacids decrease absorption. Patient should take drug 1 hour before or 2 hours after a meal and shouldn't take antacids.
• Advise patient of a possible photosensitivity reaction.
• Instruct patient to promptly report adverse reactions.

aztreonam
Azactam

Monobactam, antibiotic

Available by prescription only
Injection: 500-mg, 1-g, and 2-g vials

INDICATIONS & DOSAGE
Urinary tract, respiratory tract, intra-abdominal, gynecologic, or skin infections; septicemia caused by gram-negative bacteria; ◇ ***adjunct therapy in pelvic inflammatory disease;*** ◇ ***gonorrhea***
Adults: 500 mg to 2 g I.V. or I.M. q 8 to 12 hours. For severe systemic or life-threatening infections, 2 g q 6 to 8 hours may be given. Maximum dosage is 8 g daily. For gonorrhea, give 1 g I.M. single dose.
✦ *Dosage adjustment.* In patients with a creatinine clearance of 10 to 30 ml/minute/1.73 m^2, reduce dosage by one half after an initial dosage of 1 to 2 g. In patients with a creatinine clearance below 10 ml/minute/1.73 m^2, an initial dosage of 500 mg to 2 g should be followed by one-fourth the usual dosage at the usual intervals; give one-eighth the initial dosage after each session of hemodialysis.

PHARMACODYNAMICS
Antibiotic action: Aztreonam is a monobactam that inhibits mucopeptide synthesis of the bacterial cell wall. It preferentially binds to penicillin-binding protein 3 of susceptible organisms and often causes cell lysis and cell death.

Aztreonam has a narrow spectrum of activity and is usually bactericidal in action. Aztreonam is effective against *Escherichia coli, Enterobacter, Klebsiella pneumoniae, Proteus mirabilis,* and *Pseudomonas aeruginosa.* It has limited activity against *Citrobacter, Haemophilus influenzae, K. oxytoca, Hafnia, Serratia marcescens, E. aerogenes, Morganella morganii, Providencia, Branhamella catarrhalis, Proteus vulgaris,* and *Neisseria gonorrhoeae.*

PHARMACOKINETICS
Absorption: Aztreonam is absorbed poorly from GI tract after oral administration but is absorbed rapidly and completely after I.M. or I.V. administration; drug level peaks in 60 minutes.
Distribution: Drug is distributed rapidly and widely to all body fluids and tissues, including bile and CSF.
Metabolism: From 6% to 16% is metabolized to inactive metabolites by nonspecific hydrolysis of the beta-lactam ring; 56% to 60% is protein-bound (less if renal impairment is present).
Excretion: Drug is excreted principally in urine as unchanged drug by glomerular filtration and tubular secretion; 1.5% to 3.5% is excreted in feces as unchanged drug. Half-life averages 1.7 hours.

CONTRAINDICATIONS & PRECAUTIONS
Contraindicated in patients with hypersensitivity to aztreonam. Use cautiously in geriatric patients.

INTERACTIONS
Drug-drug. Potent inducers of beta-lactamase production such as *cefoxitin* and *imipenem* may inactivate aztreonam. Don't use together.

Use with *aminoglycosides* or *other beta-lactam antibiotics—including cefoperazone, cefotaxime, clindamycin, metronidazole,* and *piperacillin*—causes synergistic or additive effects. Use with

---

Reactions may be *common,* uncommon, *life-threatening,* or COMMON AND LIFE-THREATENING.

clavulanic acid may cause synergistic or antagonistic effects, depending on organism involved. Monitor closely.

Chloramphenicol is antagonistic. Give the two preparations several hours apart.

Use with *probenecid* may prolong the rate of tubular secretion of aztreonam.

ADVERSE REACTIONS
CNS: *seizures,* headache, insomnia, confusion.
CV: hypotension, thrombophlebitis (at I.V. site).
GI: diarrhea, nausea, vomiting.
Hematologic: *neutropenia,* anemia, *pancytopenia, thrombocytopenia,* leukocytosis, thrombocytosis.
Other: hypersensitivity reactions (rash, *anaphylaxis*), transient elevation of ALT and AST levels; discomfort, swelling (at I.M. injection site).

▣ KEY CONSIDERATIONS
• The half-life of aztreonam may be prolonged in geriatric men because of diminished renal function. Serum creatinine level may not be an accurate determinant of renal status. Estimates of creatinine clearance should be obtained and dosage adjusted accordingly.
• Drug has also been used to treat bone and joint infection caused by susceptible aerobic, gram-negative bacteria.
• To reconstitute for I.M. use, dilute with at least 3 ml of sterile water for injection, bacteriostatic water for injection, normal saline solution, or bacteriostatic normal saline solution for each gram of aztreonam (15-ml vial).
• To reconstitute for I.V. use, add 6 to 10 ml of sterile water for injection to each 15-ml vial; for I.V. infusion, prepare as for I.M. solution. May be further diluted by adding to normal saline, Ringer's, or lactated Ringer's solution; D_5W; $D_{10}W$; or other electrolyte-containing solutions. For I.V. piggyback (100-ml bottles), add at least 50 ml of diluent for each gram of aztreonam. Final concentration shouldn't exceed 20 mg/ml.
• I.V. route is preferred for dosages larger than 1 g and for patients with bacterial septicemia, localized parenchymal abscesses, peritonitis, or other life-threatening infections; administer by direct I.V. push over 3 to 5 minutes or by intermittent infusion over 20 to 60 minutes.
• After adding the diluent, shake vigorously and immediately; drug isn't intended for multiple-dose use.
• Solutions may be colorless or light straw yellow. On standing, they may develop a slightly pink tint; potency isn't affected.
• Admixtures of aztreonam and nafcillin, cephradine, or metronidazole are incompatible; in general, don't mix aztreonam with other drugs. Check with pharmacy for compatibility.
• Reduced dosage may be required in patients with impaired renal function, cirrhosis, or other hepatic impairment.
• Drug may be stored at room temperature for 48 hours or in refrigerator for 7 days.
• Aztreonam therapy alters urinary glucose determinations using cupric sulfate (Clinitest or Benedict's solution).
• Coombs' test may become positive during therapy.

Patient education
• Tell patient to call immediately if rash, redness, or itching develops.

baclofen
Lioresal

Chlorophenyl derivative, skeletal muscle relaxant

Available by prescription only
Tablets: 10 mg, 20 mg
Intrathecal kit: 500 mcg/ml,
2,000 mcg/ml

INDICATIONS & DOSAGE
Spasticity in multiple sclerosis and other spinal cord lesions
Adults: Initially, 5 mg P.O. t.i.d. for 3 days. Dosage may be increased (based on response) at 3-day intervals by 15 mg (5 mg/dose) daily up to maximum of 80 mg daily.
Intrathecal administration
Must be diluted with sterile preservative-free normal saline injection.
Adults: Screening phase: Initial intrathecal bolus of 50 mcg in 1 ml over not less than 1 minute. Observe patient over 4 to 8 hours for response. A positive response consists of a significant decrease in muscle tone or frequency or severity of spasm. If initial response is inadequate, repeat dosing at 75 mcg in 1.5 ml 24 hours after last injection. Repeat observation of patient. If there's still an inadequate response, repeat dosing at 100 mcg in 2 ml 24 hours later. If still no response, patient should not be considered for an implantable pump for continuous baclofen administration. Ranges for long-term therapy are 12 to 2,000 mcg/day.
Postimplant dose titration: If the screening dosage produced the desired effect for over 8 hours, the initial intrathecal dosage is the same as the test dosage; this dosage is infused intrathecally for 24 hours. If the screening dosage produced the desired effect for less than 8 hours, the initial intrathecal dosage is twice the test dosage, followed slowly by 10% to 30% increments at 24-hour intervals.

PHARMACODYNAMICS
Skeletal muscle relaxant action: Baclofen appears to act at the spinal cord level to inhibit transmission of monosynaptic and polysynaptic reflexes, possibly through hyperpolarization of afferent fiber terminals. It may also act at supraspinal sites because this drug at high dosages produces generalized CNS depression. Baclofen decreases the number and severity of spasms and relieves associated pain, clonus, and muscle rigidity and therefore improves mobility.

PHARMACOKINETICS
Absorption: Baclofen is rapidly and extensively absorbed from the GI tract but is subject to individual variation. Plasma levels peak in 2 to 3 hours. Also, as dosage increases, rate and extent of absorption decreases. Onset of therapeutic effect, which varies from hours to weeks, may not be immediately evident.
Distribution: Studies indicate that drug is widely distributed throughout body, with a small amount crossing the blood-brain barrier. About 30% binds to plasma proteins.
Metabolism: About 15% is metabolized in the liver via deamination.
Excretion: 70% to 80% is excreted in urine unchanged or as its metabolites; remainder, in feces.

CONTRAINDICATIONS & PRECAUTIONS
Contraindicated in patients with hypersensitivity to baclofen. Use cautiously in patients with renal impairment or seizure disorders or when spasticity is used to maintain motor function.

INTERACTIONS
Drug-drug. Use with *antipsychotics, anxiolytics, CNS depressants, general anesthetics,* or *narcotics* may add to the CNS effects of baclofen. Use with *MAO inhibitors* or *tricyclic antidepressants* may cause CNS and respiratory depression and hypotension. Monitor closely.
Drug-lifestyle. *Alcohol* may add to the CNS effects of baclofen. Don't use together.

Reactions may be *common,* uncommon, *life-threatening,* or COMMON AND LIFE-THREATENING.

ADVERSE REACTIONS

CNS: *CNS depression (potentially life-threatening with intrathecal administration),* drowsiness, dizziness, *headache, weakness, fatigue, hypotonia, confusion,* insomnia, hallucinations, dysarthria, SEIZURES.

CV: *CV collapse (secondary to CNS depression),* hypotension, hypertension.

EENT: blurred vision, nasal congestion, slurred speech.

GI: *nausea,* constipation, *vomiting.*

GU: urinary frequency.

Hepatic: increased blood glucose, AST, and alkaline phosphatase levels.

Metabolic: hyperglycemia, weight gain.

Respiratory: dyspnea, *respiratory failure (secondary to CNS depression).*

Skin: rash, pruritus.

Other: excessive perspiration.

Abrupt withdrawal after prolonged use: anxiety, agitated behavior, auditory and visual hallucinations, severe tachycardia, and acute spasticity.

🔲 KEY CONSIDERATIONS

• Geriatric patients are especially sensitive to baclofen. Observe carefully for adverse reactions, such as mental confusion, depression, and hallucinations. Lower dosages are usually indicated.

• Intrathecal administration should be performed only by qualified individuals familiar with administration techniques and patient management problems.

• To prevent adverse reactions when withdrawing the drug, slowly decrease the dosage. Abrupt withdrawal can cause hallucinations or seizures and acute exacerbation of spasticity.

• Watch for increased frequency of seizures in patients with epilepsy.

• Watch for increased blood glucose levels in diabetic patients. Baclofen may increase blood glucose levels, so the dosage of patient's antidiabetic or insulin may need to be adjusted.

• Baclofen is used investigationally to reduce choreiform movements in Huntington's chorea; to reduce rigidity in Parkinson's disease; to reduce spasticity in CVA, cerebral lesions, cerebral palsy, and rheumatic disorders; to relieve pain in trigeminal neuralgia; and to treat unstable bladder.

• In some patients, smoother response may be obtained by giving daily dosage in four divided doses.

• Patient may need supervision during walking. The initial loss of spasticity induced by baclofen may affect patient's ability to stand or walk. (In some patients, spasticity helps patient to maintain upright posture and balance.)

• Observe patient's response to drug. Signs of effective therapy may appear in a few hours to 1 week and may include diminished frequency of spasms and severity of foot and ankle clonus, increased ease and range of joint motion, and enhanced performance of daily activities.

• Discontinue drug if signs of improvement aren't evident within 1 to 2 months.

• Closely monitor patients with epilepsy by EEG, clinical observation, and interview for possible loss of seizure control.

• Implantable pump or catheter failure can result in sudden loss of effectiveness of intrathecal baclofen.

• During prolonged intrathecal baclofen therapy for spasticity, about 10% of patients become refractory to baclofen therapy requiring a drug holiday to regain sensitivity to its effects.

• Baclofen increases blood glucose, AST, and alkaline phosphatase levels.

Patient education

• Advise patient to report adverse reactions promptly. Most can be reduced by decreasing dosage. Reportedly, drowsiness, dizziness, and ataxia are more common in patients older than age 40.

• Warn patient that additive effects may occur if baclofen is used concomitantly with other CNS depressants, including alcohol.

• Caution patient to avoid hazardous activities that require mental alertness.

• Tell diabetic patient that baclofen may elevate blood glucose levels and may require adjustment of insulin dosage during treatment with baclofen. Urge patient to promptly report changes in urine or blood glucose tests.

• Caution patient against taking OTC drugs without medical approval. Explain that hazardous drug interactions are possible.

• Inform patient that drug should be withdrawn gradually over 1 to 2 weeks.

Overdose & treatment

• Signs and symptoms of overdose include absence of reflexes, vomiting, muscular hypotonia, marked salivation, drowsiness, visual disorders, seizures, respiratory depression, and coma.

• Treatment requires supportive measures, including endotracheal intubation and positive-pressure ventilation. If patient is conscious, remove drug by inducing vomiting and then performing gastric lavage.

• If patient is comatose, don't induce vomiting. You may perform gastric lavage after endotracheal tube is in place with cuff inflated. Don't use respiratory stimulants. Monitor vital signs closely.

becaplermin
Regranex Gel

Recombinant human platelet-derived growth factor, wound repair drug

Available by prescription only
Gel: 100 mcg/g in tubes of 2 g, 7.5 g, 15 g

INDICATIONS & DOSAGE
Treatment of lower-extremity diabetic neuropathic ulcers that extend into the subcutaneous tissue and beyond and have an adequate blood supply
Adults: Apply daily in ¹⁄₁₆″ even thickness to entire surface of wound. Cover site with a saline-moistened dressing. Remove after 12 hours. Rinse gel from wound with saline or water and cover wound with moist dressing. Continue treatment until complete healing occurs.

Length of gel to be applied varies with tube size and ulcer area.

Tube size	Length of gel (inches)	Length of gel (cm)
2g	Ulcer length × ulcer width × 1.3	(Ulcer length × ulcer width) ÷ 2
7.5, 15g	Ulcer length × ulcer width × 0.6	(ulcer length × ulcer width) ÷ 4

PHARMACODYNAMICS
Wound repair action: Recombinant of human platelet-derived growth factor that promotes the chemotactic recruitment and proliferation of cells involved in wound repair and enhances the formation of new granulation tissue.

PHARMACOKINETICS
Absorption: Only a minimal amount of becaplermin is absorbed systemically, less than 3% in rats.
Distribution: Unknown.
Metabolism: Unknown.
Excretion: Unknown.

CONTRAINDICATIONS & PRECAUTIONS
Contraindicated in patients with known hypersensitivity to any component of becaplermin (such as parabens or m-cresol) or in those with known neoplasms at site of application. Gel is for external use only.

INTERACTIONS
None reported.

ADVERSE REACTIONS
Skin: erythematous rash.

▣ KEY CONSIDERATIONS
• As an adjunct to—and not a substitute for—good ulcer care practices, including initial sharp debridement, pressure relief, and infection control, becaplermin increases the likelihood that a diabetic ulcer will completely heal. Its efficacy in treating diabetic neuropathic ulcers that don't extend through the dermis into subcutaneous tissue or ischemic diabetic ulcers hasn't been evaluated.

• Don't use gel in wounds that close by primary intention.

• To apply, measure the appropriate amount of gel on a clean surface, such as wax paper. Then use a cotton swab, tongue blade, or other application aid to apply it.

Reactions may be *common*, uncommon, **life-threatening**, or COMMON AND LIFE-THREATENING.

• Recalculate amount of gel to be applied weekly. If ulcer doesn't decrease by about one-third after 10 weeks or if ulcer hasn't completely healed within 20 weeks, reassess continued treatment.
• Use gel in addition to good ulcer care program, including a strict non-weight-bearing program.

Patient education

• Instruct patient to wash hands thoroughly before applying gel.
• Advise patient not to touch tip of tube against ulcer or other surfaces.
• Inform patient to use a cotton swab, tongue blade, or other application aid to apply gel evenly over the surface of the ulcer, producing a thin $\frac{1}{16}''$ continuous layer.
• Tell patient to apply drug once daily in a carefully measured quantity. Quantity will change on a weekly basis.
• Tell patient to store gel in the refrigerator, and never to freeze it.
• Inform patient not to use gel after expiration date on the bottom, crimped end of the tube.

beclomethasone dipropionate

beclomethasone dipropionate monohydrate
Nasal inhalants
Beconase, Vancenase

Nasal sprays
Beconase AQ, Vancenase AQ, Vancenase AQ double strength

Oral inhalants
Becloforte*, Beclovent, Vanceril, Vanceril double strength

Glucocorticoid, anti-inflammatory, antasthmatic

Available by prescription only
Nasal inhalant: 42 mcg/metered spray
Nasal spray: 42 mcg/metered spray
Oral inhalant: 42 mcg/metered spray, 84 mcg/metered spray

INDICATIONS & DOSAGE

For nonallergic (vasomotor) rhinitis
Adults: 1 or 2 sprays (42 to 84 mcg) in each nostril b.i.d. Usual total dosage is 168 to 336 mcg daily.

Oral inhalation
Adults: 2 inhalations of regular strength t.i.d. or q.i.d. or 4 inhalations b.i.d. Maximum of 20 inhalations daily. For double strength: 2 inhalations b.i.d., in severe asthma start with 6 to 8 inhalations daily and adjust the dosage down. Don't exceed 10 inhalations/day.

Steroid-dependent asthma
Nasal inhalation
Adults: 1 spray (42 mcg) in each nostril b.i.d. to q.i.d. Usual total dosage is 168 to 336 mcg daily.

Nasal spray
Adults: 1 or 2 sprays (42 to 84 mcg) in each nostril b.i.d. Usual total dosage is 168 to 336 mcg daily.

Perennial or seasonal rhinitis; prevention of recurrence of nasal polyps after surgical removal
Nasal inhalation
Adults: 1 spray (42 mcg) in each nostril b.i.d. to q.i.d. or 2 sprays (84 mcg) in each nostril b.i.d.

Nasal spray
Adults: 1 or 2 sprays (42 to 84 mcg) of single strength in each nostril b.i.d. or 1 or 2 sprays (84 to 168 mcg) of double strength in each nostril once daily.

PHARMACODYNAMICS

Anti-inflammatory action: Beclomethasone stimulates the synthesis of enzymes needed to decrease the inflammatory response. The anti-inflammatory and vaso-constrictor potency of topically applied beclomethasone is, on a weight basis, about 5,000 times greater than that of hydrocortisone, 500 times greater than that of betamethasone or dexamethasone, and about 5 times greater than fluocinolone or triamcinolone.

Antasthmatic action: Beclomethasone is used as a nasal inhalant to treat symptoms of seasonal or perennial rhinitis and to prevent the recurrence of nasal polyps after surgical removal, and as an oral inhalant to treat bronchial asthma in patients who require long-term administration of corticosteroids to control symptoms.

PHARMACOKINETICS

Absorption: After nasal inhalation, beclomethasone is absorbed primarily through the nasal mucosa, with minimal systemic absorption. After oral inhalation, drug is absorbed rapidly from the lungs and GI tract. Greater systemic absorption comes with oral inhalation, but systemic effects don't occur at usual dosages because of rapid metabolism in the liver and local metabolism of drug that reaches the lungs. Onset of action usually occurs in a few days but may take as long as 3 weeks in some patients.
Distribution: Distribution after intranasal administration hasn't been described. There's no evidence of tissue storage of drug or its metabolites. Ten to twenty-five percent of a nasal spray or orally inhaled dose is deposited in the respiratory tract. The remainder, deposited in the mouth and oropharynx, is swallowed. When absorbed, 87% binds to plasma proteins.
Metabolism: Swallowed drug undergoes rapid metabolism in the liver or GI tract to several metabolites, some of which have minor glucocorticoid activity. The portion that's inhaled into the respiratory tract is partially metabolized before absorption into systemic circulation. Drug is mostly metabolized in the liver.
Excretion: Excretion of inhaled drug hasn't been described; however, when drug is administered systemically, its metabolites are excreted mainly in feces via biliary elimination and to a lesser extent in urine. Biological half-life of drug averages 15 hours.

CONTRAINDICATIONS & PRECAUTIONS

Contraindicated in patients hypersensitive to beclomethasone and in those experiencing status asthmaticus or other acute episodes of asthma. Use cautiously in patients with tuberculosis, fungal or bacterial infection, herpes, or systemic viral infection.

INTERACTIONS

None reported.

ADVERSE REACTIONS

CNS: headache.
EENT: *mild transient nasal burning and stinging,* nasal congestion, sneezing, burning, stinging, dryness, epistaxis, nasopharyngeal fungal infections, hoarseness, fungal infection of throat, throat irritation.
GI: dry mouth, fungal infection of mouth.
Respiratory: *bronchospasm,* wheezing.
Skin: hypersensitivity reactions (urticaria, rash).
Other: *angioedema, suppression of hypothalamic-pituitary-adrenal function, adrenal insufficiency,* facial edema.

▣ KEY CONSIDERATIONS

• Adrenal insufficiency may accompany the replacement of systemic corticosteroid with this drug.
• Patient also receiving immunosuppressants is more prone to infection.
• Patient should be carefully instructed on the proper use of the oral or nasal inhaler or spray pump. Give patient a copy of administration instructions provided by the manufacturer.

Patient education

• Tell patient to take drug at regular intervals because its effectiveness depends on regular use.
• Tell patient to take only as directed and not to take more than prescribed.
• Inform patient 1 to 2 weeks may pass before full relief is noticeable.
• Advise patient to contact health care provider if symptoms don't improve or if they worsen.

benazepril hydrochloride
Lotensin

ACE inhibitor, antihypertensive

Available by prescription only
Tablets: 5 mg, 10 mg, 20 mg, 40 mg

INDICATIONS & DOSAGE

Hypertension

Adults: Initially, 10 mg P.O. daily. Adjust dosage as needed and tolerated; mainte-

nance dosage ranges from 20 to 40 mg daily in one or two equally divided doses.
✦ *Dosage adjustment.* In patients with renal failure and creatinine clearance below 30 ml/minute/1.73 m² or serum creatinine level above 3 mg/dl, initial dosage is 5 mg P.O. daily. Don't exceed 40 mg daily.

Note: Although rare, angioedema has been reported in patients receiving ACE inhibitors. Angioedema associated with laryngeal edema or shock may be fatal. If angioedema of the face, extremities, lips, tongue, glottis, or larynx occurs, treatment with benazepril should be discontinued and appropriate therapy instituted immediately.

PHARMACODYNAMICS
Antihypertensive action: Benazepril and its active metabolite, benazeprilat, inhibit ACE, preventing conversion of angiotensin I to angiotensin II, a potent vasoconstrictor. Reduced formation of angiotensin II decreases peripheral arterial resistance and aldosterone secretion, which reduces sodium and water retention and lowers blood pressure.

Although the primary mechanism through which benazepril lowers blood pressure is believed to be suppression of the renin-angiotensin-aldosterone system, benazepril has an antihypertensive effect even in patients with low renin levels.

PHARMACOKINETICS
Absorption: At least 37% of benazepril is absorbed. After oral administration, plasma levels peak within ½ to 1 hour.
Distribution: About 96.7% of drug and 95.3% of benazeprilat binds to serum proteins.
Metabolism: Benazepril is almost completely metabolized in the liver to benazeprilat, which has much greater ACE inhibitory activity than benazepril, and to the glucuronide conjugates of benazepril and benazeprilat.
Excretion: Drug is excreted primarily in urine.

CONTRAINDICATIONS & PRECAUTIONS
Contraindicated in patients with hypersensitivity to ACE inhibitors. Use cautiously in patients with renal or hepatic impairment.

INTERACTIONS
Drug-drug. Use with *lithium* increases serum lithium levels and lithium toxicity. Use with *potassium sparing diuretics* or *potassium supplements* increases the risk of hyperkalemia. Don't use together.

Use with *diuretics* or *other antihypertensives* increases risk of excessive hypotension. The diuretic may need to be discontinued or benazepril dosage lowered.

Use with *allopurinol* may increase risk of hypersensitivity reaction. Use with *digoxin* may increase plasma digoxin levels. Monitor closely.
Drug-food. Use with *sodium substitutes containing potassium* increases the risk of hyperkalemia. Don't use together.

ADVERSE REACTIONS
CNS: headache, dizziness, anxiety, fatigue, insomnia, nervousness, paresthesia.
CV: symptomatic hypotension, palpitations, ECG changes.
EENT: dysphagia, increased salivation.
GI: nausea, vomiting, abdominal pain, constipation.
GU: proteinuria, impotence.
Hematologic: leukopenia, eosinophilia.
Metabolic: hyperkalemia, hyponatremia.
Musculoskeletal: arthralgia, arthritis, myalgia.
Respiratory: dry, persistent, tickling, nonproductive cough; dyspnea.
Skin: hypersensitivity reactions (rash, pruritus), increased diaphoresis.
Other: *angioedema.*

▣ KEY CONSIDERATIONS
● Although no overall difference in effectiveness or safety with use in geriatric patients compared with younger adults is apparent, some geriatric patients are more sensitive to the drug.
● To verify adequate blood pressure control, blood pressure should be measured when drug levels are at peak (2 to 6 hours after a dose) and at trough (just before a dose).

• Excessive hypotension can occur when drug is given with diuretics. To decrease the risk, diuretic therapy should be discontinued 2 to 3 days before starting benazepril if possible. If benazepril doesn't adequately control blood pressure, diuretic therapy may be reinstituted with care. If the diuretic can't be discontinued, initiate benazepril therapy at 5 mg P.O. daily.
• Assess renal and hepatic function before and periodically throughout therapy. Monitor serum potassium levels.
• ACE inhibitors may cause agranulocytosis, bone marrow depression, and neutropenia. Monitor CBC with differential counts before therapy, every 2 weeks for first 3 months of therapy, and periodically thereafter.

Patient education
• Advise patient to report signs and symptoms of infection (such as fever and sore throat); easy bruising or bleeding; swelling of tongue, lips, face, eyes, mucous membranes, or extremities; difficulty swallowing or breathing; and hoarseness.
• Because light-headedness can occur, especially during the first few days of therapy, tell patient to rise slowly to minimize this effect and to report symptoms. Patients who experience syncope should stop taking drug and call immediately.
• Inadequate fluid intake, vomiting, diarrhea, and excessive perspiration can lead to light-headedness and syncope. Tell patient to use caution in hot weather and during exercise.
• Tell patient to avoid sodium substitutes; these products may contain potassium, which can cause hyperkalemia in patients taking the drug.
• A persistent dry cough may occur and usually doesn't subside unless drug is stopped. Advise patient to call if this effect becomes bothersome.

Overdose & treatment
• Hypotension is the most common sign of overdose.
• Drug is only slightly dialyzable, but dialysis might be considered in patients with severely impaired renal function. Angiotensin II could presumably serve as a specific antagonist-antidote, but angiotensin II is essentially unavailable outside of scattered research facilities. Because the hypotensive effect of the drug is achieved through vasodilation and effective hypovolemia, treatment of benazepril overdose by I.V. infusion of normal saline solution is reasonable.

---

benzonatate
Tessalon Perles

Local anesthetic (ester), nonnarcotic antitussive

Available by prescription only
Capsules: 100 mg

INDICATIONS & DOSAGE
Cough suppression
Adults: 100 mg P.O. t.i.d.; up to 600 mg daily.

PHARMACODYNAMICS
Antitussive action: Benzonatate suppresses the cough reflex at its source by anesthetizing peripheral stretch receptors located in the respiratory passages, lungs, and pleura.

PHARMACOKINETICS
Absorption: Action begins within 15 to 20 minutes and lasts for 3 to 8 hours.
Distribution: Unknown.
Metabolism: Unknown.
Excretion: Unknown.

CONTRAINDICATIONS & PRECAUTIONS
Contraindicated in patients hypersensitive to benzonatate or PABA anesthetics (such as procaine and tetracaine).

INTERACTIONS
None significant.

ADVERSE REACTIONS
CNS: dizziness, headache, sedation.
EENT: nasal congestion, burning sensation in eyes.
GI: nausea, constipation, GI upset.
Skin: hypersensitivity reactions (rash).
Other: chills.

Reactions may be *common*, uncommon, *life-threatening*, or COMMON AND LIFE-THREATENING.

◙ KEY CONSIDERATIONS
• Monitor type and frequency of cough and volume and quality of sputum. Encourage fluid intake to help liquefy sputum.

Patient education
• Instruct patient not to chew or dissolve capsules in the mouth because local anesthesia will result.
• Teach patient comfort measures for a nonproductive cough: limit talking and smoking; use a cold mist or steam vaporizer; use sugarless hard candy to increase saliva flow.

Overdose & treatment
• CNS stimulation from overdose of drug may cause restlessness and tremors, which may lead to chronic seizures followed by profound CNS depression.
• Empty stomach by gastric lavage and follow with activated charcoal. Treat seizures with a short-acting barbiturate given I.V.; don't use CNS stimulants. Mechanical respiratory support may be necessary in severe cases.

benztropine mesylate
Cogentin

Anticholinergic, antiparkinsonian

Available by prescription only
Tablets: 0.5 mg, 1 mg, 2 mg
Injection: 1 mg/ml in 2-ml ampule

INDICATIONS & DOSAGE
Acute dystonic reaction
Adults: 1 to 2 mg I.M. or I.V. followed by 1 to 2 mg P.O. b.i.d. to prevent recurrence.
Parkinsonism
Adults: 0.5 to 6 mg P.O. daily. Initially, 0.5 to 1 mg, increased 0.5 mg q 5 to 6 days. Adjust dosage to meet individual requirements. Maximum dosage, 6 mg/day.
Drug-induced extrapyramidal reactions
Adults: 1 to 4 mg P.O. or I.V. daily or b.i.d. Adjust dosage to meet individual requirements. Maximum dosage, 6 mg/day.

PHARMACODYNAMICS
Antiparkinsonian action: Benztropine blocks central cholinergic receptors, helping to balance cholinergic activity in the basal ganglia. It may also prolong effects of dopamine by blocking dopamine reuptake and storage at central receptor sites.

PHARMACOKINETICS
Absorption: Benztropine is absorbed from the GI tract.
Distribution: Unknown; however, drug crosses the blood-brain barrier.
Metabolism: Unknown.
Excretion: Like other muscarinics, drug is excreted in the urine as unchanged drug and metabolites. After oral therapy, a small amount is probably excreted in feces as unabsorbed drug.

CONTRAINDICATIONS & PRECAUTIONS
Contraindicated in patients with hypersensitivity to benztropine or its components or acute angle-closure glaucoma. Use cautiously in hot weather and in patients with mental disorders.

INTERACTIONS
Drug-drug. Use with *amantadine* may amplify such adverse anticholinergic effects as confusion and hallucinations, so benztropine dosage should be decreased before giving amantadine.

Use with *antacids* or *antidiarrheals* may decrease benztropine absorption. Administer benztropine at least 1 hour before administering these drugs.

Use with *CNS depressants* increases the sedative effects of benztropine. Use with *haloperidol* or *phenothiazines* may decrease the effect of these drugs, possibly reflecting direct CNS antagonism; concomitant use with phenothiazines increases the risk of adverse anticholinergic effects. Monitor closely.
Drug-lifestyle. *Alcohol* increases the sedative effects of benztropine. Discourage use.

ADVERSE REACTIONS
CNS: disorientation, hallucinations, depression, toxic psychosis, confusion, memory impairment, nervousness.
CV: tachycardia.

EENT: dilated pupils, blurred vision.
GI: dry mouth, *constipation,* nausea, vomiting, paralytic ileus.
GU: urine retention, dysuria.

Some adverse reactions may result from atropine-like toxicity and are dose related.

▣ KEY CONSIDERATIONS

Besides the recommendations relevant to all anticholinergics, consider the following:
• To help prevent gastric irritation, administer drug after meals.
• Never discontinue drug abruptly.
• Monitor patient for intermittent constipation and abdominal distention and pain, which may indicate paralytic ileus.

Patient education

• Explain that drug's full effect may not occur for 2 to 3 days after therapy begins.
• Caution patient not to discontinue drug suddenly; dosage should be reduced gradually.
• Advise patient to avoid alcohol while taking this drug.
• Tell patient that drug may increase sensitivity of eyes to light.
• Advise patient to avoid activities that require mental alertness until the CNS effects of the drug are known.

Overdose & treatment

• Signs and symptoms of overdose include central stimulation followed by depression and psychotic symptoms such as disorientation, confusion, hallucinations, delusions, anxiety, agitation, and restlessness. Peripheral effects may include dilated, nonreactive pupils; blurred vision; hot, flushed, dry skin; dryness of mucous membranes; dysphagia; decreased or absent bowel sounds; urine retention; hyperthermia; tachycardia; hypertension; and increased respiration.
• Treatment is primarily symptomatic and supportive, as necessary. Maintain a patent airway. If patient is alert, induce vomiting or perform gastric lavage and follow with a sodium chloride cathartic and activated charcoal to prevent further absorption. In severe cases, physostigmine may be administered to block the antimuscarinic effects of benztropine. Give fluids as needed to treat shock, diazepam to control psychotic symptoms, and pilocarpine (instilled into the eyes) to relieve mydriasis. If urine retention occurs, catheterization may be necessary.

bepridil hydrochloride
Vascor

Calcium channel blocker, antianginal

Available by prescription only
Tablets: 200 mg, 300 mg, 400 mg

INDICATIONS & DOSAGE

Treatment of chronic stable angina (classic effort-associated angina) in patients who are unresponsive or inadequately responsive to other antianginals
Adults: Initially, 200 mg P.O. daily; after 10 days, adjust dosage based on patient tolerance and response. Most common maintenance dosage is 300 mg daily. Maximum daily dosage is 400 mg.

PHARMACODYNAMICS

Antianginal action: Precise mechanism of action is unknown. Bepridil inhibits calcium ion influx into cardiac and vascular smooth muscle and also inhibits the sodium inward influx, resulting in reductions in the maximal upstroke velocity and amplitude of the action potential. It's believed to reduce heart rate and arterial pressure by dilating peripheral arterioles and reducing total peripheral resistance (afterload). The effects are dose-dependent. Bepridil has dose-related class I antiarrhythmic properties affecting electrophysiologic changes, such as prolongation of QT and QTc intervals.

PHARMACOKINETICS

Absorption: Bepridil is rapidly and completely absorbed after oral administration; levels peak in 2 to 3 hours.
Distribution: More than 99% of drug binds to plasma proteins.
Metabolism: Drug is metabolized in the liver.

Excretion: Elimination is biphasic. Drug has a distribution half-life of 2 hours. Over 10 days, 70% is excreted in urine and 22% is excreted in feces as metabolites. Terminal half-life after multiple dosing averages 42 hours (range, 26 to 64 hours).

CONTRAINDICATIONS & PRECAUTIONS

Contraindicated in patients with hypersensitivity to bepridil, uncompensated cardiac insufficiency, sick sinus syndrome or second- or third-degree AV block unless pacemaker is present; hypotension (below 90 mm Hg systolic); congenital QT interval prolongation; or history of serious ventricular arrhythmias. Also contraindicated in those receiving other drugs that prolong QT interval.

Use cautiously in patients with left bundle-branch block, sinus bradycardia, impaired renal or hepatic function, or heart failure. Drug isn't recommended for use in patients within 3 months of an MI.

INTERACTIONS

Drug-drug. *Potassium wasting diuretics* can cause hypokalemia, which increases the risk of serious ventricular arrhythmias. Use with *procainamide, quinidine,* or *tricyclic antidepressants* causes additive prolongation of the QT interval.

ADVERSE REACTIONS

CNS: *dizziness,* drowsiness, *nervousness,* headache, insomnia, paresthesia, asthenia, tremor.
CV: edema, flushing, palpitations, tachycardia, *ventricular arrhythmias, including torsades de pointes, ventricular tachycardia, ventricular fibrillation.*
EENT: tinnitus.
GI: *nausea, diarrhea,* constipation, abdominal discomfort, dry mouth, anorexia.
Hematologic: *agranulocytosis.*
Respiratory: dyspnea, shortness of breath.
Skin: rash.
Other: flulike syndrome.

⊡ KEY CONSIDERATIONS

• Once the therapeutic response has been achieved, geriatric patients may require frequent monitoring.
• Careful patient selection and monitoring are essential. Use the following selection criteria: Diagnosis of chronic stable angina with failure to respond or inadequate response to other therapies, QTc interval less than 0.44 second, absence of hypokalemia, hypotension, severe left ventricular dysfunction, serious ventricular arrhythmias, unpacked sick sinus syndrome, second- or third-degree AV block, and no concomitant use of other drugs that prolong the QT interval.
• Monitor serum potassium levels and correct hypokalemia before initiating therapy. Use potassium sparing diuretics for patients who require diuretic therapy.
• Monitor QTc interval before and during therapy. Reduced dosage is required if QTc prolongation is greater than 0.52 second or increases more than 25%. If prolongation of QTc interval persists, discontinue bepridil.
• Beta blockers, nitrates, digoxin, insulin, and oral antidiabetics may be used with bepridil.
• Food doesn't interfere with absorption of bepridil.
• Use cautiously in patients with renal or hepatic disorders. No clinical data are available.
• If infection is suspected, obtain WBC count.
• Increased ALT levels and abnormal liver function test results have been observed.

Patient education

• Instruct patient to recognize signs and symptoms of hypokalemia and the importance of compliance with prescribed potassium supplements.
• Tell patient to report signs or symptoms of infection, such as sore throat and fever.
• Instruct patient to take drug with food or at bedtime if nausea occurs.

Overdose & treatment

• Exaggerated adverse reactions, especially hypotension, high-degree AV

---

*Canada only   ◇ Unlabeled clinical use

block, and ventricular tachycardia, have been observed.

• Treat with appropriate supportive measures, including gastric lavage, beta-adrenergic stimulation, parenteral calcium solutions, vasopressors, and cardioversion, as necessary. Close observation in a cardiac care facility for a minimum of 48 hours is recommended.

betamethasone (systemic)
Betnelan*, Celestone

betamethasone sodium phosphate
Betnesol*, Celestone Phosphate, Selestoject

betamethasone sodium phosphate and betamethasone acetate
Celestone Soluspan

Glucocorticoid, anti-inflammatory

Available by prescription only
betamethasone
Tablets: 0.6 mg
Syrup: 0.6 mg/5 ml
betamethasone sodium phosphate
Tablets (effervescent): 500 mcg*
Injection: 4 mg (3-mg base)/ml in 5-ml vials
Enema:* 5 mg (base)
betamethasone sodium phosphate and betamethasone acetate suspension
Injection: betamethasone acetate 3 mg and betamethasone sodium phosphate (equivalent to 3-mg base) per ml (not for I.V. use)

INDICATIONS & DOSAGE
betamethasone
Severe inflammation or immunosuppression
Adults: 0.6 to 7.2 mg P.O. daily.
betamethasone sodium phosphate
Adults: 0.5 to 9 mg I.M., I.V., or into joint or soft tissue daily.
betamethasone sodium phosphate and betamethasone acetate suspension
Adults: 0.5 to 2 ml into joint or soft tissue q 1 to 2 weeks, p.r.n.

(*Note:* Betamethasone acetate suspension shouldn't be given I.V.)
Adrenocortical insufficiency
Adults: 0.6 to 7.2 mg P.O. daily, or up to 9 mg I.M. or I.V. daily.

PHARMACODYNAMICS
Anti-inflammatory action: Betamethasone stimulates the synthesis of enzymes needed to decrease the inflammatory response. It's a long-acting steroid with an anti-inflammatory potency 25 times that of an equal weight of hydrocortisone. It has essentially no mineralocorticoid activity. Betamethasone tablets and syrup are used as oral anti-inflammatories.

Betamethasone sodium phosphate is highly soluble, has a prompt onset of action, and may be given I.V. Betamethasone sodium phosphate and betamethasone acetate (Celestone Soluspan) combine the rapid-acting phosphate salt and the slightly soluble, slowly released acetate salt to provide rapid anti-inflammatory effects with a sustained duration of action. It's a suspension and shouldn't be given I.V. It's particularly useful as an anti-inflammatory in intra-articular, intradermal, and intralesional injections.

PHARMACOKINETICS
Absorption: Betamethasone is absorbed readily after oral administration. After oral and I.V. administration, effects peak in 1 to 2 hours. Onset and duration of action of the suspensions for injection vary, depending on their injection site (an intra-articular space or a muscle) and on the local blood supply. Systemic absorption occurs slowly following intra-articular injections.
Distribution: Drug is removed rapidly from the blood and distributed to muscle, liver, skin, intestines, and kidneys. It binds weakly to plasma proteins (transcortin and albumin). Only the unbound portion is active.
Metabolism: Metabolized in the liver to inactive glucuronide and sulfate metabolites.
Excretion: Inactive metabolites and a small amount of unmetabolized drug are excreted in urine. Insignificant quantities of drug are also excreted in feces.

Reactions may be *common*, uncommon, *life-threatening*, or COMMON AND LIFE-THREATENING.

Biological half-life of drug is 36 to 54 hours.

CONTRAINDICATIONS & PRECAUTIONS

Contraindicated in patients hypersensitive to betamethasone and in those with viral or bacterial infections (except in life-threatening situations) or systemic fungal infections.

Use with caution in patients with renal disease, hypertension, osteoporosis, diabetes mellitus, hypothyroidism, cirrhosis, diverticulitis, nonspecific ulcerative colitis, recent intestinal anastomoses, thromboembolic disorders, seizures, myasthenia gravis, heart failure, tuberculosis, ocular herpes simplex, emotional instability, and psychotic tendencies.

INTERACTIONS

Drug-drug. Use with *antacids, cholestyramine,* or *colestipol* decreases the effect of betamethasone by adsorbing the corticosteroid, decreasing the amount absorbed. Don't give together.

Betamethasone may enhance hypokalemia associated with *diuretics* and *amphotericin B.* The hypokalemia may increase the risk of toxicity in patients also receiving cardiac glycosides. Use with *barbiturates, phenytoin,* or *rifampin* may cause decreased corticosteroid effects because of increased hepatic metabolism. Use with *estrogens* may reduce the metabolism of corticosteroids by increasing transcortin levels. Use with *isoniazid* or *salicylates* increases drug metabolism. Administration with *ulcerogenics such as NSAIDs* may increase the risk of GI ulceration. Use with *oral anticoagulants* may decrease the effects of oral anticoagulants (rarely). Monitor closely.

ADVERSE REACTIONS

Most adverse reactions to corticosteroids are dose- or duration-dependent.
CNS: *euphoria, insomnia,* psychotic behavior, pseudotumor cerebri, vertigo, headache, paresthesia, *seizures.*
CV: *heart failure,* hypertension, edema, *arrhythmias,* thrombophlebitis, *thromboembolism.*
EENT: cataracts, glaucoma.

GI: *peptic ulceration,* GI irritation, increased appetite, pancreatitis, nausea, vomiting.
Metabolic: hypokalemia, hyperglycemia, and carbohydrate intolerance.
Musculoskeletal: muscle weakness, osteoporosis.
Skin: hirsutism, delayed wound healing, acne, various skin eruptions.
Other: susceptibility to infections, cushingoid state (moonface, buffalo hump, central obesity).
After abrupt withdrawal: rebound inflammation, fatigue, weakness, arthralgia, fever, dizziness, lethargy, depression, fainting, orthostatic hypotension, dyspnea, anorexia, hypoglycemia. *After prolonged use, sudden withdrawal may be fatal.*

▣ KEY CONSIDERATIONS

• Recommendations for use of betamethasone and for care and teaching of patients during therapy are the same as those for all systemic adrenocorticoids.
• Adrenocorticoid therapy suppresses reactions to skin tests; causes false-negative results in the nitroblue tetrazolium tests for systemic bacterial infections; and decreases ^{131}I uptake and protein-bound iodine levels in thyroid function tests.
• It may increase glucose and cholesterol levels; decrease serum potassium, calcium, thyroxine, and triiodothyronine levels; and increase urine glucose and calcium levels.

Patient education

• Tell patient not to stop drug abruptly or without health care provider's consent.
• Tell patient to take drug with food or milk; patients taking effervescent tablets should dissolve them in water immediately before ingestion.
• Instruct patient to report symptoms associated with corticosteroid withdrawal, including fatigue, weakness, arthralgia, dizziness, and dyspnea.

Overdose & treatment

• Acute ingestion, even in massive doses, rarely occurs. Signs and symptoms of toxic reaction rarely occur if drug is used for less than 3 weeks, even at large dosages. However, long-term use causes adverse physiological effects, including suppression of the hypothalamic-pituitary-adrenal axis, cushingoid appearance, muscle weakness, and osteoporosis.

betamethasone dipropionate
Alphatrex, Diprosone, Maxivate

betamethasone dipropionate, augmented
Diprolene, Diprolene AF

betamethasone valerate
Betacort* Betaderm*, Betatrex, Beta-Val, Betnovate*, Celestoderm-V*, Ectosone*, Metaderm*, Novobetamet*, Valisone
Topical glucocorticoid, anti-inflammatory

Available by prescription only
betamethasone dipropionate
Lotion, ointment, cream: 0.05%
Aerosol: 0.1%
betamethasone dipropionate, augmented
Cream, gel, lotion, ointment: 0.05%
betamethasone valerate
Lotion, ointment: 0.1%
Cream: 0.01%, 0.1%

INDICATIONS & DOSAGE
Inflammation of corticosteroid-responsive dermatoses
betamethasone dipropionate
Adults: Apply cream, lotion, or ointment sparingly daily or b.i.d. Dosage of augmented lotions and gels shouldn't exceed 50 g or 50 ml/week for a total of 14 days; augmented ointments and creams shouldn't exceed 45 g/week. To apply aerosol, direct spray onto affected area from a distance of 6" (15 cm) for only 3 seconds t.i.d. or q.i.d.
betamethasone valerate
Adults: Apply cream, lotion, ointment, or gel in a thin layer once daily to q.i.d.

PHARMACODYNAMICS
Anti-inflammatory action: Betamethasone stimulates the synthesis of enzymes needed to decrease the inflammatory response. Betamethasone, a fluorinated derivative, is available in various bases, so the potency can be adjusted to the condition.

PHARMACOKINETICS
Absorption: Amount absorbed depends on the potency of the preparation, amount applied, and nature of the skin at the application site. It ranges from about 1% in areas with a thick stratum corneum to as high as 36% in areas with a thin stratum corneum. Absorption increases in areas of skin damage, inflammation, or occlusion. Some of the drug may be absorbed systemically.
Distribution: After topical application, drug is distributed throughout the local skin. Drug absorbed into circulation is removed rapidly from the blood and distributed into muscle, liver, skin, intestines, and kidneys.
Metabolism: After topical administration, drug is metabolized primarily in the skin. The small amount that is absorbed into systemic circulation is metabolized primarily in the liver to inactive compounds.
Excretion: Inactive metabolites are excreted by the kidneys, primarily as glucuronides and sulfates but also as unconjugated products. A small amount of the metabolites is also excreted in feces.

CONTRAINDICATIONS & PRECAUTIONS
Contraindicated in patients hypersensitive to corticosteroids.

INTERACTIONS
None significant.

ADVERSE REACTIONS
GU: glycosuria (with betamethasone dipropionate).
Metabolic: hyperglycemia.
Skin: burning, pruritus, irritation, dryness, erythema, folliculitis, acneiform eruptions, perioral dermatitis, hypopigmentation, hypertrichosis, allergic contact dermatitis; *secondary infection,*

Reactions may be *common*, uncommon, *life-threatening*, or COMMON AND LIFE-THREATENING.

maceration, atrophy, striae, miliaria
(with occlusive dressings).
Other: *hypothalamic-pituitary-adrenal
axis suppression,* Cushing's syndrome.

▣ KEY CONSIDERATIONS
Besides the recommendations relevant to
all topical adrenocorticoids, consider the
following:
• Diprolene ointment may suppress the
hypothalamic-pituitary-adrenal axis at
dosages as low as 7 g daily. Patient
shouldn't use more than 45 g weekly and
shouldn't use occlusive dressings.

Patient education
• Advise patient to use only as directed
and not any longer than prescribed time
period.
• Tell patient this drug is for external use
only and to avoid contact with eyes.
• Tell patient to use drug only for the
disorder for which it was prescribed.
• Instruct patient not to cover affected
area with an occlusive dressing.

betaxolol hydrochloride
Betoptic, Betoptic S, Kerlone

*Beta blocker, antiglaucoma drug,
antihypertensive*

Available by prescription only
Tablets: 10 mg, 20 mg
Ophthalmic solution: 5 mg/ml (0.5%) in
2.5-ml, 5-ml, 10-ml, and 15-ml dropper
bottles
Ophthalmic suspension: 2.5 mg/ml
(0.25%) in 2.5-ml, 5-ml, 10-ml, and 15-
ml dropper bottles

INDICATIONS & DOSAGE
*Chronic open-angle glaucoma and oc-
ular hypertension*
Adults: Instill 1 or 2 gtt in eyes b.i.d.
*Management of hypertension (used
alone or with other antihypertensives)*
Adults: Initially, 10 mg P.O. once daily.
After 7 to 14 days, full antihypertensive
effect should be seen. If necessary, dou-
ble dosage to 20 mg P.O. once daily.
(Dosages up to 40 mg daily have been
used.)

Geriatric patients: Initially, 5 mg P.O.
daily. Increase by 5-mg/day increments q
2 weeks to maximum of 20 mg/day.
✦ *Dosage adjustment.* In patients with
renal impairment, initial dosage is 5 mg
P.O. daily. Increase by 5-mg/day increments q 2 weeks to maximum of
20 mg/day.

PHARMACODYNAMICS
Ocular hypotensive action: Betaxolol is
a cardioselective beta$_1$ blocker that reduces intraocular pressure (IOP), possibly by reducing production of aqueous
humor when administered as an ophthalmic solution.
Antihypertensive action: Cardioselective
adrenergic blocking effects of betaxolol
slow heart rate and decrease cardiac output.

PHARMACOKINETICS
Absorption: Betaxolol is absorbed almost completely after oral administration and minimally after ophthalmic use.
A small first-pass effect reduces
bioavailability by about 10%. Neither
food nor alcohol affects absorption.
Distribution: Plasma levels peak in
about 3 hours (range, 1.5 to 6) after a
single oral dose. About 50% of drug
binds to plasma proteins.
Metabolism: Drug is metabolized in the
liver; about 85% of drug is recovered in
the urine as metabolites. Elimination
half-life is prolonged in patients with hepatic disease, but clearance isn't affected, so dosage adjustment is unnecessary.
Excretion: About 80% of drug is from
the kidneys. Plasma half-life is 14 to 22
hours.

CONTRAINDICATIONS & PRECAUTIONS
Contraindicated in patients with hypersensitivity to betaxolol, severe bradycardia, greater than first-degree heart block,
cardiogenic shock, or uncontrolled heart
failure.

INTERACTIONS
Drug-drug. Use with *calcium channel
blockers* increases the risk of hypotension, left-sided heart failure, and AV
conduction disturbances. I.V. calcium
antagonists should be used with caution.

Use with *general anesthetics* may increase hypotensive effects. Observe carefully for excessive hypotension, bradycardia, or orthostatic hypotension.

Use of ophthalmic betaxolol and *oral beta blockers* may increase the systemic effect of the beta blockers. Use with *reserpine* or *catecholamine-depleting drugs* enhances the hypotensive and bradycardiac effect of these drugs. Monitor closely.

Use with *pilocarpine, epinephrine,* or *carbonic anhydrase inhibitors* enhances the lowering of IOP.

ADVERSE REACTIONS
Ophthalmic form
CNS: insomnia, depressive neurosis.
EENT: *eye stinging on instillation causing brief discomfort,* photophobia, erythema, itching, keratitis, pharyngitis, occasional tearing.
Systemic form
CNS: dizziness, fatigue, headache, insomnia, lethargy, anxiety.
CV: bradycardia, chest pain, *heart failure,* edema.
GI: nausea, diarrhea, dyspepsia.
GU: impotence.
Musculoskeletal: arthralgia.
Respiratory: dyspnea, *bronchospasm.*
Skin: rash.

◉ KEY CONSIDERATIONS
• Geriatric patients are especially prone to beta blocker–induced bradycardia, which may be dose related and respond to dosage reduction.
Ophthalmic use
• Betaxolol is a cardioselective beta blocker. Its pulmonary and systemic effects are considerably milder than those of timolol or levobunolol.
• Ophthalmic betaxolol is intended for twice-daily dosing. Encourage patient to comply with this regimen.
• In some patients, a few weeks' treatment may be required to stabilize pressure-lowering response. Determine IOP during the first 4 weeks of drug therapy.
Systemic use
• Withdrawal of beta blocker therapy before surgery is controversial. Some health care providers advocate withdrawal to prevent any impairment of cardiac responsiveness to reflex stimuli and to prevent any decreased responsiveness to exogenous catecholamines.
• To withdraw drug, dosage should be gradually reduced over at least 2 weeks.
• Although oral beta blockers have been reported to decrease serum glucose levels from blockage of normal glycogen release after hypoglycemia, no such effect has been reported with the use of ophthalmic beta blockers.
• Oral beta blockers may alter the results of glucose tolerance tests.

Patient education
Ophthalmic use
• Instruct patient to tilt head back and, while looking up, drop the drug into the lower lid.
• Warn patient not to touch dropper to eye or surrounding tissue.
• Instruct patient not to close eyes tightly or blink more than usual after instillation.
• Remind patient to wait at least 5 minutes before using other eyedrops.
• Advise patient to wear sunglasses or avoid exposure to bright lights.
• Tell patient to shake suspension well before use.
Systemic use
• Advise patient to take drug exactly as prescribed and warn against discontinuing it suddenly.
• Advise patient to report shortness of breath or difficulty breathing, unusually fast heartbeat, cough, or fatigue with exertion.

Overdose & treatment
• Signs and symptoms of overdose, which are extremely rare with ophthalmic use, may include diplopia, bradycardia, heart block, hypotension, shock, increased airway resistance, cyanosis, fatigue, sleepiness, headache, sedation, coma, respiratory depression, seizures, nausea, vomiting, diarrhea, hypoglycemia, hallucinations, and nightmares.
• Discontinue drug and flush eye with normal saline solution or water. For treatment of accidental substantial ingestion, emesis is most effective if initiated

---

Reactions may be *common,* uncommon, *life-threatening,* or COMMON AND LIFE-THREATENING.

within 30 minutes, providing the patient is not obtunded, comatose, or having seizures. Activated charcoal may be used. Treat bradycardia, conduction defects, and hypotension with I.V. fluids, glucagon, atropine, or isoproterenol; refractory bradycardia may require a transvenous pacemaker. Treat bronchoconstriction with I.V. aminophylline; seizures, with I.V. diazepam.

---

bethanechol chloride
Duvoid, Myotonachol, Urecholine

Cholinergic agonist, urinary tract and GI tract stimulant

Available by prescription only
Tablets: 5 mg, 10 mg, 25 mg, 50 mg
Injection: 5 mg/ml

INDICATIONS & DOSAGE
Acute postoperative urine retention, neurogenic atony of urinary bladder with retention
Adults: 10 to 50 mg P.O. t.i.d., or q.i.d. Or 2.5 to 5 mg S.C. (Use 10 mg S.C. with extreme caution.) Never give I.M. or I.V. When used for urine retention, some patients may require 50 to 100 mg P.O. per dose. Use such doses with extreme caution. Test dosage: 2.5 mg S.C. repeated at 15- to 30-minute intervals to total of four doses to determine the minimal effective dose; then use minimal effective dose q 6 to 8 hours. Adjust dosage to meet individual requirements.
◊ *Bladder dysfunction caused by phenothiazines*
Adults: 50 to 100 mg P.O. q.i.d.
◊ *To lessen the adverse effects of tricyclic antidepressants*
Adults: 25 mg P.O. t.i.d.
◊ *Chronic gastric reflux*
Adults: 25 mg P.O. q.i.d.
◊ *To diagnose flaccid or atonic neurogenic bladder*
Adults: 2.5 mg S.C.

PHARMACODYNAMICS
Urinary tract stimulant action: Bethanechol directly binds to and stimulates muscarinic receptors of the parasympathetic nervous system. That increases tone of the bladder detrusor muscle, usually resulting in contraction, decreased bladder capacity, and subsequent urination.
GI tract stimulant action: Bethanechol directly stimulates cholinergic receptors, leading to increased gastric tone and motility and peristalsis. Drug improves lower esophageal sphincter tone by directly stimulating cholinergic receptors, thereby alleviating gastric reflux.

PHARMACOKINETICS
Absorption: Bethanechol is poorly absorbed from the GI tract (absorption varies considerably among patients). After oral administration, action usually begins in 30 to 90 minutes; after S.C. administration, in 5 to 15 minutes.
Distribution: Although distribution is largely unknown, therapeutic doses don't penetrate the blood-brain barrier.
Metabolism: Unknown. Usual duration of effect after oral administration is 1 hour; after S.C. administration, up to 2 hours.
Excretion: Unknown.

CONTRAINDICATIONS & PRECAUTIONS
Contraindicated for I.M. and I.V. use and in patients with hypersensitivity to bethanechol or its components; uncertain strength or integrity of bladder wall; mechanical obstructions of GI or urinary tract; hyperthyroidism, peptic ulceration, latent or active bronchial asthma, pronounced bradycardia or hypotension, vasomotor instability, cardiac or coronary artery disease, seizure disorder, Parkinson's disease, spastic GI disturbances, acute inflammatory lesions of the GI tract, peritonitis, or marked vagotonia; or when increased muscular activity of GI or urinary tract is harmful.

INTERACTIONS
Drug-drug. Use with *ganglionic blockers such as mecamylamine* may cause a critical blood pressure decrease; this effect is usually preceded by abdominal symptoms. Use with *procainamide* or *quinidine* may reverse the cholinergic effect of bethanechol on muscle. Don't use together.

---

*Canada only   ◊ Unlabeled clinical use

Use with *cholinergics* or *cholinesterase inhibitors* may cause additive effects. Monitor closely.

ADVERSE REACTIONS
CNS: headache, malaise.
CV: hypotension, flushing, reflex tachycardia.
EENT: lacrimation, miosis.
GI: *abdominal cramps, diarrhea,* excessive salivation, nausea, belching, borborygmus.
GU: urinary urgency.
Respiratory: *bronchoconstriction,* increased bronchial secretions.
Other: diaphoresis.

◻ KEY CONSIDERATIONS
• Atropine should be readily available to counteract toxic reactions that may occur during treatment with bethanechol.
• Never give bethanechol I.M. or I.V. because that could cause circulatory collapse, hypotension, severe abdominal cramps, bloody diarrhea, shock, or cardiac arrest. Give only by S.C. route when giving parenterally.
• For administration to treat urine retention, a bedpan should be readily available.
• Give drug on an empty stomach; eating soon after drug administration may cause nausea and vomiting.
• Patients with hypertension receiving bethanechol may experience a precipitous decrease in blood pressure.
• Bethanechol increases serum levels of amylase, lipase, bilirubin, and AST and increases sulfobromophthalein retention time.

Overdose & treatment
• Signs and symptoms of overdose include nausea, vomiting, abdominal cramps, diarrhea, involuntary defecation, urinary urgency, excessive salivation, miosis, excessive tearing, bronchospasm, increased bronchial secretions, hypotension, excessive sweating, bradycardia or reflex tachycardia, and substernal pain.
• Treatment requires discontinuation of drug and administration of atropine by S.C., I.M., or I.V. route. (Atropine must be administered cautiously; an overdose

could cause bronchial plug formation.) Contact local or regional poison control center for more information.

bicalutamide
Casodex

Nonsteroidal antiandrogen, antineoplastic

Available by prescription only
Tablets: 50 mg

INDICATIONS & DOSAGE
Adjunct therapy for treatment of advanced prostate cancer
Adults: 50 mg P.O. once daily in morning or evening.

PHARMACODYNAMICS
Antineoplastic action: Bicalutamide competitively inhibits the action of androgens by binding to cytosol androgen receptors in the target tissue. Prostate cancer, known to be sensitive to androgens, responds to treatment that either counteracts the effect of androgen or removes its source.

PHARMACOKINETICS
Absorption: Bicalutamide is well absorbed from GI tract.
Distribution: 96% is protein-bound.
Metabolism: Drug—which undergoes stereospecific metabolism—is extensively metabolized by the liver. The S (inactive) isomer is metabolized primarily by glucuronidation. The R (active) isomer also undergoes glucuronidation but is predominantly oxidized to an inactive metabolite followed by glucuronidation.
Excretion: Drug is excreted in urine and feces.

CONTRAINDICATIONS & PRECAUTIONS
Contraindicated in patients with hypersensitivity to bicalutamide or to any component in the tablet. Use cautiously in patients with moderate to severe hepatic impairment.

Reactions may be *common,* uncommon, *life-threatening,* or COMMON AND LIFE-THREATENING.

INTERACTIONS

Drug-drug. Bicalutamide displaces *coumarin anticoagulants* from their protein-binding sites. Monitor PT and INR closely. The anticoagulant dosage may need to be adjusted.

ADVERSE REACTIONS

CNS: *asthenia, general pain,* headache, dizziness, paresthesia, insomnia.
CV: *hot flashes,* hypertension, chest pain, peripheral edema.
GI: constipation, *nausea, diarrhea,* abdominal pain, flatulence, vomiting.
GU: nocturia, hematuria, urinary tract infection, impotence, gynecomastia, urinary incontinence.
Hematologic: hypochromic anemia, iron-deficiency anemia.
Metabolic: increased liver enzyme levels, weight loss, hyperglycemia.
Musculoskeletal: *back or pelvic pain,* bone pain.
Respiratory: dyspnea.
Skin: rash, sweating.
Other: *infection,* flulike syndrome.

▣ KEY CONSIDERATIONS

• Bicalutamide is used in combination therapy with a luteinizing hormone–releasing hormone (LHRH) analogue for the treatment of advanced prostate cancer. Treatment should begin at the same time as that with the prescribed LHRH analogue.
• Administer bicalutamide at the same time each day.
• Monitor serum prostate specific antigen (PSA) levels regularly. PSA levels help in assessing patient's response to therapy. Elevated levels require a reevaluation of patient to determine disease progression.
• Monitor liver function studies. When a patient develops jaundice or exhibits laboratory evidence of liver injury in the absence of liver metastases, drug should be discontinued. Abnormalities are usually reversible on drug discontinuation.
• Drug isn't indicated for use in women.

Patient education

• Inform patient that drug may be taken without regard to meals.

• Advise patient to take drug at the same time each day.
• Tell patient that bicalutamide is used with other drugs. Stress importance of not interrupting or stopping any of these drugs without medical consultation.

---

biperiden hydrochloride

biperiden lactate
Akineton

Anticholinergic, antiparkinsonian

Available by prescription only
Tablets: 2 mg
Injection: 5 mg/ml in 1-ml ampule

INDICATIONS & DOSAGE

Parkinsonism
Adults: 2 mg P.O. t.i.d. or q.i.d. For prolonged therapy, adjust dosage to maximum of 16 mg daily.
Extrapyramidal disorders
Adults: 2 mg P.O. daily, b.i.d., or t.i.d., depending on severity. Usual dosage is 2 mg daily. For treatment of extrapyramidal symptoms induced by drugs, give 2 mg I.M. or slow I.V. q 30 minutes, not to exceed 8 mg in a 24-hour period.

PHARMACODYNAMICS

Antiparkinsonian action: Biperiden blocks central cholinergic receptors, helping to balance cholinergic activity in the basal ganglia. It may also prolong the effects of dopamine by blocking dopamine reuptake and storage at central receptor sites.

PHARMACOKINETICS

Absorption: Biperiden is well absorbed from the GI tract.
Distribution: Unknown.
Metabolism: Unknown.
Excretion: Excreted in the urine as unchanged drug and metabolites. After oral therapy, a small amount is probably excreted as unabsorbed drug.

CONTRAINDICATIONS & PRECAUTIONS

Contraindicated in patients with hypersensitivity to biperiden, angle-closure glaucoma, bowel obstruction, or megacolon. Use cautiously in patients with prostatic hyperplasia, arrhythmias, or seizure disorders.

INTERACTIONS

Drug-drug. *CNS depressants* increase the sedative effects of biperiden. Use may decrease the antipsychotic effectiveness of *haloperidol* or *phenothiazines*, possibly by direct CNS antagonism. Use with *phenothiazines* increases the risk of anticholinergic adverse effects. Don't use together.

Use with *amantadine* may amplify the anticholinergic adverse effects of biperiden, such as confusion and hallucinations. Decrease biperiden dosage before amantadine administration.

Antacids and antidiarrheals may decrease biperiden absorption. Administer biperiden at least 1 hour before an antacid or an antidiarrheal.

Use with *digoxin* may increase plasma levels of digoxin. Monitor closely.

Drug-lifestyle. *Alcohol* increases the sedative effects of biperiden. Don't use together. Drug increases photosensitivity to eyes. Take precautions when exposed to the *sun*.

ADVERSE REACTIONS

CNS: disorientation, euphoria, drowsiness, agitation.
CV: transient postural hypotension (with parenteral use).
EENT: blurred vision.
GI: dry mouth, *constipation*.
GU: urine retention.

Note: Adverse reactions are dose-related and may resemble atropine toxicity.

▣ KEY CONSIDERATIONS

Besides the recommendations relevant to all anticholinergics, consider the following:
• Use cautiously in geriatric patients because they're susceptible to the adverse reactions.
• When giving drug parenterally, keep patient supine; parenteral administration may cause transient postural hypotension and disturbed coordination.
• When giving biperiden I.V., inject drug slowly.

• Because biperiden may cause dizziness, patient may need assistance when walking.
• In patients with severe parkinsonism, tremors may increase when drug is administered to relieve spasticity.

Patient education
• Tell patient that tolerance to therapeutic and adverse effects can occur with long-term drug use.
• Tell patient that drug may make the eyes more sensitive to light.
• Advise patient to avoid alcohol while taking this drug.
• Tell patient to avoid activities that require mental alertness until the CNS effects of the drug are known.
• Instruct patient to take drug with food to avoid GI upset.

Overdose & treatment
• Signs and symptoms of overdose include central stimulation followed by depression and psychotic symptoms, such as disorientation, confusion, hallucinations, delusions, anxiety, agitation, and restlessness. Peripheral effects may include dilated, nonreactive pupils; blurred vision; hot, dry, flushed skin; dry mucous membranes; dysphagia; decreased or absent bowel sounds; urine retention; hyperthermia; headache; tachycardia; hypertension; and increased respiration.
• Treatment is primarily symptomatic and supportive, as necessary. Maintain patent airway. If the patient is alert, induce vomiting or perform gastric lavage and follow with a sodium chloride cathartic and activated charcoal to prevent further absorption of the drug. In severe cases, physostigmine may be administered to block antimuscarinic effects of biperiden. Give fluids, as needed, to treat shock; diazepam to control psychotic symptoms; and pilocarpine (instilled into the eyes) to relieve mydriasis. If urine retention occurs, catheterization may be necessary.

Reactions may be *common*, uncommon, *life-threatening*, or COMMON AND LIFE-THREATENING.

bisacodyl
Bisco-Lax, Dulcagen, Dulcolax, Fleet Laxative

Diphenylmethane derivative, stimulant laxative

Available without a prescription
Tablets: 5 mg
Suppositories: 10 mg
Rectal suspension: 10 mg/30 ml

INDICATIONS & DOSAGE
Constipation; preparation for delivery, surgery, or rectal or bowel examination
Adults: 10 to 15 mg P.O. daily. Up to 30 mg may be used for thorough evacuation needed for examinations or surgery. Alternatively, give one suppository (10 mg) P.R. daily.

PHARMACODYNAMICS
Laxative action: Bisacodyl directly stimulates the colon, increasing peristalsis and enhancing bowel evacuation.

PHARMACOKINETICS
Absorption: Bisacodyl is minimally absorbed; action begins 6 to 8 hours after oral administration and 15 to 60 minutes after P.R. administration.
Distribution: Drug is distributed locally.
Metabolism: Drug is metabolized in the liver.
Excretion: Most of the drug is excreted in feces; some, in urine.

CONTRAINDICATIONS & PRECAUTIONS
Contraindicated in patients with hypersensitivity, abdominal pain, nausea, vomiting, or other signs or symptoms of appendicitis or acute surgical abdomen and in those with rectal bleeding, gastroenteritis, or intestinal obstruction.

INTERACTIONS
Drug-drug. Use with *antacids* or *drugs that increase gastric pH levels* may cause the enteric coating of the drug to dissolve prematurely, resulting in intestinal or gastric irritation or cramping. Don't use together.
Drug-food. *Dairy products* may cause the enteric coating of the drug to dissolve prematurely, resulting in intestinal or gastric irritation or cramping. Don't use together.

ADVERSE REACTIONS
CNS: muscle weakness with excessive use, dizziness, faintness.
GI: *nausea, vomiting, abdominal cramps,* diarrhea (with high doses), *burning sensation in rectum (with suppositories),* laxative dependence with long-term or excessive use.
Metabolic: alkalosis, hypokalemia, fluid and electrolyte imbalance.
Other: tetany, protein-losing enteropathy with excessive use.

▣ KEY CONSIDERATIONS
• Patient should swallow tablets whole rather than crushing or chewing them, to avoid GI irritation. Administer with 8 oz (240 ml) of fluid.

Patient education
• Instruct patient not to take drug within 1 hour of consuming milk or an antacid.
• Tell patient to take only as directed to avoid laxative dependence.

bismuth subsalicylate
Pepto-Bismol

Adsorbent, antidiarrheal

Available without a prescription
Tablets (chewable): 262 mg
Suspension: 262 mg/15 ml, 524 mg/15 ml

INDICATIONS & DOSAGE
Mild, nonspecific diarrhea
Adults: 30 ml or 2 tablets q ½ to 1 hour up to a maximum of eight doses and for no more than 2 days.

PHARMACODYNAMICS
Antidiarrheal action: Bismuth adsorbs extra water in the bowel during diarrhea. It also adsorbs toxins and forms a protective coating for the intestinal mucosa.

PHARMACOKINETICS

Absorption: Bismuth is absorbed poorly; significant salicylate absorption may occur after using bismuth subsalicylate.
Distribution: Drug is distributed locally in the gut.
Metabolism: Only a small amount of drug is metabolized.
Excretion: Drug is excreted in urine.

CONTRAINDICATIONS & PRECAUTIONS

Contraindicated in patients hypersensitive to salicylates. Use cautiously in patients taking aspirin or aspirin-containing drugs.

INTERACTIONS

Drug-drug. Use with *aspirin* may cause additive effects. Use with *sulfinpyrazone* may impair the uricosuric effect of sulfinpyrazone and may increase the risk of aspirin toxicity. Don't use together.

Use with *tetracycline* may impair tetracycline absorption. Administer drugs at least 1 hour apart.

ADVERSE REACTIONS

GI: temporary darkening of tongue and stools.
Other: salicylism (with high doses).

▣ KEY CONSIDERATIONS

• Monitor hydration status and serum electrolyte levels; record number and consistency of stools.
• If administered by tube, tube should be flushed via NG tube, to clear it and make sure that drug passes into the stomach.
• If patient is also receiving tetracycline, administer drugs at least 1 hour apart; to avoid decreased drug absorption, dosages or schedules of other drugs may require adjustment.
• Bismuth subsalicylate has been used investigationally to treat peptic ulcer. Dosages of 600 mg t.i.d. may be as effective as 800 mg of cimetidine once daily.
• Because bismuth is radiopaque, it may interfere with radiologic examination of the GI tract.

Patient education

• Advise patient taking an anticoagulant or an antidiabetic or antigout drug to seek medical approval before taking bismuth.
• Instruct patient to chew tablets well or to shake suspension well before using.
• Tell patient to report persistent diarrhea.
• Warn patient that bismuth may temporarily darken stools and tongue.

---

bisoprolol fumarate
Zebeta

Beta blocker, antihypertensive

Available by prescription only
Tablets: 5 mg, 10 mg

INDICATIONS & DOSAGE

Hypertension (used alone or in combination with other antihypertensives)
Adults: Initially, 5 mg P.O. once daily. If response is inadequate, increase to 10 mg once daily. Maximum recommended dosage, 20 mg daily.
✦ *Dosage adjustment.* In adults with a creatinine clearance less than 40 ml/minute, cirrhosis, or hepatitis, start at 2.5 mg P.O.; then increase with caution.

PHARMACODYNAMICS

Antihypertensive action: Mechanism of action hasn't been completely established. Possible antihypertensive factors include decreased cardiac output, inhibition of renin release by the kidneys, and diminution of tonic sympathetic outflow from the vasomotor centers in the brain.

PHARMACOKINETICS

Absorption: Bioavailability after a 10-mg oral dose of bisoprolol is about 80%. Absorption is unaffected by food.
Distribution: About 30% of drug binds to serum proteins.
Metabolism: The first-pass metabolism of drug is about 20%.
Excretion: Drug is eliminated equally by renal and nonrenal pathways, with about 50% of dose appearing unchanged in the urine and the remainder appearing as inactive metabolites. Less than 2% of dose

---

is excreted in feces. The plasma elimination half-life of drug is 9 to 12 hours (slightly longer in geriatric patients, in part because of decreased renal function).

CONTRAINDICATIONS & PRECAUTIONS

Contraindicated in patients with hypersensitivity to bisoprolol and in those with cardiogenic shock, overt cardiac failure, marked sinus bradycardia, or second- or third-degree AV block. Use cautiously in patients with bronchospastic disease.

INTERACTIONS

Drug-drug. Bisoprolol shouldn't be combined with *other beta blockers*.

Patients taking *catecholamine-depleting drugs, such as guanethidine or reserpine,* with bisoprolol should be closely monitored because the added beta-blocking action of bisoprolol may excessively reduce sympathetic activity.

In patients taking bisoprolol with *clonidine,* bisoprolol should be discontinued for several days before clonidine is withdrawn.

ADVERSE REACTIONS

CNS: asthenia, fatigue, dizziness, *headache,* hypoesthesia, vivid dreams, depression, insomnia.
CV: *bradycardia,* peripheral edema, chest pain.
EENT: pharyngitis, rhinitis, sinusitis.
GI: nausea, vomiting, diarrhea, dry mouth.
Musculoskeletal: arthralgia.
Respiratory: cough, dyspnea.

▣ KEY CONSIDERATIONS

• A beta$_2$ agonist, or bronchodilator, should be made available to patients with bronchospastic disease.
• In patients with coronary artery disease, abrupt cessation of beta-blocker therapy has been known to exacerbate angina pectoris, MI, and ventricular arrhythmia. It's advisable, even in patients who don't have coronary artery disease, to taper bisoprolol over 1 week and keep the patient under careful observation. If withdrawal symptoms occur, bisoprolol therapy should be temporarily reinstituted.

• Drug may produce hypoglycemia and interfere with glucose or insulin tolerance tests.

Patient education
• Inform diabetic patients subject to spontaneous hypoglycemia or those requiring insulin or oral antidiabetics that bisoprolol may mask signs and symptoms of hypoglycemia, particularly tachycardia.
• Warn patient not to drive, operate machinery, or perform any other task requiring alertness until reaction to bisoprolol has been established.
• Stress importance of taking drug as prescribed, even when feeling well. Advise patient not to discontinue drug abruptly because serious consequences can occur.
• Instruct patient to call if adverse reactions occur.
• Tell patient to seek medical approval before taking OTC drugs.

Overdose & treatment
• The most common signs of overdose from a beta blocker such as bisoprolol are bradycardia, hypotension, heart failure, bronchospasm, and hypoglycemia.
• If an overdose occurs, drug therapy should be discontinued and supportive and symptomatic treatment provided.

bleomycin sulfate
Blenoxane

Antibiotic, antineoplastic (cell cycle–phase specific, G$_2$ and M phase)

Available by prescription only
Injection: 15-U and 30-U vials

INDICATIONS & DOSAGE

Dosage and indications may vary. Check current literature for recommended protocol.

Hodgkin's disease, squamous cell carcinoma, malignant lymphoma, or testicular cancer
Adults: 10 to 20 U/m^2 (0.25 to 0.5 U/kg) I.V., I.M., or S.C. one or two times weekly. After 50% response, maintenance dosage of 1 U daily or 5 U weekly.

Malignant pleural effusion, prevention of recurrent pleural effusions
Adults: 60 U in 50 to 100 ml of normal saline solution by intracavitary administration.
◊ *Tumors of the head and neck*
Adults: 10 to 20 U/m² daily by regional arterial administration for 5 to 14 days.

PHARMACODYNAMICS
Antineoplastic action: The exact mechanism of action is unknown. Bleomycin may cause scission of single- and double-stranded DNA and inhibit DNA, RNA, and protein synthesis. Drug also appears to inhibit cell progression out of the G_2 phase.

PHARMACOKINETICS
Absorption: Bleomycin is poorly absorbed across the GI tract after oral administration. I.M. administration results in lower serum levels than those occurring after equivalent I.V. doses.
Distribution: Drug distributes widely into total body water, mainly in the skin, lungs, kidneys, peritoneum, and lymphatic tissue.
Metabolism: Metabolic fate of drug is undetermined; however, extensive tissue inactivation occurs in the liver and kidney and much less in the skin and lungs.
Excretion: Bleomycin and its metabolites are excreted primarily in urine. The terminal plasma elimination phase half-life is reported at 2 hours.

CONTRAINDICATIONS & PRECAUTIONS
Contraindicated in patients hypersensitive to bleomycin. Use cautiously in patients with renal or pulmonary impairment.

INTERACTIONS
Drug-drug. Use with *digoxin* or *phenytoin* may decrease serum levels of digoxin and phenytoin. Monitor closely.

ADVERSE REACTIONS
GI: stomatitis, anorexia, nausea, vomiting, diarrhea.
Metabolic: weight loss.
Respiratory: *pulmonary fibrosis,* pulmonary toxicity such as PNEUMONITIS.

Skin: *erythema, hyperpigmentation, acne, rash, reversible alopecia, striae, skin tenderness,* pruritus.
Other: *chills,* fever, severe idiosyncratic reaction consisting of hypotension, mental confusion, fever, chills and wheezing has occurred in about 1% of lymphoma patients.

▣ KEY CONSIDERATIONS
• Use with caution in patients older than age 70 because they're at increased risk for pulmonary toxicity.
• To prepare solution for I.M. administration, reconstitute drug with 1 to 5 ml or 2 to 10 ml of normal saline solution or sterile water for injection to the 15-U or 30-U vials respectively yielding a 3 to 15 U/ml concentration.
• For I.V. administration, dilute with a minimum of 5 ml of diluent and administer over 10 minutes as I.V. push injection.
• Prepare infusions of bleomycin in glass bottles because plastic will absorb the drug over time. Plastic syringes don't interfere with bleomycin activity.
• Use precautions in preparing and handling drug; wear gloves and wash hands after preparing and administering.
• Drug can be administered by intracavitary (see manufacturer's recommendation), intra-arterial, or intratumoral injection. It can also be instilled into bladder for bladder tumors.
• Cumulative lifetime dosage shouldn't exceed 400 U.
• Response to therapy may take 2 to 3 weeks.
• Administer a 1- to 2-U test dose to lymphoma patients before the first two doses to assess hypersensitivity to bleomycin. If no reaction occurs, then follow the dosing schedule. The test dose can be incorporated as part of the total dosage for the regimen.
• Have epinephrine, diphenhydramine, I.V. corticosteroids, and oxygen available in case of anaphylactic reaction.
• Premedication with aspirin, steroids, and diphenhydramine may reduce drug fever and risk of anaphylaxis.
• Dosage should be reduced in patients with renal or pulmonary impairment.
• Drug concentrates in keratin of squamous epithelium. To prevent linear

---

Reactions may be *common,* uncommon, *life-threatening,* or COMMON AND LIFE-THREATENING.

streaking, don't use adhesive dressings on skin.

• Allergic reactions may be delayed especially in patients with lymphoma.

• Pulmonary function tests may be useful in predicting fibrosis; they should be performed to establish a baseline and then monitored periodically.

• Monitor chest X-rays and auscultate the lungs.

• Bleomycin is stable for 24 hours at room temperature and 48 hours under refrigeration. Refrigerate unopened vials containing dry powder.

Patient education
• Explain that hair should grow back after treatment is discontinued.

---

bretylium tosylate
Bretylate*, Bretylol

Adrenergic blocker, ventricular antiarrhythmic

Available by prescription only
Injection: 50 mg/ml

INDICATIONS & DOSAGE
Ventricular fibrillation and hemodynamically unstable ventricular tachycardia
Adults: 5 mg/kg undiluted by rapid I.V. injection. If ventricular fibrillation persists, increase dosage to 10 mg/kg and repeat, p.r.n. For continuous suppression, administer diluted solution by continuous I.V. infusion at 1 to 2 mg/minute, or infuse diluted solution at 5 to 10 mg/kg over more than 8 minutes q 6 hours.
Other ventricular arrhythmias
Adults: Initially, 5 to 10 mg/kg I.M., undiluted, or I.V. diluted. Repeat in 1 to 2 hours if necessary. Maintenance dose is 5 to 10 mg/kg q 6 hours I.M. or I.V. or 1 to 2 mg/minute I.V. infusion.

PHARMACODYNAMICS
Ventricular antiarrhythmic action:
Bretylium is a class III antiarrhythmic used to treat ventricular fibrillation and tachycardia. Like other class III antiarrhythmics, it widens the action potential duration (repolarization inhibition) and

increases the effective refractory period (ERP); it doesn't affect conduction velocity. These actions follow a transient increase in conduction velocity and shortening of the action potential duration and ERP.

Initial effects stem from norepinephrine release from sympathetic ganglia and postganglionic adrenergic neurons immediately after drug administration. Norepinephrine release also accounts for an increased threshold for successful defibrillation, increased blood pressure, and increased heart rate. This initial phase of drug's action is brief (up to 1 hour).

Bretylium also alters the disparity in action potential duration between ischemic and nonischemic myocardial tissue; its antiarrhythmic action may result from this activity.

Hemodynamic drug effects include increased blood pressure, heart rate, and possible cardiac irritability (all resulting from initial norepinephrine release). Drug-induced adrenergic blockade ultimately predominates, leading to vasodilation and a subsequent blood pressure drop (primarily orthostatic). This effect has been referred to as chemical sympathectomy.

PHARMACOKINETICS
Absorption: Bretylium is incompletely and erratically absorbed from the GI tract; it's well absorbed after I.M. administration. With I.M. administration, the antiarrhythmic (ventricular tachycardia and ectopy) action of the drug begins within about 20 to 60 minutes but may not reach maximal level for 6 to 9 hours when given by this route (for this reason, I.M. administration isn't recommended for treating life-threatening ventricular fibrillation).

With I.V. administration, antifibrillatory action begins within a few minutes. However, suppression of ventricular tachycardia and other ventricular arrhythmias occurs more slowly—usually within 20 minutes to 2 hours; peak antiarrhythmic effects may not occur for 6 to 9 hours.
Distribution: Drug is distributed widely throughout the body. It doesn't cross the

---

blood-brain barrier. Only about 1% to 10% binds to plasma proteins.

Metabolism: No metabolites have been identified.

Excretion: Drug is excreted in the urine mostly as unchanged drug; half-life ranges from 5 to 10 hours (longer in patients with renal impairment). Duration of effect ranges from 6 to 24 hours and may increase with continued dosage increases. (Patients with ventricular fibrillation may require continuous infusion to maintain desired effect.)

CONTRAINDICATIONS & PRECAUTIONS

Contraindicated in digitalized patients unless the arrhythmia is life-threatening, not caused by a cardiac glycoside, or is unresponsive to other antiarrhythmics. Use with caution in patients with aortic stenosis or pulmonary hypertension.

INTERACTIONS

Drug-drug. Use with *other antiarrhythmics* may cause additive toxic effects and additive or antagonistic cardiac effects. Bretylium may potentiate the action of *pressor amines (sympathomimetics).* Monitor closely.

Use with *cardiac glycosides* may exacerbate ventricular tachycardia associated with digitalis toxicity. Avoid concomitant use.

ADVERSE REACTIONS

CNS: vertigo, dizziness, syncope, lightheadedness.

CV: SEVERE HYPOTENSION, bradycardia, angina, transient arrhythmias, transient hypertension, increased PVCs.

GI: severe nausea, vomiting.

▣ KEY CONSIDERATIONS

● Administer I.V. infusion at appropriate rate to avoid or minimize adverse reactions.

● For I.M. injection, don't exceed 5-ml volume in any one site and rotate sites.

● Patient should remain in a supine position and avoid sudden postural changes until tolerance to hypotension develops.

● Monitor ECG and blood pressure throughout therapy for any significant change. If supine systolic pressure decreases to less than 75 mm Hg, norepi-

nephrine, dopamine, or volume expanders may be prescribed to elevate blood pressure.

● Monitor patient closely if patient is receiving pressor amines (sympathomimetics) to correct hypotension; bretylium potentiates the effects of these drugs.

● Observe for increased angina in susceptible patients.

● Because bretylium is excreted exclusively by the kidneys, patients with renal impairment require dosage adjustment. Dosage interval should be increased because the elimination half-life increases threefold to sixfold.

● Subtherapeutic dosages (less than 5 mg/kg) may cause hypotension.

● Drug isn't a first-line drug, according to American Heart Association advanced cardiac life-support guidelines. With ventricular fibrillation, drug should follow lidocaine; with ventricular tachycardia, drug should follow lidocaine and procainamide.

● Ventricular tachycardia and other ventricular arrhythmias respond to drug less rapidly than ventricular fibrillation.

● Drug is ineffective against atrial arrhythmias.

---

brimonidine tartrate
Alphagan

Selective alpha$_2$-adrenergic agonist, ophthalmic drug for glaucoma or ocular hypertension

Available by prescription only
Ophthalmic solution: 0.2%; 5 ml, 10 ml

INDICATIONS & DOSAGE

Lowering of intraocular pressure (IOP) in patients with open-angle glaucoma or ocular hypertension
Adults: 1 drop in affected eye t.i.d., about 8 hours apart.

PHARMACODYNAMICS

Ocular antihypertensive action: Brimonidine is an alpha$_2$-adrenergic receptor agonist that reduces aqueous humor production and increases uveoscleral outflow.

Reactions may be *common,* uncommon, *life-threatening,* or COMMON AND LIFE-THREATENING.

PHARMACOKINETICS

Absorption: After ocular administration, plasma levels peak within 1 to 4 hours and decline with a systemic half-life of about 3 hours.
Distribution: Not reported.
Metabolism: Drug is metabolized systemically, primarily in the liver.
Excretion: Drug is primarily excreted in urine.

CONTRAINDICATIONS & PRECAUTIONS

Contraindicated in patients with hypersensitivity to brimonidine or benzalkonium and in those receiving MAO inhibitor therapy. Use cautiously in patients with cerebral or coronary insufficiency, CV disease, hepatic or renal impairment, depression, Raynaud's phenomenon, orthostatic hypotension, or thromboangiitis obliterans.

INTERACTIONS

Drug-drug. Use with *antihypertensives, beta blockers,* or *cardiac glycosides* may further decrease blood pressure. Use with *CNS depressants* may potentiate drug effects or cause additive effects. Monitor closely.

Tricyclic antidepressants may interfere with the IOP-lowering effects of brimonidine. Use together cautiously.

ADVERSE REACTIONS

CNS: anxiety, asthenia, depression, dizziness, *drowsiness, fatigue, headache,* insomnia, muscular pain.
CV: hypertension, palpitations, syncope.
EENT: abnormal vision or taste; blepharitis; *blurring, burning, or stinging;* conjunctival blanching, edema, hemorrhage, discharge, or *follicles;* corneal staining or erosion; eyelid erythema or eyelid edema; *foreign body sensation;* lid crusting; nasal dryness; ocular hyperemia, *allergic reactions,* pruritus, ache or pain, dryness, tearing, or irritation; *oral dryness,* photophobia.
GI: nausea, vomiting, diarrhea.
Respiratory: cough and cold symptoms.

▣ KEY CONSIDERATIONS

• Monitor IOP because loss of effects after 1st month of therapy may occur.

Patient education

• Tell patient to wait at least 15 minutes after instilling drug to insert soft contact lenses.
• Caution patient of potential for decreased mental alertness; drug may cause fatigue or drowsiness.

bromocriptine mesylate
Parlodel

Dopamine receptor agonist, semi-synthetic ergot alkaloid, dopaminergic agonist, antiparkinsonian, inhibitor of prolactin release, inhibitor of growth hormone release

Available by prescription only
Tablets: 2.5 mg
Capsules: 5 mg

INDICATIONS & DOSAGE

Acromegaly
Adults: Initially, 1.25 to 2.5 mg P.O. with food daily h.s. for 3 days. An additional 1.25 to 2.5 mg may be added q 3 to 7 days until patient receives therapeutic benefit. Therapeutic dosage range varies from 20 to 30 mg daily in most patients. Maximum dosage shouldn't exceed 100 mg daily. Dosages of 20 to 60 mg daily have been administered as divided doses.
Parkinson's disease
Adults: Initially, 1.25 to 2.5 mg P.O. b.i.d. with meals. Dosage may be increased by 2.5 mg daily q 14 to 28 days, up to 100 mg daily or until a maximal therapeutic response is achieved. Safety in dosages over 100 mg daily hasn't been established.
◊ *Cushing's syndrome*
Adults: 1.25 to 2.5 mg P.O. b.i.d. to q.i.d.
◊ *Hepatic encephalopathy*
Adults: 1.25 mg P.O. daily, increased by 1.25 mg q 3 days until 15 mg is reached.

PHARMACODYNAMICS

Bromocriptine activates dopaminergic receptors in the neostriatum of the CNS, which may produce its antiparkinsonian activity. Drug may also affect brain serotonin activity.

PHARMACOKINETICS

Absorption: Bromocriptine is 28% absorbed when given orally and reaches peak levels in about 1 to 3 hours. Plasma levels for therapeutic effects are unknown. After an oral dose, serum prolactin level decreases within 2 hours, is decreased maximally at 8 hours, and remains decreased at 24 hours.

Distribution: Some 90% to 96% binds to serum albumin.

Metabolism: First-pass metabolism occurs with over 90% of the absorbed dose. Drug is metabolized completely in the liver, principally by hydrolysis, before excretion. The metabolites aren't active or toxic.

Excretion: Drug is excreted primarily through bile. Only 2.5% to 5.5% of dose is excreted in urine. Almost all (85%) of dose is excreted in feces within 5 days.

CONTRAINDICATIONS & PRECAUTIONS

Contraindicated in patients with hypersensitivity to ergot derivatives or with uncontrolled hypertension. Use cautiously in patients with renal or hepatic impairment and history of an MI with residual arrhythmias.

INTERACTIONS

Drug-drug. Bromocriptine may potentiate *antihypertensives,* so their dosage needs to be decreased to prevent hypotension.

The dosage of bromocriptine may need to be increased if the drug is used with *drugs that increase prolactin levels*—such as *amitriptyline, butyrophenones, imipramine, methyldopa, phenothiazines,* and *reserpine.*

Drug-lifestyle. *Alcohol* intolerance may result when high dosages of bromocriptine are administered; therefore, ingestion of alcohol should be limited.

ADVERSE REACTIONS

CNS: *dizziness, headache,* fatigue, mania, light-headedness, drowsiness, delusions, nervousness, insomnia, depression, *seizures.*

CV: *hypotension, stroke, acute MI.*

EENT: nasal congestion, blurred vision.

GI: *nausea,* vomiting, *abdominal cramps, constipation,* diarrhea, anorexia.

GU: urine retention, urinary frequency, elevated BUN levels.

Hepatic: elevated liver enzyme levels.

Skin: coolness and pallor of fingers and toes.

▣ KEY CONSIDERATIONS

● Use with caution, particularly in patients receiving long-term, high-dosage therapy. Regular physical assessment is recommended, with particular attention to changes in pulmonary function.

● Safety isn't established for long-term use at the dosages required to treat Parkinson's disease.

● First-dose phenomenon occurs in 1% of patients. Sensitive patients may experience syncope for 15 to 60 minutes but can usually tolerate subsequent treatment without ill effects. Patient should begin therapy with lowest dosage, taken at bedtime.

● Administer drug with meals, milk, or snacks to diminish GI distress.

● Alcohol intolerance may occur, especially when high dosages of bromocriptine are administered; therefore, alcohol intake should be limited.

● As an antiparkinsonian, bromocriptine is usually given with either levodopa alone or levodopa-carbidopa combination.

● Adverse reactions are more common when drug is given in high dosages, as in treating parkinsonism.

Patient education

● Tell patient to take first dose where and when he can lie down because drowsiness commonly occurs after initiation of therapy.

● Instruct patient to report visual problems, severe nausea and vomiting, or acute headaches.

● Tell patient to take drug with meals to avoid GI upset.

● Warn patient that the CNS effects of drug may impair ability to perform tasks that require alertness and coordination.

● Advise patient to limit use of alcohol during treatment.

Reactions may be *common,* uncommon, *life-threatening,* or COMMON AND LIFE-THREATENING.

brompheniramine maleate
Dimetapp Allergy

*Alkylamine antihistamine
(H_1-receptor antagonist)*

Available with or without a prescription
Liquigels: 4 mg
Elixir: 2 mg/5 ml
Injection: 10 mg/ml

INDICATIONS & DOSAGE
Rhinitis, allergies
Adults: 4 mg P.O. q 4 to 6 hours. Don't exceed 24 mg in 24 hours.
Hypersensitivity
Adults: 5 to 20 mg S.C., I.M. or I.V. b.i.d. Don't exceed 40 mg in 24 hours.

PHARMACODYNAMICS
Antihistamine action: Antihistamines compete with histamine for histamine$_1$ receptor sites on the smooth muscle of the bronchi, GI tract, uterus, and large blood vessels; by binding to cellular receptors, they prevent access of histamine and suppress histamine-induced allergic symptoms, even though they don't prevent release of histamine.

PHARMACOKINETICS
Absorption: Brompheniramine is absorbed readily from the GI tract; action begins within 15 to 30 minutes and peaks in 2 to 5 hours. A second lower peak effect exists, possibly from drug reabsorption in the distal small intestine.
Distribution: Drug is distributed widely into the body.
Metabolism: The liver metabolizes 90% to 95% of drug.
Excretion: Half-life of drug ranges from about 12 to 34½ hours. Brompheniramine and its metabolites are excreted primarily in urine; a small amount is excreted in feces. About 5% to 10% of an oral dose is excreted unchanged in urine.

CONTRAINDICATIONS & PRECAUTIONS
Contraindicated in patients with hypersensitivity to the ingredients of brompheniramine; in those with acute asthma, severe hypertension or coronary artery disease, angle-closure glaucoma, urine retention, and peptic ulcer; and within 14 days of MAO-inhibitor therapy. Use cautiously in geriatric patients, especially those with increased intraocular pressure, diabetes mellitus, ischemic heart disease, hyperthyroidism, hypertension, bronchial asthma, or prostatic hyperplasia.

INTERACTIONS
Drug-drug. Use with *other anxiolytics, barbiturates, CNS depressants, sleeping aids,* and *tranquilizers* may cause additive CNS depression. *MAO inhibitors* may interfere with the metabolism of brompheniramine and thus prolong and intensify central depressant and anticholinergic effects. Use with caution.

Brompheniramine may diminish the effects of *sulfonylureas* and may counteract the anticoagulant effects of *heparin*. Monitor closely.
Drug-lifestyle. *Alcohol* may cause additive CNS depression. Discourage use.

ADVERSE REACTIONS
CNS: dizziness, tremors, irritability, syncope, insomnia, *drowsiness, stimulation.*
CV: hypotension, palpitations.
GI: anorexia, nausea, vomiting, *dry mouth and throat.*
GU: urine retention.
Hematologic: *thrombocytopenia, agranulocytosis.*
Skin: urticaria, rash.
Other: (after parenteral administration) local stinging, diaphoresis.

▣ KEY CONSIDERATIONS
• Many geriatric patients are sensitive to adverse effects of antihistamines and are especially likely to experience dizziness, sedation, hyperexcitability, dry mouth, and urine retention. Signs and symptoms usually respond to a decrease in drug dosage.
• Drug causes less drowsiness than some antihistamines.
• Store parenteral solutions and elixirs away from light and freezing temperatures; solution may crystallize if stored below 32° F (0° C). Crystals dissolve when warmed to 86° F (30° C).

*Canada only ◊ Unlabeled clinical use

• Discontinue drug 4 days before performing diagnostic skin tests; it can prevent, reduce, or mask positive skin test response.

Patient education
• Instruct patient not to take more than 24 mg/day.
• Advise patient to avoid alcohol while taking this drug.
• Advise patient to avoid activities that require mental alertness until the CNS effects of the drug are known.

Overdose & treatment
• Signs and symptoms of overdose include those of CNS depression—such as sedation, reduced mental alertness, apnea, and CV collapse—and those of CNS stimulation—such as insomnia, hallucinations, tremors, and seizures. Anticholinergic symptoms—such as dry mouth, flushed skin, fixed and dilated pupils, and GI symptoms—are common.
• Treat overdose by inducing vomiting with ipecac syrup (in conscious patients), followed by activated charcoal to reduce further drug absorption. Perform gastric lavage if patient is unconscious or ipecac fails. Treat hypotension with vasopressors, and control seizures with diazepam or phenytoin I.V. Don't give stimulants.

budesonide
Pulmicort Turbuhaler, Rhinocort

Anti-inflammatory, glucocorticosteroid

Available by prescription only
Nasal inhaler: 32 mcg/metered dose (200 doses/container)
Oral inhalation powder: 200 mcg/dose (200 doses/container)

INDICATIONS & DOSAGE
Management of symptoms of seasonal or perennial allergic rhinitis or nonallergic perennial rhinitis
Adults: 2 sprays in each nostril in the morning and evening or 4 sprays in each nostril in the morning. Maintenance dosage should be the fewest number of sprays needed to control symptoms. Dosages exceeding 256 mcg/day (4 sprays/nostril) aren't recommended.
Note: If improvement doesn't occur within 3 weeks, discontinue treatment.
Chronic asthma
Adults: 200 to 400 mcg oral inhalation b.i.d. when previously used bronchodilators alone or inhaled corticosteroids; 400 to 800 mcg oral inhalation b.i.d. when previously used oral corticosteroids.

PHARMACODYNAMICS
Anti-inflammatory action: Precise mechanism of action is unknown. Glucocorticosteroids show a wide range of inhibitory activities against multiple cell types (such as mast cells, eosinophils, neutrophils, macrophages, and lymphocytes) and mediators (such as histamine, eicosanoids, leukotrienes, and cytokines) involved in allergic and nonallergic, irritant-mediated inflammation.

PHARMACOKINETICS
Absorption: Only 20% of an intranasal dose of budesonide reaches systemic circulation. Oral inhalation has a rapid onset of action.
Distribution: Drug is 88% protein-bound in the plasma; volume of distribution is 200 L.
Metabolism: Drug is rapidly and extensively metabolized in the liver.
Excretion: About 67% of drug is eliminated in urine; about 33%, in feces.

CONTRAINDICATIONS & PRECAUTIONS
Contraindicated in patients hypersensitive to budesonide or its components and in those who have had recent septal ulcers, nasal surgery, or nasal trauma until total healing has occurred.

Use cautiously in patients with tuberculosis infections; untreated fungal, bacterial, or systemic viral infections; or ocular herpes simplex.

INTERACTIONS
Drug-drug. Use with *other inhaled glucocorticosteroids or alternate-day prednisone therapy* may increase the risk of hypothalamic-pituitary-adrenal axis suppression. Use with *other inhaled glucocorticosteroids* may also lead to hyper-

---

Reactions may be *common*, uncommon, **life-threatening**, or COMMON AND LIFE-THREATENING.

adrenocorticism. *Ketoconazole* may increase plasma levels of budesonide. Monitor closely.

ADVERSE REACTIONS

CNS: *headache,* nervousness.
EENT: *nasal irritation, epistaxis, pharyngitis, sinusitis,* reduced sense of smell, nasal pain, hoarseness.
GI: taste perversion, dry mouth, dyspepsia, nausea, vomiting.
Metabolic: weight gain.
Musculoskeletal: myalgia.
Respiratory: *cough,* candidiasis, wheezing, dyspnea.
Skin: facial edema, rash, pruritus, contact dermatitis.
Other: hypersensitivity reactions.

▣ KEY CONSIDERATIONS

• Replacing a systemic glucocorticosteroid with a topical glucocorticosteroid can cause adrenal insufficiency; in addition, some patients may experience symptoms of withdrawal, such as joint or muscular pain, lassitude, and depression.
• Patients previously treated for prolonged periods with systemic glucocorticosteroids who are subsequently given topical glucocorticosteroids should be carefully monitored for acute adrenal insufficiency in response to stress.
• In patients with asthma or other conditions requiring long-term systemic treatment, a too-rapid decrease in systemic glucocorticosteroids may severely exacerbate symptoms.
• Excessive doses of budesonide or concomitant use with other inhaled glucocorticosteroids may lead to hyperadrenocorticism.
• Patients using budesonide for several months or longer should be examined periodically for *Candida* infection or other signs of adverse effects on the nasal mucosa.

Patient education

• Warn patient not to exceed prescribed dosage or to use drug for a long period because of risk of hypothalamic-pituitary-adrenal axis suppression.
• Have patient follow these instructions for the nasal inhaler: After opening aluminum pouch, use within 6 minutes. Shake canister well before using. Blow nose to clear nasal passages. Tilt head slightly forward; insert nozzle into nostril, pointing away from septum; hold other nostril closed; gently inhale; and spray. Shake canister again and repeat in other nostril. Store with valve downward. Don't store in high humidity. Don't break, incinerate, or store canister in extreme heat; contents under pressure.
• Instruct patient to hold the inhaler upright when loading Pulmicort Turbuhaler, not to blow or exhale into the inhaler nor shake it while loaded, and to hold inhaler upright while orally inhaling the dose. Place the mouthpiece between the lips and inhale forcefully and deeply.
• Assure patient that drug rarely causes nasal irritation or burning; advise patient to call health care provider if such symptoms recur.
• Warn patient to avoid exposure to chickenpox or measles, if at risk for contacting these diseases, and to consult health care provider immediately if exposed.
• Teach patient good nasal and oral hygiene.
• Tell patient to call health care provider if condition worsens or if symptoms don't improve within 3 weeks.
• Inform patient that effects aren't immediate; response requires regular use.
• Inform patient that with use of oral inhaler improvement in asthma control can occur within 24 hours, with maximum benefit anticipated between 1 to 2 weeks and possibly taking longer.
• Advise patient that Pulmicort Turbuhaler isn't indicated for relief of acute bronchospasm.

bumetanide
Bumex

Loop diuretic

Available by prescription only
Tablets: 0.5 mg, 1 mg, 2 mg
Injection: 0.25 mg/ml

INDICATIONS & DOSAGE
Edema (heart failure, hepatic and renal disease); ◊ *postoperative edema;* ◊ *premenstrual syndrome;* ◊ *disseminated cancer*
Adults: 0.5 to 2 mg P.O. once daily. If diuretic response is inadequate, give a second or third dose at 4- to 5-hour intervals. An alternate schedule to safely and effectively control edema, give dosage on alternate days or for 3 to 4 days with rest periods of 1 to 2 days in between doses. Maximum dosage is 10 mg/day. Give parenterally when oral route isn't feasible. Usual initial dosage is 0.5 to 1 mg I.V. over 1 to 2 minutes or I.M. If response is inadequate, give a second or third dose at 2- to 3-hour intervals. Maximum dosage is 10 mg/day.

PHARMACODYNAMICS
Diuretic action: Loop diuretics inhibit sodium and chloride reabsorption in the proximal part of the ascending loop of Henle, promoting the excretion of sodium, water, chloride, and potassium; bumetanide produces renal and peripheral vasodilation and may temporarily increase glomerular filtration rate and decrease peripheral vascular resistance.

PHARMACOKINETICS
Absorption: After oral administration, 85% to 95% of a bumetanide dose is absorbed; food delays oral absorption. I.M. bumetanide is completely absorbed. Diuresis usually begins 30 to 60 minutes after oral and 40 minutes after I.M. administration; peak diuresis occurs 1 to 2 hours after either. Diuresis begins a few minutes after I.V. administration and peaks in 15 to 30 minutes.
Distribution: Drug is 92% to 96% protein-bound; it's unknown whether bumetanide enters the CSF.
Metabolism: Drug is metabolized in the liver to at least five metabolites.
Excretion: Some 80% of drug is excreted in urine; 10% to 20%, in feces. Half-life ranges from 1 to 1½ hours; duration of effect is 2 to 4 hours.

CONTRAINDICATIONS & PRECAUTIONS
Contraindicated in patients with hypersensitivity to bumetanide or sulfonamides (possible cross-sensitivity), in those with anuria or hepatic coma, and in patients in states of severe electrolyte depletion.
Use cautiously in patients with hepatic cirrhosis and ascites and in those with depressed renal function.

INTERACTIONS
Drug-drug. Bumetanide potentiates the hypotensive effect of most *antihypertensives* and *diuretics;* both actions are used to therapeutic advantage.
Use with *indomethacin* or *probenecid* may reduce the diuretic effect of bumetanide. Don't use together; however, if no alternative exists, an increased dosage of bumetanide may be required. Use may reduce renal clearance of *lithium* and increase lithium levels; lithium dosage may need to be adjusted.
Administration with *nephrotoxic* or *ototoxic drugs* may result in enhanced toxicity. Use with *potassium sparing diuretics*—such as *amiloride, spironolactone,* and *triamterene*—may decrease bumetanide-induced potassium loss; use with other *potassium wasting drugs* such as *steroids* and *amphotericin B* may cause severe potassium loss. Monitor closely.

ADVERSE REACTIONS
CNS: dizziness, headache, vertigo, weakness.
CV: volume depletion and dehydration, orthostatic hypotension, ECG changes, chest pain.
EENT: transient deafness, tinnitus.
GI: nausea, vomiting, upset stomach, dry mouth, diarrhea, pain.
GU: *renal failure,* premature ejaculation, difficulty maintaining erection, oliguria.
Hematologic: azotemia, *thrombocytopenia.*
Metabolic: hypokalemia; hypochloremic alkalosis; fluid and electrolyte imbalances, including dilutional hyponatremia, hypocalcemia, hyperglycemia, and glucose intolerance impairment, asymptomatic hyperuricemia.
Musculoskeletal: arthritic pain, muscle pain and tenderness.
Skin: rash, pruritus, diaphoresis.

Reactions may be *common,* uncommon, *life-threatening,* or COMMON AND LIFE-THREATENING.

▣ KEY CONSIDERATIONS

Besides the recommendations relevant to all loop diuretics, consider the following:

• Geriatric patients require close observation because they're more susceptible to drug-induced diuresis. Excessive diuresis promotes rapid dehydration, hypovolemia, hypokalemia, and hyponatremia in these patients, and may cause circulatory collapse. Reduced dosages may be indicated.

• Give I.V. bumetanide slowly, over 1 to 2 minutes, for I.V. infusion; dilute bumetanide in D_5W, normal saline solution, or lactated Ringer's solution; use within 24 hours.

• Drug therapy alters electrolyte balance and liver and renal function tests.

Overdose & treatment

• Signs and symptoms of overdose include profound electrolyte and volume depletion, which may cause circulatory collapse.

• Treatment is primarily supportive; replace fluid and electrolytes as needed.

buprenorphine hydrochloride
Buprenex

Narcotic agonist-antagonist, opioid partial agonist, analgesic
Controlled substance schedule V

Available by prescription only
Injection: 0.3 mg/ml in 1-ml ampules

INDICATIONS & DOSAGE

Moderate to severe pain
Adults: 0.3 mg I.M. or slow I.V. q 6 hours, p.r.n. May repeat 0.3 mg 30 to 60 minutes after initial dosage then use p.r.n. schedule. In some patients it may be necessary to increase dosage to 0.6 mg (I.M. only) and reduce interval to q 4 hours in patients who aren't at risk for respiratory depression. S.C. administration isn't recommended.
Geriatric patients: Dosage should be reduced by about 50%.

◊ *Adults:* 25 to 250 mcg/hour via I.V. infusion (over 48 hours for postoperative pain).
◊ *Adults:* 60 to 180 mcg via epidural injection.
◊ **Reverse fentanyl-induced anesthesia**
Adults: 0.3 to 0.8 mg, I.V. or I.M., 1 to 4 hours after the induction of anesthesia and about 30 minutes before the end of surgery.

PHARMACODYNAMICS

Analgesic action: Exact mechanisms of action of buprenorphine are unknown. It's believed to be a competitive antagonist at some and an agonist at other opiate receptors, thus relieving moderate to severe pain.

PHARMACOKINETICS

Absorption: Buprenorphine is absorbed rapidly after I.M. administration. Onset of action occurs in 15 minutes, with peak effect 1 hour after dosing.
Distribution: About 96% of drug is protein-bound.
Metabolism: Drug is metabolized in the liver.
Excretion: Duration of action is 6 hours. Drug is excreted primarily in feces as unchanged drug with about 30% excreted in urine.

CONTRAINDICATIONS & PRECAUTIONS

Contraindicated in patients with hypersensitivity to buprenorphine. Use cautiously in geriatric, especially those with head injuries, increased intracranial pressure, and intracranial lesions; respiratory, kidney, or hepatic impairment; CNS depression or coma; thyroid irregularities; adrenal insufficiency; prostatic hyperplasia; urethral stricture; acute alcoholism; delirium tremens; or kyphoscoliosis.

INTERACTIONS

Drug-drug. If administered within a few hours of *barbiturate anesthetic such as thiopental,* buprenorphine may produce additive CNS and respiratory depressant effects and, possibly, apnea. Avoid this practice. *CNS depressants (antihistamines, narcotic analgesics, barbiturates, benzodiazepines, phenothiazines,* and *sedative-hypnotics), muscle relaxants,* and *tricyclic antidepressants* may potentiate the respiratory and CNS depressant, sedative, and hypotensive effects of buprenorphine, so the dosage of buprenorphine will probably need to be reduced. Use with *general anesthetics* may cause severe CV depression. Monitor closely.

Drug-lifestyle. *Alcohol* may potentiate the respiratory and CNS depressant, sedative, and hypotensive effects of the drug. Discourage use.

ADVERSE REACTIONS
CNS: *dizziness, sedation, headache, confusion, nervousness, euphoria, vertigo, increased intracranial pressure.*
CV: *hypotension,* bradycardia, tachycardia, hypertension.
EENT: *miosis,* blurred vision.
GI: *nausea,* vomiting, constipation, dry mouth.
GU: urine retention.
Respiratory: *respiratory depression,* hypoventilation, dyspnea.
Skin: pruritus.
Other: *diaphoresis.*

▣ KEY CONSIDERATIONS
Besides the recommendations relevant to all opioid (narcotic) agonist-antagonists, consider the following:
• Administer with caution to geriatric patients, who may be sensitive to the therapeutic and adverse effects of this drug.
• Adverse effects of drug may not be as readily reversed by naloxone as are those of pure agonists.
• 0.3 mg of buprenorphine is equal to 10 mg of morphine or 75 to 100 mg of meperidine in analgesic potency; duration of analgesia is longer than either.

Patient education
• Teach patient to avoid activities that require full alertness.
• Instruct patient to avoid alcohol and other CNS depressants.

bupropion hydrochloride
Wellbutrin, Wellbutrin SR

Aminoketone, antidepressant

Available by prescription only
Tablets: 75 mg, 100 mg
Tablets (sustained-release): 100 mg, 150 mg

INDICATIONS & DOSAGE
Depression
Adults: Initially, 100 mg P.O. b.i.d. If necessary, increase after 3 days to usual dosage of 100 mg P.O. t.i.d. If no response occurs after several weeks of therapy, consider increasing dosage to 150 mg t.i.d. For sustained-release tablets, start with 150 mg P.O. q morning; increase to target dosage of 150 mg P.O. b.i.d. as tolerated as early as day 4 of dosing. Maximum dosage is 400 mg/day.

PHARMACODYNAMICS
Antidepressant action: Mechanism of action is unknown. Bupropion doesn't inhibit MAO; it's a weak inhibitor of norepinephrine, dopamine, and serotonin reuptake.

PHARMACOKINETICS
Absorption: Animal studies indicate that only 5% to 20% of the drug is bioavailable. Plasma levels peak within 2 to 3 hours.
Distribution: At plasma levels up to 200 mcg/ml, about 80% appears to bind to plasma proteins.
Metabolism: Drug is probably metabolized in the liver; several active metabolites have been identified. With long-term use, the active metabolites are expected to accumulate in the plasma and their levels may exceed that of the parent compound. Drug appears to induce its own metabolism.
Excretion: Drug is primarily excreted by the kidneys; elimination half-life of parent compound in single-dose studies ranged from 8 to 24 hours.

CONTRAINDICATIONS & PRECAUTIONS

Contraindicated in patients with hypersensitivity to bupropion or seizure disorders and who have taken MAO inhibitors within the previous 14 days. Also contraindicated in patients taking Zyban, or those with history of bulimia or anorexia nervosa because of the increased risk of seizures. Use cautiously in patients with a recent MI, unstable heart disease, or renal or hepatic impairment.

INTERACTIONS

Drug-drug. Use with *levodopa, MAO inhibitors, phenothiazines,* or *tricyclic antidepressants* or *recent and rapid withdrawal of benzodiazepines* may increase the risk of adverse effects, including seizures. Monitor closely.
Drug-lifestyle. Use with *alcohol* increases the risk of seizures. Discourage use.

ADVERSE REACTIONS

CNS: *headache, **seizures,** anxiety, confusion,* delusions, euphoria, hostility, impaired sleep quality, *insomnia, sedation, tremor,* akinesia, akathisia, *agitation, dizziness,* fatigue.
CV: ***arrhythmias,*** hypertension, hypotension, palpitations, syncope, *tachycardia.*
EENT: *auditory disturbances,* blurred vision.
GI: *dry mouth,* taste disturbance, increased appetite, *constipation,* dyspepsia, *nausea, vomiting, anorexia,* diarrhea.
GU: impotence, menstrual complaints, urinary frequency, decreased libido, urine retention.
Metabolic: *weight loss, weight gain.*
Musculoskeletal: arthritis.
Skin: pruritus, rash, cutaneous temperature disturbance, *excessive diaphoresis.*
Other: fever, chills.

▣ KEY CONSIDERATIONS

● In general, geriatric patients metabolize drugs more slowly and are more sensitive to the anticholinergic, sedative, and cardiovascular adverse effects of antidepressants.
● Consider the inherent risk of suicide until significant improvement of depres-

sive state occurs. High-risk patients should be closely supervised during initial drug therapy. To reduce risk of suicidal overdose, prescribe the smallest quantity of tablets consistent with good management.
● Many patients experience a period of increased restlessness—including agitation, insomnia, and anxiety—especially when therapy is initiated. In clinical studies, these symptoms required use of a sedative-hypnotic in some patients; about 2% had to discontinue drug.
● Antidepressants can cause manic episodes during the depressed phase in patients with bipolar disorder.
● Clinical trials revealed that 28% of patients experience a weight loss of 2.3 kg (5 lb) or more. This effect should be considered if weight loss is a major factor in patient's depressive illness.

Patient education

● Advise patient to take drug regularly as scheduled and to take each day's dosage in divided doses (as instructed) to minimize risk of seizures.
● Warn patient to avoid the use of alcohol, which may contribute to the development of seizures.
● Advise patient to avoid activities that require alertness and coordination until CNS effects of drug are known.
● Tell patient not to chew, divide, or crush sustained-release tablets.
● Instruct patient not to take Zyban in combination with Wellbutrin or other drugs, including OTC drugs, without the health care provider's approval.

Overdose & treatment

● Signs and symptoms of overdose include labored breathing, salivation, arched back, ptosis, ataxia, and seizures.
● If the ingestion was recent, empty the stomach by performing gastric lavage or inducing vomiting with ipecac, as appropriate; follow with activated charcoal. Treatment should be supportive. Control seizures with I.V. benzodiazepines; if patient is stuporous or comatose or is experiencing seizures, he may need intubation. No data to evaluate the benefits of dialysis, hemoperfusion, or diuresis exists.

---

*Canada only   ◇ Unlabeled clinical use

bupropion hydrochloride
Zyban

Aminoketone, nonnicotine aid to smoking cessation

Available by prescription only
Tablets (sustained-release): 150 mg

INDICATIONS & DOSAGE
Aid to smoking cessation treatment
Adults: 150 mg daily P.O. for 3 days; increased to maximum of 300 mg daily P.O. given as 2 doses of 150 mg taken at least 8 hours apart. Course of treatment is 7 to 12 weeks.
Note: Therapy is started while patient is still smoking; about 1 week is needed to achieve steady-state blood levels of drug. Patient should set target cessation date during 2nd week of treatment.

PHARMACODYNAMICS
Smoking cessation action: The mechanism of action is unknown. Bupropion is a relatively weak inhibitor of the neuronal uptake of norepinephrine, serotonin, and dopamine, and it doesn't inhibit MAO.

PHARMACOKINETICS
Absorption: After oral administration of bupropion, plasma levels peak within 3 hours.
Distribution: Volume of distribution from a single 150-mg dose is estimated to be 1,950 L. At drug levels up to 200 mcg/ml, 84% binds to plasma proteins.
Metabolism: The P-450 2B6 isoenzyme system in the liver extensively metabolizes the drug to three active metabolites.
Excretion: Mean elimination half-life of drug is thought to be about 21 hours. After oral administration, 87% of a dose is recovered in urine and 10% in feces. 0.5% a dose is excreted unchanged.

CONTRAINDICATIONS & PRECAUTIONS
Contraindicated in patients with seizure disorders or with a current or prior diagnosis of bulimia or anorexia nervosa because of potential for seizures. Concurrent administration of MAO inhibitors is contraindicated; at least 14 days must elapse between discontinuation of an MAO inhibitor and initiation of bupropion therapy. Concurrent administration of Wellbutrin, Wellbutrin SR, or others drugs containing bupropion is contraindicated because of potential for seizures. Also contraindicated in patients known to be allergic to drug or to its formulation.

INTERACTIONS
Drug-drug. Use with *levodopa, MAO inhibitors, phenothiazines,* or *tricyclic antidepressants* or *recent and rapid withdrawal of benzodiazepines* may increase the risk of adverse effects, including seizures. Monitor closely.
Drug-lifestyle. Use with *alcohol* increases the risk of seizures. Discourage use.

ADVERSE REACTIONS
CNS: agitation, dizziness, hot flashes, *insomnia,* somnolence, tremor.
CV: *complete AV block,* edema, hypertension, hypotension, tachycardia.
EENT: *dry mouth,* taste perversion.
GI: anorexia, dyspepsia, increased appetite.
GU: impotence, polyuria, urinary frequency and urgency.
Metabolic: weight gain.
Musculoskeletal: arthralgia, leg cramps and twitching, myalgia, neck pain.
Respiratory: bronchitis, ***bronchospasm.***
Skin: dry skin, pruritus, rash, urticaria.
Other: allergic reactions.

▣ KEY CONSIDERATIONS
• In general, geriatric patients metabolize drugs more slowly and are more sensitive to the anticholinergic, sedative and cardiovascular adverse effects of antidepressants.
• Because drug use is associated with a dose-dependent risk of seizures, don't exceed 300 mg daily for smoking cessation.
• If patient hasn't made progress toward abstinence by week 7 of therapy, stop therapy because it's unlikely that he'll quit smoking.
• Dose need not be tapered when stopping treatment.

Reactions may be *common,* uncommon, *life-threatening,* or COMMON AND LIFE-THREATENING.

Patient education
• Stress the importance of combining behavioral interventions, counseling, and support services with drug therapy.
• Inform patient that risk of seizures is increased if he has a seizure or eating disorder (bulimia or anorexia nervosa), exceeds the recommended dose, or takes other drugs containing bupropion.
• Instruct patient to take doses at least 8 hours apart.
• Inform patient that drug is usually taken for 7 to 12 weeks.
• Advise patient that, although he may continue to smoke during drug therapy, it reduces his chance of breaking the smoking habit.
• Advise patient to avoid alcohol while taking the drug because of the increased risk of seizures.
• Tell patient that drug and nicotine patch should only be used together under medical supervision because his blood pressure may increase.

Overdose & treatment
• Hospitalization is recommended for overdoses. If patient is conscious, induce vomiting with ipecac. Activated charcoal may also be administered every 6 hours for first 12 hours. Perform ECG and EEG monitoring for first 48 hours. Provide adequate fluid intake and obtain baseline tests.
• If patient is stuporous or comatose or is experiencing seizures, airway intubation is recommended before undertaking gastric lavage. Gastric lavage may be beneficial within first 12 hours after ingestion because drug absorption may not be complete. Although diuresis, dialysis, or hemoperfusion is sometimes used to treat drug overdose, there's no experience with their use in managing bupropion overdose. Based on animal studies, seizures can be treated with an I.V. benzodiazepine and other supportive measures.

buspirone hydrochloride
BuSpar

Azaspirodecanedione derivative, anxiolytic

Available by prescription only
Tablets: 5 mg, 10 mg

INDICATIONS & DOSAGE
Management of anxiety disorders
Adults: Initially, 5 mg P.O. t.i.d. Dosage may be increased at 3-day intervals. Usual maintenance dosage is 20 to 30 mg daily in divided doses. Maximum daily dosage is 60 mg/day.

PHARMACODYNAMICS
Anxiolytic action: Buspirone is an azaspirodecanedione derivative with anxiolytic activity. It suppresses aggressive behavior and inhibits conditioned avoidance responses. Its precise mechanism of action is unknown, but it appears to depend on simultaneous effects on several neurotransmitters and receptor sites: decreasing serotonin neuronal activity, increasing norepinephrine metabolism, and partial action as a presynaptic dopamine antagonist. Studies suggest an indirect effect on benzodiazepine gamma-aminobutyric acid (GABA)–chloride receptor complex or GABA receptors, or on other neurotransmitter systems.

Buspirone isn't pharmacologically related to benzodiazepines, barbiturates, or other sedative or anxiolytics. It exhibits both a nontraditional clinical profile and is uniquely anxiolytic. It has no anticonvulsant or muscle relaxant activity and doesn't appear to cause physical dependence or significant sedation.

PHARMACOKINETICS
Absorption: Buspirone is absorbed rapidly and completely after oral administration, but extensive first-pass metabolism limits absolute bioavailability to 1% to 13% of the oral dose. Food slows absorption but increases the amount of unchanged drug in systemic circulation.
Distribution: Drug is 95% protein-bound; it doesn't displace other highly

protein-bound drugs such as warfarin. Onset of therapeutic effect may require 1 to 2 weeks.

Metabolism: Drug is metabolized in the liver through hydroxylation and oxidation, resulting in at least one pharmacologically active metabolite—1, pyrimidinylpiperazine (1-PP).

Excretion: 29% to 63% is excreted in urine in 24 hours, primarily as metabolites; 18% to 38%, in feces.

CONTRAINDICATIONS & PRECAUTIONS

Contraindicated in patients hypersensitive to buspirone or within 14 days of therapy with an MAO inhibitor. Use cautiously in patients with renal or hepatic impairment.

INTERACTIONS

Drug-drug. Use with *MAO inhibitors* may elevate blood pressure. Don't use together.

Use with *CNS depressants* may cause sedation, especially with dosages greater than 30 mg/day. Use with *digoxin* may displace digoxin from serum-binding sites. Use with *haloperidol* may increase serum haloperidol levels. Monitor closely.

Drug-lifestyle. Use with *alcohol* may cause sedation, especially with dosages greater than 30 mg/day. Discourage use.

ADVERSE REACTIONS

CNS: *dizziness, drowsiness,* nervousness, insomnia, headache, lightheadedness, fatigue, numbness.
EENT: blurred vision.
GI: dry mouth, nausea, diarrhea, abdominal distress.

▣ KEY CONSIDERATIONS

● Patients who have been treated with benzodiazepines previously may not show good clinical response to this drug.
● Although buspirone doesn't appear to cause tolerance or physical or psychological dependence, the possibility exists that patients prone to drug abuse may experience these effects.
● Buspirone doesn't block the withdrawal syndrome associated with benzodiazepines or other common sedative and hypnotics; therefore, these drugs should be withdrawn gradually before replacement with buspirone therapy.
● Monitor hepatic and renal function; hepatic and renal impairment impedes metabolism and excretion of drug and may lead to toxic accumulation; dosage reduction may be necessary.

Patient education

● Advise patient to take drug exactly as prescribed; explain that therapeutic effect may not occur for 2 weeks or more. Warn patient not to double-dose if one is missed, but to take a missed dose as soon as possible, unless it's almost time for next dose.
● Caution patient to avoid hazardous tasks requiring alertness until effects of the drug are known. The additive sedation and drowsiness that buspirone causes may enhance the effects of alcohol and other CNS depressants (such as antihistamines, sedatives, tranquilizers, sleeping aids, prescription pain relievers, barbiturates, seizure medicine, muscle relaxants, anesthetics, and medicines for colds, coughs, hay fever, or allergies).
● Tell patient to store drug away from heat and light and out of children's reach.
● Explain importance of regular followup visits to check progress. Urge patient to report adverse reactions immediately.
● Inform patient that results may not be seen in 3 to 4 weeks; however, an improvement may be noted within 7 to 10 days.

busulfan
Myleran

Alkylating drug (cell cycle-phase nonspecific), antineoplastic

Available by prescription only
Tablets (scored): 2 mg

INDICATIONS & DOSAGE

Dosage and indications may vary. Check current literature for recommended protocol.

Chronic myelogenous leukemia
Adults: For remission induction, usual dosage is 4 to 8 mg P.O. daily; however,

---

Reactions may be *common,* uncommon, *life-threatening,* or COMMON AND LIFE-THREATENING.

may range from 1 to 12 mg P.O. daily (0.06 mg/kg or 1.8 mg/m²). For maintenance therapy, 1 to 3 mg P.O. daily.

◇ *Myelofibrosis*
Adults: 2 to 4 mg P.O. two to three times weekly.

◇ *Polycythemia vera*
Adults: 2 to 6 mg P.O. daily

◇ *Thrombocytosis*
Adults: 4 to 6 mg P.O. daily

PHARMACODYNAMICS

Antineoplastic action: Busulfan is an alkylating drug that exerts its cytotoxic activity by interfering with DNA replication and RNA transcription, causing a disruption of nucleic acid function.

PHARMACOKINETICS

Absorption: Busulfan is well absorbed from the GI tract.
Distribution: Distribution into the brain and CSF is unknown.
Metabolism: Drug is metabolized in the liver.
Excretion: Busulfan is cleared rapidly from the plasma. Drug and its metabolites are excreted in urine.

CONTRAINDICATIONS & PRECAUTIONS

Contraindicated in patients whose chronic myelogenous leukemia has shown prior resistance to drug. Also contraindicated in patients with chronic lymphocytic leukemia or acute leukemia and in those in "blastic" crisis of chronic myelogenous leukemia.

Use cautiously in patients recently given other myelosuppressants or radiation treatment; in those with depressed neutrophil or platelet counts, head trauma, or seizures; or in those taking other drugs that reduce seizure threshold.

INTERACTIONS

None reported.

ADVERSE REACTIONS

CNS: unusual tiredness or weakness, fatigue.
EENT: cataracts.
GI: cheilosis, dry mouth, anorexia.
GU: gynecomastia.
Hematologic: *leukopenia, thrombocytopenia,* anemia, *severe pancytopenia.*

Hepatic: jaundice.
Metabolic: profound hyperuricemia caused by increased cell lysis.
Respiratory: *irreversible pulmonary fibrosis.*
Skin: alopecia, *transient hyperpigmentation,* rash, urticaria, anhidrosis.
Other: Addison-like wasting syndrome.

▣ KEY CONSIDERATIONS

• Avoid all I.M. injections when platelets are less than 100,000/mm³.
• Patient response (increased appetite, sense of well-being, decreased total leukocyte count, reduction in size of spleen) usually begins 1 to 2 weeks after initiating the drug.
• Watch for signs or symptoms of infection, including fever and sore throat.
• Pulmonary fibrosis may be delayed for 4 to 6 months.
• Persistent cough and progressive dyspnea with alveolar exudate may result from drug toxicity, not pneumonia. Instruct patient to report signs and symptoms so that dosage can be adjusted.
• Monitor uric acid, CBC, and kidney function.
• Drug-induced cellular dysplasia may interfere with interpretation of cytological studies.
• Busulfan therapy may increase blood and urine levels of uric acid as a result of increased purine catabolism that accompanies cell destruction.
• Minimize hyperuricemia by adequate hydration, alkalinization of urine, and administration of allopurinol.

Patient education

• Advise patient to use caution when taking aspirin-containing products and to promptly report any sign of bleeding.
• Tell patient to take drug at same time each day.
• Emphasize importance of continuing to take drug despite nausea and vomiting.
• Instruct patient about the signs and symptoms of infection and tell him to report them promptly if they occur.
• Advise patient to use contraception during therapy.

butabarbital sodium
Butisol

Barbiturate, sedative-hypnotic
Controlled substance schedule III

Available by prescription only
Tablets: 15 mg, 30 mg, 50 mg, 100 mg
Elixir: 30 mg/5 ml

INDICATIONS & DOSAGE
Sedation
Adults: 15 to 30 mg P.O. t.i.d. or q.i.d.
Preoperative sedation
Adults: 50 to 100 mg P.O. 60 to 90 minutes before surgery.
Insomnia
Adults: 50 to 100 mg P.O. h.s.

PHARMACODYNAMICS
Sedative-hypnotic action: The exact cellular site and mechanism of action are unknown. Butabarbital acts throughout the CNS as a nonselective depressant with an intermediate onset and duration of action. The reticular activating system, which controls CNS arousal, is particularly sensitive to the drug. Butabarbital decreases both presynaptic and postsynaptic membrane excitability by facilitating the action of gamma-aminobutyric acid.

PHARMACOKINETICS
Absorption: Butabarbital is well absorbed after oral administration, with plasma levels peaking in 3 to 4 hours. Onset of action occurs in 45 to 60 minutes. Serum levels needed for sedation and hypnosis are 2 to 3 µg/ml and 25 µg/ml, respectively.
Distribution: Drug is well distributed throughout body tissues and fluids.
Metabolism: Drug is metabolized extensively in the liver by oxidation. Its duration of action is 6 to 8 hours.
Excretion: Inactive metabolites of butabarbital are excreted in urine. Only 1% to 2% of an oral dose is excreted in urine unchanged. Terminal half-life ranges from 30 to 40 hours.

CONTRAINDICATIONS & PRECAUTIONS
Contraindicated in patients with bronchopneumonia or other severe pulmonary insufficiency, hypersensitivity to barbiturates, or porphyria. Use cautiously in patients with renal or hepatic impairment, acute or chronic pain, or history of drug abuse.

INTERACTIONS
Drug-drug. Use enhances the enzymatic degradation of *warfarin* and *other oral anticoagulants.* Patients may require increased dosages of the anticoagulants.

Use may add to or potentiate the CNS and respiratory depressant effects of *antidepressants, antihistamines, narcotics, sedative-hypnotics,* and *tranquilizers.* Use with *corticosteroids, digitoxin, oral contraceptives and other estrogens, doxycycline, rifampin, theophylline* or *other xanthines* enhances hepatic metabolism. Use with *disulfiram, MAO inhibitors,* or *valproic acid* decreases the metabolism of butabarbital and can increase its toxicity. Butabarbital impairs the effectiveness of *griseofulvin* by decreasing absorption from the GI tract. Monitor closely.
Drug-lifestyle. Butabarbital may add to or potentiate the CNS and respiratory depressant effects of *alcohol.* Discourage use.

ADVERSE REACTIONS
CNS: *drowsiness, lethargy, hangover,* paradoxical excitement, somnolence.
GI: nausea, vomiting.
Hematologic: exacerbation of porphyria.
Respiratory: *respiratory depression, apnea.*
Skin: rash, urticaria, *Stevens-Johnson syndrome.*
Other: *angioedema,* physical and psychological dependence.

▣ KEY CONSIDERATIONS
Besides the recommendations relevant to all barbiturates, consider the following:
• Geriatric patients are more susceptible to the CNS depressant effects of butabarbital. Confusion, disorientation, and excitability may occur.

Reactions may be *common,* uncommon, *life-threatening,* or COMMON AND LIFE-THREATENING.

• Geriatric patients usually require lower dosages.

• Tablet may be crushed and mixed with food or fluid if patient has difficulty swallowing. Capsule may be opened and contents mixed with food or fluids to aid in swallowing.

• Assess cardiopulmonary status frequently; monitor vital signs for significant changes.

• Monitor patient for possible allergic reaction resulting from tartrazine sensitivity.

• Periodically evaluate blood counts and renal and hepatic studies for abnormalities and adverse effects.

• Monitor PT carefully when patient on butabarbital starts or ends anticoagulant therapy. Anticoagulant dosage may need to be adjusted.

• Watch for signs of barbiturate toxicity, such as coma, pupillary constriction, cyanosis, clammy skin, and hypotension. Overdose can be fatal.

• Prolonged use isn't recommended; drug hasn't been shown to be effective after 14 days. A drug-free interval of at least 1 week is advised between dosing periods.

• Butabarbital may cause a false-positive phentolamine test. The physiological effects of drug may impair the absorption of cyanocobalamin ^{57}Co; it may decrease serum bilirubin levels in epileptic patients and patients with congenital nonhemolytic unconjugated hyperbilirubinemia. EEG patterns are altered, with a change in low-voltage, fast activity; changes persist for a time after discontinuation of therapy. Barbiturates may increase sulfobromophthalein retention.

Patient education
• Tell patient to avoid driving and other hazardous activities that require alertness because the drug may cause drowsiness.

• Warn patient that prolonged use can result in physical or psychological dependence.

• Emphasize the dangers of combining drug with alcohol. Excessive depressant effect is possible, even if drug is taken the evening before ingestion of alcohol.

Overdose & treatment
• Signs and symptoms of overdose include unsteady gait, slurred speech, sustained nystagmus, somnolence, confusion, respiratory depression, pulmonary edema, areflexia, and coma. Jaundice, hypothermia followed by fever, oliguria, and typical shock syndrome with tachycardia and hypotension may occur.

• To treat, maintain and support ventilation and pulmonary function, as necessary; support cardiac function and circulation with vasopressors and I.V. fluids, as needed. If patient is conscious with a functioning gag reflex and ingestion was recent, induce vomiting by administering ipecac syrup. If emesis is contraindicated, perform gastric lavage while a cuffed endotracheal tube is in place, to prevent aspiration. Follow by administering activated charcoal or sodium chloride cathartic. Measure intake and output, vital signs, and laboratory findings. Maintain body temperature. Alkalinization of urine may be helpful in removing drug from the body; hemodialysis may be useful in severe overdose.

butorphanol tartrate
Stadol, Stadol NS

Narcotic agonist-antagonist; opioid partial agonist, analgesic, adjunct to anesthesia

Available by prescription only
Injection: 1 mg/ml, 1-ml vials; 2 mg/ml, 1-ml, 2-ml, and 10-ml vials
Nasal spray: 10 mg/ml

INDICATIONS & DOSAGE
Moderate to severe pain
Adults: 1 to 4 mg I.M. q 3 to 4 hours, p.r.n.; or 0.5 to 2 mg I.V. q 3 to 4 hours, p.r.n., or around-the-clock. Alternatively, give 1 mg by nasal spray (1 spray in one nostril). Repeat if pain relief is inadequate after 1 to 1½ hours. Repeat q 3 to 4 hours, p.r.n.
Preoperative anesthesia
Adults: 2 mg I.M. 60 to 90 minutes before surgery or 2 mg I.V. shortly before induction.

Geriatric patients: Reduce dosage. Give 50% of the parenteral adult dosage q 6 hours, p.r.n. Initial dose of nasal solution is 1 mg. An additional 1 mg may be give nasally within 1½ to 2 hours. Repeat initial dosage sequence q 6 hours, p.r.n.

✦ *Dosage adjustment.* Patients with hepatic or renal insufficiency should receive the reduced geriatric dosage.

PHARMACODYNAMICS

Analgesic action: The exact mechanism of action is unknown. Butorphanol is believed to be a competitive antagonist at some, and an agonist at other, opiate receptors, thus relieving moderate to severe pain. Like narcotic agonists, it causes respiratory depression, sedation, and miosis.

PHARMACOKINETICS

Absorption: Butorphanol is well absorbed after I.M. administration. Onset of analgesia after parenteral administration is less than 10 minutes, with peak analgesic effect at ½ to 1 hour. Onset of analgesia usually occurs within 15 minutes after nasal administration.

Distribution: The highest levels of butorphanol and its metabolites are found in the liver, kidneys, and intestines; 80% binds to plasma proteins.

Metabolism: Metabolized extensively in the liver, primarily through hydroxylation, to inactive metabolites.

Excretion: Duration of effect is 3 to 4 hours after parenteral administration and 4 to 5 hours after nasal administration. Butorphanol is excreted in inactive form, mainly by the kidneys. 11% to 14% of a parenteral dose is excreted in feces.

CONTRAINDICATIONS & PRECAUTIONS

Contraindicated in patients who are receiving repeated doses of narcotics or who are addicted to narcotics; may precipitate withdrawal syndrome. Also contraindicated in patients with hypersensitivity to butorphanol or to the preservative benzethonium chloride.

Use cautiously in emotionally unstable patients and in those with history of drug abuse, head injuries, increased intracranial pressure, acute MI, ventricular dysfunction, coronary insufficiency, respiratory disease or depression, or renal or hepatic dysfunction.

INTERACTIONS

Drug-drug. If administered within a few hours of *barbiturate anesthetics such as thiopental,* butorphanol may produce additive CNS and respiratory depressant effects and, possibly, apnea. Monitor closely.

Use with *cimetidine* may potentiate butorphanol toxicity, causing disorientation, respiratory depression, apnea, and seizures. Because data are limited, this combination isn't contraindicated; however, be prepared to administer a narcotic antagonist if toxicity occurs.

Because *CNS depressants*—such as *antihistamines, barbiturates, benzodiazepines, muscle relaxants, narcotic analgesics, phenothiazines, sedative-hypnotics,* and *tricyclic antidepressants*—may potentiate respiratory and CNS depressant, sedative, and hypotensive effects of butorphanol, reduced dosages of butorphanol are usually necessary. Use with *general anesthetics* may also cause severe CV depression.

Drug accumulation and enhanced effects may result if drug is given with other drugs—such as *digitoxin, phenytoin,* or *rifampin*—that are extensively metabolized in the liver. Patients who are physically dependent on opioids may experience acute withdrawal syndrome if given a narcotic antagonist. Use with caution and monitor closely.

Use with *pancuronium* may increase conjunctival changes. Monitor closely.

Drug-lifestyle. *Alcohol* may increase the CNS effects of the drug.

ADVERSE REACTIONS

CNS: *confusion,* nervousness, lethargy, headache, *somnolence, dizziness, insomnia,* anxiety, paresthesia, euphoria, hallucinations, flushing, ***increased intracranial pressure.***

CV: palpitations, vasodilation, hypotension.

EENT: blurred vision, *nasal congestion* (with nasal spray), tinnitus, taste perversion.

GI: *nausea, vomiting, constipation,* anorexia.

Reactions may be *common,* uncommon, *life-threatening,* or COMMON AND LIFE-THREATENING.

Respiratory: *respiratory depression.*
Skin: rash, hives, *clamminess, excessive diaphoresis.*
Other: sensation of heat.

▣ KEY CONSIDERATIONS

Besides the recommendations relevant to all opioid (narcotic) agonist-antagonists, consider the following:
• Lower dosages are usually indicated for geriatric patients because they may be more sensitive to the therapeutic and adverse effects of the drug. Plasma half-life is increased by 25% in patients older than age 65.
• Patients who are using nasal formulation for severe pain may initiate therapy with 2 mg (one spray in each nostril) provided they remain recumbent. Dosage isn't repeated for 3 to 4 hours.
• Drug has the potential for abuse. Closely supervise use in emotionally unstable patients and in those with history of drug abuse when long-term therapy is necessary.
• Mild withdrawal symptoms have been reported with long-term use of the injectable form.

Patient education

• Teach patient how to use nasal spray. Patient should use one spray in one nostril unless otherwise directed.

---

calcifediol
Calderol

Vitamin D analogue, antihypocalcemic

Available by prescription only
Capsules: 20 mcg, 50 mcg

INDICATIONS & DOSAGE
Management of metabolic bone disease or hypocalcemia in patients on long-term renal dialysis
Adults: Initially, 300 to 350 mcg/week P.O. given daily or every other day. May increase dose at 4-week intervals based on serum levels. Most patients respond to 50 to 100 mcg/day or 100 to 200 mcg every other day. Some patients with normal calcium levels respond to doses of 20 mcg every other day.

PHARMACODYNAMICS
Antihypocalcemic action: Calcifediol is a vitamin D analogue (25-hydroxycholecalciferol) that works with parathyroid hormone to regulate serum calcium; drug must be activated for its full effect, but it appears to have some intrinsic activity.

PHARMACOKINETICS
Absorption: Calcifediol is absorbed readily from the small intestine.
Distribution: Drug is distributed widely and is highly protein-bound.
Metabolism: Drug is metabolized in the liver and kidney; half-life is 16 days. It's activated to 1,25-dihydroxycholecalciferol.
Excretion: Drug is excreted in urine and bile.

CONTRAINDICATIONS & PRECAUTIONS
Contraindicated in patients with hypercalcemia or vitamin D toxicity.

INTERACTIONS
Drug-drug. *Antacids* and *mineral oil* may alter calcifediol absorption. *Barbiturates, phenytoin,* and *primidone* may increase metabolism and reduce activity of calcifediol. Calcifediol increases calcium levels, which may potentiate the effects of *cardiac glycosides*. Use with *cholestyramine* or *colestipol hydrochloride* may reduce intestinal absorption. *Corticosteroids* counteract the effects of vitamin D analogues. *Thiazide diuretics* may cause hypercalcemia.

ADVERSE REACTIONS
CNS: headache, somnolence, weakness, irritability, psychosis (rare).
CV: hypertension, ***arrhythmias.***
EENT: conjunctivitis, photosensitivity reactions, rhinorrhea.
GI: constipation, nausea, vomiting, polydipsia, ***pancreatitis,*** metallic taste, dry mouth, anorexia, diarrhea.
GU: polyuria, nocturia, decreased libido, nephrocalcinosis.
Metabolic: weight loss.
Musculoskeletal: bone and muscle pain.
Skin: pruritus.
Other: hyperthermia.

▣ KEY CONSIDERATIONS
• Before initiating therapy, make sure serum phosphate levels are controlled. Serum calcium level (mg/dl) multiplied by serum phosphorus level (mg/dl) shouldn't exceed 70 mg/dl, to avoid ectopic calcification.
• Monitor serum calcium levels several times weekly when initiating therapy.
• Monitoring urine calcium and urine creatinine levels is helpful in screening for hypercalciuria. The ratio of urine calcium to urine creatinine should be less than or equal to 0.18. A value above 0.2 suggests hypercalciuria, so the dosage should be decreased regardless of serum calcium level.
• Calcifediol may falsely elevate cholesterol levels when using the Zlatkis-Zak reaction.

Patient education
• Explain importance of a calcium-rich diet.

Overdose & treatment
• The only sign of overdose is hypercalcemia. Treatment involves discontinuing therapy, instituting a low-calcium diet, and increasing fluid intake. Provide supportive measures. Severe overdose has led to death from cardiac and renal failure. Calcitonin administration may be useful in hypercalcemia.

---

calcipotriene
Dovonex

Synthetic vitamin D₃ analogue, topical antipsoriatic

Available by prescription only
Cream, lotion, ointment: 0.005%

INDICATIONS & DOSAGE
Moderate plaque psoriasis
Adults: Apply a thin layer to affected skin b.i.d. Rub in gently and completely.

PHARMACODYNAMICS
Antipsoriatic action: Calcipotriene is a synthetic vitamin D_3 analogue that binds to vitamin D_3 receptors in skin cells (keratinocytes), regulating skin cell production and development.

PHARMACOKINETICS
Absorption: When applied topically to psoriasis plaques, about 6% of the dose of calcipotriene is absorbed systemically; when applied to normal skin, about 5% is absorbed.
Distribution: Vitamin D and its metabolites are transported in the blood, bound to specific plasma proteins, to many parts of the body containing keratinocytes. (The scaly red patches of psoriasis are caused by the abnormal growth and production of keratinocytes.)
Metabolism: Drug metabolism after systemic uptake is rapid and occurs via a pathway similar to the natural hormone. The primary metabolites are much less potent than the parent compound.
Excretion: The active form of the vitamin—1,25-dihydroxy vitamin D_3 (calcitriol)—is recycled via the liver and is excreted in bile.

CONTRAINDICATIONS & PRECAUTIONS
Contraindicated in patients hypersensitive to calcipotriene or its components. Also contraindicated in patients with hypercalcemia or evidence of vitamin D toxicity. Use cautiously in geriatric patients. Drug should not be used on the face.

INTERACTIONS
None reported.

ADVERSE REACTIONS
Metabolic: hypercalcemia.
Skin: *burning, pruritus, irritation,* atrophy, dermatitis, dry skin, erythema, folliculitis, hyperpigmentation, peeling, rash, worsening of psoriasis.

▣ KEY CONSIDERATIONS
• Adverse dermatologic effects may be more severe in patients older than age 65.
• Drug is for topical dermatologic use only. It isn't intended for ophthalmic, oral, or intravaginal use.
• Improvement usually begins after 2 weeks of therapy. About 70% of patients show marked improvement after 8 weeks of therapy; up to 10% show complete clearing.
• It's unknown whether topical calcipotriene can be used safely and effectively in dermatoses other than psoriasis.
• Calcipotriene may irritate lesions and surrounding uninvolved skin. If irritation develops, the drug should be discontinued.
• In some patients, calcipotriene has caused a transient, rapidly reversible elevation of the serum calcium level. If the serum calcium level rises above the normal range, discontinue treatment until normal calcium levels are restored.

Patient education
• Tell patient that drug is for external use only, as directed, and to avoid contact with the face and eyes.
• Instruct patient to wash hands thoroughly after applying the drug.
• Advise patient only to use the drug for disorders for which it was prescribed.
• Tell patient to report signs of local adverse reactions.

---

calcitonin
Calcimar (salmon), Cibacalcin (human), Miacalcin (salmon)

Thyroid hormone, hypocalcemic

Available by prescription only
Injection: 200-IU/ml, 2-ml vials (salmon); 0.5 mg/vial (human)
Nasal spray: 200 IU/activation

INDICATIONS & DOSAGE
Paget's disease of bone (osteitis deformans)
Adults: Initially, 100 IU calcitonin (salmon) S.C. or I.M. daily or 0.5 mg calcitonin (human) S.C. Maintenance dosage is 50 to 100 IU calcitonin (salmon) three times weekly, 0.5 mg calcitonin (human) two or three times weekly, or 0.25 mg calcitonin (human) daily.
Hypercalcemia
Adults: 4 IU/kg calcitonin (salmon) I.M. or S.C. q 12 hours, increased by 8 IU/kg q 12 hours.
Postmenopausal osteoporosis
Adults: 100 IU calcitonin (salmon) S.C. or I.M. daily or 200 IU (1 spray) daily, alternating nostrils.
◇ Osteogenesis imperfecta
Adults: 2 IU/kg calcitonin (salmon) three times weekly combined with a daily calcium supplement.

PHARMACODYNAMICS
Hypocalcemic action: Calcitonin directly inhibits the bone resorption of calcium. This effect is mediated by drug-induced increase of cAMP levels in bone cells, which alters transport of calcium and phosphate across the plasma membrane of the osteoclast. A secondary effect occurs in the kidneys, where calcitonin directly inhibits tubular resorption of calcium, phosphate, and sodium, thereby increasing their excretion. The therapeutic effect of the drug may not be apparent for several months in patients with Paget's disease. Calcitonin salmon and calcitonin human are pharmacologically the same, but calcitonin salmon is more potent and has a longer duration of action.

PHARMACOKINETICS
Absorption: Calcitonin can be administered parenterally or nasally. Within 15 minutes of a 200-IU S.C. dose, the plasma calcitonin level ranges between 0.1 and 0.4 mg/ml. The maximum effect is seen in 2 to 4 hours; duration of action may be 8 to 24 hours for S.C. or I.M. doses, and ½ to 12 hours for I.V. doses. Peak plasma level appears 31 to 39 minutes after using the nasal form.
Distribution: It's unknown if the drug enters the CNS.
Metabolism: Drug is rapidly metabolized in the kidney, with additional activity in the blood and peripheral tissues. Calcitonin salmon has a longer half-life than calcitonin human, which has a 1-hour half-life.
Excretion: Drug is excreted in urine as inactive metabolites.

CONTRAINDICATIONS & PRECAUTIONS
Contraindicated in patients who are hypersensitive to calcitonin salmon. Calcitonin human has no contraindications.

INTERACTIONS
None reported.

ADVERSE REACTIONS
CNS: headache, weakness, dizziness, paresthesia.
CV: chest pressure, edema of feet.
EENT: eye pain, nasal congestion.
GI: transient *nausea,* unusual taste, diarrhea, anorexia, *vomiting,* epigastric discomfort, abdominal pain.
GU: *increased urinary frequency,* nocturia.
Respiratory: shortness of breath.
Skin: *facial flushing,* rash, pruritus of ear lobes, *inflammation at injection site.*
Other: hypersensitivity reactions *(anaphylaxis),* chills, tender palms and soles.

▣ KEY CONSIDERATIONS
• The S.C. route is preferred.
• Calcitonin (salmon) dosages are expressed in international units and calcitonin (human) dosages are expressed in milligrams. Don't confuse units of measurement.
• Before initiating therapy with calcitonin (salmon), consider performing a

---

Reactions may be *common*, uncommon, *life-threatening*, or COMMON AND LIFE-THREATENING.

skin test using calcitonin (salmon). If patient has allergic reactions to foreign proteins, test for hypersensitivity before therapy. Systemic allergic reactions are possible because the hormone is a protein. Epinephrine should be readily available.

• Keep parenteral calcium available during the first doses in case of hypocalcemic tetany.

• Periodically monitor serum calcium levels during therapy.

• During therapy, observe patient for signs of hypocalcemic tetany, such as muscle twitching, tetanic spasms, and convulsions if hypocalcemia is severe.

• Watch for signs and symptoms of hypercalcemic relapse: bone pain, renal calculi, polyuria, anorexia, nausea, vomiting, thirst, constipation, lethargy, bradycardia, muscle hypotonicity, pathologic fracture, psychosis, and coma. Patients with good initial response to calcitonin who suffer relapse should be evaluated for antibody formation response to the hormone protein.

• Refrigerate solution. Once activated, nasal spray should be stored upright at room temperature.

Patient education

• Instruct patient on self-administration of drug and assist him until he achieves proper technique.

• Tell patient to handle missed doses as follows: With daily dosing, take the dose as soon as possible, but don't double-dose. With every-other-day dosing, take the dose as soon as possible, then restart the alternate days from this dose.

• Stress importance of regular follow-up to assess progress.

• If drug is given for postmenopausal osteoporosis, remind patient to take calcium and vitamin D supplements.

• Instruct patient using the nasal spray to first activate pump.

• Tell patient to call if nasal irritation occurs. Periodic nasal examination should be performed.

Overdose & treatment

• Signs and symptoms of overdose include hypocalcemia and hypocalcemic tetany. Overdose usually occurs in patients at higher risk during the first few doses. Parenteral calcium corrects these signs and symptoms, so it should be readily available.

calcitriol
Calcijex, Rocaltrol

Vitamin D analogue, antihypocalcemic

Available by prescription only
Capsules: 0.25 mcg, 0.5 mcg
Injection: 1 mcg/ml, 2 mcg/ml
Oral solution: 1 mcg/ml

INDICATIONS & DOSAGE
Management of hypocalcemia in patients undergoing long-term renal dialysis
Oral
Adults: Initially, 0.25 mcg P.O. daily. Dosage may be increased by 0.25 mcg daily at 4- to 8-week intervals. Maintenance dosage is 0.25 mcg every other day up to 0.5 to 1 mcg daily.
Parenteral
Adults: 0.5 mcg I.V. three times weekly, about every other day. Dosage may be increased by 0.25 to 0.5 mcg at 2- to 4-week intervals. Maintenance dosage is 0.5 to 3 mcg I.V. three times weekly.
Management of hypoparathyroidism and pseudohypoparathyroidism
Adults: Initially, 0.25 mcg P.O. daily in the morning. Dosage may be increased at 2- to 4-week intervals. Maintenance dosage is 0.5 to 2 mcg daily.
◊ *Psoriasis vulgaris*
Adults: 0.5 mcg/day P.O. for 6 months and topically (0.5 mcg/g petroleum jelly) daily for 8 weeks.

PHARMACODYNAMICS
Antihypocalcemic action: Calcitriol, or activated cholecalciferol, is a vitamin D analogue (1,25-dihydroxycholecalciferol). It promotes absorption of calcium from the intestine by forming a calcium-binding protein. It reverses the signs of rickets and osteomalacia in patients who can't activate or use ergocalciferol or cholecalciferol. In patients with renal

failure it reduces bone pain, muscle weakness, and parathyroid serum levels.

PHARMACOKINETICS

Absorption: Calcitriol is absorbed readily after oral administration.

Distribution: Drug is distributed widely and is protein-bound.

Metabolism: Drug is metabolized in the liver and kidney, with a half-life of 3 to 8 hours. No activation step is required.

Excretion: Drug is excreted primarily in feces.

CONTRAINDICATIONS & PRECAUTIONS

Contraindicated in patients with hypercalcemia or vitamin D toxicity. Withhold all preparations containing vitamin D.

INTERACTIONS

Drug-drug. *Antacids, cholestyramine, colestipol,* and *mineral oil* may alter calcitriol absorption. *Barbiturates, phenytoin,* and *primidone* may increase metabolism of calcitriol and reduce activity. Increased calcium levels may potentiate the effects of *cardiac glycosides. Corticosteroids* may counteract the effects of vitamin D analogues. *Thiazide diuretics* may result in hypercalcemia.

ADVERSE REACTIONS

CNS: headache, somnolence, weakness, irritability, psychosis (rare).

CV: hypertension, ***arrhythmias.***

EENT: conjunctivitis, photophobia, rhinorrhea.

GI: nausea, vomiting, constipation, polydipsia, ***pancreatitis,*** metallic taste, dry mouth, anorexia.

GU: polyuria, nocturia, decreased libido, nephrocalcinosis.

Metabolic: weight loss.

Musculoskeletal: bone and muscle pain.

Skin: pruritus.

Other: hyperthermia.

▣ KEY CONSIDERATIONS

● Monitor serum calcium levels several times weekly after initiating therapy.

● Monitoring urine calcium and urine creatinine levels is helpful in screening for hypercalciuria. The ratio of urine calcium to urine creatinine should be less than or equal to 0.18. A value above 0.2 suggests hypercalciuria, so the dosage should be decreased regardless of serum calcium level.

● Calcitriol therapy may falsely elevate cholesterol determinations made using the Zlatkis-Zak reaction.

● Protect drug from heat and light.

Patient education

● Instruct patient on the importance of a calcium-rich diet.

● Advise patient to report adverse reactions immediately.

● Tell patient to avoid magnesium-containing antacids and other self-prescribed drugs.

Overdose & treatment

● A sign of overdose is hypercalcemia. Treatment requires discontinuation of drug, institution of a low-calcium diet, increased fluid intake, and supportive measures. Calcitonin may help reverse hypercalcemia. Death has followed CV and renal failure.

calcium polycarbophil
Equalactin, Fiberall, FiberCon, Fiber-Lax, Mitrolan

Hydrophilic, bulk laxative, antidiarrheal

Available without a prescription

Tablets: 500 mg (FiberCon), 625 mg (Fiber-Lax)

Tablets (chewable): 500 mg (Equalactin, Fiber-Lax, Mitrolan), 1,000 mg (Fiberall)

INDICATIONS & DOSAGE

Constipation; acute nonspecific diarrhea from irritable bowel syndrome

Adults: 1 g P.O. q.i.d. as required. Maximum dosage is 6 g/24 hours.

PHARMACODYNAMICS

Laxative action: Calcium polycarbophil absorbs water and expands, thereby increasing stool bulk and moisture and promoting normal peristalsis and bowel motility.

Antidiarrheal action: Calcium polycarbophil absorbs intestinal fluid, thereby restoring normal stool consistency and bulk.

PHARMACOKINETICS
Absorption: None.
Distribution: None.
Metabolism: None.
Excretion: Drug is excreted in feces.

CONTRAINDICATIONS & PRECAUTIONS
Contraindicated in patients with GI obstruction because calcium polycarbophil may exacerbate this condition.

INTERACTIONS
Drug-drug. Calcium polycarbophil may impair *tetracycline* absorption.

ADVERSE REACTIONS
GI: abdominal fullness and increased flatus, intestinal obstruction.
Other: laxative dependence (with long-term or excessive use).

▣ KEY CONSIDERATIONS
• Patient must chew tablets (chewable) before swallowing; administer tablets with 8 oz (240 ml) of fluid. Administer less fluid for antidiarrheal effect.
• When using drug as an antidiarrheal, don't give if the patient has a high fever.

Patient education
• *For chewable tablets:* Instruct patient to chew tablets instead of swallowing them whole. If drug is being taken as a laxative, advise patient to drink a full glass (8 oz) of fluid after each tablet; if drug is being taken as an antidiarrheal, the patient should drink less fluid.
• Warn patient not to take more than 12 tablets in 24-hour period and to take for length of time prescribed.
• If patient is taking drug as laxative, advise him to call health care provider promptly and discontinue drug if constipation persists after 1 week or if fever, nausea, vomiting, or abdominal pain occurs.
• Instruct patient that dose may be taken every 30 minutes for acute diarrhea, but not to exceed maximum daily dosage.
• Tell patient that if abdominal discomfort or fullness occurs, he may take smaller doses more frequently throughout the day, at regular intervals.

---

calcium salts

calcium acetate
Phos-Ex, PhosLo

calcium carbonate
Alka-mints, Amitone, Calciday 667, Cal-Plus, Caltrate 600, Chooz, Os-Cal 500, Rolaids, Titralac, Tums, Tums E-X

calcium chloride

calcium citrate
Citracal

calcium glubionate
Neo-Calglucon

calcium gluceptate

calcium gluconate

calcium lactate

calcium phosphate, tribasic
Posture

Calcium supplement, therapeutic drug for electrolyte balance, cardiotonic

---

Available by prescription only
calcium chloride
Injection: 10% solution (1 g/10 ml; each milliliter of solution provides 27.2 mg or 1.36 mEq of calcium) in 10-ml ampules, vials, and syringes
calcium gluceptate
Injection: 1.1 g/5 ml ampules or 50-ml vials for preparation of I.V. admixtures (each milliliter of solution provides 18 mg or 0.9 mEq of calcium)
calcium gluconate
Injection: 10% solution (1 g/10 ml; each milliliter of solution provides 9.3 mg or 0.46 mEq of calcium) in 10-ml ampules and vials, or 20-ml vials

Available without a prescription
calcium acetate
Tablets: 250 mg (62.5 mg of calcium),
668 mg (167 mg of calcium), 1,000 mg
(250 mg of calcium)
Capsules: 500 mg
calcium carbonate
Tablets: 500 mg, 650 mg, 667 mg,
1.25 g, 1.5 g
Tablets (chewable): 350 mg, 420 mg,
500 mg, 750 mg, 835 mg, 850 mg,
1.25 g
Oral suspension: 1.25 g (500 mg of calcium) per 5 ml
Capsules: 1.25 g (500 mg of calcium),
1.5 g (600 mg of calcium)
Powder: 6.5 g
calcium citrate
Tablets: 950 mg (contains 200 mg of elemental calcium/g)
Tablets (effervescent): 2,376 mg (500
mg of calcium)
calcium glubionate
Syrup: 1.8 g/5 ml (contains 115 mg of
elemental calcium/g)
calcium gluconate
Tablets: 500 mg, 650 mg, 975 mg, 1 g
(contains 90 mg of elemental calcium/g)
calcium lactate
Tablets: 325 mg, 650 mg (contains
130 mg of elemental calcium/g)
calcium phosphate, tribasic
Tablets: 600 mg

INDICATIONS & DOSAGE
Emergency treatment of hypocalcemia
calcium chloride
Adults: 500 mg to 1 g I.V. slowly (not to
exceed 1 ml/minute).
calcium gluconate
Adults: 7 to 14 mEq I.V. slowly (not to
exceed 0.7 to 1.8 mEq/minute).
Repeat above dosage based on laboratory value.
Hyperkalemia
calcium gluconate
Adults: 2.25 to 14 mEq I.V. slowly. Administration must be titrated based on
ECG response.
Hypermagnesemia
calcium chloride
Adults: 500 mg I.V. initially, repeated
based on response.
calcium gluceptate
Adults: 2 to 5 ml I.M., or 5 to 20 ml I.V.

calcium gluconate
Adults: 4.5 to 9 mEq I.V. slowly.
Hypocalcemia
calcium acetate
Adults: 2 to 4 tablets P.O. with meals.
calcium chloride
Adults: for hypocalcemic tetany, 4.5 to
16 mEq I.V. until therapeutic response is
obtained.
calcium lactate
Adults: 325 mg to 1.3 g P.O. t.i.d. with
meals.
***Hyperphosphatemia in end-stage renal
failure***
calcium acetate
Adults: 2 to 4 tablets with each meal.
Cardiotonic use
calcium chloride
Adults: 500 mg to 1 g I.V. slowly (not to
exceed 1 ml/minute); or 200 to 800 mg
intraventricularly as a single dose.
During exchange transfusions
Adults: 1.35 mEq I.V. concurrently with
each 100-ml citrated blood exchange.
Osteoporosis prevention
Adults: 1 to 1.5 g P.O. daily of elemental
calcium.

PHARMACODYNAMICS
Calcium replacement: Calcium is essential for maintaining the functional integrity of the nervous, muscular, and
skeletal systems and for ensuring cell
membrane and capillary permeability.
Calcium salts are used as a source of calcium cation to treat or prevent calcium
depletion in patients in whom dietary
measures are inadequate. Conditions associated with hypocalcemia are chronic
diarrhea, vitamin D deficiency, steatorrhea, sprue, menopause, pancreatitis, renal failure, alkalosis, hyperphosphatemia, and hypoparathyroidism.

PHARMACOKINETICS
Absorption: I.M. and I.V. calcium salts
are absorbed directly into the bloodstream. I.V. injection gives an immediate
blood level, which will decrease to previous levels in about 30 to 120 minutes.
Oral doses are absorbed actively in the
duodenum and proximal jejunum and, to
a lesser extent, in the distal part of the
small intestine. Calcium is absorbed
only in the ionized form. Vitamin D in

its active form is required for calcium absorption.

Distribution: Calcium enters the extracellular fluid and is incorporated rapidly into skeletal tissue. Bone contains 99% of the total calcium; 1% is distributed equally between the intracellular and extracellular fluids. CSF levels are about 50% of serum calcium levels.

Metabolism: None significant.

Excretion: Calcium is excreted mainly in feces as unabsorbed calcium, secreted via bile and pancreatic juice into the lumen of the GI tract. Most calcium entering the kidney is reabsorbed in the loop of Henle and the proximal and distal convoluted tubules. Only a small amount of calcium is excreted in the urine.

CONTRAINDICATIONS & PRECAUTIONS

Contraindicated in patients with ventricular fibrillation, hypercalcemia, hypophosphatemia, or renal calculi. Use cautiously in patients with sarcoidosis, renal or cardiac disease, cor pulmonale, respiratory acidosis, or respiratory failure and in patients receiving digoxin.

INTERACTIONS

Drug-drug. Administration with *atenolol, iron salts* or *quinolones* (such as *norfloxacin*) may decrease levels of these drugs. Calcium may antagonize the therapeutic effects of *calcium channel blockers,* such as *verapamil.* Calcium shouldn't be mixed with *carbonates, phosphates, sulfates,* or *tartrates,* especially at high levels. Use with *cardiac glycosides* increases *digitalis* toxicity; administer calcium very cautiously, if at all, to patients receiving digoxin. Calcium competes with *magnesium* and may compete for absorption, thus decreasing the bioavailability of *magnesium.* Administration of oral calcium decreases the therapeutic effect of *tetracycline* as a result of chelation.

Drug-food. *Oxalic acid* (found in *rhubarb* and *spinach*), *caffeine, phosphorus* (in *dairy products*), and *phytic acid* (in *bran* and *whole grain cereals*) may interfere with absorption of calcium.

Drug-lifestyle. *Alcohol* and *tobacco* may interfere with absorption of calcium.

ADVERSE REACTIONS

CNS: tingling sensations, sense of oppression or heat waves, headache, irritability, weakness (with I.V. use); syncope (with rapid I.V. injection).

CV: mild fall in blood pressure, vasodilation, bradycardia, *arrhythmias, cardiac arrest* (with rapid I.V. injection).

GI: irritation, hemorrhage, *constipation* (with oral use); chalky taste, rebound hyperacidity, *nausea* (with I.V. use); hemorrhage, nausea, vomiting, thirst, abdominal pain (with oral calcium chloride).

GU: hypercalcemia, polyuria, renal calculi.

Skin: local reactions including burning, necrosis, tissue sloughing, cellulitis, soft-tissue calcification (with I.M. use).

Other: pain and irritation (with S.C. injection), *vein irritation* (with I.V. use).

▣ KEY CONSIDERATIONS

• Calcium absorption (after oral administration) may be decreased in geriatric patients.

• Monitor ECG when giving calcium I.V. Such injections should be given slowly at a rate dependent on salt form used. Stop injection if patient complains of discomfort.

• Calcium chloride should be given I.V. only.

• I.V. calcium should be administered slowly through a small-bore needle into a large vein to avoid extravasation and necrosis.

• After I.V. injection, patient should be recumbent for 15 minutes to prevent orthostasis.

• If perivascular infiltration occurs, discontinue I.V. therapy immediately. Venospasm may be reduced by administering 1% procaine hydrochloride and hyaluronidase to the affected area.

• I.V. calcium may produce transient elevation of plasma 11-hydroxycorticosteroid levels (Glen-Nelson technique) and false-negative values for serum and urine magnesium as measured by the Titan yellow method.

• Use I.M. route only in emergencies when no I.V. route is available. Give I.M. injections in the gluteal region in adults.
• Monitor serum calcium levels frequently, especially in patients with renal impairment.
• Hypercalcemia may result when large dosages are given to patients with chronic renal failure.
• Severe necrosis and sloughing of tissue may occur after extravasation. Calcium gluconate is less irritating to veins and tissue than calcium chloride.
• Assess Chvostek's and Trousseau's signs periodically to check for tetany.
• Crash carts usually contain both calcium gluconate and calcium chloride. Be sure to specify form to be administered.
• If GI upset occurs with oral calcium, give 2 to 3 hours after meals.
• With oral product, patient may need laxatives or stool softeners to manage constipation.
• Monitor for signs and symptoms of hypercalcemia—such as nausea, vomiting, headache, mental confusion, and anorexia—and report them immediately. Calcium absorption of an oral dose is decreased in patients with certain disease states such as achlorhydria, renal osteodystrophy, steatorrhea, or uremia.

Patient education
• Tell patient not to exceed the manufacturer's recommended dosage of calcium.
• Warn patient not to use bone meal or dolomite as a source of calcium; both may contain lead.
• Advise patient to avoid tobacco and to limit intake of alcohol and caffeine-containing beverages.

Overdose & treatment
• Acute hypercalcemia syndrome is characterized by a markedly elevated plasma calcium level, lethargy, weakness, nausea and vomiting, and coma and may lead to sudden death.
• In case of overdose, calcium should be discontinued immediately. After oral ingestion of calcium overdose, treatment includes removal by emesis or gastric lavage followed by supportive therapy, as needed.

candesartan cilexetil
Atacand

Angiotensin II receptor antagonist, antihypertensive

Available by prescription only
Tablets: 4 mg, 8 mg, 16 mg, 32 mg

INDICATIONS & DOSAGE
Treatment of hypertension (used alone or in combination with other antihypertensives)
Adults: initially, 16 mg P.O. once daily when used as monotherapy; usual dosage range is 8 to 32 mg P.O. once or twice daily.
✦ *Dosage adjustment:* In patients for whom intravascular volume may be depleted, such as those treated with diuretics (particularly those with impaired renal function), consider initiating therapy with a lower dosage.

PHARMACODYNAMICS
Candesartan inhibits the vasoconstrictive and aldosterone-secreting action of angiotensin II by blocking the binding of angiotensin II to the angiotension I receptor in many tissues including vascular smooth muscle.

PHARMACOKINETICS
Absorption: Candesartan is rapidly and completely bioactivated during absorption in the GI tract. Absolute bioavailability is 15%. Peak serum level is reached after 3 to 4 hours. Peak plasma level is 50% higher in geriatric patients and the area under the curve is 80% higher; dosage doesn't need to be adjusted.
Distribution: More than 99% of the drug binds to plasma proteins.
Metabolism: A small amount of drug is metabolized in the liver to an inactive metabolite.
Excretion: Drug is excreted in both urine (26% unchanged) and feces. Elimination half-life is about 9 hours.

CONTRAINDICATIONS & PRECAUTIONS
Contraindicated in patients with hypersensitivity to candesartan or its ingredients. Use cautiously in patients who are

---

Reactions may be *common*, uncommon, *life-threatening*, or COMMON AND LIFE-THREATENING.

volume- or salt-depleted, because of the potential for symptomatic hypotension. Consider starting with a lower dosage and monitor blood pressure carefully. Use cautiously in patients whose renal function depends on the renin-angiotensin-aldosterone system (such as patients with heart failure), because of the potential for oliguria and progressive azotemia with acute renal failure or death.

INTERACTIONS
None reported.

ADVERSE REACTIONS
CNS: dizziness, fatigue, headache.
CV: chest pain, peripheral edema.
EENT: pharyngitis, rhinitis, sinusitis.
GI: abdominal pain, diarrhea, nausea, vomiting.
GU: albuminuria.
Musculoskeletal: arthralgia, back pain.
Respiratory: coughing, bronchitis, upper respiratory tract infection.

▣ KEY CONSIDERATIONS
• Carefully monitor therapeutic response and occurrence of adverse reactions in all geriatric patients, especially those with renal disease.
• If hypotension occurs after a dose of candesartan, place patient in the supine position and, if necessary, give an I.V. infusion of normal saline solution.
• Most of the antihypertensive effect is present within 2 weeks. Maximal antihypertensive effect is obtained within 4 to 6 weeks. Diuretic may be added if blood pressure isn't controlled by drug alone.

Patient education
• Instruct patient to store drug at room temperature and to keep container tightly sealed.
• Inform patient to report adverse reactions without delay.
• Inform patient that drug may be taken without regard to meals.

Overdose & treatment
• Signs and symptoms of overdose include hypotension, dizziness, and tachycardia. Treatment is supportive. Candesartan isn't removed by hemodialysis.

capsaicin
Dolorac, Zostrix, Zostrix-HP

Naturally occurring chemical derived from plants of the Solanaceae family, topical analgesic

Available without a prescription
Cream: 0.025% (Zostrix), 0.075% (Zostrix-HP), 0.25% (Dolorac)

INDICATIONS & DOSAGE
Temporary pain relief from rheumatoid arthritis, osteoarthritis, and certain neuralgias, such as pain associated with shingles (herpes zoster) or diabetic neuropathy
Dolorac
Adults: Apply thin film to affected areas b.i.d.
Zostrix
Adults: Apply to affected areas t.i.d. or q.i.d.

PHARMACODYNAMICS
Analgesic action: Although the precise mechanism of action isn't fully understood, evidence suggests that the drug renders skin and joints insensitive to pain by depleting and preventing reaccumulation of substance P in peripheral sensory neurons. Substance P is thought to be the principal chemomediator of pain impulses from the periphery to the CNS. Also, substance P is released into joint tissues and activates inflammatory mediators involved with the pathogenesis of rheumatoid arthritis.

PHARMACOKINETICS
Absorption: Unknown.
Distribution: Unknown.
Metabolism: Unknown.
Excretion: Unknown.

CONTRAINDICATIONS & PRECAUTIONS
Contraindicated in patients hypersensitive to capsaicin.

INTERACTIONS
None reported.

ADVERSE REACTIONS
Respiratory: cough, irritation.

Skin: redness, *stinging or burning on application.*

▣ KEY CONSIDERATIONS

• Although transient burning or stinging with application is normal at initial therapy, it will disappear in several days.
• Application schedules of less than three or four times daily may not provide optimum pain relief, and the burning sensation may persist.
• Capsaicin is for external use only. Avoid contact with eyes and broken or irritated skin.
• Don't bandage tightly.

Patient education

• Instruct patient how to apply cream, stressing importance of avoiding the eyes and broken or irritated skin.
• Instruct patient to wash hands after applying cream, avoiding areas where drug was applied.
• Warn patient that transient burning or stinging with application may occur but will disappear with continued use after several days.
• Tell patient not to bandage areas tightly.
• Advise patient to discontinue drug and to call health care provider if condition worsens or does not improve after 28 days.

captopril
Capoten

ACE inhibitor, antihypertensive, adjunctive treatment of heart failure

Available by prescription only
Tablets: 12.5 mg, 25 mg, 50 mg, 100 mg

INDICATIONS & DOSAGE
Mild to severe hypertension; ◇ ***idiopathic edema;*** ◇ ***Raynaud's phenomenon***
Adults: Initially, 25 mg P.O. b.i.d. or t.i.d.; if necessary, dosage may be increased to 50 mg b.i.d. or t.i.d. after 1 to 2 weeks; if control is still inadequate after 1 to 2 weeks more, a diuretic may be added. Dosage may be raised to a maximum of 150 mg t.i.d. (450 mg/day)

while continuing the diuretic. Daily dose may be given b.i.d.
Heart failure
Adults: Initially, 25 mg P.O. t.i.d.; may be increased to 50 mg t.i.d., with maximum of 450 mg/day. In a patient taking a diuretic, initial dosage is 6.25 to 12.5 mg t.i.d.
Prevention of diabetic nephropathy
Adults: 25 mg P.O. t.i.d.
Left ventricular dysfunction after an MI
Adults: Give 6.25 mg P.O. as a single dose 3 days after an MI; then 12.5 mg t.i.d. increasing dose to 25 mg t.i.d. Target dose is 50 mg t.i.d.
♦ *Dosage adjustment.* In geriatric patients, especially those with renal failure, use lower initial daily dosages and smaller increments for adjustments.

PHARMACODYNAMICS
Antihypertensive action: Captopril inhibits ACE, preventing conversion of angiotensin I to angiotensin II, a potent vasoconstrictor. Reduced formation of angiotensin II decreases peripheral arterial resistance, which results in decreased aldosterone secretion, thus reducing sodium and water retention and lowering blood pressure.
Cardiac load–reducing action: Captopril decreases systemic vascular resistance (afterload) and pulmonary capillary wedge pressure (preload), thus increasing cardiac output in patients with heart failure.

PHARMACOKINETICS
Absorption: About 60% to 75% of an oral dose of captopril is absorbed through the GI tract; food may reduce absorption by up to 40%. Antihypertensive effect begins in 15 minutes; peak blood levels occur at 1 hour. Maximum therapeutic effect may require several weeks.
Distribution: Drug is distributed into most body tissues except those of the CNS; 25% to 30% of the drug binds to proteins.
Metabolism: About 50% is metabolized in the liver.
Excretion: Captopril and its metabolites are excreted primarily in urine; a small

amount is excreted in feces. Duration of effect, which increases with higher dosages, is usually 2 to 6 hours. Elimination half-life is less than 3 hours. Duration of action may be increased in patients with renal dysfunction.

CONTRAINDICATIONS & PRECAUTIONS
Contraindicated in patients with hypersensitivity to captopril or other ACE inhibitors. Use cautiously in patients with impaired renal function, renal artery stenosis, or serious autoimmune diseases (especially lupus erythematosus) and in those taking drugs that affect WBC counts or immune response.

INTERACTIONS
Drug-drug. Captopril may increase the antihypertensive effects of *other antihypertensives* and *diuretics* and may increase serum *digoxin* levels. *Aspirin, indomethacin,* and *other NSAIDs* may decrease the antihypertensive effect of captopril; *antacids* also decrease the effects of captopril and should be given at different dose intervals. Patients with impaired renal function or heart failure and patients receiving *drugs that can increase serum potassium levels*—for example, *potassium sparing diuretics*—may develop hyperkalemia during captopril therapy. Captopril may increase *lithium* levels, which may lead to *lithium* toxicity; use together with caution and monitor *lithium* drug levels. Use with *phenothiazine* may lead to increased pharmacologic effects. *Probenecid* may increase plasma captopril levels and decrease captopril clearance.
Drug-food. Use of *potassium supplements* or *salt substitutes* during captopril therapy may lead to hyperkalemia. Because *food* may reduce absorption by up to 40%, give captopril 1 hour before meals.

ADVERSE REACTIONS
CNS: dizziness, fainting, headache, malaise, fatigue.
CV: *tachycardia, hypotension,* angina pectoris.
GI: anorexia, *dysgeusia,* nausea, vomiting, abdominal pain, constipation, dry mouth.

Hematologic: *leukopenia, agranulocytosis, pancytopenia,* anemia, *thrombocytopenia.*
Hepatic: transient increase in hepatic enzyme levels.
Metabolic: hyperkalemia.
Respiratory: *dry, persistent, tickling, nonproductive cough,* dyspnea.
Skin: *urticarial rash, maculopapular rash,* pruritus, alopecia.
Other: fever, *angioedema of face and extremities.*

KEY CONSIDERATIONS
• Geriatric patients may need lower dosages because of impaired drug clearance. They also may be more sensitive to the hypotensive effects of captopril.
• Diuretic therapy is usually discontinued 2 to 3 days before beginning ACE inhibitor therapy, to reduce risk of hypotension; if drug doesn't adequately control blood pressure, diuretics may be reinstated.
• Perform WBC and differential counts before treatment, every 2 weeks for 3 months, and periodically thereafter. Monitor serum potassium levels because potassium retention has been noted.
• Lower dosage or reduced dosing frequency is necessary in patients with impaired renal function. Adjust dosage over 1 to 2 weeks, and then reduce dosage to lowest effective level.
• The beneficial effects of captopril may not be evident for several weeks.
• Captopril may cause nephrotic syndrome and false-positive results for urine acetone proteinuria.

Patient education
• Tell patient to report light-headedness, especially in first few days, so that dosage can be adjusted; signs and symptoms of infection, such as sore throat or fever, because drug may decrease WBC count; facial swelling or difficulty breathing because drug may cause angioedema; and loss of taste because the drug may need to be discontinued.
• Advise patient to avoid sudden position changes to minimize orthostatic hypotension.
• Warn patient to seek medical approval before taking OTC cold preparations and

to call health care provider if a persistent, dry cough occurs.

Overdose & treatment
• The primary sign of overdose is severe hypotension.
• After acute ingestion, induce vomiting or perform gastric lavage. Follow with activated charcoal to reduce absorption. Subsequent treatment is usually symptomatic and supportive. In severe cases, hemodialysis may be necessary.

---

carbachol
Carboptic, Isopto Carbachol, Miostat

Cholinergic agonist, miotic

Available by prescription only
Intraocular injection: 0.01%
Ophthalmic solution: 0.75%, 1.5%, 2.25%, 3%

INDICATIONS & DOSAGE
Ocular surgery (to produce pupillary miosis)
Adults: Instill 0.5 ml of 0.01% (intraocular form) gently into the anterior chamber for production of satisfactory miosis. It may be instilled before or after securing sutures.
Open-angle or angle-closure glaucoma
Adults: Instill 2 drops of 0.75% to 3% solution up to t.i.d.

PHARMACODYNAMICS
Miotic action: The cholinergic activity of carbachol causes the sphincter muscles of the iris to contract, producing miosis, and the ciliary muscle to contract, resulting in accommodation. It also acts to deepen the anterior chamber and dilates conjunctival vessels of the outflow tract.

PHARMACOKINETICS
Absorption: Action begins within 10 to 20 minutes and peaks in less than 4 hours.
Distribution: Unknown.
Metabolism: Unknown.
Excretion: Duration of effect is usually about 8 hours.

CONTRAINDICATIONS & PRECAUTIONS
Contraindicated in patients with hypersensitivity to carbachol or in those in whom cholinergic effects, such as constriction, are undesirable (for example, acute iritis, some forms of secondary glaucoma, pupillary block glaucoma, or acute inflammatory disease of the anterior chamber of the eye).

Use cautiously in patients with acute heart failure, bronchial asthma, peptic ulcer, hyperthyroidism, GI spasm, Parkinson's disease, and urinary tract obstruction.

INTERACTIONS
Drug-drug. *Cyclopentolate* or the *ophthalmic belladonna alkaloids*—such as *atropine* and *homatropine*—may interfere with the antiglaucoma action of carbachol.

ADVERSE REACTIONS
CNS: headache, syncope.
CV: *arrhythmias,* hypotension, flushing.
EENT: spasm of eye accommodation, conjunctival vasodilation, eye and brow pain, transient stinging and burning, corneal clouding, bullous keratopathy, salivation.
GI: abdominal cramps, diarrhea.
GU: urinary urgency.
Respiratory: asthma.
Other: diaphoresis.

▣ KEY CONSIDERATIONS
• Carbachol is especially useful in glaucoma patients resistant or allergic to pilocarpine hydrochloride or nitrate.
• Premixed drugs should be used for single-dose intraocular use only.
• Discard unused portions of injectable drug.

Patient education
• Tell patient with glaucoma that long-term use may be necessary. Stress compliance, and explain importance of medical supervision for tonometer readings before and during therapy.
• Instruct patient to apply finger pressure on the lacrimal sac 1 to 2 minutes after topical instillation of the drug.
• Reassure patient that blurred vision usually diminishes with continued use.

Reactions may be *common,* uncommon, *life-threatening,* or COMMON AND LIFE-THREATENING.

- Teach patient how to instill eyedrops correctly, and warn him not to touch eye or surrounding area with dropper.
- Warn patient not to drive for 1 to 2 hours after administration until effect on vision is determined.

Overdose & treatment

- Signs and symptoms of overdose include miosis, flushing, vomiting, bradycardia, bronchospasm, increased bronchial secretion, sweating, tearing, involuntary urination, hypotension, and seizures.
- With accidental oral ingestion, vomiting is usually spontaneous; if not, induce vomiting and follow with activated charcoal or a cathartic.
- Treat dermal exposure by washing the area twice with water. Treat CV or blood pressure responses with epinephrine. Atropine has been suggested as a direct antagonist for toxicity.

carbamazepine
Atretol, Carbatrol, Epitol, Tegretol

Iminostilbene derivative; chemically related to tricyclic antidepressants, anticonvulsant, analgesic

Available by prescription only
Tablets: 200 mg
Tablets (chewable): 100 mg
Tablets (extended-release): 100 mg, 200 mg, 400 mg
Capsules (extended-release): 200 mg, 300 mg
Oral suspension: 100 mg/5 ml

INDICATIONS & DOSAGE

Generalized tonic-clonic, complex-partial, mixed seizure patterns
Adults: 200 mg P.O. b.i.d. on day 1 (if using suspension, 100 mg P.O. q.i.d.). May increase by 200 mg/day P.O. at weekly intervals, in divided doses at 6- to 8-hour intervals. Adjust to minimum effective level when control is achieved; don't exceed 1,200 mg/day. In rare instances, dosages up to 1,600 mg/day have been used in adults.

For extended-release capsules or tablets, initial dosage is 200 mg P.O.

b.i.d. Increase at weekly intervals up to 200 mg/day until optimal response obtained. Dosage shouldn't exceed 1,200 mg/day. Some adult dosages may be up to 1,600 mg/day. Maintenance dosage is usually 800 to 1,200 mg/day.
Loading dose for rapid seizure control
Adults: 8 mg/kg of oral suspension.
◊ *Bipolar affective disorder, intermittent explosive disorder*
Adults: Initially, 200 mg P.O. b.i.d.; increase, p.r.n., q 3 to 4 days. Maintenance dosage may range from 600 to 1,600 mg/day.
Trigeminal neuralgia
Adults: 100 mg P.O. b.i.d. with meals on day 1. Increase by 100 mg q 12 hours until pain is relieved. Don't exceed 1.2 g daily. Maintenance dosage is 200 to 1,200 mg P.O. daily. For extended-release capsules or tablets, 200 mg P.O. day 1. Daily dosage may be increased up to 200 mg/day q 12 hours, p.r.n., to achieve freedom from pain. Maintenance dosage is usually 400 to 800 mg/day.
◊ *Restless leg syndrome*
Adults: 100 to 300 mg h.s.

PHARMACODYNAMICS

Anticonvulsant action: Carbamazepine is chemically unrelated to other anticonvulsants and its mechanism of action is unknown. The anticonvulsant activity appears principally to involve limitations of seizure propagation by reduction of posttetanic potentiation (PTP) of synaptic transmissions.
Analgesic action: In trigeminal neuralgia, carbamazepine is a specific analgesic through its reduction of synaptic neurotransmission.

PHARMACOKINETICS

Absorption: Carbamazepine is absorbed slowly from the GI tract. With the suspension, the peak plasma level occurs at 1½ hours; with the tablets, 4 to 6 hours; and with the extended-release forms, 6 hours.
Distribution: Although drug is distributed widely throughout body, about 75% of it binds to proteins. Therapeutic serum levels in adults are 4 to 12 µg/ml. Nystagmus can occur with a level above 4 µg/ml; ataxia, dizziness, and anorexia, with a level at or above 10 µg/ml. Serum

levels may be misleading because an unmeasured active metabolite also can cause a toxic reaction.

Metabolism: Drug is metabolized in the liver to an active metabolite. It may also induce its own metabolism; over time, higher dosages are needed to maintain plasma levels. Half-life is initially 25 to 65 hours and 12 to 17 hours with multiple dosing.

Excretion: About 70% of drug is excreted in urine; 30%, in feces.

CONTRAINDICATIONS & PRECAUTIONS

Contraindicated in patients with history of previous bone marrow suppression or hypersensitivity to carbamazepine or tricyclic antidepressants and in patients who've taken an MAO inhibitor within 14 days of therapy. Use cautiously in patients with mixed-type seizure disorders.

INTERACTIONS

Drug-drug. Use with *calcium channel blockers* (such as *verapamil* and possibly *diltiazem*) may significantly increase serum carbamazepine levels; therefore, carbamazepine dosage should be decreased by 40% to 50% when given with verapamil. Use with *cimetidine, clarithromycin, erythromycin, isoniazid, propoxyphene,* or *valproic acid* also may increase serum carbamazepine levels. When used with *ethosuximide, haloperidol, phenytoin, valproic acid,* or *warfarin,* carbamazepine may increase the metabolism of these drugs. Use with *felbamate* may result in lower serum levels of either drug. *Fluoxetine* or *fluvoxamine* may increase carbamazepine levels. Use with *MAO inhibitors* may cause hypertensive crisis. Use with *phenobarbital, phenytoin,* or *primidone* lowers serum carbamazepine levels. Carbamazepine may decrease the effectiveness of *theophylline.*

ADVERSE REACTIONS

CNS: *dizziness, vertigo, drowsiness,* fatigue, *ataxia, worsening of seizures* (usually in patients with mixed-type seizure disorders, including atypical absence seizures), confusion, headache, syncope.

CV: *heart failure,* hypertension, hypotension, aggravation of coronary artery disease, *arrhythmias, AV block.*

EENT: conjunctivitis, dry mouth and pharynx, blurred vision, diplopia, nystagmus.

GI: *nausea, vomiting,* abdominal pain, diarrhea, anorexia, stomatitis, glossitis.

GU: urinary frequency, urine retention, impotence, albuminuria, glycosuria, elevated BUN level.

Hematologic: *aplastic anemia, agranulocytosis,* eosinophilia, leukocytosis, *thrombocytopenia.*

Hepatic: abnormal liver function test results, *hepatitis.*

Respiratory: pulmonary hypersensitivity.

Skin: rash, urticaria, *erythema multiforme, Stevens-Johnson syndrome.*

Other: excessive diaphoresis, fever, chills, SIADH, may decrease values of thyroid function tests.

▣ KEY CONSIDERATIONS

• Adjust drug dosage based on individual response.

• Drug is structurally similar to tricyclic antidepressants, so some risk of activating latent psychosis, confusion, or agitation in a geriatric patient exists.

• Hematologic toxicity is rare but serious. Routinely monitor CBC and liver function tests.

• Carbamazepine may be used to treat hypophyseal diabetes insipidus and certain psychiatric disorders and to manage alcohol withdrawal; however, drug isn't labeled for such use.

• For administering via an NG tube, mix with an equal volume of diluent (D_5W or normal saline solution) and administer; then flush with 100 ml of diluent.

• If using suspension, divide prescribed dosage to t.i.d. or q.i.d.

Patient education

• Remind patient to store carbamazepine in a cool, dry place, not in the medicine cabinet. Using improperly stored tablets can result in reduced bioavailability.

• Tell patient that drug may cause GI distress. Patient should take drug with food at equally spaced intervals.

• Warn patient not to stop drug abruptly.

Reactions may be *common*, uncommon, *life-threatening*, or COMMON AND LIFE-THREATENING.

• Encourage patient to promptly report unusual bleeding, bruising, jaundice, dark urine, pale stools, abdominal pain, impotence, fever, chills, sore throat, mouth ulcers, edema, or disturbances in mood, alertness, or coordination.

• Emphasize importance of follow-up laboratory tests and continued medical supervision. Periodic eye examinations are recommended.

• Warn patient that drug may cause drowsiness, dizziness, and blurred vision. Patient should avoid hazardous activities that require alertness, especially during 1st week of therapy and when dosage is increased.

• Remind patient to shake suspension well before using.

• Tell patient that a capsule can be opened, if necessary, and its contents sprinkled over food (for example, a teaspoon of applesauce), but neither the capsule nor its contents should be crushed or chewed.

Overdose & treatment

• Signs and symptoms of overdose include irregular breathing, respiratory depression, tachycardia, blood pressure changes, shock, arrhythmias, impaired consciousness (ranging to deep coma), seizures, restlessness, drowsiness, psychomotor disturbances, nausea, vomiting, anuria, or oliguria.

• Treat overdose with repeated gastric lavage, especially if patient ingested alcohol concurrently. Activated charcoal and laxatives may hasten excretion. Carefully monitor vital signs, ECG, and fluid and electrolyte balance. Diazepam may control seizures but can exacerbate respiratory depression.

---

carbamide peroxide
Auro Ear Drops, Debrox, Gly-Oxide Liquid, Murine Ear, Orajel, Orajel Perioseptic, Proxigel

Urea hydrogen peroxide, ceruminolytic, topical antiseptic

Available without a prescription
Otic solution: 6.5% carbamide in glycerin or glycerin and propylene glycol

Oral solution: 10% carbamide with glycerin and propylene glycol; 15% with anhydrous glycerin, methylparaben, and propylene glycol
Oral gel: 10% carbamide in water-free gel base

INDICATIONS & DOSAGE
Impacted cerumen
Adults: 5 to 10 gtt otic solution into ear canal b.i.d. for 3 to 4 days.
Inflammation or irritation of lips, mouth, gums
Adults: Apply several drops of undiluted oral solution to affected area or place 10 gtt on tongue (mix with saliva, swish for several minutes and expectorate after 1 to 3 minutes) after meals and h.s.

PHARMACODYNAMICS
Ceruminolytic action: Emulsifies and disperses accumulated cerumen.
Antiseptic action: Releases oxygen on contact with oral mucosa, which results in a mild anti-inflammatory action and a cleaning.

PHARMACOKINETICS
Absorption: Unknown.
Distribution: Unknown.
Metabolism: Unknown.
Excretion: Unknown.

CONTRAINDICATIONS & PRECAUTIONS
Contraindicated in patients with a perforated eardrum.

INTERACTIONS
None reported.

ADVERSE REACTIONS
GI: oral irritation or inflammation.

▣ KEY CONSIDERATIONS
• Don't use to treat swimmer's ear or itching of the ear canal or if patient has a perforated eardrum.
• The ear may need to be irrigated to help remove the cerumen.
• Tip of dropper shouldn't touch ear or ear canal when using otic preparation.
• Remove cerumen remaining after instillation by using a soft rubber-bulb otic syringe to gently irrigate the ear canal with warm water.

Patient education
- Teach patient the correct way to use product.
- Tell patient to call health care provider if inflammation or irritation persists.
- Warn patient not to use otic form for more than 4 consecutive days and to avoid contact with eyes.
- Instruct patient to keep otic solution in ear for at least 15 minutes by tilting head sideways or putting cotton in ear.
- Tell patient not to rinse mouth or drink for 5 minutes after use.

Overdose & treatment
- Signs and symptoms of overdose include mild irritation to mucosal tissue or, if swallowed, irritation, inflammation, and burns in the mouth, throat, esophagus, or stomach. Gastric distention may result from liberation of oxygen. Accidental ocular exposure causes immediate pain and irritation, but severe injury is rare.
- Irrigate eyes with a large amount of warm water for at least 15 minutes. Accidental dermal exposure bleaches the exposed area. Wash exposed skin twice with soap and water. Treat oral exposure by immediately flushing the area with water. Spontaneous vomiting may occur.

---

carbenicillin indanyl sodium
Geocillin

Extended-spectrum penicillin, alpha-carboxy-penicillin, antibiotic

---

Available by prescription only
Tablets: 382 mg

INDICATIONS & DOSAGE
Urinary tract infection and prostatitis caused by susceptible organisms
Adults: 382 to 764 mg P.O. q.i.d.

Note: To ensure adequate urine levels, use drug only in patients whose creatinine clearance is 10 ml/minute.

PHARMACODYNAMICS
Antibiotic action: Carbenicillin is bactericidal; it adheres to bacterial penicillin-binding proteins, thus inhibiting bacterial cell-wall synthesis. Extended-spectrum penicillins are resistant to inactivation by some beta-lactamases, especially those produced by gram-negative organisms.

Drug has an activity spectrum similar to that of carbenicillin disodium, including many gram-negative aerobic and anaerobic bacilli; some gram-positive aerobic and anaerobic bacilli; and many gram-positive and gram-negative aerobic cocci.

PHARMACOKINETICS
Absorption: Carbenicillin is stable in gastric acid, but only 30% to 40% of drug is absorbed from the GI tract. Plasma levels peak 30 minutes after oral dose; indanyl salt is completely hydrolyzed to carbenicillin in plasma within 90 minutes.
Distribution: Drug is distributed widely after oral administration, but levels are insufficient to treat systemic infections. About 30% to 60% of drug binds to proteins.
Metabolism: Carbenicillin indanyl sodium is hydrolyzed rapidly in plasma to carbenicillin; carbenicillin is metabolized partially.
Excretion: About 79% to 99% of drug and its metabolites are excreted in urine through renal tubular secretion and glomerular filtration. Elimination half-life in adults is about 1 hour. In patients with extensive renal impairment, half-life is 9½ to 23 hours, but urine levels in renal parenchyma and urine are insufficient for treating urinary tract infections.

CONTRAINDICATIONS & PRECAUTIONS
Contraindicated in patients with hypersensitivity to carbenicillin or other penicillins.

INTERACTIONS
Drug-drug. Use with *aminoglycoside antibiotics* results in synergistic bactericidal effects against *Citrobacter, Enterobacter, Escherichia coli, Klebsiella, Proteus mirabilis, Pseudomonas aeruginosa,* and *Serratia.* Use with *clavulanic acid* produces synergistic bactericidal effects against certain beta-lactamase–producing bacteria. Large doses of carbenicillin may interfere with renal tubular secretion of *methotrexate,* delaying

---

elimination and elevating serum methotrexate levels. Although *probenecid* may be used concomitantly to achieve higher serum drug levels, this is an undesired effect in patients with urinary tract infection.

ADVERSE REACTIONS
GI: *nausea,* vomiting, *diarrhea, flatulence, abdominal cramps, unpleasant taste,* glossitis, dry mouth, furry tongue.
Hematologic: *leukopenia, neutropenia,* eosinophilia, *hemolytic anemia, thrombocytopenia,* prolonged PT and INR.
Hepatic: transient elevations in liver function test results.
Other: hypersensitivity reactions (rash, urticaria, pruritus, *anaphylaxis*), overgrowth of nonsusceptible organisms, decreased serum aminoglycoside levels.

▣ KEY CONSIDERATIONS
Besides the recommendations relevant to all penicillins, consider the following:
• Half-life may be prolonged in geriatric patients because of decreased renal function.
• Administer drug 1 to 2 hours before and 2 to 3 hours after meals with full glass (8 oz [240 ml]) of water to obtain maximum drug levels.
• Because carbenicillin is dialyzable, patients undergoing hemodialysis may need dosage adjustments.
• Drug alters results of urine glucose tests that use cupric sulfate (Benedict's reagent or Clinitest). Make urine glucose determinations with glucose oxidase methods (Diastix or Chemstrip uG).
• Drug increases serum uric acid values (cupric sulfate method) and falsely elevates urine specific gravity in dehydrated patients with low urine output.
• Positive Coombs' tests have been reported after carbenicillin therapy; drug also interferes with some human leukocyte antigen (HLA) tests and could cause inaccurate HLA typing.

Patient education
• Inform patient of potential adverse reactions.

Overdose & treatment
• Signs and symptoms of overdose include neuromuscular hypersensitivity and seizures resulting from CNS irritation from high drug levels.
• Treatment is supportive. After recent ingestion (within 4 hours), induce vomiting or perform gastric lavage. Follow with activated charcoal to reduce absorption. Drug can be removed from circulation through hemodialysis.

carboplatin
Paraplatin

Alkylating drug (cell cycle–phase nonspecific), antineoplastic

Available by prescription only
Injection: 50-mg, 150-mg, and 450-mg vials

INDICATIONS & DOSAGE
Initial and secondary (palliative) treatment of ovarian, ◇ advanced bladder, ◇ lung, and ◇ head and neck cancers; ◇ retinoblastoma; ◇ Wilms' tumor; ◇ primary brain tumor; ◇ testicular neoplasm
Adults: Initial recommended dosage for single-drug therapy is 360 mg/m² I.V. on day 1. Dosage is repeated q 4 weeks. In combination therapy (with cyclophosphamide), give 300 mg/m² I.V. on day 1 q 4 weeks for 6 cycles.
♦ *Dosage adjustment.* Adjustments are based on the lowest posttreatment platelet or neutrophil count obtained in the patient's weekly blood count.
  In patients with impaired renal function, initial recommended dosage is 250 mg/m² for creatinine clearance levels between 41 and 59 ml/minute; for creatinine clearance levels between 16 and 40 ml/minute, dosage is 200 mg/m².

Lowest platelet count/mm³	Lowest neutrophil count/mm³	Dosage adjustment
> 100,000	> 2,000	125%
50,000-100,000	500-2,000	No adjustment
< 50,000	< 500	75%

PHARMACODYNAMICS
Antitumor action: Carboplatin causes cross-linking of DNA strands.

PHARMACOKINETICS
Absorption: Carboplatin is administered I.V.

Distribution: Volume of distribution is about equal to total body water. Although drug doesn't bind to proteins, it's degraded to platinum-containing products—87% of which bind to protein in 24 hours.

Metabolism: Drug is hydrolyzed to form hydroxylated and aquated species. The half-life of the drug is 2 to 3 hours; terminal half-life for platinum is 4 to 6 days.

Excretion: About 65% of drug is excreted by the kidneys within 12 hours; 71%, within 24 hours. Drug may recirculate through the bowel and liver.

CONTRAINDICATIONS & PRECAUTIONS
Contraindicated in patients with history of hypersensitivity to cisplatin, mannitol, or platinum-containing compounds, or with severe bone marrow suppression or bleeding.

INTERACTIONS
Drug-drug. Use with *nephrotoxic drugs* produces additive nephrotoxicity.

ADVERSE REACTIONS
CNS: dizziness, confusion, peripheral neuropathy, ototoxicity, central neurotoxicity, asthenia, paresthesia, *CVA.*

CV: *cardiac failure, embolism.*

EENT: visual disturbances, change in taste.

GI: constipation, diarrhea, *nausea, vomiting.*

GU: increased BUN and creatinine levels.

Hematologic: THROMBOCYTOPENIA, *leukopenia,* NEUTROPENIA, *anemia,* BONE MARROW SUPPRESSION.

Hepatic: elevated bilirubin, AST, or alkaline phosphatase levels.

Metabolic: decreased serum electrolyte levels.

Skin: alopecia.

Other: hypersensitivity reactions, pain, *anaphylaxis.*

▣ KEY CONSIDERATIONS
• Patients older than age 65 are at greater risk for neurotoxicity.

• Reconstitute with D_5W, normal saline solution, or sterile water for injection to make a concentration of 10 mg/ml.

• Drug can be diluted with normal saline solution or D_5W.

• Infuse over at least 15 minutes.

• Unopened vials should be stored at room temperature. Once reconstituted and diluted as directed, solution is stable at room temperature for 8 hours. Because drug doesn't contain antibacterial preservatives, unused drug should be discarded after 8 hours.

• Don't use needles or I.V. administration sets containing aluminum because drug may precipitate and lose potency.

• Although drug is promoted as causing less nausea and vomiting than cisplatin, it can cause severe vomiting. Administer an antiemetic.

• Carboplatin should only be administered under the supervision of a health care provider experienced in the use of chemotherapeutic drugs.

Patient education
• Stress importance of adequate fluid intake and increase in urine output, to facilitate uric acid excretion.

• Tell patient to report tinnitus immediately to prevent permanent hearing loss. Patient should have audiometric testing before initial and subsequent course.

• Advise patient to avoid exposure to people with infections.

• Instruct patient to promptly report unusual bleeding or bruising.

carisoprodol
Soma

Carbamate derivative, skeletal muscle relaxant

Available by prescription only
Tablets: 350 mg

INDICATIONS & DOSAGE
Adjunct for relief from discomfort in acute, painful musculoskeletal conditions

---

Reactions may be *common,* uncommon, *life-threatening,* or COMMON AND LIFE-THREATENING.

Adults: Administer 350 mg P.O. t.i.d. and h.s.

PHARMACODYNAMICS
Skeletal muscle relaxant action: Carisoprodol relaxes skeletal muscle indirectly through its sedative effects. However, the exact mechanism of action is unknown. Animal studies suggest that the drug modifies central perception of pain without eliminating peripheral pain reflexes and has slight antipyretic activity.

PHARMACOKINETICS
Absorption: With usual therapeutic dosages, onset of action occurs within 30 minutes and persists 4 to 6 hours.
Distribution: Drug is widely distributed throughout the body.
Metabolism: Drug is metabolized in the liver. Drug may cause the liver to secrete microsomal enzymes; half-life is 8 hours.
Excretion: Excreted in urine mainly as metabolites; less than 1% of a dose is excreted unchanged. Drug may be removed from circulation through hemodialysis or peritoneal dialysis.

CONTRAINDICATIONS & PRECAUTIONS
Contraindicated in patients with hypersensitivity to related compounds (for example, meprobamate or tybamate) or intermittent porphyria. Use cautiously in patients with impaired renal or hepatic function.

INTERACTIONS
Drug-drug. Use with *other CNS depressants* produces additive CNS depression. When used with other *depressants*—such as *antipsychotics, anxiolytics, general anesthetics, opioid analgesics,* or *tricyclic antidepressants*—monitor carefully to avoid overdose. Use with *MAO inhibitors* or *tricyclic antidepressants* may increase CNS depression, respiratory depression, and hypotensive effects; dosage adjustments (reduction of one or both) are required.
Drug-lifestyle. *Alcohol* produces additive CNS depression; don't use together.

ADVERSE REACTIONS
CNS: *drowsiness, dizziness,* vertigo, ataxia, tremor, agitation, irritability, headache, depressive reactions, insomnia.
CV: orthostatic hypotension, tachycardia, facial flushing.
GI: nausea, vomiting, hiccups, epigastric distress.
Hematologic: eosinophilia.
Respiratory: asthma attacks.
Skin: rash, *erythema multiforme,* pruritus.
Other: fever, *angioedema, anaphylaxis.*

▣ KEY CONSIDERATIONS
• Geriatric patients may be more sensitive to the drug's effects than patients in other age-groups.
• Use with caution with other CNS depressants because effects may be cumulative.
• Initially, allergic or idiosyncratic reactions may occur (first to the fourth dose). Symptoms usually subside after several hours; treat with supportive and symptomatic measures.
• Psychological dependence may follow long-term use.
• Patient may experience withdrawal symptoms (abdominal cramps, insomnia, chilliness, headache, and nausea) if drug is stopped abruptly after long-term use of higher-than-recommended dosages.
• Commercially available formulations may contain sodium metabisulfite, which may cause an allergic reaction.

Patient education
• Inform patient that drug may cause dizziness and faintness. Changing positions slowly and in stages may help control signs and symptoms. Patient should report persistent signs and symptoms.
• Tell patient to avoid alcoholic beverages and to use cough or cold preparations containing alcohol cautiously while taking this drug. Patient should also avoid other CNS depressants (effects may be additive) unless prescribed.
• Warn patient drug may cause drowsiness. Avoid hazardous activities that require alertness until CNS depressant effects can be determined.

• Advise patient to discontinue drug immediately and to call health care provider if rash, diplopia, dizziness, or other unusual signs or symptoms appear.
• Inform patient to store drug away from direct heat and light (not in bathroom medicine cabinet).
• Instruct patient to take a missed dose only if he remembers it within 1 hour. If he remembers it later, he should skip that dose and go back to regular schedule. Patient shouldn't double-dose.
• Instruct patient to take drug with meals if GI upset occurs.

Overdose & treatment

• Signs and symptoms of overdose include exaggerated CNS depression, stupor, coma, shock, and respiratory depression.
• When treating a conscious patient for overdose, induce vomiting or perform gastric lavage; activated charcoal may be used after gastric lavage to adsorb any remaining drug. If patient is comatose, secure an endotracheal tube with cuff inflated before gastric lavage. Provide supportive therapy by maintaining adequate airway and assisted ventilation. CNS stimulants and pressor drugs should be used cautiously. Monitor vital signs, fluid and electrolyte levels, and neurologic status closely.
• Monitor urine output and avoid overhydration. Forced diuresis using mannitol, peritoneal dialysis, or hemodialysis may be beneficial. Continue to monitor patient for relapse from incomplete gastric emptying and delayed absorption.

carmustine (BCNU)
BiCNU, Gliadel

Alkylating drug, nitrosourea (cell cycle–phase nonspecific), antineoplastic

Available by prescription only
Injection: 100-mg vial (lyophilized), with a 3-ml vial of absolute alcohol supplied as a diluent
Implant: 7.7 mg wafer

INDICATIONS & DOSAGE
Dosage and indications may vary. Check current literature for recommended protocol.
◇ *Brain,* ◇ *breast,* ◇ *GI tract,* ◇ *lung, and* ◇ *liver cancers; Hodgkin's disease; malignant lymphomas;* ◇ *malignant melanomas; multiple myeloma*
Adults: 75 to 100 mg/m² I.V. by slow infusion daily for 2 consecutive days, repeated q 6 weeks if platelet count is above 100,000/mm³ and WBC count is above 4,000/µl.
✦ *Dosage adjustment.* Reduce dosage, p.r.n., using the following guidelines.

Nadir after prior dose		% of prior dose to be given
Leukocytes/ mm³	Platelets/ mm³	
> 4,000	> 100,000	100%
3,000-3,999	75,000-99,999	100%
2,000-2,999	25,000-74,999	70%
< 2,000	< 25,000	50%

Alternative therapy: 150 to 200 mg/m² I.V. slow infusion as a single dose, repeated q 6 to 8 weeks.
Recurrent glioblastoma and recurrent metastatic brain tumors (adjunct to surgery to prolong survival)
Adults: Implant 8 wafers in the resection cavity if allowed by size and shape of cavity.

PHARMACODYNAMICS
Antineoplastic action: The cytotoxic action of carmustine is mediated through its metabolites, which inhibit several enzymes involved with DNA formation. This drug can also cause cross-linking of DNA. Cross-linking interferes with DNA, RNA, and protein synthesis. Cross-resistance between carmustine and lomustine may occur.

PHARMACOKINETICS
Absorption: Carmustine isn't absorbed across the GI tract. Implant wafers are biodegradable in the human brain when implanted into the tumor resection cavity.
Distribution: Drug is cleared rapidly from the plasma. After I.V. administration, carmustine and its metabolites distribute rapidly into the CSF.

Metabolism: Drug is metabolized extensively in the liver.

Excretion: About 60% to 70% of drug and its metabolites is excreted in urine within 96 hours, 6% to 10% is excreted as carbon dioxide from the lungs, and 1% is excreted in feces. Enterohepatic circulation and protein-binding can occur and may cause delayed hematologic toxicity.

The absorption, distribution, metabolism, and excretion of the copolymer is unknown.

CONTRAINDICATIONS & PRECAUTIONS
Contraindicated in patients with hypersensitivity to carmustine.

INTERACTIONS
Drug-drug. *Anticoagulants* and *aspirin* may increase risk of bleeding; use together cautiously. Use with *cimetidine* increases the risk of bone marrow toxicity; don't use these drugs together. *Digoxin* levels may also be decreased with concomitant use. Serum *phenytoin* levels may be decreased by a combination chemotherapy regimen including carmustine.

Drug-lifestyle. *Smoking* may increase risk of pulmonary toxicity. Avoid smoking while taking this drug.

ADVERSE REACTIONS
CNS: ataxia, drowsiness.
EENT: ocular toxicities.
GI: *nausea* beginning in 2 to 6 hours (can be severe), *vomiting.*
GU: *nephrotoxicity,* azotemia, *renal failure.*
Hematologic: *cumulative bone marrow suppression* (delayed 4 to 6 weeks, lasting 1 to 2 weeks); *leukopenia; thrombocytopenia; acute leukemia, bone marrow dysplasia* (after long-term use); anemia.
Hepatic: *hepatotoxicity,* increased AST and bilirubin levels.
Metabolic: hyperuricemia (in lymphoma patients when rapid cell lysis occurs).
Respiratory: *pulmonary fibrosis.*
Skin: facial flushing, hyperpigmentation.

Other: *intense pain at infusion site from venous spasm,* increased BUN and serum alkaline phosphatase levels.

▣ KEY CONSIDERATIONS
● When handling implant wafers, use only the instruments designated for that use and wear double gloves.
● Reconstitute 100-mg vial with the 3 ml of absolute alcohol that the manufacturer provides, then dilute further with 27 ml sterile water for injection. Resultant solution contains 3.3 mg carmustine/ml in 10% ethanol. Dilute in normal saline solution or D_5W for I.V. infusion. Give at least 250 ml over 1 to 2 hours. Discard excess drug.
● Wear gloves when infusing the drug and when changing I.V. tubing. Avoid contact with skin because carmustine will stain it brown. If drug comes into contact with skin, wash off thoroughly.
● Solution is unstable in plastic I.V. bags. Administer only in glass containers.
● Carmustine may decompose at temperatures above 80° F (26.6° C).
● If powder liquefies or appears oily, discard because both are signs of decomposition.
● Reconstituted solution may be stored in refrigerator for 24 hours.
● Don't mix with other drugs during administration.
● Avoid I.M. injections when platelet count is below 100,000/mm^3.
● To reduce pain on infusion, dilute further or slow infusion rate.
● During an I.V. infusion, intense flushing of the skin may occur, but it usually disappears within 2 to 4 hours.
● To reduce nausea, give antiemetic before administering.
● Monitor patient's CBC.
● Monitor I.V. site for extravasation, especially in patients with friable veins. At first sign of extravasation, discontinue infusion and infiltrate area with liberal injections of 0.5 mEq/ml sodium bicarbonate solution.
● To treat mycosis fungoides, drug has been applied topically in concentrations of 0.05% to 0.4%.
● Because drug crosses the blood-brain barrier, it may be used to treat primary brain tumors.

Patient education
- Warn patient to watch for signs and symptoms of infection and bone marrow toxicity, including fever, sore throat, anemia, fatigue, easy bruising, nose and gum bleeds, and melena. Patient should take his temperature daily.
- Remind patient to return for follow-up blood work weekly.
- Advise patient to avoid exposure to people with infections.
- Tell patient to avoid OTC products containing aspirin because they may precipitate bleeding. Advise patient to report signs of bleeding promptly.

Overdose & treatment
- Signs and symptoms of overdose include leukopenia, thrombocytopenia, nausea, and vomiting.
- Treatment consists of supportive measures, including transfusion of blood components, antibiotics for infections that may develop, and antiemetics.

carteolol hydrochloride
Cartrol, Ocupress

Beta blocker, antihypertensive

Available by prescription only
Tablets: 2.5 mg, 5 mg
Ophthalmic solution: 1%

INDICATIONS & DOSAGE
Hypertension
Adults: Initially, 2.5 mg as a single daily dosage. Gradually increase the dosage as required to 5 mg daily or 10 mg daily as a single dose.
◇**Angina**
Adults: 10 mg/day.
Open-angle glaucoma
Adults: 1 drop b.i.d. in eye.
✦**Dosage adjustment.** Patients with substantial renal failure should receive the usual dose of carteolol scheduled at longer intervals as shown.

Creatinine clearance (ml/min)	Dosage interval (hr)
> 60	24
20-60	48
< 20	72

PHARMACODYNAMICS
Antihypertensive action: Carteolol is a nonselective beta blocker with intrinsic sympathomimetic activity. Decreased sympathetic outflow from the brain and decreased cardiac output probably cause its antihypertensive effects. Drug doesn't have a consistent effect on renin output.

PHARMACOKINETICS
Absorption: Carteolol is absorbed rapidly, achieving peak plasma levels in 1 to 3 hours. Bioavailability is about 85%.
Distribution: About 20% to 30% of drug is bound to plasma proteins.
Metabolism: Only 30% to 50% of drug is metabolized in the liver to the active metabolite 8-hydroxycarteolol and the inactive metabolite glucuronoside.
Excretion: Drug is primarily excreted in urine. Plasma half-life is about 6 hours.

CONTRAINDICATIONS & PRECAUTIONS
Contraindicated in patients hypersensitive to any component of carteolol and in those with bronchial asthma, severe COPD, sinus bradycardia, second- or third-degree AV block, overt cardiac failure, or cardiogenic shock.
Use cautiously in patients with nonallergic bronchospastic disease, diabetes mellitus, hyperthyroidism, or decreased pulmonary function.

INTERACTIONS
Drug-drug. Use with *catecholamine-depleting drugs,* such as *reserpine,* may produce additive effects. Carteolol may potentiate the hypotension that *general anesthetics* produce; observe carefully for excessive hypotension or bradycardia and for orthostatic hypotension. The dosage of *insulin* and *oral antidiabetics* may have to be adjusted in patients receiving carteolol. Avoid administration with *oral calcium antagonists* in patients with impaired cardiac function because of the risk of hypotension, left-sided

---

Reactions may be *common,* uncommon, *life-threatening,* or COMMON AND LIFE-THREATENING.

heart failure, and AV conduction disturbances; *I.V. calcium antagonists* should be used with caution.

ADVERSE REACTIONS

CNS: lassitude, fatigue, somnolence, *asthenia, paresthesia.*
CV: *conduction disturbances.*
EENT: transient irritation, conjunctival hyperemia, *edema.*
GI: diarrhea, nausea, abdominal pain.
Musculoskeletal: *muscle cramps,* arthralgia.
Skin: rash.

▣ KEY CONSIDERATIONS

Besides the recommendations relevant to all beta blockers, consider the following:
• Dosages over 10 mg daily don't produce a greater response; they may actually decrease response.
• Food may slow the rate, but not the extent, of carteolol absorption.
• Steady-state levels are reached rapidly (within 1 to 2 days) in patients with normal renal function.

Patient education

• Advise patient to take drug exactly as prescribed and not to discontinue it suddenly.
• Advise patient to report shortness of breath or difficulty breathing, unusually fast heartbeat, cough, or fatigue with exertion.
• Inform patient that transient stinging or discomfort may occur with ophthalmic use; if reaction is severe, he should call his health care provider immediately.

Overdose & treatment

• Signs and symptoms of overdose are bradycardia, bronchospasm, heart failure, and hypotension.
• Atropine should be used to treat symptomatic bradycardia. If no response is seen, cautiously use isoproterenol. Bronchospasm should be treated with a beta$_2$-agonist, such as isoproterenol or theophylline. Cardiac glycosides or diuretics may be useful in treating heart failure. Vasopressors—such as epinephrine, dopamine, or norepinephrine—should be given to combat hypotension.

carvedilol
Coreg

Alpha$_1$-nonselective beta blocker, antihypertensive, adjunct treatment for heart failure

Available by prescription only
Tablets: 3.125 mg, 6.25 mg, 12.5 mg, 25 mg

INDICATIONS & DOSAGE
Hypertension
Adults: Dosage is individualized. Initially, 6.25 mg P.O. b.i.d. with food; obtain standing systolic pressure 1 hour after initial dose. If tolerated, continue dose for 7 to 14 days. Can increase to 12.5 mg P.O. b.i.d., repeating monitoring protocol as above. Maximum dosage is 25 mg P.O. b.i.d. as tolerated.
Heart failure
Adults: Dosage individualized and adjusted carefully. Stabilize dosing of cardiac glycosides, diuretics, and ACE inhibitors before starting therapy. Initially, 3.125 mg P.O. b.i.d. with food for 2 weeks; if tolerated, can increase to 6.25 mg P.O. b.i.d. for 2 weeks. Dosage can be doubled q 2 weeks to highest level that the patient can tolerate. When initiating a new dosage, observe patient for dizziness or light-headedness for 1 hour. Maximum dosing for patients weighing less than 187 lb (85 kg) is 25 mg P.O. b.i.d.; for those weighing more than 187 lb, give 50 mg P.O. b.i.d.

PHARMACODYNAMICS
Antihypertensive action: Mechanism of action hasn't been established. Beta blockade reduces cardiac output and tachycardia. Alpha blockade is demonstrated by the attenuated pressor effects of phenylephrine, vasodilation, and decreases in peripheral vascular resistance.
Heart failure action: Mechanism of action hasn't been fully established. Drug has been shown to decrease systemic blood pressure, pulmonary artery pressure, pressure in the right atrium, systemic vascular resistance, and heart rate while increasing stroke volume index.

PHARMACOKINETICS

Absorption: Absorption is slowed when administered with food.

Distribution: Plasma drug levels are proportional to the oral dose administered. A delay in reaching peak plasma levels occurs when drug is administered with food, but no significant difference in bioavailability exists.

Metabolism: Drug is rapidly and extensively metabolized after oral administration—primarily through aromatic ring oxidation and glucuronidation—with absolute bioavailability of 25% to 35% because of significant first-pass metabolism. The oxidative metabolites are further metabolized by conjugation via glucuronidation and sulfation. Demethylation and hydroxylation at the phenol ring produce three active metabolites with beta-blocking activity. Mean terminal elimination half-life ranges from 7 to 10 hours.

Excretion: Metabolites are primarily excreted in feces (from bile). Less than 2% of dose is excreted unchanged in urine.

CONTRAINDICATIONS & PRECAUTIONS

Contraindicated in patients with New York Heart Association class IV decompensated cardiac failure requiring I.V. inotropic therapy or having bronchial asthma or related bronchospastic conditions, second- or third-degree AV block, sick sinus syndrome (unless a permanent pacemaker is in place), cardiogenic shock, severe bradycardia, or hypersensitivity to carvedilol. Drug isn't recommended for patients with hepatic impairment.

Use cautiously in hypertensive patients with left-sided heart failure, perioperative patients who receive anesthetics that depress myocardial function (for example, ether, cyclopropane, trichloroethylene), diabetic patients receiving insulin or oral antidiabetics, and patients subject to spontaneous hypoglycemia. Also use with caution in patients with thyroid disease (may mask hyperthyroidism and drug withdrawal may precipitate thyroid storm or an exacerbation of hyperthyroidism), pheochromocytoma, Prinzmetal's variant angina, or peripheral vascular disease (may precipitate or aggravate signs and symptoms of arterial insufficiency).

INTERACTIONS

Drug-drug. Because *calcium channel blockers* can cause isolated conduction disturbances, monitor ECG and blood pressure. *Catecholamine-depleting drugs*—such as *MAO inhibitors* and *reserpine*—may cause severe bradycardia or hypotension. *Cimetidine* increases bioavailability of carvedilol by 30%. *Clonidine* may potentiate blood pressure– and heart rate–lowering effects; discontinue the beta blocker first, and then adjust the dosage of clonidine several days later. *Digoxin* levels are increased about 15% during concurrent therapy; because both drugs slow AV conduction, monitor digoxin levels. *Inhibitors of cytochrome P-2D6*—such as *fluoxetine, paroxetine, propafenone,* and *quinidine*—may increase carvedilol levels. Use with *insulin* or *oral antidiabetics* may enhance hypoglycemic properties; monitor blood glucose levels. *Rifampin* reduces plasma carvedilol levels by 70%.

ADVERSE REACTIONS

CNS: *dizziness, fatigue,* headache, hypoesthesia, insomnia, malaise, pain, paresthesia, somnolence, vertigo.

CV: aggravated angina pectoris, *AV block, bradycardia,* chest pain, fluid overload, hypertension, hypotension, postural hypertension, syncope, edema, peripheral edema.

EENT: abnormal vision, dry eyes.

GI: abdominal pain, *diarrhea,* melena, nausea, periodontitis, vomiting.

GU: abnormal renal function, albuminuria, hematuria, urinary tract infection, impotence.

Hematologic: decreased PT and INR, purpura, ***thrombocytopenia.***

Hepatic: increased ALT and AST levels.

Metabolic: dehydration; glycosuria; hypovolemia; gout; hypercholesterolemia; *hyperglycemia;* hypertriglyceridemia; hypervolemia; hyperuricemia; hypoglycemia; hyponatremia; weight gain; increased alkaline phosphatase, BUN, and nonprotein nitrogen levels.

Reactions may be *common,* uncommon, *life-threatening,* or COMMON AND LIFE-THREATENING.

Musculoskeletal: arthralgia, back pain, myalgia.
Respiratory: bronchitis, dyspnea, pharyngitis, rhinitis, sinusitis, *upper respiratory tract infection*.
Other: allergy, fever, ***sudden death***, viral infection.

▣ KEY CONSIDERATIONS

• Plasma carvedilol levels are about 50% higher in geriatric patients than in others. Monitor levels carefully.
• Dizziness is slightly more common in geriatric patients.
• Mild hepatocellular injury may occur during therapy. At first sign of hepatic dysfunction, perform tests for hepatic injury or jaundice; if present, stop drug.
• Discontinue drug gradually over 1 to 2 weeks. Decrease dosage if heart rate is below 55 beats/minute.
• Monitor patient with heart failure for worsened condition, renal dysfunction, or fluid retention; diuretics may need to be increased. Also, monitor diabetic patient because hyperglycemia may be worsened.
• Patient with history of severe anaphylactic reaction to several allergens who is taking a beta blocker may be more reactive to repeated challenge, either accidental, diagnostic, or therapeutic. They may be unresponsive to the usual dosages of epinephrine used to treat allergic reactions.

Patient education

• Tell patient not to interrupt or discontinue drug without health care provider's approval.
• Advise patient with heart failure to call if he gains weight or experiences shortness of breath.
• Inform patient that he may experience lowered blood pressure when standing. If dizziness and fainting (rare) occur, advise him to sit or lie down.
• Caution patient against performing hazardous tasks during initiation of therapy. If dizziness or fatigue occur, tell him to call health care provider for a dosage adjustment.
• Tell patient to take drug with food.

• Advise diabetic patient to report changes in his blood glucose level promptly.
• Inform patient who wears contact lenses that drug may dry his eyes.

Overdose & treatment

• Signs and symptoms of overdose include severe hypotension, bradycardia, cardiac insufficiency, cardiogenic shock, and cardiac arrest. Vomiting, lapses of consciousness, generalized seizures, and respiratory effects including bronchospasm may also occur.
• Gastric lavage or drug-induced vomiting may be effective shortly after ingestion. For bradycardia, consider using 2 mg of I.V. atropine; 5 to 10 mg of I.V. glucagon rapidly administered over 30 seconds, followed by continuous infusion at 5 mg/hour; and a sympathomimetic—such as dobutamine, isoprenaline, and adrenaline—at a dosage based on body weight and effect. For therapy-resistant bradycardia, perform pacemaker therapy. If peripheral vasodilation dominates, administer epinephrine or norepinephrine, if necessary, and continuously monitor circulatory conditions. For bronchospasm, give a beta-sympathomimetic by aerosol or I.V. or aminophylline I.V. If seizures occur, slow I.V. injection of diazepam or clonazepam may be effective. If patient experiences severe intoxication and shock, continue treatment with antidotes for a sufficiently long period of time consistent with the drug's 7- to 10-hour half-life.

cascara sagrada

cascara sagrada aromatic fluid extract

Anthraquinone glycoside mixture, laxative

Available without a prescription
Tablets: 325 mg
Aromatic fluid extract: 1 g/ml with 18% alcohol

INDICATIONS & DOSAGE
Acute constipation, preparation for bowel or rectal examination
Adults: 1 tablet P.O. h.s.

PHARMACODYNAMICS
Laxative action: Cascara sagrada, obtained from the dried bark of the buckthorn tree *(Rhamnus purshiana),* contains cascarosides A and B (barbaloin glycosides) and cascarosides C and D (chrysaloin glycosides). Drug exerts a direct irritant action on the colon that promotes peristalsis and bowel motility. Cascara sagrada also enhances colonic fluid accumulation, thus increasing the laxative effect.

PHARMACOKINETICS
Absorption: Only a small amount of cascara sagrada is absorbed in the small intestine. Onset of action usually occurs in about 6 to 12 hours but may not occur for 3 to 4 days.
Distribution: Drug may be distributed in the bile, saliva, and colonic mucosa.
Metabolism: Drug is metabolized in the liver.
Excretion: Drug is excreted in feces (from bile), in urine, or in both.

CONTRAINDICATIONS & PRECAUTIONS
Contraindicated in patients with abdominal pain, nausea, vomiting, or other signs or symptoms of appendicitis or acute surgical abdomen; acute surgical delirium; fecal impaction; or intestinal obstruction or perforation. Use cautiously in patients with rectal bleeding.

ADVERSE REACTIONS
GI: *nausea;* protein-losing enteropathy; vomiting; diarrhea; loss of normal bowel function with excessive use; *abdominal cramps,* especially in severe constipation; malabsorption of nutrients; "cathartic colon" (syndrome resembling ulcerative colitis radiologically and pathologically) with long-term misuse; discoloration of rectal mucosa after long-term use.
Metabolic: hypokalemia, electrolyte imbalance (with excessive use).
Other: laxative dependence (with long-term or excessive use).

▣ KEY CONSIDERATIONS
• Because many geriatric patients use laxatives, they're at high risk for developing laxative dependence. Urge them to use laxatives only for short periods.
• Cascara sagrada turns alkaline urine pink to red, red to violet, or red to brown and turns acidic urine yellow to brown in the phenolsulfonphthalein excretion test.
• Cascara sagrada is a common ingredient in many so-called natural laxatives available without a prescription.

Patient education
• Warn patient that drug may turn urine reddish pink or brown.
• Encourage appropriate changes in food and fluid intake to prevent constipation.

castor oil
Emulsoil, Neoloid, Purge

Glyceride, Ricinus communis derivative, stimulant laxative

Available without a prescription
Liquid: 60 ml, 120 ml
Liquid (95%): 30 ml, 60 ml
Liquid emulsion: 60 ml (95%), 90 ml (67%)

INDICATIONS & DOSAGE
Preparation for rectal or bowel examination or surgery; acute constipation (rarely)
Liquid
Adults: 15 to 60 ml (or 30 to 60 ml, 95%) P.O.
Liquid emulsion
Adults: 45 ml (67%) or 15 to 60 ml (95%) P.O. mixed with ½ to 1 glass liquid.

PHARMACODYNAMICS
Laxative action: Castor oil acts primarily in the small intestine, where it's metabolized to ricinoleic acid, which stimulates the intestine, promoting peristalsis and bowel motility.

PHARMACOKINETICS
Absorption: Unknown; action begins in 2 to 6 hours.

Distribution: Castor oil is distributed locally, primarily in the small intestine.
Metabolism: Like other fatty acids, intestinal enzymes metabolize castor oil into its active form, ricinoleic acid.
Excretion: Castor oil is excreted in feces.

CONTRAINDICATIONS & PRECAUTIONS
Contraindicated in patients with ulcerative bowel lesions or abdominal pain, nausea, vomiting, or other signs or symptoms of appendicitis or acute surgical abdomen and in patients with anal or rectal fissures, fecal impaction, or intestinal obstruction or perforation. Use cautiously in patients with rectal bleeding.

INTERACTIONS
Drug-drug. Castor oil may decrease absorption of *intestinally absorbed drugs.*

ADVERSE REACTIONS
GI: *nausea;* protein-losing enteropathy; vomiting; diarrhea; loss of normal bowel function with excessive use; *abdominal cramps,* especially in severe constipation; malabsorption of nutrients; "cathartic colon" (syndrome resembling ulcerative colitis radiologically and pathologically) with long-term misuse; laxative dependence with long-term or excessive use. May cause constipation after catharsis.
Metabolic: hypokalemia, other electrolyte imbalances (with excessive use).

▣ KEY CONSIDERATIONS
• With long-term use, geriatric patients may experience electrolyte depletion, resulting in weakness, incoordination, and orthostatic hypotension.
• Castor oil isn't recommended for routine use in constipation; it's commonly used to evacuate the bowel before diagnostic or surgical procedures.
• Don't administer drug at bedtime because of rapid onset of action.
• Drug is most effective when taken on an empty stomach; shake well.
• Observe patient for dehydration.
• Flavored preparations are available.

Patient education
• Instruct patient not to take drug at bedtime.
• Recommend that drug be chilled or taken with juice or carbonated beverage to make it more palatable.
• Instruct patient to shake emulsion well.
• Reassure patient that after response to drug he may not need to move bowels again for 1 to 2 days.

cefaclor
Ceclor, Ceclor CD

Second-generation cephalosporin, antibiotic

Available by prescription only
Tablets (extended-release): 375 mg, 500 mg
Capsules: 250 mg, 500 mg
Suspension: 125 mg/5 ml, 187 mg/5 ml, 250 mg/5 ml, 375 mg/5 ml

INDICATIONS & DOSAGE
Respiratory and urinary tract and skin infections, otitis media caused by susceptible organisms
Adults: 250 to 500 mg P.O. q 8 hours. Total daily dosage shouldn't exceed 4 g. For extended-release tablets, 375 to 500 mg P.O. q 12 hours for 7 to 10 days.
Acute uncomplicated urinary tract infection
Adults: Give 2 g as a single dose.
✦ *Dosage adjustment.* Because cefaclor is dialyzable, patients who are receiving treatment with hemodialysis or peritoneal dialysis may require dosage adjustment.

PHARMACODYNAMICS
Antibiotic action: Cefaclor is primarily bactericidal; however, it may be bacteriostatic. Activity depends on the organism and the rate at which it multiplies, tissue penetration, and drug dosage. Drug adheres to bacterial penicillin-binding proteins, thereby inhibiting cell-wall synthesis.

Drug has the same bactericidal spectrum as other second-generation cephalosporins, except that it's more active against ampicillin- or amoxicillin-resistant *Haemophilus influenzae* and *Branhamella catarrhalis*.

PHARMACOKINETICS

Absorption: Cefaclor is well absorbed from the GI tract; serum levels peak 30 to 60 minutes after an oral dose. Food delays GI tract absorption.
Distribution: Drug is distributed widely into most body tissues and fluids; CSF penetration is poor. About 25% of drug binds to proteins.
Metabolism: Drug isn't metabolized.
Excretion: Drug is excreted primarily in urine through renal tubular secretion and glomerular filtration. In patients with normal renal function, elimination half-life is ½ to 1 hour; in patients with end-stage renal disease, 3 to 5½ hours. Drug can be removed from circulation through hemodialysis.

CONTRAINDICATIONS & PRECAUTIONS

Contraindicated in patients with hypersensitivity to other cephalosporins. Use cautiously in patients with impaired renal function or penicillin allergy.

INTERACTIONS

Drug-drug. Use with *bacteriostatic drugs*—such as *chloramphenicol, erythromycin,* and *tetracyclines*—may impair its bactericidal activity. Use with *loop diuretics* or *nephrotoxic drugs*—such as *vancomycin, colistin, polymyxin B,* and *aminoglycosides*—may increase the risk of nephrotoxicity. *Probenecid* competitively inhibits renal tubular secretion of cefaclor, resulting in higher, prolonged serum cefaclor levels.

ADVERSE REACTIONS

CNS: dizziness, headache, somnolence, malaise.
GI: *nausea,* vomiting, *diarrhea,* anorexia, dyspepsia, abdominal cramps, pseudomembranous colitis, oral candidiasis.
GU: vaginal candidiasis, vaginitis.
Hematologic: transient leukopenia, anemia, eosinophilia, **thrombocytopenia,** lymphocytosis.
Hepatic: transient increases in liver enzymes.
Skin: *maculopapular rash,* dermatitis, pruritus.

Other: hypersensitivity reactions (serum sickness, ***anaphylaxis***), fever.

▣ KEY CONSIDERATIONS

Besides the recommendations relevant to all cephalosporins, consider the following:
● To prevent toxic accumulation in a patient whose creatinine clearance is below 40 ml/minute, dosage may need to be reduced.
● Cefaclor causes false-positive results in urine glucose tests using cupric sulfate (Benedict's reagent or Clinitest); use glucose oxidase tests (Chemstrip uG, Diastix, or glucose enzymatic test strip) instead. Drug may also cause false-positive Coombs' test results.
● Drug falsely elevates serum or urine creatinine levels in tests using Jaffé's reaction.
● Drug may be given with food to minimize GI distress.
● Total daily dosage may be administered b.i.d. rather than t.i.d. with similar therapeutic effect.
● Stock oral suspension is stable for 14 days if refrigerated.

Patient education
● Instruct patient to take extended-release tablets with food and not to cut, crush, or chew them.

Overdose & treatment
● Signs and symptoms of overdose include neuromuscular hypersensitivity; seizure may follow high CNS levels.
● Remove cefaclor by hemodialysis or peritoneal dialysis.

cefadroxil
Duricef

First-generation cephalosporin, antibiotic

Available by prescription only
Tablets: 1 g
Capsules: 500 mg
Suspension: 125 mg/5 ml, 250 mg/5 ml, 500 mg/5 ml

Reactions may be *common*, uncommon, *life-threatening*, or COMMON AND LIFE-THREATENING.

INDICATIONS & DOSAGE

Urinary tract, skin, and soft-tissue infections caused by susceptible organisms; pharyngitis; tonsillitis

Adults: 1 to 2 g P.O. daily, depending on the infection treated. Usually given once or twice daily.

✦ *Dosage adjustment.* In patients with creatinine clearance below 10 ml/minute, extend dosing interval to q 36 hours; if between 10 and 25 ml/minute, administer q 24 hours; and if between 25 and 50 ml/minute, give q 12 hours.

Because drug is dialyzable, patients who are receiving treatment with hemodialysis may require dosage adjustment.

PHARMACODYNAMICS

Antibiotic action: Cefadroxil is primarily bactericidal; however, it may be bacteriostatic. Activity depends on the organism and the rate at which it multiplies, tissue penetration, and drug dosage. Drug adheres to bacterial penicillin-binding proteins, thereby inhibiting cell-wall synthesis.

Drug is active against many gram-positive cocci, including penicillinase-producing *Staphylococcus aureus* and *S. epidermidis; Streptococcus pneumoniae,* group B streptococci, and group A beta-hemolytic streptococci; and susceptible gram-negative organisms, including *Klebsiella pneumoniae, Escherichia coli,* and *Proteus mirabilis.*

PHARMACOKINETICS

Absorption: Cefadroxil is absorbed rapidly and completely from the GI tract after oral administration; serum levels peak in 1 to 2 hours.

Distribution: Drug is distributed widely to most body tissues and fluids, including the gallbladder, liver, kidneys, bone, bile, sputum, and pleural and synovial fluids; CSF penetration is poor. Twenty percent of drug binds to proteins.

Metabolism: Drug isn't metabolized.

Excretion: Most of the drug is excreted unchanged in urine through glomerular filtration and renal tubular secretion. In patients with normal renal function, elimination half-life is 1 to 2 hours; in patients with end-stage renal disease, 25 hours. Drug can be removed from circulation through hemodialysis.

CONTRAINDICATIONS & PRECAUTIONS

Contraindicated in patients with hypersensitivity to cefadroxil or other cephalosporins. Use cautiously in patients with impaired renal function or penicillin allergy.

INTERACTIONS

Drug-drug. Use with *bacteriostatic drugs*—such as *chloramphenicol, erythromycin,* and *tetracyclines*—may interfere with bactericidal activity. Use with *loop diuretics* or *nephrotoxic drugs*—such as *aminoglycosides, colistin, polymyxin B,* and *vancomycin*—may increase the risk of nephrotoxicity. *Probenecid* competitively inhibits renal tubular secretion of cefadroxil, resulting in higher, prolonged serum cefadroxil levels.

ADVERSE REACTIONS

CNS: *seizures.*

GI: pseudomembranous colitis, *nausea,* vomiting, *diarrhea,* glossitis, abdominal cramps, oral candidiasis.

GU: genital pruritus, candidiasis, vaginitis, renal dysfunction.

Hematologic: *transient neutropenia,* eosinophilia, *leukopenia*, anemia, *agranulocytosis, thrombocytopenia.*

Hepatic: transient increases in liver enzyme levels.

Respiratory: dyspnea.

Skin: *maculopapular and erythematous rashes,* urticaria.

Other: hypersensitivity reactions (serum sickness, *anaphylaxis, angioedema*), fever.

▣ KEY CONSIDERATIONS

Besides the recommendations relevant to all cephalosporins, consider the following:

• Reduce dosage in geriatric patients with diminished renal function.

• Longer half-life of cefadroxil permits once- or twice-daily dosing.

• Drug causes false-positive results in urine glucose tests that use cupric sulfate (Benedict's reagent or Clinitest); use glucose oxidase test (Chemstrip uG, Di-

astix, or glucose enzymatic test strip) instead.
• Cefadroxil falsely elevates serum or urine creatinine levels in tests using Jaffé's reaction.
• Positive Coombs' test results occur in about 3% of patients taking cephalosporins.

Patient education
• Inform patient of potential adverse reactions.

Overdose & treatment
• Signs and symptoms of overdose include neuromuscular hypersensitivity; seizure may follow high CNS levels.
• Remove cefadroxil by hemodialysis. Other treatment is supportive.

---

cefamandole nafate
Mandol

Second-generation cephalosporin, antibiotic

Available by prescription only
Injectable solution: 500 mg, 1 g, 2 g

INDICATIONS & DOSAGE
Serious respiratory tract, GU, skin and soft-tissue, and bone and joint infections; septicemia; peritonitis from susceptible organisms
Adults: 500 mg to 1 g q 4 to 8 hours. In life-threatening infections, up to 2 g q 4 hours may be needed.

Total daily dosage is same for I.M. or I.V. administration and depends on susceptibility of organism and severity of infection. Drug should be injected deep I.M. into a large muscle mass, such as the gluteus or the lateral aspect of the thigh.
♦ *Dosage adjustment.* In patients with impaired renal function, doses or frequency of administration must be modified according to degree of renal impairment, severity of infection, and susceptibility of organism.

Creatinine clearance (ml/min/ 1.73 m^2)	Dosage for adults with severe infections	Dosage for adults with life-threatening infections (maximum)
> 80	1-2 g q 6 hr	2 g q 4 hr
50-80	750 mg-1.5 g q 6 hr	1.5 g q 4 hr; or 2 g q 6 hr
25-50	750 mg-1.5 g q 8 hr	1.5 g q 4 hr; or 2 g q 8 hr
10-25	500 mg-1 g q 8 hr	1 g q 6 hr; or 1.25 g q 8 hr
2-10	500-750 mg q 12 hr	670 mg q 8 hr; or 1 g q 12 hr
< 2	250-500 mg q 12 hr	500 mg q 8 hr; or 750 mg q 12 hr

PHARMACODYNAMICS
Antibiotic action: Cefamandole is primarily bactericidal; however, it may be bacteriostatic. Activity depends on the organism and the rate at which it multiplies, tissue penetration, and drug dosage. Drug adheres to bacterial penicillin-binding proteins, thereby inhibiting cell-wall synthesis.

Drug is active against *Escherichia coli* and other coliform bacteria, penicillinase- and nonpenicillinase-producing *Staphylococcus aureus, S. epidermidis,* group A beta-hemolytic streptococci, *Klebsiella, Haemophilus influenzae, Proteus mirabilis,* and *Enterobacter* as the second-generation drugs. *Bacteroides fragilis* and *Acinetobacter* are resistant to drug.

PHARMACOKINETICS
Absorption: Cefamandole isn't absorbed from the GI tract and must be given parenterally; serum levels peak ½ to 2 hours after an I.M. dose.
Distribution: Drug is distributed widely to most body tissues and fluids, including the gallbladder, liver, kidneys, bone, sputum, bile, and pleural and synovial fluids; CSF penetration is poor. About 65% to 75% of drug binds to proteins.
Metabolism: Drug isn't metabolized.
Excretion: Drug is excreted primarily in urine through renal tubular secretion and glomerular filtration. In patients with normal renal function, elimination half-life is ½ to 2 hours; in patients with se-

---

vere renal disease, 12 to 18 hours. Some of the drug can be removed from circulation through hemodialysis.

CONTRAINDICATIONS & PRECAUTIONS

Contraindicated in patients with hypersensitivity to cefamandole or other cephalosporins. Use cautiously in patients with impaired renal function or penicillin allergy.

INTERACTIONS

Drug-drug. Use with *anticoagulants* may increase risk of bleeding. Use with *bacteriostatic drugs*—such as *tetracyclines, erythromycin,* and *chloramphenicol*—may impair its bactericidal activity. Use with *loop diuretics* or *nephrotoxic drugs*—such as *aminoglycosides, colistin, polymyxin B,* and *vancomycin*—may increase the risk of nephrotoxicity. *Probenecid* competitively inhibits renal tubular secretion of cefamandole, resulting in higher, prolonged serum cefamandole levels.

Drug-lifestyle. Use with *alcohol* may cause severe disulfiram-like reactions.

ADVERSE REACTIONS

GI: pseudomembranous colitis, nausea, vomiting, *diarrhea,* oral candidiasis.
Hematologic: eosinophilia, coagulation abnormalities.
Hepatic: transient increases in liver enzyme levels.
Skin: *maculopapular and erythematous rashes, urticaria.*
Other: hypersensitivity reactions (serum sickness, **anaphylaxis**); *pain, induration, sterile abscesses,* temperature elevation, tissue sloughing (at injection site); *phlebitis, thrombophlebitis* (with I.V. injection).

🔲 KEY CONSIDERATIONS

• Dosage reduction may be required in patients with diminished renal function. Hypoprothrombinemia and bleeding have been reported mostly in geriatric, malnourished, and debilitated patients.
• For most cephalosporin-sensitive organisms, cefamandole offers little advantage over others; it's less effective than cefoxitin against anaerobic infections.

• For I.V. use, reconstitute 1 g with 10 ml of sterile water for injection, D_5W injection, or normal saline injection. Administer slowly, over 3 to 5 minutes, or by intermittent infusion or continuous infusion in compatible solutions. Check package insert.
• Don't mix with I.V. infusions containing magnesium or calcium ions, which are chemically incompatible and may cause irreversible effects.
• Cefamandole injection contains 3.3 mEq of sodium/gram of drug.
• For I.M. use, dilute 1 g of cefamandole in 3 ml of sterile or bacteriostatic water for injection, normal saline solution for injection, or bacteriostatic normal saline solution for injection.
• Administer deeply into large muscle mass to ensure maximum absorption. Rotate injection sites.
• I.M. cefamandole is less painful than cefoxitin injection; it doesn't require addition of lidocaine.
• After reconstitution, solution remains stable for 24 hours at room temperature or 96 hours under refrigeration. Solution should be light yellow to amber. Don't use solution if it's discolored or contains a precipitate.
• Monitor for signs or symptoms of bleeding. Monitor patient's PT, INR, and platelet level. Bleeding can be prevented or reversed by administering vitamin K or blood products.
• Use with alcohol causes disulfiram-like reaction. For patients who drink alcohol, consider alternative drugs if home I.V. antibiotic therapy is necessary.
• Drug causes false-positive results in urine glucose tests using cupric sulfate (Benedict's reagent or Clinitest); use glucose oxidase tests (Chemstrip uG, Diastix, or glucose enzymatic test strip) instead.
• Drug also falsely elevates serum or urine creatinine levels in tests using Jaffé's reaction.
• Drug may cause positive Coombs' test results.

Patient education

• Inform patient of potential adverse reactions.

Overdose & treatment
● Signs and symptoms of overdose include neuromuscular hypersensitivity. Seizure may follow high CNS levels. Hypoprothrombinemia and bleeding may occur; treat with vitamin K or blood products.
● Some of the drug may be removed by hemodialysis.

Creatinine clearance (ml/min/1.73 m²)	Dosage in adults
≥ 55	Usual adult dose
35-54	Full dose q 8 hr or less frequently
11-34	½ usual dose q 12 hr
≤ 10	½ usual dose q 18 to 24 hr

cefazolin sodium
Ancef, Kefzol, Zolicef

First-generation cephalosporin, antibiotic

Available by prescription only
Injection (parenteral): 250 mg, 500 mg, 1 g, 5 g, 10 g, 20 g
Infusion: 500 mg/50- or 500 mg/100-ml vial, 1 g/50- or 1 g/100-ml vial, 500-mg or 1-g Redi Vials, Faspaks, or ADD-Vantage vials

INDICATIONS & DOSAGE
Serious respiratory tract, GU, skin and soft-tissue, and bone and joint infections; biliary tract infections; septicemia, endocarditis from susceptible organisms
Adults: 250 mg I.M. or I.V. q 8 hours to 1 g q 8 hours. Maximum dosage is 12 g/day in life-threatening situations.

Total daily dosage is same for I.M. or I.V. administration and depends on the susceptibility of organism and severity of infection. Cefazolin should be injected deep I.M. into a large muscle mass, such as the gluteus or the lateral aspect of the thigh.
✦ *Dosage adjustment.* Dose or frequency of administration must be modified according to the degree of renal impairment, severity of infection, susceptibility of organism, and serum levels of drug. Because hemodialysis removes the drug from circulation, patients undergoing hemodialysis may require dosage adjustment.

PHARMACODYNAMICS
Antibiotic action: Cefazolin is primarily bactericidal; however, it may be bacteriostatic. Activity depends on the organism and the rate at which it multiplies, tissue penetration, and drug dosage. Drug adheres to bacterial penicillin-binding proteins, thereby inhibiting cell-wall synthesis.

Drug is active against *Escherichia coli, Enterobacteriaceae, Haemophilus influenzae, Klebsiella, Proteus mirabilis, Staphylococcus aureus, Streptococcus pneumoniae,* and group A beta-hemolytic streptococci.

PHARMACOKINETICS
Absorption: Cefazolin isn't well absorbed from the GI tract and must be given parenterally; serum levels peak 1 to 2 hours after an I.M. dose.
Distribution: Drug is distributed widely into most body tissues and fluids, including the gallbladder, liver, kidneys, bone, sputum, bile, and pleural and synovial fluids; CSF penetration is poor. About 74% to 86% of drug binds to proteins.
Metabolism: Drug isn't metabolized.
Excretion: Drug is excreted primarily unchanged in urine through renal tubular secretion and glomerular filtration. Elimination half-life is 1 to 2 hours in patients with normal renal function; end-stage renal disease prolongs half-life to 12 to 50 hours. Drug can be removed from circulation through hemodialysis or peritoneal dialysis.

CONTRAINDICATIONS & PRECAUTIONS
Contraindicated in patients with hypersensitivity to other cephalosporins. Use cautiously in patients with impaired renal function or penicillin allergy.

Reactions may be *common,* uncommon, ***life-threatening,*** or COMMON AND LIFE-THREATENING.

INTERACTIONS
Drug-drug. Use with *bacteriostatic drugs*—such as *chloramphenicol, erythromycin,* and *tetracyclines*—may interfere with bactericidal activity. Use with *loop diuretics* or *nephrotoxic drugs*—such as *aminoglycosides, colistin, polymyxin B,* and *vancomycin*—may increase the risk of nephrotoxicity. *Probenecid* competitively inhibits renal tubular secretion of cefazolin, resulting in higher, prolonged serum cefazolin levels.

ADVERSE REACTIONS
GI: pseudomembranous colitis, nausea, anorexia, vomiting, *diarrhea,* glossitis, dyspepsia, abdominal cramps, anal pruritus, oral candidiasis.
GU: genital pruritus, candidiasis, vaginitis.
Hematologic: *neutropenia, leukopenia,* eosinophilia, *thrombocytopenia.*
Hepatic: transient increases in liver enzyme levels.
Skin: *maculopapular and erythematous rashes, urticaria, pruritus, Stevens-Johnson syndrome.*
Other: hypersensitivity reactions (serum sickness, *anaphylaxis*); pain, *induration, sterile abscesses, tissue sloughing* (at injection site); *phlebitis, thrombophlebitis* (with I.V. injection).

▣ KEY CONSIDERATIONS
Besides the recommendations relevant to all cephalosporins, consider the following:
• For patients who must restrict their intake of sodium, know that cefazolin injection contains 2 mEq of sodium/gram of drug.
• Because of the long duration of effect, most infections can be treated with a single dose every 8 hours.
• For I.M. use, reconstitute with sterile water, bacteriostatic water, or normal saline solution: 2 ml to a 250-mg vial, 2 ml to a 500-mg vial, and 2.5 ml to a 1-g vial produces 125 mg/ml, 225 mg/ml, and 330 mg/ml respectively.
• Reconstituted solution is stable for 24 hours at room temperature; for 96 hours if refrigerated.
• I.M. cefazolin injection is less painful than that of other cephalosporins.

• Cephalosporins cause false-positive results in urine glucose tests using cupric sulfate (Benedict's reagent or Clinitest); use glucose oxidase tests (Chemstrip uG, Diastix, or glucose enzymatic test strip) instead.
• Cefazolin falsely elevates serum or urine creatinine levels in tests using Jaffé's reaction.
• Cefazolin also causes positive Coombs' test results.

Patient education
• Inform patient of potential adverse reactions.

Overdose & treatment
• Signs and symptoms of overdose include neuromuscular hypersensitivity; seizure may follow high CNS levels. Drug can be removed from circulation through hemodialysis.

---

cefdinir
Omnicef

Third-generation cephalosporin, antibiotic

Available by prescription only
Capsules: 300 mg
Suspension: 125 mg/5 ml

INDICATIONS & DOSAGE
Treatment of mild to moderate infections caused by susceptible strains of microorganisms for conditions of community-acquired pneumonia, acute exacerbations of chronic bronchitis, acute maxillary sinusitis, acute bacterial otitis media, and uncomplicated skin and skin-structure infections
Adults: 300 mg P.O. q 12 hours or 600 mg P.O. q 24 hours for 10 days. (Use q 12-hour dosages for pneumonia and skin infections.)
Treatment of pharyngitis and tonsillitis
Adults: 300 mg P.O. q 12 hours for 5 to 10 days or 600 mg P.O. q 24 hours for 10 days.
✦ **Dosage adjustment.** If creatinine clearance is below 30 ml/minute, reduce dosage to 300 mg P.O. once daily for adults.

In patients receiving long-term hemodialysis, 300 mg or 7 mg/kg P.O. at end of each dialysis session and subsequently every other day.

PHARMACODYNAMICS

Antibiotic action: Cefdinir is bactericidal; it inhibits cell-wall synthesis. Drug is stable around some beta-lactamase enzymes, causing some microorganisms resistant to penicillins and cephalosporins to be susceptible to cefdinir. Excluding *Pseudomonas, Enterobacter, Enterococcus,* and methicillin-resistant *Staphylococcus* species, the spectrum of activity of this drug includes a broad range of gram-positive and gram-negative aerobic microorganisms.

PHARMACOKINETICS

Absorption: About 21% of the 300-mg capsule dose, 16% of the 600-mg capsule dose, and 25% of the suspension is bioavailable after administration. Plasma levels peak in 2 to 4 hours; food doesn't affect absorption.
Distribution: Mean volume of distribution for adults is 0.35 L/kg, and distribution to tonsil, sinus, lung, and middle ear tissue and fluid ranges from 15% to 35% of corresponding plasma levels. About 60% to 70% of drug binds to plasma proteins.
Metabolism: Drug isn't appreciably metabolized, and its activity is due mainly to parent drug.
Excretion: Most of the drug is excreted from the kidneys; mean plasma elimination half-life is 1.7 hours. In patients with renal dysfunction, drug clearance is reduced.

CONTRAINDICATIONS & PRECAUTIONS

Contraindicated in patients allergic to cephalosporin class of antibiotics. Use cautiously in patients with known hypersensitivity to penicillin because of the possibility of cross-sensitivity with other beta-lactam antibiotics and in patients with history of colitis.

INTERACTIONS

Drug-drug. *Magnesium-* and *aluminum-containing antacids* and *iron supplements* decrease rate of absorption and bioavailability of cefdinir; administer such preparations 2 hours before or after cefdinir dose. As with other beta-lactam antibiotics, *probenecid* inhibits the renal excretion of cefdinir.
Drug-food. *Foods fortified with iron* decrease rate of absorption and bioavailability of cefdinir; eat these foods 2 hours before or after cefdinir dose.

ADVERSE REACTIONS

CNS: headache.
GI: abdominal pain, *diarrhea,* nausea, vomiting.
GU: vaginal candidiasis, vaginitis.
Skin: rash.

▣ KEY CONSIDERATIONS

• Cefdinir is well tolerated in all age-groups. Dosage adjustment isn't necessary unless patient has renal impairment.
• As with many antibiotics, prolonged drug treatment may result in possible emergence and overgrowth of resistant organisms. Alternative therapy should be considered if superinfection occurs.
• Pseudomembranous colitis has been reported with many antibiotics, including cefdinir, and should be considered in diagnosing patients who present with diarrhea subsequent to antibiotic therapy or in those with history of colitis.
• False-positive reactions for ketones (tests using nitroprusside only) and glucose (Clinitest, Benedict's solution, Fehling's solution) in the urine have been reported.
• Cephalosporins can induce a positive direct Coombs' test.

Patient education

• Instruct patient to take antacids, iron supplements, and iron-fortified foods 2 hours before or after cefdinir.
• Inform diabetic patient that each teaspoon of suspension contains 2.86 g of sucrose.
• Tell patient that drug may be taken without regard to meals.
• Advise patient to report severe diarrhea or diarrhea accompanied by abdominal pain.
• Tell patient that mild diarrhea can be treated symptomatically.

Overdose & treatment
• Signs and symptoms of overdose with other beta-lactam antibiotics include nausea, vomiting, epigastric distress, diarrhea, and seizures.
• Drug can be removed from circulation through hemodialysis.

cefepime hydrochloride
Maxipime

Semisynthetic third- or fourth-generation cephalosporin, antibiotic

Available by prescription only
Injection: 500 mg/15-ml vial, 1 g/100-ml piggyback bottle, 1 g/ADD-Vantage vial, 1 g/15-ml vial, 2 g/100-ml piggyback bottle, 2 g/20-ml vial

INDICATIONS & DOSAGE
Mild to moderate urinary tract infections caused by Escherichia coli, Klebsiella pneumoniae, *or* Proteus mirabilis, *including cases with concurrent bacteremia with these microorganisms*
Adults: 0.5 to 1 g I.M. (use I.M. route only when it's considered a more appropriate route), or I.V infused over 30 minutes q 12 hours for 7 to 10 days.
Severe urinary tract infections including pyelonephritis caused by E. coli *or* K. pneumoniae
Adults: 2 g I.V. infused over 30 minutes q 12 hours for 10 days.
Moderate to severe pneumonia caused by Streptococcus pneumoniae, Pseudomonas aeruginosa, K. pneumoniae, *or* Enterobacter *species*
Adults: 1 to 2 g I.V. infused over 30 minutes q 12 hours for 10 days.
Moderate to severe uncomplicated skin and skin-structure infections due to Staphylococcus aureus *(methicillin-susceptible strains only) or* Streptococcus pyogenes
Adults: 2 g I.V. infused over 30 minutes q 12 hours for 10 days.
✦ *Dosage adjustment.* Adjust dosage in patients with impaired renal function. Give patients a repeat dose at the end of dialysis; patients undergoing continuous ambulatory peritoneal dialysis should have doses q 48 hours.

PHARMACODYNAMICS
Antibiotic action: Cefepime is bactericidal; it inhibits cell-wall synthesis. It's usually active against gram-positive microorganisms such as *S. pneumoniae, S. aureus,* and *S. pyogenes* and gram-negative microorganisms such as *Enterobacter* species, *E. coli, K. pneumoniae, P. mirabilis,* and *P. aeruginosa.*

PHARMACOKINETICS
Absorption: Cefepime is completely absorbed after I.M. administration.
Distribution: Drug is widely distributed; 20% of it binds to plasma proteins.
Metabolism: Drug is rapidly metabolized..
Excretion: About 85% of drug is excreted in urine unchanged; less than 1% as the metabolite, 6.8% as the metabolite oxide, and 2.5% as an epimer of cefepime.

CONTRAINDICATIONS & PRECAUTIONS
Contraindicated in patients with hypersensitivity to cefepime, other cephalosporins, penicillins, or other beta-lactam antibiotics. Use cautiously in patients with history of GI disease (especially colitis), impaired renal function, or poor nutritional status and in those receiving a protracted course of antimicrobial therapy.

INTERACTIONS
Drug-drug. *Aminoglycosides* may increase risk of nephrotoxicity and ototoxicity; monitor patient's renal and hearing functions closely. *Potent diuretics* such as *furosemide* may increase risk of nephrotoxicity; monitor patient's renal function closely.

ADVERSE REACTIONS
CNS: headache.
GI: colitis, diarrhea, nausea, vomiting, oral candidiasis.
GU: vaginitis.
Skin: rash, pruritus, urticaria.
Other: phlebitis, pain, inflammation, fever.

▣ KEY CONSIDERATIONS

Besides the recommendations relevant to all cephalosporins, consider the following:

• Use caution when administering cefepime to geriatric patients with impaired renal function; dosage may need to be adjusted.

• Obtain culture and sensitivity tests before giving first dose, if appropriate. Therapy may begin pending results.

• For I.V. administration, follow the manufacturer's guidelines closely when reconstituting drug. Variations occur in constituting drug for administration and depend on concentration of drug required and how drug is packaged (piggyback vial, ADD-Vantage vial, or regular vial). Also, know that type of diluent used for constitution depends on product used. Use only solutions that the manufacturer recommends. The resulting solution should be administered over 30 minutes.

• Intermittent I.V. infusion with a Y-type administration set can be accomplished with compatible solutions. However, during infusion of a solution containing cefepime, discontinuing the other solution is recommended.

• For I.M. administration, constitute drug using sterile water for injection, normal saline solution, D_5W injection, 5% or 1% lidocaine hydrochloride, or bacteriostatic water for injection with parabens or benzyl alcohol. Follow the manufacturer's guidelines for quantity of diluent to use.

• Inspect solution for particulate matter before administration. The powder and its solutions tend to darken depending on storage conditions. However, product potency isn't adversely affected when stored as recommended.

• Monitor patient for superinfection. Drug may cause overgrowth of nonsusceptible bacteria or fungi.

• Many cephalosporins may cause a fall in prothrombin activity; patients at risk include those with renal or hepatic impairment or poor nutritional status and those receiving prolonged cefepime therapy. Monitor PT and INR in these patients. Administer exogenous vitamin K subcutaneously if necessary.

• Cefepime may result in a false-positive reaction for glucose in the urine when using Clinitest tablets. Glucose tests based on enzymatic glucose oxidase reactions (such as Chemstrip uG, Diastix, or glucose enzymatic test strip) should be used instead.

• A positive direct Coombs' test may occur during treatment with drug.

Patient education

• Warn patient receiving drug I.M. that pain may occur at injection site.

• Instruct patient to report adverse reactions promptly.

Overdose & treatment

• Signs and symptoms of overdose include seizures, encephalopathy, and neuromuscular excitability.

• Patients who receive an overdose should be carefully observed and given supportive treatment. In a patient with renal insufficiency, hemodialysis, not peritoneal dialysis, is recommended to aid in the removal of cefepime from the body.

---

cefixime
Suprax

Third-generation cephalosporin, antibiotic

Available by prescription only
Tablets: 200 mg, 400 mg
Powder for oral suspension:
100 mg/5 ml

INDICATIONS & DOSAGE

Otitis media; acute bronchitis; acute exacerbations of chronic bronchitis, pharyngitis, tonsillitis; uncomplicated urinary tract infections caused by **Escherichia coli** *and* **Proteus mirabilis;** *uncomplicated gonorrhea*
Adults: 400 mg P.O. daily in one or two divided doses; for uncomplicated gonorrhea, 400 mg as a single dose.

✦ *Dosage adjustment.* In renally impaired patients, dosages must be adjusted based on degree of renal impairment, severity of infection, and susceptibility of organism. To prevent toxic accumulation in patients with creatinine clearance below 60 ml/minute/1.73 m², dosage may need to be reduced.

Creatinine clearance (ml/min/1.73 m²)	Dosage in adults
> 60	Usual dose
20-60	75% of usual dose
< 20 or patients receiving continuous ambulatory peritoneal dialysis	50% of usual dose

PHARMACODYNAMICS

Antibacterial action: Cefixime is primarily bactericidal; it binds to penicillin-binding proteins in the bacterial cell wall, thereby inhibiting cell-wall synthesis.

It's used to treat otitis media caused by penicillinase- and nonpenicillinase-producing *Haemophilus influenzae, Moraxella (Branhamella) catarrhalis* (which is penicillinase producing), and *Streptococcus pyogenes.* Substantial drug resistance has been noted. Drug is also used to treat acute bronchitis and acute exacerbations of chronic bronchitis caused by *S. pneumoniae* and penicillinase- and nonpenicillinase-producing *H. influenzae,* pharyngitis and tonsillitis caused by *S. pyogenes,* and uncomplicated urinary tract infections caused by *E. coli* and *P. mirabilis.*

PHARMACOKINETICS

Absorption: About 30% to 50% of cefixime is absorbed after oral administration. The suspension form provides a higher serum level than the tablet form. Food delays absorption, but the total amount of drug absorbed isn't affected.
Distribution: Drug is widely distributed; about 65% of it binds to plasma proteins.
Metabolism: About 50% of drug is metabolized.
Excretion: Cefixime is excreted primarily in urine. In patients with normal renal function, elimination half-life is 3 to 4 hours; in patients with end-stage renal disease, up to 11½ hours.

CONTRAINDICATIONS & PRECAUTIONS

Contraindicated in patients with hypersensitivity to cefixime or other cephalosporins. Use cautiously in patients with impaired renal function.

INTERACTIONS

Drug-drug. *Salicylates* may increase serum cefixime levels.

ADVERSE REACTIONS

CNS: headache, dizziness.
GI: *diarrhea,* loose stools, abdominal pain, nausea, vomiting, dyspepsia, flatulence, pseudomembranous colitis.
GU: genital pruritus, vaginitis, genital candidiasis, transient increases in BUN and serum creatinine levels.
Hematologic: *thrombocytopenia, leukopenia,* eosinophilia.
Hepatic: transient increases in liver enzyme levels.
Skin: pruritus, rash, urticaria, *erythema multiforme, Stevens-Johnson syndrome.*
Other: fever, hypersensitivity reactions (serum sickness, *anaphylaxis*).

▣ KEY CONSIDERATIONS

Besides the recommendations relevant to all cephalosporins, consider the following:
● Cefixime is the first orally active, third-generation cephalosporin that's effective with once-daily dosage.
● The manufacturer suggests that the suspension, not the tablets, be used to treat otitis media.
● Patients with antibiotic-induced diarrhea should be evaluated for overgrowth of pseudomembranous colitis caused by *Clostridium difficile.* Mild cases usually respond to discontinuation of the drug; moderate to severe cases may require fluid, electrolyte, and protein supplementation. Oral vancomycin is the drug of choice for treating antibiotic-associated *C. difficile* pseudomembranous colitis.
● Acute hypersensitivity reactions should be treated immediately. Emergency measures, such as airway management, pressor amines, epinephrine, oxygen, antihistamines, and corticosteroids, may be required.
● Some cephalosporins may cause seizures, especially in patients with renal failure who receive full therapeutic dosages. If seizures occur, discontinue drug and initiate anticonvulsant therapy.
● Cefixime may cause false-positive results in urine glucose tests that use

cupric sulfate (Benedict's reagent or Clinitest); use glucose oxidase tests (Chemstrip uG, Diastix, or glucose enzymatic test strip) instead.
- Cefixime may cause false-positive results in tests for urine ketones that use nitroprusside (but not nitroferricyanide).
- Other cephalosporins cause false-positive direct Coombs' test results.

Patient education
- Instruct patient to report unpleasant effects, such as itching, rash, or severe diarrhea. Note that diarrhea is the most common adverse GI effect.
- Advise patient that oral suspension is stable for 14 days after reconstitution and doesn't require refrigeration.

Overdose & treatment
- Signs and symptoms of overdose include mild to moderate GI effects such as nausea, vomiting, and diarrhea.
- In the case of overdose, gastric lavage and supportive treatment are recommended. Peritoneal dialysis and hemodialysis will remove substantial quantities of drug.

---

cefmetazole sodium
Zefazone

Second-generation cephalosporin, antibiotic

Available by prescription only
Injection: 1 g, 2 g

INDICATIONS & DOSAGE
Serious respiratory and urinary tract, skin, soft-tissue, abdominal, and ◇pelvic infections caused by susceptible organisms
Adults: 2 g I.V. q 6 to 12 hours for 5 to 14 days.
Perioperative prophylaxis
Adults: 1 to 2 g I.V. administered 30 to 90 minutes before the procedure. Can repeat dose 8 and 16 hours after first dose for prolonged (over 4 hours) procedures.
♦ **Dosage adjustment.** In patients with creatinine clearance of 50 to 90 ml/minute, give 1 to 2 g I.V. q 12 hours; if 30 to 49 ml/minute, give 1 to 2 g I.V. q 16 hours; if 10 to 29 ml/minute, 1 to 2 g I.V. q 24 hours; and if below 10 ml/minute, give 1 to 2 g I.V. q 48 hours.

PHARMACODYNAMICS
Antibiotic action: Cefmetazole is primarily bactericidal; however, it may be bacteriostatic. Activity depends on the organism and the rate at which it multiplies, tissue penetration, and drug dosage. Drug adheres to bacterial penicillin-binding proteins, thereby inhibiting cell-wall synthesis.

Spectrum of activity resembles that of other second-generation cephalosporins. Drug is active against many gram-positive organisms and enteric gram-negative bacilli, including *Escherichia coli* and other coliform bacteria, penicillinase- and nonpenicillinase-producing *Staphylococcus aureus, S. epidermidis,* streptococci, *Klebsiella, Haemophilus influenzae,* and *Bacteroides* species (including *B. fragilis*). *Enterobacter, Pseudomonas, Acinetobacter, Serratia marcescens, Citrobacter freundii,* and methicillin-resistant *Staphylococcus* are generally resistant to cefmetazole.

PHARMACOKINETICS
Absorption: Cefmetazole isn't absorbed from the GI tract and must be given parenterally. Serum levels peak 1½ hours after an I.M. dose.
Distribution: Drug is distributed widely to most body tissues and fluids, including the gallbladder, liver, kidney, bone, sputum, bile, and pleural and synovial fluids. CSF penetration is poor. About 65% of drug binds to proteins.
Metabolism: Only about 15% of a dose is metabolized, probably in the liver.
Excretion: Drug is excreted primarily in urine through renal tubular secretion and glomerular filtration. Elimination half-life is about 1½ hours in patients with normal renal function. Patients with renal dysfunction require dosage adjustment.

CONTRAINDICATIONS & PRECAUTIONS
Contraindicated in patients with hypersensitivity to cefmetazole or other cephalosporins. Use cautiously in patients with penicillin allergy.

INTERACTIONS

Drug-drug. Use with *bacteriostatic drugs*—such as *chloramphenicol, erythromycin*, and *tetracyclines*—may interfere with bactericidal activity. Use with *loop diuretics* or *nephrotoxic drugs*—such as *aminoglycosides, colistin, polymyxin B*, and *vancomycin*—may increase the risk of nephrotoxicity. *Probenecid* competitively inhibits renal tubular secretion of cefmetazole, resulting in higher, prolonged serum cefmetazole levels.
Drug-lifestyle. Use with *alcohol* may cause disulfiram-like reactions.

ADVERSE REACTIONS

CNS: headache, hot flashes.
CV: *shock*, hypotension.
EENT: epistaxis, altered color perception.
GI: nausea, vomiting, *diarrhea*, epigastric pain, pseudomembranous colitis, candidiasis, bleeding.
GU: vaginitis.
Hepatic: may elevate liver function test results.
Musculoskeletal: joint pain and inflammation.
Respiratory: pleural effusion, dyspnea, respiratory distress.
Skin: rash, pruritus, generalized erythema, phlebitis, thrombophlebitis.
Other: fever, bacterial or fungal superinfection, hypersensitivity reactions (serum sickness, *anaphylaxis*), pain at injection site.

▣ KEY CONSIDERATIONS

• Dosage reduction may be required in patients with diminished renal function. Hypoprothrombinemia and bleeding have been reported mostly in geriatric, malnourished, and debilitated patients.
• For most cephalosporin-sensitive organisms, cefmetazole offers little advantage over other cephalosporins.
• Use with alcohol can cause disulfiram-like reactions. Use cautiously in patients who drink alcohol and receive I.V. antibiotics at home, or consider alternative drug therapy.
• Cefmetazole injection contains 2 mEq of sodium/gram of drug.

• Don't use cefmetazole I.V. solution I.M.; I.M. administration is indicated only for treatment of gonorrhea.
• Hypoprothrombinemia may occur. If bleeding occurs or if PT or INR increases, reverse the effect by administering vitamin K.
• Cefmetazole causes false-positive results of urine glucose tests that use cupric sulfate (Benedict's reagent or Clinitest); use glucose oxidase tests (Chemstrip uG, Diastix, or glucose enzymatic test strip) instead.
• Cefmetazole may cause positive Coombs' test results.

Patient education
• Inform patient of potential adverse reactions including the possible alteration of color perception.
• Instruct patient to report adverse respiratory reactions promptly.
• Advise patient to avoid alcohol while taking drug.

Overdose & treatment
• Signs and symptoms of overdose include neuromuscular hypersensitivity. Seizure may follow high CNS levels.
• Treat patients with hypoprothrombinemia or bleeding with vitamin K or blood products. Some cefmetazole may be removed by hemodialysis.

---

cefonicid sodium
Monocid

Second-generation cephalosporin, antibiotic

Available by prescription only
Injection: 1 g
Infusion: 1 g
Pharmacy bulk package: 10 g

INDICATIONS & DOSAGE
Serious lower respiratory and urinary tract, skin, and soft-tissue infections; septicemia; bone and joint infections from susceptible organisms
Adults: Usual dosage is 1 g I.V. or I.M. q 24 hours. In life-threatening infections, 2 g q 24 hours.

Preoperative prophylaxis
Adults: 1 g I.M. or I.V. 1 hour before surgery.
◊ *Uncomplicated gonorrhea*
Adults: 1 g I.M. as a single dose.

Total daily dosage is same for I.M. or I.V. administration and depends on susceptibility of organism and severity of infection. Cefonicid should be injected deep I.M. into a large muscle mass, such as the gluteus or the lateral aspect of the thigh.

♦ *Dosage adjustment.* In patients with impaired renal function, doses or frequency of administration must be modified according to degree of renal impairment, severity of infection, and susceptibility of organism. To prevent toxic accumulation, dosage may need to be reduced in patients with creatinine clearance below 80 ml/minute. Because drug is dialyzable, dosage may need to be adjusted in patients undergoing treatment with hemodialysis.

Creatinine clearance (ml/min/ 1.73 m²)	Dosage for adults with mild to moderate infections	Dosage for adults with severe infections
≥ 80	Usual adult dose	Usual adult dose
60-79	10 mg/kg q 24 hr	25 mg/kg q 24 hr
40-59	8 mg/kg q 24 hr	20 mg/kg q 24 hr
20-39	4 mg/kg q 24 hr	15 mg/kg q 24 hr
10-19	4 mg/kg q 48 hr	15 mg/kg q 48 hr
5-9	4 mg/kg q 3 to 5 days	15 mg/kg q 3 to 5 days
< 5	3 mg/kg q 3 to 5 days	4 mg/kg q 3 to 5 days

PHARMACODYNAMICS

Antibiotic action: Cefonicid is primarily bactericidal; however, it may be bacteriostatic. Activity depends on the organism and the rate at which it multiplies, tissue penetration, and drug dosage. Drug adheres to bacterial penicillin-binding proteins, thereby inhibiting cell-wall synthesis.

Cefonicid is active against many gram-positive organisms and enteric gram-negative bacilli, including *Streptococcus pneumoniae, Klebsiella pneumoniae, Escherichia coli, Haemophilus influenzae, Proteus mirabilis, Staphylococcus aureus* and *S. epidermidis,* and *Streptococcus pyogenes;* however, *Bacteroides fragilis, Pseudomonas,* and *Acinetobacter* are resistant to cefonicid. Cefonicid is less effective than cefuroxime against gram-positive cocci; it's slightly more active than cefoxitin against gonococci.

PHARMACOKINETICS

Absorption: Cefonicid isn't absorbed from the GI tract and must be given parenterally; serum levels peak 1 to 2 hours after an I.M. dose.
Distribution: Drug is distributed widely to most body tissues and fluids, including the gallbladder, liver, kidneys, bone, sputum, bile, and pleural and synovial fluids; CSF penetration is poor. About 90% to 98% binds to proteins.
Metabolism: Drug isn't metabolized.
Excretion: Most of the drug is excreted in urine through renal tubular secretion and glomerular filtration. In patients with normal renal function, elimination half-life is 3½ to 6 hours; in patients with severe renal disease, 100 hours. Some of the drug may be removed through hemodialysis.

CONTRAINDICATIONS & PRECAUTIONS

Contraindicated in patients with hypersensitivity to cefonicid or other cephalosporins. Use cautiously in patients with impaired renal function or penicillin allergy.

INTERACTIONS

Drug-drug. Use with *bacteriostatic drugs*—such as *chloramphenicol, erythromycin,* and *tetracyclines*—may interfere with bactericidal activity. Use with *loop diuretics* or *nephrotoxic drugs*—such as *aminoglycosides, colistin, polymyxin B,* and *vancomycin*—may increase the risk of nephrotoxicity. *Probenecid* competitively inhibits renal tubular secretion of cefonicid, resulting in higher, prolonged serum cefonicid levels.

ADVERSE REACTIONS

CNS: dizziness, headache, malaise, paresthesia.
GI: pseudomembranous colitis, diarrhea.
GU: *acute renal failure,* interstitial nephritis.
Hematologic: *neutropenia, leukopenia,* eosinophilia, anemia, prolonged PT and INR, thrombocytosis, *thrombocytopenia.*
Hepatic: may elevate liver function test results.
Musculoskeletal: myalgia (with I.V. injection).
Skin: *maculopapular and erythematous rashes, urticaria, phlebitis, thrombophlebitis.*
Other: hypersensitivity reactions (serum sickness, *anaphylaxis*); *pain, induration, sterile abscesses, tissue sloughing* (at injection site); fever.

⬚ KEY CONSIDERATIONS

Besides the recommendations relevant to all cephalosporins, consider the following:
● In geriatric patients with diminished renal function, dosage may need to be reduced.
● When used for surgical prophylaxis, administer drug 1 hour before surgery.
● For patients who must restrict their intake of sodium, know that cefonicid injection contains 3.7 mEq of sodium/gram of drug.
● Reconstitute I.M. or bolus I.V. dose with sterile water for injection. Shake well to ensure complete drug dissolution. Check for precipitate. Discard solution that contains a precipitate.
● Administer deep I.M. dose into a large muscle mass to decrease pain and local irritation. Rotate injection sites. Apply ice to site after administration to reduce pain. Don't inject more than 1 g into a single I.M. site.
● For I.V. infusion, further dilute drug in 50 to 100 ml of recommended fluid. Administer I.V. bolus slowly over 3 to 5 minutes directly or through I.V. tubing if solution is compatible.
● If kept at room temperature, reconstituted solution is stable for 24 hours; if refrigerated, 72 hours. Slight yellowing

of solution doesn't indicate loss of potency.
● Cefonicid causes positive Coombs' test results.
● Cefonicid causes false-positive results in urine glucose tests using cupric sulfate (Benedict's reagent or Clinitest), so use glucose oxidase tests (Chemstrip uG, Diastix, or glucose enzymatic test strip).
● Cefonicid falsely elevates serum or urine creatinine levels in tests using Jaffé's reaction.

Patient education
● Inform patient of potential adverse reactions.

Overdose & treatment
● Signs and symptoms of overdose include neuromuscular hypersensitivity. Seizure may follow high CNS levels. Some cefonicid may be removed by hemodialysis.

cefoperazone sodium
Cefobid

Third-generation cephalosporin, antibiotic

Available by prescription only
Parenteral: 1 g, 2 g
Infusion: 1 g and 2 g piggyback

INDICATIONS & DOSAGE
Serious respiratory tract, intra-abdominal, gynecologic, skin and soft-tissue, urinary tract, and enterococcal infections; bacterial septicemia caused by susceptible organisms
Adults: Usual dosage is 1 to 2 g q 12 hours I.M. or I.V. In severe infections or infections caused by less sensitive organisms, the total daily dosage or frequency may be increased up to 16 g/day in certain situations.
✦ *Dosage adjustment.* Dosage usually doesn't need to be adjusted in patients with renal impairment. However, dosages of 4 g/day should be given cautiously to patients with hepatic disease. Patients with combined hepatic and renal impairment shouldn't receive more than 1 g (base) daily without serum de-

terminations. In patients who are receiving hemodialysis treatments, a dose should follow hemodialysis.

PHARMACODYNAMICS

Antibiotic action: Cefoperazone is primarily bactericidal; however, it may be bacteriostatic. Activity depends on the organism and the rate at which it multiplies, tissue penetration, and drug dosage. Drug adheres to bacterial penicillin-binding proteins, thereby inhibiting cell-wall synthesis. Third-generation cephalosporins appear more active against some beta-lactamase–producing gram-negative organisms.

Drug is active against some gram-positive organisms and many enteric gram-negative bacilli, including *Streptococcus pneumoniae* and *S. pyogenes,* penicillinase- and nonpenicillinase-producing *Staphylococcus aureus, S. epidermidis, Escherichia coli, Klebsiella, Haemophilus influenzae, Enterobacter, Citrobacter, Proteus,* some *Pseudomonas* species (including *P. aeruginosa),* and *Bacteroides* and *Listeria* usually are resistant. Cefoperazone is less effective than cefotaxime or ceftizoxime against Enterobacteriaceae but is slightly more active than those drugs against *P. aeruginosa.*

PHARMACOKINETICS

Absorption: Cefoperazone isn't absorbed from the GI tract and must be given parenterally; serum levels peak 1 to 2 hours after an I.M. dose.
Distribution: Drug is distributed widely to most body tissues and fluids, including the gallbladder, liver, kidneys, bone, sputum, bile, and pleural and synovial fluids; in patients with inflamed meninges, drug penetrates CSF. About 82% to 93% of drug binds to proteins, but this percentage depends on the dosage and decreases as serum levels rise.
Metabolism: Drug isn't substantially metabolized.
Excretion: Drug is excreted primarily in bile; some drug is excreted in urine through renal tubular secretion and glomerular filtration. In patients with normal renal and hepatic function, elimination half-life is 1½ to 2½ hours; in pa-

tients with biliary obstruction or cirrhosis, 3½ to 7 hours. Drug may be removed from circulation through hemodialysis.

CONTRAINDICATIONS & PRECAUTIONS

Contraindicated in patients with hypersensitivity to cefoperazone or other cephalosporins. Use cautiously in patients with impaired renal or hepatic function or penicillin allergy.

INTERACTIONS

Drug-drug. Use with *aminoglycosides* results in synergistic activity against *P. aeruginosa* and *Serratia marcescens;* such combined use slightly increases the risk of nephrotoxicity. Use with *anticoagulants* may increase risk of bleeding. Use with *clavulanic acid* results in synergistic activity against many Enterobacteriaceae, *Bacteroides fragilis, S. aureus,* and *P. aeruginosa. Probenecid* competitively inhibits renal tubular secretions of cefoperazone, causing prolonged serum cefoperazone levels.
Drug-lifestyle. Use with *alcohol* may cause disulfiram-like reactions, such as flushing, sweating, tachycardia, headache, and abdominal cramping.

ADVERSE REACTIONS

GI: pseudomembranous colitis, nausea, vomiting, *diarrhea.*
Hematologic: *transient neutropenia, eosinophilia,* anemia, hypoprothrombinemia, bleeding.
Hepatic: mildly elevated liver enzyme levels.
Skin: *maculopapular and erythematous rashes, urticaria.*
Other: hypersensitivity reactions (serum sickness, **anaphylaxis**); *pain, induration, sterile abscesses, temperature elevation, tissue sloughing* (at injection site); *phlebitis, thrombophlebitis,* drug fever (with I.V. injection).

▣ KEY CONSIDERATIONS

Besides the recommendations relevant to all cephalosporins, consider the following:
• Hypoprothrombinemia and bleeding are more common in geriatric patients.

Reactions may be *common,* uncommon, *life-threatening,* or **COMMON AND LIFE-THREATENING.**

Use with caution, monitor PT and INR, and check for abnormal bleeding.
• Diarrhea may be more common with this drug than with other cephalosporins because it's primarily excreted in bile.
• Patients with biliary disease may need lower dosages.
• For patients who must restrict their intake of sodium, know that cefoperazone injection contains 1.5 mEq of sodium/gram of drug.
• To prepare I.M. injection, use the appropriate diluent, including sterile water for injection or bacteriostatic water for injection. Follow manufacturer's recommendations for mixing drug with sterile water for injection and lidocaine 2% injection. Final solution for I.M. injection will contain 0.5% lidocaine and will be produce less pain on administration (recommended for concentrations of 250 mg/ml or greater). Cefoperazone should be injected deep I.M. into a large muscle mass, such as the gluteus or the lateral aspect of the thigh.
• Store drug in refrigerator and away from light before reconstituting.
• Allow solution to stand after reconstituting to allow foam to dissipate and solution to clear. Solution can be shaken vigorously to ensure complete drug dissolution.
• If stored at room temperature, reconstituted solution is stable for 24 hours; if refrigerated, 3 days. Protecting drug from light is unnecessary.
• Cephalosporins cause false-positive results in urine glucose tests using cupric sulfate (Benedict's reagent or Clinitest); use glucose oxidase (Chemstrip uG, Diastix, or glucose enzymatic test strip) instead.
• Cefoperazone may cause positive Coombs' test results.
• Because cefoperazone is dialyzable, patients undergoing treatment with hemodialysis may require dosage adjustment.
• Use with alcohol can cause disulfiram-like reaction. Use cautiously in patients who drink alcohol and receive I.V. antibiotics at home, or consider alternative drug therapy.

Patient education
• Inform patient of potential adverse reactions.
• Caution patient against the use of alcohol.

Overdose & treatment
• Signs and symptoms of overdose include neuromuscular hypersensitivity. Seizure may follow high CNS levels. Hypoprothrombinemia and bleeding may occur and may require treatment with vitamin K or blood products.
• Drug can be removed from circulation through hemodialysis.

cefotaxime sodium
Claforan

Third-generation cephalosporin, antibiotic

Available by prescription only
Injection: 500 mg, 1 g, 2 g
Pharmacy bulk package: 10-g vial
Infusion: 1 g, 2 g

INDICATIONS & DOSAGE
Serious lower respiratory and urinary tract, CNS, bone and joint, intra-abdominal, gynecologic, and skin infections; bacteremia; septicemia caused by susceptible organisms; ◊ ***pelvic inflammatory disease***
Adults: Usual dosage is 1 g I.V. or I.M. q 6 to 12 hours. Up to 12 g daily can be administered in life-threatening infections.
   Total daily dosage is same for I.M. or I.V. administration and depends on susceptibility of organism and severity of infection. Cefotaxime should be injected deep I.M. into a large muscle mass, such as the lateral aspect of the thigh.
Uncomplicated gonorrhea
Adults: 1 g I.M. as a single dose.
Perioperative prophylaxis
Adults: 1 g I.V. or I.M. 30 to 90 minutes before surgery.
◊ ***Disseminated gonococcal infection***
Adults: 1 g I.V. q 8 hours.
✦ ***Dosage adjustment.*** In patients with impaired renal function, modify dosage or frequency of administration based on

degree of renal impairment, severity of infection, and susceptibility of organism. Reduced dosage may be needed in patients with creatinine clearance below 20 ml/minute to prevent toxicity.

PHARMACODYNAMICS

Antibiotic action: Cefotaxime is primarily bactericidal; however, it may be bacteriostatic. Activity depends on the organism and the rate at which it multiplies, tissue penetration, and drug dosage. Drug adheres to bacterial penicillin-binding proteins, thereby inhibiting cell-wall synthesis.

Third-generation cephalosporins appear more active against some beta-lactamase producing gram-negative organisms.

Drug is active against some gram-positive organisms and many enteric gram-negative bacilli, including streptococci (*Streptococcus pneumoniae* and *S. pyogenes*), penicillinase- and nonpenicillinase-producing *Staphylococcus aureus*, *S. epidermidis*, *Escherichia coli*, *Klebsiella* species, *Haemophilus influenzae*, *Enterobacter* species, *Proteus* species, and *Peptostreptococcus* species, and some strains of *Pseudomonas aeruginosa*. *Listeria* and *Acinetobacter* are often resistant. The active metabolite of cefotaxime, desacetylcefotaxime, may act synergistically with the parent drug against some bacterial strains.

PHARMACOKINETICS

Absorption: Cefotaxime isn't absorbed from the GI tract and must be given parenterally; serum levels peak 30 minutes after an I.M. dose.
Distribution: Drug is distributed widely to most body tissues and fluids, including the gallbladder, liver, kidneys, bone, sputum, bile, and pleural and synovial fluids. Unlike most cephalosporins, drug adequately penetrates CSF when meninges are inflamed; 13% to 38% of drug binds to protein.
Metabolism: Drug is metabolized partially to desacetylcefotaxime, which is an active metabolite.
Excretion: Most of the drug and its metabolites are excreted in urine through renal tubular secretion. About 25% of cefotaxime is excreted in urine as the active metabolite. In patients with normal renal function, elimination half-life is 1 to 1½ hours for cefotaxime and 1½ to 2 hours for desacetylcefotaxime; in patients with severe renal impairment, 11½ hours and up to 56 hours, respectively. Both drug and its metabolites can be removed from circulation through hemodialysis.

CONTRAINDICATIONS & PRECAUTIONS

Contraindicated in patients with hypersensitivity to cefotaxime or other cephalosporins. Use cautiously in patients with impaired renal function or penicillin allergies.

INTERACTIONS

Drug-drug. Use with *aminoglycosides* results in apparent synergistic activity against Enterobacteriaceae and some strains of *P. aeruginosa* and *Serratia marcescens;* such combined use may increase risk of nephrotoxicity. *Probenecid* may block renal tubular secretion of cefotaxime and prolong its half-life.

ADVERSE REACTIONS

CNS: headache.
GI: pseudomembranous colitis, nausea, vomiting, *diarrhea.*
GU: vaginitis, candidiasis, interstitial nephritis.
Hematologic: *transient neutropenia,* eosinophilia, *hemolytic anemia, thrombocytopenia, agranulocytosis.*
Hepatic: transient increases in liver enzyme levels.
Skin: *maculopapular and erythematous rashes, urticaria; phlebitis, thrombophlebitis* (with I.V. injection).
Other: hypersensitivity reactions (serum sickness, *anaphylaxis*); elevated temperature; *pain, induration, sterile abscesses, temperature elevation, tissue sloughing* (at injection site).

⊡ KEY CONSIDERATIONS

Besides the recommendations relevant to all cephalosporins, consider the following:
• Use with caution in geriatric patients with diminished renal function.

Reactions may be *common*, uncommon, *life-threatening*, or COMMON AND LIFE-THREATENING.

• For patients who must restrict their intake of sodium, note that cefotaxime contains 2.2 mEq of sodium/gram of drug.

• For I.M. injection, add 2 ml, 3 ml, or 5 ml of sterile or bacteriostatic water for injection to each 500-mg, 1-g, or 2-g vial. Shake well to dissolve drug completely. Check solution for particles and discoloration. Color ranges from light yellow to amber.

• To prevent pain and tissue reaction, don't inject more than 1 g into a single I.M. site.

• Don't mix with aminoglycosides or sodium bicarbonate or fluids with a pH above 7.5.

• For I.V. use, reconstitute all strengths of an I.V. dose with 10 ml of sterile water for injection. For infusion bottles, add 50 to 100 ml of normal saline solution injection or D_5W injection. May further reconstitute to 50 to 1,000 ml with fluids the manufacturer has recommended.

• Administer drug by direct intermittent I.V. infusion over 3 to 5 minutes. Cefotaxime also may be given more slowly into a flowing I.V. line of compatible solution.

• Solution is stable for 24 hours at room temperature or for at least 5 days under refrigeration. Cefotaxime may be stored in disposable glass or plastic syringes.

• Because drug is hemodialyzable, patients undergoing treatment with hemodialysis may need the dosage adjusted.

• Cephalosporins cause false-positive results in urine glucose tests using cupric sulfate (Benedict's reagent or Clinitest); use glucose oxidase (Chemstrip uG, Diastix, or glucose enzymatic test strip) instead. Cefotaxime also falsely elevates in urine creatinine levels in tests using Jaffé's reaction.

• Cefotaxime may cause positive Coombs' tests results.

Patient education

• Inform patient of potential adverse reactions.

Overdose & treatment

• Signs and symptoms of overdose include neuromuscular hypersensitivity. Seizure may follow high CNS levels.

• Drug may be removed through hemodialysis.

cefotetan disodium
Cefotan

Second-generation cephalosporin, cephamycin, antibiotic

Available by prescription only
Injection: 1 g, 2 g, and 10 g (pharmacy bulk package)
Infusion: 1 g and 2 g piggyback

INDICATIONS & DOSAGE

Serious urinary and lower respiratory tract, gynecologic, skin, intra-abdominal, and bone and joint infections caused by susceptible organisms
Adults: 500 mg to 3 g I.V. or I.M. q 12 hours for 5 to 10 days. Up to 6 g daily in life-threatening infections.
Preoperative prophylaxis
Adults: 1 to 2 g I.V. 30 to 60 minutes before surgery.
Postcesarean treatment
Adults: 1 to 2 g I.V. as soon as umbilical cord is clamped.

Total daily dosage is same for I.M. or I.V. administration and depends on the susceptibility of the organism and severity of infection. Cefotetan should be injected deep I.M. into a large muscle mass, such as the gluteus or the lateral aspect of the thigh.

✦*Dosage adjustment.* In patients with impaired renal function, doses or frequency of administration must be modified based on degree of renal impairment, severity of infection, and susceptibility of organism. Reduced dosage may be necessary in patients with creatinine clearance below 30 ml/minute to prevent toxic reaction. Because drug is hemodialyzable, hemodialysis patients may require dosage adjustment of one-quarter the usual adult dose every 24 hours between hemodialysis sessions and one-half the usual adult dose the day of the hemodialysis session.

Creatinine clearance (ml/min/1.73 m²)	Dosage in adults
> 30	Usual adult dose
10-30	Usual adult dose q 24 hr; or ½ usual adult dose q 12 hr
< 10	Usual adult dose q 48 hr; or ¼ usual adult dose q 12 hr

PHARMACODYNAMICS

Antibiotic action: Cefotetan is primarily bactericidal; however, it may be bacteriostatic. Activity depends on the organism and the rate at which it multiplies, tissue penetration, and drug dosage. Drug adheres to bacterial penicillin-binding proteins, thereby inhibiting cell-wall synthesis.

Cefotetan is active against many gram-positive organisms and enteric gram-negative bacilli, including streptococci, penicillinase- and nonpenicillinase-producing *Staphylococcus aureus*, *S. epidermidis, Escherichia coli, Klebsiella* species, *Enterobacter* species, *Proteus* species, *Haemophilus influenzae, Neisseria gonorrhoeae,* and *Bacteroides* species (including some strains of *B. fragilis*); however, some *B. fragilis* strains, *Pseudomonas,* and *Acinetobacter* are resistant to cefotetan. Most Enterobacteriaceae are more susceptible to cefotetan than to other second-generation cephalosporins.

PHARMACOKINETICS

Absorption: Cefotetan isn't absorbed from the GI tract and must be given parenterally; serum levels peak 1½ to 3 hours after an I.M. dose.
Distribution: Drug is distributed widely to most body tissues and fluids, including the gallbladder, liver, kidneys, bone, sputum, bile, and pleural and synovial fluids; CSF penetration is poor. In patients with normal gallbladder function, biliary cefotetan levels can be up to 20 times higher than serum levels. About 75% to 90% of drug binds to proteins.
Metabolism: Drug isn't metabolized.
Excretion: Drug is excreted primarily in urine through glomerular filtration and some renal tubular secretion; 20% is excreted in bile. In patients with normal re-

nal function, elimination half-life is 3 to 4½ hours.

CONTRAINDICATIONS & PRECAUTIONS

Contraindicated in patients with hypersensitivity to cefotetan or other cephalosporins. Use cautiously in patients with impaired renal function or penicillin allergy.

INTERACTIONS

Drug-drug. Use with *anticoagulants* may increase risk of bleeding. Use with *loop diuretics* or *nephrotoxic drugs*— such as *aminoglycosides, colistin, polymyxin B,* and *vancomycin*—may increase the risk of nephrotoxicity.
Drug-lifestyle. Use with *alcohol* may cause disulfiram-like reactions, such as flushing, sweating, tachycardia, headache, and abdominal cramping.

ADVERSE REACTIONS

GI: pseudomembranous colitis, nausea, *diarrhea.*
GU: *nephrotoxicity.*
Hematologic: *transient neutropenia,* eosinophilia, *hemolytic anemia,* hypoprothrombinemia, bleeding, thrombocytosis, *agranulocytosis, thrombocytopenia.*
Hepatic: transient increases in liver enzyme levels.
Skin: *maculopapular and erythematous rashes, urticaria, phlebitis, thrombophlebitis* (with I.V. injection).
Other: hypersensitivity reactions (serum sickness, *anaphylaxis*); elevated temperature; *pain, induration, sterile abscesses, tissue sloughing* (at injection site).

▣ KEY CONSIDERATIONS

Besides the recommendations relevant to all cephalosporins, consider the following:
• Hypoprothrombinemia and bleeding are more common in geriatric and debilitated patients.
• For I.V. use, reconstitute with sterile water for injection. Then it may be mixed with 50 to 100 ml D_5W or normal saline solution. Infuse intermittently over 30 to 60 minutes.
• For I.M. injection, cefotetan may be reconstituted with sterile water or bacterio-

static water for injection or with normal saline or 0.5% or 1% lidocaine hydrochloride. Shake to dissolve and let solution stand until clear.
• Reconstituted solution remains stable for 24 hours at room temperature or for 96 hours when refrigerated.
• Check for overt and occult bleeding. Monitor vital signs. Check CBC with differential and platelet counts and PT and INR for abnormalities.
• Bleeding can be reversed promptly by administering vitamin K.
• Use with alcohol may cause severe disulfiram-like reactions.
• Cefotetan also causes false-positive results in urine glucose tests using cupric sulfate (Benedict's reagent or Clinitest); use glucose oxidase tests (Chemstrip uG, Diastix, or glucose enzymatic test strip) instead.
• Cefotetan falsely elevates serum or urine creatinine levels in tests using Jaffé's reaction.
• Drug may cause positive Coombs' test results.

Patient education
• Inform patient of potential adverse reactions.
• Caution patient against use of alcohol during therapy.
• Instruct patient to promptly report bleeding, such as blood in the stool or urine, nosebleeds, or bruising.

Overdose & treatment
• Signs and symptoms of overdose include neuromuscular hypersensitivity. Seizure may follow high CNS levels. Hypoprothrombinemia and bleeding may occur; they may be treated with vitamin K or blood products.
• Drug may be removed by hemodialysis.

---

cefoxitin sodium
Mefoxin

Second-generation cephalosporin, cephamycin, antibiotic

Available by prescription only
Injection: 1 g, 2 g
Pharmacy bulk package: 10 g

Infusion: 1 g and 2 g in 50-ml containers

INDICATIONS & DOSAGE
Serious respiratory tract, GU, gynecologic, skin, soft-tissue, bone and joint, blood, and intra-abdominal infections caused by susceptible organisms
Adults: 1 to 2 g q 6 to 8 hours for uncomplicated forms of infection. Up to 12 g daily in life-threatening infections.

Total daily dosage is same for I.M. or I.V. administration and depends on susceptibility of organism and severity of infection. Cefoxitin should be injected deep I.M. into a large muscle mass, such as the gluteus or lateral aspect of the thigh.
Preoperative prophylaxis
Adults: 2 g I.V. 30 to 60 minutes before surgery; then 2 g I.V. q 6 hours for 24 hours postoperatively.
Uncomplicated gonorrhea
Adults: Give 2 g I.M. as a single dose with 1 g probenecid P.O. at the same time or up to 30 minutes beforehand.
Pelvic inflammatory disease
Adults: 2 g I.V. q 6 hours. (If *Chlamydia trachomatis* is suspected, additional antichlamydial coverage should be given.)
♦ ***Dosage adjustment.*** In patients with impaired renal function, dosage and frequency of administration must be modified based on degree of renal impairment, severity of infection, and susceptibility of organism. To prevent toxic accumulation, dosage may need to be reduced in patients with creatinine clearance below 50 ml/minute/1.73 m^2.

Creatinine clearance (ml/min/1.73 m^2)	Dosage in adults
> 50	Usual adult dose
30-50	1-2 g q 8 to 12 hr
10-29	1-2 g q 12 to 24 hr
5-9	500 mg to 1 g q 12-24 hr
< 5	500 mg to 1 g q 24-48 hr

PHARMACODYNAMICS
Antibiotic action: Cefoxitin is primarily bactericidal; however, it may be bacteriostatic. Activity depends on the organism and the rate at which it multiplies, tissue penetration, and drug dosage.

Drug adheres to bacterial penicillin-binding proteins, thereby inhibiting cell-wall synthesis.

Drug is active against many gram-positive organisms and enteric gram-negative bacilli, including *Escherichia coli* and other coliform bacteria, penicillinase- and nonpenicillinase-producing *Staphylococcus aureus*, *S. epidermidis*, streptococci, *Klebsiella*, *Haemophilus influenzae*, and *Bacteroides* species (including *B. fragilis*). *Enterobacter*, *Pseudomonas*, and *Acinetobacter* are resistant to cefoxitin.

PHARMACOKINETICS

Absorption: Cefoxitin isn't absorbed from the GI tract and must be given parenterally; serum levels peak 20 to 30 minutes after an I.M. dose.
Distribution: Drug is distributed widely to most body tissues and fluids, including the gallbladder, liver, kidneys, bone, sputum, bile, and pleural and synovial fluids; CSF penetration is poor. About 50% to 80% of drug binds to proteins.
Metabolism: About 2% of a cefoxitin dose is metabolized.
Excretion: Most of the drug is excreted in urine through renal tubular secretion and glomerular filtration. In patients with normal renal function, elimination half-life is ½ to 1 hour; in patients with severe renal dysfunction, 6½ to 21½ hours. Drug can be removed from circulation through hemodialysis but not through peritoneal dialysis.

CONTRAINDICATIONS & PRECAUTIONS

Contraindicated in patients with hypersensitivity to cefoxitin or other cephalosporins. Use cautiously in patients with impaired renal function or penicillin allergy.

INTERACTIONS

Drug-drug. Use with *bacteriostatic drugs*—such as *chloramphenicol, erythromycin*, and *tetracyclines*—may impair bactericidal activity of the drug. Use with *loop diuretics* or *nephrotoxic drugs*—such as *aminoglycosides, colistin, polymyxin B*, and *vancomycin*—may increase the risk of nephrotoxicity. *Probenecid* competitively inhibits renal tubular secretion of cefoxitin, resulting in higher, prolonged serum cefoxitin levels.

ADVERSE REACTIONS

CV: hypotension.
GI: pseudomembranous colitis, nausea, vomiting, *diarrhea.*
GU: *acute renal failure.*
Hematologic: *transient neutropenia,* eosinophilia, *hemolytic anemia,* anemia, *thrombocytopenia.*
Hepatic: transient increases in liver enzyme levels.
Respiratory: dyspnea (with I.V. injection).
Skin: *maculopapular and erythematous rash, urticaria,* exfoliative dermatitis, *phlebitis, thrombophlebitis* (with I.V. injection).
Other: hypersensitivity reactions (serum sickness, *anaphylaxis*); elevated temperature; *pain, induration, sterile abscesses, tissue sloughing* (at injection site).

◙ KEY CONSIDERATIONS

Besides the recommendations relevant to all cephalosporins, consider the following:
● Dosage may need to be reduced in geriatric patients with diminished renal function.
● For I.V. use, reconstitute 1 g of cefoxitin with at least 10 ml of sterile water for injection, or 2 g of cefoxitin with 10 to 20 ml. Solutions of D_5W and normal saline solution for injection can also be used.
● Cefoxitin has been associated with thrombophlebitis. Assess I.V. site frequently for infiltration or phlebitis. Change I.V. site every 48 to 72 hours.
● For I.M. injection, reconstitute with 0.5% to 1% lidocaine hydrochloride (without epinephrine) to minimize pain at injection site.
● Administer I.M. dose deep into a large muscle mass. To prevent inadvertent injection into a blood vessel, aspirate before injecting. Rotate injection sites to prevent tissue damage.
● To ensure complete drug dissolution after reconstituting, shake vial and then let stand until clear. Solution is stable for 24 hours at room temperature, for 1 week if refrigerated, or 26 weeks if frozen.

Reactions may be *common*, uncommon, *life-threatening*, or COMMON AND LIFE-THREATENING.

- Solution may range from colorless to light amber and may darken during storage. Slight color change doesn't indicate loss of potency.
- Cefoxitin injection contains 2.3 mEq of sodium/gram of drug.
- Because drug is hemodialyzable, patients undergoing treatment with hemodialysis may require dosage adjustments.
- Cefoxitin causes false-positive results in urine glucose tests using cupric sulfate (Benedict's reagent or Clinitest); use glucose oxidase tests (Chemstrip uG, Diastix, or glucose enzymatic test strip) instead.
- Cefoxitin also falsely elevates in serum or urine creatinine levels in tests using Jaffé's reaction.
- Cefoxitin may cause positive Coombs' test results.

Patient education
- Inform patient of potential adverse reactions.

Overdose & treatment
- Signs and symptoms of overdose include neuromuscular hypersensitivity. Seizure may follow high CNS levels.
- Drug may be removed through hemodialysis.

cefpodoxime proxetil
Vantin

Third-generation cephalosporin, antibiotic

Available by prescription only
Tablets (film-coated): 100 mg, 200 mg
Oral suspension: 50 mg/5 ml, 100 mg/5 ml

INDICATIONS & DOSAGE
Acute, community-acquired pneumonia caused by non-beta-lactamase–producing strains of Haemophilus influenzae *or* Streptococcus pneumoniae
Adults: 200 mg P.O. q 12 hours for 14 days.
Acute bacterial exacerbations of chronic bronchitis caused by non-beta-lactamase–producing strains of H. influenzae, S. pneumoniae, *or* Moraxella catarrhalis
Adults: 200 mg P.O. q 12 hours for 10 days.
Uncomplicated gonorrhea in men and women; rectal gonococcal infections in women
Adults: 200 mg P.O. as a single dose. Follow with doxycycline 100 mg P.O. b.i.d. for 7 days.
Uncomplicated skin and soft-tissue infections caused by Staphylococcus aureus *or* Streptococcus pyogenes
Adults: 400 mg P.O. q 12 hours for 7 to 14 days.
Pharyngitis or tonsillitis caused by S. pyogenes
Adults: 100 mg P.O. q 12 hours for 7 to 10 days.
Uncomplicated urinary tract infections caused by Escherichia coli, Klebsiella pneumoniae, Proteus mirabilis, *or* Staphylococcus saprophyticus
Adults: 100 mg P.O. q 12 hours for 7 days.
✦ *Dosage adjustment.* In patients with renal impairment when creatinine clearance is below 30 ml/minute, dosage interval should be increased to q 24 hours. Patients receiving hemodialysis should receive drug three times weekly, after dialysis.

PHARMACODYNAMICS
Antibiotic action: A second-generation cephalosporin, cefpodoxime is a bactericide that inhibits cell-wall synthesis. It's usually active against gram-positive aerobes, such as *S. aureus* (including penicillinase-producing strains), *S. saprophyticus, S. pneumoniae,* and *S. pyogenes,* and gram-negative aerobes, such as *E. coli, H. influenzae* (including beta-lactamase–producing strains), *K. pneumoniae, M. (Branhamella) catarrhalis, Neisseria gonorrhoeae* (including penicillinase-producing strains), and *P. mirabilis.*

PHARMACOKINETICS
Absorption: Cefpodoxime is absorbed in the GI tract. Food increases absorption and mean peak plasma levels.
Distribution: Cephalosporins are widely distributed to most tissues and fluids.

Second-generation cephalosporins don't enter CSF even when the meninges are inflamed, although data on cefpodoxime aren't available. About 22% to 33% of the drug binds to serum proteins, and 21% to 29% binds to plasma proteins. *Metabolism:* Cefpodoxime proxetil is de-esterified to its active metabolite, cefpodoxime.
Excretion: Most of the drug is excreted in urine.

CONTRAINDICATIONS & PRECAUTIONS

Contraindicated in patients with hypersensitivity to cefpodoxime or other cephalosporins. Use cautiously in patients with impaired renal function or penicillin allergy.

INTERACTIONS

Drug-drug. *Antacids* and *H_2 antagonists* decrease absorption of cefpodoxime and shouldn't be administered concurrently. *Probenecid* decreases the excretion of cefpodoxime; monitor patient for a toxic reaction to the drug. Although nephrotoxicity isn't an adverse effect of cefpodoxime, patient's renal function should be monitored closely if he's taking a *drug that causes nephrotoxicity.*

ADVERSE REACTIONS

CNS: headache.
GI: *diarrhea,* nausea, vomiting, abdominal pain.
GU: vaginal fungal infections.
Skin: rash.
Other: hypersensitivity reactions *(anaphylaxis).*

◙ KEY CONSIDERATIONS

● Cefpodoxime is highly stable in presence of beta-lactamase enzymes. As a result, many organisms resistant to penicillins and some cephalosporins, because of presence of beta-lactamases, may be susceptible to cefpodoxime.
● Drug is inactive against most strains of *Pseudomonas, Enterobacter,* and *Enterococcus.*
● As with other antibiotics, long-term use of drug may result in overgrowth of nonsusceptible organisms. Patient's condition must be evaluated repeatedly, and

appropriate measures should be taken if superinfection occurs during therapy.
● Obtain specimen for culture and sensitivity tests before giving first dose. Therapy may begin pending test results.
● Drug may induce a positive direct Coombs' test.
● Store suspension in refrigerator (36° to 46° F [2° to 8° C]). Shake well before using. Discard unused portion after 14 days.

Patient education

● Instruct patient to take drug with food to enhance absorption.
● Inform patient that oral suspension of drug should be refrigerated.
● Instruct patient to shake container well before using and to discard unused portion after 14 days.
● Tell patient to continue taking drug for the prescribed course of therapy, even after feeling better.

Overdose & treatment

● No information on cefpodoxime overdose is available. Signs and symptoms of overdose of other beta-lactam antibiotics include nausea, vomiting, epigastric distress, and diarrhea. If patient experiences any of these signs or symptoms while taking cefpodoxime, it may be from an overdose.
● Hemodialysis or peritoneal dialysis may aid in removing drug from the body, particularly if renal function is compromised.

cefprozil
Cefzil

Second-generation cephalosporin, antibiotic

Available by prescription only
Tablets: 250 mg, 500 mg
Oral suspension: 125 mg/5 ml, 250 mg/5 ml

INDICATIONS & DOSAGE

Pharyngitis or tonsillitis caused by **Streptococcus pyogenes**
Adults: 500 mg P.O. daily for at least 10 days.

Secondary bacterial infections of acute bronchitis and acute bacterial exacerbation of chronic bronchitis caused by **Streptococcus pneumoniae, Haemophilus influenzae,** *and* **Moraxella (Branhamella) catarrhalis**
Adults: 500 mg P.O. q 12 hours for 10 days.
Uncomplicated skin and soft-tissue infections caused by **Staphylococcus aureus** *and* **S. pyogenes**
Adults: 250 mg P.O. b.i.d., or 500 mg daily to b.i.d. for 10 days.
✦ *Dosage adjustment.* For patients with creatinine clearance over 30 ml/minute, dosage doesn't have to be adjusted. For patients with creatinine clearance of 30 ml/minute or under, dosage should be reduced by 50%; however, dosing interval remains unchanged. Because drug is partially removed by hemodialysis, it should be administered after the hemodialysis session.

PHARMACODYNAMICS
Antibiotic action: Cefprozil interferes with bacterial cell-wall synthesis during cell replication, leading to osmotic instability and cell lysis. Bactericidal or bacteriostatic, depending on concentration.

PHARMACOKINETICS
Absorption: About 95% of cefprozil is absorbed from the GI tract. Drug levels peak within 1½ hours of a dose. Although food doesn't interfere with absorption of the cefprozil capsule, it's unknown if food interferes with absorption of the tablet or oral suspension.
Distribution: About 36% of the drug binds to proteins.
Metabolism: Drug is probably metabolized in the liver. In patients with impaired hepatic function, plasma half-life increases only slightly.
Excretion: About 60% of a dose is recovered unchanged in the urine. In patients with normal renal function, plasma half-life is 1.3 hours; in those with impaired hepatic function, 2 hours; and in those with end-stage renal disease, 5.2 to 5.9 hours. Drug may be removed from circulation through hemodialysis.
  Note: Data for this section come from investigational studies that used an oral capsule form of the drug that isn't commercially available.

CONTRAINDICATIONS & PRECAUTIONS
Contraindicated in patients with hypersensitivity to cefprozil or other cephalosporins. Use cautiously in patients with impaired renal function or penicillin allergy.

INTERACTIONS
Drug-drug. Use with *aminoglycosides* may increase the risk of nephrotoxicity. *Probenecid* may decrease excretion of cefprozil.

ADVERSE REACTIONS
CNS: dizziness, hyperactivity, headache, nervousness, insomnia, confusion, somnolence.
GI: *diarrhea, nausea,* vomiting, abdominal pain.
GU: elevated BUN level, elevated serum creatinine level, genital pruritus, vaginitis.
Hematologic: decreased leukocyte count, eosinophilia.
Hepatic: elevated liver enzyme levels, cholestatic jaundice (rare).
Skin: rash, urticaria, diaper rash.
Other: superinfection, hypersensitivity reactions (serum sickness, *anaphylaxis*).

▣ KEY CONSIDERATIONS
Besides the recommendations relevant to all cephalosporins, consider the following:
● Patients ages 65 and older exhibited a higher area under the plasma-level-versus-time curve and lower renal clearance compared with younger patients.
● Pseudomembranous colitis has been reported with nearly all antibacterials. Consider this diagnosis in patients who develop diarrhea secondary to antibiotic therapy. Although most patients respond to withdrawal of drug therapy alone, it may be necessary to institute treatment with an antibacterial that's effective against *Clostridium difficile,* an organism linked to this disorder.
● Obtain specimen for culture and sensitivity tests before giving first dose. Therapy may begin pending test results.

---

*Canada only   ◇ Unlabeled clinical use

- Drug may cause overgrowth of nonsusceptible bacteria or fungi. Monitor for signs and symptoms of superinfection.
- Advise patients with phenylketonuria that oral suspension contains 28 mg/5 ml phenylalanine.
- Cephalosporins may produce a false-positive test for urine glucose with tests that use copper reduction method (Benedict's test, Fehling's solution, or Clinitest tablets). Instead, use enzymatic methods (such as glucose enzymatic test strip).
- A false-negative result is possible with the ferricyanide test for blood glucose.

Patient education

- Tell patient to take all of drug as prescribed, even if he feels better.

Overdose & treatment

- Because the kidneys eliminate most of the drug, the manufacturer states that in cases of extreme overdose—especially in patients with decreased renal function—the drug may be removed through hemodialysis.

---

ceftazidime
Ceptaz, Fortaz, Tazicef, Tazidime

Third-generation cephalosporin, antibiotic

Available by prescription only
Injection: 500 mg, 1 g, 2 g
Pharmacy bulk package: 6 g, 10 g
Infusion: 1 g and 2 g in 20-, 50-, and 100-ml vials and bags

INDICATIONS & DOSAGE
Bacteremia, septicemia, and serious respiratory and urinary tract, gynecologic, bone and joint, intra-abdominal, CNS, and skin infections from susceptible organisms
Adults: 1 g I.V. or I.M. q 8 to 12 hours; up to 6 g daily in life-threatening infections. Total daily dosage is the same for I.M. or I.V. administration and depends on susceptibility of organism and severity of infection. Ceftazidime should be injected deep I.M. into a large muscle mass, such as the gluteus or lateral aspect of the thigh.

✦ *Dosage adjustment.* In patients with impaired renal function, doses or frequency of administration must be modified according to the degree of renal impairment, severity of infection, and susceptibility of organism. In hemodialysis patients, give 1 g after each hemodialysis period; in peritoneal dialysis patients, 500 mg q 24 hours. To prevent toxic accumulation, reduced dosage may be required in patients with creatinine clearance below 50 ml/minute/1.73 m^2.

Creatinine clearance (ml/min/1.73 m^2)	Dosage in adults
> 50	Usual adult dose
31-50	1 g q 12 hr
16-30	1 g q 24 hr
6-15	500 mg q 24 hr
≤ 5	500 mg q 48 hr

PHARMACODYNAMICS
Antibiotic action: Ceftazidime is primarily bactericidal; however, it may be bacteriostatic. Activity depends on the organism and the rate at which it multiplies, tissue penetration, and drug dosage. It acts by adhering to bacterial penicillin-binding proteins, thereby inhibiting cell-wall synthesis. Third-generation cephalosporins appear more active against some beta-lactamase–producing gram-negative organisms.

Drug is active against some gram-positive organisms and many enteric gram-negative bacilli as well as streptococci (*Streptococcus pneumoniae* and *S. pyogenes*), penicillinase- and nonpenicillinase-producing *Staphylococcus aureus, Escherichia coli, Klebsiella* species, *Proteus* species, *Enterobacter species, Haemophilus influenzae, Pseudomonas* species, and some strains of *Bacteroides* species. It's more effective than any cephalosporin or penicillin derivative against *Pseudomonas.* Some other third-generation cephalosporins are more active against gram-positive organisms and anaerobes.

PHARMACOKINETICS
Absorption: Ceftazidime isn't absorbed from the GI tract and must be given parenterally; serum levels peak 1 hour after an I.M. dose.

Distribution: Drug is distributed widely to most body tissues and fluids, including the gallbladder, liver, kidneys, bone, sputum, bile, and pleural and synovial fluids; unlike most other cephalosporins, drug penetrates CSF well. About 5% to 24% of the drug binds to proteins.
Metabolism: Drug isn't metabolized.
Excretion: Drug is excreted primarily in urine through glomerular filtration. In patients with normal renal function, elimination half-life is 1½ to 2 hours; in patients with severe renal disease, up to 35 hours. Drug may be removed through hemodialysis or peritoneal dialysis.

CONTRAINDICATIONS & PRECAUTIONS

Contraindicated in patients with hypersensitivity to ceftazidime or other cephalosporins. Use cautiously in patients with impaired renal function or penicillin allergy.

INTERACTIONS

Drug-drug. Use with *aminoglycosides* results in synergistic activity against *P. aeruginosa* and some strains of *Enterobacter;* such combined use may slightly increase the risk of nephrotoxicity. Use with *clavulanic acid* results in synergistic activity against some strains of *Bacteroides fragilis.*

ADVERSE REACTIONS

CNS: headache, dizziness, paresthesia, *seizures.*
GI: pseudomembranous colitis, nausea, vomiting, diarrhea, candidiasis, abdominal cramps.
GU: vaginitis.
Hematologic: eosinophilia, thrombocytosis, *leukopenia, hemolytic anemia, agranulocytosis, thrombocytopenia.*
Hepatic: transient elevation in liver enzyme levels.
Skin: *maculopapular and erythematous rash, urticaria, phlebitis, thrombophlebitis* (with I.V. injection).
Other: hypersensitivity reactions (serum sickness, *anaphylaxis*); *pain, induration, sterile abscesses, tissue sloughing* (at injection site).

▣ KEY CONSIDERATIONS

Besides the recommendations relevant to all cephalosporins, consider the following:
● Reduced dosage may be necessary in geriatric patients with diminished renal function.
● For patients on sodium restriction, note that ceftazidime contains 2.3 mEq of sodium/gram of drug.
● Ceftazidime powders (excluding Ceptaz) for injection contain 118 mg sodium carbonate/gram of drug; ceftazidime sodium is more water-soluble and is formed in situ on reconstitution.
● Vials are supplied under reduced pressure. When the antibiotic is dissolved, carbon dioxide is released and a positive pressure develops. Each brand of ceftazidime includes specific instructions for reconstitution. Read and follow these instructions carefully.
● Because drug is hemodialyzable, patients undergoing hemodialysis or peritoneal dialysis may require dosage adjustment.
● Separate I.V. sites should be used for aminoglycosides and ceftazidime.
● Ceftazidime causes false-positive results in urine glucose tests using cupric sulfate (Benedict's reagent or Clinitest); use glucose oxidase (Chemstrip uG, Diastix, or glucose enzymatic test strip) instead.
● Ceftazidime causes falsely elevates urine creatinine levels in tests using Jaffé's reaction.
● Ceftazidime may cause positive Coombs' test results.

Patient education

● Inform patient of potential adverse reactions.

Overdose & treatment

● Signs and symptoms of overdose include neuromuscular hypersensitivity. Seizure may follow high CNS levels.
● Drug may be removed through hemodialysis or peritoneal dialysis.

ceftibuten
Cedax

Third-generation cephalosporin, antibiotic

Available by prescription only
Capsules: 400 mg
Oral suspension: 90 mg/5 ml, 180 mg/5 ml

INDICATIONS & DOSAGE
***Acute exacerbations of chronic bronchitis from* Haemophilus influenzae, Moraxella catarrhalis, *or* Streptococcus pneumoniae; *pharyngitis and tonsillitis from* S. pyogenes; *acute otitis media from* H. influenzae, M. catarrhalis, *or* S. pyogenes**
Adults: 400 mg P.O. daily for 10 days.
♦ *Dosage adjustment.* For patients with creatinine clearance over 50 ml/minute, dosage doesn't need to be adjusted. Give 4.5 mg/kg (or 200 mg) daily to patients with creatinine clearance between 30 and 49 ml/minute and 2.25 mg/kg (or 100 mg) daily for those with creatinine clearance of 5 to 29 ml/minute. For patients undergoing hemodialysis two or three times weekly, give a single 400-mg dose (capsule form) or administer a single dose of 9 mg/kg (maximum dose, 400 mg) using oral suspension at the end of each hemodialysis session.

PHARMACODYNAMICS
Antibiotic action: Ceftibuten exerts its bactericidal action by binding to essential target proteins of the bacterial cell wall. This binding leads to inhibition of cell-wall synthesis. It's usually active against gram-positive aerobes (*S. pneumoniae, S. pyogenes*) and gram-negative aerobes (*H. influenzae, M. catarrhalis*).

PHARMACOKINETICS
Absorption: Ceftibuten is rapidly absorbed from GI tract. Food decreases bioavailability of drug.
Distribution: About 65% of drug binds to plasma proteins.
Metabolism: Drug is metabolized to its predominant component, cis-ceftibuten.

About 10% of ceftibuten is converted to the transisomer.
Excretion: Drug is excreted in urine and in feces.

CONTRAINDICATIONS & PRECAUTIONS
Contraindicated in patients with hypersensitivity to cephalosporins. Use cautiously if administering to patients with history of hypersensitivity to penicillin because up to 10% of these patients exhibit cross-sensitivity to a cephalosporin. Also use cautiously in patients with impaired renal function and GI disease (especially colitis).

INTERACTIONS
Drug-food. *Food* decreases the bioavailability of the drug; give 2 hours before or 1 hour after a meal.

ADVERSE REACTIONS
CNS: headache, dizziness, fatigue, paresthesia, somnolence, taste perversion, agitation, hyperkinesia, insomnia, irritability, rigors.
EENT: nasal congestion.
GI: nausea, dyspepsia, abdominal pain, vomiting, anorexia, constipation, dry mouth, eructation, flatulence, loose stools.
GU: dysuria, hematuria, elevated BUN and serum creatinine levels, vaginitis, candidiasis.
Hematologic: elevated eosinophil count, decreased hemoglobin level, altered platelet count, decreased leukocyte count.
Hepatic: elevated liver enzyme, bilirubin, and alkaline phosphatase levels.
Respiratory: dyspnea.
Skin: rash, pruritus, urticaria.
Other: dehydration, fever.

▣ KEY CONSIDERATIONS
Besides the recommendations relevant to all cephalosporins, consider the following:
• Use with caution when administering drug to geriatric patients. Dosage adjustment may be necessary if patient has impaired renal function.
• Pseudomembranous colitis has been reported with nearly all antibacterials; consider this diagnosis in patients who

develop diarrhea secondary to antibiotic therapy. Although most patients respond to withdrawal of drug therapy alone, it may be necessary to institute treatment with an antibacterial that's effective against *Clostridium difficile,* an organism linked to this disorder.

• Obtain specimen for culture and sensitivity tests before giving first dose. Therapy may begin pending test results.

• When preparing oral suspension, first tap the bottle to loosen powder. Follow chart supplied by manufacturer for amount of water to add to powder when mixing oral suspension. Add water in two portions, shaking well after each portion is added. After mixing, the suspension may be kept for 14 days and must be stored in the refrigerator.

• Drug may cause overgrowth of nonsusceptible bacteria or fungi. Monitor patient for superinfection.

• Other cephalosporins have caused a false-positive direct Coombs' test.

Patient education

• Tell patient to take all of drug as prescribed, even if he's feeling better.

• Instruct patient using oral suspension to take it at least 2 hours before or 1 hour after a meal.

• Inform diabetic patient that oral suspension contains 1 g of sucrose/tsp of suspension.

• Instruct patient using oral suspension to shake bottle well before measuring dose.

• Tell patient to keep oral suspension in the refrigerator with lid tightly closed and to discard unused drug after 14 days.

Overdose & treatment

• An overdose of cephalosporins can cause cerebral irritation leading to seizures.

• Ceftibuten is readily dialyzable and significant quantities (65% of plasma level) can be removed from the circulation in a single hemodialysis session.

ceftizoxime sodium
Cefizox

Third-generation cephalosporin, antibiotic

Available by prescription only
Injection: 500 mg, 1 g, 2 g, 10 g
Infusion: 1 g and 2 g in 100-ml vials; 50 ml in D_5W

INDICATIONS & DOSAGE
Bacteremia, septicemia, meningitis, pelvic inflammatory disease, and serious respiratory and urinary tract, gynecologic, intra-abdominal, bone and joint, and skin infections from susceptible organisms

Adults: Usual dosage is 500 mg to 2 g I.V. or I.M. q 8 to 12 hours. In life-threatening infections, 3 to 4 g I.V. q 8 hours. Total daily dosage is same for I.M. or I.V. administration and depends on susceptibility of organism and severity of infection. Ceftizoxime should be injected deep I.M. into a large muscle mass, such as the gluteus or lateral aspect of the thigh.

Uncomplicated gonorrhea

Adults: 1 g I.M. given as a single dose.

✦ *Dosage adjustment.* In patients with impaired renal function, modify doses or frequency of administration according to degree of renal impairment, severity of infection, and susceptibility of organism. To prevent toxic accumulation in patients with creatinine clearance below 80 ml/minute, dosage may need to be reduced.

Creatinine clearance (ml/min/ 1.73 m²)	Adults with less severe infections	Adults with life-threatening infections
> 80	Usual adult dose	Usual adult dose
50-79	500 mg q 8 hr	750 mg-1.5 g q 8 hr
5-49	250-500 mg q 12 hr	500 mg-1 g q 12 hr
≤ 4	500 mg q 48 hr; or 250 mg q 24 hr	500 mg-1 g q 48 hr; or 500 mg q 24 hr

PHARMACODYNAMICS

Antibiotic action: Ceftizoxime is primarily bactericidal; however, it may be bacteriostatic. Activity depends on the organism and the rate at which it multiplies, tissue penetration, and drug dosage. Drug adheres to bacterial penicillin-binding proteins, thereby inhibiting cell-wall synthesis. Third-generation cephalosporins appear more active against some beta-lactamase-producing gram-negative organisms.

Drug is active against some gram-positive organisms, many enteric gram-negative bacilli, and streptococci (*Streptococcus pneumoniae* and *S. pyogenes),* penicillinase- and nonpenicillinase-producing *Staphylococcus aureus, S. epidermidis, Escherichia coli, Klebsiella* species, *Haemophilus influenzae, Enterobacter* species, *Proteus* species, *Bacteroides* species (including *Bacteroides fragilis), Peptostreptococcus* species, and some strains of *Pseudomonas* and *Acinetobacter.* Cefotaxime is slightly more active than ceftizoxime against gram-positive organisms but is less active against gram-negative organisms.

PHARMACOKINETICS

Absorption: Ceftizoxime isn't absorbed from the GI tract and must be given parenterally; serum levels peak ½ to 1½ hours after an I.M. dose.
Distribution: Drug is distributed widely to most body tissues and fluids, including the gallbladder, liver, kidneys, bone, sputum, bile, and pleural and synovial fluids; unlike most cephalosporins, ceftizoxime penetrates CSF well and achieves adequate levels in inflamed meninges. About 30% of drug binds to proteins.
Metabolism: Drug isn't metabolized.
Excretion: Most of the drug is excreted in urine through renal tubular secretion and glomerular filtration. In patients with normal renal function, elimination half-life is about 1½ to 2 hours; in patients with severe renal disease, up to 30 hours. Some of the drug can be removed from circulation through hemodialysis or peritoneal dialysis.

CONTRAINDICATIONS & PRECAUTIONS

Contraindicated in patients with hypersensitivity to ceftizoxime or other cephalosporins. Use cautiously in patients with impaired renal function or penicillin allergy.

INTERACTIONS

Drug-drug. Use with *aminoglycosides* may slightly increase the risk of nephrotoxicity. *Probenecid* competitively inhibits renal tubular secretion of ceftizoxime, causing higher, prolonged serum ceftizoxime levels.

ADVERSE REACTIONS

GI: pseudomembranous colitis, nausea, anorexia, vomiting, *diarrhea.*
GU: vaginitis.
Hematologic: *transient neutropenia,* eosinophilia, ***hemolytic anemia,*** thrombocytosis, anemia, ***thrombocytopenia.***
Hepatic: transient elevation in liver enzyme levels (with I.V. injection).
Respiratory: dyspnea.
Skin: *maculopapular and erythematous rash, urticaria, phlebitis, thrombophlebitis* (with I.V. injection).
Other: hypersensitivity reactions (serum sickness, *anaphylaxis*); elevated temperature; *pain, induration, sterile abscesses, tissue sloughing* (at injection site).

◉ KEY CONSIDERATIONS

Besides the recommendations relevant to all cephalosporins, consider the following:
● Reduced dosage may be necessary in geriatric patients with diminished renal function.
● For patients who must restrict their sodium intake, note that ceftizoxime contains 2.6 mEq of sodium/gram of drug.
● Drug may be supplied as frozen, sterile solution in plastic containers. Thaw at room temperature. Thawed solution is stable for 24 hours at room temperature or for 10 days if refrigerated. Don't refreeze.
● For I.M. use, reconstitute with sterile water for injection. Shake vial well to ensure drug is completely dissolved. To administer a dose that exceeds 1 g, di-

---

Reactions may be *common*, uncommon, *life-threatening*, or COMMON AND LIFE-THREATENING.

vide the dose and inject it into separate sites to prevent tissue injury.
• For I.V. use, reconstitute I.V. dose with sterile water for injection. Solution should clear after shaking well and range in color from yellow to amber. If particles are visible, discard solution. Reconstituted solution is stable for 24 hours at room temperature or 96 hours if refrigerated.
• Administer I.V. as a direct injection slowly over 3 to 5 minutes directly or through tubing of compatible infusion fluid. If given as intermittent infusion, dilute reconstituted drug in 50 to 100 ml of compatible fluid. Check package insert.
• Ceftizoxime causes false-positive results in urine glucose tests using cupric sulfate (Benedict's reagent or Clinitest); use glucose oxidase (Chemstrip uG, Diastix, or glucose enzymatic test strip) instead.
• Ceftizoxime falsely elevates urine creatinine levels using Jaffé's reaction.
• Ceftizoxime may cause positive Coombs' test results.

Patient education
• Inform patient of potential adverse reactions.

Overdose & treatment
• Signs and symptoms of overdose include neuromuscular hypersensitivity. Seizure may follow high CNS levels.
• Drug may be removed from circulation through hemodialysis.

ceftriaxone sodium
Rocephin

Third-generation cephalosporin, antibiotic

Available by prescription only
Injection: 250 mg, 500 mg, 1 g, 2 g
Infusion: 1 g, 2 g

INDICATIONS & DOSAGE
Bacteremia, septicemia, and serious respiratory and urinary tract, bone, joint, gynecologic, intra-abdominal, **and skin infections from susceptible organisms**
Adults: 1 to 2 g I.M. or I.V. once daily or in equally divided doses b.i.d. Total daily dosage shouldn't exceed 4 g.
Gonococcal meningitis, endocarditis
Adults: 1 to 2 g I.V. q 12 hours for 10 to 14 days for meningitis and 3 to 4 weeks for endocarditis. May give an initial dosage of 100 mg/kg (not to exceed 4 g) to initiate therapy. Total daily dosage is same for I.M. or I.V. administration and depends on susceptibility of organism and severity of infection. Ceftriaxone should be injected deep I.M. into a large muscle mass, such as the gluteus or lateral aspect of the thigh.
Preoperative prophylaxis
Adults: 1 g I.M. or I.V. 30 minutes to 2 hours before surgery.
Uncomplicated gonorrhea
Adults: 125 to 250 mg I.M. given as a single dose; ◇ 1 to 2 g I.M. or I.V. daily until improvement occurs.
◇ **Haemophilus ducreyi** *infection*
Adults: 250 mg I.M. as a single dose.
◇ **Sexually transmitted epididymitis, pelvic inflammatory disease**
Adults: 250 mg I.M. as a single dose; follow up with other antibiotics.
◇ **Anti-infective for sexual assault victims**
Adults: 125 mg I.M. as a single dose in conjunction with other antibiotics.
◇ **Lyme disease**
Adults: 1 to 2 g I.M. or I.V. q 12 to 24 hours.
✦ **Dosage adjustment.** In patients with impaired hepatic and renal function, dosage shouldn't exceed 2 g/day without monitoring serum drug levels.

PHARMACODYNAMICS
Antibiotic action: Ceftriaxone is primarily bactericidal; however, it may be bacteriostatic. Activity depends on organism and the rate at which it multiplies, tissue penetration, and drug dosage. Drug adheres to bacterial penicillin-binding proteins, thereby inhibiting cell-wall synthesis. Third-generation cephalosporins appear more active against some beta-lactamase-producing gram-negative organisms.

Ceftriaxone is active against some gram-positive organisms, many enteric gram-negative bacilli, as well as streptococci, *Streptococcus pneumoniae* and *S. pyogenes,* penicillinase- and nonpenicillinase-producing *Staphylococcus aureus, S. epidermidis, Escherichia coli, Klebsiella* species, *Haemophilus influenzae, Enterobacter, Proteus,* some strains of *Pseudomonas* and *Peptostreptococcus,* and spirochetes such as *Borrelia burgdorferi* (the causative organism of Lyme disease). Most strains of *Listeria, Pseudomonas,* and *Acinetobacter* are resistant. Generally, ceftriaxone is most like cefotaxime and ceftizoxime in terms of activity.

PHARMACOKINETICS
Absorption: Ceftriaxone isn't absorbed from the GI tract and must be given parenterally; serum levels peak 2 to 3 hours after an I.M. dose.
Distribution: Drug is distributed widely to most body tissues and fluids, including the gallbladder, liver, kidneys, bone, sputum, bile, and pleural and synovial fluids; unlike most other cephalosporins, ceftriaxone penetrates CSF well. About 84% to 96% of the drug binds to proteins, but this percentage depends on the dosage and decreases as serum levels rise.
Metabolism: Drug is partially metabolized.
Excretion: Most of the drug is excreted in urine; some drug is excreted in bile. In patients with normal renal function, elimination half-life is 5½ to 11 hours; in patients with severe renal disease, half-life is prolonged only moderately. Neither hemodialysis nor peritoneal dialysis removes ceftriaxone.

CONTRAINDICATIONS & PRECAUTIONS
Contraindicated in patients with hypersensitivity to ceftriaxone or other cephalosporins. Use cautiously in patients with penicillin allergy.

INTERACTIONS
Drug-drug. Use with *aminoglycosides* produces synergistic antimicrobial activity against *P. aeruginosa* and some strains of Enterobacteriaceae. High dosages of *probenecid* may increase clearance by blocking biliary secretion and displacement of ceftriaxone from plasma proteins.

ADVERSE REACTIONS
CNS: headache, dizziness.
GI: pseudomembranous colitis, nausea, vomiting, diarrhea, urolithiasis.
GU: genital pruritus, candidiasis, elevated BUN levels.
Hematologic: eosinophilia, thrombocytosis, *leukopenia.*
Hepatic: elevations in liver function test results, jaundice.
Skin: pain, induration, tenderness (at injection site); phlebitis; *rash;* pruritus.
Other: hypersensitivity reactions (serum sickness, *anaphylaxis*), elevated temperature, chills.

▣ KEY CONSIDERATIONS
Besides the recommendations relevant to all cephalosporins, consider the following:
● For patients who must restrict their sodium intake, note that ceftriaxone injection contains 3.6 mEq of sodium/gram of drug.
● Ceftriaxone is used commonly in home care programs to manage serious infections, such as osteomyelitis.
● In patients with renal insufficiency, dosage usually doesn't need to be adjusted because of partial biliary excretion.
● Ceftriaxone causes false-positive results in urine glucose tests utilizing cupric sulfate (Benedict's reagent or Clinitest); use glucose oxidase (Chemstrip uG, Diastix, or glucose enzymatic test strip) instead.
● Ceftriaxone falsely elevates urine creatinine levels in tests using Jaffé's reaction.
● Ceftriaxone may cause positive Coombs' test results.

Patient education
● Inform patient of potential adverse reactions.

Overdose & treatment
● Signs and symptoms of overdose include neuromuscular hypersensitivity. Seizure may follow high CNS levels.
● Treatment is supportive.

Reactions may be *common,* uncommon, *life-threatening,* or COMMON AND LIFE-THREATENING.

cefuroxime axetil
Ceftin

cefuroxime sodium
Kefurox, Zinacef

Second-generation cephalosporin, antibiotic

Available by prescription only
cefuroxime axetil
Tablets: 125 mg, 250 mg, 500 mg
Suspension: 125 mg/5 ml, 250 mg/5ml
cefuroxime sodium
Injection: 750 mg, 1.5 g
Infusion: 750 mg, 1.5-g infusion, 7.5-g bulk

INDICATIONS & DOSAGE
Serious lower respiratory and urinary tract, skin and soft-tissue infections, septicemia, meningitis caused by susceptible organisms
Adults: Usual dosage is 750 mg to 1.5 g I.M. or I.V. q 8 hours, usually for 5 to 10 days. For life-threatening infections and infections caused by less susceptible organisms, 1.5 g I.M. or I.V. q 6 hours; for bacterial meningitis, up to 3 g I.V. q 8 hours.

Total daily dosage is same for I.M. or I.V. administration and depends on susceptibility of organism and severity of infection. Cefuroxime should be injected deep I.M. into a large muscle mass, such as the gluteus or lateral aspect of the thigh.
Pharyngitis, tonsillitis, lower respiratory tract and urinary tract infection
Adults: 125 to 500 mg P.O. b.i.d. for 10 days.
Preoperative prophylaxis
Adults: 1.5 g I.V. 30 to 60 minutes before surgery; then 750 mg I.M. or I.V. q 8 hours intraoperatively for a prolonged procedure.
◊ *Gonorrhea (urethral, endocervical,* ◊ *rectal)*
Adults: 1.5 g I.M. given as a single dose, alone or with other antibiotics.
Lyme disease (erythema migrans) caused by **Borrelia burgdorferi**
Adults: 500 mg P.O. b.i.d. for 20 days.

✦ *Dosage adjustment.* It's unknown whether the drug is safe for patients with impaired renal function to use. In these patients, dosage and frequency of administration must be modified based on degree of renal impairment, severity of infection, and susceptibility of organism. In hemodialysis patients, give 750 mg at the end of each hemodialysis period with the regular dose. To prevent toxic accumulation, reduced I.M. or I.V. dosage may be required in patients with creatinine clearance below 20 ml/minute/1.73 m².

Creatinine clearance (ml/min/1.73 m²)	Dosage in adults
> 20	750 mg-1.5 g q 8 hr
10-20	750 mg q 12 hr
< 10	750 mg q 24 hr

PHARMACODYNAMICS
Antibiotic action: Cefuroxime is primarily bactericidal; however, it may be bacteriostatic. Activity depends on the organism and the rate at which it multiplies, tissue penetration, and drug dosage. Drug adheres to bacterial penicillin-binding proteins, thereby inhibiting cell-wall synthesis.

Cefuroxime is active against many gram-positive organisms and enteric gram-negative bacilli, including *Streptococcus pneumoniae* and *S. pyogenes, Haemophilus influenzae, Klebsiella* species, *Staphylococcus aureus, Escherichia coli, Enterobacter,* and *Neisseria gonorrhoeae; Bacteroides fragilis, Pseudomonas,* and *Acinetobacter* are resistant to cefuroxime.

PHARMACOKINETICS
Absorption: Cefuroxime sodium isn't well absorbed from the GI tract and must be given parenterally; peak serum levels occur 15 to 60 minutes after an I.M. dose.

Cefuroxime axetil is better absorbed orally, with between 37% to 52% of an oral dose reaching systemic circulation. After oral administration, serum levels peak in about 2 hours. Food appears to enhance absorption. Tablets and suspension aren't bioequivalent.

Distribution: Drug is distributed widely into most body tissues and fluids, including the gallbladder, liver, kidneys, bone, bile, and pleural and synovial fluids; CSF penetration is greater than that of most first- and second-generation cephalosporins and achieves adequate therapeutic levels in inflamed meninges. About 33% to 50% of drug binds to proteins.

Metabolism: Cefuroxime isn't metabolized.

Excretion: Drug is primarily excreted in urine through renal tubular secretion and glomerular filtration. In patients with normal renal function, elimination half-life is 1 to 2 hours; in patients with end-stage renal disease, 15 to 22 hours. Drug may be removed from circulation through hemodialysis.

CONTRAINDICATIONS & PRECAUTIONS
Contraindicated in patients with hypersensitivity to cefuroxime or other cephalosporins. Use cautiously in those with impaired renal function or penicillin allergy.

INTERACTIONS
Drug-drug. Use with *loop diuretics* or *nephrotoxic drugs*—such as *aminoglycosides, colistin, polymyxin B,* and *vancomycin*—may increase the risk of nephrotoxicity. *Probenecid* competitively inhibits renal tubular secretion of cefuroxime, resulting in higher, prolonged serum cefuroxime levels.

ADVERSE REACTIONS
GI: pseudomembranous colitis, nausea, anorexia, vomiting, *diarrhea.*
Hematologic: *transient neutropenia,* eosinophilia, *hemolytic anemia, thrombocytopenia,* decreased hemoglobin levels and hematocrit.
Hepatic: transient increases in liver enzyme levels.
Skin: *maculopapular and erythematous rash, urticaria, phlebitis, thrombophlebitis* (with I.V. injection).
Other: hypersensitivity reactions (serum sickness, *anaphylaxis*); *pain, induration, sterile abscesses, temperature elevation, tissue sloughing* (at injection site).

🔲 KEY CONSIDERATIONS
Besides the recommendations relevant to all cephalosporins, consider the following:
- Use with caution in geriatric patients with renal compromise.
- Unlike many second-generation cephalosporins, drug isn't known to cause prothrombin deficiency and bleeding, and it's effective in treating meningitis.
- Tablets and suspension aren't bioequivalent and can't be substituted on a milligram-per-milligram basis.
- For patients who must restrict their sodium intake, note that cefuroxime sodium contains 2.4 mEq of sodium/ gram of drug.
- Check solutions for particulate matter and discoloration. Solution may range in color from light yellow to amber without affecting potency.
- Shake I.M. solution gently before administration to ensure complete drug dissolution. Administer deep I.M. in a large muscle mass, preferably the gluteus area. Aspirate before injecting to prevent inadvertent injection into a blood vessel. Rotate injection sites to prevent tissue damage. Apply ice to injection site to relieve pain.
- For direct intermittent I.V., inject solution slowly into vein over 3 to 5 minutes or slowly through tubing of free-running, compatible I.V. solution.
- Reconstituted solution retains potency for 24 hours at room temperature or for 48 hours if refrigerated.
- Because drug is hemodialyzable, patients undergoing treatment with hemodialysis or peritoneal dialysis may require dosage adjustments.
- Reconstituted suspension can be stored at room temperature or in refrigerator. Unused portion should be discarded after 10 days. Shake well before each dose.
- Drug causes false-positive results in urine glucose tests using cupric sulfate (Benedict's reagent or Clinitest); use glucose oxidase tests (Chemstrip uG, Diastix, or glucose enzymatic test strip) instead.
- Cefuroxime falsely elevates serum or urine creatinine levels in tests using Jaffé's reaction.

Reactions may be *common,* uncommon, *life-threatening,* or COMMON AND LIFE-THREATENING.

• Cefuroxime may cause positive Coombs' test results.

Patient education
• Inform patient of potential adverse reactions.

Overdose & treatment
• Signs and symptoms of overdose include neuromuscular hypersensitivity. Seizure may follow high CNS levels.
• Hemodialysis or peritoneal dialysis will remove cefuroxime.

---

celecoxib
Celebrex

Cyclooxygenase-2 (COX-2) inhibitor, analgesic, antipyretic, selective nonsteroidal anti-inflammatory

Available by prescription only.
Capsules: 100 mg, 200 mg

INDICATIONS & DOSAGE
Osteoarthritis
Adults: 200 mg daily as a single dose or 100 mg b.i.d. with or without food.
Rheumatoid arthritis
Adults: 100 to 200 mg b.i.d. with or without food as tolerated.
◆ *Dosage adjustment.* In geriatric patients weighing less than 50 kg (110 lb), the lowest recommended initial dosage should be given. In patients with moderate hepatic impairment, dosage should be reduced. Drug shouldn't be given to patients with severe hepatic impairment.

PHARMACODYNAMICS
Anti-inflammatory, analgesic, and antipyretic action: Celecoxib is thought to selectively inhibit cyclooxygenase-2 (COX-2), resulting in decreased prostaglandin synthesis. Because celecoxib doesn't inhibit COX-1 at therapeutic levels, the reduction in signs and symptoms of osteoarthritis and rheumatoid arthritis may result from a lower incidence of peripheral adverse effects.

PHARMACOKINETICS
Absorption: After oral administration, plasma levels peak in about 3 hours. If celecoxib is given in multiple dosages, steady-state plasma levels can be expected within 5 days. Although a high-fat meal may delay absorption by 1 to 2 hours, drug can be administered without regard to meals. Geriatric patients may have higher serum levels than younger adults.
Distribution: Drug is highly protein bound, primarily to albumin, which is important when administered with other highly protein-bound drugs or to a patient who's severely malnourished. It's also distributed extensively into the tissues.
Metabolism: Cytochrome P-450 2C9 metabolizes most of the drug. In vitro studies indicate that drug is a cytochrome P-450 2D6 inhibitor, although the significance of this hasn't been established. No active metabolites of drug have been identified.
Excretion: Drug is eliminated primarily through hepatic metabolism; 27% is excreted in urine. In a patient who's fasting, elimination half-life is about 11 hours.

CONTRAINDICATIONS & PRECAUTIONS
Contraindicated in patients with hypersensitivity to celecoxib, sulfonamides, aspirin, or other NSAIDs.

Use cautiously in geriatric patients, especially those with a history of ulcers or GI bleeding, advanced renal disease, anemia, symptomatic liver disease, hypertension, edema, heart failure, or asthma; debilitated patients; patients who smoke or use alcohol; and patients taking oral corticosteroids or anticoagulants.

INTERACTIONS
Drug-drug. Use with *ACE inhibitors* can diminish antihypertensive effects; monitor the patient's blood pressure. *Aluminum* and *magnesium antacids* can decrease plasma celecoxib levels; administer these drugs at least 1 hour apart. Although use with *aspirin* can increase the risk of GI ulceration, low doses of aspirin can be used safely to prevent cardiovascular events; monitor the patient for signs and symptoms of GI bleeding. *Drugs that inhibit cytochrome*

P-450 isoenzymes 2C9 and 2D6 increase celecoxib levels; use caution when administering other drugs that induce or inhibit these same enzymes. *Fluconazole* can increase celecoxib levels; reduce the dose of celecoxib to the minimal effective dose. Use can reduce sodium excretion from *diuretics* such as *furosemide*, leading to sodium retention; monitor the patient for swelling and increased blood pressure. Use with *lithium* may increase plasma lithium levels; monitor levels closely during treatment. A direct interaction with *warfarin* hasn't been reported; however, close monitoring of signs and symptoms of bleeding is necessary because of the increased risk with warfarin.

Drug-lifestyle. *Alcohol* can increase the risk of GI irritation or bleeding if it's used excessively or long-term; monitor patient for signs and symptoms of bleeding.

ADVERSE REACTIONS
CNS: dizziness, *headache,* insomnia.
GI: abdominal pain, diarrhea, dyspepsia, flatulence, nausea, vomiting.
GU: elevated BUN levels.
Hematologic: anemia.
Metabolic: hyperchloremia, hypophosphatemia.
Musculoskeletal: back pain.
Respiratory: pharyngitis, rhinitis, sinusitis, upper respiratory tract infection.
Skin: rash.
Other: peripheral edema, accidental injury.

⊡ KEY CONSIDERATIONS
• Geriatric patients experience more adverse reactions overall. Closely observe patient for elevated blood pressure, fluid retention, and mental status changes.
• Patients with a history of ulcers or GI bleeding are at higher risk for GI bleeding. Assess patient for overt and occult bleeding. Other risk factors for GI bleeding include treatment with corticosteroids or anticoagulants, long-term NSAID therapy, smoking, alcoholism, older age, and poor overall health.
• Patients may be allergic to celecoxib if they have an allergy to sulfonamides, aspirin, or other NSAIDs.

• Assess patient for hepatic and renal toxicity, especially if the patient is dehydrated.
• Food may decrease the incidence of GI upset.
• Aluminum and magnesium antacids may decrease the effect of celecoxib, so they should be administered at least an hour apart.

Patient education
• Educate the patient on the cross-sensitivity of celecoxib with sulfonamides, aspirin, or other NSAIDs.
• Instruct the patient to report signs and symptoms of bleeding, swelling, hepatotoxicity, or anaphylaxis to the health care provider immediately.
• If stomach upset occurs, instruct the patient to take drug with food.
• Antacids with aluminum or magnesium should be taken at least an hour apart from celecoxib.
• Inform the patient that it may take several days before he feels consistent pain relief.
• Advise patient to avoid alcohol while taking drug.

Overdose & treatment
• Common signs and symptoms of overdose include lethargy, drowsiness, nausea, vomiting, epigastric pain, and GI bleeding. Other signs include hypertension, acute renal failure, respiratory depression, and coma.
• Although no antidote for overdose exists, symptomatic and supportive care is usually sufficient. If it's within 4 hours of the overdose, induce vomiting and/or administer activated charcoal and/or an osmotic cathartic. Because drug is highly protein bound, dialysis is unlikely to be effective.

Reactions may be *common,* uncommon, *life-threatening,* or COMMON AND LIFE-THREATENING.

cephalexin hydrochloride
Keftab

cephalexin monohydrate
Biocef, Keflex, Novo-Lexin*

First-generation cephalosporin, antibiotic

Available by prescription only
cephalexin hydrochloride
Tablets: 500 mg
cephalexin monohydrate
Tablets: 250 mg, 500 mg, 1 g
Capsules: 250 mg, 500 mg
Suspension: 125 mg/5 ml, 250 mg/5 ml

INDICATIONS & DOSAGE
Respiratory tract, GU, skin and soft-tissue, and bone and joint infections caused by susceptible organisms; otitis media
Adults: 250 mg to 1 g P.O. q 6 hours
✦ *Dosage adjustment.* To prevent toxic accumulation in patients with impaired renal function and creatinine clearance below 40 ml/minute, give reduced dosage. If creatinine clearance is below 5 ml/minute, give 250 mg q 12 to 24 hours; between 5 ml/minute and 10 ml/minute, 250 mg q 12 hours; and between 11 ml/minute and 40 ml/minute, 500 mg q 8 to 12 hours.

PHARMACODYNAMICS
Antibacterial action: Cephalexin is primarily bactericidal; however, it may be bacteriostatic. Activity depends on the organism and the rate at which it multiplies, tissue penetration, and drug dosage. Drug adheres to bacterial penicillin-binding proteins, thereby inhibiting cell-wall synthesis.

Drug is active against many gram-positive organisms, including penicillinase-producing *Staphylococcus aureus* and *S. epidermidis, Streptococcus pneumoniae,* group B streptococci, and group A beta-hemolytic streptococci; susceptible gram-negative organisms include *Klebsiella pneumoniae, Escherichia coli, Proteus mirabilis,* and *Shigella.*

PHARMACOKINETICS
Absorption: Cephalexin is absorbed rapidly and completely from the GI tract after oral administration; serum levels peak within 1 hour. The base monohydrate is probably converted to the hydrochloride in the stomach before absorption. Food delays absorption.
Distribution: Drug is distributed widely into most body tissues and fluids, including the gallbladder, liver, kidneys, bone, sputum, bile, and pleural and synovial fluids; CSF penetration is poor. About 6% to 15% of drug binds to proteins.
Metabolism: Drug isn't metabolized.
Excretion: Drug is excreted primarily unchanged in urine through glomerular filtration and renal tubular secretion. In patients with normal renal function, elimination half-life is ½ to 1 hour; in patients with severe renal impairment, 7½ to 14 hours. Drug can be removed from circulation through hemodialysis or peritoneal dialysis.

CONTRAINDICATIONS & PRECAUTIONS
Contraindicated in patients with hypersensitivity to cephalosporins. Use cautiously in patients with impaired renal function or penicillin allergy.

INTERACTIONS
Drug-drug. Use with *loop diuretics* or *nephrotoxic drugs*—such as *aminoglycosides, colistin, polymyxin B,* and *vancomycin*—may increase the risk of nephrotoxicity. *Probenecid* competitively inhibits renal tubular secretion of cephalexin, resulting in higher, prolonged serum cephalexin levels.

ADVERSE REACTIONS
CNS: dizziness, headache, fatigue, agitation, confusion, hallucinations.
GI: pseudomembranous colitis, *nausea, anorexia,* vomiting, *diarrhea,* gastritis, glossitis, dyspepsia, abdominal pain, anal pruritus, tenesmus, oral candidiasis.
GU: genital pruritus and candidiasis, vaginitis, interstitial nephritis.
Hematologic: *neutropenia,* eosinophilia, anemia, *thrombocytopenia.*
Hepatic: transient increases in liver enzyme levels.

Musculoskeletal: arthritis, arthralgia, joint pain.
Skin: *maculopapular and erythematous rash, urticaria.*
Other: hypersensitivity reactions (serum sickness, *anaphylaxis*).

▣ KEY CONSIDERATIONS

Besides the recommendations relevant to all cephalosporins, consider the following:

• Reduce dosage in geriatric patients with diminished renal function.

• To prepare the oral suspension, add the required amount of water to the powder in two portions. Shake well after each addition. After mixing, store in refrigerator. Suspension is stable for 14 days without significant loss of potency. Store mixture in tightly closed container. Shake well before using.

• Because cephalexin is dialyzable, dosage may need to be adjusted in patients undergoing hemodialysis or peritoneal dialysis.

• Drug causes false-positive results in urine glucose tests using cupric sulfate (Benedict's reagent or Clinitest); use glucose oxidase test (Chemstrip uG, Diastix, or glucose enzymatic test strip) instead.

• Cephalexin falsely elevates serum or urine creatinine levels in tests using Jaffé's reaction.

• Positive Coombs' test results occur in about 3% of patients taking cephalexin.

Patient education

• Inform patient of potential adverse reactions.

Overdose & treatment

• Signs and symptoms of overdose include neuromuscular hypersensitivity; seizure may follow high CNS levels.

• Remove cephalexin through hemodialysis or peritoneal dialysis. Other treatment is supportive.

cerivastatin sodium
Baycol

3-Hydroxy-3-methylglutaryl-coenzyme A (HMG-CoA) reductase inhibitor, antilipemic

Available by prescription only
Tablets: 0.2 mg, 0.3 mg

INDICATIONS & DOSAGE

Adjunct to diet for reducing elevated total and low-density lipoprotein (LDL) cholesterol levels in patients with primary hypercholesterolemia and mixed dyslipidemia when diet and other non-pharmacologic measures have been inadequate
Adults: 0.3 mg, P.O., once daily in the evening.
♦ *Dosage adjustment.* In patients with significant renal impairment (creatinine clearance 60 ml/minute/1.73 m^2 or less), 0.2 mg P.O. once daily in the evening.

PHARMACODYNAMICS

Antilipemic action: Competitive inhibitor of HMG-CoA reductase that's responsible for converting HMG-CoA to mevalonate, a precursor of sterols including cholesterol. Reducing the level of cholesterol in hepatic cells stimulates synthesis of LDL receptors, leading to an increase in uptake of LDL particles.

PHARMACOKINETICS

Absorption: Cerivastatin is absorbed in the active form. Mean absolute bioavailability of 0.2-mg tablet is 60%, with levels peaking about 2.5 hours after a dose. Food doesn't affect absorption.
Distribution: Mean volume of distribution is 0.3 L/kg. More than 99% of circulating drug binds to plasma proteins (80% binds to albumin).
Metabolism: Drug is extensively metabolized to two active metabolites, M1 and M23. A demethylation reaction forms M1, and a hydroxylation reaction forms M23. The relative potencies of M1 and M23 are 50% and 80% of the active compound, respectively. Because metabolite levels are significantly lower than those of the parent compound, the

---

Reactions may be *common,* uncommon, *life-threatening,* or COMMON AND LIFE-THREATENING.

cholesterol-lowering effect of the drug comes from the parent compound. *Excretion:* M1 and M23 are excreted in urine and in feces. After an oral dose of 0.4 mg of ^{14}C-cerivastatin, healthy patients excrete about 24% of radioactivity in urine and 70% in feces. The parent compound, cerivastatin, accounts for less than 2% of total radioactivity excreted.

CONTRAINDICATIONS & PRECAUTIONS
Contraindicated in patients with active liver disease, unexplained persistent elevations of serum transaminase levels, or known hypersensitivity to cerivastatin. Use cautiously in patients with history of liver disease or long-term alcohol use.

INTERACTIONS
Drug-drug. *Azole antifungals, cyclosporine, erythromycin, fibric acid derivatives,* and *niacin* may increase the risk of myopathy. *Cholestyramine* given within 4 hours of cerivastatin results in decreased absorption and decreased peak plasma levels of cerivastatin; however, administration of cerivastatin at bedtime and cholestyramine 1 hour before the evening meal doesn't significantly decrease the effect of cerivastatin. *Erythromycin* decreases hepatic metabolism of drug and increases serum cerivastatin levels up to 50%.

ADVERSE REACTIONS
CNS: asthenia, dizziness, *headache,* insomnia.
CV: chest pain, peripheral edema.
EENT: *pharyngitis, rhinitis,* sinusitis.
GI: abdominal pain, constipation, diarrhea, dyspepsia, flatulence, nausea.
GU: urinary tract infection.
Hepatic: may elevate transaminase, gamma glutamyl transpeptidase, and bilirubin levels.
Musculoskeletal: arthralgia, back or leg pain, myalgia.
Respiratory: increased cough.
Skin: rash.
Other: flulike syndrome, possible elevations of CK and alkaline phosphatase levels, and thyroid function abnormalities.

▣ KEY CONSIDERATIONS
• Plasma drug levels are similar in healthy geriatric male patients older than age 65 and in young male patients younger than age 40.
• Withhold drug temporarily in patients with conditions predisposing them to renal failure secondary to rhabdomyolysis—for example, trauma; major surgery; severe metabolic, endocrine, and electrolyte disorders; severe acute infection; hypotension; and uncontrolled seizures. Rare cases of rhabdomyolysis have been reported with other HMG-CoA reductase inhibitors.
• Therapy with antilipemics should be a component of multiple risk factor intervention program and attempts should be made to control cholesterol with diet, exercise, and weight reduction before initiating therapy with antilipemics.
• Before initiating treatment, exclude secondary causes for hypercholesterolemia and perform a baseline lipid profile. Periodic liver function tests and lipid levels should be done before starting treatment, at 6 and 12 weeks after initiation, or after an increase in dosage and periodically thereafter.
• Because maximal effect of drug is seen within 4 weeks, lipid determinations should be performed at this time.
• Drug may be taken with or without food.

Patient education
• Teach patient proper dietary management, weight control, and exercise.
• Explain importance of controlling elevated serum lipid levels.
• Tell patient to take drug in the evening with or without food.
• Warn patient to avoid heavy alcohol use.
• Inform patient that it may take up to 4 weeks for full therapeutic effect to occur.
• Tell patient to immediately report unexplained muscle pain, tenderness, or weakness, especially if accompanied by fever or malaise.

cetirizine hydrochloride
Zyrtec

Selective H₁-receptor antagonist, antihistamine

Available by prescription only
Tablets: 5 mg, 10 mg
Syrup: 5 mg/ml

INDICATIONS & DOSAGE
Seasonal allergic rhinitis, perennial allergic rhinitis, chronic urticaria
Adults: 5 or 10 mg P.O. daily.
✦ *Dosage adjustment.* In hemodialysis patients or those with hepatic impairment or creatinine clearance below 31 ml/minute, 5 mg P.O. daily.

PHARMACODYNAMICS
Antihistamine action: The principal effects of cetirizine are mediated via selective inhibition of peripheral H₁ receptors.

PHARMACOKINETICS
Absorption: Cetirizine is rapidly absorbed.
Distribution: About 93% of drug binds to plasma proteins.
Metabolism: Drug is metabolized to a very limited extent by oxidative O-dealkylation to a metabolite with negligible antihistaminic activity.
Excretion: Drug is primarily excreted in urine, with 50% as unchanged drug. A small amount is excreted in feces.

CONTRAINDICATIONS & PRECAUTIONS
Contraindicated in patients with hypersensitivity to cetirizine or hydroxyzine. Use cautiously in patients with impaired renal function.

INTERACTIONS
Drug-drug. *CNS depressants* and *anticholinergics* may cause a possible additive effect; avoid concomitant use. *Theophylline* may cause decreased clearance of cetirizine; monitor patient closely.
Drug-lifestyle. *Alcohol* may cause additive CNS effects.

ADVERSE REACTIONS
CNS: somnolence, fatigue, dizziness.
EENT: pharyngitis, dry mouth.

▣ KEY CONSIDERATIONS
● It's unknown whether abuse or dependency occurs with cetirizine use.

Patient education
● Caution patient not to perform hazardous activities if somnolence occurs with drug use.
● Instruct patient not to consume alcohol or other CNS depressants while taking drug because of additive effect.

Overdose & treatment
● Signs and symptoms of overdose include somnolence.
● Treatment for overdose should be symptomatic or supportive.

---

chloral hydrate
Aquachloral Supprettes, Noctec, Novo-Chlorhydrate*

General CNS depressant, sedative-hypnotic
Controlled substance schedule IV

Available by prescription only
Capsules: 250 mg, 500 mg
Syrup: 250 mg/5 ml, 500 mg/5 ml
Suppositories: 325 mg, 500 mg, 650 mg

INDICATIONS & DOSAGE
Sedation
Adults: 250 mg P.O. t.i.d. after meals.
Management of alcohol withdrawal symptoms
Adults: 500 to 1,000 mg; may repeat q 6 hours, p.r.n.
Insomnia
Adults: 500 mg to 1 g P.O. or P.R. 15 to 30 minutes before bedtime.

PHARMACODYNAMICS
Sedative-hypnotic action: Chloral hydrate has CNS depressant activities similar to those of the barbiturates. Nonspecific CNS depression occurs at hypnotic dosages; however, respiratory drive is only slightly affected. Drug's primary site of action is the reticular activating

---

Reactions may be *common*, uncommon, ***life-threatening***, or COMMON AND LIFE-THREATENING.

system, which controls arousal. The cellular site of action is not known.

PHARMACOKINETICS
Absorption: Chloral hydrate is absorbed well after oral and rectal administration. Sleep occurs 30 to 60 minutes after a 500-mg to 1-g dose.
Distribution: Drug and its active metabolite, trichloroethanol, are distributed throughout the body tissue and fluids. About 35% to 41% of drug binds to proteins.
Metabolism: Drug is metabolized rapidly and nearly completely in the liver and erythrocytes to the active metabolite trichloroethanol, which is further metabolized in the liver and kidneys to trichloroacetic acid and other inactive metabolites.
Excretion: Inactive metabolites of drug hydrate are excreted primarily in urine. A small amount is excreted in bile. Half-life of trichloroethanol is 8 to 10 hours.

CONTRAINDICATIONS & PRECAUTIONS
Contraindicated in patients with impaired hepatic or renal function, severe cardiac disease, or hypersensitivity to chloral hydrate. Oral administration is contraindicated in patients with gastric disorders. Use with extreme caution in patients with mental depression, suicidal tendencies, or history of drug abuse.

INTERACTIONS
Drug-drug. Use with *antihistamines, narcotics, other CNS depressants, sedative-hypnotics, tranquilizers,* or *tricyclic antidepressants* can add to or potentiate their effects. Administration of drug followed by *I.V. furosemide* may cause a hypermetabolic state by displacing thyroid hormone from binding sites, resulting in sweating, hot flashes, tachycardia, and variable blood pressure. Chloral hydrate may displace *oral anticoagulants* such as *warfarin* from protein-binding sites, causing increased hypoprothrombinemic effects. Elimination of *phenytoin* may be increased with concomitant use.
Drug-lifestyle. *Alcohol* can add to or potentiate effects of chloral hydrate. Also, use with *alcohol* may cause va-

sodilation, tachycardia, sweating, and flushing in some patients.

ADVERSE REACTIONS
CNS: drowsiness, nightmares, dizziness, ataxia, paradoxical excitement, hangover, somnolence, disorientation, delirium, light-headedness, hallucinations, confusion, vertigo, malaise.
GI: *nausea, vomiting, diarrhea,* flatulence.
Hematologic: eosinophilia, *leukopenia.*
Skin: hypersensitivity reactions (rash, urticaria).
Other: physical and psychological dependence.

▣ KEY CONSIDERATIONS
• Geriatric patients may be more susceptible to the CNS depressant effects of the drug because of decreased elimination. Lower dosages are indicated.
• Chloral hydrate isn't a first-line drug because of potential for adverse or toxic adverse effects.
• Some brands contain tartrazine, which may cause allergic reactions in susceptible individuals.
• Assess level of consciousness before administering drug to ensure appropriate baseline level.
• To lessen GI upset, give drug capsules with a full glass (8 oz [240 ml]) of water; to improve taste, dilute syrup in a half glass of water or juice before administration.
• Monitor vital signs frequently.
• To prevent breakdown of medicine, store in dark container away from heat and moisture. Store suppositories in refrigerator.
• Drug may produce false-positive results for urine glucose with tests using cupric sulfate, such as Benedict's reagent and possibly Clinitest. Drug doesn't interfere with Chemstrip uG, Diastix, or glucose enzymatic test strip results. Because drug interferes with fluorometric tests for urine catecholamines, don't use it for 48 hours before the test. Drug may also interfere with Reddy-Jenkins-Thorn test for urine 17-hydroxycorticosteroid levels.
• Drug also may cause a false-positive phentolamine test.

Patient education

- Advise patient to take drug with a full glass (8 oz [240 ml]) of water and to dilute syrup with juice or water before use.
- Instruct patient in proper administration of drug form prescribed.
- Warn patient not to attempt tasks that require mental alertness or physical coordination until the CNS effects of drug are known.
- Tell patient to avoid alcohol and other CNS depressants.
- Instruct patient to call before using OTC allergy or cold preparations.
- Warn patient not to increase dosage and not to stop drug except as prescribed.

Overdose & treatment

- Signs and symptoms of overdose include stupor, coma, respiratory depression, pinpoint pupils, hypotension, and hypothermia. Esophageal stricture may follow gastric necrosis and perforation. GI hemorrhage has also been reported. Hepatic damage and jaundice may occur.
- Treatment is supportive of respiration (including mechanical ventilation if needed), blood pressure, and body temperature. If patient is conscious, empty stomach by inducing vomiting or performing gastric lavage. Hemodialysis will remove drug and its metabolite. Peritoneal dialysis may be effective.

---

chlorambucil
Leukeran

Alkylating agent (cell cycle–phase nonspecific), antineoplastic

---

Available by prescription only
Tablets (sugar-coated): 2 mg

INDICATIONS & DOSAGE

Dosage and indications may vary. Check current literature for recommended protocol.
Chronic lymphocytic leukemia, malignant lymphomas including lymphosarcoma, giant follicular lymphomas, Hodgkin's disease, ◊ autoimmune hemolytic anemias, ◊ nephrotic syndrome, ◊ polycythemia vera, ◊ macroglobulinemia, ◊ ovarian neoplasms
Adults: 100 to 200 mcg/kg P.O. daily or 3 to 6 mg/m² P.O. daily as a single dose or in divided doses; for 3 to 6 weeks. Usual dosage is 4 to 10 mg daily. Reduce dosage if within 4 weeks of a full course of radiation therapy.
◊ Macroglobulinemia
Adults: 2 to 10 mg P.O. daily.
◊ Metastatic trophoblastic neoplasia
Adults: 6 to 10 mg P.O. daily for 5 days; repeat q 1 to 2 weeks.
◊ Idiopathic uveitis
Adults: 6 to 12 mg P.O. daily for 1 year.
◊ Rheumatoid arthritis
Adults: 0.1 to 0.3 mg/kg P.O. daily.

PHARMACODYNAMICS

Antineoplastic action: Drug exerts its cytotoxic activity by cross-linking strands of cellular DNA and RNA, disrupting normal nucleic acid function.

PHARMACOKINETICS

Absorption: Chlorambucil is well absorbed from the GI tract.
Distribution: Not well understood. However, drug and its metabolites have been shown to be highly bound to plasma and tissue proteins.
Metabolism: Drug is metabolized in the liver. Its primary metabolite, phenylacetic acid mustard, also possesses cytotoxic activity.
Excretion: Metabolites of the drug are excreted in urine. Half-life of parent compound is 2 hours; the phenylacetic acid metabolite, 2½ hours. Drug probably isn't dialyzable.

CONTRAINDICATIONS & PRECAUTIONS

Contraindicated in patients with hypersensitivity or resistance to previous therapy. Patients hypersensitive to other alkylating drugs also may be hypersensitive to chlorambucil.
   Use cautiously in patients with history of head trauma or seizures and in those receiving other drugs that lower seizure threshold.

INTERACTIONS

None reported.

ADVERSE REACTIONS

CNS: *seizures,* peripheral neuropathy, tremor, muscle twitching, confusion, agitation, ataxia, flaccid paresis.

GI: *nausea, vomiting, stomatitis,* diarrhea.

GU: *azoospermia, infertility.*

Hematologic: *neutropenia,* delayed up to 3 weeks, lasting up to 10 days after last dose; *bone marrow suppression; thrombocytopenia; anemia.*

Hepatic: *hepatotoxicity,* increased AST levels.

Respiratory: interstitial pneumonitis, *pulmonary fibrosis* (rare).

Skin: rash, *hypersensitivity.*

Other: allergic febrile reaction; may increase serum alkaline phosphatase and blood and urine uric acid levels.

▣ KEY CONSIDERATIONS

• Oral suspension can be prepared in the pharmacy by crushing tablets and mixing powder with a suspending agent and simple syrup.

• Avoid all I.M. injections when platelet count is below 100,000/mm³.

• Anticoagulants and aspirin products should be used cautiously. Watch closely for bleeding.

• Drug-induced pancytopenia generally lasts 1 to 2 weeks but may persist for 3 to 4 weeks. It's reversible up to a cumulative dose of 6.5 mg/kg in a single course.

• To prevent hyperuricemia with resulting uric acid nephropathy, allopurinol may be used with adequate hydration. Monitor uric acid.

• Store tablets in a tightly closed, light-resistant container.

Patient education

• Emphasize importance of continuing drug, despite nausea and vomiting, and of keeping appointments for periodic blood work.

• Advise patient to call health care provider if vomiting occurs shortly after taking dose or if symptoms of infection or bleeding are present.

• Tell patient to avoid people with infections.

• Instruct patient to avoid OTC products containing aspirin.

Overdose & treatment

• Signs and symptoms of overdose include reversible pancytopenia.

• Treatment is usually supportive with transfusion of blood components, if necessary, and appropriate anticonvulsant therapy if seizures occur. To remove unabsorbed drug, induce vomiting, administer activated charcoal, or perform gastric lavage.

chloramphenicol
Chloromycetin, Chloroptic, Econochlor, Fenicol*, Ophthochlor, Pentamycetin*

chloramphenicol sodium succinate
Chloromycetin Sodium Succinate, Pentamycetin*

Dichloroacetic acid derivative, antibiotic

Available by prescription only
Powder for solution: 25 mg/vial
Injection: 1-g and 10-g vials
Ophthalmic solution: 0.5%
Ophthalmic ointment: 1%
Otic solution: 0.5%, 4.5%*

INDICATIONS & DOSAGE

Severe meningitis, brain abscesses, bacteremia, or other serious infections
Adults: 50 to 100 mg/kg I.V. daily, divided q 6 hours. Maximum dosage is 100 mg/kg daily.

Superficial infections of the skin caused by susceptible bacteria
Adults: Rub into affected area b.i.d. or t.i.d.

External ear canal infection
Adults: Instill 2 or 3 gtt into ear canal t.i.d or q.i.d.

Surface bacterial infection involving conjunctiva or cornea
Adults: Instill 2 gtt of solution in eye every hour until condition improves, or instill q.i.d., depending on severity of infection. Apply small amount of ointment to lower conjunctival sac at bedtime as supplement to drops. To use ointment alone, apply small amount to lower conjunctival sac every 3 to 6 hours or more

frequently if necessary. Continue with treatment up to 48 hours after condition improves.

PHARMACODYNAMICS

Antibiotic action: Chloramphenicol palmitate and chloramphenicol sodium succinate must be hydrolyzed to chloramphenicol before antimicrobial activity can take place. The active compound then inhibits bacterial protein synthesis by binding to the ribosome's 50S subunit, thus inhibiting peptide bond formation.

Drug usually produces bacteriostatic effects on susceptible bacteria, including *Rickettsia, Chlamydia, Mycoplasma,* and certain *Salmonella* strains as well as most gram-positive and gram-negative organisms. Chloramphenicol is used to treat *Haemophilus influenzae,* Rocky Mountain spotted fever, meningitis, lymphogranuloma, psittacosis, severe meningitis, and bacteremia.

PHARMACOKINETICS

Absorption: With I.V. administration, serum levels vary greatly, depending on patient's metabolism.
Distribution: Drug is distributed widely to most body tissues and fluids, including CSF, liver, and kidneys. About 50% to 60% of drug binds to plasma proteins.
Metabolism: Parent drug is metabolized primarily by hepatic glucuronyl transferase to inactive metabolites.
Excretion: About 8% to 12% of dose is excreted from the kidneys as unchanged drug; the remainder is excreted as inactive metabolites. Plasma half-life ranges from 1½ to 4½ hours in adults with normal hepatic and renal function. Plasma half-life of parent drug is prolonged in patients with hepatic dysfunction. Peritoneal hemodialysis doesn't remove a significant amount of drug. Plasma chloramphenicol levels may be elevated in patients with renal impairment after I.V. chloramphenicol administration.

CONTRAINDICATIONS & PRECAUTIONS

Contraindicated in patients with hypersensitivity to chloramphenicol.

Use cautiously in patients who have impaired renal or hepatic function, acute intermittent porphyria, or G6PD deficiency or take drugs that suppress bone marrow function.

INTERACTIONS

Drug-drug. Use with *acetaminophen* elevates the serum chloramphenicol level by an unknown mechanism, possibly resulting in an enhanced pharmacologic effect. Chloramphenicol inhibits hepatic metabolism of *chlorpropamide, cyclophosphamide, dicumarol, phenobarbital, phenytoin,* and *tolbutamide* by inhibiting microsomal enzyme activity, leading to prolonged plasma half-life of these drugs and possible toxic reactions from increased serum drug levels. Use with *folic acid, iron salts,* and *vitamin B₂* reduces the hematologic response to these substances. Chloramphenicol may antagonize the bactericidal activity of *penicillin.*

ADVERSE REACTIONS

CNS: headache, mild depression, confusion, delirium, peripheral neuropathy with prolonged therapy.
EENT: optic neuritis (in patients with cystic fibrosis), glossitis, decreased visual acuity, stinging or burning of eye after instillation, blurred vision (with ointment).
GI: nausea, vomiting, stomatitis, diarrhea, enterocolitis.
Hematologic: *aplastic anemia, hypoplastic anemia, agranulocytosis, thrombocytopenia,* decreased erythrocyte and leukocyte counts, hemoglobinuria.
Hepatic: jaundice.
Skin: possible contact sensitivity; burning, urticaria, pruritus, angioedema in hypersensitive patients.
Other: hypersensitivity reactions (fever, rash, urticaria, *anaphylaxis*), lactic acidosis.

⬚ KEY CONSIDERATIONS

● Administer drug cautiously to geriatric patients with impaired liver function.
● Culture and sensitivity tests may be performed when the first dose is administered and may be repeated as needed.
● Use drug only when clearly indicated for severe infection. Because the drug can cause severe toxic reactions, it should be reserved for potentially life-threatening infections.

• Refrigerate ophthalmic solution.
• If administering drug concomitantly with penicillin, give penicillin 1 hour or more before chloramphenicol to avoid reducing the bactericidal activity of penicillin.
• For I.V. administration, reconstitute 1-g vial of powder for injection with 10 ml of sterile water for injection; concentration will be 100 mg/ml. Solution remains stable for 30 days at room temperature; however, refrigeration is recommended. Don't use cloudy solutions. Administer I.V. infusion slowly, over at least 1 minute. Check injection site daily for phlebitis and irritation.
• Therapeutic range is 10 to 20 µg/ml for peak levels and 5 to 10 µg/ml for trough levels.
• Monitor CBC, platelet count, reticulocyte count, and serum iron level before therapy begins and every 2 days during therapy. Discontinue immediately if test results indicate anemia, reticulocytopenia, leukopenia, or thrombocytopenia.
• Observe patient for signs and symptoms of superinfection by nonsusceptible organisms.
• False elevation of urine PABA levels will result if chloramphenicol is administered during a bentiromide test for pancreatic function. Drug therapy will cause false-positive results on tests for urine glucose level using cupric sulfate (Clinitest).

Patient education
• Instruct patient to report adverse reactions, especially nausea, vomiting, diarrhea, bleeding, fever, confusion, sore throat, or mouth sores.
• Tell patient to take drug for prescribed period and to take it exactly as directed, even after he feels better.
• Instruct patient to wash hands before and after applying topical ointment or solution.
• Warn patient using otic solution not to touch ear with dropper.
• Caution patient using topical cream to avoid sharing washcloths and towels with family members.
• Tell patient using ophthalmic drug to clean eye area of excess exudate before applying drug, and show him how to in-

still drug in eye. Warn him not to touch applicator tip to eye or surrounding tissue. Instruct him to observe for signs and symptoms of sensitivity, such as itchy eyelids or constant burning, and to discontinue drug and call health care provider immediately should any occur.

Overdose & treatment
• Signs and symptoms of parenterally administered overdose include anemia and metabolic acidosis followed by hypotension, hypothermia, abdominal distention, and possible death.
• Initial treatment is symptomatic and supportive. Drug may be removed by charcoal hemoperfusion.

---

chlordiazepoxide
Libritabs

chlordiazepoxide hydrochloride
Librium, Mitran, Reposans-10

Benzodiazepine, anxiolytic, anticonvulsant, sedative-hypnotic
Controlled substance schedule IV

Available by prescription only
Tablets: 5 mg, 10 mg, 25 mg
Capsules: 5 mg, 10 mg, 25 mg
Powder for injection: 100 mg/ampule

INDICATIONS & DOSAGE
Mild to moderate anxiety and tension
Adults: 5 to 10 mg t.i.d. or q.i.d.
Geriatric patients: 5 mg P.O. b.i.d. to q.i.d. Maximum dosage is 10 mg P.O. b.i.d. or t.i.d.
✦ *Dosage adjustment. Geriatric patients, debilitated patients or patients with hepatic or renal dysfunction:* 5 mg P.O. b.i.d. to q.i.d. Maximum dosage is 10 mg P.O. b.i.d. or t.i.d.
Severe anxiety and tension
Adults: 20 to 25 mg P.O. t.i.d. or q.i.d.
Preoperative apprehension and anxiety
Adults: 5 to 10 mg P.O. t.i.d. or q.i.d. on day before surgery; or 50 to 100 mg I.M. 1 hour before surgery.
Withdrawal symptoms of acute alcoholism

Adults: 50 to 100 mg P.O., I.M., or I.V. Maximum dosage is 300 mg/day.

PHARMACODYNAMICS

Anxiolytic action: Chlordiazepoxide depresses the CNS at the limbic and subcortical levels of the brain. It produces an anxiolytic effect by influencing the effect of the neurotransmitter gamma-aminobutyric acid (GABA) on its receptor in the ascending reticular activating system, which increases inhibition and blocks both cortical and limbic arousal after stimulation of the reticular formation.

Anticonvulsant action: Drug suppresses the spread of seizure activity produced by the epileptogenic foci in the cortex, thalamus, and limbic structures by enhancing presynaptic inhibition.

PHARMACOKINETICS

Absorption: When given orally, chlordiazepoxide is absorbed well through the GI tract. Action begins within 30 to 45 minutes, with peak action in 1 to 3 hours. I.M. administration results in erratic absorption of drug; onset of action usually occurs in 15 to 30 minutes. After I.V. administration, rapid onset of action occurs in 1 to 5 minutes after injection.

Distribution: Drug is distributed widely throughout the body; 90% to 98% binds to proteins.

Metabolism: Drug is metabolized in the liver to several active metabolites.

Excretion: Most metabolites are excreted in urine as glucuronide conjugates. Half-life of drug is 5 to 30 hours.

CONTRAINDICATIONS & PRECAUTIONS

Contraindicated in patients hypersensitive to chlordiazepoxide. Use cautiously in patients with impaired renal or hepatic function, mental depression, or porphyria.

INTERACTIONS

Drug-drug. *Antacids* may delay the absorption of chlordiazepoxide. Chlordiazepoxide potentiates the CNS depressant effects of *antidepressants, antihistamines, barbiturates, general anesthetics, MAO inhibitors, narcotics,* and *phenothiazines.* Use with *cimetidine* and possibly *disulfiram* diminishes hepatic metabolism of chlordiazepoxide, which increases its plasma levels. Use with *digoxin* or *phenytoin* may increase levels of these drugs. Use with *haloperidol* may decrease serum haloperidol levels. Use with *levodopa* may decrease therapeutic effects of levodopa.

Drug-lifestyle. Chlordiazepoxide potentiates the CNS depressant effects of *alcohol. Heavy smoking* accelerates metabolism of chlordiazepoxide, making the drug less effective.

ADVERSE REACTIONS

CNS: *drowsiness, lethargy,* ataxia, confusion, extrapyramidal symptoms, EEG changes.

CV: edema.

GI: nausea, constipation.

GU: increased or decreased libido, menstrual irregularities.

Hematologic: *agranulocytosis.*

Hepatic: jaundice, elevated liver function tests.

Skin: *swelling, pain at injection site,* skin eruptions.

▣ KEY CONSIDERATIONS

Besides the recommendations relevant to all benzodiazepines, consider the following:

● Geriatric patients are more sensitive to the CNS depressant effects of drug. Some may require supervision with ambulation and activities of daily living during initiation of therapy or after an increase in dosage.

● Lower dosages are usually effective in geriatric patients because of decreased elimination.

● Parenteral administration of drug is more likely to cause apnea, hypotension, and bradycardia in geriatric patients.

● I.M. administration isn't recommended because of erratic and slow absorption. However, if I.M. route is used, reconstitute with special diluent only. Don't use diluent if hazy. Discard unused portion. Inject I.M. deep into large muscle mass.

● For I.V. administration, drug should be reconstituted with sterile water or normal saline solution and infused slowly, directly into a large vein, at a rate not exceeding 50 mg/minute for adults. Don't

infuse chlordiazepoxide into small veins. Avoid extravasation into subcutaneous tissue. Observe infusion site for phlebitis. Keep resuscitation equipment nearby in case of an emergency.
• Prepare solutions for I.V. or I.M. use immediately before administration. Discard unused portions.
• Patients should remain in bed under observation for at least 3 hours after parenteral administration of chlordiazepoxide.
• Lower dosages are effective in patients with renal or hepatic dysfunction. Closely monitor renal and hepatic studies for signs of dysfunction.
• Chlordiazepoxide may also alter urine 17-ketosteroid (Zimmerman reaction), urine alkaloid (Frings thin-layer chromatography method), and urine glucose levels (with Chemstrip uG and Diastix, but not glucose enzymatic test strip).

Patient education
• Warn patient that sudden changes in position may cause dizziness. Advise patient to dangle legs a few minutes before getting out of bed to prevent falls and injury.
• Advise patient to avoid driving or performing other tasks that require alertness because drug may cause drowsiness.
• Tell patient to avoid alcohol consumption and smoking.

Overdose & treatment
• Signs and symptoms of overdose include somnolence, confusion, coma, hypoactive reflexes, dyspnea, labored breathing, hypotension, bradycardia, slurred speech, and unsteady gait or impaired coordination.
• Support blood pressure and respiration until drug effects subside; monitor vital signs. Flumazenil, a specific benzodiazepine antagonist, may be useful. Mechanical ventilatory assistance via endotracheal tube may be required to maintain a patent airway and support adequate oxygenation. To treat hypotension, use I.V. fluids and vasopressors, such as dopamine and phenylephrine. Perform gastric lavage if ingestion was recent, but only if an endotracheal tube is in place to prevent aspiration, or induce vomiting if the patient is conscious. Then, administer activated charcoal with a cathartic as a single dose. Don't administer barbiturates if excitation occurs. Dialysis is of limited value.

---

chlorpheniramine maleate
Aller-Chlor, Chlo-Amine, Chlor-100, Chlor-Pro, Chlorspan-12, Chlortab-4, Chlortab-8, Chlor-Trimeton, Chlor-Tripolon*, Novo-Pheniram*, Pfeiffer's Allergy, Phenetron, Teldrin

Propylamine-derivative antihistamine, H₁-receptor antagonist

Available with or without a prescription
Tablets: 4 mg, 8 mg, 12 mg
Tablets (chewable): 2 mg
Tablets (timed-release): 8 mg, 12 mg
Capsules (timed-release): 8 mg, 12 mg
Syrup: 2 mg/5 ml
Injection: 10 mg/ml, 100 mg/ml

INDICATIONS & DOSAGE
Rhinitis, allergy symptoms
Adults: 4 mg of tablets or syrup q 4 to 6 hours; or 8 to 12 mg of timed-release tablets b.i.d. or t.i.d. Maximum dosage is 24 mg/day; 10 to 20 mg S.C., I.V., or I.M. also may be used.

PHARMACODYNAMICS
Antihistamine action: Antihistamines compete with histamine for histamine H_1-receptor sites on smooth muscle of the bronchi, GI tract, uterus, and large blood vessels; they bind to cellular receptors, preventing access of histamine, thereby suppressing histamine-induced allergic symptoms. They don't directly alter histamine or its release.

PHARMACOKINETICS
Absorption: Chlorpheniramine is well absorbed from the GI tract; action begins within 30 to 60 minutes, and peaks in 2 to 6 hours. Food in the stomach delays absorption but doesn't affect bioavailability.
Distribution: Drug is distributed extensively into the body; about 72% binds to proteins.

Metabolism: Drug is metabolized largely in GI mucosal cells and liver (first-pass effect).

Excretion: Half-life is 12 to 43 hours in adults; drug and metabolites are excreted in urine.

CONTRAINDICATIONS & PRECAUTIONS

Contraindicated in patients having acute asthma attacks.

Use cautiously in geriatric patients and in patients with increased intraocular pressure, hyperthyroidism, CV or renal disease, hypertension, bronchial asthma, urine retention, prostatic hyperplasia, bladder neck obstruction, or stenosing peptic ulcers.

INTERACTIONS

Drug-drug. Use with *other CNS depressants*—such as *anxiolytics, barbiturates, sleeping aids,* or *tranquilizers*—may cause additive sedation. Chlorpheniramine enhances the effects of *epinephrine,* may diminish the effects of *sulfonylureas,* and partially counteracts the anticoagulant action of *heparin. MAO inhibitors* interfere with the detoxification of chlorpheniramine and thus prolong and intensify its central depressant and anticholinergic effects.

Drug-lifestyle. Use with *alcohol* leads to additive sedation.

ADVERSE REACTIONS

CNS: *stimulation,* sedation, *drowsiness,* excitability.

CV: hypotension, palpitations, weak pulse, pallor.

GI: epigastric distress, *dry mouth.*

GU: urine retention.

Respiratory: thick bronchial secretions.

Skin: rash, urticaria.

Other: local stinging, burning sensation (after parenteral administration).

▣ KEY CONSIDERATIONS

Besides the recommendations relevant to all antihistamines, consider the following:

● Geriatric patients are usually more sensitive to adverse effects of antihistamines and are especially likely to experience a greater degree of dizziness, sedation, hyperexcitability, dry mouth, and urine re-

tention than younger patients. Signs and symptoms usually respond to a decrease in dosage.

● Give 100 mg/ml of injectable form S.C. or I.M. *only.* Do not give I.V.; I.V. preparation contains preservatives.

● Don't use parenteral solutions I.D.

● Administer I.V. solution slowly, over 1 minute.

● Antihistamines can prevent, reduce, or mask positive skin test response. Discontinue drug 4 days before diagnostic skin tests.

Patient education

● Instruct patient to swallow sustained-release tablets whole; they shouldn't be crushed or chewed.

● Inform patient to store syrup and parenteral solution away from light.

● Advise patient to avoid alcohol while taking drug.

Overdose & treatment

● Signs and symptoms of overdose include those of CNS depression—such as sedation, reduced mental alertness, apnea, and CV collapse—and those of CNS stimulation—such as insomnia, hallucinations, tremors, and seizures. Atropine-like signs and symptoms—such as dry mouth, flushed skin, fixed and dilated pupils, and GI symptoms—are common.

● Treat overdose by inducing vomiting with ipecac syrup (in conscious patient), followed by activated charcoal to reduce further drug absorption. Use gastric lavage if patient is unconscious or ipecac fails. Treat hypotension with vasopressors, and control seizures with diazepam or phenytoin. Don't give stimulants. Administering ammonium chloride or vitamin C to acidify urine promotes drug excretion.

Reactions may be *common*, uncommon, *life-threatening*, or COMMON AND LIFE-THREATENING.

chlorpromazine hydrochloride

Chlorpromanyl-5*, Chlorpromanyl-
20*, Largactil*, Novo-
Chlorpromazine*, Ormazine,
Thorazine, Thor-Prom

*Aliphatic phenothiazine, antiemetic,
antipsychotic*

Available by prescription only
Tablets: 10 mg, 25 mg, 50 mg, 100 mg,
200 mg
Capsules (sustained-release): 30 mg,
75 mg, 150 mg, 200 mg, 300 mg
Syrup: 10 mg/5 ml
Oral concentrate: 30 mg/ml, 100 mg/ml
Suppositories: 25 mg, 100 mg
Injection: 25 mg/ml

INDICATIONS & DOSAGE

Psychosis
Adults: 30 to 75 mg P.O. daily in two to
four divided doses. Dosage may be increased twice weekly by 20 to 50 mg until symptoms are controlled. Most patients respond to 200 mg daily, but
dosages up to 800 mg may be necessary.
*Acute management of psychosis in se-
verely agitated patients*
Adults: 25 mg I.M.; may give additional
25 to 50 mg in 1 hour if necessary. Increase dosage gradually, up to 400 mg q
4 to 6 hours until symptoms are controlled.
Nausea, vomiting
Adults: 10 to 25 mg P.O. or 25 mg I.M. q
4 to 6 hours, p.r.n.; or 100 mg rectally q
6 to 8 hours, p.r.n.
Intractable hiccups
Adults: 25 to 50 mg P.O. or I.M. t.i.d. or
q.i.d.
*Mild alcohol withdrawal, acute inter-
mittent porphyria, tetanus*
Adults: 25 mg to 50 mg I.M. t.i.d. or
q.i.d.

PHARMACODYNAMICS

Antipsychotic action: Chlorpromazine is
thought to exert its antipsychotic effects
by postsynaptic blockade of CNS
dopamine receptors, thereby inhibiting
dopamine-mediated effects.

Antiemetic action: Antiemetic effects are
attributed to dopamine receptor blockade
in the medullary chemoreceptor trigger
zone. Drug has many other central and
peripheral effects; it produces both alpha
and ganglionic blockade and counteracts
histamine- and serotonin-mediated activity. Its most prominent adverse reactions
are antimuscarinic effects and sedation.

PHARMACOKINETICS

Absorption: Rate and extent of absorption vary with route of administration.
Oral tablet is absorbed erratically and
variably, with onset ranging from ½ to
1 hour; effects peak in 2 to 4 hours and
duration of action is 4 to 6 hours.
Sustained-release preparations have similar absorption, but action lasts for 10 to
12 hours. Suppositories act in 60 minutes and last 3 to 4 hours. Oral concentrates and syrups are much more predictable; I.M. drug is absorbed rapidly.
Distribution: Drug is distributed widely
into the body; drug level is usually higher in CNS than plasma. Steady-state
serum level is achieved within 4 to 7
days. About 91% to 99% of drug binds
to proteins.
Metabolism: Drug is metabolized extensively in the liver and forms 10 to 12
metabolites; some are pharmacologically
active.
Excretion: Drug is mostly excreted as
metabolites in urine; some is excreted in
feces via the biliary tract. Drug may undergo enterohepatic circulation.

CONTRAINDICATIONS & PRECAUTIONS

Contraindicated in patients with hypersensitivity to chlorpromazine or in patients experiencing CNS depression,
bone marrow suppression, subcortical
damage, and coma.

Use cautiously in geriatric or debilitated patients and in patients with impaired
renal or hepatic function, severe CV disease, glaucoma, prostatic hyperplasia,
respiratory or seizure disorders, hypocalcemia, reaction to insulin or electroconvulsive therapy, or exposure to heat,
cold, or organophosphate insecticides.

INTERACTIONS

Drug-drug. Use of chlorpromazine and *aluminum- or magnesium-containing antacids, antidiarrheals,* or *phenobarbital* may cause pharmacokinetic alterations and subsequent decreased therapeutic response to chlorpromazine. *Aluminum- and magnesium-containing antacids* and *antidiarrheals* decrease absorption of chlorpromazine and *phenobarbital* enhances renal excretion of it. Use with *appetite suppressants* may decrease their stimulatory and pressor effects and *sympathomimetics,* including *ephedrine* (commonly found in *nasal sprays*), *epinephrine, phenylephrine,* and *phenylpropanolamine. Beta blockers* may inhibit chlorpromazine metabolism, increasing blood levels. Chlorpromazine may antagonize the therapeutic effect of *bromocriptine* on prolactin secretion. Chlorpromazine may inhibit blood pressure response to *centrally acting antihypertensives* such as *clonidine, guanabenz, guanadrel, guanethidine, methyldopa,* and *reserpine.*

Use with the following drugs may cause additive effects: *CNS depressants*—including *analgesics, barbiturates,* and *epidural, general,* or *spinal anesthetics, narcotics,* or *tranquilizers*—or *parenteral magnesium sulfate* (oversedation, respiratory depression, and hypotension); *antiarrhythmics, disopyramide, procainamide,* or *quinidine* (increased frequency of arrhythmias and conduction defects); *atropine* or other *anticholinergics,* including *antidepressants, MAO inhibitors* (increased risk of seizures). Chlorpromazine may decrease the vasoconstrictive effects of high-dose *dopamine* and may decrease effectiveness and increase toxicity of *levodopa* through dopamine blockade.

Chlorpromazine may cause *epinephrine* reversal: The beta agonist activity of *epinephrine* is evident whereas its alpha effects are blocked, leading to decreased diastolic and increased systolic pressures and tachycardia. Use with *lithium* may cause a decreased therapeutic response to chlorpromazine and severe toxicity with an encephalitis-like syndrome. Chlorpromazine may inhibit metabolism and increase toxic levels of *phenytoin.*

Use with *propylthiouracil* increases risk of agranulocytosis.

Drug-food. Decreased therapeutic response to chlorpromazine may follow use with *caffeine.*

Drug-lifestyle. *Alcohol* may cause additive CNS effects. *Heavy smoking* decreases therapeutic response to chlorpromazine by increasing drug metabolism. *Sun exposure* increases the risk of photosensitivity reactions.

ADVERSE REACTIONS

CNS: *extrapyramidal reactions,* drowsiness, *sedation, seizures, tardive dyskinesia,* pseudoparkinsonism, dizziness.
CV: *orthostatic hypotension,* tachycardia, ECG changes.
EENT: ocular changes, blurred vision, nasal congestion, sore throat.
GI: *dry mouth, constipation,* nausea.
GU: *urine retention,* menstrual irregularities, gynecomastia, inhibited ejaculation, priapism.
Hematologic: *leukopenia, agranulocytosis,* eosinophilia, *hemolytic anemia, aplastic anemia, thrombocytopenia.*
Hepatic: jaundice, abnormal liver function test results.
Skin: *mild photosensitivity,* allergic reactions, *pain at I.M. injection site,* sterile abscess, skin pigmentation.
Other: *neuroleptic malignant syndrome,* fever.
After abrupt withdrawal of long-term therapy: gastritis, nausea, vomiting, dizziness, tremor.

▣ KEY CONSIDERATIONS

Besides the recommendations relevant to all phenothiazines, consider the following:

● Geriatric patients tend to require lower dosages and individual adjustments. They're also more likely to develop adverse reactions, especially tardive dyskinesia and other extrapyramidal effects.
● Drug may discolor urine to a pink-brown.
● Because photosensitivity reactions are a common adverse effect of the drug, patient should avoid exposure to sunlight or heat lamps.
● Sustained-release preparations should be swallowed whole.

Reactions may be *common,* uncommon, *life-threatening,* or COMMON AND LIFE-THREATENING.

• Oral formulations may cause stomach upset and may be administered with food or fluid.

• Dilute concentrate in 2 to 4 oz (60 to 120 ml) of liquid, preferably water, carbonated drinks, fruit juice, tomato juice, milk, pudding, or applesauce.

• Store suppository form in a cool place.

• If tissue irritation occurs, chlorpromazine injection may be diluted with normal saline solution or 2% procaine.

• I.V. form should be used only during surgery or for severe hiccups. Dilute injection to 1 mg/ml with normal saline solution and administer at a rate of 1 mg/minute for adults.

• I.M. injection should be given deep in the outer upper quadrant of the buttocks. Injection is usually painful; massaging the area after administration may prevent abscess formation.

• Liquid and injectable forms may cause a rash if skin contact occurs.

• Solution for injection may be slightly discolored. Don't use if drug is excessively discolored or if it has a precipitate. Monitor blood pressure before and after parenteral administration.

• Drug causes false-positive test results for urine porphyrins, urobilinogen, amylase, and 5-hydroxyindoleacetic acid because metabolites darken urine.

Patient education
• Explain risks of dystonic reactions and tardive dyskinesia, and tell patient to report abnormal body movements.

• To prevent photosensitivity reactions, tell patient to avoid sun exposure and to wear sunscreen when going outdoors. (Note that sunlamps and tanning beds also may cause the skin to burn or discolor.)

• Warn patient to avoid extremely hot or cold baths or exposure to temperature extremes, sunlamps, or tanning beds. Drug may cause thermoregulatory changes.

• Tell patient not to spill the liquid preparation on the skin because rash and irritation may result.

• Instruct patient to take drug exactly as prescribed and not to double-dose to compensate for missed doses.

• Explain that many drug interactions are possible. Patient should seek health care provider's approval before taking any self-prescribed drugs.

• Tell patient not to stop taking drug suddenly.

• Encourage patient to report difficulty urinating, sore throat, dizziness, fainting, or fever.

• Advise patient to avoid hazardous activities that require alertness until the effect of the drug is established. Excessive sedative effects tend to subside after several weeks.

• Tell patient to avoid alcohol and drugs that may cause excessive sedation.

• Explain what fluids are appropriate for diluting the concentrate and the dropper technique for measuring dose. Teach patient how to use suppository form.

• Inform patient that sugarless chewing gum or hard candy, ice chips, or artificial saliva may help to alleviate dry mouth.

Overdose & treatment
• CNS depression is characterized by deep, unarousable sleep and possibly coma; hypotension or hypertension; extrapyramidal symptoms; abnormal involuntary muscle movements; agitation; seizures; arrhythmias; ECG changes; hypothermia or hyperthermia; and autonomic nervous system dysfunction.

• Treatment is symptomatic and supportive, including maintaining vital signs, airway, stable body temperature, and fluid and electrolyte balance.

• Don't induce vomiting: Drug inhibits cough reflex, and aspiration may occur. Perform gastric lavage, then administer activated charcoal and sodium chloride cathartics; dialysis doesn't help. Regulate body temperature as needed. Treat hypotension with I.V. fluids: Don't give epinephrine. Treat seizures with parenteral diazepam or barbiturates; arrhythmias with parenteral phenytoin (1 mg/kg with rate titrated to blood pressure); extrapyramidal reactions with 1 to 2 mg of benztropine or 10 to 50 mg of parenteral diphenhydramine.

chlorpropamide
Diabinese, Novo-Propamide*

Sulfonylurea, antidiabetic

Available by prescription only
Tablets: 100 mg, 250 mg

INDICATIONS & DOSAGE
Adjunct to diet to lower blood glucose levels in patients with type 2 diabetes mellitus
Adults: 250 mg P.O. daily with breakfast or in divided doses if GI disturbances occur. First dosage increase may be made after 5 to 7 days because of extended duration of action, then dosage may be increased q 3 to 5 days by 50 to 125 mg, if needed, to a maximum of 750 mg daily.
Geriatric patients: initial dosage should be 100 to 125 mg/day.
To change from insulin to oral therapy
Adults: If insulin dosage is less than 40 U/day, insulin may be stopped and oral therapy started as above. If insulin dosage is 40 U or more daily, start oral therapy as above, with insulin dose reduced 50% the first few days. Further insulin reductions should be made based on patient response.

PHARMACODYNAMICS
Antidiabetic action: Chlorpropamide lowers blood glucose levels by stimulating insulin release from beta cells in the pancreas. After long-term therapy, it produces hypoglycemic effects through extrapancreatic mechanisms, including reduced basal hepatic glucose production and enhanced peripheral sensitivity to insulin; the latter may result either from an increased number of insulin receptors or from changes in events that follow insulin binding.
Antidiuretic action: Drug appears to potentiate the effects of minimal levels of ADH.

PHARMACOKINETICS
Absorption: Chlorpropamide is absorbed readily from the GI tract. Onset of action occurs within 1 hour, with a maximum decrease in serum glucose levels at 3 to 6 hours.
Distribution: Not fully understood, but is probably similar to that of the other sulfonylureas. It's highly protein-bound.
Metabolism: Liver metabolizes about 80% of drug. It's unknown whether the metabolites have hypoglycemic activity.
Excretion: Drug and its metabolites are excreted in urine. Rate of excretion depends on urine pH; it increases in alkaline urine and decreases in acidic urine. Duration of action is up to 60 hours; half-life is 36 hours.

CONTRAINDICATIONS & PRECAUTIONS
Contraindicated for treating type 1 diabetes mellitus or diabetes that can be adequately controlled by diet. Also contraindicated in patients with type 2 diabetes mellitus complicated by ketosis, acidosis, diabetic coma, major surgery, severe infections, or severe trauma and in patients with hypersensitivity to drug.

Use cautiously in geriatric, debilitated, or malnourished patients and those with porphyria or impaired renal or hepatic function.

INTERACTIONS
Drug-drug. Use with *anticoagulants* may increase plasma levels of both drugs and, after continued therapy, may reduce plasma levels and anticoagulant effects. Use with *drugs that may increase blood glucose levels*—such as *acetazolamide, adrenocorticoids, glucocorticoids, amphetamines, baclofen, corticotropin, epinephrine, estrogens, ethacrynic acid, furosemide, phenytoin, thiazide diuretics, thyroid hormones* or *triamterene*—may require dosage adjustments. Use with *nonspecific beta blockers*, including *ophthalmics*, may increase the risk of hypoglycemia by masking its signs, such as rising pulse rate and blood pressure.

Use with *chloramphenicol, guanethidine, insulin, MAO inhibitors, probenecid, salicylates,* or *sulfonamides* may enhance hypoglycemic effects by displacing chlorpropamide from its protein-binding sites.
Drug-lifestyle. Use with *alcohol* may produce a disulfiram-like reaction con-

sisting of nausea, vomiting, abdominal cramps, and headaches. *Smoking* increases corticosteroid release; patients who smoke may require higher dosages of chlorpropamide.

ADVERSE REACTIONS
CNS: paresthesia, fatigue, dizziness, vertigo, malaise, headache.
EENT: tinnitus.
GI: nausea, heartburn, epigastric distress.
GU: hematuria, dysuria, anuria.
Hematologic: *leukopenia, thrombocytopenia, aplastic anemia, agranulocytosis, hemolytic anemia.*
Metabolic: *prolonged hypoglycemia, dilutional hyponatremia.*
Skin: rash, pruritus, erythema, urticaria.
Other: *hypersensitivity reactions.*

▣ KEY CONSIDERATIONS
Besides the recommendations relevant to all sulfonylureas, consider the following:
• Geriatric patients may be more sensitive to the effects of drug because of reduced metabolism and elimination. They are more likely to develop neurological symptoms of hypoglycemia and usually require a lower initial dosage because the drug has a longer duration of action.
• To avoid GI intolerance in those patients who require dosages of 250 mg/day or more and to improve control of hyperglycemia, divided doses are recommended. These are given before the morning and evening meals.
• Chlorpropamide appears to potentiate the effects of minimal levels of ADH.
• Patients switching from chlorpropamide to another sulfonylurea should be monitored closely for 1 week because the body retains chlorpropamide for a prolonged period.
• Because drug has a long duration of action, adverse reactions, especially hypoglycemia, may be more frequent or severe than with some other sulfonylureas.
• Patients with severe diabetes who don't respond to 500 mg usually won't respond to higher dosages.
• Drug may accumulate in patients with renal insufficiency. Watch for such signs as dysuria, anuria, and hematuria.

• Chlorpropamide may potentiate antidiuretic effects of vasopressin. Watch for drowsiness, muscle cramps, seizures, unconsciousness, water retention, and weakness.
• Compared with diet or diet and insulin treatments, oral antidiabetics increase the risk of CV mortality.

Patient education
• Emphasize the importance of following the prescribed diet and medical regimen and exercising.
• Instruct patient to take drug at the same time each day. If a dose is missed, it should be taken immediately, unless it's almost time for the next dose. Patient should never double-dose.
• Tell patient to avoid alcohol, and remind him that many foods and OTC drugs contain alcohol. Alcohol may cause a disulfiram-like reaction.
• Encourage patient to wear a medical identification bracelet or necklace.
• Instruct patient to take drug with food if it causes GI upset.
• Teach patient how to monitor blood glucose, urine glucose, and ketone levels, as needed.
• Teach patient the signs and symptoms of hypoglycemia and hyperglycemia and the appropriate steps to take if they occur.
• Reassure patient that skin reactions are transient and usually subside as therapy continues.

Overdose & treatment
• Signs and symptoms of overdose include low blood glucose levels, tingling of lips and tongue, hunger, nausea, decreased cerebral function (lethargy, yawning, confusion, agitation, and nervousness), increased sympathetic activity (tachycardia, sweating, and tremor), and ultimately seizures, stupor, and coma.
• Mild hypoglycemia, without loss of consciousness or neurological findings, can be treated with oral glucose and dosage adjustments. If patient loses consciousness or experiences neurological symptoms, he should receive rapid injection of dextrose 50%, followed by a continuous infusion of $D_{10}W$ at a rate to maintain blood glucose levels greater than 100 mg/dl. Because chlorpropa-

mide has long half-life, monitor patient for 3 to 5 days.

cholera vaccine

Vaccine, cholera prophylaxis

Available by prescription only
Injection: suspension of killed *Vibrio cholerae* (each milliliter contains 8 U of Inaba and Ogawa serotypes) in 1.5-ml and 20-ml vials

INDICATIONS & DOSAGE
Primary immunization
Adults: 2 doses of 0.5 ml I.M. or S.C., 1 week to 1 month apart, before traveling in cholera-infected area. Booster dosage is 0.5 ml q 6 months for as long as protection is needed.

PHARMACODYNAMICS
Cholera prophylaxis action: Vaccine promotes active immunity to cholera in about 50% of those immunized.

PHARMACOKINETICS
Absorption: Unknown.
Distribution: Unknown. Virus-induced immunity begins to taper off within 3 to 6 months.
Metabolism: Unknown.
Excretion: Unknown.

CONTRAINDICATIONS & PRECAUTIONS
Contraindicated in patients with acute illness or history of severe systemic reaction or allergic response to vaccine.

INTERACTIONS
Drug-drug. Use with *corticosteroids* or *immunosuppressants* may impair the immune response to cholera vaccine and therefore should be avoided. Use with *yellow fever vaccine* may decrease the response to both.

ADVERSE REACTIONS
CNS: headache, malaise.
Other: *erythema, swelling, pain, induration (at injection site);* fever.

KEY CONSIDERATIONS
● Obtain a thorough history of allergies and reactions to immunizations.
● Epinephrine solution 1:1,000 should be available to treat allergic reactions.
● When possible, cholera and yellow fever vaccines should be administered at least 3 weeks apart; however, they may be administered simultaneously if necessary.
● Cholera vaccine may be given I.D. (0.2 ml) in adults.
● Shake vial well before removing a dose.
● Administer I.M. in deltoid muscle.
● Don't use I.M. route in patients with thrombocytopenia or other coagulation disorders that would contraindicate I.M. injection. Cholera vaccine shouldn't be administered I.V. Aspirate before S.C. or I.M. injection.
● Store vaccine at 36° to 46° F (2° to 8°C). Don't freeze.

Patient education
● Tell patient to report skin changes, difficulty breathing, fever, or joint pain.
● Inform patient that acetaminophen may be taken to relieve minor adverse effects, such as pain and tenderness at injection site.
● Tell patient that use of vaccine doesn't prevent infection.
● Advise patient to avoid consumption of contaminated food or water.

cholestyramine
Questran, Questran Light

Anion exchange resin, antilipemic, bile acid sequestrant

Available by prescription only
Powder: 378-g cans, 9-g single-dose packets (Questran); 5-g single dose packets (Questran Light). Each scoop of powder or single-dose packet contains 4 g of cholestyramine resin.

INDICATIONS & DOSAGE
Primary hyperlipidemia and hypercholesterolemia unresponsive to dietary measures alone; to reduce the risks of atherosclerotic coronary artery disease

---

Reactions may be *common*, uncommon, **life-threatening**, OR COMMON AND LIFE-THREATENING.

and MI; to relieve pruritus from partial biliary obstruction; ◊ cardiac glycoside toxicity

Adults: 4 g before meals and h.s. not to exceed 32 g daily. Can be given in one to six divided doses.

PHARMACODYNAMICS

Antilipemic action: Bile is normally excreted into the intestine to facilitate absorption of fat and other lipid materials. Cholestyramine binds with bile acid, forming an insoluble compound that's excreted in feces. With less bile available in the digestive system, fewer fat and lipid materials in food are absorbed, the liver uses more cholesterol to replace its supply of bile acids, and the serum cholesterol level decreases. In partial biliary obstruction, excess bile acids accumulate in dermal tissue, resulting in pruritus; by reducing levels of dermal bile acids, cholestyramine combats pruritus.

Drug can also act as an antidiarrheal in postoperative diarrhea caused by bile acids in the colon.

PHARMACOKINETICS

Absorption: Cholestyramine isn't absorbed. Cholesterol levels may begin to decrease 24 to 48 hours after the start of therapy and may continue to fall for up to 12 months. In some patients, the initial decrease is followed by a return to or above baseline cholesterol levels on continued therapy. Relief of pruritus associated with cholestasis occurs 1 to 3 weeks after initiation of therapy. Diarrhea caused by bile acids may cease in 24 hours.

Distribution: None.
Metabolism: None.
Excretion: Insoluble cholestyramine with bile acid complex is excreted in feces.

CONTRAINDICATIONS & PRECAUTIONS

Contraindicated in patients with hypersensitivity to bile-acid sequestering resins and in those with complete biliary obstruction. Use cautiously in patients who have coronary artery disease or are predisposed to constipation.

INTERACTIONS

Drug-drug. Cholestyramine may reduce absorption of other oral drugs, such as *acetaminophen, cardiac glycosides, corticosteroids, thiazide diuretics,* and *thyroid preparations* thus decreasing their therapeutic effects. Dosage of oral drugs may require adjustment to compensate for possible binding with cholestyramine, so give them at least 1 hour before or 4 to 6 hours after cholestyramine (longer if possible). To prevent high-dose toxicity, readjustment must also be made when cholestyramine is withdrawn.

Cholestyramine may decrease anticoagulant effects of *warfarin;* concurrent depletion of vitamin K may either negate this effect or increase anticoagulant activity. Careful monitoring of PT and INR is mandatory.

ADVERSE REACTIONS

CNS: headache, anxiety, vertigo, dizziness, insomnia, fatigue, syncope, tinnitus.
GI: *constipation,* **fecal impaction,** hemorrhoids, *abdominal discomfort,* flatulence, *nausea,* vomiting, steatorrhea, GI bleeding, diarrhea, anorexia.
GU: hematuria, dysuria.
Hematologic: anemia, ecchymoses, bleeding tendencies.
Hepatic: altered serum levels of ALT, AST.
Metabolic: altered serum levels of chloride, phosphorus, potassium, calcium, and sodium; hyperchloremic acidosis (with long-term use or very high dosages).
Musculoskeletal: backache, muscle and joint pain, osteoporosis.
Skin: *rash;* irritation of skin, tongue, and perianal area.
Other: *vitamin A, D, E, and K deficiencies from decreased absorption.*

▣ KEY CONSIDERATIONS

• Patients older than age 60 are more likely to experience adverse GI effects and adverse nutritional effects.
• To mix, sprinkle powder on surface of preferred beverage or wet food, let stand a few minutes and stir to obtain uniform suspension; avoid excess foaming by using large glass and mixing slowly. Use at

least 3 oz (90 ml) of water or other fluid, soup, milk, or pulpy fruit; rinse container and have patient drink this liquid to be sure he ingests entire dose.
• Because cholestyramine binds cardiac glycosides and prevents enterohepatic recycling, it has been used to treat cardiac glycoside overdose. When used as an adjunct to hyperlipidemia, monitor levels of cardiac glycosides and other drugs to ensure appropriate dosage during and after therapy with cholestyramine.
• Determine serum cholesterol level frequently during first few months of therapy and periodically thereafter.
• Monitor bowel function. Treat constipation promptly by decreasing dosage, adding a stool softener, or discontinuing drug.
• Monitor patient for vitamin A, D, or K deficiency.
• Questran Light contains aspartame and provides 1.6 calories per packet or scoop.
• Cholecystography using iopanoic acid yields abnormal results because iopanoic acid is also bound by cholestyramine.

Patient education
• Explain disease process and rationale for therapy, and encourage patient to comply with continued blood testing and special diet; although therapy isn't curative, it helps control serum cholesterol level.
• To increase awareness of other cardiac risk factors, encourage patient to control his weight and to stop smoking.
• Tell patient not to take the powder in dry form; teach him to mix drug with fluids or pulpy fruits.

choline magnesium trisalicylates
Tricosal, Trilisate

choline salicylate
Arthropan

Salicylate, nonnarcotic analgesic, antipyretic, anti-inflammatory

Available by prescription only

Tablets: 500 mg, 750 mg, 1,000 mg of salicylate (as choline and magnesium salicylate)
Solution: 500 mg of salicylate/5 ml (as choline and magnesium salicylate); 870 mg/5 ml (as choline salicylate)

INDICATIONS & DOSAGE
Rheumatoid arthritis, osteoarthritis
Adults: 1,500 mg P.O. b.i.d. or 3,000 mg h.s.
◆ *Dosage adjustment.* In geriatric patients, give 750 mg t.i.d.
Arthritis, mild; antipyresis
Adults: 2,000 to 3,000 mg P.O. daily in divided doses b.i.d.

PHARMACODYNAMICS
Analgesic action: Choline salicylates exert an ill-defined effect on the hypothalamus (central action) and by blocking production of pain impulses (peripheral action), possibly by inhibiting prostaglandin synthesis.
Antipyretic action: Choline salicylates act on the hypothalamic heat-regulating center to produce peripheral vasodilation. This increases peripheral blood supply and promotes sweating, which leads to loss of heat and to cooling by evaporation. These drugs don't affect platelet aggregation and shouldn't be used to prevent thrombosis.
Anti-inflammatory action: Choline salicylates inhibit prostaglandin synthesis; they may also inhibit the synthesis or action of other inflammation mediators.

PHARMACOKINETICS
Absorption: Choline salicylates are absorbed rapidly and completely from the GI tract. Peak therapeutic effect occurs in 2 hours.
Distribution: Protein binding depends on drug level and ranges from 75% to 90%, decreasing as serum levels increase. Severe toxic effects may occur at serum levels greater than 400 µg/ml.
Metabolism: Drug is hydrolyzed to salicylate in the liver.
Excretion: Metabolites are excreted in urine.

Reactions may be *common*, uncommon, *life-threatening*, or COMMON AND LIFE-THREATENING.

CONTRAINDICATIONS & PRECAUTIONS

Contraindicated in patients hypersensitive to choline salicylates. Also contraindicated in patients who have hemophilia or bleeding ulcers, who are in a hemorrhagic state, or who consume three or more alcoholic beverages per day. Use cautiously in patients with impaired renal or hepatic function, peptic ulcer disease, or gastritis.

INTERACTIONS

Drug-drug. *Ammonium chloride* and *other urine acidifiers* increase blood choline salicylate levels; monitor blood drug levels for toxicity. *Antacids* delay and decrease absorption of choline salicylates; monitor patient for decreased salicylate effect. *Corticosteroids* enhance salicylate elimination; monitor patient for decreased effect. Use with *drugs that are highly protein-bound*—such as *phenytoin, sulfonylureas,* and *warfarin*—may displace either drug and cause adverse effects; monitor therapy closely. Use with *methotrexate* may displace bound methotrexate and inhibit renal excretion. Use of other *GI irritants*—such as *antibiotics, other NSAIDs,* and *steroids*—may potentiate the adverse effects of choline salicylates; use together with caution. Choline salicylates decrease renal clearance of *lithium carbonate,* thus increasing serum lithium levels and the risk of adverse effects. Choline salicylates may enhance the hypoglycemic effects of *sulfonylureas.* Use with other *urine alkalizers* decreases choline salicylate blood levels; monitor patient for decreased salicylate effect. Choline salicylates enhance the hypoprothrombinemic effects of *warfarin.*
Drug-food. *Food* delays and decreases absorption of choline salicylates.

ADVERSE REACTIONS

EENT: tinnitus, hearing loss.
GI: GI distress, nausea, vomiting.
GU: *acute tubular necrosis with renal failure.*
Skin: rash.
Other: *hypersensitivity reactions (anaphylaxis), Reye's syndrome.*

▣ KEY CONSIDERATIONS

Besides the recommendations relevant to all salicylates, consider the following:
● Patients older than age 60 may be more susceptible to the toxic effects of these drugs.
● Don't mix choline salicylates with antacids.
● Administer oral solution of choline salicylate mixed with fruit juice. To ensure passage into stomach, follow with a full 8-oz (240 ml) glass of water.
● To prevent possible magnesium toxicity, monitor serum magnesium levels.
● Choline salicylates may interfere with urine glucose analysis performed via Chemstrip uG, Diastix, glucose enzymatic test strip, Clinitest, and Benedict's solution. These drugs also interfere with urine 5-hydroxyindole acetic acid and vanillylmandelic acid levels.
● Be aware that free T4 levels may be elevated.

Patient education

● Advise patient to avoid alcohol while taking drug.
● Instruct patient to take drug mixed with fruit juice, followed by a full 8-oz (240 ml) glass of water and to avoid taking drug with food, because it decreases and delays absorption of drug.
● Instruct patient on importance of periodic blood tests.

Overdose & treatment

● Signs and symptoms of overdose include metabolic acidosis with respiratory alkalosis, hyperpnea, and tachypnea from increased carbon dioxide production and direct stimulation of the respiratory center.
● To treat overdose of choline salicylates, empty stomach immediately by inducing vomiting with ipecac syrup, if patient is conscious, or by gastric lavage. Administer activated charcoal via NG tube. Provide symptomatic and supportive measures (respiratory support and correction of fluid and electrolyte imbalances). Monitor laboratory parameters and vital signs closely. Hemodialysis is effective in removing choline salicylates but is used only in severe poisoning. Forced di-

uresis with alkalinizing drug accelerates salicylate excretion.

---

cimetidine
Tagamet, Tagamet HB

H₂-receptor antagonist, antiulcerative

Available by prescription only
Tablets: 200 mg, 300 mg, 400 mg, 800 mg
Injection: 150 mg/ml, 300 mg/50 ml (premixed)
Liquid: 300 mg/5 ml
Available without a prescription
Tablets: 100 mg

INDICATIONS & DOSAGE
Duodenal ulcer (short-term treatment)
Adults: 800 mg h.s. for maximum of 8 weeks. Alternatively, give 400 mg P.O. b.i.d. or 300 mg P.O. q.i.d. with meals and h.s. When healing occurs, stop treatment or give h.s. dose only to control nocturnal hypersecretion.
Parenteral
300 mg diluted to 20 ml with normal saline solution or other compatible I.V. solution by I.V. push over 5 minutes q 6 hours. Or 300 mg diluted in 50 ml D₅W solution or other compatible I.V. solution by I.V. infusion over 15 to 20 minutes q 6 to 8 hours. Or 300 mg I.M. q 6 to 8 hours (no dilution necessary). To increase dosage, give more frequently to maximum daily dosage of 2,400 mg.
Duodenal ulcer prophylaxis
Adults: 400 mg h.s.
Active benign gastric ulcer
Adults: 800 mg h.s., or 300 mg q.i.d. with meals and h.s. for up to 8 weeks.
Pathological hypersecretory conditions (such as Zollinger-Ellison syndrome, systemic mastocytosis, and multiple endocrine adenomas); ◊ *short-bowel syndrome*
Adults: 300 mg P.O. q.i.d. with meals and h.s. Adjust to patient's needs. Maximum daily dosage is 2,400 mg.
Parenteral
300 mg diluted to 20 ml with normal saline solution or other compatible I.V. solution by I.V. push over 5 minutes q 6

to 8 hours. Or 300 mg diluted in 50 ml D₅W solution or other compatible I.V. solution by I.V. infusion over 15 to 20 minutes q 6 to 8 hours. To increase dosage, give 300 mg doses more frequently to maximum daily dosage of 2,400 mg.
Symptomatic relief of gastroesophageal reflux
Adults: 800 mg P.O. b.i.d. or 400 mg q.i.d., before meals and h.s.
◊ *Active upper GI bleeding, peptic esophagitis, stress ulcer*
Adults: 1 to 2 g I.V. or P.O. daily, in four divided doses.
Continuous infusion for patients unable to tolerate oral drugs
Adults: 37.5 mg/hour (900 mg/day) by continuous I.V. infusion. Use an infusion pump if total volume is less than 250 ml/day.
Heartburn, acid indigestion, sour stomach
Adults: 200 mg P.O. up to a maximum of b.i.d. (400 mg).
✦ *Dosage adjustment.* In patients with renal failure, recommended dose is 300 mg P.O. or I.V. q 8 to 12 hours at end of dialysis. Dosage may be decreased further if hepatic failure is also present.

PHARMACODYNAMICS
Antiulcer action: Cimetidine competitively inhibits histamine's action at H₂ receptors in gastric parietal cells, inhibiting basal and nocturnal gastric acid secretion (such as from stimulation by food, caffeine, insulin, histamine, betazole, or pentagastrin). Cimetidine may also enhance gastromucosal defense and healing.
   A 300-mg oral or parenteral dose inhibits about 80% of gastric acid secretion for 4 to 5 hours.

PHARMACOKINETICS
Absorption: About 60% to 75% of oral dose is absorbed. Food may affect absorption rate, but not extent.
Distribution: Drug is distributed to many body tissues. About 15% to 20% of drug binds to proteins.
Metabolism: About 30% to 40% of dose is metabolized in the liver. Drug has a

---

Reactions may be *common*, uncommon, *life-threatening*, or COMMON AND LIFE-THREATENING.

half-life of 2 hours in patients with normal renal function; half-life increases with decreasing renal function.
Excretion: About 48% of oral dose and 75% of parenteral dose is excreted in urine; 10% of oral dose is excreted in feces.

CONTRAINDICATIONS & PRECAUTIONS
Contraindicated in patients hypersensitive to cimetidine. Use with caution in geriatric or debilitated patients.

INTERACTIONS
Drug-drug. Cimetidine decreases the metabolism of the following drugs, thus increasing potential toxicity and possibly necessitating dosage reduction: *benzodiazepines, beta blockers* (such as *propranolol*), *carmustine, disulfiram, isoniazid, lidocaine, metronidazole, phenytoin, procainamide, quinidine, triamterene, xanthines, tricyclic antidepressants,* and *warfarin.* Serum *digoxin* levels may be reduced with concomitant use. Cimetidine may also affect the absorption of *ferrous salts, indomethacin, ketoconazole,* and *tetracyclines* by altering gastric pH. Administration with *flecainide* may increase serum *flecainide* levels and pharmacological effects.

ADVERSE REACTIONS
CNS: confusion, dizziness, headache, peripheral neuropathy, somnolence, hallucinations.
GI: *mild and transient diarrhea.*
GU: transient elevations in serum creatinine levels, impotence, mild gynecomastia if used for over 1 month.
Hematologic: *agranulocytosis* (rare), *neutropenia, thrombocytopenia* (rare), *aplastic anemia* (rare).
Hepatic: jaundice (rare), increased serum alkaline phosphatase levels.
Musculoskeletal: muscle pain, arthralgia.
Other: *hypersensitivity reactions,* increased prolactin levels.

KEY CONSIDERATIONS
Besides the recommendations relevant to all H_2-receptor antagonists, consider the following:
• Use caution when administering cimetidine to geriatric patients because of the potential for adverse reactions affecting the CNS.
• I.V. cimetidine must be diluted before it's administered. Don't dilute drug with sterile water for injection; use normal saline solution, D_5W or $D_{10}W$, lactated Ringer's solution, or 5% sodium bicarbonate injection to a total volume of 20 ml. I.M. administration may be painful.
• After administration of the liquid via NG tube, tube should be flushed to clear it and to make sure that drug has passed to the stomach.
• Hemodialysis removes drug; schedule dose after dialysis session.
• Other unlabeled uses of drug include pancreatic insufficiency, hives, and hirsutism.
• Cimetidine may antagonize the effect of pentagastrin during gastric acid secretion tests; it may cause false-negative results in skin tests using allergen extracts.
• Be aware that FD&C blue dye #2 used in Tagamet tablets may impair interpretation of Hemoccult and Gastroccult tests on gastric content aspirate. Be sure to wait at least 15 minutes after tablet administration before drawing the sample, and follow test manufacturer's instructions closely.

Patient education
• Warn patient to take drug as directed and to continue taking it even after pain subsides, to allow for adequate healing. Urge patient to avoid smoking, because it may increase gastric acid secretion and worsen disease.

Overdose & treatment
• Signs and symptoms of overdose include respiratory failure and tachycardia.
• Support respiration and maintain a patent airway. Induce vomiting or use gastric lavage; to prevent further absorption, follow with activated charcoal. Treat tachycardia with propranolol if necessary.

ciprofloxacin (systemic)
Cipro

Fluoroquinolone antibiotic

Available by prescription only
Tablets: 250 mg, 500 mg, 750 mg
Injection: 200 mg/20-ml vial;
400 mg/40-ml vial; 200 mg in 100 ml
D_5W; 400 mg in 200 ml D_5W

INDICATIONS & DOSAGE
Mild to moderate urinary tract infection caused by susceptible bacteria
Adults: 250 mg P.O. or 200 mg I.V. q 12 hours.
Infectious diarrhea, mild to moderate respiratory tract infections, bone and joint infections, severe or complicated urinary tract infections
Adults: 500 mg P.O. q 12 hours or 400 mg I.V. q 12 hours.
Severe or complicated infections of the respiratory tract, bones, joints, skin, or skin-structures; ◇ mycobacterial infections
Adults: 750 mg P.O. q 12 hours or 400 mg I.V. q 12 hours.
Typhoid fever
Adults: 500 mg P.O. q 12 hours.
Intra-abdominal infection (in combination with metronidazole)
Adults: 500 mg P.O. q 12 hours
◇ Uncomplicated gonorrhea
Adults: 250 mg P.O. as a single dose
◇ Neisseria meningitidis in nasal passages
Adults: 500 to 750 mg P.O. as a single dose, or 250 mg P.O. b.i.d. for 2 days, or 500 mg P.O. b.i.d. for 5 days.
✦ *Dosage adjustment.* For patients on hemodialysis or peritoneal dialysis, use 250 to 500 mg/day after dialysis. For patients with renal failure, refer to following table.

Oral ciprofloxacin

Creatinine clearance (ml/min/1.73 m²)	Dosage in adults
> 50	No adjustment
30-50	250-500 mg q 12 hr
5-29	250-500 mg q 18 hr

I.V. ciprofloxacin

Creatinine clearance (ml/min/1.73 m²)	Dosage in adults
>30	No adjustment
5-29	250-400 mg I.V. q 18-24 hr

PHARMACODYNAMICS
Antibiotic action: Ciprofloxacin inhibits DNA gyrase, preventing bacterial DNA replication. The following organisms are susceptible (in vitro) to ciprofloxacin: *Campylobacter jejuni, Citrobacter diversus, C. freundii, Enterobacter cloacae, Escherichia coli* (including enterotoxigenic strains), *Haemophilus parainfluenzae, Klebsiella pneumoniae, Morganella morganii, Proteus mirabilis, P. vulgaris, Providencia stuartii, P. rettgeri, Pseudomonas aeruginosa, Serratia marcescens, Shigella flexneri, S. sonnei,* penicillinase– and nonpenicillinase–producing strains of *Staphylococcus aureus, S. epidermidis, Streptococcus faecalis,* and *S. pyogenes.*

PHARMACOKINETICS
Absorption: About 70% of ciprofloxacin is absorbed after oral administration. Food delays the rate but not the extent of absorption.
Distribution: Serum levels peak within 1 to 2 hours after oral dosing. About 20% to 40% of drug binds to proteins; CSF levels are only about 10% of plasma levels.
Metabolism: Drug is probably metabolized in the liver. Four metabolites have been identified; each has less antimicrobial activity than the parent compound.
Excretion: Drug is primarily excreted by the kidneys. Serum half-life is about 4 hours in adults with normal renal function.

CONTRAINDICATIONS & PRECAUTIONS
Contraindicated in patients sensitive to fluoroquinolone antibiotics. Use cautiously in patients with CNS disorders or those at risk for seizures.

INTERACTIONS
Drug-drug. *Aluminum-, calcium-,* and *magnesium-containing antacids* may in-

---

Reactions may be *common*, uncommon, *life-threatening*, or COMMON AND LIFE-THREATENING.

terfere with ciprofloxacin absorption; antacids may be safely administered 2 hours before or 6 hours after ciprofloxacin. Use with *aminoglycosides* or *beta-lactams* causes synergistic effects. *Iron, minerals,* and *vitamins* may interfere with absorption of ciprofloxacin. Use with *probenecid* interferes with renal tubular secretion and results in higher plasma ciprofloxacin levels. Use with *sucralfate* reduces absorption of ciprofloxacin by 50%. Ciprofloxacin may attenuate elimination of *theophylline,* increasing the risk of theophylline toxicity. Use with *warfarin* increases PT and INR.

Drug-food. Ciprofloxacin prolongs elimination half-life of *caffeine.*

ADVERSE REACTIONS

CNS: headache, restlessness, tremor, dizziness, fatigue, drowsiness, insomnia, depression, light-headedness, confusion, hallucinations, *seizures,* paresthesia.
CV: thrombophlebitis (with I.V. administration).
GI: *nausea, diarrhea,* vomiting, abdominal pain or discomfort, oral candidiasis, pseudomembranous colitis, dyspepsia, flatulence, constipation.
GU: crystalluria, increased serum creatinine and BUN levels, interstitial nephritis.
Hepatic: elevated liver enzyme levels.
Musculoskeletal: arthralgia, joint or back pain, joint inflammation, joint stiffness, aching, neck or chest pain.
Skin: *rash;* photosensitivity; *toxic epidermal necrolysis;* exfoliative dermatitis; *Stevens-Johnson syndrome;* pruritus, erythema (with I.V. administration).
Other: *hypersensitivity;* burning, edema (with I.V. administration).

KEY CONSIDERATIONS

• Duration of therapy depends on type and severity of infection. Therapy should continue for 2 days after symptoms have abated. Most infections are well controlled in 1 to 2 weeks, but bone or joint infections may require therapy for 4 weeks or longer.
• Closer monitoring of theophylline levels may be necessary because of increased risk of theophylline toxicity in patient receiving ciprofloxacin.

Patient education

• Tell patient that although drug may be taken without regard to food, the preferred time is 2 hours after a meal.
• Advise patient to avoid taking drug with antacids, iron, or calcium and to drink plenty of fluids during therapy. If antacids are used, take them 2 hours before or 6 hours after ciprofloxacin.
• Inform patient that because dizziness, light-headedness, or drowsiness may occur, he should avoid hazardous activities that require mental alertness until CNS effects of drug are determined.

Overdose & treatment

• Limited experience with overdose is reported. If patient reports taking an overdose, induce vomiting or perform gastric lavage. Provide general supportive measures and maintain hydration. Peritoneal dialysis or hemodialysis may be helpful, particularly if patient's renal function is compromised.

ciprofloxacin hydrochloride (ophthalmic)
Ciloxan

Fluoroquinolone, antibacterial

Available by prescription only
Ophthalmic solution: 0.3% in 2.5- and 5-ml containers

INDICATIONS & DOSAGE

Corneal ulcers caused by Pseudomonas aeruginosa, Staphylococcus aureus, S. epidermidis, Streptococcus pneumoniae, and possibly Serratia marcescens and S. viridans
Adults: Instill 2 drops in the affected eye q 15 minutes for first 6 hours, then 2 drops q 30 minutes for remainder of first day. On day 2, instill 2 drops hourly. On days 3 to 14, instill 2 drops q 4 hours.
Bacterial conjunctivitis caused by S. aureus and S. epidermidis and possibly S. pneumoniae
Adults: Instill 1 or 2 drops into the conjunctival sac of affected eye q 2 hours

while awake, for first 2 days. Then 1 or 2 drops q 4 hours while awake, for next 5 days.

PHARMACODYNAMICS
Antibacterial action: Inhibits bacterial DNA gyrase, an enzyme necessary for bacterial replication. Bacteriostatic or bactericidal, depending on concentration.

PHARMACOKINETICS
Absorption: Systemic absorption is limited. In a study where the drug was administered in each eye every 2 hours for 2 days while the patient was awake, followed by every 4 hours for 5 more days while the patient was awake, showed that the maximum plasma level was below 5 ng/ml, and the mean plasma level was below 2.5 ng/ml.
Distribution: Unknown.
Metabolism: Unknown.
Excretion: Unknown.

CONTRAINDICATIONS & PRECAUTIONS
Contraindicated in patients with history of hypersensitivity to ciprofloxacin or other fluoroquinolone antibiotics.

INTERACTIONS
None reported.

ADVERSE REACTIONS
EENT: *local burning or discomfort, white crystalline precipitate* (in the superficial portion of the corneal defect in patients with corneal ulcers), *margin crusting, crystals or scales, foreign body sensation, itching, conjunctival hyperemia,* bad or bitter taste in mouth, corneal staining, allergic reactions, keratopathy, lid edema, tearing, photophobia, decreased vision.
GI: nausea.

▣ KEY CONSIDERATIONS
• If corneal epithelium is still compromised after 14 days of treatment, continue therapy.

Patient education
• Teach patient how to instill drug correctly. Remind him not to touch the tip of the bottle with his hands and to avoid contact of the tip with the eye or surrounding tissue.
• Remind patient not to share washcloths or towels with other family members to avoid spreading infection.
• Advise patient to wash hands before and after instilling solution.

Overdose & treatment
• A topical overdose of drug may be flushed from the eye with warm tap water.

---

cisapride
Propulsid

Serotonin-4 receptor agonist, GI prokinetic

Available by prescription only
Tablets: 10 mg, 20 mg
Suspension: 1 mg/ml

INDICATIONS & DOSAGE
Symptomatic treatment of nocturnal heartburn due to gastroesophageal reflux disease that doesn't respond adequately to lifestyle modifications, antacids, and gastric acid–reducing drugs
Adults: 10 mg P.O. q.i.d. at least 15 minutes before meals and h.s. Dosage may be increased to 20 mg q.i.d., if needed.

PHARMACODYNAMICS
GI prokinetic action: Cisapride is thought to enhance release of acetylcholine at the myenteric plexus, increasing GI motility. Cisapride doesn't induce muscarinic or nicotinic receptor stimulation, nor does it inhibit acetylcholinesterase activity. It also doesn't increase or decrease basal- or pentagastrin-induced gastric acid secretion.

PHARMACOKINETICS
Absorption: Cisapride is rapidly absorbed; onset of action is 30 to 60 minutes after oral administration. Plasma levels peak 1 to 1½ hours after administration.
Distribution: Drug is extensively distributed (the volume of distribution is about

---

Reactions may be *common,* uncommon, *life-threatening,* or COMMON AND LIFE-THREATENING.

180 L). About 97.5% to 98% binds to plasma proteins, mainly albumin.
Metabolism: Drug is extensively metabolized in the liver. Norcisapride, formed by N-dealkylation, is the principal metabolite in plasma, feces, and urine.
Excretion: Drug is excreted in urine and feces. Unchanged drug accounts for less than 10% of urinary and fecal recovery after oral administration. The mean terminal half-life ranges from 6 to 12 hours.

CONTRAINDICATIONS & PRECAUTIONS

Contraindicated in patients hypersensitive to cisapride. Also contraindicated in patients for whom increased GI motility may be harmful, such as those with mechanical obstruction, hemorrhage, or perforation of the GI tract.

Use with macrolides, antifungals, protease inhibitors, and nefazodone is contraindicated. Also contraindicated in patients with history of prolonged QT intervals, ventricular arrhythmias, ischemic heart disease, uncorrected electrolyte disorders (such as hypokalemia and hypomagnesemia), and heart, renal, or respiratory failure.

INTERACTIONS

Drug-drug. *Anticholinergics* may decrease therapeutic effects of cisapride. Administration of cisapride during *anticoagulant* therapy has led to increased coagulation times; check coagulation time 1 week after the start and discontinuation of cisapride therapy, with an appropriate adjustment of the anticoagulant dose, if necessary. Use with *benzodiazepines* accelerates the sedative effects. Administration with *cimetidine* leads to increased peak plasma cisapride levels. GI absorption of *cimetidine* and *ranitidine* is accelerated when they are coadministered with cisapride. Administration with *clarithromycin, erthromycin, fluconazole, indinavir, itraconazole, ketoconazole, miconazole, nefazodone, ritonavir, troleandomycin,* and *drugs that inhibit cytochrome P-450 IIIA4* is contraindicated because of the increased risk of prolonged QT intervals and arrhythmias. Cisapride may increase the absorption of *digoxin.* Cisapride may af-

fect the absorption of *other drugs* by accelerating gastric emptying, so patients receiving *narrow therapeutic ratio drugs* or other *drugs that require careful adjustment* should be monitored closely and plasma levels reassessed.
Drug-lifestyle. *Alcohol* accelerates sedative effects; don't use together.

ADVERSE REACTIONS

CNS: *headache,* insomnia, anxiety, nervousness.
EENT: abnormal vision.
GI: *diarrhea, abdominal pain,* nausea, constipation, flatulence, dyspepsia.
GU: frequency, urinary tract infection, vaginitis.
Musculoskeletal: arthralgia.
Respiratory: rhinitis, sinusitis, cough, upper respiratory tract infection.
Skin: rash, pruritus.
Other: pain, fever, viral infections.

◼ KEY CONSIDERATIONS

• Steady-state plasma cisapride levels are generally higher in older patients than in younger ones because of a moderately prolonged elimination half-life. Patient should be monitored closely for adverse reactions. Therapeutic doses are similar to those used in younger adults.
• Be aware that cisapride may accelerate the sedative effects of benzodiazepines and alcohol.

Patient education

• Instruct patient to take cisapride at least 15 minutes before meals and at bedtime.
• Warn patient that drug may accelerate the sedative effects of benzodiazepines and alcohol.
• Caution patient against use of oral fluconazole, ketoconazole, itraconazole, miconazole, erythromycin, clarithromycin, indinavir, nefazodone, ritonavir, troleandomycin because of potential for serious adverse reactions.

Overdose & treatment

• Signs and symptoms of overdose include retching, borborygmi, flatulence, and increased stool and urinary frequency.

• Treatment should include gastric lavage or activated charcoal, close observation, and general supportive measures.

cisplatin (cis-platinum)
Platinol, Platinol AQ

Alkylating agent (cell cycle–phase nonspecific), antineoplastic

Available by prescription only
Injection: 10-mg and 50-mg vials (lyophilized), 50-mg and 100-mg vials (aqueous)

INDICATIONS & DOSAGE
Dosage and indications may vary. Check current literature for recommended protocol.

Adjunctive therapy in metastatic testicular cancer
Adults: 20 mg/m^2 I.V. daily for 5 days. Repeat q 3 weeks for three cycles or more. Usually used in therapeutic regimen with bleomycin and vinblastine.

Adjunctive therapy in metastatic ovarian cancer
Adults: 75 to 100 mg/m^2 I.V. Repeat q 4 weeks. Or 50 mg/m^2 I.V. q 3 weeks with concurrent doxorubicin hydrochloride therapy.

Treatment of advanced bladder cancer
Adults: 50 to 70 mg/m^2 I.V. once q 3 to 4 weeks. Patients who have received other antineoplastics or radiation therapy should receive 50 mg/m^2 q 4 weeks.

◊ ***Head and neck cancer***
Adults: 80 to 120 mg/m^2 I.V. once q 3 weeks.

◊ ***Cervical cancer***
Adults: 50 mg/m^2 I.V. once q 3 weeks.

◊ ***Non-small-cell lung cancer***
Adults: 70 to 120 mg/m^2 I.V. once q 3 to 6 weeks.

Note: Prehydration and mannitol diuresis may significantly reduce renal toxicity and ototoxicity.

PHARMACODYNAMICS
Antineoplastic action: Cisplatin exerts its cytotoxic effects by binding with DNA and inhibiting DNA synthesis and, to a lesser extent, by inhibiting protein and RNA synthesis. Cisplatin also acts as a bifunctional alkylating drug, causing intrastrand and interstrand cross-links of DNA. Interstrand cross-linking appears to correlate well with the cytotoxicity of drug.

PHARMACOKINETICS
Absorption: Cisplatin isn't administered orally or I.M.
Distribution: Drug distributes widely into tissues, with the highest levels found in the kidneys, liver, and prostate. Drug can accumulate in body tissues, with drug being detected up to 6 months after the last dose. Drug doesn't readily cross the blood-brain barrier. Drug extensively and irreversibly binds to plasma proteins and tissue proteins.
Metabolism: Metabolic fate of drug is unclear.
Excretion: Drug is excreted primarily unchanged in urine. In patients with normal renal function, the half-life of the initial elimination phase is 25 to 79 minutes and the terminal phase 58 to 78 hours. The terminal half-life of total cisplatin is up to 10 days.

CONTRAINDICATIONS & PRECAUTIONS
Contraindicated in patients with hypersensitivity to cisplatin or to other platinum-containing compounds and in those with severe renal disease, hearing impairment, or myelosuppression.

INTERACTIONS
Drug-drug. Use with *aminoglycosides* potentiates the nephrotoxic effects of cisplatin; therefore, aminoglycosides shouldn't be used within 2 weeks of cisplatin therapy. Use with *loop diuretics* increases the risk of ototoxicity; closely monitor patient's audiologic status. Use with *phenytoin* may decrease serum phenytoin levels.

ADVERSE REACTIONS
CNS: *peripheral neuritis*, loss of taste, *seizures.*
EENT: *tinnitus, hearing loss, ototoxicity*, vestibular toxicity.
GI: *nausea, vomiting* (beginning 1 to 4 hours after dose and lasting 24 hours).
GU: more prolonged and SEVERE RENAL TOXICITY with repeated courses of thera-

py; increased BUN and serum creatinine levels.

Hematologic: MYELOSUPPRESSION, *leukopenia, thrombocytopenia, anemia,* nadirs in circulating platelet and WBC counts on days 18 to 23, with recovery by day 39.

Metabolic: *hypomagnesemia,* hypokalemia, hypocalcemia, hyponatremia, hypophosphatemia, hyperuricemia.

Other: *anaphylactoid reaction.*

▣ KEY CONSIDERATIONS

• Review hematologic status and creatinine clearance before therapy.

• Reconstitute 10-mg vial with 10 ml of sterile water for injection and 50-mg vial with 50 ml of sterile water for injection to yield a concentration of 1 mg/ml. The drug may be diluted further in a sodium chloride–containing solution for I.V. infusion.

• Don't use aluminum needles to reconstitute or administer cisplatin; a black precipitate may form. Use stainless steel needles.

• Drug is stable for 24 hours in normal saline solution at room temperature. Don't refrigerate because precipitation may occur. Discard solution containing precipitate.

• Infusions are most stable in chloride-containing solutions, such as normal saline solution, half-normal saline solution, or 0.225% NaCl.

• Mannitol may be given as a 12.5-g I.V. bolus before starting cisplatin infusion. Follow by infusion of mannitol at rate of up to 10 g/hour, as necessary, to maintain urine output during cisplatin infusion and for 6 to 24 hours after infusion.

• To decrease risk of nephrotoxicity, I.V. sodium thiosulfate may be administered with cisplatin infusion.

• Hydrate patient with normal saline solution before giving drug. Maintain urine output of 100 ml/hour for 4 consecutive hours before and for 24 hours after infusion.

• Hydrate patient by encouraging oral fluid intake when possible.

• Avoid all I.M. injections when platelet count is low.

• Nausea and vomiting may be severe and protracted (up to 24 hours).

Antiemetics can be started 24 hours before therapy. Monitor fluid intake and output. Continue I.V. hydration until patient can tolerate adequate oral intake.

• High-dose metoclopramide (2 mg/kg I.V.) has been used to prevent and treat nausea and vomiting. Dexamethasone 10 to 20 mg has been administered I.V. with metoclopramide to help alleviate nausea and vomiting. Many patients respond favorably to treatment with ondansetron (Zofran). Pretreatment with this 5-HT$_3$ antagonist should begin 30 minutes before cisplatin therapy is started.

• Treat extravasation with local injections of a 1/6 M sodium thiosulfate solution (prepared by mixing 4 ml of sodium thiosulfate 10% and 6 ml of sterile water for injection).

• Monitor CBC, platelet count, and renal function studies before initial and subsequent doses. Don't repeat dose unless platelet count is over 100,000/mm^3, WBC count is over 4,000/μl, serum creatinine level is under 1.5 mg/dl, or BUN level is under 25 mg/dl.

• Renal toxicity becomes more severe with repeated doses. Renal function must return to normal before next dose can be given.

• Monitor electrolytes extensively; aggressive supplementation is often required after a course of therapy.

• Anaphylactoid reaction usually responds to immediate treatment with epinephrine, corticosteroids, or antihistamines.

• Avoid contact with skin. If contact occurs, wash drug off immediately with soap and water.

Patient education

• Stress importance of adequate fluid intake and increase in urine output, to facilitate uric acid excretion.

• Tell patient to report tinnitus immediately, to prevent permanent hearing loss. Patient should have audiometric tests before initial and subsequent courses.

• Advise patient to avoid exposure to people with infections.

• Inform patient to promptly report unusual bleeding or bruising.

---

*Canada only   ◇ Unlabeled clinical use

Overdose & treatment
● Signs and symptoms of overdose include leukopenia, thrombocytopenia, nausea, and vomiting.
● Treatment is generally supportive and includes transfusion of blood components, antibiotics for possible infections, and antiemetics. Cisplatin can be removed by dialysis, but only within 3 hours after administration.

---

citalopram hydrobromide
Celexa

Selective serotonin reuptake inhibitor (SSRI), antidepressant

---

Available by prescription only
Tablets: 20 mg, 40 mg

INDICATIONS & DOSAGE
Depression
Adults: initially, 20 mg P.O. once daily, increasing to 40 mg daily after no less than 1 week. Maximum recommended dosage is 40 mg daily.
Geriatric patients: 20 mg/day P.O. with dosage adjusted to 40 mg/day for nonresponding patients.
✦ *Dosage adjustment.* For patients with hepatic impairment, use 20 mg/day P.O. with dosage adjusted to 40 mg/day only for nonresponding patients.

PHARMACODYNAMICS
Antidepressant action: Action of citalopram is presumed to be linked to potentiation of serotonergic activity in the CNS resulting from inhibition of neuronal reuptake of serotonin.

PHARMACOKINETICS
Absorption: Absolute bioavailability is 80% after oral administration. Serum levels peak in 4 hours.
Distribution: About 80% binds to plasma proteins.
Metabolism: Cytochrome P-450 3A4 and cytochrome P-450 2C19 metabolize the drug extensively to inactive metabolites.
Excretion: About 20% is excreted in the urine. Elimination half-life is about 35 hours. In patients older than age 60, the half-life is increased to 30%.

CONTRAINDICATIONS & PRECAUTIONS
Contraindicated in patients also taking MAO inhibitors or within 14 days of MAO inhibitor therapy and in those with hypersensitivity to citalopram or its inactive ingredients.

INTERACTIONS
Drug-drug. *Carbamazepine* may increase citalopram clearance; monitor for effects. Use with *CNS drugs* may produce additive effects; use together cautiously. Use with *drugs that inhibit cytochrome P-450 isoenzymes 3A4 and 2C19* decreases clearance of citalopram; monitor closely. Use with *imipramine or other tricyclic antidepressants* increases levels of imipramine metabolite desipramine by about 50%; use together cautiously. *Lithium* may enhance serotonergic effect of citalopram; use with caution, and monitor lithium levels. Use with *MAO inhibitors* can cause serious, sometimes fatal, reactions; don't use drug within 14 days of an MAO inhibitor. Use with *warfarin* increases prothrombin time by 5%; monitor closely.
Drug-lifestyle. *Alcohol* may increase CNS effects; don't use together.

ADVERSE REACTIONS
CNS: tremor, *somnolence, insomnia,* anxiety, agitation, dizziness, paresthesia, migraine, impaired concentration, amnesia, depression, apathy, ***suicide attempt,*** confusion, fatigue.
CV: tachycardia, orthostatic hypotension, hypotension.
EENT: rhinitis, sinusitis, abnormal accommodation.
GI: *dry mouth, nausea,* diarrhea, anorexia, dyspepsia, vomiting, abdominal pain, taste perversion, increased saliva, flatulence, decreased and increased weight, increased appetite.
GU: dysmenorrhea, amenorrhea, ejaculation disorder, impotence, polyuria.
Musculoskeletal: arthralgia, myalgia.
Respiratory: upper respiratory tract infection, coughing.
Skin: rash, pruritus.

Reactions may be *common,* uncommon, *life-threatening,* or COMMON AND LIFE-THREATENING.

Other: *increased sweating,* fever, yawning, decreased libido.

◙ KEY CONSIDERATIONS

• Use cautiously in patients with history of mania, seizures, suicidal ideation, or hepatic or renal impairment.
• Although drug hasn't been shown to impair psychomotor performance, any psychoactive drug has the potential to impair judgment, thinking, and motor skills.
• The possibility of a suicide attempt is inherent in depression and may persist until significant remission occurs. Closely supervise high-risk patients at the start of drug therapy. Reduce risk of overdose by limiting the amount of drug available per refill.
• At least 14 days should elapse between MAO inhibitor therapy and citalopram therapy.

Patient education

• Inform patient that although improvement may occur within 1 to 4 weeks, he should continue therapy as prescribed.
• Instruct patient to exercise caution when operating hazardous machinery, including automobiles, because of the potential of psychoactive drugs to impair judgment, thinking, and motor skills.
• Advise patient to consult health care provider before taking other prescription or OTC drugs.
• Warn patient to avoid concomitant use of alcohol.
• Caution patient against use of MAO inhibitors while taking citalopram.
• Tell patient that drug may be taken in the morning or evening without regard to food.

---

clarithromycin
Biaxin

Macrolide, antibiotic

Available by prescription only
Tablets: 250 mg, 500 mg
Suspension: 125 mg/5 ml, 250 mg/5 ml

INDICATIONS & DOSAGE

***Pharyngitis or tonsillitis caused by* Streptococcus pyogenes**
Adults: 250 mg P.O. q 12 hours for 10 days.
***Acute maxillary sinusitis caused by* S. pneumoniae, Haemophilus influenzae, *or* Moraxella catarrhalis**
Adults: 500 mg P.O. q 12 hours for 14 days.
***Acute exacerbations of chronic bronchitis caused by* M. (Branhamella) catarrhalis *or* S. pneumoniae; *pneumonia caused by* S. pneumoniae *or* Mycoplasma pneumoniae**
Adults: 250 mg P.O. q 12 hours for 7 to 14 days.
***Acute exacerbations of chronic bronchitis caused by* H. influenzae**
Adults: 500 mg P.O. q 12 hours for 7 to 14 days.
***Uncomplicated skin and skin-structure infections caused by* Staphylococcus aureus *or* S. pyogenes**
Adults: 250 mg P.O. q 12 hours for 7 to 14 days.
***Prophylaxis and treatment of disseminated infection due to* Mycobacterium avium complex**
Adults: 500 mg P.O. b.i.d.
✦ *Dosage adjustment.* In patients with creatinine clearance of less than 30 ml/minute, dosage should be decreased or dosing interval prolonged.

PHARMACODYNAMICS

Antibiotic action: Clarithromycin, a macrolide antibiotic that's a derivative of erythromycin, binds to the 50S subunit of bacterial ribosomes, blocking protein synthesis. It's bacteriostatic or bactericidal, depending on the concentration.

PHARMACOKINETICS

Absorption: Clarithromycin is rapidly absorbed from the GI tract; absolute bioavailability is about 50%. Serum levels peak within 2 hours of dosing. Although food slightly delays onset of absorption and formation of the active metabolite, it doesn't alter the total amount of drug absorbed, so drug may be taken without regard to food.
Distribution: Drug is widely distributed; because it readily penetrates cells, tissue

levels are higher than plasma levels. Plasma half-life is dose-dependent; half-life is 3 to 4 hours at doses of 250 mg q 12 hours and increases to 5 to 7 hours at doses of 500 mg q 12 hours.

Metabolism: The major metabolite of clarithromycin, 14-hydroxy clarithromycin, has significant antimicrobial activity. It's about twice as active against *H. influenzae* as the parent drug.

Excretion: In patients taking 250 mg q 12 hours, about 20% is eliminated in the urine unchanged; this increases to 30% in patients taking 500 mg q 12 hours. The major metabolite accounts for about 15% of drug in urine. Elimination half-life of the active metabolite is dose-dependent: 5 to 6 hours with 250 mg q 12 hours; 7 hours with 500 mg q 12 hours.

CONTRAINDICATIONS & PRECAUTIONS

Contraindicated in patients with hypersensitivity to erythromycin or other macrolides who have preexisting cardiac abnormalities or electrolyte disturbances. Use cautiously in patients with impaired renal or hepatic function.

INTERACTIONS

Drug-drug. Use may increase serum levels of *carbamazepine* and *theophylline;* monitor plasma levels of these drugs carefully. Use with *digoxin* increases digoxin levels.Use with *dihydroergotamine* or *ergotamine* can cause ergot toxicity. Use with *cyclosporine*, *phenytoin*, or *triazolam* decreases metabolism of these drugs. Use with *warfarin* increases PT and INR.

ADVERSE REACTIONS

CNS: headache.
GI: *diarrhea, nausea, abnormal taste,* dyspepsia, abdominal pain or discomfort.
Hematologic: increased PT and INR; decreased WBC count; elevated liver function test results and BUN and creatinine levels.

⬚ KEY CONSIDERATIONS

• Because of age-related decreases in renal function, drug may need to be given once daily in geriatric patients to avoid adverse reactions.

• Obtain specimen for culture and sensitivity tests before giving first dose. Therapy may begin pending test results.
• Drug may be taken without regard to food.
• Drug may cause overgrowth of nonsusceptible bacteria or fungi. Monitor for signs and symptoms of superinfection.
• Reconstituted suspension shouldn't be refrigerated; discard any unused portion after 14 days.

Patient education

• Tell patient to take all of drug as prescribed, even if he feels better.
• Inform patient that he may take drug without regard to food.
• Instruct patient to shake suspension well before use and not to refrigerate.

clindamycin hydrochloride
Cleocin

clindamycin phosphate
Cleocin Phosphate, Cleocin T

Lincomycin derivative, antibiotic

Available by prescription only
Capsules: 75 mg, 150 mg, 300 mg
Solution: 75 mg/5 ml
Injection: 150 mg/ml
Infusion for I.V. use: 300 mg, 600 mg, 900 mg
Gel, lotion, topical solution: 1%
Vaginal cream: 2%

INDICATIONS & DOSAGE

Infections caused by sensitive organisms
Adults: 150 to 450 mg P.O. q 6 hours; or 600 to 2,700 mg/day I.M. or I.V. divided into two to four equal doses.
Bacterial vaginosis
Adults: 100 mg intravaginally h.s. for 7 days.
Acne vulgaris
Adults: Apply thin film of topical solution to affected areas b.i.d.
◊ *Toxoplasmosis (cerebral or ocular) in immunocompromised patients*
Adults: 1,200 to 4,800 mg/day I.V. or P.O. Also administered with

---

Reactions may be *common*, uncommon, **life-threatening**, or COMMON AND LIFE-THREATENING.

pyrimethamine in dosages up to 75 mg/day P.O. and with folinic acid in a dosage of 10 mg/day P.O.
◊ **Pneumocystis carinii** *pneumonia*
Adults: 600 mg I.V. q 6 hours or 300 to 450 mg P.O. q.i.d. With primaquine, give 15 to 30 mg P.O. daily.

PHARMACODYNAMICS
Antibiotic action: Clindamycin inhibits bacterial protein synthesis by binding to ribosome's 50S subunit. It may produce bacteriostatic or bactericidal effects on susceptible bacteria, including most aerobic gram-positive cocci and anaerobic gram-negative and gram-positive organisms. It's considered a first-line drug in the treatment of *Bacteroides fragilis* and most other gram-positive and gram-negative anaerobes. It's also effective against *Mycoplasma pneumoniae, Leptotrichia buccalis,* and some gram-positive cocci and bacilli.

PHARMACOKINETICS
Absorption: When administered orally, clindamycin is absorbed rapidly and almost completely from the GI tract, regardless of formulation. Levels peak (at 1.9 to 3.9 μg/ml) in 45 to 60 minutes. Drug may also be given I.M. with good absorption. Levels peak in about 3 hours. With a 300-mg dose, levels peak at about 6 μg/ml; with a 600-mg dose, about 10 μg/ml.
Distribution: Distributed widely to most body tissues and fluids (except CSF). About 93% binds to plasma proteins.
Metabolism: Drug is metabolized partially to inactive metabolites.
Excretion: About 10% of dose is excreted unchanged in urine; remainder is excreted as inactive metabolites. Plasma half-life is 2½ to 3 hours in patients with normal renal function; 3½ to 5 hours in anephric patients; and 7 to 14 hours in patients with hepatic disease. Peritoneal dialysis and hemodialysis don't remove drug from circulation.

CONTRAINDICATIONS & PRECAUTIONS
Contraindicated in patients with hypersensitivity to the antibiotic congener lincomycin; in those with a history of ulcerative colitis, regional enteritis, or antibiotic-associated colitis; and in those with a history of atopic reactions.
Use cautiously in patients with asthma, impaired renal or hepatic function, or history of GI diseases or significant allergies.

INTERACTIONS
Drug-drug. When used with other *acne preparations* (such as *benzoyl peroxide* or *tretinoin*), topical clindamycin may cause a cumulative irritant or drying effect. Use with such *antidiarrheals* as *diphenoxylate* and *opiates* may prolong or worsen clindamycin-induced diarrhea by reducing excretion of bacterial toxins. *Erythromycin* may act as an antagonist, blocking clindamycin from reaching its site of action. Use with *kaolin products* may reduce GI absorption of clindamycin. Clindamycin may potentiate the action of *neuromuscular blockers* (such as *pancuronium* and *tubocurarine*).

ADVERSE REACTIONS
GI: *nausea,* vomiting, abdominal pain, *diarrhea, pseudomembranous colitis.*
GU: *cervicitis, vaginitis, Candida albicans* overgrowth, *vulvar irritation.*
Hematologic: *transient leukopenia,* eosinophilia, *thrombocytopenia.*
Hepatic: abnormal liver function test results, jaundice.
Skin: maculopapular rash, urticaria, dryness, *redness,* pruritus, swelling, irritation, contact dermatitis, burning.
Other: *anaphylaxis.*

▣ KEY CONSIDERATIONS
• Geriatric patients may tolerate drug-induced diarrhea poorly. Monitor closely for change in bowel frequency.
• Culture and sensitivity tests should be done before treatment starts and should be repeated as needed.
• Don't refrigerate reconstituted oral solution, because it will thicken. Drug remains stable for 2 weeks at room temperature.
• I.M. preparation should be given deep I.M. Rotate sites. Dosages exceeding 600 mg aren't recommended.

• I.M. injection may increase creatinine phosphokinase levels because of muscle irritation.

• For I.V. infusion, dilute each 300 mg in 50 ml of D₅W, normal saline solution, or lactated Ringer's solution and give no faster than 30 mg/minute. Don't administer more than 1.2 g/hour.

• Topical form may produce adverse systemic effects.

• Monitor renal, hepatic, and hematopoietic functions during prolonged therapy.

• Don't administer diphenoxylate compound (Lomotil) to treat drug-induced diarrhea because this may worsen and prolong diarrhea.

Patient education

• Warn patient that I.M. injection may be painful.

• Instruct patient to report adverse effects, especially diarrhea. Warn patient not to self-treat diarrhea.

• Advise patient to take capsules with full glass (8 oz [240 ml]) of water to prevent dysphagia.

• Instruct patient using topical solution to wash, rinse, and dry affected areas before application. Warn patient not to use topical solution near eyes, nose, mouth, or other mucous membranes, and caution about sharing washcloths and towels with family members.

clofibrate
Atromid-S

Fibric acid derivative, antilipemic

Available by prescription only
Capsules: 500 mg

INDICATIONS & DOSAGE
Hyperlipidemia and xanthoma tuberosum; type III hyperlipidemia that doesn't respond adequately to diet
Adults: 2 g P.O. daily in two to four divided doses. Some patients may respond to lower dosages as assessed by serum lipid monitoring.
◇ ***Diabetes insipidus***
Adults: 1.5 to 2 g P.O. daily in divided doses.

PHARMACODYNAMICS
Antilipemic action: Clofibrate may lower serum triglyceride levels by accelerating catabolism of very low-density lipoproteins; drug lowers serum cholesterol levels (to a lesser degree) by inhibiting cholesterol biosynthesis. Both mechanisms are unknown. Drug is closely related to gemfibrozil.

PHARMACOKINETICS
Absorption: Clofibrate is absorbed slowly but completely from GI tract. Plasma levels peak 2 to 6 hours after a single dose. Serum triglyceride levels decrease in 2 to 5 days, with peak effect at 21 days.
Distribution: Clofibrate is distributed into extracellular space as its active form, clofibric acid, 98% of which binds to proteins.
Metabolism: Clofibrate is hydrolyzed by serum enzymes to clofibric acid, which the liver metabolizes.
Excretion: About 20% of clofibric acid is excreted unchanged in urine; 70% is eliminated in urine as conjugated metabolite. Plasma half-life after a single dose ranges from 6 to 25 hours; in patients with renal impairment and cirrhosis, half-life can be as long as 113 hours.

CONTRAINDICATIONS & PRECAUTIONS
Contraindicated in patients with significant hepatic or renal dysfunction, primary biliary cirrhosis, or hypersensitivity to clofibrate. Use cautiously in patients with peptic ulcer or history of gallbladder disease.

INTERACTIONS
Drug-drug. Administration with *cholestyramine* decreases absorption rate of clofibrate. Use with *furosemide* may cause increased diuresis as both drugs compete for albumin binding sites; use cautiously. Clofibrate potentiates the effects of *oral anticoagulants,* which may cause fatal hemorrhage; if such a combination is necessary, reduce *oral anticoagulant* dosage by 50%, and evaluate PT and INR frequently. Clofibrate may also enhance the effects of *sulfonylureas,* causing hypoglycemia; a dosage adjustment may be needed.

ADVERSE REACTIONS

CNS: fatigue, weakness, drowsiness, dizziness, headache.
CV: *arrhythmias,* angina, *thromboembolic events,* intermittent claudication.
GI: *nausea, diarrhea, vomiting,* stomatitis, *dyspepsia,* flatulence, increased serum amylase level, *cholelithiasis, cholecystitis.*
GU: impotence and decreased libido, renal dysfunction (dysuria, hematuria, proteinuria, decreased urine output).
Hematologic: *leukopenia,* anemia, eosinophilia.
Hepatic: gallstones, *transient and reversible elevations of liver function test results,* hepatomegaly.
Metabolic: *weight gain,* increased serum creatine kinase level; decreased plasma beta-lipoprotein and plasma fibrinogen levels.
Musculoskeletal: myalgia and arthralgia, resembling a flulike syndrome.
Skin: rash, urticaria, pruritus, dry skin and hair.
Other: *polyphagia.*

◫ KEY CONSIDERATIONS

• Clofibrate shouldn't be used indiscriminately; it may pose an increased risk of gallstones, heart disease, and cancer.
• Use cautiously in geriatric patients with potential hepatic or renal dysfunction.
• Monitor serum cholesterol and triglyceride levels regularly during clofibrate therapy.
• Observe patient for following serious adverse reactions: thrombophlebitis, pulmonary embolism, angina, and arrhythmias; monitor renal and hepatic function, blood counts, and serum electrolyte and blood glucose levels.
• Clofibrate may increase risk of death from cancer, postcholecystectomy complications, and pancreatitis.

Patient education

• Warn patient to report flulike symptoms immediately.
• Stress importance of close medical supervision and of reporting adverse reactions; encourage patient to comply with prescribed regimen and diet.

• Warn patient not to exceed prescribed dosage.
• Advise patient to take drug with food to minimize GI discomfort.
• Emphasize that drug therapy won't replace diet, exercise, and weight reduction for the control of hyperlipidemia.

---

clomipramine hydrochloride
Anafranil

Tricyclic antidepressant, anti-obsessive-compulsive drug

Available by prescription only
Capsules: 25 mg, 50 mg, 75 mg

INDICATIONS & DOSAGE
Treatment of obsessive-compulsive disorder
Adults: Initially, 25 mg P.O. daily, gradually increasing to 100 mg P.O. daily (in divided doses, with meals) during the first 2 weeks. Maximum dosage is 250 mg daily. After adjustment, entire daily dosage may be given h.s.

PHARMACODYNAMICS
Anti-obsessive-compulsive action: A selective inhibitor of serotonin (5-HT) reuptake into neurons within the CNS. It may also have some blocking activity at postsynaptic dopamine receptors. The exact mechanism by which clomipramine treats obsessive-compulsive disorder is unknown.

PHARMACOKINETICS
Absorption: Clomipramine is well absorbed from GI tract, but extensive first-pass metabolism limits bioavailablity to about 50%.
Distribution: Drug distributes well into lipophilic tissues; the volume of distribution is about 12 L/kg; 98% binds to plasma proteins.
Metabolism: Drug is metabolized primarily in the liver. Several metabolites have been identified; desmethyl-clomipramine is the primary active metabolite.
Excretion: About 66% is excreted in urine and the remainder in feces. Mean elimination half-life of the parent com-

pound is about 36 hours; the elimination half-life of desmethylclomipramine has a mean of 69 hours. After multiple dosing, the half-life may increase.

CONTRAINDICATIONS & PRECAUTIONS

Contraindicated in patients with hypersensitivity to clomipramine or other tricyclic antidepressants; in patients who have taken MAO inhibitors within the previous 14 days; and in patients during acute recovery period after an MI.

Use cautiously in patients with urine retention, suicidal tendencies, glaucoma, increased intraocular pressure, brain damage, or seizure disorders and in patients taking drugs that may lower the seizure threshold. Also use cautiously in patients with impaired renal or hepatic function, hyperthyroidism, or tumors of the adrenal medulla and in those undergoing elective surgery or receiving thyroid drugs or electroconvulsive treatment.

INTERACTIONS

Drug-drug. Use of *barbiturates* increases the activity of hepatic microsomal enzymes with repeated doses and may decrease blood clomipramine levels; monitor for decreased effectiveness. *Barbiturates* or other *CNS depressants* may cause an exaggerated depressant effect when used concomitantly. Use with *epinephrine* or *norepinephrine* may produce an increased hypertensive effect. Administration with *MAO inhibitors* may cause hyperpyretic crisis, seizures, coma, and death. *Methylphenidate* may increase blood clomipramine levels.
Drug-lifestyle. Use with *alcohol* may cause an exaggerated depressant effect.

ADVERSE REACTIONS

CNS: *somnolence, tremor, dizziness, headache, insomnia, nervousness, myoclonus, fatigue,* EEG changes, **seizures,** mania, hypomania.
CV: *postural hypotension, palpitations, tachycardia.*
EENT: *pharyngitis, rhinitis, visual changes.*
GI: *dry mouth, constipation, nausea, dyspepsia, increased appetite,* diarrhea, *anorexia, abdominal pain.*

GU: *urinary hesitancy,* urinary tract infection, *dysmenorrhea, ejaculation failure, impotence, altered libido.*
Hematologic: purpura, anemia.
Metabolic: *weight gain.*
Musculoskeletal: *myalgia.*
Skin: *diaphoresis,* rash, pruritus, dry skin.

▣ KEY CONSIDERATIONS

● To minimize risk of overdose, dispense drug in small quantities.
● Monitor for urine retention and constipation. Suggest stool softener or high-fiber diet, as needed, and encourage adequate fluid intake.
● Don't withdraw drug abruptly.
● Drug may cause mania or hypomania.

Patient education

● Warn patient to avoid hazardous activities that require alertness or good psychomotor coordination until adverse CNS effects are known. This is especially important during the dosage adjustment period when daytime sedation and dizziness may occur.
● Instruct patient to avoid alcohol and other depressants.
● Suggest that dry mouth may be relieved with saliva substitutes or sugarless candy or gum.
● Tell patient adverse GI effects can be minimized by taking drug with meals during the dosage adjustment period. Later, the entire daily dose may be taken at bedtime to limit daytime drowsiness.
● Inform patient to avoid using OTC drugs, particularly antihistamines and decongestants, unless a health care provider or pharmacist recommends them.
● Encourage patient to continue therapy and not to discontinue drug abruptly, even if adverse reactions are troublesome.

Overdose & treatment

● Signs and symptoms of clomipramine overdose are similar to those of other tricyclic antidepressants and have included sinus tachycardia, intraventricular block, hypotension, irritability, fixed and dilated pupils, drowsiness, delirium, stupor, hyperreflexia, and hyperpyrexia.

Reactions may be *common,* uncommon, *life-threatening,* or COMMON AND LIFE-THREATENING.

• Treatment should include gastric lavage with large quantities of fluid. Lavage should be continued for 12 hours because the anticholinergic effects of the drug slow gastric emptying. Hemodialysis, peritoneal dialysis, and forced diuresis are ineffective because of the high degree of plasma protein binding. Support respiration and monitor cardiac function. Treat shock with plasma expanders or corticosteroids; treat seizures with diazepam.

clonazepam
Klonopin, Rivotril*

Benzodiazepine, anticonvulsant
Controlled substance schedule IV

Available by prescription only
Tablets: 0.5 mg, 1 mg, 2 mg

INDICATIONS & DOSAGE
Absence and atypical absence seizures; akinetic and myoclonic seizures;* ◊ *generalized tonic-clonic seizures
Adults: Initial dosage should not exceed 1.5 mg P.O. daily, divided into three doses. May be increased by 0.5 to 1 mg q 3 days until seizures are controlled. Maximum recommended daily dosage is 20 mg.
◊ Leg movements during sleep;* ◊ *adjunct treatment in schizophrenia
Adults: 0.5 to 2 mg P.O. h.s.
◊ Parkinsonian dysarthria
Adults: 0.25 to 0.5 mg P.O. daily.
◊ Acute manic episodes
Adults: 0.75 to 16 mg P.O. daily.
◊ Multifocal tic disorders
Adults: 1.5 to 12 mg P.O. daily.
◊ Neuralgia
Adults: 2 to 4 mg P.O. daily.

PHARMACODYNAMICS
Anticonvulsant action: Clonazepam facilitates binding of gamma aminobutyric acid, the major neurotransmitter in the CNS; drug appears to act in the limbic system, thalamus, and hypothalamus.

Drug is used to treat myoclonic, atonic, and absence seizures resistant to other anticonvulsants and to suppress or eliminate attacks of sleep-related nocturnal myoclonus (restless legs syndrome).

PHARMACOKINETICS
Absorption: Clonazepam is well absorbed from the GI tract; action begins in 20 to 60 minutes and persists for up to 12 hours in adults.
Distribution: Drug is distributed widely throughout the body; about 85% binds to proteins.
Metabolism: The liver metabolizes drug to several metabolites. The half-life of drug is 18 to 39 hours.
Excretion: Drug is excreted in urine.

CONTRAINDICATIONS & PRECAUTIONS
Contraindicated in patients with significant hepatic disease; in those with sensitivity to benzodiazepines; and in patients with acute angle-closure glaucoma. Use cautiously in patients with mixed-type seizures, respiratory disease, or glaucoma.

INTERACTIONS
Drug-drug. Use with other *CNS depressants*—such as *anxiolytics, barbiturates, narcotics,* and *tranquilizers*—and other *anticonvulsants* produces additive CNS depressant effects. Use with *ritonavir* may significantly increase levels of clonazepam. Use with *valproic acid* may induce absence seizures.
Drug-lifestyle. *Alcohol* leads to additive CNS depressant effects.

ADVERSE REACTIONS
CNS: *drowsiness, ataxia, behavioral disturbances,* slurred speech, tremor, confusion, psychosis, agitation.
CV: palpitations.
EENT: nystagmus, abnormal eye movements, sore gums.
GI: constipation, gastritis, change in appetite, nausea, anorexia, diarrhea.
GU: dysuria, enuresis, nocturia, urine retention.
Hematologic: *leukopenia, thrombocytopenia,* eosinophilia.
Hepatic: elevate phenytoin levels and liver function test values.
Respiratory: *respiratory depression,* chest congestion, shortness of breath.
Skin: rash.

KEY CONSIDERATIONS

- Geriatric patients may require lower dosages because of diminished renal function; such patients also are at greater risk for oversedation from CNS depressants.
- Abrupt withdrawal may precipitate status epilepticus; after long-term use, lower dosage gradually.
- Use with barbiturates or other CNS depressants may impair ability to perform tasks requiring mental alertness, such as driving a car. Warn patient to avoid such combined use.
- Monitor CBC and liver function tests periodically.
- Monitor for oversedation, especially in geriatric patients.
- Phenytoin levels may be elevated.

Patient education

- Explain rationale for therapy as well as its risks and benefits.
- Teach patient signs and symptoms of adverse reactions and need to report them promptly.
- Tell patient to avoid alcohol and other sedatives to prevent added CNS depression.
- Warn patient not to discontinue drug or change dosage unless prescribed.
- Advise patient to avoid tasks that require mental alertness until degree of sedative effect is determined.

Overdose & treatment

- Signs and symptoms of overdose include ataxia, confusion, coma, decreased reflexes, and hypotension.
- Treat overdose with gastric lavage and supportive therapy. Flumazenil, a specific benzodiazepine antagonist, may be useful. Vasopressors should be used to treat hypotension. Carefully monitor vital signs, ECG, and fluid and electrolyte balance. Clonazepam isn't dialyzable.

clonidine hydrochloride
Catapres, Catapres-TTS, Dixarit*

Centrally acting alpha-adrenergic agonist antiadrenergic, antihypertensive

Available by prescription only
Tablets: 0.1 mg, 0.2 mg, 0.3 mg
Transdermal: TTS-1 (releases 0.1 mg/24 hours), TTS-3 (releases 0.3 mg/24 hours)

INDICATIONS & DOSAGE
Hypertension
Adults: Initially, 0.1 mg P.O. b.i.d.; then increased by 0.1 to 0.2 mg daily or every few days until desired response is achieved. Usual dosage range is 0.2 to 0.6 mg daily in divided doses. Maximum effective dosage is 2.4 mg/day. If transdermal patch is used, apply to an area of hairless intact skin once q 7 days.
◊ *Adjunctive therapy in nicotine withdrawal*
Adults: Initially, 0.15 mg P.O. daily, gradually increased to 0.4 mg P.O. daily as tolerated. Alternatively, apply transdermal patch (0.2 mg/24 hours) and replace weekly for the first 2 to 3 weeks after smoking cessation.
◊ *Prophylaxis for vascular headache*
Adults: 0.025 mg P.O. b.i.d. to q.i.d. up to 0.15 mg P.O. daily in divided doses.
◊ *Adjunctive treatment of menopausal symptoms*
Adults: 0.025 to 0.075 mg P.O. b.i.d.
◊ *Adjunctive therapy in opiate withdrawal*
Adults: 5 to 17 mcg/kg P.O. daily in divided doses for up to 10 days. To avoid hypotension and excessive sedation, adjust dosage and slowly withdraw drug.
◊ *Ulcerative colitis*
Adults: 0.3 mg P.O. t.i.d.
◊ *Neuralgia*
Adults: 0.2 mg P.O. daily.
◊ *Tourette syndrome*
Adults: 0.15 to 0.2 mg P.O. daily.
◊ *Diabetic diarrhea*
Adults: 0.15 to 1.2 mg/day P.O. or 1 or 2 patches/week (0.3 mg/24 hours).
◊ *To diagnose pheochromocytoma*
Adults: 0.3 mg given once.

Reactions may be *common*, uncommon, *life-threatening*, or COMMON AND LIFE-THREATENING.

PHARMACODYNAMICS

Antihypertensive action: Clonidine decreases peripheral vascular resistance by stimulating central alpha-adrenergic receptors, thus decreasing cerebral sympathetic outflow; drug may also inhibit renin release. Initially, clonidine may stimulate peripheral alpha-adrenergic receptors, producing transient vasoconstriction.

PHARMACOKINETICS

Absorption: After oral administration, clonidine is absorbed well from the GI tract; then, blood pressure begins to decline in 30 to 60 minutes, with maximal effect occurring in 2 to 4 hours. After transdermal administration, drug is absorbed well through the skin; transdermal therapeutic plasma levels are achieved 2 to 3 days after initial application.
Distribution: Drug is distributed widely into the body.
Metabolism: Drug is metabolized in the liver, where nearly 50% is transformed to inactive metabolites.
Excretion: About 65% of a given dose is excreted in urine; 20% is excreted in feces. Half-life of clonidine ranges from 6 to 20 hours in patients with normal renal function. After oral administration, the antihypertensive effect lasts up to 8 hours; after transdermal administration, the antihypertensive effect lasts up to 7 days.

CONTRAINDICATIONS & PRECAUTIONS

Contraindicated in patients with hypersensitivity to clonidine. Transdermal form is contraindicated in patients with hypersensitivity to any component of the adhesive layer of the transdermal system. Use cautiously in patients with severe coronary disease, a recent MI, cerebrovascular disease, and impaired hepatic or renal function.

INTERACTIONS

Drug-drug. Clonidine may increase CNS depressant effects of *barbiturates* and other *sedatives*. Use with *other beta blockers* or *propranolol* may have an additive effect, producing bradycardia; this may increase rebound hypertension on withdrawal. *MAO inhibitors, tolazoline,*

and *tricyclic antidepressants* may inhibit the antihypertensive effects of clonidine.
Drug-lifestyle. Use with *alcohol* leads to increased CNS depressant effects.

ADVERSE REACTIONS

CNS: *drowsiness, dizziness,* fatigue, *sedation, weakness,* malaise, agitation, depression.
CV: orthostatic hypotension, bradycardia, severe rebound hypertension.
GI: *constipation, dry mouth,* nausea, vomiting, anorexia.
GU: urine retention, impotence, loss of libido.
Metabolic: slightly increased blood or serum glucose levels, weight gain.
Skin: *pruritus, dermatitis* (with transdermal patch), rash.

▣ KEY CONSIDERATIONS

• Geriatric patients may require lower dosages because they may be more sensitive to the hypotensive effects of clonidine.
• In geriatric patients, monitor renal function carefully.
• Monitor pulse and blood pressure frequently; dosage is usually adjusted to patient's response and tolerance.
• To prevent severe rebound hypertension, don't discontinue drug abruptly; reduce dosage gradually over 2 to 4 days.
• Patients with renal impairment may respond to smaller dosages of drug.
• Give 4 to 6 hours before scheduled surgery.
• Clonidine may be used to lower blood pressure quickly in some hypertensive emergencies.
• Monitor fluid retention by checking the patient's weight daily during initiation of therapy.
• Therapeutic plasma levels are achieved 2 to 3 days after applying transdermal form. Patient may need an oral antihypertensive during this interim period.
• Transdermal systems should be removed when attempting defibrillation or synchronized cardioversion because of electrical conductivity.
• Clonidine may decrease urine excretion of vanillylmandelic acid and catecholamines.

• Drug may cause a weakly positive Coombs' test.

Patient education

• Explain disease and rationale for therapy; emphasize importance of follow-up visits in establishing therapeutic regimen.
• Teach patient signs and symptoms of adverse effects and need to report them; patient should also report excessive weight gain (more than 11 kg [5 lb] weekly).
• Warn patient to avoid hazardous activities that require mental alertness until his body becomes tolerant to the sedation, drowsiness, and other CNS effects that the drug can cause.
• To minimize orthostatic hypotension, advise patient to avoid sudden position changes.
• Inform patient that ice chips, hard candy, or gum will relieve dry mouth.
• Warn patient to call for instructions before taking OTC cold preparations.
• To ensure nighttime blood pressure control, advise taking last dose at bedtime.
• Tell patient not to discontinue drug suddenly; rebound hypertension may develop.

Overdose & treatment

• Signs and symptoms of overdose include bradycardia, CNS depression, respiratory depression, hypothermia, apnea, seizures, lethargy, agitation, irritability, diarrhea, and hypotension; hypertension has also been reported.
• After overdose with oral clonidine, don't induce vomiting because rapid onset of CNS depression can lead to aspiration. After ensuring an adequate airway, perform gastric lavage to empty the stomach and then administer activated charcoal. After overdose with transdermal therapy, remove transdermal patch.

clopidrogrel bisulfate
Plavix

Inhibitor of ADP-induced platelet aggregation, antiplatelet drug

Available by prescription only
Tablets: 75 mg

INDICATIONS & DOSAGE
To reduce atherosclerotic events (MI, CVA, vascular death) in patients with atherosclerosis documented by a recent MI, CVA, or peripheral arterial disease
Adults: 75 mg P.O. once daily with or without food.

PHARMACODYNAMICS
Antiplatelet action: Clopidrogrel inhibits the binding of adenosine diphosphate (ADP) to its platelet receptor and the subsequent ADP-mediated activation of glycoprotein IIb/IIIa complex, thereby inhibiting platelet aggregation. Because clopidrogrel acts by irreversibly modifying the platelet ADP receptor, platelets exposed to the drug are affected for their life span. Dose-dependent inhibition of platelet aggregation can be seen 2 hours after single doses, and becomes maximal after 3 to 7 days of repeated dosing. After the drug is discontinued, platelet aggregation and bleeding time return to baseline in about 5 days.

PHARMACOKINETICS
Absorption: After repeated oral doses, plasma levels of parent compound, which has no platelet-inhibiting effect, are very low and generally below quantification limit. Pharmacokinetic evaluations are generally stated in terms of the main circulating metabolite. After oral administration, about 50% of dose is rapidly absorbed, with plasma levels of the main circulating metabolite peaking about 1 hour after dosing.
Distribution: About 98% of clopidrogrel and 94% of main circulating metabolite bind reversibly to human plasma proteins.
Metabolism: Drug is extensively metabolized in the liver. Main circulating metabolite is the carboxylic acid derivative that has no effect on platelet aggregation. It represents about 85% of circulating drug. Elimination half-life of main circulating metabolite is 8 hours after single and repeated doses.
Excretion: After oral administration, about 50% is excreted in urine and 46% in feces.

CONTRAINDICATIONS & PRECAUTIONS

Contraindicated in patients with pathological bleeding, such as peptic ulcer or intracranial hemorrhage, and in those with known hypersensitivity to clopidrogrel or its components.

Use with caution in patients at risk for increased bleeding from trauma, surgery, or other pathological conditions and in those with hepatic impairment or severe hepatic disease.

INTERACTIONS

Drug-drug. *Aspirin* may increase risk for GI bleeding; it doesn't modify the clopidrogrel-mediated inhibition of ADP-induced platelet aggregation. Safe use with *heparin* or *warfarin* hasn't been established; use together cautiously. (Clopidrogrel doesn't alter the heparin dose or the effect of heparin on coagulation; coadministration of heparin doesn't affect the ability of clopidrogrel to inhibit platelet aggregation.) Administration with *NSAIDs* may increase occult GI blood loss. Use with caution.

ADVERSE REACTIONS

CNS: asthenia, depression, dizziness, fatigue, headache, paresthesia, syncope.
CV: chest pain, edema, hypertension, palpitations.
EENT: epistaxis, rhinitis.
GI: abdominal pain, constipation, diarrhea, dyspepsia, gastritis, hemorrhage, nausea, vomiting.
GU: urinary tract infection.
Hematologic: purpura.
Musculoskeletal: arthralgia.
Respiratory: bronchitis, coughing, dyspnea, upper respiratory tract infection.
Skin: rash, pruritus.
Other: flulike syndrome, pain.

▣ KEY CONSIDERATIONS

• Clopidrogrel is usually used in patients who are hypersensitive or intolerant to aspirin.
• If patient is to undergo surgery and an antiplatelet effect isn't desired, drug should be stopped 7 days before surgery.

Patient education

• Inform patient it may take longer than usual to stop bleeding; therefore, advise him to refrain from activities in which trauma and bleeding may occur. Encourage use of seat belts.
• Instruct patient to report unusual bleeding or bruising.
• Tell patient to inform health care provider or dentist that he's taking clopidrogrel before scheduling surgery or taking new drugs.
• Inform patient that drug may be taken without regard to food.

Overdose & treatment

• Signs and symptoms of acute toxicity in animal studies include vomiting, prostration, GI hemorrhage, and difficulty breathing.
• Based on biological plausibility, platelet transfusion may be appropriate to reverse the pharmacologic effects of clopidrogrel if quick reversal is required.

---

clorazepate dipotassium
Novo-Clopate*, Tranxene*, Tranxene-SD, Tranxene-SD Half Strength

Benzodiazepine, anxiolytic, anticonvulsant, sedative-hypnotic
Controlled substance schedule IV

Available by prescription only
Tablets: 3.75 mg, 7.5 mg, 11.25 mg, 15 mg, 22.5 mg
Capsules: 3.75 mg, 7.5 mg, 15 mg

INDICATIONS & DOSAGE
Anxiety
Adults: 15 to 60 mg P.O. daily.
As an adjunct in treatment of partial seizures
Adults: Maximum recommended initial dosage is 7.5 mg P.O. t.i.d. Dosage increases shouldn't exceed 7.5 mg/week. Maximum daily dosage shouldn't exceed 90 mg.
Acute alcohol withdrawal
Adults: Day 1—30 mg P.O., followed by 30 to 60 mg P.O. in divided doses; day 2—45 to 90 mg P.O. in divided doses; day 3—22.5 to 45 mg P.O. in divided doses; day 4—15 to 30 mg P.O. in divided doses; gradually reduce daily dosage to 7.5 to 15 mg.

PHARMACODYNAMICS

Anxiolytic and sedative actions: Clorazepate depresses the CNS at the limbic and subcortical levels of the brain. It produces an anxiolytic effect by enhancing the effect of the neurotransmitter gamma-aminobutyric acid (GABA) on its receptor in the ascending reticular activating system, which increases inhibition and blocks both cortical and limbic arousal.

Anticonvulsant action: By enhancing presynaptic inhibition, drug suppresses spread of seizure activity that epileptogenic foci in the cortex, thalamus, and limbic structures produce.

PHARMACOKINETICS

Absorption: After oral administration, clorazepate is hydrolyzed in the stomach to desmethyldiazepam, which is absorbed completely and rapidly. Serum levels peak in 1 to 2 hours.

Distribution: Drug is distributed widely throughout the body. About 80% to 95% of an administered dose binds to plasma protein.

Metabolism: Desmethyldiazepam is metabolized in the liver to conjugated oxazepam.

Excretion: Inactive glucuronide metabolites are excreted in urine. The half-life of desmethyldiazepam ranges from 30 to 100 hours.

CONTRAINDICATIONS & PRECAUTIONS

Contraindicated in patients who are hypersensitive to clorazepate or other benzodiazepines and in patients who have acute angle-closure glaucoma.

Use cautiously in patients with impaired renal or hepatic function, suicidal tendencies, or history of drug abuse.

INTERACTIONS

Drug-drug. *Antacids* delay absorption of clorazepate and reduce the total amount absorbed. Clorazepate potentiates the CNS depressant effects of *antidepressants, barbiturates, general anesthetics, MAO inhibitors, narcotics,* and *phenothiazines.* Use with *cimetidine* and possibly *disulfiram* causes diminished hepatic metabolism of clorazepate, which increases its plasma level. Clor-

azepate may reduce serum levels of *haloperidol* and may decrease the therapeutic effectiveness of *levodopa.*

Drug-lifestyle. Clorazepate potentiates the CNS depressant effects of *alcohol. Heavy smoking* accelerates metabolism of the drug, thus lowering its effectiveness.

ADVERSE REACTIONS

CNS: *drowsiness,* dizziness, nervousness, confusion, headache, insomnia, depression, irritability, tremor, changes in EEG patterns.

CV: hypotension.

EENT: blurred vision, diplopia.

GI: nausea, vomiting, abdominal discomfort, dry mouth.

GU: urine retention, incontinence.

Hepatic: elevated liver function test results.

Skin: rash.

KEY CONSIDERATIONS

Besides the recommendations relevant to all benzodiazepines, consider the following:

• Lower dosages are usually effective in geriatric patients, especially in those with renal or hepatic dysfunction, because of decreased elimination. Use with caution.

• Geriatric patients who receive this drug require supervision with ambulation and activities of daily living during initiation of therapy or after dosage increase.

• Store in a cool, dry place away from direct light.

Patient education

• Advise patient of potential for physical and psychological dependence with long-term use of clorazepate.

• Instruct patient not to alter drug regimen without health care provider's approval.

• Warn patient that sudden position changes may cause dizziness. Advise patient to dangle legs for a few minutes before getting out of bed to prevent falls and injury.

• Advise patient to take antacids 1 hour before or after clorazepate.

• Inform patient not to suddenly stop taking drug.

Reactions may be *common,* uncommon, *life-threatening,* or COMMON AND LIFE-THREATENING.

- Advise patient to avoid alcohol use and smoking while taking drug.

Overdose & treatment

- Signs and symptoms of overdose include somnolence, confusion, coma, hypoactive reflexes, dyspnea, labored breathing, hypotension, bradycardia, slurred speech, unsteady gait, and impaired coordination.
- Support blood pressure and respiration until drug effects subside; monitor vital signs. Flumazenil, a specific benzodiazepine antagonist, may be useful. Mechanical ventilatory assistance via endotracheal tube may be required to maintain a patent airway and support adequate oxygenation. Treat hypotension with I.V. fluids and vasopressors such as dopamine and phenylephrine as needed. Induce vomiting if patient is conscious, or perform gastric lavage if ingestion was recent, but only if an endotracheal tube is present, to prevent aspiration. Then, administer activated charcoal with a cathartic as a single dose. Dialysis is of limited value. Don't use barbiturates because they may worsen CNS adverse effects.

---

clotrimazole
FemCare, Gyne-Lotrimin, Lotrimin, Lotrimin AF, Mycelex, Mycelex-G, Mycelex OTC, Mycelex-7

Synthetic imidazole derivative, topical antifungal

Available by prescription only
Vaginal tablets: 500 mg
Topical cream: 1%
Topical lotion: 1%
Topical solution: 1%
Lozenges: 10 mg
Available without a prescription
Vaginal tablets: 100 mg
Vaginal cream: 1%
Combination pack: Vaginal tablets 500 mg/topical cream 1%

INDICATIONS & DOSAGE

Tinea pedis, tinea cruris, tinea versicolor, tinea corporis, cutaneous candidiasis

Adults: Apply a thin layer and massage into the cleaned affected and surrounding area, morning and evening, for prescribed period (usually 1 to 4 weeks; however, therapy may take up to 8 weeks).
Vulvovaginal candidiasis
Adults: Insert 1 tablet intravaginally h.s. for 7 consecutive days. If vaginal cream is used, insert 1 applicatorful intravaginally h.s. for 7 to 14 consecutive days.
Oropharyngeal candidiasis
Adults: Administer orally and dissolve slowly (15 to 30 minutes) in mouth; usual dosage is 1 lozenge five times daily for 14 consecutive days.
◊ *Keratitis*
Adults: 1% ointment in sterile peanut oil q 2 to 4 hours for up to 6 weeks.

PHARMACODYNAMICS

Antifungal action: Clotrimazole alters cell membrane permeability by binding with phospholipids in the fungal cell membrane. Clotrimazole inhibits or kills many fungi, including yeast and dermatophytes, and also is active against some gram-positive bacteria.

PHARMACOKINETICS

Absorption: Absorption of clotrimazole is limited with topical administration. Absorption after dissolution of a lozenge in the mouth hasn't been determined.
Distribution: Minimal with local application.
Metabolism: Unknown.
Excretion: Unknown.

CONTRAINDICATIONS & PRECAUTIONS

Contraindicated in patients hypersensitive to clotrimazole. Also contraindicated for ophthalmic use.

INTERACTIONS
None reported.

ADVERSE REACTIONS

GI: nausea, vomiting (with lozenges); lower abdominal cramps.
GU: *mild vaginal burning or irritation* (with vaginal use), cramping, urinary frequency.
Hepatic: abnormal liver function test results

Skin: blistering, *erythema,* edema, blistering, pruritus, burning, stinging, peeling, urticaria, skin fissures, general irritation.

▣ KEY CONSIDERATIONS
• Patients treated with clotrimazole lozenges, especially those who have pre-existing liver dysfunction, should have periodic liver function tests.
• Abnormal liver function tests have been reported in patients receiving clotrimazole lozenges.

Patient education
• Advise patient that lozenges must dissolve slowly in the mouth to achieve maximum effect. Tell patient not to chew lozenges.
• Instruct patients using intravaginal application to insert drug high into the vagina and to refrain from sexual contact during treatment period to avoid reinfection. Also, tell patient to use a sanitary napkin to prevent staining of clothing and to absorb discharge.
• Tell patient to complete the full course of therapy. Improvement usually will be noted within 1 week. Patient should call health care provider if no improvement occurs in 4 weeks or if condition worsens.
• Advise patient to watch for and report irritation or sensitivity and, if this occurs, to discontinue use.

cloxacillin sodium
Cloxapen, Tegopen

Penicillinase-resistant penicillin, antibiotic

Available by prescription only
Capsules: 250 mg, 500 mg
Oral solution: 125 mg/5 ml (after reconstitution)

INDICATIONS & DOSAGE
Systemic infections caused by penicillinase-producing staphylococci organisms
Adults: 250 to 500 mg q 6 hours.

PHARMACODYNAMICS
Antibiotic action: Cloxacillin is bactericidal; it adheres to bacterial penicillin-binding proteins, thereby inhibiting bacterial cell-wall synthesis.
   Drug resists the effects of penicillinases—enzymes that inactivate penicillin—and therefore is active against many strains of penicillinase-producing bacteria; this activity is most pronounced against penicillinase-producing staphylococci; some strains may remain resistant. Cloxacillin is also active against gram-positive aerobic and anaerobic bacilli but has no significant effect on gram-negative bacilli.

PHARMACOKINETICS
Absorption: Cloxacillin is absorbed rapidly but incompletely (37% to 60%) from the GI tract; it's relatively acid stable. Plasma levels peak ½ to 2 hours after an oral dose. Food may decrease both rate and extent of absorption.
Distribution: Drug is distributed widely. CSF penetration is poor but enhanced in meningeal inflammation. About 90% to 96% binds to proteins.
Metabolism: Drug is only partially metabolized.
Excretion: Cloxacillin and metabolites are excreted in urine through renal tubular secretion and glomerular filtration. Elimination half-life in adults is ½ to 1 hour, extended minimally to 2½ hours in patients with renal impairment.

CONTRAINDICATIONS & PRECAUTIONS
Contraindicated in patients with hypersensitivity to cloxacillin or other penicillins.

INTERACTIONS
Drug-drug. Use with *aminoglycosides* produces synergistic bactericidal effects against *Staphylococcus aureus.* However, the drugs are physically and chemically incompatible and are inactivated when mixed or given together. In vivo inactivation has been reported when *aminoglycosides* and penicillins are used concomitantly.
   Probenecid blocks renal tubular secretion of carbenicillin, raising its serum levels.

Reactions may be *common,* uncommon, *life-threatening,* or COMMON AND LIFE-THREATENING.

Drug-food. Acid in *carbonated beverages* or *fruit juice* may inactivate drug. *Food* decreases absorption of drug.

ADVERSE REACTIONS
CNS: lethargy, hallucinations, *seizures*, anxiety, confusion, agitation, depression, dizziness, fatigue.
GI: *nausea,* vomiting, *epigastric distress, diarrhea,* enterocolitis, pseudomembranous colitis, black "hairy" tongue, abdominal pain.
GU: interstitial nephritis, nephropathy.
Hematologic: eosinophilia, anemia, *thrombocytopenia, leukopenia, hemolytic anemia, agranulocytosis.*
Hepatic: transient elevations in liver function test results, drug-induced cholestasis or hepatitis.
Other: hypersensitivity reactions (rash, urticaria, chills, fever, sneezing, wheezing, *anaphylaxis*), overgrowth of nonsusceptible organisms.

▣ KEY CONSIDERATIONS
Besides the recommendations relevant to all penicillins, consider the following:
• Give drug with water only; acid in fruit juice or carbonated beverage may inactivate drug.
• Give dose on empty stomach; food decreases absorption.
• Refrigerate oral suspension and discard any unused drug after 14 days. Unrefrigerated suspension is stable for 3 days.
• Cloxacillin alters test results for urine and serum proteins; it produces false-positive or elevated results in turbidimetric urine and serum protein tests using sulfosalicylic acid or trichloroacetic acid; it also reportedly produces false results on the Bradshaw screening test for Bence Jones protein.
• Cloxacillin may falsely decrease serum aminoglycoside levels.

Patient education
• Inform patient of potential adverse reactions.
• Instruct patient to take on an empty stomach and take with water only.
• Tell patient to refrigerate oral suspension and to discard any unused suspension after the course of treatment.

Overdose & treatment
• Signs and symptoms of overdose include neuromuscular irritability and seizures.
• Treatment is symptomatic. After recent ingestion (within 4 hours), induce vomiting or perform gastric lavage; to reduce absorption, follow with activated charcoal. Cloxacillin isn't appreciably removed through hemodialysis or peritoneal dialysis.

clozapine
Clozaril

Tricyclic dibenzodiazepine derivative, antipsychotic

Available by prescription only
Tablets: 25 mg, 100 mg

INDICATIONS & DOSAGE
Treatment of schizophrenia in severely ill patients unresponsive to other therapies
Adults: Initially, 12.5 mg P.O. once or twice daily, adjusted upward at 25 to 50 mg daily (if tolerated) to a daily dosage of 300 to 450 mg by end of 2 weeks. Individual dosage is based on patient's response, tolerance, and adverse reactions. Subsequent increases of dosage should occur no more than once or twice weekly and shouldn't exceed 100 mg. Many patients respond to dosages of 300 to 600 mg daily, but some patients require as much as 900 mg daily. Don't exceed 900 mg/day.

PHARMACODYNAMICS
Antipsychotic action: Clozapine binds to dopamine receptors (D-1, D-2, D-3, D-4, and D-5) within the limbic system of the CNS. It also may interfere with adrenergic, cholinergic, histaminergic, and serotoninergic receptors.

PHARMACOKINETICS
Absorption: Drug levels peak about 2½ hours after oral administration. Food doesn't appear to interfere with bioavailability. Only 27% to 50% of the dose reaches systemic circulation.

---

*Canada only   ◊ Unlabeled clinical use

Distribution: About 95% binds to serum proteins.

Metabolism: Drug metabolizes nearly completely; very little unchanged drug appears in the urine.

Excretion: About 50% of drug appears in urine and 30% in feces, mostly as metabolites. Elimination half-life appears proportional to dose and may range from 4 to 66 hours.

CONTRAINDICATIONS & PRECAUTIONS

Contraindicated in patients with uncontrolled epilepsy or history of clozapine-induced agranulocytosis; in patients with a WBC count below 3,500/µl; in patients with severe CNS depression or coma; in patients taking other drugs that suppress bone marrow function; and in those with myelosuppressive disorders.

Use cautiously in patients with renal, hepatic, or cardiac disease, prostatic hyperplasia, or angle-closure glaucoma and in those receiving general anesthesia.

INTERACTIONS

Drug-drug. Clozapine may potentiate the hypotensive effects of *antihypertensives. Anticholinergics* may potentiate the anticholinergic effects of clozapine. Administration of clozapine to a patient taking a *benzodiazepine* may pose a risk of respiratory arrest and severe hypotension; avoid concomitant use. Use cautiously with other *CNS-active drugs* because of the potential for additive effects. Use may increase serum levels of *digoxin, other highly protein-bound drugs,* and *warfarin;* monitor closely for adverse reactions. Use cautiously with other *drugs metabolized by cytochrome P-450 2D6,* including *antidepressants, carbamazepine, phenothiazines,* and *type IC antiarrhythmics*—such as *encainide, flecainide,* and *propafenone*—or *drugs that inhibit this enzyme,* such as *quinidine.* Increased bone marrow toxicity may follow concomitant use with *drugs that suppress bone marrow function.* Clozapine may decrease *phenytoin* levels and may lower the seizure threshold; therefore, avoid use with other drugs that have the same effect.

Drug-lifestyle. *Alcohol* leads to increased CNS depression; don't use together.

ADVERSE REACTIONS

CNS: *drowsiness, sedation, seizures,* dizziness, syncope, vertigo, headache, tremor, disturbed sleep or nightmares, restlessness, hypokinesia or akinesia, agitation, rigidity, akathisia, confusion, fatigue, insomnia, hyperkinesia, weakness, lethargy, ataxia, slurred speech, depression, myoclonus, anxiety, *neuroleptic malignant syndrome.*

CV: *tachycardia, hypotension,* hypertension, chest pain, ECG changes, orthostatic hypotension.

EENT: visual disturbances.

GI: *dry mouth, constipation,* nausea, vomiting, *excessive salivation,* heartburn, constipation, diarrhea.

GU: urinary abnormalities (urinary frequency or urgency, urine retention), incontinence, abnormal ejaculation.

Hematologic: *leukopenia, agranulocytosis.*

Metabolic: weight gain.

Musculoskeletal: muscle pain or spasm, muscle weakness.

Skin: rash.

Other: fever, diaphoresis.

▣ KEY CONSIDERATIONS

• Geriatric patients may require lower dosages because they are potentially more sensitive to the adverse effects of clozapine, especially orthostatic hypotension, dry mouth, and constipation.

• Clozapine therapy must be given with a monitoring program that ensures weekly testing of WBC counts for the first 6 months and then every other week thereafter. Blood tests must be performed weekly, and no more than a 1-week supply of drug should be distributed.

• To discontinue clozapine therapy, withdraw drug gradually (over 1 to 2 weeks). However, changes in the patient's status (including the development of leukopenia) may require abrupt discontinuation of the drug. If so, monitor closely for recurrence of psychotic symptoms.

• To reinstate therapy in patients withdrawn from drug, follow usual guidelines for increasing dosage. However, re-

---

exposure of the patient may increase the risk and severity of adverse reactions. If therapy was terminated for WBC counts below 2,000/µl or granulocyte counts below 1,000/mm³, drug shouldn't be continued.
• Some patients experience transient fevers (temperature above 100.4° F [38° C]), especially in the first 3 weeks of therapy. Monitor patients closely.
• Assess patient periodically for abnormal body movement.

Patient education

• Warn patient about risk of developing agranulocytosis. He should know that safe use of drug requires weekly blood tests for 6 months to monitor for agranulocytosis. Advise patient to promptly report flulike symptoms, fever, sore throat, lethargy, malaise, or other signs or symptoms of infection.
• Advise patient to call before taking OTC drugs.
• Advise patient to avoid alcohol while taking drug.
• Tell patient that ice chips or sugarless candy or gum may help to relieve dry mouth.
• Warn patient to rise slowly to upright position to avoid orthostatic hypotension.

Overdose & treatment

• Fatalities have occurred at doses exceeding 2.5 g. Signs and symptoms include drowsiness, delirium, coma, hypotension, hypersalivation, tachycardia, respiratory depression and, rarely, seizures.
• Treat symptomatically. Establish an airway and ensure adequate ventilation. Gastric lavage with activated charcoal and sorbitol may be effective. Monitor vital signs. Avoid epinephrine (and derivatives), quinidine, and procainamide when treating hypotension and arrhythmias.

codeine phosphate

codeine sulfate

Opioid, analgesic, antitussive
Controlled substance schedule II

Available by prescription only
Tablets: 15 mg, 30 mg, 60 mg; 15 mg, 30 mg, 60 mg (soluble)
Oral solution: 15 mg/5 ml codeine phosphate
Injection: 15 mg/ml, 30 mg/ml, 60 mg/ml codeine phosphate

INDICATIONS & DOSAGE
Mild to moderate pain
Adults: 15 to 60 mg P.O. or 15 to 60 mg (phosphate) S.C. or I.M. q 4 to 6 hours, p.r.n., or around-the-clock.
Nonproductive cough
Adults: 10 to 20 mg P.O. q 4 to 6 hours. Maximum dosage is 120 mg/day.

PHARMACODYNAMICS
Analgesic action: Codeine (methylmorphine) has analgesic properties that result from its agonist activity at the opiate receptors.
Antitussive action: Codeine has a direct suppressant action on the cough reflex center.

PHARMACOKINETICS
Absorption: Codeine is well absorbed after oral or parenteral administration. It's about two-thirds as potent orally as it is parenterally. After oral or subcutaneous administration, action occurs in less than 30 minutes. Analgesic effect peaks in ½ to 1 hour, and the duration of action is 4 to 6 hours.
Distribution: Drug is distributed widely throughout the body.
Metabolism: Drug is metabolized mainly in the liver, through demethylation or conjugation with glucuronic acid.
Excretion: Drug is excreted mainly in the urine as norcodeine and free and conjugated morphine.

CONTRAINDICATIONS & PRECAUTIONS

Contraindicated in patients with hypersensitivity to codeine. Use cautiously in geriatric patients, especially those who have impaired renal or hepatic function, head injuries, increased intracranial pressure, increased CSF pressure, hypothyroidism, Addison's disease, acute alcoholism, CNS depression, bronchial asthma, COPD, respiratory depression, or shock or who are debilitated.

INTERACTIONS

Drug-drug. Use with *anticholinergics* may cause paralytic ileus. Use with *cimetidine* may increase respiratory and CNS depression, causing confusion, disorientation, apnea, or seizures. Use with other *CNS depressants*—such as *antihistamines, barbiturates, benzodiazepines, general anesthetics, MAO inhibitors, muscle relaxants, narcotic analgesics, phenothiazines, sedative-hypnotics,* and *tricyclic antidepressants*—potentiates the respiratory and CNS depression, sedation, and hypotensive effects that the drug can cause. Drug accumulation and enhanced effects may result from concomitant use with other *drugs that are extensively metabolized in the liver*—such as *digitoxin, phenytoin,* and *rifampin.* Use with *drugs that induce P-450 enzymes* results in increased clearance and decreased effect of codeine. Use with *general anesthetics* may cause severe CV depression. Patients who become physically dependent on drug may experience acute withdrawal syndrome if given a *narcotic antagonist.*
Drug-lifestyle. *Alcohol* potentiates the respiratory and CNS depression, sedation, and hypotensive effects that drug can cause.

ADVERSE REACTIONS

CNS: *sedation, clouded sensorium, euphoria, dizziness, light-headedness.*
CV: *hypotension, **bradycardia.***
GI: *nausea, vomiting, constipation, dry mouth,* ileus, increase plasma amylase and lipase levels.
GU: *urine retention.*
Respiratory: *respiratory depression.*
Skin: pruritus, flushing, *diaphoresis.*
Other: *physical dependence.*

▣ KEY CONSIDERATIONS

Besides the recommendations relevant to all opioids, consider the following:
● Lower dosages are usually indicated for geriatric patients, who may be more sensitive to the therapeutic and adverse effects of drug.
● Codeine and aspirin have additive analgesic effects. Give together for maximum pain relief.
● Codeine is less likely to be abused than morphine.
● Drug may increase biliary tract pressure resulting from contraction of the sphincter of Oddi, and may interfere with hepatobiliary imaging studies.

Patient education

● Inform patient that codeine may cause drowsiness, dizziness, or blurring of vision; tell him to use caution while driving or performing tasks that require mental alertness.
● Advise patient to avoid consumption of alcohol and other CNS depressants and to take drug with food if GI upset occurs.

Overdose & treatment

● The most common signs and symptoms of overdose are CNS depression, respiratory depression, and miosis (pinpoint pupils). Other acute toxic effects include hypotension, bradycardia, hypothermia, shock, apnea, cardiopulmonary arrest, circulatory collapse, pulmonary edema, and seizures.
● To treat acute overdose, first establish adequate respiratory exchange via a patent airway and ventilation as needed; to reverse respiratory depression, administer a narcotic antagonist (naloxone). (Because the duration of action of codeine is longer than that of naloxone, repeated naloxone dosing is necessary.) Naloxone shouldn't be given unless the patient has significant respiratory or CV depression. Monitor vital signs closely.
● Within 2 hours of an oral overdose, empty the stomach immediately by inducing vomiting with ipecac syrup or performing gastric lavage. Use caution to avoid risk of aspiration. Administer activated charcoal via an NG tube to further prevent absorption.

Reactions may be *common,* uncommon, *life-threatening,* or COMMON AND LIFE-THREATENING.

colchicine

Colchicum autumnale *alkaloid, antigout drug*

Available by prescription only
Injection: 1 mg (1/60 grain)/2-ml ampule
Tablets: 0.6 mg (1/100 grain), 0.5 mg (1/120 grain) as sugar-coated granules

INDICATIONS & DOSAGE
To prevent acute attacks of gout as prophylactic or maintenance therapy
Adults: 0.5 or 0.6 mg P.O. one to four times weekly.
To prevent attacks of gout in patients undergoing surgery
Adults: 0.5 to 0.6 mg P.O. t.i.d. 3 days before and 3 days after surgery.
Acute gout, acute gouty arthritis
Adults: Initially, 0.5 to 1.3 mg P.O., followed by 0.5 to 0.65 mg P.O. q 1 to 2 hours or 1 to 1.3 mg P.O. q 2 hours; total daily dosage is usually 4 to 8 mg P.O.; give until pain is relieved or until nausea, vomiting, or diarrhea ensues. Or 2 mg I.V. followed by 0.5 mg I.V. q 6 hours if necessary. Total I.V. dosage over 24 hours (one course of treatment) shouldn't exceed 4 mg.
◇ ***Familial Mediterranean fever***
Colchicine has been used effectively to treat familial Mediterranean fever (hereditary disorder characterized by acute episodes of fever, peritonitis, and pleuritis).
Adults: 1 to 2 mg/day in divided doses.
◇ ***Amyloidosis suppressant***
Adults: 500 to 600 mcg P.O. once daily to b.i.d.
◇ ***Dermatitis herpetiformis suppressant***
Adults: 600 mcg P.O. b.i.d. or t.i.d.
◇ ***Hepatic cirrhosis***
Adults: 1 mg 5 days weekly.
◇ ***Primary biliary cirrhosis***
Adults: 0.6 mg b.i.d.

PHARMACODYNAMICS
Antigout action: Although the exact mechanism of action is unknown, colchicine helps inhibit leukocyte migration; reduces lactic acid production by leukocytes, resulting in decreased deposits of uric acid; and interferes with kinin formation.
Anti-inflammatory action: Colchicine reduces the inflammatory response to deposited uric acid crystals and diminishes phagocytosis.

PHARMACOKINETICS
Absorption: When administered P.O., colchicine is rapidly absorbed from the GI tract. Unchanged drug may be reabsorbed from the intestine by biliary processes.
Distribution: Drug is distributed rapidly into various tissues after reabsorption from the intestine. It's concentrated in leukocytes and distributed into the kidneys, liver, spleen, and intestinal tract, but is absent in the heart, skeletal muscle, and brain.
Metabolism: Drug is metabolized partially in the liver and also slowly metabolized in other tissues.
Excretion: Drug and its metabolites are excreted primarily in feces, with lesser amounts excreted in urine.

CONTRAINDICATIONS & PRECAUTIONS
Contraindicated in patients with hypersensitivity to colchicine; blood dyscrasias; or serious CV, renal, or GI disease. Use cautiously in geriatric patients, especially those who are debilitated or have early signs of CV, renal, or GI disease.

INTERACTIONS
Drug-drug. *Acidifying drugs* inhibit colchicine; *alkalizing drugs* increase its action. Colchicine may increase sensitivity to *CNS depressants,* may enhance the response to *sympathomimetics,* and induces reversible malabsorption of *vitamin B₁₂.* Use with *cyclosporine* may cause GI dysfunction, hepatonephropathy, and neuromyopathy.
Drug-lifestyle. *Alcohol* inhibits colchicine.

ADVERSE REACTIONS
CNS: peripheral neuritis.
GI: *nausea, vomiting, abdominal pain, diarrhea.*
GU: reversible azoospermia.

Hematologic: *aplastic anemia, thrombocytopenia, and agranulocytosis* (with long-term use); nonthrombocytopenic purpura.
Hepatic: increased alkaline phosphatase, AST, and ALT levels.
Musculoskeletal: myopathy.
Skin: alopecia, urticaria, dermatitis, hypersensitivity reactions.
Other: severe local irritation if extravasation occurs, may decrease serum carotene and cholesterol levels.

▣ KEY CONSIDERATIONS
• Administer with caution to geriatric patients, especially those who are debilitated or who have renal, GI, or heart disease or hematologic disorders. Reduce dosage or consider discontinuing if patient experiences weakness, anorexia, nausea, vomiting, or diarrhea.
• To avoid cumulative toxicity, don't repeat a course of oral colchicine for at least 3 days; a course of I.V. colchicine shouldn't be repeated for several weeks.
• Don't administer I.M. or S.C.; severe local irritation occurs.
• Obtain baseline laboratory studies, including CBC, before initiating therapy and periodically thereafter.
• Give I.V. by slow I.V. push over 2 to 5 minutes by direct I.V. injection or into tubing of a free-flowing I.V. with compatible I.V. fluid. Avoid extravasation. Don't dilute colchicine injection with bacteriostatic normal saline solution, D_5W injection, or any other fluid that might change pH of colchicine solution. If lower concentration of colchicine injection is needed, dilute with sterile water or normal saline solution. However, if diluted solution becomes turbid, don't inject.
• Store drug in a tightly closed, light-resistant container, away from moisture and high temperatures.
• Colchicine may cause false-positive results of urine tests for RBCs or hemoglobin.

Patient education
• Advise patient to report rash, sore throat, fever, unusual bleeding, bruising, tiredness, weakness, numbness, or tingling.

• Tell patient to discontinue drug as soon as gout pain is relieved or at the first sign of nausea, vomiting, abdominal pain, or diarrhea. Advise patient to report persistent symptoms.
• Instruct patient to avoid alcohol during drug therapy, because alcohol may inhibit drug action.

Overdose & treatment
• First sign of acute overdosage may be GI symptoms, followed by vascular damage, muscle weakness, and ascending paralysis. Delirium and convulsions may occur without loss of consciousness.
• Signs and symptoms of overdose include nausea, vomiting, abdominal pain, and diarrhea. Diarrhea may be severe and bloody from hemorrhagic gastroenteritis. Burning sensations in the throat, stomach, and skin also may occur. Extensive vascular damage may result in shock, hematuria, and oliguria, indicating kidney damage. Patient develops severe dehydration, hypotension, and muscle weakness with an ascending paralysis of the CNS. Death may result from respiratory depression.
• Treatment begins with gastric lavage and preventive measures for shock. Recent studies support the use of hemodialysis and peritoneal dialysis; atropine and morphine may relieve abdominal pain; paregoric usually is administered to control diarrhea and cramps. Respiratory assistance may be needed.

colestipol hydrochloride
Colestid

Anion exchange resin, antilipemic

Available by prescription only
Tablets: 1 g
Granules: 300-g and 500-g multidose bottles, 5-g packets

INDICATIONS & DOSAGE
Primary hypercholesterolemia and xanthomas
Adults: **Tablets:** Initially, 2 g P.O. once daily or b.i.d., then increase in 2-g incre-

---

ments at 1- to 2-month intervals. Usual dosage is 2 to 16 g P.O. daily given as a single dose or in divided doses.

Granules: Initially, 5 g P.O. once daily or b.i.d., then increase in 5-g increments at 1- to 2-month intervals. Usual dosage is 5 to 30 g P.O. daily given as a single dose or in divided doses.

◊ *Digitoxin overdose*
Adults: Initially, 10 g P.O. followed by 5 g P.O. q 6 to 8 hours.

PHARMACODYNAMICS

Antilipemic action: Bile is normally excreted into the intestine to facilitate absorption of fat and other lipid materials. Colestipol binds with bile acid, forming an insoluble compound that is excreted in feces. With less bile available in the digestive system, less fat and lipid materials in food are absorbed, more cholesterol is used by the liver to replace its supply of bile acids, and the serum cholesterol level decreases.

PHARMACOKINETICS

Absorption: Colestipol isn't absorbed. Cholesterol levels may decrease in 24 to 48 hours, with peak effect occurring at 1 month. In some patients, the initial decrease is followed by a return to or above baseline cholesterol levels on continued therapy.
Distribution: None.
Metabolism: None.
Excretion: Drug is excreted in feces; cholesterol levels return to baseline within 1 month after therapy stops.

CONTRAINDICATIONS & PRECAUTIONS

Contraindicated in patients with hypersensitivity reactions to bile-acid sequestering resins. Use cautiously in patients prone to constipation and in those with conditions aggravated by constipation, such as symptomatic coronary artery disease.

INTERACTIONS

Drug-drug. Colestipol impairs absorption of *cardiac glycosides* (including *digitoxin* and *digoxin*), *chenodiol, penicillin G, tetracycline,* and *thiazide diuretics,* thus decreasing their therapeutic effect. Dosage of any *oral drug* may re-

quire adjustment to compensate for possible binding with colestipol; give other drugs at least 1 hour before or 4 to 6 hours after colestipol (longer if possible); to prevent high-dose toxicity, readjustment must also be made when colestipol is withdrawn. Colestipol may interfere with *oral phosphate supplements* and may decrease GI absorption of *propranolol.*

ADVERSE REACTIONS

CNS: headache, dizziness, anxiety, vertigo, insomnia, fatigue, syncope, tinnitus.
GI: *constipation,* **fecal impaction,** hemorrhoids, abdominal discomfort, flatulence, nausea, vomiting, steatorrhea, **GI bleeding,** diarrhea, anorexia.
GU: dysuria, hematuria.
Hematologic: anemia, ecchymoses, bleeding tendencies.
Hepatic: altered serum levels of alkaline phosphatase, ALT, and AST.
Metabolic: altered levels of chloride, phosphorus, potassium, and sodium; hyperchloremic acidosis with long-term use or high dosage.
Musculoskeletal: backache, muscle and joint pain, osteoporosis.
Skin: rash, irritation of tongue and perianal area.
Other: vitamin A, D, E, and K deficiencies from decreased absorption.

▣ KEY CONSIDERATIONS

• Geriatric patients are more likely to experience adverse GI effects and adverse nutritional effects.
• To mix, sprinkle granules on surface of preferred beverage or wet food, let stand a few minutes, and stir to obtain uniform suspension; avoid excess foaming by using large glass and mixing slowly. Use at least 3 oz (90 ml) of water or other fluid, soups, milk, or pulpy fruit; rinse container and have patient drink this to be sure he ingests entire dose. Tablets should be swallowed whole.
• To ensure appropriate dosage during and after therapy with colestipol, monitor levels of cardiac glycosides and other drugs.

• Determine serum cholesterol level frequently during first few months of therapy and periodically thereafter.
• Drug therapy is most successful if used concomitantly with a diet and exercise program.
• Monitor bowel habits; treat constipation promptly by decreasing dosage, increasing fluid intake, adding a stool softener, or discontinuing drug.
• Monitor for signs of vitamin A, D, or K deficiency.

Patient education
• Explain disease process and rationale for therapy and encourage patient to comply with continued blood testing and special diet; although therapy isn't curative, it helps control serum cholesterol level.
• Teach patient how to administer drug. Other drugs should be taken at least 1 hour before or 4 hours after colestipol.

Overdose & treatment
• In the case of overdose, the chief risk is intestinal obstruction; treatment depends on location and degree of obstruction and on amount of gut motility.

co-trimoxazole (trimethoprim-sulfamethoxazole)
Apo-Sulfatrim*, Bactrim, Bactrim DS, Bactrim I.V., Cotrim, Cotrim D.S., Novo-Trimel*, Roubac*, Septra, Septra DS, Septra I.V., SMZ-TMP, Sulfatrim

Sulfonamide and folate antagonist, antibiotic

Available by prescription only
Tablets: trimethoprim 80 mg and sulfamethoxazole 400 mg; trimethoprim 160 mg and sulfamethoxazole 800 mg
Suspension: trimethoprim 40 mg and sulfamethoxazole 200 mg/5 ml
Injectable: trimethoprim 80 mg and sulfamethoxazole 400 mg/5 ml

INDICATIONS & DOSAGE
Urinary tract infections and shigellosis

Adults: 1 double-strength tablet or 2 regular-strength tablets P.O. q 12 hours for 10 to 14 days or 5 days for shigellosis. Or, 8 to 10 mg/kg (based on trimethoprim) I.V. daily given in 2 to 4 equally divided doses for up to 14 days (5 days for shigellosis). Maximum daily dosage is 960 mg.
Pneumocystis carinii *pneumonitis*
Adults: 15 to 20 mg/kg trimethoprim and 75 to 100 mg/kg sulfamethoxazole P.O. daily, in equally divided doses, q 6 to 8 hours for 14 to 21 days.
Chronic bronchitis
Adults: 1 double-strength tablet or 2 regular-strength tablets q 12 hours for 14 days.
Traveler's diarrhea
Adults: 1 double-strength tablet or 2 regular-strength tablets q 12 hours for 5 days.
   Note: For the following unlabeled uses, dosages refer to oral trimethoprim (as co-trimoxazole).
◊ *Septic agranulocytosis*
Adults: 2.5 mg/kg I.V. q.i.d.; for prophylaxis, 80 to 160 mg b.i.d.
◊ *Nocardia infection*
Adults: 640 mg P.O. daily for 7 months.
◊ *Pharyngeal gonococcal infections*
Adults: 720 mg P.O. daily for 5 days.
◊ *Chancroid*
Adults: 160 mg P.O. b.i.d for 7 days.
◊ *Pertussis*
Adults: 320 mg P.O. daily in two divided doses.
◊ *Cholera*
Adults: 160 mg P.O. b.i.d for 3 days.
◊ *Isosporiasis*
Adults: 160 mg P.O. q.i.d. for 10 days, followed by 160 mg b.i.d. for 3 weeks.
✦ *Dosage adjustment.* In patients with impaired renal function, adjust dosage or frequency of administration of parenteral form according to degree of renal impairment, severity of infection, and susceptibility of organism.

Creatinine clearance (ml/min/1.73 m^2)	Dosage in adults
> 30	Usual regimen
15-30	½ usual regimen
< 15	Use isn't recommended

PHARMACODYNAMICS

Antibacterial action: Co-trimoxazole is generally bactericidal; it sequentially blocks folic acid enzymes in the synthesis pathway. The sulfamethoxazole component inhibits formation of dihydrofolic acid from para-aminobenzoic (PABA), whereas trimethoprim inhibits dihydrofolate reductase. Both drugs block folic acid synthesis, preventing bacterial cell synthesis of essential nucleic acids.

Co-trimoxazole is effective against *Escherichia coli, Klebsiella, Enterobacter, Proteus mirabilis, Haemophilus influenzae, Streptococcus pneumoniae, Staphylococcus aureus, Acinetobacter, Salmonella, Shigella,* and *Pneumocystis carinii.*

PHARMACOKINETICS

Absorption: Co-trimoxazole is well absorbed from the GI tract after oral administration; serum levels peak in 1 to 4 hours.
Distribution: Drug is distributed widely into body tissues and fluids, including middle ear fluid, prostatic fluid, bile, aqueous humor, and CSF. About 44% of trimethoprim and 70% of sulfamethoxazole bind to protein.
Metabolism: Co-trimoxazole is metabolized in the liver.
Excretion: Both components of co-trimoxazole are excreted primarily in urine through glomerular filtration and renal tubular secretion. In patients with normal renal function, half-life of trimethoprim is 8 to 11 hours; in patients with severe renal dysfunction, 26 hours. In patients with normal renal function, plasma half-life of sulfamethoxazole is normally 10 to 13 hours; in patients with severe renal dysfunction, 30 to 40 hours. Hemodialysis removes some co-trimoxazole.

CONTRAINDICATIONS & PRECAUTIONS

Contraindicated in patients with hypersensitivity to trimethoprim or sulfonamides, severe renal impairment (creatinine clearance below 15 ml/minute), or porphyria and in patients with megaloblastic anemia caused by folate deficiency.

Use cautiously in patients with impaired renal or hepatic function, severe allergies, severe bronchial asthma, G6PD deficiency, or blood dyscrasia.

INTERACTIONS

Drug-drug. Use with *cyclosporine* may decrease the therapeutic effect of cyclosporine and increase risk of nephrotoxicity. Use with *methotrexate* can displace it from plasma-binding sites and increase drug levels. Co-trimoxazole may inhibit hepatic metabolism of *oral anticoagulants,* displacing them from binding sites and enhancing anticoagulant effects. Use with *oral sulfonylureas* enhances their hypoglycemic effects, probably by displacement of sulfonylureas from protein-binding sites. Use with *PABA* antagonizes sulfonamide effects. Use may decrease hepatic clearance of *phenytoin* (27%) and prolong the half-life (39%). Serum levels of *zidovudine* may be increased as a result of reduced renal clearance.

ADVERSE REACTIONS

CNS: headache, mental depression, aseptic meningitis, tinnitus, apathy, *seizures,* hallucinations, ataxia, nervousness, fatigue, muscle weakness, vertigo, insomnia.
CV: thrombophlebitis.
GI: *nausea, vomiting, diarrhea,* abdominal pain, anorexia, stomatitis, *pancreatitis,* pseudomembranous colitis.
GU: *toxic nephrosis with oliguria and anuria,* crystalluria, hematuria, interstitial nephritis.
Hematologic: *agranulocytosis, aplastic anemia,* megaloblastic anemia, *thrombocytopenia, leukopenia, hemolytic anemia.*
Hepatic: jaundice, *hepatic necrosis,* elevated liver function test results.
Musculoskeletal: arthralgia, myalgia.
Respiratory: pulmonary infiltrates.
Skin: *erythema multiforme (Stevens-Johnson syndrome),* generalized skin eruptions, *epidermal necrolysis, exfoliative dermatitis,* photosensitivity, urticaria, pruritus.
Other: hypersensitivity reactions (*serum sickness, drug fever, anaphylaxis*).

◫ KEY CONSIDERATIONS

Besides the recommendations relevant to all sulfonamides, consider the following:

• In geriatric patients, diminished renal function may prolong half-life. Such patients also have an increased risk of adverse reactions. Therefore, the drug may need to be given at a lower dosage and/or less frequently.

• Co-trimoxazole has been used effectively to treat chronic bacterial prostatitis and traveler's diarrhea and to prevent recurrent urinary tract infection in women.

• For I.V. use, dilute infusion in D_5W. Don't mix with other drugs. Don't administer by rapid infusion or bolus injection. Infuse slowly over 60 to 90 minutes. Change infusion site every 48 to 72 hours.

• I.V. infusion must be diluted before use. Each 5 ml should be added to 125 ml D_5W. Don't refrigerate solution; diluted solutions must be used within 6 hours. A dilution of 5 ml /75 ml D_5W may be prepared for patients requiring fluid restriction, but these solutions should be used within 2 hours.

• Check solution carefully for precipitate before starting infusion. Don't use solution containing a precipitate.

• Assess I.V. site for signs of phlebitis or infiltration.

• Shake oral suspension thoroughly before administering.

• Note that DS means double-strength.

• Trimethoprim can interfere with serum methotrexate assay as determined by the competitive binding protein technique. No interference occurs if radioimmunoassay is used.

Patient education

• Inform patient of potential adverse reactions.

Overdose & treatment

• Signs and symptoms of overdose include mental depression, drowsiness, anorexia, jaundice, confusion, headache, nausea, vomiting, diarrhea, facial swelling, slight elevations in liver function test results, and bone marrow depression.

• Treat by inducing vomiting or by administering gastric lavage, followed by supportive care (correction of acidosis, forced oral fluid, and I.V. fluids). Treatment of renal failure may be required; transfuse appropriate blood products in severe hematologic toxicity; use folinic acid to rescue bone marrow. Hemodialysis has limited ability to remove co-trimoxazole.

---

cromolyn sodium

Gastrocrom, Intal Aerosol Spray, Intal Nebulizer Solution, Nasalcrom, Opticrom

Chromone derivative, mast cell stabilizer, antasthmatic

Available by prescription only
Capsules: 100 mg
Aerosol: 800 mcg/metered spray
Solution: 20 mg/2 ml for nebulization
Ophthalmic solution: 4%
Nasal solution: 5.2 mg/metered spray (40 mg/ml)
Powder for inhalation: 20 mg (in capsules)

INDICATIONS & DOSAGE

Adjunct in treatment of severe perennial bronchial asthma

Adults: 2 inhalations q.i.d. at regular intervals; aqueous solution administered through a nebulizer, 1 ampule q.i.d; or, 1 capsule (20 mg) of powder for inhalation q.i.d.

Prevention and treatment of allergic rhinitis

Adults: 1 spray (5.2 mg) of nasal solution in each nostril t.i.d or q.i.d. May give up to six times daily.

Prevention of exercise-induced bronchospasm

Adults: 2 metered sprays using inhaler, or 1 capsule (20 mg) of powder for inhalation no more than 1 hour before anticipated exercise.

Inhalation of 20 mg of oral inhalation solution may be used in adults. Repeat inhalation as required for protection during long exercise.

Allergic ocular disorders (giant papillary conjunctivitis, vernal keratoconjunctivitis, vernal keratitis, allergic keratoconjunctivitis)

Adults: Instill 1 or 2 drops in each eye four to six times daily at regular intervals. 1 drop contains about 1.6 mg cromolyn sodium.

Systemic mastocytosis
Adults: 200 mg P.O. q.i.d.

◊ **Food allergy, inflammatory bowel disease**
Adults: 200 mg P.O. q.i.d. 15 to 20 minutes before meals.

PHARMACODYNAMICS

Antasthmatic action: Cromolyn prevents release of the mediators of type I allergic reactions, including histamine and slow-reacting substance of anaphylaxis (SRS-A), from sensitized mast cells after the antigen-antibody union has taken place. Cromolyn doesn't inhibit the binding of the immunoglobulin E (IgE) to the mast cell nor the interaction between the cell-bound IgE and the specific antigen. It does inhibit the release of substances (such as histamine and SRS-A) in response to the IgE binding to the mast cell. The main site of action occurs locally on the lung mucosa, nasal mucosa, and eyes.

Bronchodilating action: Besides the mast cell stabilization, recent evidence suggests that drug may have a bronchodilating effect by an unknown mechanism. Comparative studies have shown cromolyn and theophylline to be equally efficacious but less effective than orally inhaled beta$_2$ agonists in preventing this bronchospasm.

Ocular antiallergy action: Cromolyn inhibits the degranulation of sensitized mast cells that occurs after exposure to specific antigens, preventing the release of histamine and SRS-A.

Cromolyn has no direct antihistamine, anti-inflammatory, vasoconstrictor, antiserotonin, or corticosteroid-like properties.

Cromolyn dissolved in water and given orally has been found to be effective in managing food allergy, inflammatory bowel disease (Crohn's disease, ulcerative colitis), and systemic mastocytosis.

PHARMACOKINETICS

Absorption: Only 0.5% to 2% of an oral dose is absorbed. The amount reaching the lungs depends on patient's ability to use inhaler correctly, amount of bronchoconstriction, and size or presence of mucus plugs. The degree of absorption depends on method of administration; most absorption occurs with the aerosol via metered-dose inhaler, and least occurs with the administration of the solution via power-operated nebulizer. Less than 7% of an intranasal dose of cromolyn as a solution is absorbed systemically. Only minimal absorption (0.03%) of an ophthalmic dose occurs after instillation into the eye. Absorption half-life from the lung is 1 hour. A plasma level of 9 ng/ml can be achieved 15 minutes after following a 20-mg dose.

Distribution: Drug doesn't cross most biological membranes because it's ionized and lipid-insoluble at the body's pH.

Metabolism: None significant.

Excretion: About 50% of drug is excreted unchanged in urine; about 50%, in bile. A small amount may be excreted in feces or exhaled. Elimination half-life is 81 minutes.

CONTRAINDICATIONS & PRECAUTIONS

Contraindicated in patients experiencing acute asthma attacks or status asthmaticus and in patients with hypersensitivity to cromolyn. Use inhalation form cautiously in patients with cardiac disease or arrhythmias.

INTERACTIONS

None reported.

ADVERSE REACTIONS

CNS: dizziness, headache.

EENT: *irritated throat and trachea,* nasal congestion, pharyngeal irritation, *sneezing,* nasal burning and irritation, epistaxis, lacrimation, swollen parotid gland, bad taste in mouth.

GI: nausea, esophagitis, abdominal pain.

GU: dysuria, urinary frequency.

Musculoskeletal: joint swelling and pain.

Respiratory: *bronchospasm* (after inhalation of dry powder), *cough,* wheezing, *eosinophilic pneumonia.*

Skin: rash, urticaria.

Other: *angioedema.*

KEY CONSIDERATIONS
• Monitor pulmonary status before and immediately after therapy.
• Bronchospasm or cough occasionally occur after inhalation and may require stopping therapy. Prior bronchodilation may help but it may still be necessary to stop the cromolyn therapy.
• Asthma symptoms may recur if cromolyn dosage is reduced below the recommended dosage.
• Use reduced dosage in patients with impaired renal or hepatic function.
• Eosinophilic pneumonia or pulmonary infiltrates with eosinophilia requires stopping drug.
• Nasal solution may cause nasal stinging or sneezing immediately after instillation of drug but this reaction rarely requires discontinuation of drug.
• Watch for recurrence of asthmatic symptoms when corticosteroids are also used. Use only when acute episode has been controlled, airway is cleared, and patient is able to inhale.
• Perform pulmonary function tests to confirm significant bronchodilator-reversible component of airway obstruction in patients considered for cromolyn therapy.
• Protect oral solution and ophthalmic solution from direct sunlight.
• Therapeutic effects may not be seen for 2 to 4 weeks after initiating therapy.

Patient education
• Teach correct use of metered-dose inhaler: Exhale completely before placing mouthpiece between lips, then inhale deeply and slowly with steady, even breath; remove inhaler from mouth, hold breath for 5 to 10 seconds, and exhale.
• Urge patient to call health care provider if drug causes wheezing or coughing.
• Instruct patient with asthma or seasonal or perennial allergic rhinitis to administer drug at regular intervals to ensure effectiveness.
• Advise patient that gargling and rinsing mouth after administration can help reduce mouth dryness.
• Tell patient taking prescribed adrenocorticoids to continue taking them during therapy, if appropriate.

• Instruct patient who uses a bronchodilator inhaler to administer dose 5 minutes before taking cromolyn (unless otherwise indicated); explain that this step helps reduce adverse reactions.

cyanocobalamin (vitamin B$_{12}$)
Bedoz,* Cobex, Crystamine, Cyanoject, Cyomin, Rubesol-1000, Rubramin PC, Vibal

hydroxocobalamin (vitamin B$_{12}$)
Hydrobexan, Hydro-Cobex, LA-12

Water-soluble vitamin, nutrition supplement

Available by prescription only
Injection: 30-ml vials (30 mcg/ml, 100 mcg/ml, 120 mcg/ml with benzyl alcohol, 1,000 mcg/ml, 1,000 mcg/ml with benzyl alcohol), 10-ml vials (100 mcg/ml, 100 mcg/ml with benzyl alcohol, 1,000 mcg/ml, 1,000 mcg/ml with benzyl alcohol, 1,000 mcg/ml with methyl and propyl parabens), 5-ml vials (1,000 mcg/ml with benzyl alcohol), 1-ml vials (1,000 mcg/ml with benzyl alcohol), 1-ml unimatic (1,000 mcg/ml with benzyl alcohol)
Tablets: 25 mcg, 50 mcg, 100 mcg, 250 mcg, 500 mcg, 1,000 mcg

INDICATIONS & DOSAGE
Vitamin B$_{12}$ deficiency from any cause except malabsorption related to pernicious anemia or other GI disease
Adults: 25 mcg P.O. daily as dietary supplement, or 30 to 100 mcg S.C. or I.M. daily for 5 to 10 days, depending on severity of deficiency. (I.M. route recommended for pernicious anemia.)
    Maintenance dosage is 100 to 200 mcg I.M. monthly. For subsequent prophylaxis, advise adequate nutrition and daily RDA vitamin B$_{12}$ supplements.
Diagnostic test for vitamin B$_{12}$ deficiency without concealing folate deficiency in patients with megaloblastic anemias
Adults: 1 mcg I.M. daily for 10 days with diet low in vitamin B$_{12}$ and folate. Reticulocytosis between days 3 and 10

confirms diagnosis of vitamin B_{12} deficiency.
Schilling test flushing dose
Adults: 1,000 mcg I.M. in a single dose.

PHARMACODYNAMICS
Nutritional action: Vitamin B_{12} can be converted to coenzyme B_{12} in tissues and, as such, is essential for conversion of methylmalonate to succinate and synthesis of methionine from homocystine, a reaction that also requires folate. Without coenzyme B_{12}, folate deficiency occurs. Vitamin B_{12} is also associated with fat and carbohydrate metabolism and protein synthesis. Cells characterized by rapid division (epithelial cells, bone marrow, and myeloid cells) appear to have the greatest requirement for vitamin B_{12}.

Vitamin B_{12} deficiency may cause megaloblastic anemia, GI lesions, and neurologic damage; it begins with an inability to produce myelin followed by gradual degeneration of the axon and nerve. Parenteral administration of vitamin B_{12} completely reverses the megaloblastic anemia and GI symptoms of vitamin B_{12} deficiency.

PHARMACOKINETICS
Absorption: After oral administration, vitamin B_{12} is absorbed irregularly from the distal small intestine. Vitamin B_{12} binds to proteins, and this bond must be split by proteolysis and gastric acid before absorption. Absorption depends on sufficient intrinsic factor and calcium. Vitamin B_{12} is inadequate in malabsorptive states and in pernicious anemia. Vitamin B_{12} is absorbed rapidly from I.M. and S.C. injection sites; the plasma level peaks within 1 hour. After oral administration of doses below 3 mcg, plasma levels don't peak for 8 to 12 hours.
Distribution: Vitamin B_{12} is distributed into the liver, bone marrow, and other tissues. Unlike cyanocobalamin, hydroxocobalamin is absorbed more slowly parenterally and may be taken up by the liver in larger quantities; it also produces a greater increase in serum cobalamin levels and less urine excretion.

Metabolism: Cyanocobalamin and hydroxocobalamin are metabolized in the liver.
Excretion: In healthy persons receiving only dietary vitamin B_{12}, 3 to 8 mcg of the vitamin is secreted into the GI tract daily, mainly from bile, and all but about 1 mcg is reabsorbed; less than 0.25 mcg is usually excreted in the urine daily. When vitamin B_{12} is administered in amounts that exceed the binding capacity of plasma, the liver, and other tissues, it's free in the blood for urine excretion.

CONTRAINDICATIONS & PRECAUTIONS
Contraindicated in patients hypersensitive to vitamin B_{12} or cobalt and in patients with early Leber's disease. Use cautiously in anemic patients with coexisting cardiac, pulmonary, or hypertensive disease and in those with severe vitamin B_{12}–dependent deficiencies.

INTERACTIONS
Drug-drug. Use of the following drugs decreases vitamin B_{12} absorption from the GI tract: *aminoglycosides, aminosalicylic acid and its salts, anticonvulsants, cobalt irradiation* of the small bowel, *colchicine,* and *extended-release potassium preparations.* A large amount of *ascorbic acid* shouldn't be administered within 1 hour of taking vitamin B_{12} because ascorbic acid may destroy vitamin B_{12}; in patients with pernicious anemia, vitamin B_{12} absorption and intrinsic factor secretion may be increased. Vitamin B_{12} and *chloramphenicol* shouldn't be given concurrently because of an antagonized hematopoietic response; careful monitoring of the hematologic response and alternate therapy is necessary. Administration with *colchicine* may increase *neomycin*-induced malabsorption of vitamin B_{12}.
Drug-lifestyle. *Alcohol* decreases vitamin B_{12} absorption from the GI tract. *Smoking* increases requirement for vitamin B_{12}.

ADVERSE REACTIONS
CV: peripheral vascular thrombosis, ***pulmonary edema, heart failure.***
GI: transient diarrhea.

Skin: itching, transitory exanthema, urticaria.

Other: ***anaphylaxis, anaphylactoid reactions*** (with parenteral administration); pain, burning (at S.C. or I.M. injection sites).

▣ KEY CONSIDERATIONS

• Recommended RDA for vitamin B_{12} is 2 mcg in adults.

• To identify poor nutritional habits, obtain patient's diet and drug history, including patterns of alcohol use.

• Oral solution should be administered promptly after mixing with fruit juice. Ascorbic acid makes vitamin B_{12} unstable.

• To increase absorption, administer oral vitamin B_{12} with food.

• Monitor bowel function because regularity is essential for consistent absorption of oral preparations.

• Don't mix the parenteral form with dextrose solutions, alkaline or strongly acidic solutions, or oxidizing and reducing drugs, because anaphylactic reactions may occur with I.V. use. Check compatibility with pharmacist.

• Protect solutions from light.

• Parenteral therapy is preferred for patients with pernicious anemia because oral administration may be unreliable. In patients with neurologic complications, prolonged inadequate oral therapy may lead to permanent spinal cord damage. Oral therapy is appropriate for mild conditions without neurologic signs and for those patients who refuse or are sensitive to the parenteral form.

• Monitor vital signs in patients with cardiac disease and those receiving parenteral vitamin B_{12}. Watch for symptoms of pulmonary edema, which tend to develop early in therapy.

• Patients with a history of sensitivities and those suspected of being sensitive to vitamin B_{12} should receive an intradermal test dose before therapy begins. Sensitization to vitamin B_{12} may develop after as many as 8 years of treatment.

• Expect therapeutic response to occur within 48 hours; it's measured by laboratory values and effect on fatigue, GI symptoms, anorexia, pallid or yellow complexion, glossitis, distaste for meat,

dyspnea on exertion, palpitation, neurologic degeneration (paresthesia, loss of vibratory and position sense and deep reflexes, incoordination), psychotic behavior, anosmia, and visual disturbances.

• Therapeutic response to vitamin B_{12} may be impaired by concurrent infection, uremia, folic acid or iron deficiency, or drugs having bone marrow suppressant effects. Large doses of vitamin B_{12} may improve folate-deficient megaloblastic anemia.

• Expect reticulocyte count to rise in 3 to 4 days, peak in 5 to 8 days, and then gradually decline as erythrocyte count and hemoglobin level rise to normal (in 4 to 6 weeks).

• Monitor potassium levels during the first 48 hours, especially in patients with pernicious anemia or megaloblastic anemia. Potassium supplements may be required. Conversion to normal erythropoiesis increases erythrocyte potassium requirement and can result in fatal hypokalemia in these patients.

• Patients with mild peripheral neurological defects may respond to concomitant physical therapy. Usually, neurologic damage that doesn't improve after 12 to 18 months of therapy is considered irreversible. Severe vitamin B_{12} deficiency that persists for 3 months or longer may cause permanent spinal cord degeneration.

• Continue periodic hematologic evaluations throughout patient's lifetime.

• Vitamin B_{12} therapy may cause false-positive results for intrinsic factor antibodies, which are present in the blood of half of all patients with pernicious anemia.

• Methotrexate, pyrimethamine, and most anti-infectives invalidate diagnostic blood assays for vitamin B_{12}.

Patient education

• Emphasize importance of a well-balanced diet. To prevent progression of subacute combined degeneration, don't use folic acid instead of vitamin B_{12} to prevent anemia.

• Tell patient to avoid smoking, which appears to increase requirement for vita-

---

Reactions may be *common*, uncommon, ***life-threatening***, or COMMON AND LIFE-THREATENING.

min B$_{12}$, and alcohol use, which decreases absorption of vitamin B$_{12}$.
• Instruct patient to report infection or disease in case his condition requires increased dosage of vitamin B$_{12}$.
• Tell patient with pernicious anemia that he must have lifelong treatment with vitamin B$_{12}$ to prevent recurring symptoms and the risk of incapacitating and irreversible spinal cord damage.
• Inform patient to store tablets in a tightly closed container at room temperature.

cyclobenzaprine hydrochloride
Flexeril

Tricyclic antidepressant derivative, skeletal muscle relaxant

Available by prescription only
Tablets: 10 mg

INDICATIONS & DOSAGE
Adjunct in acute, painful musculoskeletal conditions
Adults: 20 to 40 mg P.O. divided b.i.d. to q.i.d.; maximum dosage, 60 mg daily. Drug shouldn't be administered for more than 2 weeks.
◊ *Fibrositis*
Adults: 10 to 40 mg P.O. daily.

PHARMACODYNAMICS
Skeletal muscle relaxant action: Cyclobenzaprine relaxes skeletal muscles through an unknown mechanism of action. Cyclobenzaprine is a CNS depressant.

Drug also potentiates the effects of norepinephrine and exhibits anticholinergic effects similar to those of tricyclic antidepressants, including central and peripheral antimuscarinic actions, sedation, and increased heart rate.

PHARMACOKINETICS
Absorption: Cyclobenzaprine is almost completely absorbed during first pass through GI tract. Onset of action occurs within 1 hour, with levels peaking in 3 to 8 hours. Duration of action is 12 to 24 hours.

Distribution: About 93% binds to plasma proteins.
Metabolism: During first pass through GI tract and liver, drug and metabolites undergo enterohepatic recycling. The half-life of cyclobenzaprine is 1 to 3 days.
Excretion: Drug is excreted primarily in urine as conjugated metabolites; also in feces via bile as unchanged drug.

CONTRAINDICATIONS & PRECAUTIONS
Contraindicated in patients who have received MAO inhibitors within 14 days, who are in the acute recovery phase of an MI, or who have hyperthyroidism, hypersensitivity to drug, heart block, arrhythmias, conduction disturbances, or heart failure. Use cautiously in geriatric patients, especially those who are debilitated or who have increased intraocular pressure, glaucoma, or urine retention.

INTERACTIONS
Drug-drug. Antimuscarinic effects may be potentiated when cyclobenzaprine is used with *antidyskinetics* or *antimuscarinics* (especially *atropine and related compounds*). Use with *CNS depressants*—including *antipsychotics, anxiolytics, narcotics, parenteral magnesium salts,* and *tricyclic antidepressants*—may potentiate the effects of the CNS depressant. Cyclobenzaprine may decrease or block the antihypertensive effects of *guanadrel* or *guanethidine.*

Use with *MAO inhibitors* isn't recommended for outpatients. Hyperpyretic crisis, severe seizures, and death have resulted from the tricyclic antidepressant–like effect of cyclobenzaprine. Wait 14 days after discontinuing *MAO inhibitor* therapy before starting cyclobenzaprine and 5 to 7 days after discontinuing cyclobenzaprine therapy before starting an MAO inhibitor.
Drug-lifestyle. *Alcohol* use may potentiate the CNS depressant effects.

ADVERSE REACTIONS
CNS: *drowsiness,* headache, insomnia, fatigue, asthenia, nervousness, confusion, paresthesia, *dizziness,* depression, visual disturbances, ***seizures.***

CV: tachycardia, syncope, *arrhythmias,* palpitations, hypotension, vasodilation.
EENT: blurred vision, *dry mouth.*
GI: dyspepsia, abnormal taste, constipation, nausea.
GU: urine retention, urinary frequency.
Skin: rash, urticaria, pruritus.
Other: with high dosages, watch for adverse reactions similar to those of other tricyclic antidepressants.

◻ **KEY CONSIDERATIONS**
• Geriatric patients are more sensitive to drug's effects; monitor closely.
• Drug may cause effects and adverse reactions similar to those of tricyclic antidepressants.
• Note that drug's antimuscarinic effect may inhibit salivary flow, resulting in development of dental caries, periodontal disease, oral candidiasis, and mouth discomfort.
• Allow 14 days to elapse after discontinuance of MAO inhibitors before starting cyclobenzaprine; 5 to 7 days after discontinuing cyclobenzaprine before starting MAO inhibitors.
• Monitor patient for GI problems.
• Drug is intended for short-term (2- to 3-week) treatment, because risk-benefit ratio associated with prolonged use is unknown. Additionally, muscle spasm accompanying acute musculoskeletal conditions is usually transient.
• Spasmolytic effect usually begins within 1 to 2 days, with a lessening of pain and tenderness and an increase in range of motion and ability to perform activities of daily living.

Patient education
• Warn patient about possible drowsiness and dizziness. Tell him to avoid hazardous activities that require alertness until reaction to drug is known.
• Instruct patient to avoid alcohol and other CNS depressants (unless prescribed), because combined use with drug causes additive effects.
• Advise patient to relieve dry mouth (anticholinergic effect) with frequent clear water rinses, extra fluid intake, or with sugarless gum or candy.
• Tell patient to report discomfort immediately.

• Inform patient to use cough and cold preparations cautiously because some products contain alcohol.
• Instruct patient to check with dentist to minimize risk of dental disease (tooth decay, fungal infections, or gum disease) if treatment lasts longer than 2 weeks.

Overdose & treatment
• Signs and symptoms of overdose include severe drowsiness, troubled breathing, syncope, seizures, tachycardia, arrhythmias, hallucinations, altered body temperature, and vomiting.
• To treat overdose, induce vomiting or perform gastric lavage. As ordered, give 20 to 30 g activated charcoal every 4 to 6 hours for 24 to 48 hours. Take ECG and monitor cardiac functions for arrhythmias. Monitor vital signs, especially body temperature and ECG. Maintain adequate airway and fluid intake. If needed, 1 to 3 mg I.V. physostigmine may be given to combat severe life-threatening antimuscarinic effects. Provide supportive therapy for arrhythmias, cardiac failure, circulatory shock, seizures, and metabolic acidosis as necessary.

cyclophosphamide
Cytoxan, Neosar

Alkylating drug (cell cycle–phase nonspecific), antineoplastic

Available by prescription only
Tablets: 25 mg, 50 mg
Injection: 100-mg, 200-mg, 500-mg, 1-g, and 2-g vials

INDICATIONS & DOSAGE
Dosage and indications may vary. Check literature for recommended protocols.
Breast, head, neck, lung, and ovarian cancer; Hodgkin's disease; chronic lymphocytic or myelocytic and acute lymphoblastic leukemia; neuroblastoma; retinoblastoma; malignant lymphomas; multiple myeloma; mycosis fungoides; sarcomas; severe rheumatoid disorders; immunosuppression after transplants

---

Reactions may be *common,* uncommon, *life-threatening,* or COMMON AND LIFE-THREATENING.

Adults: 40 to 50 mg/kg I.V. in divided doses over 2 to 5 days. Oral dosing for initial and maintenance dosage is 1 to 5 mg/kg P.O. daily.

◇ *Polymyositis*
Adults: 1 to 2 mg/kg P.O. daily.

◇ *Rheumatoid arthritis*
Adults: 1.5 to 3 mg/kg P.O. daily.

◇ *Wegener's granulomatosis*
Adults: 1 to 2 mg/kg P.O. daily (usually administered with prednisone).

PHARMACODYNAMICS

Antineoplastic action: Cytotoxic action of cyclophosphamide is mediated by its two active metabolites. These metabolites function as alkylating agents, preventing cell division by cross-linking DNA strands. This results in an imbalance of growth within the cell, leading to cell death. Cyclophosphamide also has significant immunosuppressive activity.

PHARMACOKINETICS

Absorption: Cyclophosphamide is almost completely absorbed from the GI tract at doses of 100 mg or less. Higher doses (300 mg) are about 75% absorbed.
Distribution: Drug is distributed throughout the body, although only minimal amounts have been found in saliva, sweat, and synovial fluid. The drug level in the CSF is too low for treatment of meningeal leukemia. The active metabolites are about 50% bound to plasma proteins.
Metabolism: Metabolized to its active form by hepatic microsomal enzymes. The activity of these metabolites is terminated by metabolism to inactive forms.
Excretion: Drug and its metabolites are eliminated primarily in urine, with 15% to 30% excreted as unchanged drug. The elimination half-life ranges from 3 to 12 hours.

CONTRAINDICATIONS & PRECAUTIONS

Contraindicated in patients with hypersensitivity to cyclophosphamide or with severe bone marrow suppression. Use cautiously in patients with impaired renal or hepatic function, leukopenia, thrombocytopenia, or malignant cell infiltration of bone marrow and in those who have recently undergone radiation therapy or chemotherapy.

INTERACTIONS

Drug-drug. *Allopurinol, chloramphenicol, chloroquine, imipramine, phenothiazines, potassium iodide,* and *vitamin A* may inhibit cyclophosphamide metabolism. Use with *barbiturates, chloral hydrate,* or *phenytoin* increases the rate at which cyclophosphamide is metabolized; these drugs are known to induce hepatic microsomal enzymes. *Corticosteroids* are known to initially inhibit the metabolism of cyclophosphamide, reducing its effect; eventual reduction of dose or discontinuation of steroids may increase metabolism of cyclophosphamide to a toxic level. Use may potentiate the cardiotoxic effects of *doxorubicin.*

Because cyclophosphamide depresses the activity of pseudocholinesterases, the enzyme responsible for the inactivation of succinylcholine, patients on cyclophosphamide therapy who receive *succinylcholine* as an adjunct to anesthesia may experience prolonged respiratory distress and apnea up to several days after the discontinuation of cyclophosphamide. Use succinylcholine with caution or not at all.

ADVERSE REACTIONS

CV: *cardiotoxicity* (with very high doses and with doxorubicin).
GI: anorexia, *nausea, vomiting* (within 6 hours); abdominal pain, stomatitis, mucositis.
GU: HEMORRHAGIC CYSTITIS, fertility impairment.
Hematologic: *leukopenia,* nadir between days 8 to 15, recovery in 17 to 28 days; *thrombocytopenia, anemia.*
Hepatic: *hepatotoxicity.*
Metabolic: increased serum uric acid levels, decreased serum pseudocholinesterase levels.
Respiratory: *pulmonary fibrosis* (with high doses).
Skin: *reversible alopecia.*
Other: *secondary malignant disease, anaphylaxis, hypersensitivity reactions.*

▣ KEY CONSIDERATIONS

- Follow institutional guidelines for safe preparation, administration, and disposal of chemotherapeutic drugs.
- Reconstitute vials with appropriate volume of bacteriostatic or sterile water for injection to give a concentration of 20 mg/ml.
- Reconstituted solution is stable 6 days if refrigerated or 24 hours at room temperature.
- Drug can be given by direct I.V. push into a running I.V. line or by infusion in normal saline solution or D₅W.
- Avoid all I.M. injections when platelet counts are low.
- Oral drugs should be taken with or after a meal. Higher oral doses (400 mg) may be tolerated better if divided into smaller doses.
- Administration with cold foods such as ice cream may improve toleration of oral dose.
- To prevent hemorrhagic cystitis, push fluid (3 qt [3 L] daily). Some health care providers use uroprotective agents such as mesna. Drug shouldn't be given at bedtime, because voiding afterward is too infrequent to avoid cystitis. If hemorrhagic cystitis occurs, discontinue drug. Cystitis can occur months after therapy has been discontinued.
- Reduce drug dosage if patient is also receiving corticosteroid therapy and develops viral or bacterial infections.
- Monitor for cyclophosphamide toxicity if patient's corticosteroid therapy is discontinued.
- Monitor uric acid, CBC, and renal and hepatic functions.
- Observe for hematuria and ask patient if he has dysuria.
- Nausea and vomiting are most common with high doses of I.V. cyclophosphamide.
- Drug has been used successfully to treat many nonmalignant conditions (for example, multiple sclerosis) because of its immunosuppressive activity.
- Drug may suppress positive reaction to *Candida*, mumps, trichophytin, and tuberculin TB skin tests.
- A false-positive result for the Papanicolaou test may occur.

Patient education

- Emphasize importance of continuing drug therapy despite nausea and vomiting.
- Advise patient to report vomiting that occurs shortly after an oral dose.
- Warn patient that alopecia is likely to occur, but that it's reversible.
- Encourage adequate fluid intake to prevent hemorrhagic cystitis and to facilitate uric acid excretion.
- Tell patient to promptly report unusual bleeding or bruising.
- Advise patient to avoid individuals with infections and to call immediately if fever, chills, or signs or symptoms of infection occur.

Overdose & treatment

- Signs and symptoms of overdose include myelosuppression, alopecia, nausea, vomiting, and anorexia.
- Treatment is generally supportive and includes transfusion of blood components and antiemetics. Drug is dialyzable.

cyclosporine
Neoral, Sandimmune

Polypeptide antibiotic, immunosuppressant

Available by prescription only
Capsules: 25 mg, 50 mg, 100 mg
Oral solution: 100 mg/ml
Capsules for microemulsion: 25 mg, 100 mg
Injection: 50 mg/ml

INDICATIONS & DOSAGE

Prophylaxis of organ rejection in kidney, liver, heart, bone marrow, ◊ pancreas, ◊ cornea transplants
Adults: 15 mg/kg P.O. daily 4 to 12 hours before transplantation. Continue daily dose postoperatively for 1 to 2 weeks. Then, gradually reduce dosage by 5% weekly to maintenance level of 5 to 10 mg/kg/day. Alternatively, administer an I.V. concentrate of 5 to 6 mg/kg 4 to 12 hours before transplantation.
    Postoperatively, administer 5 to 6 mg/kg daily as an I.V. dilute solution

infusion (50 mg/20 to 100 ml infused over 2 to 6 hours) until patient can tolerate oral forms.

Note: Sandimmune and Neoral aren't bioequivalent and can't be used interchangeably without health care provider's supervision. When converting to Neoral from Sandimmune, start with same daily dose (1:1) and follow serum trough levels frequently.

PHARMACODYNAMICS

Immunosuppressant action: Exact mechanism is unknown; purportedly, cyclosporine inhibits the induction of interleukin II, which plays a role in both cellular and humoral immune responses.

PHARMACOKINETICS

Absorption: Absorption after oral administration varies widely between patients and in the same individual. Only 30% of an oral dose reaches systemic circulation; levels peak in 3 to 4 hours. Neoral has a greater bioavailability than Sandimmune.

Distribution: Drug is distributed widely outside the blood volume. About 33% to 47% is found in plasma; 4% to 9%, in leukocytes; 5% to 12%, in granulocytes; and 41% to 58%, in erythrocytes. In plasma, about 90% binds to proteins, primarily lipoproteins.

Metabolism: Drug is metabolized extensively in the liver.

Excretion: Drug is primarily excreted in feces (biliary excretion) with only 6% of drug found in urine.

CONTRAINDICATIONS & PRECAUTIONS

Contraindicated in patients hypersensitive to cyclosporine or to polyoxyethylated castor oil (found in injectable form).

INTERACTIONS

Drug-drug. Use with *aminoglycosides* or *amphotericin B* is likely to increase nephrotoxicity because both drugs are nephrotoxic. *Amphotericin* may increase cyclosporine blood levels. Except for *corticosteroids*, cyclosporine shouldn't be used with *immunosuppressants* because of the increased risk of malignancy (lymphoma) and susceptibility to infection. *Diltiazem, erythromycin, flu-*

conazole, itraconazole, ketoconazole, ve-rapamil, and possibly *corticosteroids* impair hepatic enzyme metabolism and increase plasma cyclosporine levels; reduced dosage of cyclosporine may be necessary. *Co-trimoxazole, phenobarbital, phenytoin, rifampin* and increase hepatic metabolism and may lower plasma levels of cyclosporine.

Drug-food. Administration with *food* decreases the area under the curve and maximum cyclosporine levels. *Grapefruit juice* can increase trough levels of cyclosporine.

ADVERSE REACTIONS

CNS: *tremor, headache,* **seizures,** confusion, paresthesia.
CV: *hypertension.*
EENT: *gum hyperplasia,* oral candidiasis, sinusitis.
GI: *nausea, vomiting,* diarrhea, abdominal discomfort.
GU: NEPHROTOXICITY, gynecomastia.
Hematologic: anemia, *leukopenia, thrombocytopenia,* hemolytic anemia.
Hepatic: *hepatotoxicity.*
Skin: acne, flushing.
Other: increased low-density lipoprotein levels, *infections,* hirsutism, *anaphylaxis.*

▣ KEY CONSIDERATIONS

• Cyclosporine usually is prescribed with corticosteroids.
• Possible kidney rejection should be considered before drug is discontinued because of suspected nephrotoxicity.
• Monitor hepatic and renal function tests routinely; hepatotoxicity may occur in first month after transplantation, but renal toxicity may be delayed for 2 to 3 months.
• Dose should be given at same time each day. Oral solution should be measured carefully in oral syringe and mixed with plain or chocolate milk or fruit juice to increase palatability; it should be served in a glass to minimize drug adherence to container walls. Drug can be taken with food to minimize nausea.
• Neoral capsules and oral solution are bioequivalent. Sandimmune capsules and oral solution have decreased bioavailability compared with Neoral.

Patient education
• Teach patient about rationale for therapy; explain possible adverse effects and importance of reporting them, especially fever, sore throat, mouth sores, abdominal pain, unusual bleeding or bruising, pale stools, or dark urine.
• Encourage compliance with therapy and follow-up visits.
• Teach patient how and when to take drug for optimal benefit and minimal discomfort; caution against discontinuing drug without health care provider's approval.
• Advise patient to make oral solution more palatable by diluting with room temperature milk, chocolate milk, or orange juice. Don't use grapefruit juice or food when taking Neoral.
• Tell patient not to rinse syringe with water.

Overdose & treatment
• Signs and symptoms of overdose include extensions of common adverse effects. Hepatotoxicity and nephrotoxicity often accompany nausea and vomiting; tremor and seizures may occur.
• Up to 2 hours after ingestion, empty stomach by inducing vomiting or performing lavage; thereafter, treat supportively. Monitor vital signs and fluid and electrolyte levels closely. Neither hemodialysis nor charcoal hemoperfusion removes the drug.

cyproheptadine hydrochloride
Periactin

Piperidine-derivative antihistamine, H₁-receptor antagonist, antipruritic

Available by prescription only
Tablets: 4 mg
Syrup: 2 mg/5 ml

INDICATIONS & DOSAGE
Allergy symptoms, pruritus, cold urticaria, allergic conjunctivitis, appetite stimulant, vascular cluster headaches
Adults: 4 mg P.O. t.i.d. or q.i.d. Maximum dosage, 0.5 mg/kg daily.

◇ *Cushing's syndrome*
Adults: 8 to 24 mg P.O. daily in divided doses.

PHARMACODYNAMICS
Antihistamine action: Antihistamines compete with histamine for histamine H₁-receptor sites on smooth muscle of the bronchi, GI tract, uterus, and large blood vessels; they bind to cellular receptors, preventing access of histamine, thereby suppressing histamine-induced allergy symptoms. They don't directly alter histamine or its release.
   Drug also displays significant anticholinergic and antiserotonin activity.

PHARMACOKINETICS
Absorption: Cyproheptadine is well absorbed from the GI tract; peak action occurs in 6 to 9 hours.
Distribution: Unknown.
Metabolism: Drug appears to be almost completely metabolized in the liver.
Excretion: Drug's metabolites are excreted primarily in urine; unchanged drug isn't excreted in urine. A small amount of unchanged cyproheptadine and metabolites are excreted in feces.

CONTRAINDICATIONS & PRECAUTIONS
Contraindicated in patients with hypersensitivity to cyproheptadine or other drugs of similar chemical structure; in patients with acute asthma, angle-closure glaucoma, stenosing peptic ulcer, symptomatic prostatic hyperplasia, bladder neck obstruction, or pyloroduodenal obstruction; and in patients undergoing concurrent therapy with MAO inhibitors. Use cautiously in patients with increased intraocular pressure, hyperthyroidism, CV disease, hypertension, or bronchial asthma.

INTERACTIONS
Drug-drug. Additive sedative effects result when cyproheptadine is used concomitantly with other *CNS depressants,* such as *anxiolytics, barbiturates, sleeping aids,* and *tranquilizers. MAO inhibitors* interfere with the detoxification of cyproheptadine and thus prolong and intensify its central depressant and anticholinergic effects. Administration with

---

Reactions may be *common*, uncommon, *life-threatening*, or COMMON AND LIFE-THREATENING.

thyrotropin-releasing hormone may increase serum amylase and prolactin levels.

Drug-lifestyle. Use with *alcohol* causes additive sedative effects.

ADVERSE REACTIONS

CNS: *drowsiness,* dizziness, headache, fatigue, sedation, sleepiness, incoordination, confusion, restlessness, insomnia, nervousness, tremor, *seizures.*
CV: hypotension, palpitations, tachycardia.
GI: nausea, vomiting, epigastric distress, *dry mouth,* diarrhea, constipation.
GU: urine retention, urinary frequency.
Hematologic: *hemolytic anemia, leukopenia, agranulocytosis, thrombocytopenia.*
Metabolic: weight gain.
Skin: rash, urticaria, photosensitivity.
Other: *anaphylactic shock.*

▣ KEY CONSIDERATIONS

Besides the recommendations relevant to all antihistamines, consider the following:
• Geriatric patients are more susceptible to the sedative effect of drug. Instruct patient to change positions slowly and gradually. Geriatric patients may experience dizziness or hypotension more readily than younger patients.
• Drug can cause weight gain. Monitor weight.
• In some patients, sedative effect disappears within 3 to 4 days.
• Be aware to discontinue drug 4 days before diagnostic skin tests. Antihistamines can prevent, reduce, or mask positive skin test response.

Patient education
• Inform patient about potential adverse reactions.
• Advise patient to avoid alcohol while taking drug.

Overdose & treatment
• Signs and symptoms of overdose include those of CNS depression—such as sedation, reduced mental alertness, apnea, and CV collapse—and those of CNS stimulation—such as insomnia, hallucinations, tremors, and seizures.

Anticholinergic signs and symptoms—such as dry mouth, flushed skin, fixed and dilated pupils, and GI symptoms—are common.
• Treat overdose by inducing vomiting with ipecac syrup (in conscious patient), followed by activated charcoal to reduce further drug absorption. Use gastric lavage if patient is unconscious or ipecac fails. Treat hypotension with vasopressors, and control seizures with diazepam or phenytoin. Don't give stimulants.

daclizumab
Zenapax

Humanized immunoglobulin G1 monoclonal antibody, immunosuppressant

Available by prescription only
Injection (for I.V. use): 25 mg/5 ml

INDICATIONS & DOSAGE
Prophylaxis of acute organ rejection in patients receiving renal transplants
Adults: 1.0 mg/kg in 50 ml normal saline solution given I.V. over 15 minutes via a central or peripheral line. The standard course of therapy is five doses. Administer first dose no more than 24 hours before transplantation and the remaining four doses at 14-day intervals.

Drug is used as part of an immunosuppressive regimen that includes corticosteroids and cyclosporine.

PHARMACODYNAMICS
Immunosuppressive action: Daclizumab is an interleukin (IL)–2 receptor antagonist that binds to the 1-alpha Tac subunit of the IL-2 receptor complex and inhibits IL-2 binding. This effect prevents IL-2–mediated activation of lymphocytes, a critical pathway in the cellular immune response against allografts. Once in circulation, drug impairs the ability of the immune system to respond to antigenic challenges. After drug administration, the Tac subunit of the IL-2 receptor is saturated for about 120 days after transplantation.

PHARMACOKINETICS
Absorption: Serum daclizumab levels increase between first and fifth doses.
Distribution: Unknown.
Metabolism: Unknown, but given a known relationship between body weight and systemic clearance, dosing is based on mg/kg.
Excretion: Estimated terminal elimination half-life is 20 days (480 hours).

CONTRAINDICATIONS & PRECAUTIONS
Contraindicated in patients with a known hypersensitivity to daclizumab or any of its components.

It's unknown if drug has a long-term effect on the immune response to antigens first encountered during therapy. Readministration of drug after initial course of treatment hasn't been studied. The possible risks of prolonged immunosuppression, anaphylaxis, or anaphylactoid reactions haven't been identified.

INTERACTIONS
None reported.

ADVERSE REACTIONS
CNS: *tremor, headache, dizziness, insomnia,* generalized weakness, prickly sensation, *fever, pain, fatigue,* depression, anxiety.
CV: tachycardia, hypertension, *pulmonary edema,* hypotension, aggravated hypertension, *edema,* fluid overload, chest pain.
EENT: blurred vision, pharyngitis, rhinitis.
GI: constipation, nausea, diarrhea, vomiting, abdominal pain, dyspepsia, pyrosis, abdominal distention, epigastric pain, flatulence, gastritis, hemorrhoids.
GU: *oliguria, dysuria, renal tubular necrosis, renal damage,* urine retention, hydronephrosis, urinary tract bleeding, urinary tract disorder, *renal insufficiency.*
Hematologic: *lymphocele.*
Metabolic: diabetes mellitus, dehydration.
Musculoskeletal: *musculoskeletal or back pain,* arthralgia, myalgia, leg cramps.
Respiratory: *dyspnea, coughing,* atelectasis, congestion, **hypoxia,** crackles, abnormal breath sounds, pleural effusion.
Skin: *acne, impaired wound healing without infection,* pruritus, hirsutism, rash, night sweats, increased sweating.
Other: *posttraumatic pain,* shivering, extremity edema.

Reactions may be *common,* uncommon, *life-threatening,* or COMMON AND LIFE-THREATENING.

▣ KEY CONSIDERATIONS

• Use daclizumab cautiously in geriatric patients because of potential for prolonged immunosuppression and multiple adverse reactions.

• Only health care providers experienced in immunosuppressive therapy and management and follow-up of organ transplant patients should prescribe drug. Patients receiving drug should be managed in facilities equipped and staffed with adequate laboratory and supportive medical care.

• In clinical trials, lipoproliferative disorders and opportunistic infections occurred the same as with placebo. However, patients undergoing immunosuppressive therapy are at increased risk; monitor carefully.

• Drug isn't for direct injection.

• Other drugs shouldn't be added or infused simultaneously through the same I.V. line.

Patient education

• Tell patient to consult health care provider before taking other drugs during daclizumab therapy.

• Advise patient to take precautions to prevent infection.

• Inform patient that neither he nor any household member should receive vaccinations without health care provider's approval.

• Tell patient to immediately report wounds that fail to heal, unusual bruising or bleeding, or fever.

• Advise patient to drink plenty of fluids during drug therapy and to report painful urination, blood in the urine, or a decrease in urine amount.

dalteparin sodium
Fragmin

Low-molecular-weight heparin derivative, anticoagulant

Available by prescription only
Injection: 2,500 anti-factor Xa IU/0.2 ml, 5,000 anti-factor Xa IU/0.2 ml

INDICATIONS & DOSAGE

Prophylaxis against deep vein thrombosis (DVT) in patients undergoing abdominal surgery who aren't at risk for thromboembolic complications (including those who are older than age 40, obese, and undergoing general anesthesia lasting longer than 30 minutes and those who have a history of DVT or pulmonary embolism)

Adults: 2,500 IU S.C. daily, starting 1 to 2 hours before surgery and repeated once daily for 5 to 10 days postoperatively.

PHARMACODYNAMICS

Anticoagulant action: Dalteparin enhances the ability of antithrombin to inhibit factor Xa and thrombin.

PHARMACOKINETICS

Absorption: Absolute bioavailability of dalteparin measured in anti-factor Xa activity is about 87%.

Distribution: Volume of distribution for dalteparin anti-factor Xa activity is 40 to 60 ml/kg.

Metabolism: Unknown.

Excretion: Unknown.

CONTRAINDICATIONS & PRECAUTIONS

Contraindicated in patients with hypersensitivity to dalteparin, heparin, or pork products; active major bleeding; or thrombocytopenia associated with positive in vitro tests for antiplatelet antibody in the presence of drug.

Use with extreme caution in patients with history of heparin-induced thrombocytopenia and in those with increased risk of hemorrhage, such as those who have severe uncontrolled hypertension, bacterial endocarditis, congenital or acquired bleeding disorders, active ulceration and angiodysplastic GI disease, or hemorrhagic stroke or those who have recently undergone brain, spinal, or ophthalmic surgery. Use cautiously in patients with bleeding diathesis, thrombocytopenia, or platelet defects; severe liver or kidney insufficiency; hypertensive or diabetic retinopathy; and recent GI bleeding.

INTERACTIONS

Drug-drug. *Oral anticoagulants* or *platelet inhibitors* may increase risk of bleeding; use together with caution.

ADVERSE REACTIONS

Hematologic: *thrombocytopenia.*
Hepatic: falsely elevated AST and ALT levels.
Skin: pruritus, rash, *hematoma,* pain or skin necrosis (rare) (at injection site).
Other: hemorrhage, ecchymoses, bleeding complications, fever, *anaphylactoid reactions* (rare).

▣ KEY CONSIDERATIONS

• Patient should either sit or lie down when drug is administered. Drug should be injected deeply S.C. Injection sites include a U-shaped area around the navel, the upper outer side of the thigh, or the outer upper quadrant of the buttock. Sites should be rotated daily. Before injecting drug into the area around the navel or the thigh, lift up a fold of skin with the thumb and forefinger. The entire length of the needle should be inserted at a 45- to 90-degree angle.
• Dalteparin should never be administered I.M.
• Don't mix drug with other injections or infusions unless specific compatibility data are available that support such mixing.
• Drug isn't interchangeable (unit for unit) with unfractionated heparin or other low-molecular-weight heparins.
• Periodic routine CBC, including platelet count, and stool occult blood tests are recommended during therapy. PT, INR, and PTT don't have to be regularly monitored.
• Monitor patient closely for thrombocytopenia.
• Discontinue drug if a thromboembolic event occurs despite dalteparin prophylaxis.

Patient education

• Instruct patient and his family to watch for signs of bleeding and report them immediately.
• Tell patient to avoid OTC drugs containing aspirin or other salicylates.

Overdose & treatment

• An overdose may cause hemorrhagic complications.
• To treat an overdose, slowly inject protamine sulfate (1% solution) I.V., at a dose of 1 mg protamine for every 100 anti-factor Xa IU of dalteparin given. A second infusion of 0.5 mg protamine sulfate/100 anti-factor Xa IU of dalteparin may be administered if the PTT measured 2 to 4 hours after the first infusion remains prolonged. Even with these additional doses of protamine sulfate, the PTT may remain more prolonged than would usually be found after administration of conventional heparin.

---

danaparoid sodium
Orgaran Injection

Glycosaminoglycuronan, antithrombotic

Available by prescription only
Ampule: 750 anti-Xa U/0.6 ml
Syringe: 750 anti-Xa U/0.6 ml

INDICATIONS & DOSAGE

Prophylaxis against postoperative deep vein thrombosis (DVT), which may lead to pulmonary embolism in patients undergoing elective hip replacement surgery
Adults: 750 anti-Xa U S.C. b.i.d. beginning 1 to 4 hours preoperatively; then no sooner than 2 hours after surgery. Continue treatment for 7 to 10 days postoperatively or until risk of DVT has diminished.

PHARMACODYNAMICS

Antithrombotic action: Danaparoid prevents fibrin formation by inhibiting generation of thrombin by anti-Xa and anti-IIa. Because of its predominant anti-Xa activity, danaparoid injection has little effect on clotting assays such as PT and PTT. Drug has only a minor effect on platelet function and platelet aggregability.

PHARMACOKINETICS

Because no specific chemical assay methods are available, the information in

---

this section describes the biological activity (plasma anti-Xa activity) of danaparoid.

Absorption: After S.C. administration, about 100% is bioavailable, compared with same dose administered I.V. Onset and duration are unknown. Peak anti-Xa activity occurs in 2 to 5 hours.

Distribution: Unknown.

Metabolism: Unknown.

Excretion: Drug is mainly eliminated through the kidneys. Mean value for the terminal half-life is about 24 hours. In patients with severely impaired renal function, elimination half-life of plasma anti-Xa activity may be prolonged.

CONTRAINDICATIONS & PRECAUTIONS

Contraindicated in patients with hypersensitivity to danaparoid or to pork products, severe hemorrhagic diathesis (such as hemophilia or idiopathic thrombocytopenic purpura), active major bleeding (including hemorrhagic stroke in the acute phase), or type II thrombocytopenia associated with positive in vitro tests for antiplatelet antibody in the presence of the drug.

Use with extreme caution in patients at increased risk for hemorrhage, such as those with severe uncontrolled hypertension, acute bacterial endocarditis, congenital or acquired bleeding disorders, active ulcerative or angiodysplastic GI disease, or nonhemorrhagic stroke; those who are using an indwelling epidural catheter postoperatively; and those who have recently had brain, spinal, or ophthalmic surgery.

Use cautiously in patients with impaired renal function and in those receiving oral anticoagulants or platelet inhibitors.

INTERACTIONS

Drug-drug. *Oral anticoagulants* or *platelet inhibitors* may increase the risk of bleeding; use together cautiously.

ADVERSE REACTIONS

CNS: insomnia, headache, asthenia, dizziness.

CV: peripheral edema, *hemorrhage.*

GI: *nausea, constipation,* vomiting.

GU: urinary tract infection, urine retention.

Hematologic: anemia.

Musculoskeletal: joint disorder, pain.

Skin: rash, pruritus.

Other: *fever,* pain at injection site, infection, edema.

◙ KEY CONSIDERATIONS

• Danaparoid contains sodium sulfite, which may cause allergic-type reactions, including anaphylactic symptoms and life-threatening or less-severe asthmatic episodes in certain patients. The overall prevalence of sulfite allergy in the general population is unknown and probably low. Sulfite sensitivity is seen more frequently in asthmatic than in nonasthmatic patients.

• Risks and benefits of danaparoid injection should be carefully considered before use in patients with severely impaired renal function or hemorrhagic disorders.

• Don't give drug I.M. To administer drug, have patient lie down. Give S.C. injection deeply, using a 25G to 26G needle. Alternate injection sites between the left and right anterolateral and posterolateral abdominal wall. Gently pull up a skinfold with thumb and forefinger and insert entire length of the needle into tissue. Don't rub or pinch afterward.

• Drug isn't interchangeable (unit for unit) with heparin or low-molecular-weight heparins.

• Periodic, routine CBCs (including platelet count) and fecal occult blood tests are recommended during therapy. PT, INR, and PTT don't have to be regularly monitored.

• Drug has little effect on PT, INR, PTT, fibrinolytic activity, and bleeding time.

• Monitor patient's hematocrit and blood pressure closely; a decrease in either may signal hemorrhage. If serious bleeding occurs, stop drug and transfuse blood products if needed.

• Monitor patient with severely impaired renal function carefully.

• Carefully monitor patients with serum creatinine level 2 mg/dl or greater.

• PT and Thrombotest are unreliable for monitoring anticoagulant activity of oral anticoagulants if used within 5 hours of danaparoid administration.

Patient education
• Instruct patient and family to watch for and report signs of bleeding.
• Tell patient to avoid OTC drugs containing aspirin or other salicylates.

Overdose & treatment
• Overdose of danaparoid injection may lead to bleeding complications. No agents antagonize the effects of danaparoid on anti-Xa activity. Although protamine sulfate partially neutralizes the anti-Xa activity of danaparoid and can be safely coadministered, no evidence that protamine sulfate is capable of reducing severe nonsurgical bleeding during treatment with danaparoid. If serious bleeding occurs, stop drug and administer blood or blood products as needed.
• Signs and symptoms of acute toxicity after I.V. dosing include respiratory depression, prostration, and twitching.

danazol
Cyclomen*, Danocrine

Androgen, antiestrogen

Available by prescription only
Capsules: 50 mg, 100 mg, 200 mg

INDICATIONS & DOSAGE
Mild endometriosis
Adults: Initially, 100 to 200 mg P.O. b.i.d. uninterrupted for 3 to 6 months; may continue for 9 months. Subsequent dosage based on patient response.
Moderate to severe endometriosis
Adults: 400 mg P.O. b.i.d. uninterrupted for 3 to 6 months; may continue for 9 months.
Fibrocystic breast disease
Adults: 100 to 400 mg P.O. daily in two divided doses uninterrupted for 2 to 6 months.
Prevention of hereditary angioedema
Adults: 200 mg P.O. b.i.d. or t.i.d., continued until favorable response is achieved. Then, dosage should be decreased by half at 1- to 3-month intervals.

PHARMACODYNAMICS
Antiestrogenic action: Danazol causes regression and atrophy of normal and ectopic endometrial tissue. Drug also decreases the rate of growth and nodularity of abnormal breast tissue in fibrocystic breast disease.
Androgenic action: Danazol increases levels of the C1 and C4 components of complement, which reduces the frequency and severity of attacks associated with hereditary angioedema.

PHARMACOKINETICS
Absorption: Amount of danazol absorbed by the body isn't proportional to the administered dose; doubling drug dose increases drug absorption by only 35% to 40%.
Distribution: Unknown.
Metabolism: Drug is metabolized to 2-hydroxymethylethisterone.
Excretion: Unknown.

CONTRAINDICATIONS & PRECAUTIONS
Contraindicated in patients with undiagnosed abnormal genital bleeding or prostatic hyperplasia; porphyria; or impaired renal, cardiac, or hepatic function.
Use cautiously in geriatric patients and those with seizure disorders or migraine headaches.

INTERACTIONS
Drug-drug. Danazol may increase the plasma *carbamazepine* levels in patients taking both drugs. In patients with diabetes, danazol may decrease blood glucose levels, so dosages of *insulin* or *oral antidiabetics* may need to be adjusted. Danazol may also potentiate the action of *warfarin-type anticoagulants,* prolonging PT and INR.

ADVERSE REACTIONS
CNS: dizziness, headache, sleep disorders, fatigue, tremor, irritability, excitation, lethargy, mental depression, chills, paresthesia.
CV: elevated blood pressure.
EENT: visual disturbances.
GI: gastric irritation, nausea, vomiting, diarrhea, constipation, change in appetite.

GU: hematuria, *hypoestrogenic effects (flushing, diaphoresis, vaginitis [including itching, dryness, and burning], vaginal bleeding, nervousness, emotional lability, menstrual irregularities),* androgenic effects in women *(weight gain, hirsutism,* hoarseness, clitoral enlargement, *decreased breast size,* acne, edema, changes in libido, *oily skin or hair,* voice deepening).

Hematologic: prolonged PT and INR.

Hepatic: reversible jaundice, elevated liver enzyme levels, hepatic dysfunction.

Metabolic: abnormal glucose tolerance test results, decreased total serum T_4 levels, increased total serum T_3 levels.

Musculoskeletal: muscle cramps or spasms.

◙ KEY CONSIDERATIONS

Besides the recommendations relevant to all androgens, consider the following:

• Use with caution in the geriatric patients. Observe geriatric male patients for prostatic hyperplasia; if patient develops symptomatic prostatic hyperplasia or prostate cancer, danazol must be discontinued.

• Because drug may cause hepatic dysfunction, periodic liver function studies should be performed.

• Danazol provides alternative therapy for patients who can't tolerate or fail to respond to other means of therapy. (It isn't indicated in cases in which surgery is the best choice).

Patient education

• Advise patient to report voice changes or other signs of virilization promptly. Some androgenic effects such as voice deepening may be irreversible.

• Instruct patient to immediately report nausea, vomiting, headache, and visual disturbances, which may suggest pseudotumor cerebri.

• Advise patient who is taking danazol for fibrocystic disease to examine breasts regularly. If breast nodule enlarges during treatment, she should call immediately.

• Advise male patient that he may need to have his semen evaluated periodically.

dantrolene sodium
Dantrium

Hydantoin derivative, skeletal muscle relaxant

Available by prescription only
Capsules: 25 mg, 50 mg, 100 mg
Injection: 20 mg parenteral (contains 3 g mannitol)

INDICATIONS & DOSAGE

Spasticity resulting from upper motor neuron disorders
Adults: 25 mg P.O. daily, increased gradually in increments of 25 mg at 4- to 7-day intervals, up to 100 mg b.i.d. to q.i.d., to maximum of 400 mg daily.

Prevention of malignant hyperthermia in susceptible patients who require surgery
Adults: 4 to 8 mg/kg/day P.O. given in three or four divided doses for 1 to 2 days before procedure; administer last dose 3 to 4 hours before procedure. Alternatively, give 2.5 mg/kg I.V. over 1 hour about 75 minutes before anesthesia.

Management of malignant hyperthermia crisis
Adults: Initially, 1 mg/kg I.V.; then continue until symptoms subside or maximum cumulative dose of 10 mg/kg has been reached.

Prevention of recurrence of malignant hyperthermia after crisis
Adults: 4 to 8 mg/kg/day P.O. given in four divided doses for up to 3 days after crisis. Alternatively, give 1 mg/kg or more I.V. based on the situation.

◊ *To reduce succinylcholine-induced muscle fasciculations and postoperative muscle pain*
Adults under 45 kg (99 lb): 100 mg P.O. 2 hours before succinylcholine.
Adults over 45 kg: 150 mg P.O. 2 hours before succinylcholine.

PHARMACODYNAMICS

Skeletal muscle relaxant action: A hydantoin derivative, dantrolene is chemically and pharmacologically unrelated to other skeletal muscle relaxants. It directly affects skeletal muscle, reducing muscle tension. It interferes with the release of calcium ions from the sarcoplasmic reticulum, resulting in decreased muscle contraction. This mechanism is of particular importance in malignant hyperthermia when increased myoplasmic calcium ion levels activate acute catabolism in the skeletal muscle cell. Dantrolene prevents or reduces the increase in myoplasmic calcium levels associated with malignant hyperthermia crises.

PHARMACOKINETICS
Absorption: About 35% of oral dose is absorbed through GI tract, with serum half-life reached within 8 to 9 hours after oral administration and 5 hours after I.V. administration. Therapeutic effect in patients with upper motor neuron disorders may take 1 week or more.
Distribution: Drug is substantially plasma protein-bound, mainly to albumin.
Metabolism: Drug is metabolized in the liver to its less active 5-hydroxy derivative and by the reductive pathways to its amino derivative.
Excretion: Drug is excreted in urine as metabolites.

CONTRAINDICATIONS & PRECAUTIONS
Contraindicated in patients in whom spasticity is used to maintain motor function and in patients with upper motor neuron disorders, active hepatic disease, or spasms from rheumatic disorders. Combination with verapamil to manage malignant hyperthermia is contraindicated. Use cautiously in women (especially those taking estrogen), in patients older than age 35, and in patients with severely impaired cardiac or pulmonary function or preexisting hepatic disease.

INTERACTIONS
Drug-drug. Use with other *CNS depressants*—including *antipsychotics, anxiolytics, narcotics,* and *tricyclic antidepressants*—may increase CNS depression; reduce dosage of one or both. Use with *estrogen* therapy in women older than age 35 may increase incidence of hepatotoxicity. Administration with *verapamil* has resulted in rare reports of cardiac collapse.

Drug-lifestyle. *Alcohol* causes increased CNS depression; *sun exposure,* photosensitivity reactions.

ADVERSE REACTIONS
CNS: *muscle weakness, drowsiness, dizziness, light-headedness, malaise, fatigue, headache, confusion, nervousness, insomnia, **seizures.***
CV: tachycardia, blood pressure changes.
EENT: excessive lacrimation, speech disturbance, altered taste, diplopia, visual disturbances.
GI: anorexia, constipation, cramping, dysphagia, metallic taste, severe diarrhea, GI bleeding.
GU: urinary frequency, hematuria, incontinence, nocturia, dysuria, crystalluria, difficult erection, urine retention, altered BUN level.
Hepatic: *hepatitis;* increased ALT, AST, alkaline phosphatase, and LD levels; altered total serum bilirubin level.
Musculoskeletal: myalgia, back pain.
Respiratory: pleural effusion with pericarditis.
Skin: eczematous eruption, pruritus, urticaria.
Other: abnormal hair growth, diaphoresis, chills, fever.

▣ KEY CONSIDERATIONS
• Administer dantrolene with extreme caution to geriatric patients because of cardiopulmonary and hepatic adverse effects.
• To prepare suspension for single oral dose, dissolve contents of appropriate number of capsules in fruit juice or other suitable liquid.
• Before therapy begins, check patient's baseline neuromuscular functions—posture, gait, coordination, range of motion, muscle strength and tone, abnormal muscle movements, and reflexes—for later comparisons.
• Drug may cause muscle weakness and impaired walking ability. Use with caution and carefully supervise patients receiving drug for prophylactic treatment for malignant hyperthermia.
• Walking should be supervised until patient's reaction to drug is known. With

---

Reactions may be *common,* uncommon, *life-threatening,* or COMMON AND LIFE-THREATENING.

relief from spasticity, patient may lose ability to maintain balance.

• Improvement may require 1 week or more of drug therapy.

• Because of the risk of hepatic injury, discontinue drug if no improvement is evident within 45 days.

• Perform baseline and regularly scheduled liver function tests (alkaline phosphatase, ALT, AST, and total bilirubin levels), blood cell counts, and renal function tests.

• Risk of hepatotoxicity may be greater in women, in patients older than age 35, and in those taking other drugs (especially estrogen) or high dantrolene dosages (400 mg or more daily) for prolonged periods.

• Signs and symptoms of malignant hyperthermia include skeletal muscle rigidity (often the first sign), sudden tachycardia, cardiac arrhythmias, cyanosis, tachypnea, severe hypercarbia, unstable blood pressure, rapidly rising temperature, acidosis, and shock.

• In malignant hyperthermia crisis, drug should be given by rapid I.V. injection as soon as reaction is recognized.

• To reconstitute, add 60 ml sterile water for injection to 20-mg vial. Don't use bacteriostatic water, D_5W, or normal saline solution for injection. Reconstituted solution should be stored away from direct sunlight at room temperature and should be discarded after 6 hours.

• Treating malignant hyperthermia requires continual monitoring of body temperature, management of fever, correction of acidosis, maintenance of fluid and electrolyte balance, monitoring of intake and output, adequate oxygenation, and seizure precautions.

Patient education

• Instruct patient to report promptly the onset of jaundice: yellow skin or sclerae, dark urine, clay-colored stools, itching, and abdominal discomfort. Hepatotoxicity occurs more frequently between the 3rd and 12th month of therapy.

• Advise patient susceptible to malignant hyperthermia to wear a medical identification bracelet indicating diagnosis, health care provider's name and telephone number, drug causing reaction, and treatment used.

• Because hepatotoxicity is more common after other drugs are used concurrently with dantrolene, warn patient to avoid OTC drugs, alcoholic beverages, and other CNS depressants except as prescribed.

• To guard against photosensitivity reactions, advise patient to avoid excessive or unnecessary exposure to sunlight and to use protective clothing and sunscreen.

• Warn patient to avoid hazardous activities that require alertness until CNS depressant effects are determined. Drug may cause drowsiness.

• Advise patient to report adverse reactions immediately.

• Tell patient to store drug away from heat and direct light (not in bathroom medicine cabinet). Keep out of reach of children.

• If patient misses a dose, tell him to take it within 1 hour; otherwise, he should omit the dose and return to regular dosing schedule. Tell him not to double-dose.

Overdose & treatment

• Signs and symptoms of overdose include exaggeration of adverse reactions, particularly CNS depression, and nausea and vomiting.

• Treatment includes supportive measures, gastric lavage, and observation of signs and symptoms. Maintain adequate airway, have emergency ventilation equipment on hand, monitor ECG, and administer large quantities of I.V. solutions to prevent crystalluria. Monitor vital signs closely. The benefit of dialysis is unknown.

daunorubicin hydrochloride
Cerubidine

Antibiotic antineoplastic (cell cycle–phase nonspecific)

Available by prescription only
Injection: 20-mg vials (with 100 mg of mannitol)

INDICATIONS & DOSAGE

Dosage and indications may vary. Check current literature for recommended protocols.

Remission induction in acute nonlymphocytic leukemia (myelogenous, monocytic, erythroid)

Adults younger than age 60: 45 mg/m^2 I.V. daily on days 1 to 3 of first course and on days 1 and 2 of subsequent courses. Give all courses in combination with cytosine arabinoside infusions.

Adults age 60 and older: 30 mg/m^2 I.V. daily on days 1 to 3 of first course and on days 1 and 2 of subsequent courses. Give all courses in combination with cytosine arabinoside infusions.

Remission induction in acute lymphocytic leukemia

Adults: 45 mg/m^2/day I.V. on days 1 to 3; give in combination with vincristine, prednisone, and l-asparaginase.

✦ *Dosage adjustment.* Use reduced dosage if patient has hepatic or renal impairment. In patients with serum bilirubin level of 1.2 to 3 mg/dl, reduce dose by 25%; with serum bilirubin or creatinine levels over 3 mg/dl, reduce dose by 50%.

PHARMACODYNAMICS

Antineoplastic action: Daunorubicin exerts its cytotoxic activity by intercalating between DNA base pairs and uncoiling the DNA helix, which inhibits DNA synthesis and DNA-dependent RNA synthesis. Drug may also inhibit polymerase activity.

PHARMACOKINETICS

Absorption: Because daunorubicin can cause blistering, it must be given I.V.

Distribution: Drug is widely distributed into body tissues, with the highest levels found in the spleen, kidneys, liver, lungs, and heart. It doesn't cross the blood-brain barrier.

Metabolism: Microsomal enzymes in the liver extensively metabolize the drug. One of the metabolites has cytotoxic activity.

Excretion: Drug and its metabolites are primarily excreted in bile, with a small portion excreted in urine. Plasma elimination has been described as biphasic, with an initial phase half-life of 45 minutes and a terminal phase half-life of 18½ hours.

CONTRAINDICATIONS & PRECAUTIONS

No known contraindications. Use cautiously in patients with myelosuppression or impaired cardiac, renal, or hepatic function.

INTERACTIONS

Drug-drug. Don't mix daunorubicin with either *dexamethasone phosphate* or *heparin sodium;* admixture of these drugs results in the formation of a precipitate. Other *hepatotoxic drugs* may increase the risk of hepatotoxicity with daunorubicin.

ADVERSE REACTIONS

CV: *irreversible cardiomyopathy* (dose-related), ECG changes.

GI: *nausea, vomiting,* diarrhea, *mucositis* (may occur 3 to 7 days after administration).

GU: red urine (transient).

Hematologic: *bone marrow suppression* (lowest blood counts 10 to 14 days after administration).

Hepatic: *hepatotoxicity,* increase in serum alkaline phosphatase, AST, and bilirubin levels.

Skin: rash, *alopecia.*

Other: *severe cellulitis, tissue sloughing* (if drug extravasates), fever, chills, hyperuricemia.

▣ KEY CONSIDERATIONS

● Geriatric patients have an increased incidence of drug-induced cardiotoxicity.

● Monitor for hematologic toxicity because some geriatric patients have poor bone marrow reserve.

● To reconstitute drug for I.V. administration, add 4 ml of sterile water for injection to a 20-mg vial to give a concentration of 5 mg/ml.

● Drug may be diluted further into 100 ml of D$_5$W or normal saline solution and infused over 30 to 45 minutes.

● For I.V. push administration, withdraw reconstituted drug into syringe containing 10 to 15 ml of normal saline solution or D$_5$W and inject over 2 to 3 minutes into the tubing of a freely flowing I.V.

Reactions may be *common*, uncommon, *life-threatening*, or COMMON AND LIFE-THREATENING.

infusion. Reconstituted solution is stable for 24 hours at room temperature and 48 hours in refrigeration.

• Reddish color of drug looks similar to that of doxorubicin. Don't confuse the two drugs.

• Erythematous streaking along the vein or flushing in the face indicate that the drug is being administered too rapidly.

• Extravasation may be treated by applying topical dimethyl sulfoxide and ice packs to the site.

• Antiemetics may be used to prevent or treat nausea and vomiting.

• Darkening or redness of the skin may occur in prior radiation fields.

• ECG monitoring or monitoring of systolic injection fraction may help identify early changes associated with drug-induced cardiomyopathy. An ECG or determination of systolic injection fraction should be performed before each course of therapy.

• To prevent cardiomyopathy, limit cumulative dose in adults to 500 to 600 mg/m^2 (400 to 450 mg/m^2 when patient has been receiving other cardiotoxic drugs, such as cyclophosphamide, or radiation therapy that encompasses the heart).

• Monitor CBC and hepatic function.

• Note if resting pulse rate is high (a sign of cardiac adverse reactions).

• Don't use a scalp tourniquet or apply ice to prevent alopecia because this may compromise effectiveness of drug.

• Nausea and vomiting may be very severe and last 24 to 48 hours.

Patient education

• Warn patient that urine may be red for 1 to 2 days and that this is a drug effect, not bleeding.

• Advise patient that alopecia may occur, but that it's usually reversible.

• Tell patient to avoid exposure to people with infections.

• Encourage adequate fluid intake to increase urine output and facilitate excretion of uric acid.

• Warn patient that nausea and vomiting may be severe and may last for 24 to 48 hours.

• Instruct patient to call health care provider if sore throat, fever, or signs of bleeding occur.

Overdose & treatment

• Signs and symptoms of overdose include myelosuppression, nausea, vomiting, and stomatitis.

• Treatment is usually supportive and includes transfusion of blood components and antiemetics.

---

deferoxamine mesylate
Desferal

Chelating drug, heavy metal antagonist

Available by prescription only
Injectable powder for injection: 500-mg vial

INDICATIONS & DOSAGE

Acute iron intoxication
Adults: 1 g I.M. or I.V. (I.M. injection is preferred route for all patients in shock), followed by 500 mg I.M. or I.V. q 4 hours for two doses; then 500 mg I.M. or I.V. q 4 to 12 hours if needed. I.V. infusion rate shouldn't exceed 15 mg/kg/hour. Don't exceed 6 g in 24 hours. (I.V. infusion should be reserved for patients in CV collapse.)

Chronic iron overload resulting from multiple transfusions
Adults: 500 mg to 1 g I.M. daily and 2 g slow I.V. infusion in separate solutions along with each unit of blood transfused. I.V. infusion rate shouldn't exceed 15 mg/kg/hour. Alternatively, give 1 to 2 g via a S.C. infusion pump over 8 to 24 hours.

PHARMACODYNAMICS

Chelating action: Deferoxamine chelates iron by binding ferric ions to the 3-hydroxamic groups of the molecule, preventing it from entering into further chemical reactions. It also chelates aluminum to a lesser extent.

PHARMACOKINETICS

Absorption: Deferoxamine is absorbed poorly after oral administration; however, absorption may occur in patients with acute iron toxicity.

Distribution: Distributes widely into the body after parenteral administration.

Metabolism: Plasma enzymes metabolize a small amount of drug.

Excretion: Drug is excreted in urine as unchanged drug or as ferrioxamine, the deferoxamine-iron complex.

INTERACTIONS
None reported.

ADVERSE REACTIONS
CV: tachycardia (with long-term use).
EENT: blurred vision, cataracts, hearing loss.
GI: diarrhea, abdominal discomfort (with long-term use).
GU: dysuria (with long-term use).
Musculoskeletal: leg cramps.
Other: hypersensitivity reactions (cutaneous wheal formation, pruritus, rash, **anaphylaxis**), pain and induration at injection site, fever, *erythema, urticaria, hypotension, shock* (after too-rapid I.V. administration). Acute intoxication is anticipated to include extension and exacerbation of adverse reactions. Treat symptomatically.

▣ KEY CONSIDERATIONS
• Deferoxamine should be used with caution because geriatric patients are more likely to have visual or hearing impairment and renal dysfunction than younger patients.
• Observe closely, and be prepared to treat hypersensitivity reactions; monitor renal, vision, and hearing function throughout therapy.
• If patient isn't in shock, use I.M. route for acute iron intoxication. If patient is in shock, administer I.V. *slowly;* avoid S.C. route.
• Drug has been used to treat iron overload from congenital anemias and to diagnose and treat primary hemochromatosis. It also has been applied topically to remove corneal rust rings and has been used I.V. or intraperitoneally to promote aluminum excretion or removal.
• Drug has also been used experimentally as a chelator to reduce aluminum levels in bones of patients with renal failure

and in patients presenting with dialysis-induced encephalopathy. It has also been shown to slow cognitive deterioration by 50% in long-term clinical trials.
• Drug can be removed through hemodialysis.

Patient education
• Advise patient that ophthalmic and, possibly, audiometric examinations are needed every 3 to 6 months during continuous therapy; stress importance of reporting changes in vision or hearing.
• Explain that drug may turn urine red.

delavirdine mesylate
Rescriptor

Antiviral, nonnucleoside reverse-transcriptase inhibitor of HIV-1

Available by prescription only
Tablets: 100 mg

INDICATIONS & DOSAGE
HIV infection
Adults: 400 mg P.O. t.i.d.; use with other antiretrovirals as appropriate.

PHARMACODYNAMICS
Antiviral action: Delavirdine is a nonnucleoside reverse transcriptase (RT) inhibitor of HIV-1. It binds directly to RT and blocks RNA- and DNA-dependent DNA polymerase activities.

PHARMACOKINETICS
Absorption: Rapidly absorbed after oral administration, with drug level peaking in about 1 hour.
Distribution: About 98% binds to plasma proteins, primarily albumin. Distribution into CSF, saliva, and semen is about 0.4%, 6%, and 2%, respectively, of the corresponding plasma levels.
Metabolism: Drug is converted to several inactive metabolites and is primarily metabolized in liver by cytochrome P-450 3A (CYP3A) enzyme system. However, in vitro data also suggest that CYP2D6 may also be involved. Delavirdine can reduce CYP3A activity and can inhibit its own metabolism; this is usually reversed within 1 week after the drug

---

is discontinued. In vitro data also suggest that CYP2C9 and CYP2C19 activity are also reduced by delavirdine. *Excretion:* After multiple doses, 44% of the dose was recovered in feces, and 51% was excreted in urine. Less than 5% of the dose was recovered unchanged in urine. Mean elimination half-life was 5.8 hours.

CONTRAINDICATIONS & PRECAUTIONS

Contraindicated in patients with hypersensitivity to delavirdine. Use caution when administering to patients with impaired hepatic function. Nonnucleoside RT inhibitors, when used alone or in combination, may confer cross-resistance to other drugs in that class.

INTERACTIONS

Drug-drug. Administration with *amphetamines, benzodiazepines, calcium channel blockers, cisapride, clarithromycin, dapsone, ergot alkaloid preparations, indinavir, nonsedating antihistamines, quinidine, rifabutin, saquinavir, sedative hypnotics,* or *warfarin* may increase plasma levels of these drugs. Higher plasma levels of these drugs could increase or prolong both therapeutic and adverse effects; therefore, drug dosages may need to be reduced.

Because absorption of delavirdine is reduced when administered with *antacids,* separate doses by at least 1 hour. *Carbamazepine, phenobarbital, phenytoin, rifabutin,* and *rifampin* decrease plasma delavirdine levels, so use with caution. *Clarithromycin, fluoxetine,* and *ketoconazole* increase bioavailability of delavirdine by 50%. Administration with *didanosine* should be separated by at least 1 hour because bioavailability of both drugs is reduced by 20%. H_2 receptor antagonists increase gastric pH and may reduce the absorption of delavirdine, so long-term concomitant use isn't recommended. Use caution when administering delavirdine to patients receiving enzyme-inducing or inhibiting drugs such as *phenobarbital* and *rifampin.*

Use with *saquinavir* increases bioavailability of saquinavir fivefold. In a small, preliminary study, liver enzyme levels increased in 13% of patients treated with both drugs. Monitor AST and ALT levels frequently.

ADVERSE REACTIONS

CNS: headache, abnormal coordination, agitation, amnesia, anxiety, change in dreams, cognitive impairment, confusion, depression, disorientation, emotional lability, hallucinations, hyperesthesia, hyperreflexia, hypesthesia, impaired concentration, insomnia, manic symptoms, *fatigue,* nervousness, neuropathy, nightmares, nystagmus, paralysis, paranoid symptoms, paresthesia, restlessness, somnolence, tingling, tremor, vertigo, weakness, pallor.
CV: *bradycardia,* palpitations, postural hypotension, syncope, tachycardia, vasodilation, chest pain, edema (generalized or localized).
EENT: blepharitis, conjunctivitis, diplopia, dry eyes, ear pain, photophobia, taste perversion, tinnitus.
GI: *nausea,* vomiting, diarrhea, anorexia, aphthous stomatitis, bloody stools, colitis, constipation, decreased appetite, diverticulitis, duodenitis, dry mouth, dyspepsia, dysphagia, enteritis, esophagitis, fecal incontinence, flatulence, gagging, gastritis, gastroesophageal reflux, *GI bleeding,* gingivitis, gum hemorrhage, increased thirst and appetite, increased saliva, mouth ulcer, nonspecific hepatitis, *pancreatitis,* sialadenitis, stomatitis, tongue edema or ulceration, abdominal cramps, distention, pain (generalized or localized).
GU: breast enlargement, renal calculi, epididymitis, hematuria, hemospermia, impotence, renal pain, metrorrhagia, nocturia, polyuria, proteinuria, vaginal candidiasis, decreased libido.
Hematologic: *anemia,* ecchymosis, eosinophilia, *granulocytosis, neutropenia, pancytopenia,* petechia, prolonged PTT, purpura, spleen disorder, *thrombocytopenia.*
Hepatic: *increased ALT and AST levels.*
Metabolic: alcohol intolerance; bilirubinemia; hyperkalemia; hyperuricemia; hypocalcemia; hyponatremia; hypophosphatemia; increased gamma-glutamyltransferase, lipase, serum alkaline phosphatase, serum amylase, and serum CK

levels; peripheral edema; weight gain or loss.

Musculoskeletal: asthenia, back pain, neck rigidity, arthralgia or arthritis of single and multiple joints, bone pain, leg cramps, muscular weakness, muscle cramps, myalgia, tendon disorder, tenosynovitis, tetany.

Respiratory: upper respiratory tract infection, bronchitis, chest congestion, cough, dyspnea, epistaxis, laryngismus, pharyngitis, rhinitis, sinusitis.

Skin: *rash, pruritus, angioedema,* dermal leukocytoblastic vasculitis, dermatitis, desquamation, diaphoresis, dry skin, *erythema multiforme,* folliculitis, fungal dermatitis, alopecia, nail disorder, petechial rash, seborrhea, skin nodule, *Stevens-Johnson syndrome,* urticaria.

Other: bruise, allergic reaction, chills, epidermal cyst, fever, flank pain, flulike syndrome, lethargy, lip edema, malaise, pain (generalized or localized), sebaceous cyst, trauma.

◉ KEY CONSIDERATIONS

● Monitor the geriatric patient closely because safety and effectiveness haven't been studied in patients older than age 65.

● Drug-induced rash—typically diffuse, maculopapular, erythematous and often pruritic—occurs commonly; its incidence doesn't appear to be significantly reduced when drug dosage is adjusted.

● Rash is more common in patients with lower CD4+ cell counts and usually occurs within the first 3 weeks of treatment. Severe rash occurred in 3.6% of patients. In most cases, rash lasted less than 2 weeks and didn't require dose reduction or drug discontinuation. Most patients were able to resume therapy after treatment interruption caused by rash.

● Rash occurred mainly on the upper body and proximal arms, with decreasing lesion intensity on the neck and face and less on the rest of the trunk and limbs. Erythema multiforme and Stevens-Johnson syndrome were rarely seen, and resolved after drug was stopped. Occurrence of drug-related rash after 1 month of therapy is uncommon unless prolonged interruption of drug treatment occurs.

● Patient taking delavirdine may develop neutropenia (absolute neutrophil count < 750/mm^3), anemia (hemoglobin level < 7 g/dl), or thrombocytopenia (platelet count < 50,000/mm^3) or altered ALT and AST levels (> 5 times upper limit of normal), bilirubin level (> 2½ times upper limit of normal) or amylase level (> twice upper limit of normal). Monitor patient carefully.

● Symptomatic relief may be obtained by using diphenhydramine, hydroxyzine, or topical corticosteroids.

● Monitor patients with hepatic or renal impairment because drug effect hasn't been studied.

● Drug hasn't been shown to reduce risk of HIV-1 transmission.

Patient education

● Instruct patient to discontinue drug and call health care provider if severe rash or signs or symptoms such as fever, blistering, oral lesions, conjunctivitis, swelling, or muscle or joint aches occur.

● Tell patient that drug isn't a cure for HIV-1 infection. He may continue to acquire illnesses associated with HIV-1 infection, including opportunistic infections. Therapy hasn't been shown to reduce the frequency of such illnesses.

● Advise patient to remain under medical supervision when taking drug because long-term effects are unknown.

● Inform patient to take drug as prescribed and not to alter doses without medical approval. If a dose is missed, tell him to take the next dose as soon as possible; he should not double the next dose.

● Inform patient that drug may be dispersed in water before ingestion. Add tablets to at least 3 oz (90 ml) of water, allow to stand for a few minutes, and stir until a uniform dispersion occurs. Tell patient to drink dispersion promptly, rinse glass, and swallow the rinse to ensure that entire dose is consumed.

● Tell patient that drug may be taken with or without food.

● Advise patient with achlorhydria to take drug with an acidic beverage such as orange or cranberry juice.

● Instruct patient to take drug and antacids at least 1 hour apart.

Reactions may be *common,* uncommon, *life-threatening,* or COMMON AND LIFE-THREATENING.

• Advise patient to report the use of other prescription or OTC drugs.

demeclocycline hydrochloride
Declomycin

Tetracycline antibiotic

Available by prescription only
Tablets: 150 mg, 300 mg
Capsules: 150 mg

INDICATIONS & DOSAGE
Infections caused by susceptible organisms
Adults: 150 mg P.O. q 6 hours or 300 mg P.O. q 12 hours.
Gonorrhea
Adults: 600 mg P.O. initially, then 300 mg P.O. q 12 hours for 4 days (total, 3 g).
◊*SIADH secretion (a hyperosmolar state)*
Adults: 600 to 1,200 mg P.O. daily in three or four divided doses.

PHARMACODYNAMICS
Antibiotic action: Demeclocycline is bacteriostatic. Tetracyclines bind reversibly to ribosomal subunits, thereby inhibiting bacterial protein synthesis. Demeclocycline is active against many gram-negative and gram-positive organisms, *Mycoplasma, Rickettsia, Chlamydia,* and spirochetes.

PHARMACOKINETICS
Absorption: About 60% to 80% of demeclocycline is absorbed from the GI tract after oral administration; serum levels peak in 3 to 4 hours. Food or milk reduces absorption by 50%; antacids chelate with tetracyclines and further reduce absorption. Drug has the greatest affinity of all tetracyclines for calcium ions.
Distribution: Drug is distributed widely into body tissues and fluids, including synovial, pleural, prostatic, and seminal fluids; bronchial secretions; saliva; and aqueous humor; CSF penetration is poor. About 36% to 91% binds to protein.
Metabolism: Drug isn't metabolized.

Excretion: Drug is excreted primarily unchanged in urine through glomerular filtration. Plasma half-life is 10 to 17 hours in adults with normal renal function. Hemodialysis and peritoneal dialysis remove only a small amount of demeclocycline.

CONTRAINDICATIONS & PRECAUTIONS
Contraindicated in patients with hypersensitivity to demeclocycline or other tetracyclines. Use cautiously in patients with impaired renal or hepatic function.

INTERACTIONS
Drug-drug. Use with *antacids containing aluminum, calcium,* or *magnesium; laxatives containing magnesium; iron products;* or *sodium bicarbonate* impairs absorption of oral demeclocycline. Use with *oral anticoagulants* necessitates lowered dosages of oral anticoagulants because of enhanced effects. Use with *digoxin* necessitates lowered dosages of digoxin because of increased bioavailability. Use with *methoxyflurane* increases the risk of nephrotoxicity. Demeclocycline may antagonize bactericidal effects of *penicillin,* inhibiting cell growth because of bacteriostatic action; administer penicillin 2 to 3 hours before demeclocycline.
Drug-food. *Food* and *dairy products* impair absorption of demeclocycline.
Drug-lifestyle. Increased photosensitivity reactions may occur with *sun exposure.*

ADVERSE REACTIONS
CNS: *intracranial hypertension (pseudotumor cerebri),* dizziness.
CV: pericarditis.
EENT: dysphagia, glossitis, tinnitus, visual disturbances.
GI: anorexia, *nausea, vomiting, diarrhea,* enterocolitis, anogenital inflammation, *pancreatitis.*
GU: *increased BUN level.*
Hematologic: *neutropenia,* eosinophilia, *thrombocytopenia, hemolytic anemia.*
Hepatic: elevated liver enzyme levels.
Skin: *maculopapular and erythematous rash, photosensitivity, increased pigmentation, urticaria.*

---

*Canada only   ◊ Unlabeled clinical use

Other: hypersensitivity reactions *(anaphylaxis)*, diabetes insipidus syndrome (polyuria, polydipsia, weakness).

▣ KEY CONSIDERATIONS

Besides the recommendations relevant to all tetracyclines, consider the following:
• As an anti-infective, drug is usually reserved for patients intolerant of other antibiotics.
• A reversible diabetes insipidus syndrome has been reported with long-term use of demeclocycline; monitor patient for signs and symptoms, including weakness, polyuria, and polydipsia.
• Drug causes false-negative results in urine tests using glucose oxidase reagent (Diastix, Chemstrip uG, or glucose enzymatic test strip). It also falsely elevates urine catecholamine levels in fluorometric tests.

Patient education

• Advise patient to take drug at least 1 hour before or 2 hours after meals. Drug shouldn't be taken with dairy products.
• Tell patient to avoid prolonged exposure to sunlight.

Overdose & treatment

• Signs and symptoms of overdose are usually limited to the GI tract.
• Treatment may include antacids or gastric lavage if drug was ingested within the preceding 4 hours.

---

desipramine hydrochloride
Norpramin

Dibenzazepine tricyclic antidepressant

Available by prescription only
Tablets: 10 mg, 25 mg, 50 mg, 75 mg, 100 mg, 150 mg

INDICATIONS & DOSAGE
Depression
Adults: 100 to 200 mg P.O. daily in divided doses, increasing to maximum of 300 mg daily. Alternatively, the entire dosage can be given once daily, usually h.s.

✦ *Dosage adjustment.* 25 to 100 mg P.O. daily, increasing gradually to a maximum of 100 mg daily (maximum of 150 mg/daily only for the severely ill in this age-group).

PHARMACODYNAMICS
Antidepressant action: Desipramine is thought to inhibit reuptake of norepinephrine and serotonin in CNS nerve terminals (presynaptic neurons), which results in increased levels and enhanced activity of these neurotransmitters in the synaptic cleft. Desipramine more strongly inhibits reuptake of norepinephrine than serotonin; it has a lesser incidence of sedative effects and less anticholinergic and hypotensive activity than its parent compound, imipramine.

PHARMACOKINETICS
Absorption: Desipramine is absorbed rapidly from the GI tract after oral administration.
Distribution: Drug is distributed widely into the body, including the CNS. About 90% binds to proteins. Peak effect occurs in 4 to 6 hours; steady state, within 2 to 11 days; and full therapeutic effect, in 2 to 4 weeks. Proposed therapeutic plasma levels (parent drug and metabolite) range from 125 to 300 ng/ml.
Metabolism: Drug is metabolized in the liver; a significant first-pass effect may explain variability of serum levels in different patients taking the same dosage.
Excretion: Drug is excreted primarily in urine.

CONTRAINDICATIONS & PRECAUTIONS
Contraindicated in patients with hypersensitivity to desipramine, in those who have taken MAO inhibitors within the previous 14 days, and in patients who are in the acute recovery phase of an MI. Use with extreme caution in patients with history of seizure disorders or urine retention, CV or thyroid disease, or glaucoma and in those taking thyroid drugs.

INTERACTIONS
Drug-drug. Use with *antiarrhythmics, pimozide,* or *thyroid drugs*—such as *disopyramide, procainamide,* and *quinidine*—may increase incidence of cardiac

---

arrhythmias and conduction defects. *Barbiturates* induce desipramine metabolism and decrease therapeutic efficacy. *Beta blockers, cimetidine, methylphenidate,* and *propoxyphene* may inhibit desipramine metabolism, increasing plasma levels and toxicity. Desipramine may decrease hypotensive effects of *centrally acting antihypertensives,* such as *clonidine, guanabenz, guanadrel, guanethidine, methyldopa,* and *reserpine.* Use with *disulfiram* or *ethchlorvynol* may cause delirium and tachycardia.

Additive effects are likely when used with the following drugs: *CNS depressants,* including *analgesics, anesthetics barbiturates, narcotics,* and *tranquilizers* (oversedation); *atropine* or *other anticholinergics,* including *antihistamines, antiparkinsonians, meperidine,* and *phenothiazines* (oversedation, paralytic ileus, visual changes, and severe constipation); or *metrizamide* (increased risk of seizures).

Haloperidol and *phenothiazines* decrease desipramine metabolism, decreasing therapeutic efficacy. Use caution when using concomitantly with *selective serotonin-uptake inhibitors* because patient may experience toxic reaction to desipramine at much lower dosages. Use with *sympathomimetics*—including *epinephrine, ephedrine* (found in many nasal sprays), *phenylephrine,* and *phenylpropanolamine*—may increase blood pressure; use with *warfarin* may increase PT and INR and cause bleeding. **Drug-lifestyle.** Use with *alcohol* can lead to additive effects. *Heavy smoking* induces desipramine metabolism and decreased therapeutic efficacy. Photosensitivity reactions are possible with *sun exposure.*

ADVERSE REACTIONS
CNS: *drowsiness, dizziness,* excitation, tremor, weakness, confusion, anxiety, restlessness, agitation, headache, nervousness, EEG changes, *seizures,* extrapyramidal reactions.
CV: orthostatic hypotension, *tachycardia, ECG changes* (elongation of QT and PR intervals, flattened T waves on ECG), hypertension, *sudden death.*

EENT: *blurred vision,* tinnitus, mydriasis.
GI: *dry mouth, constipation,* nausea, vomiting, anorexia, paralytic ileus.
GU: *urine retention.*
Hematologic: decreased WBC counts.
Hepatic: elevated liver function tests.
Metabolic: decreased or increased serum glucose levels.
Skin: rash, urticaria, photosensitivity.
Other: *diaphoresis,* *hypersensitivity reaction.*
After abrupt withdrawal of long-term therapy: nausea, headache, malaise (doesn't indicate addiction).

▣ KEY CONSIDERATIONS
Besides the recommendations relevant to all tricyclic antidepressants, consider the following:
● Geriatric patients may be more susceptible to adverse cardiovascular and anticholinergic effects.
● To decrease the risk of a suicidal overdose, dispense drug in the smallest possible quantities to depressed outpatients.
● Before administering desipramine, check standing and sitting blood pressure to assess orthostasis.
● Drug isn't as likely to cause sedative effects and produces fewer anticholinergic and hypotensive effects than its parent compound imipramine.
● To help offset daytime sedation, the full dose may be given at bedtime.
● Tolerance usually develops to the sedative effects of drug during initial weeks of therapy.
● Don't withdraw drug abruptly; taper gradually over 3 to 6 weeks.
● Discontinue drug at least 48 hours before surgical procedures.
● Drug therapy in patients with bipolar illness may induce a hypomanic state.

Patient education
● Tell patient to take the full dose at bedtime to alleviate daytime sedation.
● Explain that full effects of drug may not become apparent for 4 weeks or more after initiation of therapy.
● Tell patient to take the drug exactly as prescribed and not to double-dose if he misses a dose.

• To prevent dizziness, advise patient to lie down for about 30 minutes after each dose at start of therapy and to avoid sudden postural changes, especially when rising to upright position.

• Warn patient not to stop taking drug suddenly.

• Encourage patient to report unusual or troublesome effects, especially confusion, movement disorders, rapid heartbeat, dizziness, fainting, or difficulty urinating.

• Tell patient sugarless chewing gum, hard candy, or ice may alleviate dry mouth.

• Stress importance of regular dental hygiene to avoid caries.

• Warn patient to avoid alcohol and prolonged sunlight while taking this drug.

• Advise patient that heavy smoking will decrease drug effectiveness.

• Tell patient to store drug safely away from children.

Overdose & treatment

• The first 12 hours after acute ingestion are a stimulatory phase characterized by excessive anticholinergic activity—agitation, irritation, confusion, hallucinations, parkinsonian symptoms, hyperthermia, seizures, urine retention, dry mucous membranes, pupillary dilation, constipation, and ileus. This is followed by CNS depressant effects, including hypothermia, decreased or absent reflexes, sedation, hypotension, cyanosis, and cardiac irregularities, including tachycardia, conduction disturbances, and quinidine-like effects on the ECG.

• Severity of overdose is best indicated by widening of the QRS complex, which usually represents a serum level over 1,000 ng/ml; serum levels generally aren't helpful. Metabolic acidosis may follow hypotension, hypoventilation, and seizures.

• Treatment is symptomatic and supportive, including maintaining airway, stable body temperature, and fluid and electrolyte balance. Induce vomiting with ipecac if patient is conscious; follow with gastric lavage and activated charcoal to prevent further absorption. Dialysis is of little use. Physostigmine may be used with caution to reverse CV abnor-malities or coma; too rapid administration may cause seizures. Treat seizures with parenteral diazepam or phenytoin; arrhythmias, with parenteral phenytoin or lidocaine; and acidosis, with sodium bicarbonate. Don't give barbiturates; these may enhance CNS and respiratory depressant effects.

dexamethasone (ophthalmic suspension)
Maxidex

dexamethasone sodium phosphate
AK-Dex, Decadron, Dexair, I-Methasone, Ocu-Dex

Corticosteroid, ophthalmic anti-inflammatory

Available by prescription only
dexamethasone
Ophthalmic suspension: 0.1%
dexamethasone sodium phosphate
Ophthalmic ointment: 0.05%
Ophthalmic solution: 0.1%

INDICATIONS & DOSAGE

Uveitis; iridocyclitis; inflammation of eyelids, conjunctiva, cornea, anterior segment of globe; corneal injury from burns or penetration by foreign bodies; allergic conjunctivitis; suppression of graft rejection after keratoplasty
Adults: Instill 1 or 2 drops of suspension or solution or apply 1.25 to 2.5 cm of ointment into conjunctival sac. For initial therapy of severe cases, instill the solution or suspension into the conjunctival sac every hour, gradually discontinue dose as patient's condition improves. In mild condition, use drops up to six times daily or apply ointment t.i.d. or q.i.d. As patient's condition improves, taper dose to b.i.d. then once daily. Treatment may extend from a few days to several weeks.

PHARMACODYNAMICS

Anti-inflammatory action: Corticosteroids stimulate the synthesis of enzymes needed to decrease the inflammatory response. Dexamethasone, a long-acting fluorinated synthetic adrenocorticoid

---

Reactions may be *common,* uncommon, *life-threatening,* or COMMON AND LIFE-THREATENING.

with strong anti-inflammatory activity and minimal mineralocorticoid activity, is 25 to 30 times more potent than an equal weight of hydrocortisone.

Drug is poorly soluble and therefore has a slower onset of action but a longer duration of action when applied in a liquid suspension. The sodium phosphate salt is highly soluble and has a rapid onset but short duration of action.

PHARMACOKINETICS

Absorption: After ophthalmic administration, dexamethasone is absorbed through the aqueous humor. Because only low doses are administered, little if any systemic absorption occurs.

Distribution: Drug is distributed throughout the local tissue layers. Drug absorbed into circulation is rapidly removed from the blood and distributed into muscle, liver, skin, intestines, and kidneys.

Metabolism: Drug is primarily metabolized locally. The small amount that's absorbed into systemic circulation is metabolized primarily in the liver to inactive compounds.

Excretion: Inactive metabolites are excreted from the kidneys, primarily as glucuronides and sulfates, but also as unconjugated products. A small amount of metabolites is also excreted in feces.

CONTRAINDICATIONS & PRECAUTIONS

Contraindicated in patients with acute superficial herpes simplex (dendritic keratitis), vaccinia, varicella, or other fungal or viral diseases of cornea and conjunctiva; ocular tuberculosis; or acute, purulent, untreated infections of the eye.

Use cautiously in patients with corneal abrasions that may be infected (especially with herpes). Also use cautiously in patients with glaucoma because intraocular pressure may increase. Antiglaucoma drugs may need to be increased to compensate.

INTERACTIONS

None reported.

ADVERSE REACTIONS

EENT: increased intraocular pressure; thinning of cornea; interference with corneal wound healing; increased susceptibility to viral or fungal corneal infection; corneal ulceration; glaucoma exacerbation; cataracts; defects in visual acuity and visual field; optic nerve damage; mild blurred vision; burning, stinging, or redness of eyes; watery eyes; discharge; discomfort; ocular pain; foreign body sensation (with excessive or long-term use).

Other: systemic effects and adrenal suppression (with excessive or long-term use).

▣ KEY CONSIDERATIONS

• Watch for corneal ulceration; may require stopping drug.
• Shake suspension well before use.
• Drug is not recommended for long-term use.

Patient education

• Teach patient proper procedure for using drug.
• Advise patient of potential adverse reactions.

dexamethasone (systemic)
Decadron, Deronil*, Dexasone*, Dexone, Hexadrol

dexamethasone acetate
Dalalone D.P., Decadron-L.A., Decaject-L.A., Dexasone-L.A., Dexone L.A., Solurex L.A.

dexamethasone sodium phosphate
AK-Dex, Dalalone, Decadrol, Decadron, Decaject, Dexameth, Dexasone, Dexone, Hexadrol Phosphate, Oradexon*, Solurex

Glucocorticoid, anti-inflammatory, immunosuppressant

Available by prescription only
dexamethasone
Tablets: 0.25 mg, 0.5 mg, 0.75 mg, 1 mg, 1.5 mg, 2 mg, 4 mg, 6 mg
Elixir: 0.5 mg/5 ml

Oral solution: 0.5 mg/0.5 ml,
0.5 mg/5 ml
dexamethasone acetate
Injection: 8-mg/ml and 16-mg/ml suspension
dexamethasone sodium phosphate
Injection: 4 mg/ml, 10 mg/ml,
20 mg/ml, 24 mg/ml

INDICATIONS & DOSAGE
Cerebral edema
dexamethasone sodium phosphate
Adults: Initially, 10 mg I.V., then 4 mg
I.M. q 6 hours for 2 to 4 days, then taper
over 5 to 7 days.
Inflammatory conditions, allergic reactions, neoplasias
Adults: 0.75 to 9 mg P.O. daily divided
b.i.d., t.i.d., or q.i.d.
dexamethasone acetate
Adults: 4 to 16 mg intra-articularly or
into soft tissue q 1 to 3 weeks; 0.8 to
1.6 mg into lesions q 1 to 3 weeks; or 8
to 16 mg I.M. q 1 to 3 weeks, p.r.n.
dexamethasone sodium phosphate
Adults: 0.2 to 6 mg intra-articularly, intralesionally, or into soft tissue; or 0.5 to
9 mg I.M.
Shock (other than adrenal crisis)
dexamethasone sodium phosphate
Adults: 1 to 6 mg/kg I.V. daily as a single dose; or 40 mg I.V. q 2 to 6 hours,
p.r.n.
Dexamethasone suppression test
Adults: 0.5 mg P.O. q 6 hours for 48
hours.
Adrenal insufficiency
Adults: 0.75 to 9 mg P.O. daily in divided doses.
dexamethasone sodium phosphate
Adults: 0.5 to 9 mg I.M. or I.V. daily.
◊ *Prevention of cancer chemotherapy-induced nausea and vomiting*
Adults: 10 to 20 mg I.V. before administration of chemotherapy. Additional doses (individualized for each patient and
usually lower than initial dose) may be
administered I.V. or P.O. for 24 to 72
hours after cancer chemotherapy, if
needed.

PHARMACODYNAMICS
Anti-inflammatory action: Dexamethasone stimulates the synthesis of enzymes
needed to decrease the inflammatory response. It causes suppression of the immune system by reducing activity and
volume of the lymphatic system,
producing lymphocytopenia (primarily
T-lymphocytes), decreasing passage of
immune complexes through basement
membranes, and possibly depressing reactivity of tissue to antigen-antibody interactions.

Drug is a long-acting synthetic adrenocorticoid with strong anti-inflammatory
activity and minimal mineralocorticoid
properties. It's 25 to 30 times more potent than an equal weight of hydrocortisone.

The acetate salt is a suspension and
shouldn't be used I.V. It's particularly
useful as an anti-inflammatory in intra-articular, intradermal, and intralesional
injections.

The sodium phosphate salt is highly
soluble and has a more rapid onset and a
shorter duration of action than does the
acetate salt. It's most commonly used for
cerebral edema and unresponsive shock.
It can also be used in intra-articular, intralesional, or soft-tissue inflammation.
Other uses for dexamethasone are symptomatic treatment of bronchial asthma
and chemotherapy-induced nausea and
diagnostic test for Cushing's syndrome.

PHARMACOKINETICS
Absorption: After oral administration,
drug is absorbed readily, and peak effects occur in 1 to 2 hours. The suspension for injection has a variable onset
and duration of action (ranging from 2 to
21 days), depending on whether it is injected into an intra-articular space, a
muscle, or the blood supply to the muscle. After I.V. injection, dexamethasone
is rapidly and completely absorbed into
the tissues.
Distribution: Drug is removed rapidly
from the blood and distributed to muscle, liver, skin, intestines, and kidneys.
Dexamethasone binds weakly to plasma
proteins (transcortin and albumin). Only
the unbound portion is active.
Metabolism: Metabolized in the liver to
inactive glucuronide and sulfate metabolites.
Excretion: The inactive metabolites and
a small amount of unmetabolized drug

Reactions may be *common*, uncommon, *life-threatening*, or COMMON AND LIFE-THREATENING.

are excreted by the kidneys. Insignificant quantities of drug are also excreted in feces; biological half-life is 36 to 54 hours.

CONTRAINDICATIONS & PRECAUTIONS

Contraindicated in patients hypersensitive to any component of dexamethasone and in those with systemic fungal infections.

Use cautiously in patients with recent MI, GI ulcer, renal disease, hypertension, osteoporosis, diabetes mellitus, hypothyroidism, cirrhosis, diverticulitis, nonspecific ulcerative colitis, recent intestinal anastomoses, thromboembolic disorders, seizures, myasthenia gravis, heart failure, tuberculosis, ocular herpes simplex, emotional instability, and psychotic tendencies. Because some formulations contain sulfite preservatives, also use cautiously in patients sensitive to sulfites.

INTERACTIONS

Drug-drug. Dexamethasone may enhance hypokalemia from *amphotericin B* or *diuretic* therapy. *Antacids, cholestyramine,* and *colestipol* decrease the corticosteroid effect by adsorbing the corticosteroid, decreasing the amount absorbed. Dexamethasone may in rare cases decrease the effects of *oral anticoagulants* by unknown mechanisms. Use with *barbiturates, phenytoin,* and *rifampin* may decrease the effects of dexamethasone because of increased hepatic metabolism. Dexamethasone causes hyperglycemia, requiring dosage adjustment of *insulin* or *oral antidiabetics* in diabetic patients. Use with *estrogens* may reduce metabolism of dexamethasone by increasing transcortin levels; the half-life of dexamethasone is then prolonged because of increased protein-binding. Dexamethasone increases the metabolism of *isoniazid* and *salicylates;* the hypokalemia may increase the risk of toxicity in patients concurrently receiving *cardiac glycosides.* Administration with *ulcerogenic drugs,* such as *NSAIDs,* may increase the risk of GI ulceration.

ADVERSE REACTIONS

Most adverse reactions to corticosteroids depend on drug dose or duration.

CNS: *euphoria, insomnia,* psychotic behavior, pseudotumor cerebri, vertigo, headache, paresthesia, *seizures.*

CV: *heart failure,* hypertension, edema, *arrhythmias,* thrombophlebitis, *thromboembolism.*

EENT: cataracts, glaucoma.

Endocrine: menstrual irregularities, cushingoid state (moonface, buffalo hump, central obesity).

GI: *peptic ulceration,* GI irritation, increased appetite, *pancreatitis,* nausea, vomiting.

Metabolic: hypokalemia, hypocalcemia, hyperglycemia, carbohydrate intolerance, decreased T_4 and T_3, increased urine glucose and calcium levels.

Musculoskeletal: muscle weakness, osteoporosis.

Skin: delayed wound healing, acne, various skin eruptions, atrophy (at I.M. injection sites).

Other: susceptibility to infections, hirsutism, acute adrenal insufficiency after increased stress (infection, surgery, or trauma) or abrupt withdrawal after long-term therapy.

After abrupt withdrawal: rebound inflammation, fatigue, weakness, arthralgia, fever, dizziness, lethargy, depression, fainting, orthostatic hypotension, dyspnea, anorexia, hypoglycemia. *After prolonged use, sudden withdrawal may be fatal.*

▣ KEY CONSIDERATIONS

• Recommendations for use of dexamethasone, for care and teaching of patients during therapy, and for use in geriatric patients are the same as those for all systemic adrenocorticoids.

• Long-term use causes adverse physiological effects, including suppression of the hypothalamic-pituitary-adrenal axis, cushingoid appearance, muscle weakness, and osteoporosis.

• Dexamethasone suppresses reactions to skin tests; causes false-negative results in the nitroblue tetrazolium test for systemic bacterial infections; and decreases ^{131}I uptake and protein-bound iodine levels in thyroid function tests.

Patient education
• Advise patient of potential adverse reactions.

---

dexamethasone (topical)
Aeroseb-Dex, Decaspray

dexamethasone sodium phosphate
Decadron Phosphate

Corticosteroid, anti-inflammatory

Available by prescription only
dexamethasone
Aerosol: 0.01%, 0.04%
Gel: 0.1%
dexamethasone sodium phosphate
Cream: 0.1%

INDICATIONS & DOSAGE
Inflammation of corticosteroid-responsive dermatoses
Adults: Apply sparingly t.i.d. or q.i.d. For aerosol use on scalp, shake can well and apply to dry scalp after shampooing. Hold can upright. Slide applicator tube under hair so that it touches scalp. Spray while moving tube to all affected areas, keeping tube under hair and in contact with scalp throughout spraying, which should take about 2 seconds. Inadequately covered areas may be spot sprayed. Slide applicator tube through hair to touch scalp, press and immediately release spray button. Don't massage drug into scalp or spray forehead or eyes.

PHARMACODYNAMICS
Anti-inflammatory action: Dexamethasone is a synthetic fluorinated corticosteroid. It's usually classed as a group VII potency anti-inflammatory. Occlusive dressings may be used in severe cases. The aerosol spray is usually used for dermatologic conditions of the scalp.

PHARMACOKINETICS
Absorption: Dexamethasone absorption depends on the potency of the preparation, the amount applied, the vehicle used, and the skin at the application site. It ranges from about 1% in areas with a thick stratum corneum (such as the palms, soles, elbows, and knees) to 25% in areas of the thinnest stratum corneum (face, eyelids, and genitals). Inflamed or damaged skin may absorb more than 33%. Absorption increases in areas of skin damage, inflammation, or occlusion. Some systemic absorption occurs, especially through the oral mucosa.
Distribution: After topical application, dexamethasone is distributed throughout the local skin layer. If absorbed into circulation, the drug is distributed rapidly into muscle, liver, skin, intestines, and kidneys.
Metabolism: After topical administration, dexamethasone is metabolized primarily in the skin. The small amount that's absorbed into systemic circulation is primarily metabolized in the liver to inactive compounds.
Excretion: Inactive metabolites are excreted from the kidneys, primarily as glucuronides and sulfates, but also as unconjugated products. A small amount of metabolites is also excreted in feces.

CONTRAINDICATIONS & PRECAUTIONS
Contraindicated in patients hypersensitive to dexamethasone.

INTERACTIONS
None significant.

ADVERSE REACTIONS
Metabolic: hyperglycemia, glycosuria.
Skin: burning, pruritus, irritation, dryness, erythema, folliculitis, hypertrichosis, acneiform eruptions, perioral dermatitis, hypopigmentation, allergic contact dermatitis; *maceration, secondary infection, atrophy, striae, miliaria* (with occlusive dressings).
Other: *hypothalamic-pituitary-adrenal axis suppression,* Cushing's syndrome.

⊡ KEY CONSIDERATIONS
• Recommendations for use of dexamethasone, for care and teaching of patients during therapy and for use in geriatric patients are the same as those for all topical adrenocorticoids.

Patient education
• Teach patient to properly administer drug.

Reactions may be *common,* uncommon, *life-threatening,* or COMMON AND LIFE-THREATENING.

dexamethasone sodium phosphate

Nasal inhalant
Dexacort Phosphate Turbinaire

Oral inhalant
Dexacort Phosphate in Respihaler

Glucocorticoid, anti-inflammatory, antasthmatic

Available by prescription only
Nasal aerosol: 100 mcg of dexamethasone sodium phosphate/metered spray (equivalent to 84 mcg of dexamethasone); 170 doses/canister
Oral inhalation aerosol: 100 mcg of dexamethasone sodium phosphate/metered spray (equivalent to 84 mcg of dexamethasone); 170 doses/canister

INDICATIONS & DOSAGE

Allergic or inflammatory conditions, nasal polyps (excluding polyps originating within the sinuses)
Nasal inhaler
Adults: 2 sprays (168 mcg) into each nostril b.i.d. or t.i.d. Maximum daily dosage is 12 sprays (1,008 mcg).
Control of bronchial asthma in patients with steroid-dependent asthma
Oral inhaler
Adults: 3 inhalations t.i.d. or q.i.d., to a maximum dosage of 12 inhalations daily.

PHARMACODYNAMICS

Anti-inflammatory action: Dexamethasone stimulates the synthesis of enzymes needed to decrease the inflammatory response.
Antasthmatic action: Used as a nasal inhalant for the symptomatic treatment of seasonal or perennial rhinitis and nasal polyposis. It's used as an oral inhalant to treat bronchial asthma in patients who require corticosteroids to control symptoms.

PHARMACOKINETICS

Absorption: About 30% to 50% of an orally inhaled dose is systemically absorbed. Onset of action usually occurs within a few days, but may take as long as 7 days in some patients.
Distribution: Distribution after intranasal aerosol administration hasn't been described. After oral aerosol administration, drug is mostly distributed into the mouth and throat; the remainder is distributed through the trachea and bronchial tissue. When absorbed systemically, drug is distributed rapidly to muscle, liver, skin, intestines, and kidneys. Dexamethasone binds weakly to plasma proteins (transcortin and albumin). Only the unbound portion is active.
Metabolism: Drug is metabolized primarily in the liver to inactive glucuronide and sulfate metabolites. Some drug may be metabolized locally in the lung tissue.
Excretion: The inactive metabolites and a small amount of unmetabolized drug are excreted from the kidneys. Insignificant quantities of drug are excreted in feces. The biological half-life of dexamethasone is 36 to 54 hours.

CONTRAINDICATIONS & PRECAUTIONS

Oral inhalant is contraindicated in patients hypersensitive to any component of the formulation (fluorocarbons, ethanol) and in those with status asthmaticus, persistent positive sputum cultures for *Candida albicans,* or systemic fungal infections. Use oral inhalant cautiously in patients with ocular herpes simplex, nonspecific ulcerative colitis, diverticulitis, recent intestinal anastomoses, peptic ulcer, renal insufficiency, hypertension, osteoporosis, and myasthenia gravis. Dexamethasone shouldn't be added to therapy if bronchodilators or noncorticosteroids are controlling the asthma or if patient has nonasthmatic bronchial disease.

Nasal inhalant is contraindicated in patients with hypersensitivity to dexamethasone or in patients with systemic fungal infections, tuberculosis, viral and fungal nasal conditions, or ocular herpes simplex. Use nasal inhalant cautiously in patients with diabetes mellitus, peptic ulcer, ulcerative colitis, abscess or other pyrogenic infection, diverticulitis, recent intestinal anastomoses, renal insufficiency, hypertension, osteoporosis, and myasthenia gravis.

INTERACTIONS
None reported.

ADVERSE REACTIONS
EENT: nasal irritation, dryness, rebound nasal congestion, pharyngeal candidiasis (with use of oral inhalant).
Other: *hypersensitivity reactions,* systemic effects with prolonged use (pituitary-adrenal suppression, sodium retention, *heart failure,* hypertension, peptic ulceration, ecchymoses, petechiae, masking of infection).

▣ KEY CONSIDERATIONS
• Recommendations for use of inhalant dexamethasone and for care and teaching of the patient during therapy are the same as those for all inhalant adrenocorticoids.

Patient education
• Instruct patient on proper use of inhaler.

dexrazoxane
Zinecard

Intracellular chelating drug, cardioprotective drug

Available by prescription only
Injection: 250 mg and 500 mg in single-dose vials

INDICATIONS & DOSAGE
Reduction of incidence and severity of doxorubicin-induced cardiomyopathy in women with metastatic breast cancer who have received a cumulative doxorubicin dose of 300 mg/m² but would benefit from continued therapy with doxorubicin
Adults: Dosage ratio of dexrazoxane to doxorubicin must be 10:1 such as 500 mg/m² dexrazoxane:50 mg/m² doxorubicin. After reconstitution, dexrazoxane should be administered by slow I.V. push or rapid drip I.V. infusion. After dexrazoxane has been administered and before a total elapsed time of 30 minutes

from the beginning of the dexrazoxane administration, the I.V. injection of the doxorubicin dose should be given.

PHARMACODYNAMICS
Cardioprotective action: The specific mechanism of action is unknown. Dexrazoxane is a cyclic derivative of ethylenediaminetetraacetic that readily penetrates cell membranes. Studies suggest that drug is converted intracellularly to a ring-opened chelating agent that interferes with iron-mediated free radical generation believed to be responsible, in part, for anthracycline-induced cardiomyopathy.

PHARMACOKINETICS
Absorption: Dexrazoxane is given I.V.
Distribution: Unknown. Drug doesn't bind to plasma proteins.
Metabolism: Drug probably isn't metabolized.
Excretion: Drug is primarily excreted in urine.

CONTRAINDICATIONS & PRECAUTIONS
Contraindicated in patients who aren't receiving doxorubicin as part of the chemotherapy regimen. Use cautiously in all patients because additive effects of immunosuppression may occur from concomitant administration of cytotoxic drugs.

INTERACTIONS
None reported.

ADVERSE REACTIONS
The following reactions (except for pain on injection) may be attributed to the FAC regimen (fluorouracil, doxorubicin, cyclophosphamide) given shortly after dexrazoxane.
CNS: *fatigue, malaise, neurotoxicity.*
GI: *nausea, vomiting, anorexia, stomatitis, diarrhea,* esophagitis, dysphagia.
Hematologic: *hemorrhage.*
Skin: urticaria, *alopecia.*
Other: *fever, infection, pain on injection, sepsis,* streaking at I.V. insertion site, erythema, phlebitis, extravasation.

Reactions may be *common*, uncommon, *life-threatening*, or COMMON AND LIFE-THREATENING.

▣ KEY CONSIDERATIONS

• Doxorubicin shouldn't be given before dexrazoxane. Also, dexrazoxane isn't recommended for use with the initiation of doxorubicin therapy. Use only after 300 mg/m² of doxorubicin has been given and continuation of doxorubicin is desired.

• Drug must be diluted with the diluent supplied with drug (0.167 M sodium lactate injection) to give a concentration of 10 mg dexrazoxane for each ml of sodium lactate. Reconstituted solution should be given by slow I.V. push or rapid drip I.V. infusion from a bag.

• Reconstituted solution, when transferred to an empty infusion bag, is stable for 6 hours from the time of reconstitution when stored at controlled room temperature (36° to 46° F [2° to 8° C]) or under refrigeration. Discard unused solution.

• Reconstituted drug may be diluted with either normal saline solution or D₅W injection to a concentration range of 1.3 to 5.0 mg/ml in I.V. infusion bags. The resultant solution is also stable for 6 hours under the same storage conditions as the diluted drug.

• Dexrazoxane shouldn't be mixed with other drugs because of possible incompatibility.

• Use caution when handling and preparing the reconstituted solution; follow same precautions as handling antineoplastics. Be sure to use gloves. If drug powder or solution touches the skin or mucosa, immediately wash thoroughly with soap and water.

• Monitor CBC closely because drug is always used with other cytotoxic drugs and it may add to the myelosuppressive effects of cytotoxic drugs itself.

• The administration of dexrazoxane with doxorubicin doesn't eliminate the possibility of cardiac toxicity. Therefore cardiac function should be carefully monitored.

Patient education

• Inform patient of need for drug during continued doxorubicin therapy.

• Warn patient to watch for signs of and symptoms of infection (such as fever, sore throat, and fatigue) and bleeding

(such as easy bruising, nose bleeds, bleeding gums, and melena). Tell patient to take temperature daily and teach him infection control and bleeding precautions.

• Inform patient that alopecia may occur but that it's usually reversible.

Overdose and treatment

• Suspected overdose should be managed with good supportive care until resolution of myelosuppression and related conditions is complete.

• Management of overdose should include treatment of infections, fluid regulation, and maintenance of nutritional requirements.

---

dextromethorphan hydrobromide

Balminil D.M.*, Benylin DM Cough, Broncho-Grippol-DM*, Delsym, DM Syrup*, Hold, Koffex*, Mediquell, Neo-DM*, Robidex*, Sedatuss*, St. Joseph Cough Suppressant for Children, Sucrets Cough Control Formula, Suppress, Trocal, Vicks Formula 44

Levorphanol derivative (dextro-rotatory methyl ether), antitussive (nonnarcotic)

Available without a prescription
Syrup: 10 mg/5 ml, 15 mg/15 ml
Liquid (sustained-action): 30 mg/5 ml
Liquid: 3.5 mg/5 ml, 7.5 mg/5 ml, 15 mg/5 ml
Lozenges: 2.5 mg, 5 mg, 7.5 mg
Chewable pieces: 15 mg

INDICATIONS & DOSAGE

Nonproductive cough (chronic)
Adults: 10 to 20 mg q 4 hours, or 30 mg q 6 to 8 hours. Or the controlled-release liquid b.i.d. (60 mg b.i.d.). Maximum dose is 120 mg daily.

PHARMACODYNAMICS

Antitussive action: Dextromethorphan suppresses the cough reflex by directly acting on the cough center in the medulla. It's almost equal in antitussive potency to codeine, but causes no analgesia or

---

*Canada only   ◇ Unlabeled clinical use

addiction and little or no CNS depression and has no expectorant action; it also produces fewer subjective and GI adverse effects than codeine. Treatment is intended to relieve cough frequency without abolishing protective cough reflex. In therapeutic doses, drug doesn't inhibit ciliary activity.

PHARMACOKINETICS
Absorption: Dextromethorphan is absorbed readily from the GI tract; action begins within 15 to 30 minutes.
Distribution: Unknown.
Metabolism: Drug is metabolized extensively in the liver. Plasma half-life is about 11 hours.
Excretion: Little drug is excreted unchanged. Metabolites are excreted primarily in urine; 7% to 10% is excreted in feces. Antitussive effect persists for 5 to 6 hours.

CONTRAINDICATIONS & PRECAUTIONS
Contraindicated in patients who are taking MAO inhibitors or who have discontinued them within the past 2 weeks. Use cautiously with sedated or debilitated patients and those confined to the supine position. Also use cautiously in patients with sensitivity to aspirin.

INTERACTIONS
Use with *MAO inhibitors* may cause nausea, hypotension, excitation, hyperpyrexia, and coma; don't give dextromethorphan to patients at any interval less than 2 weeks after MAO inhibitors are discontinued.

ADVERSE REACTIONS
CNS: drowsiness, dizziness.
GI: nausea, vomiting, stomach pain.

▣ KEY CONSIDERATIONS
• Treatment is intended to relieve cough intensity and frequency, without completely abolishing the protective cough reflex.
• Use with percussion and chest vibration.
• Monitor nature and frequency of coughing.

Patient education
• Tell patient to call if cough persists more than 7 days.
• Instruct patient to use sugarless throat lozenges for throat irritation and resulting cough.
• Recommend a humidifier to filter dust, smoke, and air pollutants.

Overdose & treatment
• Signs and symptoms of overdose include nausea, vomiting, drowsiness, dizziness, blurred vision, nystagmus, shallow respirations, urine retention, toxic psychosis, stupor, and coma.
• Treatment of overdose involves administering activated charcoal to reduce drug absorption and administering I.V. naloxone to support respiration. Other symptoms are treated supportively.

diazepam
Apo-Diazepam*, Dizac, Novo-Dipam*, Valium, Vivol*, Zetran

Benzodiazepine, anxiolytic, skeletal muscle relaxant, antiamnesia drug, anticonvulsant, sedative-hypnotic
Controlled substance schedule IV

Available by prescription only
Tablets: 2 mg, 5 mg, 10 mg
Capsules (extended-release): 15 mg
Oral solution: 5 mg/ml; 5 mg/5 ml
Oral suspension: 5 mg/5 ml
Injection: 5 mg/ml in 2-ml ampules or 10-ml vials
Disposable syringe: 2-ml Tel-E-Ject

INDICATIONS & DOSAGE
Anxiety
Adults: Depending on severity, 2 to 10 mg P.O. b.i.d. to q.i.d. or 15 to 30 mg extended-release capsules P.O. once daily. Alternatively, 2 to 10 mg I.M. or I.V. q 3 to 4 hours p.r.n.
Muscle spasm
Adults: 2 to 10 mg P.O. b.i.d. to q.i.d.; or 15 to 30 mg extended-release capsules once daily. Alternatively, 5 to 10 mg I.M. or I.V. q 3 to 4 hours, p.r.n.
Adjunct to convulsive disorders
Adults: 2 to 10 mg P.O. b.i.d. to q.i.d.

Status epilepticus
Adults: 5 to 10 mg I.V. (preferred) or
I.M. initially, repeated at 10- to 15-
minute intervals up to a maximum dose
of 30 mg. Repeat q 2 to 4 hours, p.r.n.
Adjunct to anesthesia; endoscopic pro-
cedures
Adults: 5 to 10 mg I.M. before surgery;
or administer I.V. slowly just before procedure, titrating dose to effect. Usually,
less than 10 mg is used, but up to 20 mg
may be given.
Cardioversion
Adults: Administer 5 to 15 mg I.V. 5 to
10 minutes before procedure.
Acute alcohol withdrawal
Adults: 10 mg P.O. t.i.d. or q.i.d. for the
first 24 hours; reduce to 5 mg t.i.d. or
q.i.d., p.r.n.; or 10 mg I.M. or I.V. initially, followed by 5 to 10 mg q 3 to 4 hours,
p.r.n.

PHARMACODYNAMICS

Anxiolytic and sedative-hypnotic ac-
tions: Diazepam depresses the CNS at
the limbic and subcortical levels of the
brain. It produces an anxiolytic effect by
facilitating the binding of the neurotransmitter gamma-aminobutyric acid on
its receptor in the ascending reticular activating system, which increases inhibition and blocks cortical and limbic
arousal.
Skeletal muscle relaxant action: The exact mechanism is unknown, but it's believed to involve inhibiting polysynaptic
afferent pathways.
Antiamnesia action: The exact mechanism of action is unknown.
Anticonvulsant action: Diazepam suppresses the spread of seizure activity
produced by epileptogenic foci in the
cortex, thalamus, and limbic structures
by enhancing presynaptic inhibition.

PHARMACOKINETICS

Absorption: When administered orally,
diazepam is absorbed through the GI
tract. Onset of action occurs within 30 to
60 minutes, with peak action in 1 to 2
hours. I.M. administration results in erratic absorption of the drug; onset of action usually occurs in 15 to 30 minutes.
After I.V. administration, rapid onset of

action occurs 1 to 5 minutes after injection.
Distribution: Distributed widely
throughout the body. About 85% to 95%
of an administered dose binds to plasma
protein.
Metabolism: Drug is metabolized in the
liver to the active metabolite desmethyldiazepam.
Excretion: Most metabolites of diazepam are excreted in urine, with only
a small amount excreted in feces. Half-
life of desmethyldiazepam is 30 to 200
hours. Duration of sedative effect is 3
hours; this may be prolonged up to 90
hours in geriatric patients, especially
those with hepatic or renal dysfunction.
Anticonvulsant effect is 30 to 60 minutes
after I.V. administration.

CONTRAINDICATIONS & PRECAUTIONS

Contraindicated in patients with hypersensitivity or angle-closure glaucoma; in
patients experiencing shock, coma, or
acute alcohol intoxication (parenteral
form). Use cautiously in geriatric patients, in debilitated patients, and in
those with impaired hepatic or renal
function, depression, or chronic open-
angle glaucoma.

INTERACTIONS

Drug-drug. *Antacids* may decrease the
rate of absorption of diazepam. Diazepam potentiates the CNS depressant effects of *antidepressants, antihistamines,*
barbiturates, general anesthetics, MAO
inhibitors, narcotics, and *phenothia-*
zines. Use with *cimetidine* or possibly
disulfiram causes diminished hepatic
metabolism of diazepam, which increases its plasma level. Diazepam reportedly
can decrease *digoxin* clearance; monitor
patients for digoxin toxicity. *Haloperidol*
may change the seizure patterns of patients treated with diazepam, and diazepam may reduce the serum haloperidol
levels. Diazepam may inhibit the therapeutic effect of *levodopa.* Use with *non-*
depolarizing neuromuscular blockers
such as *pancuronium* and *succinyl-*
choline can cause intensified and prolonged respiratory depression.
Drug-lifestyle. Diazepam potentiates the
CNS depressant effects of *alcohol.*

Heavy smoking accelerates metabolism of diazepam, thus lowering drug effectiveness.

ADVERSE REACTIONS

CNS: *drowsiness,* slurred speech, tremor, transient amnesia, fatigue, ataxia, headache, insomnia, paradoxical anxiety, hallucinations, minor changes in EEG patterns.
CV: hypotension, *CV collapse,* bradycardia.
EENT: diplopia, blurred vision, nystagmus.
GI: nausea, constipation.
GU: incontinence, urine retention, altered libido.
Hematologic: *neutropenia.*
Hepatic: elevated liver function tests, *jaundice.*
Musculoskeletal: *dysarthria.*
Respiratory: *respiratory depression.*
Skin: rash.
Other: physical or psychological dependence, *acute withdrawal syndrome* after sudden discontinuation in physically dependent persons, *pain, phlebitis* (at injection site).

▣ KEY CONSIDERATIONS

Besides the recommendations relevant to all benzodiazepines, consider the following:
• Geriatric patients are more sensitive to the CNS depressant effects of diazepam. Use with caution.
• Lower dosages are usually effective in geriatric patients because of decreased elimination.
• Geriatric patients who receive this drug require assistance with walking and activities of daily living during initiation of therapy or after an increase in dosage.
• Parenteral administration of this drug is more likely to cause apnea, hypotension, and bradycardia in geriatric patients.
• Don't discontinue drug suddenly; decrease dosage slowly over 8 to 12 weeks after long-term therapy.
• To enhance taste, oral solution can be mixed with liquids or semisolid foods, such as applesauce or puddings, immediately before administration.

• Extended-release capsule should be swallowed whole; don't let patient crush or chew capsule.
• Shake oral suspension well before administering.
• When prescribing with opiates for endoscopic procedures, reduce opiate dosage by at least one-third.
• Parenteral forms of diazepam may be diluted in normal saline solution; a slight precipitate may form, but the solution can still be used.
• Diazepam interacts with plastic. Don't store diazepam in plastic syringes or administer it in plastic administration sets, which will decrease availability of the infused drug.
• I.V. route is preferred because of rapid and more uniform absorption.
• For I.V. administration, drug should be infused slowly, directly into a large vein, at a rate not exceeding 5 mg/minute for adults. To avoid extravasation into subcutaneous tissue, don't inject diazepam into small veins. Observe infusion site for phlebitis. If direct I.V. administration is impossible, inject diazepam directly into I.V. tubing at point closest to vein insertion site to prevent extravasation.
• Administration by continuous I.V. infusion isn't recommended.
• Inject I.M. dose deep into deltoid muscle. To prevent inadvertent intra-arterial administration aspirate for backflow. Use I.M. route only if I.V. or oral routes are unavailable.
• Patient should remain in bed under observation for at least 3 hours after parenteral administration of diazepam to prevent potential hazards; keep resuscitation equipment nearby.
• During prolonged therapy, periodically monitor blood counts and liver function studies.
• Lower dosages are effective in patients with renal or hepatic dysfunction.
• To prevent aspiration, assess gag reflex after performing endoscopy and before resuming oral intake.
• Anticipate possible transient increase in frequency or severity of seizures when diazepam is used as adjunctive treatment of convulsive disorders. Impose seizure precautions.

Reactions may be *common,* uncommon, *life-threatening,* or COMMON AND LIFE-THREATENING.

• Don't mix diazepam with other drugs in a syringe or infusion container.

Patient education

• Advise patient of the potential for physical and psychological dependence with long-term use.
• Warn patient that sudden changes of position can cause dizziness. Advise patient to dangle legs for a few minutes before getting out of bed to prevent falls and injury.
• Encourage patient to avoid or limit smoking to prevent increased diazepam metabolism.
• Caution patient to avoid alcohol while taking diazepam.
• Advise patient not to suddenly discontinue drug.

Overdose & treatment

• Signs and symptoms of overdose include somnolence, confusion, coma, hypoactive reflexes, dyspnea, labored breathing, hypotension, bradycardia, slurred speech, and unsteady gait or impaired coordination.
• Support blood pressure and respiration until drug effects subside; monitor vital signs. Mechanical ventilatory assistance via endotracheal tube may be required to maintain a patent airway and support adequate oxygenation. Flumazenil, a specific benzodiazepine antagonist, may be useful; however, it shouldn't be used in a patient with status epilepticus. Use I.V. fluids and vasopressors such as dopamine and phenylephrine to treat hypotension as needed. If the patient is conscious, induce vomiting; use gastric lavage if ingestion was recent, but only if an endotracheal tube is present to prevent aspiration. Then, administer activated charcoal with a cathartic as a single dose. Dialysis is of limited value.

diazoxide
Hyperstat IV, Proglycem

Peripheral vasodilator, antihypertensive, antidiabetic

Available by prescription only
Capsules: 50 mg

Oral suspension: 50 mg/ml in 30-ml bottle
Injection: 300 mg/20-ml ampule

INDICATIONS & DOSAGE
Hypertensive crisis
Adults: 1 to 3 mg/kg I.V. (up to a maximum of 150 mg) q 5 to 15 minutes until blood pressure is adequately reduced.
  Note: The use of 300-mg I.V. bolus push is no longer recommended. Switch to therapy with oral antihypertensives as soon as possible.
Hypoglycemia from hyperinsulinism
Adults: Usual daily dosage is 3 to 8 mg/kg/day P.O. divided in two or three equal doses.

PHARMACODYNAMICS
Antihypertensive action: Diazoxide directly relaxes arteriolar smooth muscle, causing vasodilation and reducing peripheral vascular resistance, thus reducing blood pressure.
Antidiabetic action: Drug increases blood glucose levels by inhibiting pancreatic secretion of insulin, stimulating catecholamine release, and increasing hepatic release of glucose.
  Diazoxide is a nondiuretic congener of thiazide diuretics.

PHARMACOKINETICS
Absorption: After I.V. administration, blood pressure should decrease promptly, with maximum decrease in under 5 minutes. After oral administration, hyperglycemic effect begins in 1 hour.
Distribution: Diazoxide is distributed throughout the body; highest levels found in kidneys, liver, and adrenal glands. Drug crosses blood-brain barrier; about 90% binds to proteins.
Metabolism: Drug is metabolized partially in the liver.
Excretion: Drug and its metabolites are excreted slowly from the kidneys. Duration of antihypertensive effect varies widely, ranging from 30 minutes to 72 hours (average 3 to 12 hours) after I.V. administration; after oral administration, antihypoglycemic effect persists for about 8 hours. Antihypertensive and antihypoglycemic effects may be pro-

longed in patients with renal dysfunction.

CONTRAINDICATIONS & PRECAUTIONS

Parenteral form is contraindicated in patients with hypersensitivity to diazoxide, other thiazides, or sulfonamide-derived drugs and in the treatment of compensatory hypertension (such as that associated with coarctation of the aorta or arteriovenous shunt). Oral form is contraindicated in patients with functional hypoglycemia.

Use cautiously in patients with uremia or impaired cerebral or cardiac function.

INTERACTIONS

Drug-drug. Diazoxide may potentiate antihypertensive effects of other *antihypertensives,* especially if I.V. diazoxide is administered within 6 hours after patient has received another antihypertensive. Diazoxide may displace *bilirubin, other highly protein-bound substances,* or *warfarin* from protein-binding sites. Diazoxide may alter *insulin* and *oral antidiabetic* requirements in diabetic patients with previously stable conditions. Use with *diuretics* may potentiate antihypoglycemic, hyperuricemic, or antihypertensive effects of diazoxide. Use with *phenytoin* may increase metabolism and decrease the plasma protein binding of phenytoin. Use with other *thiazides* may enhance effects of diazoxide.

ADVERSE REACTIONS

CNS: dizziness, weakness, headache, malaise, anxiety, insomnia, paresthesia (with oral form); headache, *seizures, paralysis, cerebral ischemia,* lightheadedness, euphoria (with parenteral form).
CV: *arrhythmias,* tachycardia, hypotension, hypertension (with oral form); *sodium and water retention, orthostatic hypotension,* diaphoresis, flushing, warmth, angina, myocardial ischemia, *arrhythmias,* ECG changes, *shock, MI* (with parenteral form).
EENT: diplopia, transient cataracts, blurred vision, lacrimation (with oral form); optic nerve infarction (with parenteral form).

GI: abdominal discomfort, diarrhea, nausea, vomiting, anorexia, taste alteration (with oral form); *nausea, vomiting,* dry mouth, constipation (with parenteral form).
GU: azotemia, reversible nephrotic syndrome, decreased urine output, hematuria, albuminuria (with oral form).
Hematologic: *leukopenia, thrombocytopenia,* anemia, eosinophilia, excessive bleeding (with oral form).
Metabolic: *sodium and fluid retention, ketoacidosis and hyperosmolar nonketotic syndrome, hyperuricemia, hyperglycemia.*
Skin: rash, pruritus (with oral form).
Other: hirsutism, fever (with oral form), inflammation and pain resulting from extravasation.

▣ KEY CONSIDERATIONS

● Geriatric patients may have a more pronounced hypotensive response.
● Diazoxide is used to treat only hypoglycemia resulting from hyperinsulinism; it isn't used to treat functional hypoglycemia. It may be used temporarily to control preoperative or postoperative hypoglycemia in patients with hyperinsulinism.
● Diazoxide inhibits glucose-stimulated insulin release and may cause falsenegative insulin response to glucagon. Prolonged use of oral diazoxide may decrease hemoglobin levels and hematocrit.
● I.V. use of diazoxide is seldom necessary for more than 4 to 5 days.
● After I.V. injection, monitor blood pressure every 5 minutes for 15 to 30 minutes, then hourly when patient's condition is stable. Discontinue if severe hypotension develops or if blood pressure continues to fall 30 minutes after drug infusion; keep patient recumbent during this time and have norepinephrine available. Monitor I.V. site for infiltration or extravasation.
● Monitor patient's intake and output carefully. If fluid or sodium retention develops, diuretics may be given 30 to 60 minutes after diazoxide. Keep patient recumbent for 8 to 10 hours after diuretic administration.

Reactions may be *common,* uncommon, *life-threatening*, or COMMON AND LIFE-THREATENING.

• Monitor daily blood glucose and electrolyte levels, watching diabetic patients closely for severe hyperglycemia or hyperosmolar hyperglycemic nonketotic syndrome; also monitor daily urine glucose and ketone levels, intake and output, and weight. Check serum uric acid levels frequently.

• Protect solutions from light, heat, or freezing; don't administer solutions that have darkened or that contain particulate matter.

• Significant hypotension doesn't occur after oral administration in doses used to treat hypoglycemia.

• Drug may be given by constant I.V. infusion (7.5 to 30 mg/minute) until blood pressure is adequately reduced.

Patient education

• Explain that orthostatic hypotension can be minimized by rising slowly and avoiding sudden position changes.

• Tell patient to report adverse effects immediately, including pain and redness at injection site, which may indicate infiltration.

• Instruct patient to check weight daily and report gains of more than 2.3 kg (5 lb)/week; diazoxide causes sodium and water retention.

• Reassure patient that excessive hair growth is a common reaction that subsides when drug treatment is completed.

Overdose & treatment

• Hyperglycemia is the primary sign of overdose; ketoacidosis and hypotension may occur.

• Treat acute overdose supportively and symptomatically. If hyperglycemia develops, give insulin and replace fluid and electrolyte losses; use vasopressors if hypotension fails to respond to conservative treatment. Prolonged monitoring may be necessary because diazoxide has a long half-life.

diclofenac potassium
Cataflam

diclofenac sodium
Voltaren, Voltaren Ophthalmic, Voltaren-XR

NSAID, antarthritic, antipyretic, anti-inflammatory

Available by prescription only
Tablets: 25 mg*, 50 mg
Tablets (enteric-coated): 25 mg, 50 mg, 75 mg, 100 mg
Ophthalmic solution: 0.1%

INDICATIONS & DOSAGE
Osteoarthritis
Adults: 50 mg P.O. b.i.d. or t.i.d., or 75 mg P.O. b.i.d. (diclofenac sodium only).
Ankylosing spondylitis
Adults: 25 mg P.O. q.i.d. An additional 25 mg dose may be needed h.s.
Rheumatoid arthritis
Adults: 50 mg P.O. t.i.d. or q.i.d. Alternatively, 75 mg P.O. b.i.d. (diclofenac sodium only).
Analgesia and primary dysmenorrhea
Adults: 50 mg (diclofenac potassium only) P.O. t.i.d. Alternatively, 100 mg (diclofenac potassium only) P.O. initially, followed by 50-mg doses, up to a maximum dosage of 200 mg in first 24 hours; subsequent dosing should follow 50-mg t.i.d. regimen.
Postoperative inflammation after cataract removal
Adults: 1 drop in the conjunctival sac q.i.d. beginning 24 hours after surgery and continuing throughout the first 2 weeks of the postoperative period.

PHARMACODYNAMICS
Antiarthritic, anti-inflammatory, and antipyretic actions: Diclofenac produces its effects through an unknown mechanism that may involve inhibition of prostaglandin synthesis.

PHARMACOKINETICS
Absorption: After oral administration, diclofenac is rapidly and almost completely absorbed, with plasma levels

peaking in 10 to 30 minutes. Food delays absorption, with plasma levels peaking in 2½ to 12 hours; however, bioavailability is unchanged.

Distribution: Nearly 100% of drug binds to proteins.

Metabolism: Drug undergoes first-pass metabolism, with 60% of unchanged drug reaching systemic circulation. The principal active metabolite, 4'-hydroxydiclofenac, has about 3% the activity of the parent compound. Mean terminal half-life is 1.2 to 1.8 hours after an oral dose.

Excretion: About 40% to 60% of diclofenac is excreted in the urine; the balance is excreted in the bile. The 4'-hydroxy metabolite accounts for 20% to 30% of the dose excreted in the urine; the other metabolites account for 10% to 20%; 5% to 10% excreted unchanged in the urine. More than 90% is excreted within 72 hours. Moderate renal impairment doesn't alter the elimination rate of unchanged diclofenac but may reduce the elimination rate of the metabolites. Hepatic impairment doesn't appear to affect the pharmacokinetics of diclofenac.

CONTRAINDICATIONS & PRECAUTIONS

Oral form is contraindicated in patients with hypersensitivity to diclofenac and in those with hepatic porphyria or a history of asthma, urticaria, or other allergic reactions after taking aspirin or other NSAIDs. Ophthalmic solution is contraindicated in patients with hypersensitivity to any component of the drug and in those wearing soft contact lenses.

Use oral form cautiously in patients with history of peptic ulcer disease, hepatic or renal dysfunction, cardiac disease, hypertension, or conditions associated with fluid retention.

Use ophthalmic solution cautiously in patients with hypersensitivity to aspirin, phenylacetic acid derivatives, and other NSAIDs and in surgical patients with known bleeding tendencies or in those receiving drugs that may prolong bleeding time.

INTERACTIONS

Drug-drug. Administration with *aspirin* lowers plasma levels of diclofenac and isn't recommended. Use with *cyclosporine, digoxin,* or *methotrexate* may increase toxicity of these drugs. Diclofenac may inhibit the action of *diuretics.* Use with *insulin* or *oral antidiabetics* may alter the patient's response to these drugs. Use with *lithium* decreases renal clearance of lithium and therefore increases its plasma levels and may lead to lithium toxicity. Administration with *other drugs that produce adverse GI effects,* such as *glucocorticoids,* may aggravate such effects. Use with *potassium sparing diuretics* may increase serum potassium levels. Use with *warfarin* requires close monitoring of anticoagulant dosage because diclofenac, like other NSAIDs, affects platelet function.

ADVERSE REACTIONS

Unless noted, adverse reactions refer to oral form of drug.

CNS: anxiety, depression, dizziness, drowsiness, insomnia, irritability, headache.

CV: *heart failure,* hypertension, edema.

EENT: *tinnitus,* laryngeal edema, swelling of the lips and tongue, blurred vision, eye pain, night blindness, epistaxis, taste disorder, reversible hearing loss, *transient stinging and burning, increased intraocular pressure, keratitis,* anterior chamber reaction, ocular allergy (with ophthalmic solution).

GI: *abdominal pain or cramps, constipation, diarrhea, indigestion, nausea,* vomiting, abdominal distention, flatulence, peptic ulceration, *bleeding,* melena, bloody diarrhea, appetite change, colitis.

GU: proteinuria, *acute renal failure,* oliguria, interstitial nephritis, papillary necrosis, *nephrotic syndrome,* fluid retention.

Hepatic: elevated liver enzyme levels, jaundice, hepatitis, *hepatotoxicity.*

Hematologic: increased platelet aggregation time.

Metabolic: hypoglycemia, hyperglycemia.

Musculoskeletal: back, leg, or joint pain.

Reactions may be *common,* uncommon, *life-threatening,* or COMMON AND LIFE-THREATENING.

Respiratory: asthma.

Skin: rash, pruritus, urticaria, eczema, dermatitis, alopecia, photosensitivity, bullous eruption, *Stevens-Johnson syndrome* (rare), allergic purpura.

Other: *anaphylaxis, anaphylactoid reactions, angioedema,* viral infection (with ophthalmic solution).

☑ KEY CONSIDERATIONS

• Use with caution in geriatric patients. They may be more susceptible to adverse reactions, especially GI toxicity and nephrotoxicity. Reduce dosage to lowest level that controls symptoms.

• Periodic evaluation of hematopoietic function is recommended because bone marrow abnormalities have occurred. To detect toxic effects on the GI tract, regularly check patient's hemoglobin level.

• Because the anti-inflammatory, antipyretic, and analgesic effects of diclofenac may mask the usual signs of infection, monitor carefully for infection.

• Monitor renal function during treatment. Use with caution and at reduced dosage in patients with renal impairment.

• Periodic ophthalmologic examinations are recommended during long-term therapy.

• Monitor liver function during therapy. Abnormal liver function test results and severe hepatic reactions may occur.

Patient education

• Advise patient to take drug with meals or milk to avoid GI upset.

• Teach patient to restrict salt intake, as diclofenac may cause edema, especially if patient is hypertensive.

• Instruct patient to report signs and symptoms that may be related to GI ulceration, such as epigastric pain and black or tarry stools, as well as other unusual signs and symptoms such as rash, pruritus, or significant edema or weight gain.

Overdose & treatment

• Supportive and symptomatic treatment may include inducing vomiting and performing gastric lavage. Administering activated charcoal and performing dialysis may also be appropriate.

dicloxacillin sodium
Dycill, Dynapen, Pathocil

Penicillinase-resistant penicillin, antibiotic

Available by prescription only
Capsules: 125 mg, 250 mg, 500 mg
Oral suspension: 62.5 mg/5 ml (after reconstitution)

INDICATIONS & DOSAGE

Systemic infections caused by penicillinase-producing staphylococci
Adults: 125 to 250 mg P.O. q 6 hours.

PHARMACODYNAMICS

Antibiotic action: Dicloxacillin is bactericidal; it adheres to bacterial penicillin-binding proteins, thus inhibiting bacterial cell wall synthesis. It resists the effects of penicillinases—enzymes that inactivate penicillin—and is thus active against many strains of penicillinase-producing bacteria; this activity is most important against penicillinase-producing staphylococci; some strains may remain resistant. And dicloxacillin is active against a few gram-positive aerobic and anaerobic bacilli but has no significant effect on gram-negative bacilli.

PHARMACOKINETICS

Absorption: Dicloxacillin is absorbed rapidly but incompletely (35% to 76%) from the GI tract; it's relatively acid stable. Plasma levels peak ½ to 2 hours after an oral dose. Food may decrease both rate and extent of absorption.

Distribution: Distributed widely into bone, bile, and pleural and synovial fluids. CSF penetration is poor but is enhanced by meningeal inflammation. About 95% to 99% binds to proteins.

Metabolism: Drug is only partially metabolized.

Excretion: Drug and metabolites are excreted in urine through renal tubular secretion and glomerular filtration. Elimination half-life in adults is ½ to 1 hour, extended minimally to 2.2 hours in patients with renal impairment.

---

*Canada only ◊ Unlabeled clinical use

CONTRAINDICATIONS & PRECAUTIONS

Contraindicated in patients with hypersensitivity to dicloxacillin or other penicillins. Use cautiously in patients with other drug allergies, especially to cephalosporins, and in those with mononucleosis.

INTERACTIONS

Drug-drug. Use with *aminoglycosides* produces synergistic bactericidal effects against *Staphylococcus aureus;* however, the drugs are physically and chemically incompatible and are inactivated when mixed or given together. *Probenecid* blocks renal tubular secretion of dicloxacillin, raising its serum levels.
Drug-food. Acid in *carbonated beverages* or *fruit juices* may inactivate drug. *Food* decreases absorption of drug.

ADVERSE REACTIONS

CNS: neuromuscular irritability, *seizures,* lethargy, hallucinations, anxiety, confusion, agitation, depression, dizziness, fatigue.
GI: *nausea,* vomiting, *epigastric distress,* flatulence, *diarrhea,* enterocolitis, pseudomembranous colitis, black "hairy" tongue, abdominal pain.
GU: interstitial nephritis, nephropathy.
Hematologic: eosinophilia, anemia, *thrombocytopenia, leukopenia, hemolytic anemia, agranulocytosis.*
Hepatic: transient elevations in liver function tests indicating drug-induced cholestasis or *hepatitis.*
Other: hypersensitivity reactions (pruritus, urticaria, rash, *anaphylaxis*), overgrowth of nonsusceptible organisms.

▣ KEY CONSIDERATIONS

Besides the recommendations relevant to all penicillins, consider the following:
• Half-life may be prolonged in geriatric patients because of impaired renal function.
• Give drug with water only; acid in fruit juice or carbonated beverages may inactivate drug.
• Give dose on empty stomach; food decreases absorption.
• Regularly assess renal, hepatic, and hematopoietic function during prolonged therapy.

• Dicloxacillin alters test results for urine and serum proteins; it produces false-positive or elevated results in turbidimetric urine and serum protein tests using sulfosalicylic acid or trichloroacetic acid; it also reportedly produces false results on the Bradshaw screening test for Bence Jones protein.
• Dicloxacillin may falsely decrease serum aminoglycoside levels.

Patient education

• Tell patient to report severe diarrhea promptly. He should also report rash or itching.
• Instruct patient to complete full course of therapy.
• Advise patient to take drug with water on empty stomach, and avoid taking with fruit juice or carbonated beverages, which may inactivate drug.

Overdose & treatment

• Signs and symptoms of overdose include neuromuscular irritability or seizures.
• Treatment is supportive. After recent ingestion (4 hours or less), induce vomiting or perform gastric lavage; follow with activated charcoal to reduce absorption. Drug isn't appreciably dialyzable.

dicyclomine hydrochloride

Antispas, A-Spas, Bentyl, Bentylol*, Byclomine, Dibent, Formulex*, Lomine*, Neoquess, Or-Tyl, Spasmoban*, Spasmoject

Anticholinergic, GI antispasmodic

Available by prescription only
Tablets: 20 mg
Capsules: 10 mg, 20 mg
Syrup: 10 mg/5 ml
Injection: 10 mg/ml in 2-ml vials, 10-ml vials, 2-ml ampules

INDICATIONS & DOSAGE

Irritable bowel syndrome and other functional GI disorders
Adults: Initially, 20 mg P.O. q.i.d., then increase to 40 mg P.O. q.i.d. during first week of therapy unless precluded by ad-

verse reactions. Alternatively, give 20 mg I.M. q 4 to 6 hours.

Note: High environmental temperatures may induce heatstroke during drug use. If symptoms occur, the drug should be discontinued.

PHARMACODYNAMICS

Antispasmodic action: Dicyclomine exerts a nonspecific, direct spasmolytic action on smooth muscle. It also has some local anesthetic properties that may contribute to spasmolysis in the GI and biliary tracts.

PHARMACOKINETICS

Absorption: About 67% of an oral dose is absorbed from the GI tract.
Distribution: Largely unknown.
Metabolism: Unknown.
Excretion: After oral administration, 80% of a dose is excreted in urine and 10% in feces.

CONTRAINDICATIONS & PRECAUTIONS

Contraindicated in patients with obstructive uropathy, obstructive disease of the GI tract, reflux esophagitis, severe ulcerative colitis, myasthenia gravis, hypersensitivity to anticholinergics, unstable CV status in acute hemorrhage, or glaucoma.

Use cautiously in patients with autonomic neuropathy, hyperthyroidism, coronary artery disease, arrhythmias, heart failure, hypertension, hiatal hernia, hepatic or renal disease, prostatic hyperplasia, and ulcerative colitis.

INTERACTIONS

Drug-drug. Administration with *antacids* decreases oral absorption of anticholinergics; administer dicyclomine at least 1 hour before antacids. *Anticholinergics*—such as *ketoconazole* and *levodopa*—may decrease GI absorption of digoxin. Conversely, slowly dissolving *digoxin* tablets may yield higher serum digoxin levels when administered with anticholinergics. Administration with *drugs with anticholinergic effects* may cause additive toxicity. Use cautiously with *oral potassium supplements* (especially *wax-matrix formulations*) because the risk of potassium-induced GI ulcerations may be increased.

ADVERSE REACTIONS

CNS: *headache, dizziness,* insomnia, light-headedness, drowsiness, nervousness, confusion, excitement (in geriatric patients).
CV: *palpitations,* tachycardia.
EENT: blurred vision, increased intraocular pressure, mydriasis.
GI: nausea, vomiting, *constipation, dry mouth,* abdominal distention, heartburn, paralytic ileus.
GU: *urinary hesitancy, urine retention,* impotence.
Skin: urticaria, decreased sweating or possible anhidrosis, other dermal effects, local irritation.
Other: fever, *allergic reactions.*

Dicyclomine is a synthetic tertiary derivative that may have atropine-like adverse reactions.

🔲 KEY CONSIDERATIONS

Besides the recommendations relevant to all anticholinergics, consider the following:
• Dicyclomine should be administered cautiously to geriatric patients because adverse reactions may be more severe in this population. Lower dosages are indicated.
• Never give dicyclomine I.V. or S.C.

Patient education

• Tell patient that syrup formulation may be diluted with water.
• Warn patient that high environmental temperatures may induce heatstroke while drug is being used; tell patient to avoid exposure to such temperatures.

Overdose & treatment

• Signs and symptoms of overdose include symptoms of CNS stimulation (followed by depression) and such psychotic symptoms as disorientation, confusion, hallucinations, delusions, anxiety, agitation, and restlessness. Peripheral effects may include dilated, nonreactive pupils; hot, flushed, dry skin; tachycardia; hypertension; and increased respiration.

• Treatment is primarily symptomatic and supportive, as necessary. Maintain patent airway. If patient is alert, induce vomiting (or perform gastric lavage) and follow with a saline cathartic and activated charcoal to prevent further drug absorption. In severe cases, physostigmine may be administered to block the antimuscarinic effects of dicyclomine. Give fluids, as needed, to treat shock, diazepam to control psychotic symptoms, and pilocarpine (instilled into the eyes) to relieve mydriasis. If urine retention occurs, catheterization may be necessary.

didanosine (ddI)
Videx

Purine analogue, antiviral

Available by prescription only
Tablets (chewable): 25 mg, 50 mg, 100 mg, 150 mg
Powder for solution (buffered): 100 mg/packet, 167 mg/packet, 250 mg/packet, 375 mg/packet

INDICATIONS & DOSAGE
Treatment of HIV infection when antiretroviral therapy is warranted
Adults weighing 132 lb (60 kg) or more: 200 mg (tablets) P.O. q 12 hours, or 250 mg buffered powder P.O. q 12 hours.
Adults weighing less than 132 lb: 125 mg (tablets) P.O. q 12 hours, or 167 mg buffered powder P.O. q 12 hours.
◆ *Dosage adjustment.* Patients with renal or hepatic impairment may need their dosage adjusted; however, insufficient data exist to provide specific recommendations.

PHARMACODYNAMICS
Antiviral action: Didanosine is a synthetic purine analogue of deoxyadenosine. After didanosine enters the cell, it's converted to its active form dideoxyadenosine triphosphate (ddATP), which inhibits replication of HIV by preventing DNA replication. In addition, ddATP inhibits the enzyme HIV-RNA dependent DNA polymerase (reverse transcriptase).

PHARMACOKINETICS
Absorption: Didanosine degrades rapidly in gastric acid. Commercially available preparations contain buffers to raise stomach pH. Bioavailability averages about 33%; tablets may exhibit better bioavailability than buffered powder for oral solution. Food can decrease absorption by 50%.
Distribution: Drug is widely distributed; drug penetration into the CNS varies, but CSF levels average 46% of concurrent plasma levels.
Metabolism: Drug metabolism isn't fully understood, but it's probably similar to that of endogenous purines.
Excretion: Drug is excreted in urine as allantoin, hypoxanthine, xanthine, and uric acid. Serum half-life averages 0.8 hour.

CONTRAINDICATIONS & PRECAUTIONS
Contraindicated in patients with history of hypersensitivity to any component of didanosine.
  Use cautiously in patients with history of pancreatitis. Also use cautiously in patients with peripheral neuropathy, impaired renal or hepatic function, or hyperuricemia.

INTERACTIONS
Drug-drug. Use with *antacids containing magnesium or aluminum hydroxide* may produce enhanced adverse effects, such as diarrhea or constipation. *Dapsone, ketoconazole,* and other *drugs that require gastric acid for adequate absorption* may be rendered ineffective because of the buffering action of didanosine on gastric acid; administer such drugs 2 hours before didanosine. *Fluoroquinolones* and *tetracyclines* may show decreased absorption because of buffering agents in didanosine tablets.
Drug-food. Taking drug with *food* decreases absorption. *Fruit juices* or other *acidic beverages* cause drug to degrade rapidly.

ADVERSE REACTIONS
CNS: *headache, seizures,* confusion, anxiety, nervousness, abnormal thinking, twitching, depression, *peripheral neuropathy.*

Reactions may be *common,* uncommon, *life-threatening,* or COMMON AND LIFE-THREATENING.

GI: *diarrhea, nausea, vomiting, abdominal pain,* **pancreatitis,** dry mouth, anorexia.
Hematologic: *leukopenia,* granulocytosis, **thrombocytopenia,** anemia.
Hepatic: *hepatic failure,* elevated liver enzyme levels.
Metabolic: increased serum uric acid levels.
Musculoskeletal: asthenia, myopathy.
Respiratory: dyspnea.
Skin: rash, pruritus.
Other: pain, pneumonia, infection, sarcoma, *allergic reactions, chills, fever.*

◻ KEY CONSIDERATIONS
• The major toxicity of didanosine use is pancreatitis, which must be considered when a patient develops abdominal pain, nausea, and vomiting or biochemical markers are elevated. Discontinue use of drug until pancreatitis is excluded.
• Administer didanosine on an empty stomach, regardless of dosage form used, because food can decrease absorption by 50%.
• Tablets contain buffers that raise stomach pH to levels that prevent degradation of the active drug. Tablets should be thoroughly chewed before swallowing, and the patient should drink at least 1 oz (30 ml) water with each dose. If tablets are manually crushed, mix drug in 1 oz water; stir to disperse uniformly, then have patient drink it immediately. Know that single-dose packets containing buffered powder for oral solution are available.
• To administer buffered powder for oral solution, carefully open the packet and pour the contents into 4 oz (120 ml) water. Don't use fruit juice or other acidic beverages. Stir for 2 to 3 minutes until the powder dissolves completely. Administer immediately.
• In early clinical trials, about one-third of patients taking buffered powder for oral solution developed diarrhea. Although no evidence exists that other formulations have a lower incidence of diarrhea, consider substituting the chewable tablets if diarrhea occurs.
• When preparing powder or crushing tablets, avoid dispersing an excessive amount of drug particles into the air.

Patient education
• Tell patient to take drug on an empty stomach to ensure adequate absorption, to chew tablets thoroughly before swallowing, and to drink at least 1 oz (30 ml) water with each dose.
• Remind patient using buffered powder for oral solution not to use fruit juice or other acidic beverages. Allow 3 minutes for powder to dissolve completely, and take immediately. Make sure he understands how to mix the solution.

Overdose & treatment
• Signs and symptoms of overdose include diarrhea, pancreatitis, peripheral neuropathy, hyperuricemia, and hepatic dysfunction.
• Treatment is supportive. No specific antidote is available, and it's unknown if drug is dialyzable.

diflunisal
Dolobid

NSAID, salicylic acid derivative, nonnarcotic analgesic, antipyretic, anti-inflammatory

Available by prescription only
Tablets: 250 mg, 500 mg

INDICATIONS & DOSAGE
Mild to moderate pain
Adults: Initiate therapy with 1 g, then 500 mg daily in two or three divided doses, usually q 8 to 12 hours. Maximum dose is 1,500 mg daily.
✦ *Dosage adjustment.* In adults older than age 65, start with one-half the usual adult dose.
Rheumatoid arthritis and osteoarthritis
Adults: 500 to 1,000 mg P.O. daily in two divided doses, usually q 12 hours. Maximum dose is 1,500 mg daily.
✦ *Dosage adjustment.* In adults older than age 65, start with one-half the usual dose.

PHARMACODYNAMICS
Analgesic, antipyretic, and anti-inflammatory actions: Mechanisms of action are unknown, but are probably related to inhibition of prostaglandin syn-

thesis. Diflunisal is a salicylic acid derivative, but isn't hydrolyzed to free salicylate in vivo.

PHARMACOKINETICS

Absorption: Diflunisal is absorbed rapidly and completely via the GI tract. Plasma levels peak in 2 to 3 hours. Analgesia is achieved within 1 hour and peaks within 2 to 3 hours.

Distribution: Drug is highly protein-bound.

Metabolism: Drug is metabolized in the liver; it isn't metabolized to salicylic acid.

Excretion: Drug is excreted in urine. Half-life is 8 to 12 hours.

CONTRAINDICATIONS & PRECAUTIONS

Contraindicated in patients who are hypersensitive to the drug or in whom aspirin or other NSAIDs cause acute asthmatic attacks, urticaria, or rhinitis. Use cautiously in patients with GI bleeding, history of peptic ulcer disease, renal impairment, and compromised cardiac function, hypertension, or other conditions predisposing patient to fluid retention.

INTERACTIONS

Drug-drug. Use with *acetaminophen* may increase serum acetaminophen levels by as much as 50%, leading to potential hepatotoxicity; this interaction may also be nephrotoxic. *Antacids* delay and decrease the absorption of diflunisal. Use with *anticoagulants* or *thrombolytics* may potentiate their anticoagulant effects as a result of the platelet-inhibiting effect of diflunisal. Use with *antihypertensives* may decrease their effect on blood pressure. *Aspirin* may decrease the bioavailability of diflunisal. Use with *diuretics* or *gold compounds* may increase nephrotoxic potential. Use with *furosemide* may decrease the hyperuricemic effect of furosemide. Use of diflunisal with other *GI irritants*—such as *antibiotics, corticosteroids,* and other *NSAIDs*—may potentiate the adverse GI effects of diflunisal; use together cautiously. Use with other *highly protein-bound drugs*—such as *phenytoin, sulfonylureas,* and *warfarin*—may displace

either drug and cause adverse effects; monitor therapy closely. Use with *hydrochlorothiazide* may increase plasma levels of hydrochlorothiazide but decrease its hyperuricemic, diuretic, antihypertensive, and natriuretic effects. Use with *indomethacin* may decrease renal clearance of indomethacin and cause fatal GI hemorrhage. Use with *lithium* may increase serum lithium levels. Diflunisal may decrease renal clearance of *methotrexate, nifedipine,* and *verapamil.* *Probenecid* may decrease the renal clearance of diflunisal.

Drug-food. *Food* delays and decreases the absorption of diflunisal.

Drug-lifestyle. *Alcohol* may potentiate the adverse GI effects of diflunisal.

ADVERSE REACTIONS

CNS: *dizziness,* somnolence, insomnia, *headache,* fatigue.

EENT: *tinnitus,* visual disturbances (rare).

GI: *nausea, dyspepsia, GI pain, diarrhea,* vomiting, constipation, flatulence.

GU: renal impairment, hematuria, interstitial nephritis.

Hematologic: prolonged bleeding time.

Hepatic: increased liver function tests (serum transaminase, alkaline phosphatase, and LD levels).

Metabolic: increased serum BUN, creatinine, and potassium levels; decreased serum uric acid level.

Skin: *rash,* pruritus, sweating, stomatitis, **erythema multiforme, Stevens-Johnson syndrome.**

🔲 KEY CONSIDERATIONS

Besides the recommendations relevant to all NSAIDs, consider the following:

• Patients older than age 60 may be more susceptible to the toxic effects (particularly GI toxicity) of diflunisal.

• Drug may affect renal prostaglandins and cause fluid retention and edema, a significant drawback for geriatric patients, especially those with heart failure or hypertension.

• Similar to aspirin, diflunisal is a salicylic acid derivative but is metabolized differently.

Reactions may be *common,* uncommon, *life-threatening,* or COMMON AND LIFE-THREATENING.

- Diflunisal is recommended for twice-daily dosing for added patient convenience and compliance.
- Don't break, crush, or allow patient to chew diflunisal. Patient should swallow the drug whole.
- Administer diflunisal with water, milk, or food to minimize GI upset.
- Don't administer concurrently with aspirin or acetaminophen.
- Monitor results of laboratory tests, especially renal and liver function studies. Assess presence and amount of peripheral edema. Monitor weight frequently.
- Evaluate patient's response to diflunisal therapy as evidenced by a reduction in pain or inflammation. Monitor vital signs frequently, especially temperature.
- Assess patient for signs and symptoms of potential hemorrhage, such as bruising, petechiae, coffee-ground vomitus, and black, tarry stools.
- If patient experiences CNS effects, institute safety measures to prevent injury.

Patient education
- Instruct patient on diflunisal regimen and need for compliance. Advise him to report adverse reactions.
- Tell patient to take diflunisal with food to minimize GI upset and to swallow capsule whole.
- Caution patient to avoid activities requiring alertness or concentration, such as driving, until CNS effects are known.
- Instruct patient in safety measures to prevent injury.
- Advise patient to avoid alcohol while taking drug.

Overdose & treatment
- Signs and symptoms of overdose include drowsiness, nausea, vomiting, hyperventilation, tachycardia, sweating, tinnitus, disorientation, stupor, and coma.
- To treat overdose of diflunisal, empty stomach immediately by inducing vomiting with ipecac syrup if patient is conscious or by performing gastric lavage. Administer activated charcoal via NG tube. Provide symptomatic and supportive measures (respiratory support and correction of fluid and electrolyte imbalances). Monitor laboratory parameters and vital signs closely. Hemodialysis has little effect on removing drug from circulation.

---

digoxin
Lanoxicaps, Lanoxin, Novodigoxin*

Cardiac glycoside, antiarrhythmic, inotropic

Available by prescription only
Tablets: 0.125 mg, 0.25 mg, 0.5 mg
Capsules: 0.05 mg, 0.10 mg, 0.20 mg
Elixir: 0.05 mg/ml
Injection: 0.05 mg/ml*, 0.1 mg/ml (pediatric), 0.25 mg/ml

INDICATIONS & DOSAGE
Heart failure, atrial fibrillation and flutter, paroxysmal atrial tachycardia
Tablets, elixir
Adults: For rapid digitalization, give 0.75 to 1.25 mg P.O. over 24 hours in two or more divided doses q 6 to 8 hours. For slow digitalization, give 0.125 to 0.5 mg daily for 5 to 7 days. Maintenance dosage is 0.125 to 0.5 mg/day.
Capsules
Adults: For rapid digitalization, give 0.4 to 0.6 mg P.O. initially, followed by 0.1 to 0.3 mg q 6 to 8 hours, as needed and tolerated, for 24 hours. For slow digitalization, give 0.05 to 0.35 mg daily in two divided doses for 7 to 22 days, p.r.n., until therapeutic serum levels are reached. Maintenance dosage is 0.05 to 0.35 mg/day in one or two divided doses.
Injection
Adults: For rapid digitalization, give 0.4 to 0.6 mg I.V. initially, followed by 0.1 to 0.3 mg I.V. q 4 to 8 hours, as needed and tolerated, for 24 hours. For slow digitalization, give appropriate daily maintenance dose for 7 to 22 days as needed until therapeutic serum levels are reached. Maintenance dosage is 0.125 to 0.5 mg/day I.V. in one or two divided doses.
♦ *Dosage adjustment.* Reduce dosage in patients with impaired renal function. Hypothyroid patients are highly sensitive to glycosides; hyperthyroid patients may need larger dosages.

PHARMACODYNAMICS

Inotropic action: The effect of digoxin on the myocardium is dose-related and involves both direct and indirect mechanisms. It directly increases the force and velocity of myocardial contraction, AV node refractory period, and total peripheral resistance; at higher dosages, it also increases sympathetic outflow. It indirectly depresses the SA node and prolongs conduction to the AV node. In patients with heart failure, increased contractile force boosts cardiac output, improves systolic emptying, and decreases diastolic heart size. It also reduces ventricular end-diastolic pressure and, consequently, pulmonary and systemic venous pressures. Increased myocardial contractility and cardiac output in these patients reflexively reduce sympathetic tone. This compensates for drug's direct vasoconstrictive action, thereby reducing total peripheral resistance. In edematous patients, it also slows increased heart rate and causes diuresis.

Antiarrhythmic action: Digoxin-induced heart-rate slowing in patients without heart failure is negligible and stems mainly from vagal (cholinergic) and sympatholytic effects on the SA node; however, with toxic doses, heart-rate slowing results from direct depression of SA node automaticity. Therapeutic doses produce little effect on the action potential, but toxic doses increase the automaticity (spontaneous diastolic depolarization) of all cardiac regions except the SA node.

PHARMACOKINETICS

Absorption: With tablet or elixir administration, 60% to 85% of dose is absorbed. With capsule form, bioavailability increases. About 90% to 100% of a dose is absorbed. With I.M. administration, about 80% of dose is absorbed. With oral administration, onset of action occurs in 30 minutes to 2 hours; peak effects, in 6 to 8 hours. With I.M. administration, onset of action occurs in 30 minutes; peak effects, in 4 to 6 hours. With I.V. administration, action occurs in 5 to 30 minutes; peak effects, in 1 to 5 hours.

Distribution: Digoxin is distributed widely in body tissues; highest levels are in the heart, kidneys, intestine, stomach, liver, and skeletal muscle; lowest levels are in the plasma and brain. Digoxin crosses the blood-brain barrier. About 20% to 30% binds to plasma proteins. Usual therapeutic range for steady-state serum levels is 0.5 to 2 ng/ml. In treatment of atrial tachyarrhythmias, higher serum levels (such as 2 to 4 ng/ml) may be needed. Because of drug's long half-life, achievement of steady-state levels may take 7 days or longer, depending on patient's renal function. Toxic symptoms may appear within the usual therapeutic range; however, these are more frequent and serious with levels above 2.5 ng/ml.

Metabolism: In most patients, a small amount of digoxin apparently is metabolized in the liver and gut by bacteria. This metabolism varies and may be substantial in some patients. Drug undergoes some enterohepatic recirculation (also variable). Metabolites have minimal cardiac activity.

Excretion: Most of dose is excreted by the kidneys as unchanged drug. Some patients excrete a substantial amount of metabolized or reduced drug. In patients with renal failure, biliary excretion is more important. In healthy patients, terminal half-life is 30 to 40 hours. In patients lacking functioning kidneys, half-life is at least 4 days.

CONTRAINDICATIONS & PRECAUTIONS

Contraindicated in patients with hypersensitivity to digoxin, digoxin toxicity, ventricular fibrillation, or ventricular tachycardia unless caused by heart failure.

Use very cautiously in geriatric patients, especially those with an acute MI, an incomplete AV block, sinus bradycardia, PVCs, chronic constrictive pericarditis, hypertrophic cardiomyopathy, renal insufficiency, severe pulmonary disease, or hypothyroidism.

INTERACTIONS

Drug-drug. Use with *amiodarone, diltiazem, nifedipine, quinidine,* or *verapamil* may cause increased serum digoxin levels, predisposing the patient to toxicity.

Amphotericin B, corticosteroids, corticotropin, edetate disodium, laxatives, and *sodium polystyrene sulfonate* deplete total body potassium, possibly causing digoxin toxicity. Use with *antacids containing aluminum or magnesium hydroxide, aminosalicylic acid, kaolin-pectin, magnesium trisilicate,* or *sulfasalazine* decreases absorption of orally administered digoxin. Certain *antibiotics* may interfere with bacterial flora that allow formation of inactive reduction products in the GI tract, possibly causing a significant increase in digoxin bioavailability and, consequently, increased serum digoxin levels. Use with *cardiac drugs affecting AV conduction*—such as *procainamide, propranolol,* and *verapamil*—may cause additive cardiac effects. *Cholestyramine* and *colestipol* may bind digoxin in the GI tract and impair absorption. Use with *cytotoxic drugs* or *radiation therapy* may decrease digoxin absorption if the intestinal mucosa is damaged; digoxin elixir or capsules are recommended in this situation. *Dextrose-insulin infusions, glucagon,* and *large dextrose doses* reduce extracellular potassium, possibly leading to digoxin toxicity.

Use with *electrolyte-altering drugs* may increase or decrease serum electrolyte levels, predisposing the patient to digoxin toxicity. For example, such *diuretics* as *bumetanide, ethacrynic acid, furosemide,* and *thiazides* may cause hypokalemia and hypomagnesemia; thiazides may cause hypercalcemia. Fatal cardiac arrhythmias may result. Use with *I.V. calcium preparations* may cause synergistic effects that precipitate arrhythmias.

Use with *succinylcholine* may precipitate cardiac arrhythmias by potentiating the effects of digoxin. Use with *sympathomimetics*—such as *ephedrine, epinephrine,* and *isoproterenol*—or *rauwolfia alkaloids* may increase the risk of arrhythmias.

ADVERSE REACTIONS

CNS: *fatigue, generalized muscle weakness, agitation, hallucinations,* headache, malaise, dizziness, vertigo, stupor, paresthesia.

CV: *arrhythmias* (most commonly, conduction disturbances with or without AV block, PVCs, and supraventricular arrhythmias) that may lead to increased severity of *heart failure* and hypotension. *Toxic effects on the heart may be life-threatening and may require immediate attention.*
EENT: *yellow-green halos around visual images, blurred vision,* light flashes, photophobia, diplopia.
GI: *anorexia, nausea,* vomiting, diarrhea.

▣ KEY CONSIDERATIONS

• Digoxin should be used with caution in geriatric patients, especially those with compromised renal function; to prevent systemic accumulation, adjust dosage.
• Digoxin is the most widely used cardiac glycoside.
• Obtain baseline heart rate and rhythm, blood pressure, and serum electrolyte levels before giving first dose.
• Question patient about use of cardiac glycosides within the previous 2 to 3 weeks before administering a loading dose. Always divide loading dose over first 24 hours unless situation indicates otherwise.
• Adjust dosage to patient's condition and renal function; monitor ECG and serum levels of digoxin, calcium, potassium, magnesium, and creatinine. Therapeutic serum digoxin levels range from 0.5 to 2 ng/ml. Take corrective action before hypokalemia occurs.
• Monitor patient's status. Take apical-radial pulse for a full minute. Watch for significant changes (sudden rate increase or decrease, pulse deficit, irregular beats, and especially regularization of a previously irregular rhythm). Check blood pressure and obtain 12-lead ECG if these changes occur.
• GI absorption may be reduced in patients with heart failure, especially right-sided heart failure.
• Digoxin dosage generally should be reduced and serum level monitored if patient is receiving digoxin concomitantly with amiodarone, diltiazem, nifedipine, verapamil, or quinidine. Also, monitor patient closely for signs and symptoms

of digoxin toxicity. Obtain serum digoxin levels if you suspect toxicity.

• Because digoxin may predispose patients to postcardioversion asystole, most health care providers withhold digoxin 1 to 2 days before elective cardioversion in patients with atrial fibrillation. (However, consider consequences of increased ventricular response to atrial fibrillation if drug is withheld.)

• In patients with signs of digoxin toxicity, elective cardioversion should be postponed.

• Don't administer calcium rapidly by the I.V. route to patient receiving digoxin. Calcium affects cardiac contractility and excitability in much the same way that digoxin does and may lead to serious arrhythmias.

• Monitor patient's eating patterns. Ask about nausea, vomiting, anorexia, visual disturbances, and other evidence of toxicity.

• Consider that different brands may not be therapeutically interchangeable.

• Digoxin solution is enclosed in newly available soft capsule (Lanoxicaps). Because these capsules are better absorbed than tablets, dosage is usually slightly lower.

Patient education

• Inform patient and responsible family member about drug action, drug regimen, method for measuring pulse rate, reportable signs, and follow-up plans. Patient must understand importance of follow-up laboratory tests and have access to outpatient laboratory facilities.

• Instruct patient not to take an "extra" dose of digoxin if dose is missed.

• Tell patient to call health care provider if severe nausea, vomiting, or diarrhea occurs because these conditions may make patient more prone to toxicity.

• Advise patient to use the same brand consistently.

• Tell patient to call his health care provider before using OTC preparations, especially those high in sodium.

Overdose & treatment

• Signs and symptoms of overdose are primarily GI, CNS, and cardiac reactions.

• Severe intoxication may cause hyperkalemia, which may develop rapidly and result in life-threatening cardiac effects. Cardiac signs of digoxin toxicity may occur with or without (and may commonly precede) other signs and symptoms of toxicity. Digoxin has caused almost every kind of arrhythmia; various combinations of arrhythmias may occur in the same patient. Patients with chronic digoxin toxicity commonly have ventricular arrhythmias or AV conduction disturbances. Patients with digoxin-induced ventricular tachycardia have a high mortality because ventricular fibrillation or asystole may result.

• If toxicity is suspected, discontinue drug and obtain serum drug levels. Usually, drug takes at least 6 hours to distribute between plasma and tissue and reach equilibrium. Other treatment measures include immediately inducing vomiting, performing gastric lavage, and administering activated charcoal to reduce absorption of drug remaining in the gut. Multiple doses of activated charcoal (such as 50 g q 6 hours) may help reduce further absorption, especially of any drug undergoing enterohepatic recirculation.

• Some health care providers advocate cholestyramine administration if digoxin was recently ingested; however, it may not be useful if the ingestion is life-threatening. Interacting drugs probably should be discontinued. Ventricular arrhythmias may be treated with I.V. potassium (replacement dose; but not in patients with significant AV block), I.V. phenytoin, I.V. lidocaine, or I.V. propranolol. Refractory ventricular tachyarrhythmias may be controlled with overdrive pacing. Procainamide may be used for ventricular arrhythmias that don't respond to the above treatments. In severe AV block, asystole, and hemodynamically significant sinus bradycardia, atropine restores a normal rate.

• Administration of digoxin-specific antibody fragments (digoxin immune Fab) is a treatment for life-threatening digoxin toxicity. Each 40 mg of digoxin immune Fab binds about 0.6 mg of digoxin in the bloodstream. The complex is then excreted in the urine, rapidly decreasing

---

Reactions may be *common*, uncommon, *life-threatening*, or **COMMON AND LIFE-THREATENING**.

serum levels and therefore cardiac drug levels.

digoxin immune Fab (ovine)
Digibind

Antibody fragment, cardiac glyco-side antidote

Available by prescription only
Injection: 38-mg vial

INDICATIONS & DOSAGE
Potentially life-threatening digoxin or digitoxin intoxication
Adults: Administered I.V. over 30 minutes or as a bolus if cardiac arrest is imminent. Dosage varies based on amount of drug to be neutralized; average dosage for adults is 6 vials (228 mg). However, if toxicity resulted from acute digoxin ingestion, and neither a serum digoxin level nor an estimated ingestion amount is known, 10 to 20 vials (380 to 760 mg) should be administered. See package insert for complete, specific dosage instructions.

PHARMACODYNAMICS
Cardiac glycoside antidote: Specific antigen-binding fragments bind to free digoxin in extracellular fluid and intravascularly, preventing and reversing pharmacologic and toxic effects of the cardiac glycoside. This binding is preferential for digoxin and digitoxin; preliminary evidence suggests some binding to other digoxin derivatives and cardioactive metabolites.

Once free, digoxin is bound and removed from serum, tissue-bound digoxin is released into the serum to maintain efflux-influx balance. As digoxin is released, it, too, is bound and removed by digoxin immune Fab, resulting in a reduction of serum and tissue digoxin. Cardiac glycoside toxicity begins to subside within 30 minutes after completion of a 15- to 30-minute I.V. infusion of digoxin immune Fab. The onset of action and response is variable and appears to depend on rate of infusion, dose administered relative to body load of glycoside, and possibly other, as yet unidentified factors. Reversal of toxicity, including hyperkalemia, is usually complete within 2 to 6 hours after administration of digoxin immune Fab.

PHARMACOKINETICS
Absorption: Serum levels peak when I.V. infusion is complete. Digoxin immune Fab has a serum half-life of 15 to 20 hours. The association reaction between Fab fragments and glycoside molecules appears to occur rapidly; data are limited.
Distribution: Not fully characterized. After I.V. administration, drug appears to distribute rapidly throughout extracellular space, into both plasma and interstitial fluid.
Metabolism: Unknown.
Excretion: Drug is excreted in urine through glomerular filtration.

CONTRAINDICATIONS & PRECAUTIONS
No known contraindications. Use cautiously in patients known to be allergic to ovine proteins. In these high-risk patients, skin testing is recommended because the drug is derived from digoxin-specific antibody fragments obtained from immunized sheep.

INTERACTIONS
Drug-drug. Digoxin immune Fab binds *cardiac glycosides*—including *digitoxin, digoxin,* and *lanatoside C*. This binding will also occur if redigitalization is attempted before digoxin immune Fab is completely eliminated (several days for patients with normal renal function; 1 week or longer for patients with renal impairment).

ADVERSE REACTIONS
CV: *heart failure,* rapid ventricular rate (both caused by reversal of cardiac glycoside's therapeutic effects).
Metabolic: hypokalemia.
Other: hypersensitivity reactions *(anaphylaxis).*

▣ KEY CONSIDERATIONS
• Give I.V. using a 0.22-micron filter needle over 30 minutes or as a bolus injection when cardiac arrest is imminent. Dose depends on amount of digoxin to

be neutralized. Each 38-mg vial binds about 0.5 mg of digoxin or digitoxin. Reconstitute vial with 4 ml of sterile water for injection, mix gently, and use immediately. May be stored in refrigerator up to 4 hours.

• To determine appropriate dosage, divide the total digitalis glycoside body load by 0.5; the resultant number estimates the number of vials required for appropriate dosage. Alternatively, in cases of acute ingestion of a known quantity of digitalis glycoside, multiply the amount of digitalis glycoside ingested in milligrams by 0.80 (to account for incomplete absorption).

• Skin testing may be appropriate for high-risk patients. One of two methods may be used:

Intradermal test—Dilute 0.1 ml of reconstituted solution in 9.9 ml of sterile saline for injection; then withdraw and inject 0.1 ml of this solution I.D. Inspect site after 20 minutes for signs of erythema or urticaria.

Scratch test—Dilute as for I.D. test. Place 1 drop of diluted solution on skin and make a ¼" scratch through the drop with a sterile needle. Inspect site after 20 minutes for signs of erythema or urticaria. If results are positive, avoid use of digoxin immune Fab unless necessary. If systemic reaction occurs, treat symptomatically.

• Pretreat patients who are sensitive or allergic to sheep or ovine products or who have positive skin test results with an antihistamine such as diphenhydramine and a corticosteroid before administering digoxin immune Fab.

• For patients who respond poorly to withdrawal of digoxin's inotropic effects, keep drugs and equipment for cardiopulmonary resuscitation readily available during administration of digoxin immune Fab. Dopamine, dobutamine, or other cardiac load–reducing drugs may be used. Catecholamines may aggravate arrhythmias induced by digoxin toxicity and should be used with caution.

• Measure serum digoxin or digitoxin levels before giving antidote, because serum levels may be difficult to interpret after therapy with antidote.

• Closely monitor temperature, blood pressure, ECG, and potassium level before, during, and after administration of antidote.

• Potassium levels must be checked repeatedly because severe digitalis intoxication can cause life-threatening hyperkalemia, and reversal by digoxin immune Fab may lead to rapid hypokalemia.

• Suicidal ingestion often involves more than one drug. Be alert for possible toxic effects secondary to these other drugs.

• Delay redigitalization until Fab fragments are completely eliminated, which could take several days in patients with normal renal function and a week or longer in patients with impaired renal function.

• Digoxin immune Fab therapy alters standard cardiac glycoside determinations by radioimmunoassay procedures. Results may be falsely increased or decreased, depending on separation method used.

• Serum potassium levels may decrease rapidly.

Overdose & treatment
• Limited information is available; however, administration of doses larger than needed for neutralizing the cardiac glycoside may subject the patient to increased risk of allergic or febrile reaction or delayed serum sickness. Large doses may also prolong the time span required before redigitalization.

dihydroergotamine mesylate
D.H.E. 45, Migranal

Ergot alkaloid, vasoconstrictor

Available by prescription only
Injection: 1 mg/ml
Nasal spray: 4 mg/ml

INDICATIONS & DOSAGE
To prevent or abort vascular headaches, including migraine headaches
Adults: 1 mg I.M. or I.V., repeated at 1-hour intervals, up to total of 3 mg I.M. or 2 mg I.V. Maximum weekly dosage is 6 mg.

Reactions may be *common*, uncommon, **life-threatening**, or COMMON AND LIFE-THREATENING.

*To acutely treat migraine headaches
with or without aura*
Adults: 1 spray (0.5 mg) administered in
each nostril, then another spray in each
nostril in 15 minutes for a total of 4
sprays (2 mg).

PHARMACODYNAMICS

Vasoconstrictor action: By stimulating
alpha-adrenergic receptors, dihydroergotamine causes peripheral vasoconstriction (if vascular tone is low). However, it
causes vasodilation in hypertonic blood
vessels. At high dosages, it's a competitive alpha-adrenergic blocker. In therapeutic doses, drug inhibits the reuptake
of norepinephrine. A weak antagonist of
serotonin, drug reduces the rate of
platelet aggregation after serotonin has
increased it.

In the treatment of vascular headaches,
drug probably causes direct vasoconstriction of the dilated carotid artery bed
while decreasing the amplitude of pulsations. Its serotoninergic and catecholamine effects also appear to be involved.

Effects on blood pressure are minimal.
The vasoconstrictor effect is more pronounced on veins and venules than on
arteries and arterioles.

PHARMACOKINETICS

Absorption: Onset of action depends on
how promptly after onset of headache dihydroergotamine is given. After I.M. injection or intranasal administration, onset of action occurs within 15 to 30 minutes, and after I.V. injection, within a
few minutes. Duration of action persists
3 to 4 hours after I.M. injection.
Distribution: About 90% of a dose binds
to plasma proteins.
Metabolism: Drug is extensively metabolized, probably in the liver.
Excretion: About 10% of a dose is excreted in urine within 72 hours as
metabolites; the rest, in feces.

CONTRAINDICATIONS & PRECAUTIONS

Contraindicated in patients with hypersensitivity to dihydroergotamine and in
those with peripheral and occlusive vascular disease, coronary artery disease,
uncontrolled hypertension, sepsis, hemiplegic or basilar migraine, and severe

hepatic or renal dysfunction. Avoid use
of drug in patients with uncontrolled hypertension or within 24 hours of 5-HT_1
agonists, ergotamine-containing or
ergot-type drugs, or methysergide.

INTERACTIONS

Drug-drug. Use with *antihypertensives*
may antagonize their antihypertensive
effects. Use with *erythromycin* may
cause ergot toxicity. Use with *vasodilators* may result in pressor effects and
dangerous hypertension.
Drug-lifestyle. *Cold temperatures* and
smoking may increase adverse effects of
drug.

ADVERSE REACTIONS

CV: numbness and tingling in fingers
and toes, transient tachycardia or **bradycardia**, precordial distress and pain, increased arterial pressure.
GI: *nausea, vomiting.*
Musculoskeletal: weakness in legs,
muscle pain in extremities.
Skin: itching.
Other: localized edema.

▣ KEY CONSIDERATIONS

Besides the recommendations relevant to
all ergot alkaloids, consider the following:
• Use drug cautiously in geriatric patients because they're more likely to
have preexisting cardiac and vascular
conditions.
• Drug is most effective when used at
first sign of migraine, or as soon after
onset as possible.
• If severe vasospasm occurs, keep extremities warm. To prevent tissue damage, provide supportive treatment. Give
vasodilators if needed.
• Protect ampules from heat and light.
Don't use if discolored.
• For short-term use only. Don't exceed
recommended dose.
• Ergotamine rebound or an increase in
frequency or duration of headaches may
occur when drug is stopped.
• Drug has also been used to treat postural hypotension as an unlabeled use.

Patient education
• Advise patient to lie down and relax in a quiet, darkened room after dose is administered.
• Urge patient to report immediately feelings of numbness or tingling in fingers and toes, or red or violet blisters on hands or feet.
• Warn patient to avoid alcoholic beverages during drug therapy.
• Caution patient to avoid smoking during drug therapy because it can increase the adverse effects of the drug.
• Tell patient to avoid prolonged exposure to very cold temperatures while taking this drug. Cold may increase adverse reactions.
• Advise patient to report illness or infection, which may increase sensitivity to drug reactions.
• Tell patient that Migranal solution is for nasal use only and shouldn't be injected.
• Instruct patient to prime the pump before using nasal spray.
• Instruct patient to discard nasal spray applicator after use and any unused drug after 8 hours.

Overdose & treatment
• Signs and symptoms of overdose include those of ergot toxicity, including peripheral ischemia, paresthesia, headache, nausea, and vomiting.
• Treatment requires prolonged and careful monitoring. Provide respiratory support, treat seizures if necessary, and apply warmth (not direct heat) to ischemic extremities if vasospasm occurs. Administer vasodilators, if needed.

---

diltiazem hydrochloride
Cardizem, Cardizem CD, Cardizem SR, Dilacor XR

Calcium channel blocker, antianginal, antihypertensive

Available by prescription only
Tablets: 30 mg, 60 mg, 90 mg, 120 mg
Capsules (extended-release): 120 mg, 180 mg, 240 mg, 300 mg (Cardizem CD); 120 mg, 180 mg, 240 mg (Dilacor XR)

Capsules (sustained-release): 60 mg, 90 mg, 120 mg (Cardizem SR)
Injection: 5 mg/ml 5-ml vials, Lyo-ject 25-mg syringe

INDICATIONS & DOSAGE
Management of Prinzmetal's or variant angina or chronic stable angina pectoris
Adults: 30 mg P.O. q.i.d. before meals and h.s. Increase dose gradually to maximum of 360 mg/day divided into three or four doses, p.r.n. Alternatively, give 120 or 180 mg (extended-release) P.O. once daily. Adjust dosage over a 7- to 14-day period as needed and tolerated up to a maximum dosage of 480 mg daily.
Hypertension
Adults: 60 to 120 mg P.O. b.i.d. (sustained-release). Adjust dosage up to maximum recommended dosage of 360 mg/day, p.r.n. Alternatively, give 180 to 240 mg (extended-release) P.O. once daily. Adjust dosage based on patient response to a maximum dosage of 480 mg/day.
Atrial fibrillation or flutter; paroxysmal supraventricular tachycardia
Adults: 0.25 mg/kg I.V. as a bolus injection over 2 minutes. Repeat after 15 minutes if response isn't adequate with a dosage of 0.35 mg/kg I.V. over 2 minutes. Follow bolus with continuous I.V. infusion at 5 to 15 mg/hour (for up to 24 hours).

PHARMACODYNAMICS
Antianginal or antihypertensive action: By dilating systemic arteries, diltiazem decreases total peripheral resistance and afterload, slightly reduces blood pressure, and increases cardiac index, when given in high doses (over 200 mg). Afterload reduction, which occurs at rest and with exercise, and the resulting decrease in myocardial oxygen consumption make diltiazem effective in controlling chronic stable angina.

Diltiazem also decreases myocardial oxygen demand and cardiac work by reducing heart rate, relieving coronary artery spasm (through coronary artery vasodilation), and dilating peripheral vessels. These effects relieve ischemia and pain. In patients with Prinzmetal's

---

Reactions may be *common*, uncommon, **life-threatening**, or COMMON AND LIFE-THREATENING.

angina, diltiazem inhibits coronary artery spasm, increasing myocardial oxygen delivery.

Antiarrhythmic action: By impeding the slow inward influx of calcium at the AV node, diltiazem decreases conduction velocity and increases refractory period, thereby decreasing the impulses transmitted to the ventricles in atrial fibrillation or flutter. The end result is a decreased ventricular rate.

PHARMACOKINETICS

Absorption: About 80% of a diltiazem dose is absorbed rapidly from the GI tract. However, only about 40% of drug enters systemic circulation because of a significant first-pass effect in the liver. Serum levels peak in 2 to 3 hours.
Distribution: About 70% to 85% of circulating drug binds to plasma proteins.
Metabolism: Drug is metabolized in the liver.
Excretion: About 35% of drug is excreted in urine and about 65% in bile as unchanged drug and inactive and active metabolites. Elimination half-life is 3 to 9 hours. Half-life may increase in geriatric patients; however, renal dysfunction doesn't appear to affect half-life.

CONTRAINDICATIONS & PRECAUTIONS

Contraindicated in patients with sick sinus syndrome or second- or third-degree AV block in the absence of an artificial pacemaker, in supraventricular tachycardias associated with a bypass tract such as in Wolfe-Parkinson-White syndrome or Lown-Ganong-Levine syndrome, left-sided heart failure, hypotension (systolic blood pressure < 90 mm Hg), hypersensitivity to diltiazem, an acute MI, and pulmonary congestion (documented by X-ray). Use cautiously in geriatric patients, especially those with heart failure or impaired hepatic or renal function.

INTERACTIONS

Drug-drug. *Beta blockers* may cause combined effects that result in heart failure, conduction disturbances, arrhythmias, and hypotension. *Cimetidine* may increase plasma diltiazem levels; patient should be carefully monitored for a change in the effects of diltiazem when initiating and discontinuing therapy with cimetidine. Use with *cyclosporine* may cause increased serum cyclosporine levels and subsequent cyclosporine-induced nephrotoxicity.

ADVERSE REACTIONS

CNS: *headache,* dizziness, asthenia, somnolence.
CV: *edema,* **arrhythmias,** flushing, **bradycardia,** hypotension, conduction abnormalities, **heart failure,** AV block, abnormal ECG.
GI: *nausea, constipation,* abdominal discomfort.
Hepatic: acute hepatic injury.
Skin: *rash.*

▣ KEY CONSIDERATIONS

Besides the recommendations relevant to all calcium channel blockers, consider the following:
● Use drug with caution in geriatric patients because the half-life may be prolonged.
● If diltiazem is added to therapy of patient receiving digoxin, monitor serum digoxin levels and observe patient closely for signs of toxicity, especially if the patient's renal function is unstable or his serum digoxin levels in the upper therapeutic range.
● Sublingual nitroglycerin may be administered concomitantly, as needed, if patient has signs or symptoms of acute angina.
● Diltiazem has been used investigationally to prevent reinfarction after a non–Q-wave MI and adjunctly to treat peripheral vascular disorders as well as to treat several spastic smooth muscle disorders, including esophageal spasm.

Patient education
● Tell patient that nitrate therapy prescribed during titration of diltiazem dosage may cause dizziness. Urge patient to comply with drug regimen.
● Inform patient of proper use, dosage, and adverse effects associated with diltiazem use.
● Instruct patient to continue taking drug even when feeling better.

• Tell patient to report feelings of light-headedness or dizziness and to avoid sudden position changes.

Overdose & treatment

• Signs and symptoms of overdose primarily are extensions of the adverse effects of the drug. Heart block, asystole, and hypotension are the most serious effects and require immediate attention.

• Treatment may involve I.V. isoproterenol, norepinephrine, epinephrine, atropine, or calcium gluconate administered in usual doses. Ensure adequate hydration. Inotropic drugs, including dobutamine and dopamine, may be used, if necessary. If the patient develops severe conduction disturbances (such as heart block and asystole) with hypotension that doesn't respond to drug therapy, cardiac pacing should be initiated immediately with cardiopulmonary resuscitation measures, as indicated.

dimenhydrinate

Apo-Dimenhydrinate*, Calm-X, Dimetabs, Dinate, Dommanate, Dramamine, Dramocen, Dramoject, Dymenate, Gravol*, Hydrate, Nauseatrol*, PMS-Dimenhydrinate*, Wehamine

Ethanol-amine-derivative antihistamine, H_1-receptor antagonist, antiemetic, antivertigo drug

Available with or without a prescription
Tablets: 50 mg
Capsules: 50 mg
Liquid: 12.5 mg/4 ml, 15 mg/5 ml*
Injection: 50 mg/ml

INDICATIONS & DOSAGE

Prophylaxis and treatment of nausea, vomiting, and dizziness associated with motion sickness
Adults: 50 to 100 mg q 4 to 6 hours P.O., I.V., or I.M. For I.V. administration, dilute each 50-mg dose in 10 ml of normal saline solution and inject slowly over 2 minutes.

◇ **Meniere's disease**
Adults: 50 mg I.M. for acute attack; maintenance dosage is 25 to 50 mg P.O. t.i.d.

PHARMACODYNAMICS

Antiemetic and antivertigo action: Dimenhydrinate probably inhibits nausea and vomiting by centrally depressing sensitivity of the labyrinth apparatus that relays stimuli to the chemoreceptor trigger zone and stimulates the vomiting center in the brain.

PHARMACOKINETICS

Absorption: Dimenhydrinate is well absorbed. Action begins within 15 to 30 minutes after oral administration, 20 to 30 minutes after I.M. administration, and almost immediately after I.V. administration. Its duration of action is 3 to 6 hours.
Distribution: Drug is well distributed throughout the body.
Metabolism: Drug is metabolized in the liver.
Excretion: Metabolites are excreted in urine.

CONTRAINDICATIONS & PRECAUTIONS

Contraindicated in patients hypersensitive to dimenhydrinate or its components; I.V. product contains benzyl alcohol.

Use cautiously in patients who have seizures, acute angle-closure glaucoma, or enlarged prostate gland and in those who take ototoxic drugs.

INTERACTIONS

Drug-drug. Additive CNS sedation and depression may occur when drug is used with other *CNS depressants,* such as *anxiolytics, barbiturates, sleeping drugs,* and *tranquilizers.* Dimenhydrinate may mask the signs of ototoxicity caused by known *ototoxic drugs,* including *aminoglycosides, cisplatin, loop diuretics, salicylates,* and *vancomycin.*
Drug-lifestyle. *Alcohol* use leads to additive CNS sedation and depression.

ADVERSE REACTIONS

CNS: *drowsiness,* headache, dizziness, confusion, nervousness, insomnia, verti-

---

Reactions may be *common,* uncommon, **life-threatening,** or **COMMON AND LIFE-THREATENING.**

go, tingling and weakness of hands, lassitude, excitation.
CV: palpitations, hypotension, tachycardia, tightness of chest.
EENT: blurred vision, dry respiratory passages, diplopia, nasal congestion.
GI: dry mouth, nausea, vomiting, diarrhea, epigastric distress, constipation, anorexia.
Respiratory: wheezing, thickened bronchial secretions.
Skin: photosensitivity, urticaria, rash.
Other: *anaphylaxis.*

▣ KEY CONSIDERATIONS
Besides the recommendations relevant to all antihistamines, consider the following:
● Geriatric patients are usually more sensitive to adverse effects of antihistamines and are especially likely to experience a greater degree of dizziness, sedation, hyperexcitability, dry mouth, and urine retention than younger patients.
● Incorrectly administered or undiluted I.V. solution can irritate the veins and cause sclerosis.
● Parenteral solution is incompatible with many drugs; don't mix other drugs in the same syringe.
● Advise safety measures for all patients; dimenhydrinate causes drowsiness in many patients. Tolerance to CNS depressant effects usually develops within a few days.
● To prevent motion sickness, patient should take drug 30 minutes before traveling and again before meals and at bedtime.
● Antiemetic effect may diminish with long-term use.
● Dimenhydrinate may alter or confuse test results for xanthines (caffeine, aminophylline) because of its 8-chlorotheophylline content; discontinue dimenhydrinate 4 days before diagnostic skin tests to avoid preventing, reducing, or masking test response.

Patient education
● Tell patient to avoid hazardous activities, such as driving or operating heavy machinery, until adverse CNS effects of drug are known.

● For motion sickness, tell patient to take drug 30 minutes before exposure.
● Advise patient to avoid alcohol while taking drug.

Overdose & treatment
● Signs and symptoms of overdose include those of CNS depression—such as sedation, reduced mental alertness, apnea, and CV collapse—and those of CNS stimulation—such as insomnia, hallucinations, tremors, and seizures. Anticholinergic signs and symptoms, such as dry mouth, flushed skin, fixed and dilated pupils, and GI symptoms, are likely to occur.
● Use gastric lavage to empty stomach contents; emetics may be ineffective. Diazepam or phenytoin may be used to control seizures. Provide supportive treatment.

---

diphenhydramine hydrochloride
Benadryl, Benadryl Allergy, Benylin, Compoz, Diphen AF, Diphen Cough, Hydramine, Nervine Nighttime Sleep-Aid, Nytol with DPH, Sleep-Eze 3, Sominex, Tusstat, Twilite

Ethanolamine-derivative antihistamine, H_1-receptor antagonist, antiemetic, antivertigo drug, antitussive, sedative-hypnotic, topical anesthetic, antidyskinetic (anticholinergic)

Available with or without a prescription
Tablets: 25 mg, 50 mg
Capsules: 25 mg, 50 mg
Capsules (chewable): 12.5 mg
Elixir: 12.5 mg/5 ml (14% alcohol)
Syrup: 12.5 mg/5 ml (5% alcohol)
Injection: 50 mg/ml
Cream: 1%, 2%
Gel: 1%, 2%
Spray: 1%, 2%

INDICATIONS & DOSAGE
Rhinitis, allergy symptoms, motion sickness, Parkinson's disease
Adults: 25 to 50 mg P.O. t.i.d. or q.i.d.; or 10 to 50 mg I.V. or deep I.M. Maximum I.M. or I.V. dosage is 400 mg daily.

Nonproductive cough
Adults: 25 mg P.O. q 4 to 6 hours. Maximum dosage is 150 mg daily.
Insomnia
Adults: 50 mg P.O. h.s.
Sedation
Adults: 25 to 50 mg P.O., or deep I.M., p.r.n.

PHARMACODYNAMICS
Antihistamine action: Antihistamines compete for H_1-receptor sites on the smooth muscle of the bronchi, GI tract, uterus, and large blood vessels; by binding to cellular receptors, they prevent access of histamine and suppress histamine-induced allergic symptoms, even though they don't prevent its release.
Antiemetic, antivertigo, and antidyskinetic action: Central antimuscarinic actions of antihistamines probably are responsible for these effects of diphenhydramine.
Antitussive action: Drug suppresses the cough reflex by directly affecting the cough center.
Sedative-hypnotic action: Mechanism of the CNS depressant effects is unknown.
Anesthetic action: Drug is structurally related to local anesthetics, which prevent initiation and transmission of nerve impulses; this is the probable source of its topical and local anesthetic effects.

PHARMACOKINETICS
Absorption: Diphenhydramine is well absorbed from the GI tract. Action begins within 15 to 30 minutes and peaks in 1 to 4 hours.
Distribution: Drug is distributed widely throughout the body, including the CNS. About 82% binds to proteins.
Metabolism: About 50% to 60% of an oral dose is metabolized in the liver before reaching the systemic circulation (first-pass effect); virtually all available drug is metabolized in the liver within 24 to 48 hours.
Excretion: Plasma elimination half-life of drug is 2½ to 9 hours; drug and metabolites are excreted primarily in urine.

CONTRAINDICATIONS & PRECAUTIONS
Contraindicated in patients who are hypersensitive to the drug or who are experiencing an acute asthmatic attack.

Use with extreme caution in patients with angle-closure glaucoma, prostatic hyperplasia, pyloroduodenal and bladder neck obstruction, asthma or COPD, increased intraocular pressure, hyperthyroidism, CV disease, hypertension, and stenosing peptic ulcer.

INTERACTIONS
Drug-drug. Use with other *CNS depressants*—such as *anxiolytics, barbiturates, sleeping aids,* and *tranquilizers*—may cause additive CNS depression. Diphenhydramine may enhance the effects of *epinephrine,* partially counteract the anticoagulant effects of *heparin,* and diminish the effects of *sulfonylureas. MAO inhibitors* interfere with the detoxification of diphenhydramine, thus prolonging their central depressant and anticholinergic effects.
Drug-lifestyle. Additive CNS depression may occur when diphenhydramine is given with *alcohol.*

ADVERSE REACTIONS
CNS: *drowsiness,* confusion, insomnia, headache, vertigo, *sedation, sleepiness, dizziness, incoordination,* fatigue, restlessness, tremor, nervousness, **seizures.**
CV: palpitations, hypotension, tachycardia.
EENT: diplopia, blurred vision, tinnitus.
GI: *nausea,* vomiting, diarrhea, *dry mouth,* constipation, *epigastric distress,* anorexia.
GU: dysuria, urine retention, urinary frequency.
Hematologic: *hemolytic anemia, thrombocytopenia, agranulocytosis.*
Respiratory: nasal congestion, *thickening of bronchial secretions.*
Skin: urticaria, photosensitivity, rash.
Other: *anaphylactic shock.*

▣ KEY CONSIDERATIONS
Besides the recommendations relevant to all antihistamines, consider the following:
• Geriatric patients are usually more sensitive to adverse effects of antihistamines

---

Reactions may be *common,* uncommon, *life-threatening,* or **COMMON AND LIFE-THREATENING.**

and are especially likely to experience a greater degree of dizziness, sedation, hyperexcitability, dry mouth, and urine retention than younger patients. Signs and symptoms usually respond to a decrease in dosage.

• Diphenhydramine injection is compatible with most I.V. solutions but is incompatible with some drugs; check compatibility before mixing in the same I.V. line.

• To prevent irritation, alternate injection sites. Administer deep I.M. into large muscle.

• Drowsiness is the most common adverse effect during initial therapy but usually disappears with continued use of drug.

• Injectable and elixir solutions are light-sensitive; protect them from light.

• Discontinue drug 4 days before diagnostic skin tests; antihistamines can prevent, reduce, or mask positive skin test response.

Patient education
• Advise patient that drowsiness is very common initially, but may be reduced with continued use of drug.

• Warn patient to avoid alcohol during therapy.

• Advise patient undergoing skin testing for allergies to notify health care provider of current drug therapy.

Overdose & treatment
• The most common symptom of overdose is drowsiness. Seizures, coma, and respiratory depression may occur with profound overdose. Anticholinergic signs and symptoms—such as dry mouth, flushed skin, fixed and dilated pupils, and GI symptoms—are common.

• To treat overdose, induce vomiting with ipecac syrup (in conscious patient); then administer activated charcoal to reduce further drug absorption. Use gastric lavage if patient is unconscious or ipecac fails. Treat hypotension with vasopressors, and control seizures with diazepam or phenytoin. *Don't give stimulants.*

diphenoxylate hydrochloride
(with atropine sulfate)
Lofene, Logen, Lomanate, Lomotil, Lonox

Opiate, antidiarrheal
Controlled substance schedule V

Available by prescription only
Tablets: 2.5 mg diphenoxylate hydrochloride and 0.025 mg atropine sulfate/tablet
Liquid: 2.5 mg diphenoxylate hydrochloride and 0.025 mg atropine sulfate/5 ml

INDICATIONS & DOSAGE
Acute, nonspecific diarrhea
Adults: 5 mg diphenoxylate component P.O. q.i.d., then adjust, p.r.n.

PHARMACODYNAMICS
Antidiarrheal action: Diphenoxylate is a meperidine analogue that inhibits GI motility locally and centrally. In high dosages, it may produce an opiate effect. To prevent abuse and deliberate overdose, atropine is added in subtherapeutic dosages.

PHARMACOKINETICS
Absorption: About 90% of an oral dose is absorbed. Action begins in 45 to 60 minutes.
Distribution: Unknown.
Metabolism: Diphenoxylate is metabolized extensively in the liver.
Excretion: Metabolites are excreted mainly in feces via the biliary tract, with lesser amounts excreted in urine. Duration of effect is 3 to 4 hours.

CONTRAINDICATIONS & PRECAUTIONS
Contraindicated in patients with hypersensitivity to diphenoxylate or atropine, acute diarrhea resulting from poison until toxic material is eliminated from GI tract, acute diarrhea caused by organisms that penetrate intestinal mucosa, or diarrhea resulting from antibiotic-induced pseudomembranous enterocolitis or enterotoxin-producing bacteria; also contraindicated in patients with obstructive jaundice.

Use cautiously in patients with hepatic disease, narcotic dependence, or acute ulcerative colitis. Stop therapy immediately if abdominal distention or other signs of toxic megacolon develop.

INTERACTIONS
Drug-drug. Use with such *CNS depressants* as *barbiturates* and *tranquilizers* may result in an increased depressant effect. Diphenoxylate may precipitate hypertensive crisis in patients receiving *MAO inhibitors.*
Drug-lifestyle. *Alcohol* may increase the depressant effect of diphenoxylate.

ADVERSE REACTIONS
CNS: *sedation, dizziness,* headache, drowsiness, lethargy, restlessness, depression, euphoria, malaise, confusion, numbness in extremities.
CV: tachycardia.
EENT: mydriasis.
GI: *dry mouth,* nausea, vomiting, abdominal discomfort or distention, *paralytic ileus,* anorexia, fluid retention in bowel or megacolon (may mask depletion of extracellular fluid and electrolytes), increase serum amylase levels, *pancreatitis,* swollen gums, possible physical dependence with long-term use.
GU: urine retention.
Respiratory: *respiratory depression.*
Skin: pruritus, rash, dry skin.
Other: *angioedema, anaphylaxis.*

◉ KEY CONSIDERATIONS
• Geriatric patients may be more susceptible to respiratory depression and to exacerbation of preexisting glaucoma.
• Monitor vital signs and intake and output; observe patient for adverse reactions, especially CNS reactions.
• Monitor bowel function.
• Drug is usually ineffective in treating antibiotic-induced diarrhea.
• Reduce dosage as soon as symptoms are controlled.
• Diphenoxylate may decrease urine excretion of phenolsulfonphthalein (PSP) during the PSP excretion test.

Patient education
• Warn patient to take drug exactly as ordered and not to exceed recommended dose.
• Advise patient to maintain adequate fluid intake during course of diarrhea and teach him about diet and fluid replacement.
• Caution patient to avoid driving during drug therapy because drowsiness and dizziness may occur; warn patient to avoid alcohol while taking drug because additive depressant effect may occur.
• Advise patient to call health care provider if drug isn't effective within 48 hours.
• Warn patient that prolonged use may result in tolerance and that use of larger-than-recommended doses may result in drug dependence.

Overdose & treatment
• Signs and symptoms of overdose include drowsiness, low blood pressure, marked seizures, apnea, blurred vision, miosis, flushing, dry mouth and mucous membranes, and psychotic episodes.
• Treatment is supportive; maintain airway and support vital functions. A narcotic antagonist, such as naloxone, may be given. Gastric lavage may be performed. Monitor patient for 48 to 72 hours.

diphtheria and tetanus toxoids, adsorbed (Td)

Toxoid, diphtheria and tetanus prophylaxis

Available by prescription only
Injection: 2 limited flocculation (Lf) U of inactivated diphtheria and 2 to 10 Lf U of inactivated tetanus per 0.5 ml, in 5-ml vials

INDICATIONS & DOSAGE
Primary immunization
Adults: Give 0.5 ml I.M. 4 to 8 weeks apart for two doses and a third dose 6 to 12 months later. Booster dosage is 0.5 ml I.M. q 10 years.

PHARMACODYNAMICS
Diphtheria and tetanus prophylaxis:
Diphtheria and tetanus toxoids promote active immunization to diphtheria and tetanus by inducing production of antitoxins.

PHARMACOKINETICS
No information available.

CONTRAINDICATIONS & PRECAUTIONS
Contraindicated in immunosuppressed patients and in those receiving radiation or corticosteroid therapy. Vaccination should be deferred in patients with respiratory illness or acute illness (except during emergency) and during polio outbreaks. When polio is a risk, a single antigen is used. Diphtheria and tetanus toxoids also contraindicated in patients with history of adverse reactions to constituents of drug.

INTERACTIONS
Drug-drug. Concomitant use with *corticosteroids* or *immunosuppressants* may impair the immune response to diphtheria and tetanus toxoids; avoid elective immunization under these circumstances.

ADVERSE REACTIONS
CV: flushing, tachycardia, hypotension, **shock.**
Skin: *pain, stinging, edema, erythema, induration at injection site,* urticaria, pruritus.
Other: *anaphylaxis,* chills, fever, malaise, headache.

▣ KEY CONSIDERATIONS
• Obtain a thorough history of allergies and reactions to immunizations.
• Epinephrine solution 1:1,000 should be available to treat allergic reactions.
• These toxoids aren't used to treat active tetanus or diphtheria infections.
• To prevent sciatic nerve damage, avoid administration in gluteal muscle. During primary immunization, don't inject same site more than once.
• Store toxoids between 36° and 46° F (2° and 8° C). Don't freeze. Shake well before withdrawing each dose.

Patient education
• Inform patient that he may experience discomfort at the injection site and that a nodule may develop there and persist for several weeks after immunization. He also may develop fever, headache, upset stomach, general malaise, or body aches and pains. Tell patient to relieve such effects with acetaminophen.
• Tell patient to report distressing adverse reactions.
• Stress importance of keeping all scheduled appointments for subsequent doses because full immunization requires a series of injections.

dipivefrin hydrochloride
Propine

Sympathomimetic, antiglaucoma drug

Available by prescription only
Ophthalmic solution: 0.1%

INDICATIONS & DOSAGE
To reduce intraocular pressure in chronic open-angle glaucoma
Adults: For initial glaucoma therapy, 1 drop in eye q 12 hours; then adjust dose based on patient response as determined by tonometric readings.

PHARMACODYNAMICS
Antiglaucoma action: Dipivefrin is a pro-drug converted to epinephrine in the eye. It decreases aqueous humor production and enhances outflow. It's commonly used with a miotic.

PHARMACOKINETICS
Absorption: Action begins in about 30 minutes, with peak effect in 1 hour.
Distribution: Unknown.
Metabolism: Unknown.
Excretion: Unknown.

CONTRAINDICATIONS & PRECAUTIONS
Contraindicated in patients with angle-closure glaucoma or hypersensitivity to dipivefrin. Use cautiously in patients with asthma, hypersensitivity to epinephrine, and aphakia or CV disease.

INTERACTIONS
Drug-drug. When used with *carbonic anhydrase inhibitors* or *miotics,* dipivefrin may enhance the lowering of intraocular pressure. Depending on the extent of systemic absorption and the amount present, use with *sympathomimetics* may produce additive toxic effects and use with *anesthetics, digoxin,* or *tricyclic antidepressants* may increase the risk of cardiac arrhythmias.

ADVERSE REACTIONS
CV: tachycardia, hypertension, *arrhythmias.*
EENT: eye burning or stinging, conjunctival injection, conjunctivitis, mydriasis, allergic reaction, photophobia.

▣ KEY CONSIDERATIONS
• To avoid precipitating angle-closure glaucoma, use dipivefrin with caution in geriatric patients.
• Drug may cause fewer adverse reactions than with conventional epinephrine therapy; it's commonly used concomitantly with other antiglaucoma drugs.
• Store away from heat and light.

Patient education
• Teach patient the correct way to instill drops and warn him not to touch eye with dropper.
• Teach patient that if also using other eyedrops, he should instill dipivefrin first, then wait at least 5 minutes before using the other drops.
• Instruct patient not to blink more than usual and not to close his eyes tightly after instillation.
• Tell patient instillation of drug may cause transient burning or stinging.

Overdose & treatment
• Overdose is quite rare with ophthalmic use but may cause the following effects after accidental ingestion: hypertension with tachycardia or bradycardia, arrhythmias, precordial pain, anxiety, nervousness, insomnia, muscle tremor, cerebral hemorrhage, seizures, altered mental status, anorexia, nausea and vomiting, and acute renal failure. To treat oral overdose, dilute immediately then induce vomiting and administer activated charcoal and a cathartic, unless the patient is comatose or obtunded. Monitor urine output. As ordered, treat seizures with I.V. diazepam, and hypertension with nitroprusside; treat arrhythmias appropriately, depending on the type of arrhythmia. Preparations containing sulfites may cause GI or cardiac toxicities and hypotension.

---

dipyridamole
Persantine

Pyrimidine analogue, coronary vasodilator, platelet aggregation inhibitor

---

Available by prescription only
Tablets: 25 mg, 50 mg, 75 mg
Injection: 10 mg/ampule

INDICATIONS & DOSAGE
Alternative to exercise in thallium myocardial perfusion imaging
Adults: 0.142 mg/kg/minute infused over 4 minutes (0.57 mg/kg total).
Inhibition of platelet adhesion in patients with prosthetic heart valves, in combination with warfarin or aspirin
Adults: 75 to 100 mg P.O. q.i.d.
◊ *Chronic angina pectoris*
Adults: 50 mg P.O. t.i.d. at least 1 hour before meals; 2 to 3 months of therapy may be required before response to therapy is apparent.
◊ *Prevention of thromboembolic complications in patients with various thromboembolic disorders other than prosthetic heart valves*
Adults: 150 to 400 mg P.O. daily (in combination with warfarin or aspirin).

PHARMACODYNAMICS
Coronary vasodilating action: Dipyridamole increases coronary blood flow by selectively dilating the coronary arteries. Coronary vasodilator effect follows inhibition of serum adenosine deaminase, which allows accumulation of adenosine, a potent vasodilator. Dipyridamole inhibits platelet adhesion by increasing effects of prostacyclin or by inhibiting phosphodiesterase.

Reactions may be *common*, uncommon, *life-threatening*, or COMMON AND LIFE-THREATENING.

PHARMACOKINETICS

Absorption: Absorption is variable and slow; bioavailability ranges from 27% to 59%. Serum dipyridamole levels peak 45 minutes to 2½ hours after oral administration.
Distribution: Animal studies indicate wide distribution in body tissues. About 91% to 97% binds to proteins.
Metabolism: Drug is metabolized by the liver.
Excretion: Elimination occurs via biliary excretion of glucuronide conjugates. Some dipyridamole and conjugates may undergo enterohepatic circulation and fecal excretion; a small amount is excreted in urine. Half-life varies from 1 to 12 hours.

CONTRAINDICATIONS & PRECAUTIONS

No known contraindications. Use cautiously in patients with hypotension.

INTERACTIONS

Drug-drug. *Aminophylline* inhibits the action of dipyridamole. Dipyridamole can enhance the effects of *heparin* and *oral anticoagulants.*

ADVERSE REACTIONS

CNS: *headache, dizziness.*
CV: flushing, fainting, *hypotension,* angina, chest pain, *blood pressure lability, hypertension* (with I.V. infusion).
GI: *nausea,* vomiting, diarrhea, abdominal distress.
Hematologic: bleeding, increased bleeding time.
Skin: rash, irritation (with undiluted injection), pruritus.

▣ KEY CONSIDERATIONS

• Be alert for adverse reactions, including signs of bleeding and increased bleeding time, especially at high dosages and during long-term therapy.
• Monitor blood pressure.
• Give drug at least 1 hour before meals.
• When used as a pharmacologic "stress test," total dosages need not exceed 60 mg.
• Dilute I.V. form to at least a 1:2 ratio with half-normal saline injection, normal saline injection, or D_5W to a total

volume of 20 to 50 ml. Inject thallium within 5 minutes of dipyridamole.

Patient education

• Explain that response may require 2 to 3 months of continuous therapy; encourage patient compliance.
• Discuss adverse reactions and how to manage therapy.

Overdose & treatment

• Signs and symptoms of overdose include peripheral vasodilation and hypotension.
• Maintain blood pressure and treat symptomatically.

dirithromycin
Dynabac

Macrolide, antibiotic

Available by prescription only
Tablets: 250 mg

INDICATIONS & DOSAGE

Acute bacterial exacerbations of chronic bronchitis caused by **Moraxella catarrhalis** *or* **Streptococcus pneumoniae,** *secondary bacterial infection of acute bronchitis caused by*
M. catarrhalis *or* **S. pneumoniae,** *uncomplicated skin and soft-tissue infections caused by* **Staphylococcus aureus (methicillin susceptible)**
Adults: 500 mg P.O. daily with food for 7 days.
Community-acquired pneumonia caused by **Legionella pneumophila, Mycoplasma pneumoniae,** *or* **Streptococcus pneumoniae**
Adults: 500 mg P.O. daily with food for 14 days.
Pharyngitis or tonsillitis caused by **Streptococcus pyogenes**
Adults: 500 mg P.O. daily with food for 10 days.

PHARMACODYNAMICS

Antibiotic action: Dirithromycin inhibits bacterial RNA-dependent protein synthesis by binding to the 50S subunit of the ribosome. Its spectrum of activity includes gram-positive aerobes such as

S. aureus (methicillin-susceptible strains only), *S. pneumoniae, S. pyogenes;* gram-negative aerobes such as *L. pneumophila* and *Moraxella catarrhalis;* and other bacteria such as *M. pneumoniae.*

PHARMACOKINETICS
Absorption: Dirithromycin is rapidly absorbed from GI tract and converted by nonenzymatic hydrolysis to the microbiologically active compound erythromycylamine. Food slightly increases bioavailability of drug.
Distribution: Drug is widely distributed throughout the body. The protein binding of erythromycylamine ranges from 15% to 30%.
Metabolism: Dirithromycin undergoes little to no hepatic metabolism.
Excretion: Drug is primarily eliminated in bile or feces, with a small amount eliminated in urine. Mean half-life of erythromycylamine is about 8 hours.

CONTRAINDICATIONS & PRECAUTIONS
Contraindicated in patients with hypersensitivity to dirithromycin, erythromycin, or other macrolide antibiotics.

Use cautiously in patients with hepatic insufficiency.

INTERACTIONS
Drug-drug. The following drugs interact with erythromycin; however, it's unknown whether they interact with dirithromycin. Until further data are available, use caution when coadministering *alfentanil, anticoagulants, bromocriptine, carbamazepine, cyclosporine, digoxin, disopyramide, ergotamine, hexobarbital, lovastatin, phenytoin, triazolam,* or *valproate* with dirithromycin. The absorption of *antacids* and *H₂ antagonists* may be slightly enhanced when dirithromycin is administered immediately after these drugs. Dirithromycin may alter steady-state plasma *theophylline* levels; monitor levels and adjust dosage as needed.

ADVERSE REACTIONS
CNS: headache, dizziness, vertigo, insomnia, asthenia.

GI: abdominal pain, nausea, diarrhea, vomiting, dyspepsia, GI disorder, flatulence.
Hematologic: increased platelet, eosinophil, and neutrophil counts.
Metabolic: hyperkalemia, decreased bicarbonate levels, increased CK levels.
Respiratory: increased cough, dyspnea.
Skin: rash, pruritus, urticaria.
Other: pain (nonspecific).

▣ KEY CONSIDERATIONS
• Obtain culture and sensitivity tests before initiating dirithromycin therapy. Therapy may begin pending results.
• Don't use drug in patients with known, suspected, or potential bacteremias because serum levels are inadequate to provide antibacterial coverage of the bloodstream.
• Administer drug with food or within 1 hour of eating.
• Monitor patient for superinfection. Drug may cause overgrowth of nonsusceptible bacteria or fungi.

Patient education
• Tell patient to take all of drug as prescribed, even after he feels better.
• Instruct patient to take drug with food or within 1 hour of having eaten. Tell him not to cut, chew, or crush the tablet.

Overdose & treatment
• Signs and symptoms of a macrolide antibiotic overdose may include nausea, vomiting, epigastric distress, and diarrhea.
• Treatment should be supportive. Forced diuresis, dialysis, and hemoperfusion haven't proven helpful for dirithromycin overdose.

disopyramide phosphate
Norpace, Norpace CR, Rythmodan*, Rythmodan-LA*

Pyridine derivative antiarrhythmic, group IA antiarrhythmic, ventricular antiarrhythmic, supraventricular antiarrhythmic, atrial antitachyarrhythmic

Available by prescription only

Capsules: 100 mg, 150 mg
Capsules (extended-release): 100 mg, 150 mg

INDICATIONS & DOSAGE

PVCs (unifocal, multifocal, or coupled), ventricular tachycardia, and ◊ conversion of atrial fibrillation, atrial flutter, and paroxysmal atrial tachycardia to normal sinus rhythm

Adults: Initially, 200 to 300 mg loading dose. Usual maintenance dosage is 150 mg P.O. q 6 hours or 300 mg (extended-release) P.O. q 12 hours; for patients weighing under 110 lb (50 kg), give 100 mg P.O. q 6 hours or 200 mg (extended-release) P.O. q 12 hours; and for patients with cardiomyopathy or possible cardiac decompensation, give 100 mg P.O. q 6 to 8 hours initially and then adjust, p.r.n.

✦ *Dosage adjustment.* Geriatric patients may need dosage reduction. Adults with hepatic insufficiency or moderately impaired renal function should receive 100 mg P.O. q 6 hours or 200 mg (extended-release) q 12 hours. Patients with severe impaired renal function should receive only 100 mg (regular-release) at the following intervals:

Creatinine clearance (ml/minute)	Dosage interval
30-40	q 8 hr
15-30	q 12 hr
< 15	q 24 hr

PHARMACODYNAMICS

A class IA antiarrhythmic, disopyramide depresses phase O of the action potential. It's considered a myocardial depressant because it decreases myocardial excitability and conduction velocity and may depress myocardial contractility. It also possesses anticholinergic activity that may modify the drug's direct myocardial effects. In therapeutic doses, disopyramide reduces conduction velocity in the atria, ventricles, and His-Purkinje system. By prolonging the effective refractory period, it helps control atrial tachyarrhythmias (however, this indication is unapproved in the United States). Its anticholinergic action, which

is much greater than that of quinidine, may increase AV node conductivity.

Disopyramide also has a greater myocardial depressant (negative inotropic) effect than quinidine. It helps manage premature ventricular beats by suppressing automaticity in the His-Purkinje system and ectopic pacemakers. At therapeutic doses, it usually doesn't prolong the QRS segment duration and PR interval but may prolong the QT interval.

PHARMACOKINETICS

Absorption: Disopyramide is rapidly and well absorbed from the GI tract; 60% to 80% of drug reaches systemic circulation. Onset of action usually occurs in 30 minutes; peak blood levels occur about 2 hours after administration of conventional capsules and 5 hours after administration of extended-release capsules.

Distribution: Drug is well distributed throughout extracellular fluid but isn't extensively bound to tissues. Plasma protein binding varies, depending on drug levels, but generally ranges from 50% to 65%. Usual therapeutic serum level ranges from 2 to 4 µg/ml, although some patients may require levels up to 7 µg/ml. Levels above 9 µg/ml generally are considered toxic.

Metabolism: Drug is metabolized in the liver to one major metabolite that possesses little antiarrhythmic activity but greater anticholinergic activity than the parent compound.

Excretion: About 90% of an orally administered dose is excreted in the urine as unchanged drug and metabolites; 40% to 60% is excreted as unchanged drug. Usual elimination half-life is about 7 hours, but it's longer in patients with renal or hepatic insufficiency. Duration of effect is usually 6 to 7 hours.

CONTRAINDICATIONS & PRECAUTIONS

Contraindicated in patients with hypersensitivity to disopyramide, cardiogenic shock, or second- or third-degree heart block in the absence of an artificial pacemaker.

Use very cautiously and avoid, if possible, in patients with heart failure. Use cautiously in patients with underlying conduction abnormalities, urinary tract diseases (especially prostatic hyperplasia), hepatic or renal impairment, myasthenia gravis, or acute angle-closure glaucoma.

INTERACTIONS

Drug-drug. Use with *anticholinergics* may cause additive anticholinergic effects. Use with *enzyme inducers,* such as *rifampin,* may impair antiarrhythmic activity of disopyramide. *Erythromycin* may increase disopyramide levels causing arrhythmias and increased QT intervals. *Insulin* or *oral antidiabetics* may cause additive hypoglycemia. Use with *other antiarrhythmics* may cause additive or antagonistic cardiac effects and additive toxicity. Use with *warfarin* may potentiate anticoagulant effects.

ADVERSE REACTIONS

CNS: dizziness, agitation, depression, fatigue, muscle weakness, syncope.
CV: *hypotension, heart failure, heart block,* edema, weight gain, **arrhythmias,** shortness of breath, chest pain.
EENT: *blurred vision, dry eyes or nose.*
GI: nausea, vomiting, anorexia, bloating, abdominal pain, diarrhea.
Hepatic: cholestatic jaundice.
Metabolic: hypoglycemia (rare).
Musculoskeletal: aches, muscle weakness.
Skin: rash, pruritus, dermatosis.
Other: pain.

▣ KEY CONSIDERATIONS

• Monitor geriatric patients closely for signs of toxicity; also monitor serum electrolyte and drug levels.
• Correct underlying electrolyte abnormalities, especially hypokalemia, before administering drug, because disopyramide may be ineffective in patients with these problems.
• Don't give sustained-release capsules for rapid control of ventricular arrhythmias if therapeutic blood drug levels must be attained rapidly or if patient has cardiomyopathy, possible cardiac decompensation, or severe renal impairment.
• Watch for signs of developing heart block, such as QRS complex widening

by more than 25% or QT interval lengthening by more than 25% above baseline.
• Drug may cause hypoglycemia in some patients; monitor serum glucose levels in patients with altered serum glucose regulatory mechanisms.
• If drug causes constipation, administer laxatives and ensure proper diet.
• Drug is commonly prescribed for patients who can't tolerate quinidine or procainamide.
• To ensure that enhanced AV conduction doesn't lead to ventricular tachycardia, patients with atrial flutter or fibrillation should be digitalized before disopyramide is administered.
• Pharmacist may prepare disopyramide suspension.
• Drug is removed by hemodialysis. Dosage adjustments may be necessary in patients undergoing dialysis.

Patient education

• When changing from immediate-release to sustained-release capsules, advise patient to begin taking sustained-release capsule 6 hours after last immediate-release capsule.
• Teach patient importance of taking drug on time, exactly as prescribed. To do this, he may have to use an alarm clock for night doses.
• Advise patient to use sugarless gum or hard candy to relieve dry mouth.

Overdose & treatment

• Signs and symptoms of overdose include anticholinergic effects, severe hypotension, widening of QRS complex and QT interval, ventricular arrhythmias, cardiac conduction disturbances, bradycardia, heart failure, asystole, loss of consciousness, seizures, apnea episodes, and respiratory arrest.
• Treatment involves general supportive measures (including respiratory and CV support) and hemodynamic and ECG monitoring. If ingestion was recent, induce vomiting (or perform gastric lavage) and administer activated charcoal to decrease absorption. After patient has been adequately hydrated, isoproterenol or dopamine may be administered to correct hypotension. Digoxin and diuretics may be administered to

treat heart failure. Hemodialysis and charcoal hemoperfusion may effectively remove disopyramide. Some patients may require intra-aortic balloon counter-pulsation, mechanically assisted respiration, or endocardial pacing.

disulfiram
Antabuse

Aldehyde dehydrogenase inhibitor, antialcoholic drug

Available by prescription only
Tablets: 250 mg, 500 mg

INDICATIONS & DOSAGE
Adjunct in management of chronic alcoholism
Adults: Give maximum dosage of 500 mg P.O. as a single dose in the morning for 1 to 2 weeks. Can be taken in evening if drowsiness occurs. Maintenance dosage is 125 to 500 mg/day (average dosage is 250 mg/day) until permanent self-control is established. Treatment may continue for months or years.

PHARMACODYNAMICS
Antialcoholic action: Disulfiram irreversibly inhibits aldehyde dehydrogenase, which prevents the oxidation of alcohol after the acetaldehyde stage. It interacts with ingested alcohol to produce acetaldehyde levels five to ten times higher than are produced by normal alcohol metabolism. Excess acetaldehyde produces a highly unpleasant reaction (nausea and vomiting) to even a small amount of alcohol. Patient doesn't develop tolerance to disulfiram; rather, he becomes more sensitive to alcohol as disulfiram therapy continues.

PHARMACOKINETICS
Absorption: Disulfiram is absorbed completely after oral administration, but 3 to 12 hours may be required before effects occur. Toxic reactions to alcohol may occur up to 2 weeks after the last dose of disulfiram.
Distribution: Drug is highly lipid-soluble and is initially localized in adipose tissue.

Metabolism: Drug is mostly oxidized in the liver and excreted in urine as free drug and metabolites (for example, diethyldithiocarbamate, diethylamine, and carbon disulfide).
Excretion: About 5% to 20% is unabsorbed and is eliminated in feces. A small amount is eliminated through the lungs, but most is excreted in urine. It may take several days for all of the drug to be eliminated.

CONTRAINDICATIONS & PRECAUTIONS
Contraindicated in patients intoxicated by alcohol and within 12 hours of alcohol ingestion; in patients with psychoses, myocardial disease, coronary occlusion, or hypersensitivity to disulfiram or to other thiuram derivatives used in pesticides and rubber vulcanization; and in patients receiving metronidazole, paraldehyde, alcohol, or alcohol-containing preparations.
    Use with extreme caution in patients with diabetes mellitus, hypothyroidism, seizure disorder, cerebral damage, or nephritis or hepatic cirrhosis or insufficiency and in patients taking phenytoin.

INTERACTIONS
Drug-drug. Disulfiram interferes with the metabolism of *anticoagulants, barbiturates, chlordiazepoxide, coumarin diazepam, paraldehyde,* and *phenytoin;* therefore, it may increase the blood levels of these drugs. Use with *isoniazid* may produce ataxia, unsteady gait, or marked behavioral changes and should be avoided. Use with *metronidazole* can produce psychosis or confusion and should be avoided.
Drug-food. Disulfiram inhibits the metabolism of *caffeine,* greatly increasing its half-life. Exaggerated or prolonged effects of caffeine may occur.
Drug-lifestyle. Disulfiram interferes with the metabolism of *alcohol.* Also, disulfiram reaction will occur. Disulfiram has been reported to produce a synergistic CNS stimulation when used with *marijuana.*

ADVERSE REACTIONS
CNS: drowsiness, headache, fatigue, delirium, depression, neuritis, peripheral

---

neuritis, polyneuritis, restlessness, psychotic reactions.
EENT: optic neuritis.
GI: metallic or garlic aftertaste.
GU: impotence.
Metabolic: decreased ^{131}I uptake levels or protein-bound iodine levels may occur rarely, elevated serum cholesterol levels.
Skin: acneiform or allergic dermatitis, occasional eruptions.
Other: disulfiram reaction (precipitated by ethanol use), which may include flushing, throbbing headache, dyspnea, nausea, copious vomiting, diaphoresis, thirst, chest pain, palpitations, hyperventilation, hypotension, syncope, anxiety, weakness, blurred vision, confusion, arthropathy.
In severe reactions: *respiratory depression, CV collapse, arrhythmias, MI, acute heart failure, seizures, unconsciousness, or death.*

▣ **KEY CONSIDERATIONS**
● Disulfiram use requires close medical supervision. Patients should clearly understand consequences of disulfiram therapy and give informed consent before use.
● Use drug only in patients who are cooperative and well motivated and are receiving supportive psychiatric therapy.
● Complete physical examination and laboratory studies (CBC and electrolyte and transaminase levels) should precede therapy and be repeated regularly.
● Disulfiram shouldn't be administered for at least 12 hours after the last alcohol ingestion.
● Disulfiram may decrease urine vanillylmandelic acid excretion and increase urine homovanillic acid levels.

Patient education
● Explain that although disulfiram can help discourage use of alcohol, it isn't a cure for alcoholism.
● Inform patient of seriousness of disulfiram-alcohol reaction and the consequences of alcohol use.
● Warn patient to avoid all sources of alcohol: sauces or soups made with sherry or other wines or alcohol (even "cooking alcohol") and cough syrups. External application of aftershave, liniments, or other topical preparations may cause disulfiram reaction (because of the products' alcohol content).
● Tell patient that alcohol reaction may occur for up to 2 weeks after a single dose of disulfiram. The longer the disulfiram therapy, the more sensitive patient will be to alcohol.
● Warn patient that drug may cause drowsiness.
● Instruct patient to carry identification card stating that disulfiram is being used and including the phone number of the health care provider or clinic to contact if a reaction occurs.

Overdose & treatment
● Signs and symptoms include GI upset and vomiting, abnormal EEG findings, drowsiness, altered consciousness, hallucinations, speech impairment, incoordination, and coma. Treat overdose or accidental overingestion by gastric aspiration or lavage along with supportive therapy.
● Treatment of alcohol-induced disulfiram reaction is supportive and symptomatic. These reactions aren't usually life-threatening. Emergency equipment and drugs should be available because arrhythmias and severe hypotension may occur. Treat severe reactions like shock by administering plasma or electrolyte solutions as needed. Large I.V. doses of ascorbic acid, iron, and antihistamines have been used but are of questionable value. Hypokalemia has been reported; it requires careful monitoring and potassium supplements.

dobutamine hydrochloride
Dobutrex

Adrenergic, beta₁ agonist, inotropic

Available by prescription only
Injection: 12.5 mg/ml in 20-ml vials (parenteral)

INDICATIONS & DOSAGE
To increase cardiac output in short-term treatment of cardiac decompensation caused by depressed contractility

---

Reactions may be *common,* uncommon, *life-threatening,* or COMMON AND LIFE-THREATENING.

Adults: 2.5 to 15 mcg/kg/minute as an I.V. infusion. Rarely, infusion rates up to 40 mcg/kg/minute may be needed. Titrate dosage carefully to patient response.

✦ *Dosage adjustment.* Geriatric patients require lower dosages because they may be more sensitive to the effects of the drug.

PHARMACODYNAMICS

Inotropic action: Dobutamine selectively stimulates beta$_1$ receptors to increase myocardial contractility and stroke volume, resulting in increased cardiac output (a positive inotropic effect in patients who have a normal heart or who are experiencing heart failure). At therapeutic doses, dobutamine decreases peripheral resistance (afterload), reduces ventricular filling pressure (preload), and may facilitate AV node conduction. Systolic blood pressure and pulse pressure may remain unchanged or increased from increased cardiac output. Increased myocardial contractility results in increased coronary blood flow and myocardial oxygen consumption. Heart rate usually remains unchanged; however, excessive doses do have chronotropic effects. Dobutamine doesn't appear to affect dopaminergic receptors, nor does it cause renal or mesenteric vasodilation; however, urine flow may increase because of increased cardiac output.

PHARMACOKINETICS

Absorption: After I.V. administration, onset of action occurs within 2 minutes, with dobutamine levels peaking within 10 minutes. Effects persist a few minutes after I.V. is discontinued.
Distribution: Drug is widely distributed throughout the body.
Metabolism: Drug is metabolized in the liver, where it's conjugated to inactive metabolites.
Excretion: Drug is excreted mainly in urine, with a small amount in feces, as metabolites and conjugates.

CONTRAINDICATIONS & PRECAUTIONS

Contraindicated in patients with hypersensitivity to dobutamine or its formulation or hypertrophic cardiomyopathy.

Use cautiously in patients with a history of hypertension or after recent MI. Drug may precipitate an exaggerated pressor response.

INTERACTIONS

Drug-drug. *Beta blockers* may antagonize the cardiac effects of dobutamine, resulting in increased peripheral resistance and predominance of alpha-adrenergic effects. Dobutamine may decrease the hypotensive effects of *guanadrel* and *guanethidine;* however, these drugs may potentiate the pressor effects of dobutamine, possibly resulting in hypertension and cardiac arrhythmias. Use with *inhalation hydrocarbon anesthetics,* especially *cyclopropane* and *halothane,* may trigger ventricular arrhythmias. Use with *nitroprusside* may cause higher cardiac output and lower pulmonary artery wedge pressure (PAWP). Theoretically, *rauwolfia alkaloids* may prolong the actions of dobutamine (a denervation supersensitivity response).

ADVERSE REACTIONS

CNS: headache.
CV: *increased heart rate,* **hypertension,** **PVCs,** angina, nonspecific chest pain, palpitations, hypotension.
GI: nausea, vomiting.
Respiratory: shortness of breath, **asthmatic episodes.**
Other: phlebitis, hypersensitivity reactions **(anaphylaxis).**

▣ KEY CONSIDERATIONS

Besides the recommendations relevant to all adrenergics, consider the following:
• Use with caution in geriatric patients; they require lower dosages because they may be more sensitive to the effects of the drug.
• Before administration of dobutamine, correct hypovolemia with appropriate plasma volume expanders.
• Monitor ECG, blood pressure, cardiac output, and PAWP.
• Before giving dobutamine, administer a cardiac glycoside if patient has atrial fibrillation (dobutamine increases AV conduction).

• Most patients experience an increase of 10 to 20 mm Hg in systolic blood pressure; some show an increase of 50 mm Hg or more. Most also experience an increase in heart rate of 5 to 15 beats/minute; some show increases of 30 or more beats/minute. Premature ventricular arrhythmias may also occur in about 5% of patients. Dosage reduction may be necessary when these occur.

• Dosage should be adjusted to meet individual needs and achieve desired response. Drug must be administered by I.V. infusion using an infusion pump or other device to control flow rate.

• Concentration of infusion solution shouldn't exceed 5,000 mcg/ml; the solution should be used within 24 hours. Rate and duration of infusion depend on patient response.

• Pink discoloration of solution indicates slight oxidation but no significant loss of potency.

• Dobutamine is incompatible with alkaline solution (sodium bicarbonate). Also, don't mix with or give through same I.V. line as heparin, hydrocortisone, cefazolin, cefamandole, or penicillin.

Patient education
• Advise patient to report adverse reactions.
• Inform patient that he'll need frequent monitoring of vital signs.

Overdose & treatment
• Signs and symptoms of overdose include nervousness and fatigue.
• No treatment is necessary beyond dosage reduction or withdrawal of drug.

---

docetaxel
Taxotere

Taxoid, antineoplastic

Available by prescription only
Injection: 20 mg, 80 mg

INDICATIONS & DOSAGE
Treatment of patients with locally advanced or metastatic breast cancer who have progressed during anthracycline-based therapy or have relapsed during anthracycline-based adjuvant therapy
Adults: 60 to 100 mg/m² I.V. over 1 hour q 3 weeks.

PHARMACODYNAMICS
Antineoplastic action: Docetaxel acts by disrupting the microtubular network in cells that's essential for mitotic and interphase cellular functions.

PHARMACOKINETICS
Absorption: Docetaxel is administered I.V.
Distribution: About 94% binds to proteins.
Metabolism: Drug undergoes oxidative metabolism.
Excretion: Drug is eliminated primarily in feces, with a small amount eliminated in urine.

CONTRAINDICATIONS & PRECAUTIONS
Contraindicated in patients with history of severe hypersensitivity to docetaxel or other drugs formulated with polysorbate 80. Docetaxel shouldn't be used in patients with neutrophil counts below 1,500/mm³.

INTERACTIONS
Drug-drug. *Compounds that induce, inhibit, or are metabolized by cytochrome P-450 3A4*—such as *cyclosporine, erythromycin, ketoconazole,* and *troleandomycin*—can alter metabolism of docetaxel; use caution when administering these drugs concomitantly.

ADVERSE REACTIONS
CNS: paresthesia, dysesthesia, pain (including burning sensation), weakness.
CV: fluid retention, hypotension, chest tightness.
GI: *stomatitis,* nausea, vomiting, diarrhea.
Hematologic: *anemia,* NEUTROPENIA, FEBRILE NEUTROPENIA, *myelosuppression* (dose-limiting), LEUKOPENIA, *thrombocytopenia.*
Musculoskeletal: back pain.
Respiratory: dyspnea.
Skin: *alopecia,* maculopapular eruptions, desquamation, nail pigmentation

---

alteration, onycholysis, nail pain, flushing, rash.
Other: *hypersensitivity reactions, infections,* drug fever, chills.

▣ KEY CONSIDERATIONS

• Patients with an above-normal bilirubin level generally shouldn't receive docetaxel. Also, patients with ALT or AST levels that exceed 1.5 times the upper limits of normal and alkaline phosphatase level greater than 2.5 times the upper limits of normal generally shouldn't receive drug.

• To reduce the incidence and severity of fluid retention and hypersensitivity reactions, all patients should be premedicated with oral corticosteroids such as 16 mg dexamethasone daily for 5 days starting 1 day before docetaxel administration.

• Docetaxel requires dilution before administration using the diluent supplied with drug. Allow drug and diluent to stand at room temperature for about 5 minutes before mixing. After adding all the diluent to the vial of docetaxel, gently rotate the vial for about 15 seconds. Then allow solution to stand for a few minutes to allow any foam that appeared to dissipate. All of the foam doesn't need to dissipate before continuing the preparation.

• To prepare the docetaxel infusion solution, aseptically withdraw the required amount of premix solution from the vial and inject into a 250-ml infusion bag or bottle of normal saline solution or D_5W solution to produce a final concentration of 0.3 to 0.9 mg/ml. Doses exceeding 240 mg require a larger volume of infusion solution so that a concentration of 0.9 mg/ml of docetaxel isn't exceeded. Thoroughly mix the infusion by rotating the infusion bag or bottle.

• Caution should be used during preparation and administration of docetaxel. Use of gloves is recommended. If solution touches the skin, wash skin immediately and thoroughly with soap and water. If docetaxel touches the mucous membranes, the membranes should be flushed thoroughly with water. Mark all waste materials with "Chemotherapy Hazard" labels.

• Make sure that the undiluted concentrate doesn't come in contact with plasticized polyvinyl chloride equipment or devices used to prepare solutions for infusion. Prepare and store infusion solutions in glass or polypropylene bottles or polypropylene or polyolefin bags and administer through polyethylene-lined administration sets.

• Patients who are dosed initially at 100 mg/m² and who experience either febrile neutropenia, a neutrophil count under 500/mm³ for more than 1 week, severe or cumulative cutaneous reactions, or severe peripheral neuropathy during docetaxel therapy should have dosage adjusted from 100 to 75 mg/m². If the patient continues to experience these reactions, dosage should either be decreased from 75 to 55 mg/m² or the treatment discontinued.

• Patients who are dosed initially at 60 mg/m² and who don't experience febrile neutropenia, a neutrophil count below 500/mm³ for more than 1 week, severe or cumulative cutaneous reactions, or severe peripheral neuropathy during docetaxel therapy may tolerate higher dosages.

• Bone marrow toxicity is the most frequent and dose-limiting toxicity. Frequent blood count monitoring is necessary during therapy.

• Monitor patient closely for hypersensitivity reactions, especially during the first and second infusions. If minor reactions such as flushing or localized skin reactions occur, interruption of therapy is not required. More severe reactions require the immediate discontinuation of docetaxel and aggressive treatment.

Patient education

• Warn patient that alopecia occurs in almost 80% of all patients.
• Tell patient to promptly report a sore throat or fever or unusual bruising or bleeding.

Overdose & treatment

• Signs and symptoms of overdose may include bone marrow suppression, peripheral neurotoxicity, and mucositis.
• No known antidote for docetaxel exists. Patient should be kept in a special-

ized unit where vital functions can be closely monitored.

docusate calcium
Pro-Cal-Sof, Surfak

docusate potassium
Dialose, Diocto-K, Kasof

docusate sodium
Colace, Diocto, Dioeze, Diosuccin, Disonate, DOK, DOS, Doxinate, D-S-S, Duosol, Modane Soft, Pro-Sof, Regulax SS, Regulex*, Regutol, Theravac-SB

Surfactant, emollient laxative

Available without a prescription
Tablets: 50 mg, 100 mg
Capsules: 50 mg, 60 mg, 100 mg, 120 mg, 240 mg, 250 mg, 300 mg
Syrup: 50 mg/15 ml, 60 mg/15 ml
Liquid: 150 mg/15 ml
Solution: 50 mg/ml

INDICATIONS & DOSAGE
Stool softener
docusate sodium
Adults: 50 to 200 mg P.O. daily until bowel movements are normal. Alternatively, add 50 to 100 mg to saline or oil retention enema to treat fecal impaction.
docusate calcium or potassium
Adults: 240 mg (calcium) or 100 to 300 mg (potassium) P.O. daily until bowel movements are normal. Higher dosages are for initial therapy. Adjust dosage to individual response.

PHARMACODYNAMICS
Laxative action: Docusate salts act as detergents in the intestine, reducing surface tension of interfacing liquids; this promotes incorporation of fat and additional liquid, softening the stool.

PHARMACOKINETICS
Absorption: Docusate salts are absorbed minimally in the duodenum and jejunum; drug acts in 1 to 3 days.
Distribution: Drug is distributed primarily locally, in the gut.
Metabolism: None.

Excretion: Drug is excreted in feces.

CONTRAINDICATIONS & PRECAUTIONS
Contraindicated in patients hypersensitive to docusate salts and in those with intestinal obstruction, undiagnosed abdominal pain, vomiting or other signs or symptoms of appendicitis, fecal impaction, or acute surgical abdomen.

INTERACTIONS
Drug-drug. Docusate salts may increase absorption of *mineral oil*.

ADVERSE REACTIONS
GI: bitter taste, mild abdominal cramping, diarrhea, laxative dependence (with long-term or excessive use).

▣ KEY CONSIDERATIONS
• Docusate salts are good choices for geriatric patients because they rarely cause laxative dependence and cause fewer adverse effects and are gentler than some other laxatives.
• To prevent throat irritation, liquid or syrup must be given in 6 to 8 oz (180 to 240 ml) of milk or fruit juice.
• After administration of liquid through an NG tube, flush the tube to clear it and to ensure that all drug has been dispersed into the stomach.
• Avoid using docusate sodium in sodium-restricted patients.
• Docusate salts are available in combination with casanthranol (Peri-Colace), senna (Senokot, Gentlax), and phenolphthalein (Ex-Lax, Feen-a-Mint, Correctol).
• Docusate salts are the preferred laxative for most patients who must avoid straining during bowel movements, such as those recovering from an MI or rectal surgery.
• Docusate salts are less likely than other laxatives to cause laxative dependence; however, their effectiveness may decrease with long-term use.

Patient education
• Docusate salts lose their effectiveness over time; advise patient to report if drug stops working.

Reactions may be *common*, uncommon, *life-threatening*, or COMMON AND LIFE-THREATENING.

• Advise patient to take liquid or syrup with 6 to 8 oz (180 to 240 ml) of milk or fruit juice to prevent throat irritation.

dolasetron mesylate
Anzemet

Selective serotonin 5-HT₃ receptor antagonist, antinauseant, antiemetic

Available by prescription only
Tablets: 50 mg, 100 mg
Injection: 20 mg/ml as 12.5 mg/0.625-ml ampules or 100 mg/5-ml vials

INDICATIONS & DOSAGE
Prevention of nausea and vomiting associated with cancer chemotherapy
Adults: 100 mg P.O. given as a single dose 1 hour before chemotherapy, or 1.8 mg/kg as a single I.V. dose given 30 minutes before chemotherapy, or a fixed dose of 100 mg I.V. given 30 minutes before chemotherapy.
Prevention of postoperative nausea and vomiting
Adults: 100 mg P.O. within 2 hours before surgery; 12.5 mg as a single I.V. dose about 15 minutes before cessation of anesthesia.
Treatment of postoperative nausea and vomiting (I.V. form only)
Adults: 12.5 mg as a single I.V. dose as soon as nausea or vomiting presents.

PHARMACODYNAMICS
Antinauseant and antiemetic action:
Dolasetron is a selective serotonin 5-HT₃ receptor antagonist that blocks the action of serotonin. 5-HT₃ receptors are located on the nerve terminals of the vagus nerve in the periphery and in the central chemoreceptor trigger zone. Blocking the activity of the serotonin receptors prevents serotonin from stimulating the vomiting reflex.

PHARMACOKINETICS
Absorption: All forms of dolasetron are bioequivalent. The oral form is well absorbed; however, the parent drug is rarely detected in plasma because the drug is rapidly and completely metabo-

lized to its most relevant metabolite, hydrodolasetron.
Distribution: Drug is widely distributed in the body, with a mean apparent volume of distribution of 5.8 L/kg; 69% to 77% of hydrodolasetron binds to plasma proteins.
Metabolism: A ubiquitous enzyme, carbonyl reductase mediates the reduction of dolasetron to hydrodolasetron. Cytochrome P-450 (CYP) 2D6 and CYP3A are responsible for subsequent hydroxylation and N-oxidation of hydrodolasetron, respectively.
Excretion: Two-thirds of dose is excreted in urine and one-third in feces. Mean elimination half-life of hydrodolasetron is 8.1 hours.

CONTRAINDICATIONS & PRECAUTIONS
Contraindicated in patients hypersensitive to dolasetron.
Use drug cautiously in patients who have or who are at risk for developing prolonged cardiac conduction intervals, particularly QTc. These include patients taking antiarrhythmics or other drugs that lead to QT prolongation, hypokalemia or hypomagnesemia, electrolyte abnormalities (for example, diuretics), or congenital QT syndrome, and in patients who have received cumulative high-dosage anthracycline therapy.

INTERACTIONS
Drug-drug. *Drugs that induce the P-450 enzymes* such as *rifampin* may decrease hydrodolasetron levels; monitor patient for decreased efficacy of antiemetic. *Drugs that inhibit the P-450 enzymes* (such as *cimetidine*) can increase hydrodolasetron levels; monitor patient for adverse effects. *Drugs that prolong ECG intervals* such as *antiarrhythmics* can increase the risk of arrhythmias; monitor patient closely.

ADVERSE REACTIONS
CNS: *headache,* dizziness, drowsiness, fatigue.
CV: *arrhythmias,* ECG changes, hypotension, hypertension, tachycardia, bradycardia.
GI: *diarrhea,* dyspepsia, abdominal pain, constipation, anorexia.

---

*Canada only   ◊ Unlabeled clinical use

GU: oliguria, urine retention.
Hepatic: elevated liver function tests.
Skin: pruritus, rash.
Other: fever, chills, pain at injection site.

▣ KEY CONSIDERATIONS

• Dosage adjustment isn't needed in patients older than age 65.
• Safety and efficacy of multiple drug doses haven't been evaluated. Efficacy studies have all been conducted with single doses of drug.
• Injection for oral administration is stable in apple or apple-grape juice for 2 hours at room temperature.
• I.V. injection can be infused as rapidly as 100 mg/30 seconds or diluted in 50 ml compatible solution and infused over 15 minutes.

Patient education

• Inform patient that oral doses of drug must be taken 1 to 2 hours before surgery or 1 hour before chemotherapy to be effective.
• Teach patient about potential adverse effects.
• Instruct patient not to mix injection in juice for oral administration until just before dosing.
• Tell patient to report if nausea or vomiting occurs.

---

donepezil hydrochloride
Aricept

Acetylcholinesterase inhibitor, cholinomimetic

Available by prescription only
Tablets: 5 mg, 10 mg

INDICATIONS & DOSAGE
Mild to moderate dementia of the Alzheimer's type
Adults: Initially, 5 mg P.O. daily h.s. After 4 to 6 weeks, dosage may be increased to 10 mg daily.

PHARMACODYNAMICS
Anticholinesterase action: Donepezil is believed to inhibit the enzyme acetylcholinesterase in the CNS, increasing acetylcholine levels and temporarily improving cognitive function in patients with Alzheimer's disease. Drug doesn't alter the course of the underlying disease.

PHARMACOKINETICS
Absorption: Donepezil is well absorbed with a relative bioavailability of 100%; plasma levels peak in 3 to 4 hours. Steady state is reached within 15 days.
Distribution: Steady state volume of distribution is 12 L/kg. About 96% binds to plasma proteins, mainly to albumin (about 75%) and alpha$_1$-acid glycoprotein (about 21%) over the concentration range of 2 to 1,000 ng/ml.
Metabolism: Extensively metabolized in the liver to four major metabolites (two are known to be active) and several minor metabolites (not all have been identified). Drug is metabolized by cytochrome P-450 isoenzymes 2D6 and 3A4 and undergoes glucuronidation.
Excretion: Elimination half-life is about 70 hours and mean apparent plasma clearance is 0.13 L/hour/kg. About 17% of drug is eliminated from the kidneys as unchanged drug.

CONTRAINDICATIONS & PRECAUTIONS
Contraindicated in patients with known hypersensitivity to donepezil or to piperidine derivatives. Use very cautiously in patients with sick sinus syndrome or other supraventricular cardiac conduction conditions because drug may cause bradycardia. Use cautiously in patients with CV disease, asthma, or history of ulcer disease and in those taking NSAIDs.

INTERACTIONS
Drug-drug. Use with *anticholinergics* may interfere with anticholinergic activity. Use with *bethanechol* or *succinylcholine* may produce additive effects. *Carbamazepine, dexamethasone, phenobarbital, phenytoin,* and *rifampin* may increase rate of elimination of donepezil. *Cholinomimetics* and *cholinesterase inhibitors* may produce synergistic effect. Monitor the patient closely when using any of these drugs with donepezil.

ADVERSE REACTIONS
CNS: abnormal dreams or crying, aggression, aphasia, ataxia, dizziness, depression, *headache, insomnia,* irritability, nervousness, paresthesia, restlessness, somnolence, seizures, tremor, vertigo.
CV: atrial fibrillation, chest pain, hypertension, vasodilation, hypotension, syncope.
EENT: blurred vision, cataract, eye irritation.
GI: anorexia, bloating, *diarrhea,* epigastric pain, fecal incontinence, GI bleeding, *nausea,* vomiting.
GU: frequent urination, hot flashes, nocturia, increased libido.
Hematologic: ecchymosis.
Musculoskeletal: arthritis, bone fracture, muscle cramps, toothache.
Respiratory: bronchitis, dyspnea, sore throat.
Skin: diaphoresis, pruritus, urticaria.
Other: accident, dehydration, fatigue, influenza, pain, weight loss.

▣ KEY CONSIDERATIONS
• Syncopal episodes have been reported with drug use.
• Drug may increase gastric acid secretion owing to increased cholinergic activity. Closely monitor patients at increased risk for developing ulcers (such as those with history of ulcer disease or those receiving NSAIDs) for symptoms of active or occult GI bleeding.
• Diarrhea, nausea, and vomiting occur more frequently with the 10-mg dose than with the 5-mg dose. These effects are mostly mild and transient, sometimes lasting 1 to 3 weeks, and resolve during continued drug therapy.
• Although not observed in clinical trials, drug may cause bladder outflow obstruction.
• Cholinomimetics can cause generalized seizures. However, seizure activity also may result from Alzheimer's disease.

Patient education
• Explain to patient and caregiver that drug doesn't alter disease but can alleviate or stabilize symptoms. Effects of therapy depend on drug administration at regular intervals.

• Tell caregiver to give drug in the evening, before bedtime.
• Advise patient and caregiver to immediately report significant adverse effects or changes in overall health status.
• If patient is to receive anesthesia, tell patient and caregiver to inform health care team that patient takes donepezil.

Overdose & treatment
• An overdose can result in cholinergic crisis, which is characterized by severe nausea, vomiting, salivation, sweating, bradycardia, hypotension, respiratory depression, collapse, and seizures. Increasing muscle weakness may also occur and may result in death if respiratory muscles are involved.
• Tertiary anticholinergics such as atropine may be used as an antidote for drug overdosage. I.V. atropine sulfate titrated to effect is recommended; give an initial dose of 1 to 2 mg I.V. and base subsequent doses on response. Atypical responses in blood pressure and heart rate have been reported with other cholinomimetics when coadministered with quaternary anticholinergics such as glycopyrrolate. It's unknown if dialysis can remove donepezil or its metabolites from circulation.

---

dopamine hydrochloride
Intropin

Adrenergic, inotropic, vasopressor

Available by prescription only
Injection: 40 mg/ml, 80 mg/ml, and 160 mg/ml parenteral concentrate for injection for I.V. infusion; 0.8 mg/ml (200 or 400 mg) in D_5W 1.6 mg/ml (400 or 800 mg) in D_5W, and 3.2 mg/ml (800 mg) in D_5W parenteral injection for I.V. infusion

INDICATIONS & DOSAGE
Adjunct in shock to increase cardiac output, blood pressure, and urine flow
Adults: 1 to 5 mcg/kg/minute I.V. infusion, up to 20 to 50 mcg/kg/minute. Infusion rate may be increased by 1 to 4 mcg/kg/minute at 10- to 30-minute intervals until optimum response is

achieved. In severely ill patient, infusion may begin at 5 mcg/kg/minute and gradually increase by increments of 5 to 10 mcg/kg/minute until optimum response is achieved.

Short-term treatment of severe, refractory, chronic heart failure

Adults: Initially, 0.5 to 2 mcg/kg/minute I.V. infusion. Dosage may be increased until desired renal response occurs. Average dosage is 1 to 3 mcg/kg/minute.

PHARMACODYNAMICS

Inotropic action: Low to moderate dosages result in cardiac stimulation (positive inotropic effects) and renal and mesenteric vasodilation (dopaminergic response). High dosages result in increased peripheral resistance and renal vasoconstriction.

Vasopressor action: An immediate precursor of norepinephrine, dopamine stimulates dopaminergic, beta, and alpha-adrenergic receptors of the sympathetic nervous system. The main effects produced are dose-dependent. It has a direct stimulating effect on $beta_1$ receptors (in I.V. doses of 2 to 10 mcg/kg/minute) and little or no effect on $beta_2$ receptors. In I.V. doses of 0.5 to 2 mcg/kg/minute, it acts on dopaminergic receptors, causing vasodilation in the renal, mesenteric, coronary, and intracerebral vascular beds; in I.V. doses above 10 mcg/kg/minute, it stimulates alpha receptors.

PHARMACOKINETICS

Absorption: Onset of action after I.V. administration occurs within 5 minutes and persists for less than 10 minutes.

Distribution: Dopamine is widely distributed throughout the body; however, it doesn't cross the blood-brain barrier.

Metabolism: In the liver, kidneys, and plasma, MAO and catechol-O-methyltransferase metabolize the drug to inactive compounds. About 25% is metabolized to norepinephrine within adrenergic nerve terminals.

Excretion: Drug is excreted in urine, mainly as metabolites.

CONTRAINDICATIONS & PRECAUTIONS

Contraindicated in patients with uncorrected tachyarrhythmias, pheochromocytoma, or ventricular fibrillation. Use cautiously in patients who have occlusive vascular disease, cold injuries, diabetic endarteritis, or arterial embolism or who are taking an MAO inhibitor.

INTERACTIONS

Drug-drug. Use with *alpha-adrenergic blockers* may antagonize the peripheral vasoconstriction that high doses of dopamine cause. Use with *beta blockers* antagonizes the cardiac effects of dopamine. Use with *diuretics* increases diuretic effects of both drugs. Use with *general anesthetics,* especially *cyclopropane* and *halothane*, may cause ventricular arrhythmias and hypertension. Use with *MAO inhibitors* may prolong and intensify the effects of dopamine. Use with I.V. *phenytoin* may cause hypotension and bradycardia.

ADVERSE REACTIONS

CNS: headache.

CV: ectopic beats, tachycardia, anginal pain, palpitations, *hypotension;* ***bradycardia,*** conduction disturbances, hypertension, vasoconstriction, widening of QRS complex (less frequently).

GI: nausea, vomiting.

Metabolic: azotemia, elevated urine catecholamine levels.

Respiratory: dyspnea, ***asthmatic episodes.***

Other: necrosis and tissue sloughing with extravasation, piloerection, ***anaphylactic reactions.***

▣ KEY CONSIDERATIONS

Besides the recommendations relevant to all adrenergics, consider the following:

● Lower dosages are indicated because geriatric patients may be more sensitive to drug's effects.

● Hypovolemia should be corrected with appropriate plasma volume expanders before dopamine is administered.

● Dopamine is administered by I.V. infusion using an infusion device to control rate of flow.

● To prevent extravasation, administer drug into a large vein. If necessary to ad-

---

Reactions may be *common*, uncommon, *life-threatening*, or COMMON AND LIFE-THREATENING.

minister in hand or ankle veins, change injection site to larger vein as soon as possible. Monitor continuously for free flow. Central venous access is recommended.

• Adjust dosage to meet individual needs of patient and to achieve desired response. If dosage required to obtain desired systolic blood pressure exceeds optimum rate of renal response, reduce dosage as soon as hemodynamic condition is stabilized.

• Severe hypotension may result if the infusion is abruptly withdrawn; therefore, reduce dose gradually.

• If extravasation occurs, stop infusion and infiltrate site promptly with 10 to 15 ml normal saline injection containing 5 to 10 mg of phentolamine. Use syringe with a fine needle, and infiltrate area liberally with phentolamine solution.

• Don't mix other drugs in dopamine solutions. Discard solutions after 24 hours.

• Monitor blood pressure, cardiac output, ECG, and intake and output during infusion, especially if dose exceeds 20 mcg/kg/minute. Watch for cold extremities.

Patient education
• Advise patient to report adverse reactions.
• Inform patient of need for frequent monitoring of his vital signs and condition.

Overdose & treatment
• Signs and symptoms of overdose include excessive, severe hypertension.
• No treatment is necessary beyond dosage reduction or withdrawal of drug. If that fails to lower blood pressure, a short-acting alpha-adrenergic blocker may be helpful.

---

dorzolamide hydrochloride
Trusopt

Sulfonamide, antiglaucoma drug

Available by prescription only
Ophthalmic solution: 2%

INDICATIONS & DOSAGE
Treatment of increased intraocular pressure in patients with ocular hypertension or open-angle glaucoma
Adults: Instill 1 gtt in the conjunctival sac of affected eye t.i.d.

PHARMACODYNAMICS
Antiglaucoma action: Dorzolamide inhibits carbonic anhydrase in the ciliary processes of the eye, which decreases aqueous humor secretion, presumably by slowing the formation of bicarbonate ions with subsequent reduction in sodium and fluid transport. The result is a reduction in intraocular pressure.

PHARMACOKINETICS
Absorption: Dorzolamide reaches the systemic circulation when applied topically.
Distribution: Drug accumulates in RBCs during long-term treatment as a result of binding to carbonic anhydrase II.
Metabolism: Unknown.
Excretion: Drug is primarily excreted unchanged in urine.

CONTRAINDICATIONS & PRECAUTIONS
Contraindicated in patients with hypersensitivity to any component of dorzolamide or in those with impaired renal function. Use cautiously in patients with impaired hepatic function.

INTERACTIONS
Drug-drug. *Oral carbonic anhydrase inhibitors* may cause additive effects; don't administer concomitantly.

ADVERSE REACTIONS
CNS: headache, asthenia, fatigue.
GI: nausea.
GU: urolithiasis.
EENT: *ocular burning, stinging, or discomfort; superficial punctate keratitis; ocular allergic reactions; blurred vision; lacrimation; dryness; photophobia;* iridocyclitis; *bitter taste.*
Skin: rash.

▣ KEY CONSIDERATIONS
• Use with caution in geriatric patients because they may be more sensitive to

---

dorzolamide than patients in other age-groups.

• Because dorzolamide is a sulfonamide and is absorbed systemically, topical dorzolamide may produce the same adverse effects as other sulfonamides.

• If signs of serious adverse reactions or hypersensitivity occur, drug should be discontinued.

Patient education

• Instruct patient that if more than one topical ophthalmic drug is being used, he should apply them at least 10 minutes apart.

• Teach patient how to instill drops. Advise him to wash hands before and after instilling solution, and warn him not to touch dropper or tip to eye or surrounding tissue.

• Advise patient to apply light finger pressure on lacrimal sac for 1 minute after instillation to minimize systemic absorption of drug.

• Tell patient that topical dorzolamide may produce the same adverse effects as other sulfonamides. If signs of serious adverse reactions or hypersensitivity occur, tell patient to stop the drug and call immediately.

• Inform patient to report ocular reactions, particularly conjunctivitis and lid reactions, and discontinue drug.

• Tell patient not to wear soft contact lenses while using drug.

• Stress importance of complying with recommended therapy.

Overdose & treatment

• An overdose may result in electrolyte imbalance, acidosis, and possible CNS effects.

• Serum electrolyte levels (especially potassium) and blood pH levels should be monitored. Treatment is supportive.

doxazosin mesylate
Cardura

Alpha-adrenergic blocker, antihypertensive, smooth-muscle relaxant

Available by prescription only
Tablets: 1 mg, 2 mg, 4 mg, 8 mg

INDICATIONS & DOSAGE
Essential hypertension
Adult: Dosage must be individualized. Initially, administer 1 mg P.O. daily and determine effect on standing and supine blood pressure at 2 to 6 hours and 24 hours after dosing. If necessary, increase dose to 2 mg daily. To minimize adverse reactions, adjust dosage slowly (dosage typically increased only q 2 weeks). If necessary, increase dose to 4 mg daily, then 8 mg. Although maximum daily dosage is 16 mg, doses exceeding 4 mg daily increase the risk of adverse reactions.
Benign prostatic hyperplasia
Adults: Initially, 1 mg P.O. once daily in the morning or evening; increase to 2 mg and, thereafter, to 4 mg and 8 mg once daily. Recommended dosage adjustment interval is 1 to 2 weeks.

PHARMACODYNAMICS
Antihypertensive action: Doxazosin selectively blocks postsynaptic alpha$_1$-adrenergic receptors, dilating both resistance (arterioles) and capacitance (veins) vessels. It lowers both supine and standing blood pressure, producing more pronounced effects on diastolic pressure. Maximum reductions occur 2 to 6 hours after dosing and are associated with a small increase in standing heart rate. Doxazosin has a greater effect on blood pressure and heart rate in the standing position.
Smooth-muscle relaxant: Doxazosin improves urine flow related to relaxation of smooth muscles produced by blockade of alpha adrenoreceptors in the bladder neck and prostate.

PHARMACOKINETICS
Absorption: Doxazosin is readily absorbed from the GI tract after oral administration. Plasma levels peak in 2 to 3 hours.
Distribution: About 98% binds to proteins.
Metabolism: Drug is extensively metabolized in the liver through hydroxylation or O-demethylation. Secondary peaking of plasma levels suggests enterohepatic recycling.

Reactions may be *common*, uncommon, *life-threatening*, or COMMON AND LIFE-THREATENING.

Excretion: About 63% is excreted in bile and feces (4.8% as unchanged drug); 9% is excreted in urine.

CONTRAINDICATIONS & PRECAUTIONS
Contraindicated in patients with hypersensitivity to doxazosin and quinazoline derivatives (including prazosin and terazosin). Use cautiously in patients with impaired hepatic function.

INTERACTIONS
Drug-drug. Antihypertensive effects of *clonidine* may be decreased with concomitant use.

ADVERSE REACTIONS
CNS: *dizziness,* vertigo, somnolence, drowsiness, *asthenia, headache.*
CV: *orthostatic hypotension,* hypotension, edema, palpitations, *arrhythmias,* tachycardia.
EENT: rhinitis, pharyngitis, abnormal vision.
GI: nausea, vomiting, diarrhea, constipation.
Hematologic: decreased WBC and neutrophil counts.
Musculoskeletal: arthralgia, myalgia.
Respiratory: dyspnea.
Skin: rash, pruritus.
Other: pain.

▣ KEY CONSIDERATIONS
• Use with caution in geriatric patients with underlying autonomic dysfunction or cardiac arrhythmias.
• Geriatric patients may be more susceptible to the postural effects of alpha-adrenergic blockers than patients in other age-groups.
• Postural effects are most likely to occur 2 to 6 hours after dose. Monitor blood pressure during this time after the first dose and after subsequent increases in dosage. Daily doses exceeding 4 mg increase the potential for excessive postural effects.
• First-dose effect (orthostatic hypotension) occurs with doxazosin but is less pronounced than with prazosin or terazosin.

Patient education
• Tell patient that orthostatic hypotension and syncope may occur, especially after first few doses and with dosage changes. To prevent orthostatic hypertension, patient should arise slowly.
• Caution patient that drug may cause drowsiness and somnolence. Patient should avoid driving and performing other hazardous tasks that require alertness for 12 to 24 hours after first dose, after dosage increases, and after resumption of interrupted therapy.
• Tell patient to report bothersome palpitations or dizziness.
• Tell patient drug may be taken with food if nausea occurs. Inform patient that nausea should improve as therapy continues.

Overdose & treatment
• Keep patient supine to restore blood pressure and heart rate. If necessary, treat shock with volume expanders. Administer vasopressors and monitor and support renal function.

---

doxepin hydrochloride
Adapin, Sinequan, Triadapin*

Tricyclic antidepressant, anxiolytic

Available by prescription only
Capsules: 10 mg, 25 mg, 50 mg, 75 mg, 100 mg, 150 mg
Oral concentrate: 10 mg/ml

INDICATIONS & DOSAGE
Depression or anxiety
Adults: Initially, 25 to 75 mg P.O. daily in divided doses, to a maximum of 300 mg daily. Alternatively, give entire maintenance dosage once daily with a maximum dosage of 150 mg P.O.
✦ **Dosage adjustment.** Reduce dosage in geriatric patients, especially those who are debilitated or are receiving other drugs (especially anticholinergics).

PHARMACODYNAMICS
Antidepressant action: Doxepin is thought to exert its antidepressant effects by inhibiting reuptake of norepinephrine and serotonin in CNS nerve

terminals (presynaptic neurons), which results in increased levels and enhanced activity of these neurotransmitters in the synaptic cleft. Doxepin more actively inhibits reuptake of serotonin than norepinephrine. Anxiolytic effects of this drug usually precede antidepressant effects. Doxepin also may be used as an anxiolytic. Doxepin has the greatest sedative effect of all tricyclic antidepressants; tolerance to this effect usually develops in a few weeks.

PHARMACOKINETICS

Absorption: Doxepin is absorbed rapidly from the GI tract after oral administration.

Distribution: Drug is distributed widely into the body, including the CNS. About 90% binds to proteins. Peak effect occurs in 2 to 4 hours; steady state is achieved within 7 days. Therapeutic levels (parent drug and metabolite) are thought to range from 150 to 250 ng/ml.

Metabolism: Drug is metabolized in the liver to the active metabolite desmethyldoxepin. A significant first-pass effect may explain variability of serum levels in different patients taking the same dosage.

Excretion: Drug is mostly excreted in urine.

CONTRAINDICATIONS & PRECAUTIONS

Contraindicated in patients with glaucoma, urine retention, or hypersensitivity to doxepin.

INTERACTIONS

Drug-drug. Use with the following drugs is likely to cause additive effects: *CNS depressants*—including *analgesics, anesthetics, barbiturates, narcotics,* and *tranquilizers* (oversedation); *atropine* and other *anticholinergics,* including *antiparkinsonians, antihistamines, meperidine,* and *phenothiazines* (oversedation, paralytic ileus, visual changes, and severe constipation); and *metrizamide* (increased risk of seizures). Use with *antiarrhythmics*—such as *disopyramide, procainamide,* and *quinidine-pimozide,* or *thyroid drugs* may increase the risk of cardiac arrhythmias and conduction defects. *Barbiturates* induce doxepin me-

tabolism and decrease therapeutic efficacy. *Beta blockers, cimetidine, methylphenidate,* and *propoxyphene* may inhibit doxepin metabolism, increasing plasma levels and toxicity. Doxepin may decrease hypotensive effects of *centrally acting antihypertensives,* such as *guanethidine, clonidine, guanadrel, guanabenz, methyldopa,* and *reserpine*. Use with *disulfiram* or *ethchlorvynol* may cause delirium and tachycardia. *Haloperidol* and *phenothiazines* decrease metabolism of doxepin, decreasing therapeutic efficacy. Use with *sympathomimetics*—including *ephedrine* (found in many nasal sprays), *epinephrine, phenylephrine,* and *phenylpropanolamine*—may increase blood pressure. Use with *warfarin* may increase PT and INR and cause bleeding.

Drug-food. Drug is incompatible with *carbonated beverages.*

Drug-lifestyle. Additive effects are likely after use with *alcohol. Heavy smoking* induces metabolism of doxepin and decreases its therapeutic efficacy.

ADVERSE REACTIONS

CNS: *drowsiness, dizziness,* confusion, numbness, hallucinations, paresthesia, ataxia, weakness, headache, **seizures,** extrapyramidal reactions.

CV: *orthostatic hypotension, tachycardia,* elongation of QT and PR intervals, flattened T waves on ECG.

EENT: *blurred vision,* tinnitus.

GI: *dry mouth, constipation,* nausea, vomiting, anorexia.

GU: urine retention.

Hematologic*: eosinophilia,* **bone marrow depression,** decreased WBC counts.

Hepatic: elevated liver function tests.

Metabolic: hypoglycemia, hyperglycemia.

Skin: rash, urticaria, photosensitivity.

Other: *diaphoresis,* **hypersensitivity reaction.**

After abrupt withdrawal of long-term therapy: nausea, headache, malaise (doesn't indicate addiction).

▣ KEY CONSIDERATIONS

• Geriatric patients are at increased risk for developing adverse CNS reactions,

---

Reactions may be *common,* uncommon, *life-threatening,* or **COMMON AND LIFE-THREATENING.**

hypotension, and GI and GU disturbances.

• Recommendations for administration of doxepin and care of patients during therapy are the same as those for all tricyclic antidepressants.

Patient education

• Teach patient to dilute oral concentrate with 4 oz (120 ml) water, milk, or juice (grapefruit, orange, pineapple, prune, or tomato). Drug is incompatible with carbonated beverages.

• To treat dry mouth, tell patient to use ice chips, sugarless gum or hard candy, or saliva substitutes.

• Advise patient to avoid alcohol or other sedatives while taking doxepin. Drug has a strong sedative effect and such combinations can cause excessive sedation.

• Advise patient that heavy smoking decreases the effectiveness of the drug.

• Warn patient to avoid taking other drugs while taking doxepin unless they have been prescribed.

• Instruct patient to take full dose at bedtime.

• Tell patient to store drug safely away from children.

Overdose & treatment

• The first 12 hours after acute ingestion are a stimulatory phase characterized by excessive anticholinergic activity (agitation, irritation, confusion, hallucinations, hyperthermia, parkinsonian symptoms, seizures, urine retention, dry mucous membranes, pupillary dilatation, constipation, and ileus). This is followed by CNS depressant effects, including hypothermia, decreased or absent reflexes, sedation, hypotension, cyanosis, and cardiac irregularities, including tachycardia, conduction disturbances, and quinidine-like effects on the ECG.

• Severity of overdose is best indicated by widening of QRS complex, which usually represents a serum level exceeding 1,000 ng/ml. Serum levels generally aren't helpful. Metabolic acidosis may follow hypotension, hypoventilation, and seizures.

• Treatment is symptomatic and supportive, including maintaining airway, stable body temperature, and fluid and electrolyte balance. Induce vomiting with ipecac if patient is conscious; follow with gastric lavage and activated charcoal to prevent further absorption. Dialysis is of little use. Physostigmine may be cautiously used to reverse central anticholinergic effects. Treat seizures with parenteral diazepam or phenytoin; arrhythmias with parenteral phenytoin or lidocaine; and acidosis with sodium bicarbonate. Don't give barbiturates: these may enhance CNS and respiratory depressant effects.

doxorubicin hydrochloride
Adriamycin PFS, Adriamycin RDF, Rubex

Antineoplastic antibiotic (cell cycle–phase nonspecific)

Available by prescription only
Injection: 10-mg, 20-mg, 50-mg, 100-mg, and 150-mg vials
Injection (preservative-free): 2 mg/ml

INDICATIONS & DOSAGE
Dosage and indications may vary. Check current literature for recommended protocol or for information on liposomal doxorubicin.
Bladder, breast, lung, ovarian, stomach, and thyroid cancers; Hodgkin's disease; acute lymphoblastic and myeloblastic leukemia; Wilms' tumor; neuroblastoma; lymphoma; sarcoma
Adults: 60 to 75 mg/m^2 I.V. as a single dose q 21 days; or 25 to 30 mg/m^2 I.V. as a single daily dose on days 1 to 3 of 4-week cycle. Alternatively, 20 mg/m^2 I.V. once weekly. Maximum cumulative dosage is 550 mg/m^2 (450 mg/m^2 in patients who have received chest irradiation).

PHARMACODYNAMICS
Antineoplastic action: Doxorubicin exerts its cytotoxic activity by intercalating between DNA base pairs and uncoiling the DNA helix. The result is inhibition of DNA synthesis and DNA-dependent RNA synthesis. Doxorubicin also inhibits protein synthesis.

PHARMACOKINETICS

Absorption: Because of its vesicant effects, doxorubicin must be administered I.V.

Distribution: Drug distributes widely into body tissues, with the highest levels found in the liver, heart, and kidneys. However, it doesn't cross the blood-brain barrier.

Metabolism: Drug is extensively metabolized in the liver to several metabolites, one of which possesses cytotoxic activity.

Excretion: Drug and its metabolites are excreted primarily in bile. A minute amount is eliminated in urine. The plasma elimination of doxorubicin is described as biphasic with a half-life of 15 to 30 minutes in the initial phase and 16½ hours in the terminal phase.

CONTRAINDICATIONS & PRECAUTIONS

Contraindicated in patients with marked myelosuppression from previous treatment with other antitumorigenic drugs or by radiotherapy and in those who have received lifetime cumulative dosage of 550 mg/m^2.

INTERACTIONS

Drug-drug. Doxorubicin shouldn't be mixed with *aminophylline, cephalosporins, dexamethasone phosphate, fluorouracil, heparin sodium,* or *hydrocortisone sodium phosphate* because it will result in a precipitate. Use with *cyclophosphamide* or *daunorubicin* may potentiate the cardiotoxicity of doxorubicin through additive effects on the heart. Doxorubicin may worsen *cyclophosphamide*-induced hemorrhagic cystitis and *mercaptopurine*-induced hepatotoxicity. Serum *digoxin* levels may be decreased if used concomitantly. Use with *streptozocin* may increase the plasma half-life of doxorubicin by an unknown mechanism, increasing the activity of doxorubicin.

ADVERSE REACTIONS

CV: cardiac depression, seen in such ECG changes as sinus tachycardia, T-wave flattening, ST-segment depression, voltage reduction; *arrhythmias; acute left-sided failure; irreversible cardiomyopathy.*

EENT: conjunctivitis.

GI: *nausea, vomiting,* diarrhea, *stomatitis,* esophagitis, anorexia.

GU: red urine (transient).

Hematologic: *leukopenia* during days 10 to 15 with recovery by day 21, *thrombocytopenia,* MYELOSUPPRESSION.

Metabolic: hyperuricemia.

Skin: urticaria, facial flushing, *complete alopecia within 3 to 4 weeks* (hair may regrow 2 to 5 months after drug is stopped).

Other: *severe cellulitis or tissue sloughing* (if drug extravasates), fever, chills, *anaphylaxis.*

◻ KEY CONSIDERATIONS

● Patients older than age 70 have an increased incidence of drug-induced cardiotoxicity. Caution should be taken in geriatric patients with low bone marrow reserve to prevent serious hematologic toxicity.

● To reconstitute to a concentration of 2 mg/ml, add 5 ml of normal saline injection, USP, to the 10-mg vial, 10 ml to the 20-mg vial, or 25 ml to the 50-mg vial.

● Drug may be further diluted with normal saline solution or D$_5$W and administered by I.V. infusion.

● Drug may be administered by I.V. push injection over 5 to 10 minutes into the tubing of a freely flowing I.V. infusion.

● The alternative dosage schedule (once-weekly dosing) has been found to reduce the risk of cardiomyopathy.

● If cumulative dose exceeds 550 mg/m^2 body surface area, 30% of patients develop cardiac adverse reactions, which begin 2 weeks to 6 months after stopping drug. With high doses of doxorubicin, consider concomitant dosing with the cardioprotective drug dexrazoxane.

● Streaking along a vein or facial flushing indicates that drug is being administered too rapidly.

● Applying a scalp tourniquet or ice may decrease alopecia. However, don't use these if treating leukemias or other neoplasms where tumor stem cells may be present in scalp.

• Drug should be discontinued or rate of infusion slowed if tachycardia develops. Treat extravasation with topical application of dimethyl sulfoxide and ice packs.
• Monitor CBC and hepatic function.
• Decrease dosage as follows if serum bilirubin level increases: 50% of dose when bilirubin level is 1.2 to 3 mg/100 ml; 25% of dose when bilirubin level exceeds 3 mg/100 ml.
• Esophagitis is very common in patients who have also received radiation therapy.

Patient education
• Encourage adequate fluid intake to increase urine output and facilitate excretion of uric acid.
• Advise patient to avoid exposure to people with infections.
• Warn patient that alopecia will occur. Explain that hair growth should resume 2 to 5 months after drug is stopped.
• Advise patient that urine will appear red for 1 to 2 days after the dose and doesn't indicate bleeding. The urine may stain clothes.
• Instruct patient not to receive immunizations during therapy and for several weeks after. Other members of the patient's household shouldn't receive immunizations during the same period.
• Tell patient to call health care provider if he experiences unusual bruising or bleeding or signs of an infection.

Overdose & treatment
• Signs and symptoms of overdose include myelosuppression, nausea, vomiting, mucositis, and irreversible myocardial toxicity.
• Treatment is usually supportive and includes transfusion of blood components, antiemetics, antibiotics for infections which may develop, symptomatic treatment of mucositis, and cardiac glycoside preparations.

doxycycline
Vibramycin

doxycycline calcium
Vibramycin

doxycycline hyclate
Doryx, Doxy-100, Doxy-200, Doxy-Caps, Vibramycin, Vibra-Tabs

doxycycline monohydrate
Monodox, Vibramycin

Tetracycline, antibiotic

Available by prescription only
doxycycline
Oral suspension: 25 mg/5 ml
doxycycline calcium
Oral suspension: 50 mg/5 ml
doxycycline hyclate
Tablets: 100 mg
Capsules: 50 mg, 100 mg
Injection: 100 mg, 200 mg
doxycycline monohydrate
Capsules: 50 mg, 100 mg
Oral suspension: 25 mg/5 ml

INDICATIONS & DOSAGE
Infections caused by sensitive organisms
Adults weighing 99 lb (45 kg) and over: 100 mg P.O. q 12 hours on day 1, then 100 mg P.O. daily; or 200 mg I.V. on day 1 in one or two infusions, then 100 to 200 mg I.V. daily.
Give I.V. infusion slowly (minimum 1 hour). Infusion must be completed within 12 hours (within 6 hours in lactated Ringer's solution or D₅W in lactated Ringer's solution).
Gonorrhea in patients allergic to penicillin
Adults: 100 mg P.O. b.i.d. for 7 days; or 300 mg P.O. initially and repeat dose in 1 hour.
◊*Syphilis in patients allergic to penicillin*
Adults: 100 mg P.O. b.i.d. for 2 weeks (early detection) or 4 weeks (if more than 1 year duration).
Chlamydia trachomatis, *nongonococcal urethritis, and uncomplicated urethral, endocervical, or rectal infections*

Adults: 100 mg P.O. b.i.d. for at least 7 days.
Acute pelvic inflammatory disease (PID)
Adults: 250 mg I.M. ceftriaxone, followed by 100 mg doxycycline P.O. b.i.d. for 10 to 14 days.
Acute epididymo-orchitis caused by C. trachomatis *or* Neisseria gonorrhoeae
Adults: 100 mg P.O. b.i.d for at least 10 days.
◇ *To prevent traveler's diarrhea commonly caused by enterotoxigenic* **Escherichia coli**
Adults: 100 mg P.O. daily for up to 3 days.
◇ *Prophylaxis for rape victims*
Adults: 100 mg P.O. b.i.d. for 7 days after a single 2-g oral dose of metronidazole is given in conjunction with a single 125-mg I.M. dose of ceftriaxone.
Chemoprophylaxis for malaria in travelers to areas where chloroquine-resistant Plasmodium falciparum *is* endemic and mefloquine is contraindicated
Adults: 100 mg P.O. once daily. Begin prophylaxis 1 to 2 days before travel to malarious areas; continue daily while in affected area, and continue for 4 weeks after return from malarious area.
◇ *Lyme disease*
Adults: 100 mg P.O. b.i.d. or t.i.d. for 10 to 30 days.
◇ *Pleural effusions associated with cancer*
Adults: 500 mg of doxycycline diluted in 250 ml of normal saline and instilled into pleural space via a chest tube.

PHARMACODYNAMICS
Antibacterial action: Doxycycline is bacteriostatic; it binds reversibly to ribosomal units, thereby inhibiting bacterial protein synthesis. Spectrum of activity includes many gram-negative and gram-positive organisms, *Mycoplasma, Rickettsia, Chlamydia,* and spirochetes.

PHARMACOKINETICS
Absorption: About 90% to 100% of doxycycline is absorbed after oral administration; serum levels peak in 1½ to 4 hours. Doxycycline has the least affinity for calcium of all tetracyclines; milk

and other dairy products alter absorption, but insignificantly.
Distribution: Drug is distributed widely into body tissues and fluids, including synovial, pleural, prostatic, and seminal fluids; bronchial secretions; saliva; and aqueous humor. CSF penetration is poor. About 25% to 93% bind to proteins.
Metabolism: Drug is insignificantly metabolized; some hepatic degradation occurs.
Excretion: Drug is excreted primarily unchanged in urine through glomerular filtration. In adults with normal renal function, plasma half-life is 22 to 24 hours after multiple dosing; in patients with severe renal impairment, 20 to 30 hours. Some drug is excreted in feces.

CONTRAINDICATIONS & PRECAUTIONS
Contraindicated in patients with hypersensitivity to doxycycline or other tetracyclines. Use cautiously in patients with impaired renal or hepatic function.

INTERACTIONS
Drug-drug. Use with *antacids containing aluminum, calcium, or magnesium* or *laxatives containing magnesium* decreases oral absorption of doxycycline because of chelation. Use with *oral anticoagulants* necessitates lowered dosage of oral anticoagulants because of enhanced effects; with *digoxin,* lowered dosages of digoxin are needed because of increased bioavailability. Use with *oral iron products* or *sodium bicarbonate* also impairs absorption of doxycycline. Doxycycline may antagonize bactericidal effects of *penicillin,* inhibiting cell growth because of bacteriostatic action; administer penicillin 2 to 3 hours before doxycycline.

ADVERSE REACTIONS
CNS: *intracranial hypertension (pseudotumor cerebri).*
CV: pericarditis, thrombophlebitis.
EENT: glossitis, dysphagia.
GI: anorexia, *epigastric distress, nausea,* vomiting, *diarrhea,* oral candidiasis, enterocolitis, anogenital inflammation.
Hematologic: *neutropenia,* eosinophilia, ***thrombocytopenia,*** hemolytic anemia.

Reactions may be *common,* uncommon, *life-threatening,* or COMMON AND LIFE-THREATENING.

Hepatic: elevated liver enzyme levels.
Skin: *maculopapular and erythematous rashes, photosensitivity, increased pigmentation, urticaria.*
Other: hypersensitivity reactions *(anaphylaxis),* superinfection.

▣ KEY CONSIDERATIONS

Besides the recommendations relevant to all tetracyclines, consider the following:
• Reconstitute powder for injection with sterile water for injection. Use 10 ml in a 100-mg vial and 20 ml in a 200-mg vial. Dilute solution to 100 to 1,000 ml for I.V. infusion. Don't infuse solutions more concentrated than 1 mg/ml.
• Reconstituted solution is stable for 72 hours if refrigerated and protected from light.
• Don't inject S.C. or I.M.
• Drug may be used in patients with impaired renal function; it doesn't accumulate or cause a significant rise in BUN levels.
• Doxycycline causes false-negative results in urine tests using glucose oxidase reagent (Diastix, Chemstrip uG, or glucose enzymatic test strip); parenteral dosage form may cause false-negative Clinitest results.
• Doxycycline causes falsely elevated urine catecholamine levels in fluorometric tests.

Patient teaching

• Tell patient that drug may be taken with food to prevent GI upset.

Overdose & treatment

• Signs and symptoms of overdose are usually limited to the GI tract.
• Give antacids or perform gastric lavage to empty stomach if ingestion occurred within the preceding 4 hours.

◊ Unlabeled clinical use

enalaprilat
Vasotec I.V.

enalapril maleate
Vasotec

ACE inhibitor, antihypertensive

Available by prescription only
Tablets: 2.5 mg, 5 mg, 10 mg, 20 mg
Injection: 1.25 mg/ml in 2-ml vials

INDICATIONS & DOSAGE
Hypertension
Adults: For patient not receiving diuretics, initially 5 mg P.O. once daily, then adjusted according to response. Usual dosage range is 10 to 40 mg daily as a single dose or two divided doses. Alternatively, 1.25 mg I.V. infusion q 6 hours over 5 minutes. For patient taking diuretics, initially 2.5 mg P.O. once daily. Alternatively, administer 0.625 mg I.V. over 5 minutes, repeat in 1 hour if needed, then follow with 1.25 mg I.V. q 6 hours.
To convert from I.V. therapy to oral therapy
Adults: If patient wasn't treated with diuretics and was receiving 1.25 mg q 6 hours, then initially, 5 mg P.O. once daily. If patient is being treated with diuretics and was receiving 0.625 mg I.V. q 6 hours, then 2.5 mg P.O. once daily. Adjust dosage according to response.
To convert from oral therapy to I.V. therapy
Adults: 1.25 mg I.V. over 5 minutes q 6 hours. Higher doses haven't demonstrated greater efficacy.
✦ *Dosage adjustment.* In hypertensive patients with renal failure who have a creatinine clearance less than 30 ml/minute, begin therapy at 2.5 mg/day. Gradually titrate dosage according to response. Patients undergoing hemodialysis should receive a supplemental dose of 2.5 mg on days of dialysis.
Heart failure
Adults: Initially, 2.5 mg P.O. Recommended dosing range is 2.5 to 20 mg b.i.d. adjust dosage upward, as tolerated, over a few days or weeks. Maximum daily dose is 40 mg P.O. in divided doses.
Asymptomatic left ventricular dysfunction
Adults: Initially, 2.5 mg P.O. b.i.d.; titrate dosage to targeted daily dose of 20 mg (in divided doses) as tolerated.
✦ *Dosage adjustment.* For patients with heart failure and renal impairment or hyponatremia (serum sodium level less than 130 mEq/L or serum creatinine level above 1.6 mg/dl), begin therapy with 2.5 mg P.O. daily. Increase dosage to 2.5 mg b.i.d., then 5 mg b.i.d. and higher, p.r.n., usually at intervals of 4 days or more.

PHARMACODYNAMICS
Antihypertensive action: Enalapril inhibits ACE, preventing angiotensin I from converting to angiotensin II, a potent vasoconstrictor. Reduced angiotensin II levels decrease peripheral arterial resistance, lowering blood pressure, and decrease aldosterone secretion, thus reducing sodium and water retention.

PHARMACOKINETICS
Absorption: About 60% of a given dose of enalapril is absorbed from the GI tract; blood pressure decreases within 1 hour, with the antihypertensive effect peaking in 4 to 6 hours.
Distribution: Full distribution pattern of enalapril is unknown; drug doesn't appear to cross the blood-brain barrier.
Metabolism: Drug is metabolized extensively to the active metabolite enalaprilat.
Excretion: About 94% of a dose of enalapril is excreted in urine and feces as enalaprilat and enalapril.

CONTRAINDICATIONS & PRECAUTIONS
Contraindicated in patients with hypersensitivity to enalapril or history of angioedema related to previous treatment with an ACE inhibitor. Use cautiously in patients with impaired renal function.

INTERACTIONS
Drug-drug. Enalapril, similar to other *ACE inhibitors,* may cause a dry hacking

cough. Use of *aspirin* or *indomethacin* may decrease the antihypertensive effect of enalapril. Enalapril may increase antihypertensive effects of *diuretics, other antihypertensives,* or *phenothiazines.* Enalapril may decrease the renal clearance of *lithium* and may decrease the pharmacologic effects of *rifampin.* Enalapril may enhance effects of *potassium sparing diuretics, potassium supplements,* and *salt substitutes,* thereby causing hyperkalemia; such products should be used cautiously.

ADVERSE REACTIONS
CNS: *headache, dizziness, fatigue,* vertigo, asthenia, syncope.
CV: *hypotension,* chest pain.
GI: diarrhea, nausea, abdominal pain, vomiting.
GU: decreased renal function (in patients with bilateral renal artery stenosis or heart failure), proteinuria, nephrotic syndrome.
Hematologic: *neutropenia, agranulocytosis.*
Respiratory: *dry, persistent, tickling, nonproductive cough;* dyspnea.
Skin: rash.
Other: *angioedema.*

◙ KEY CONSIDERATIONS
• Geriatric patients may need lower dosages of enalapril because of impaired drug clearance.
• To reduce risk of hypotension, discontinue diuretic therapy 2 to 3 days before beginning enalapril therapy; if drug doesn't adequately control blood pressure, reinstate diuretics.
• Perform WBC and differential counts before treatment, every 2 weeks for 3 months, and periodically thereafter.
• Give drug before, during, or after meals because food doesn't appear to affect absorption.
• Enalapril may elevate BUN and serum creatinine levels and, less commonly, liver enzyme and bilirubin levels; it may slightly decrease hemoglobin level and hematocrit. Rare cases of neutropenia, thrombocytopenia, and bone marrow depression have been reported.

Patient education
• Tell patient to report feelings of lightheadedness, especially in the first few days, so dosage can be adjusted; signs and symptoms of infection, such as sore throat and fever, because drug may decrease WBC count; facial swelling or difficulty breathing because drug may cause angioedema; and loss of taste because drug may need to be discontinued.
• Advise patient not to change position suddenly, to minimize orthostatic hypotension.
• Warn patient to seek health care provider's approval before taking OTC cold preparations, particularly antitussives.

enoxaparin sodium
Lovenox

Low-molecular-weight heparin, anticoagulant

Available by prescription only
Ampules: 30 mg/0.3 ml
Syringes (prefilled): 30 mg/0.3 ml, 40 mg/0.4 ml
Syringes (graduated prefilled): 60 mg/0.6 ml, 80 mg/0.8 ml, 100 mg/1 ml

INDICATIONS & DOSAGE
Prevention of deep vein thrombosis (DVT), which may lead to pulmonary embolism, after hip or knee replacement surgery
Adults: 30 mg S.C. q 12 hours for 7 to 10 days. Give initial dose between 12 and 24 hours postoperatively, provided hemostasis has been established.
Prevention of DVT, which may lead to pulmonary embolism, after abdominal surgery
Adults: 40 mg S.C. once daily for 7 to 10 days. Give initial dose 2 hours before surgery.
Prevention of ischemic complications of unstable angina and non-Q-wave MI, when concurrently administered with aspirin
Adults: 1 mg/kg S.C. q 12 hours for 2 to 8 days in conjunction with oral aspirin therapy (100 to 325 mg once daily).

Note: To minimize risk of bleeding after vascular instrumentation during the treatment of unstable angina, adhere precisely to the intervals recommended between enoxaparin doses.

PHARMACODYNAMICS

Anticoagulant action: Enoxaparin is a low-molecular-weight heparin that accelerates the formation of antithrombin III-thrombin complex and deactivates thrombin, preventing fibrinogen from converting to fibrin. It has a higher antifactor Xa to anti-factor IIa activity than unfractionated heparin.

PHARMACOKINETICS

Absorption: Maximum anti-factor Xa and anti-factor IIa (antithrombin) activities occur 3 to 5 hours after S.C. injection of enoxaparin.
Distribution: Volume of distribution of anti-factor Xa activity is about 6 L.
Metabolism: No information available.
Excretion: Elimination half-life based on anti-factor Xa activity is about 4½ hours after S.C. administration.

CONTRAINDICATIONS & PRECAUTIONS

Contraindicated in patients with hypersensitivity to enoxaparin or heparin or pork products; in patients with active, major bleeding or thrombocytopenia; and in those who demonstrate antiplatelet antibodies in the presence of drug.

Use with extreme caution in patients with history of heparin-induced thrombocytopenia. Use cautiously in patients with conditions that put them at increased risk for hemorrhage, such as bacterial endocarditis; congenital or acquired bleeding disorders; ulcer disease; angiodysplastic GI disease; hemorrhagic stroke; recent spinal, eye, or brain surgery; or in those treated concomitantly with NSAIDs, platelet inhibitors, or other anticoagulants that affect hemostasis. Also, use cautiously in patients with a bleeding diathesis, uncontrolled arterial hypertension, recent GI ulceration, diabetic retinopathy, and hemorrhage. Use with care in geriatric patients and patients with renal insufficiency who may show delayed elimination of enoxaparin.

Use with extreme caution in patients with postoperative indwelling epidural catheters. Cases of epidural or spinal hematomas have been reported with the use of enoxaparin and spinal or epidural anesthesia or spinal puncture, resulting in long-term or permanent paralysis.

INTERACTIONS

Drug-drug. Use of *antiplatelets* or *other anticoagulants* increases the risk of bleeding.

ADVERSE REACTIONS

CNS: confusion.
CV: edema, peripheral edema.
GI: nausea.
Hematologic: hypochromic anemia, ***thrombocytopenia,*** ecchymoses, bleeding complications, ***hemorrhage.***
Other: irritation, pain, hematoma, erythema (at injection site); fever; pain.

▣ KEY CONSIDERATIONS

• Enoxaparin isn't intended for I.M. administration.
• Don't use drug interchangeably (unit for unit) with unfractionated heparin or other low-molecular-weight heparins.
• Don't mix drug with other injections or infusions.
• To rule out a bleeding disorder, screen all patients before enoxaparin prophylaxis.
• Daily monitoring of the effect of enoxaparin usually isn't needed in patients with normal presurgical coagulation parameters.
• Administer drug by deep S.C. injection with patient lying down. Introduce the full length of the needle into a skin fold held between the thumb and forefinger, and hold the skin fold throughout the injection. Alternate administration sites exist between the left and right anterolateral and left and right posterolateral abdominal wall.
• Don't expel air bubble from syringe before injection because drug may be lost.
• Discontinue drug and initiate appropriate therapy if thromboembolic events occur despite enoxaparin prophylaxis.
• Consider the potential benefit versus risk before neuraxial intervention in patients who are or will be anticoagulated

for thromboprophylaxis. When epidural or spinal anesthesia or spinal puncture is used, patients taking enoxaparin to prevent coagulation are at risk for developing an epidural or spinal hematoma. Monitor patients frequently for signs and symptoms of neurologic impairment. If neurologic compromise is noted, urgent treatment is necessary.

• Enoxaparin therapy may decrease the patient's platelet count and increase his AST and ALT levels.

Overdose & treatment

• Enoxaparin overdose may lead to hemorrhagic complications.

• To treat overdose, slowly inject protamine sulfate (1%) solution I.V. The dose of protamine sulfate should be equal to the dose of enoxaparin injection (1 mg of protamine neutralizes 1 mg of enoxaparin).

ephedrine

ephedrine hydrochloride

ephedrine sulfate
Ephedrine Sulfate Capsules,
Ephedrine Sulfate Injection

Adrenergic, bronchodilator, vasopressor (parenteral form), nasal decongestant

Available with and without a prescription
Capsules: 25 mg, 50 mg
Nasal preparations: 1% jelly; 0.25% spray; 0.5% drops
Injection: 25 mg/ml, 50 mg/ml (parenteral)

INDICATIONS & DOSAGE
To correct hypotensive states
Adults: 25 to 50 mg I.M. or S.C., or 10 to 25 mg slow I.V. bolus. If necessary, a second I.M. dose of 50 mg or I.V. dose of 25 mg may be administered. Additional I.V. doses may be given in 5 to 10 minutes. Maximum dose is 150 mg daily.
Orthostatic hypotension
Adults: 25 mg P.O. once daily to q.i.d.
Bronchodilator or nasal decongestant
Adults: 25 to 50 mg q 3 to 4 hours,

p.r.n.; 12.5 to 25 mg I.M., I.V., or S.C., repeated based on patient response.
As nasal decongestant, 2 or 3 drops instilled into each nostril or on a nasal pack. Instill no more often than q 4 hours.
Severe, acute bronchospasm
Adults: 12.5 to 25 mg I.M., S.C., or I.V.
Enuresis
Adults: 25 to 50 mg P.O. h.s.
Myasthenia gravis
Adults: 25 mg t.i.d. or q.i.d.

PHARMACODYNAMICS
Ephedrine is both a direct- and indirect-acting sympathomimetic that stimulates alpha-adrenergic and beta receptors. Release of norepinephrine from its storage sites is one of its indirect effects. In therapeutic doses, ephedrine relaxes bronchial smooth muscle and produces cardiac stimulation with increased systolic and diastolic blood pressure when norepinephrine stores aren't depleted.
Bronchodilator action: Ephedrine relaxes bronchial smooth muscle by stimulating $beta_2$ receptors, resulting in increased vital capacity, relief of mild bronchospasm, improved air exchange, and decreased residual volume.
Vasopressor action: Drug produces positive inotropic effects with low doses by acting on the $beta_1$ receptors in the heart. Vasodilation results from its effects on $beta_2$ receptors; vasoconstriction, from its alpha-adrenergic effects. Pressor effects may result from vasoconstriction or cardiac stimulation; however, when peripheral vascular resistance is decreased, blood pressure elevates because of increased cardiac output.
Nasal decongestant action: Ephedrine stimulates alpha-adrenergic receptors in blood vessels of the nasal mucosa, producing vasoconstriction and nasal decongestion.

PHARMACOKINETICS
Absorption: Ephedrine is rapidly and completely absorbed after oral, S.C., or I.M. administration. After oral administration, onset of action occurs within 15 to 60 minutes and persists for 2 to 4 hours. Pressor and cardiac effects last 1 hour after I.V. dose of 10 to 25 mg or I.M. or S.C. dose of 25 to 50 mg; they

last up to 4 hours after oral dose of 15 to 50 mg.

Distribution: Drug is widely distributed throughout the body.

Metabolism: Drug is slowly metabolized in the liver through oxidative deamination, demethylation, aromatic hydroxylation, and conjugation.

Excretion: Dose is mostly excreted unchanged in urine; rate of excretion depends on urine pH.

CONTRAINDICATIONS & PRECAUTIONS

Contraindicated in patients with hypersensitivity to ephedrine and other sympathomimetics; in those with porphyria, severe coronary artery disease, arrhythmias, angle-closure glaucoma, psychoneurosis, angina pectoris, substantial organic heart disease, and CV disease; and in those taking MAO inhibitors.

Nasal solution is contraindicated in patients with angle-closure glaucoma, psychoneurosis, angina pectoris, substantial organic heart disease, CV disease, and hypersensitivity to drug or other sympathomimetics.

Use with extreme caution in geriatric men and in those with hypertension, hyperthyroidism, nervous or excitable states, diabetes, and prostatic hyperplasia. Use nasal solution cautiously in patients with hyperthyroidism, hypertension, diabetes mellitus, or prostatic hyperplasia.

INTERACTIONS

Drug-drug. Use with *alpha-adrenergic blockers* may decrease vasopressor effects of ephedrine. Administration with a theophylline derivative such as *aminophylline* reportedly produces a greater incidence of adverse reactions than either drug when used alone. Use with *atropine* blocks reflex bradycardia and enhances pressor effects. Use of *beta blockers* may block CV and bronchodilating effects of ephedrine. Use with *cardiac glycosides* and *general anesthetics* (especially *cyclopropane* or *halothane*) may sensitize myocardium to the effects of ephedrine, causing arrhythmias. *Diuretics, guanethidine, methyldopa,* and *reserpine* may decrease ephedrine's pressor effects. *MAO inhibitors* may potenti-

ate the pressor effects of ephedrine, possibly resulting in hypertensive crisis. Allow 14 days to lapse after withdrawal of MAO inhibitor before using ephedrine. Use of other *sympathomimetics* may add to their effects and toxicity.

ADVERSE REACTIONS

CNS: *insomnia, nervousness,* dizziness, headache, muscle weakness, diaphoresis, euphoria, confusion, delirium, nervousness, excitation (with nasal solution).

CV: *palpitations,* tachycardia, hypertension, precordial pain; *tachycardia* (with nasal solution).

EENT: dry nose and throat, rebound nasal congestion with long-term or excessive use, mucosal irritation (with nasal solution).

GI: nausea, vomiting, anorexia.

GU: urine retention, painful urination due to visceral sphincter spasm.

▣ KEY CONSIDERATIONS

Besides the recommendations relevant to all adrenergics, consider the following:

• Administer ephedrine cautiously because geriatric patients may be more sensitive to the effects of the drug. Lower dose may be recommended.

• Correct fluid volume depletion before administration. As a pressor agent, ephedrine isn't a substitute for blood, plasma, fluids, or electrolytes.

• Increase dose if tolerance develops after prolonged or excessive use. If drug is discontinued for a few days and readministered, effectiveness may be restored.

• To prevent insomnia, administer last dose at least 2 hours before bedtime.

• Monitor vital signs closely during parenteral dosing. Tachycardia is common.

Patient education

• Tell patient using an OTC product to follow directions on the label, to take last dose a few hours before bedtime to reduce the possibility of insomnia, to take only as directed, and not to increase dose or frequency.

• Advise patient to store drug away from heat and light (not in bathroom medicine cabinet) and to keep out of reach of children.

Reactions may be *common,* uncommon, *life-threatening,* or **COMMON AND LIFE-THREATENING.**

- Instruct patient who misses a dose to take it as soon as remembered if within 1 hour. If beyond 1 hour, patient should skip dose and return to regular schedule.
- Teach patient to be aware of palpitations and significant pulse rate changes.
- Instruct patient to clear nose before instilling nasal solutions.

Overdose & treatment

- Signs and symptoms of overdose include exaggeration of common adverse reactions, especially arrhythmias, extreme tremor or seizures, nausea and vomiting, fever, and CNS and respiratory depression.
- Treatment is supportive and symptomatic. If patient is conscious, induce vomiting with ipecac and follow with activated charcoal. If patient is depressed or hyperactive, perform gastric lavage. Maintain airway and blood pressure. Don't administer vasopressors. Monitor vital signs closely.
- A beta blocker (such as propranolol) may be used to treat arrhythmias. A cardioselective beta blocker is recommended in asthmatic patients. Phentolamine may be used for hypertension, paraldehyde or diazepam for seizures, and dexamethasone for pyrexia.

epinephrine
Bronkaid Mist, Bronkaid Mistometer*, EpiPen, EpiPen Jr., Primatene Mist, Sus-Phrine

epinephrine bitartrate
AsthmaHaler

epinephrine hydrochloride
Adrenalin Chloride, AsthmaNefrin, Epifrin, Glaucon, MicroNefrin, Vaponefrin

epinephryl borate
Epinal

Adrenergic, bronchodilator, vasopressor, cardiac stimulant, local anesthetic (adjunct), topical antihemorrhagic, antiglaucoma drug

Available by prescription only

Injection: 0.01 mg/ml (1:100,000), 0.1 mg/ml (1:10,000), 0.5 mg/ml (1:2,000), 1 mg/ml (1:1,000) parenteral; 5 mg/ml (1:200) parenteral suspension
Ophthalmic: 0.1%, 0.25%, 0.5%, 1%, 2% solution
Available without a prescription
Nebulizer inhaler: 1% (1:100), 1.25%, 2.25%
Aerosol inhaler: 160 mcg, 200 mcg, 250 mcg/metered spray
Nasal solution: 0.1%

INDICATIONS & DOSAGE
Bronchospasm, hypersensitivity reactions, anaphylaxis
Adults: Initially, 0.1 to 0.5 mg (0.1 to 0.5 ml of a 1:1,000 solution) S.C. or I.M.; may be repeated at 10- to 15-minute intervals, p.r.n. Alternatively, 0.1 to 0.25 mg (1 to 2.5 ml of a 1:10,000 solution) I.V. slowly over 5 to 10 minutes. May be repeated q 5 to 15 minutes if needed or followed by a 1- to 4-mcg/minute I.V. infusion.
Bronchodilation
Adults: 1 inhalation via metered aerosol, repeated once if needed after 1 minute; subsequent doses shouldn't be repeated for at least 3 hours. Alternatively, 1 or 2 deep inhalations via hand-bulb nebulizer of a 1% (1:100) solution; may be repeated at 1- to 2-minute intervals. Alternatively, 0.03 ml (0.3 mg) of a 1% solution via intermittent positive-pressure breathing.
To restore cardiac rhythm in cardiac arrest
Adults: Initially, 0.5 to 1 mg (range, 0.1 to 1 mg to 10 ml of a 1:10,000 solution) I.V. bolus; may be repeated q 3 to 5 minutes, p.r.n. Alternatively, initial dose followed by 0.3 mg S.C. or 1 to 4 mcg/minute I.V. infusion. Alternatively, 1 mg (10 ml of a 1:10,000 solution) intratracheally or 0.1 to 1 mg (1 to 10 ml of a 1:10,000 solution) by intracardiac injection.
Hemostasis
Adults: 1:50,000 to 1:1,000, applied topically.
To prolong local anesthetic effect
Adults: 1:500,000 to 1:50,000 mixed with local anesthetic.

Open-angle glaucoma
Adults: 1 or 2 gtt of 1% to 2% solution instilled daily or b.i.d.
Nasal congestion, local superficial bleeding
Adults: Instill 1 or 2 gtt of solution.

PHARMACODYNAMICS

Epinephrine acts directly by stimulating alpha-adrenergic and beta receptors in the sympathetic nervous system. It primarily relaxes bronchial smooth muscle, stimulates the heart, and dilates skeletal muscle vasculature.
Bronchodilator action: Epinephrine relaxes bronchial smooth muscle by stimulating beta$_2$ receptors. Epinephrine constricts bronchial arterioles by stimulating alpha-adrenergic receptors, relieving bronchospasm, reducing congestion and edema, and increasing tidal volume and vital capacity. By inhibiting histamine release, it may reverse bronchiolar constriction, vasodilation, and edema.
CV and vasopressor actions: As a cardiac stimulant, epinephrine produces positive chronotropic and inotropic effects by acting on beta$_1$ receptors in the heart: It increases cardiac output, myocardial oxygen consumption, and force of contraction and decreases cardiac efficiency. Vasodilation results from its effects on beta$_2$ receptors; vasoconstriction, from its alpha-adrenergic effects.
Local anesthetic (adjunct) action: Epinephrine acts on alpha receptors in the skin, mucous membranes, and viscera. Drug produces vasoconstriction, which reduces absorption of local anesthetic, thus prolonging its duration of action, localizing anesthesia, and decreasing risk of anesthetic toxicity.
Topical antihemorrhagic action: Epinephrine acts on alpha receptors in the skin, mucous membranes, and viscera, which produces vasoconstriction and hemostasis in small vessels.
Antiglaucoma action: It's unknown exactly how epinephrine lowers intraocular pressure. When applied topically to the conjunctiva or injected into the interior chamber of the eye, epinephrine constricts conjunctival blood vessels, contracts the dilator muscle of the pupil, and may dilate the pupil.

PHARMACOKINETICS

Absorption: Well absorbed after S.C. or I.M. injection, epinephrine has a rapid onset of action and short duration of action. Bronchodilation occurs within 5 to 10 minutes and peaks in 20 minutes after S.C. injection; onset after oral inhalation is within 1 minute.

Topical administration or intraocular injection usually produces local vasoconstriction within 5 minutes and lasts less than 1 hour. After topical application to the conjunctiva, reduction of intraocular pressure occurs within 1 hour, peaks in 4 to 8 hours, and persists up to 24 hours.
Distribution: Drug is distributed widely throughout the body.
Metabolism: Drug is metabolized at sympathetic nerve endings, liver, and other tissues to inactive metabolites.
Excretion: Drug is excreted in the urine, mainly as its metabolites and conjugates.

CONTRAINDICATIONS & PRECAUTIONS

Contraindicated in patients with angle-closure glaucoma, shock (other than anaphylactic shock), organic brain damage, cardiac dilation, arrhythmias, coronary insufficiency, or cerebral arteriosclerosis. Also contraindicated in patients during general anesthesia with halogenated hydrocarbons or cyclopropane and in patients in labor (may delay second stage).

Some commercial products contain sulfites; drug is contraindicated in patients with sulfite allergies except when epinephrine is being used to treat serious allergic reactions or other emergencies.

In conjunction with local anesthetics, epinephrine is contraindicated for use in fingers, toes, ears, nose, or genitalia.

Ophthalmic preparation is contraindicated in patients with angle-closure glaucoma or when nature of the glaucoma hasn't been established and in patients with hypersensitivity to the drug, organic mental syndrome, or cardiac dilation and coronary insufficiency. Nasal solution is contraindicated in patients with hypersensitivity to drug.

Use with extreme caution in patients with long-standing bronchial asthma and emphysema who've developed degenerative heart disease. Also, use cautiously in geriatric patients, especially those with hyperthyroidism, CV disease, hypertension, psychoneurosis, and diabetes.

Use ophthalmic preparation cautiously in geriatric patients and in patients with diabetes, hypertension, Parkinson's disease, hyperthyroidism, aphakia (eye without lens), cardiac disease, cerebral arteriosclerosis, or bronchial asthma.

INTERACTIONS
Drug-drug. *Alpha-adrenergic blockers* antagonize vasoconstriction and hypertension. Use with *antidiabetics* may decrease their effects. Dosage adjustments may be necessary. Use with *antihistamines, thyroid hormones,* and *tricyclic antidepressants* may potentiate adverse cardiac effects of epinephrine. *Beta blockers* antagonize cardiac and bronchodilating effects of epinephrine. Use of *carbonic anhydrase inhibitors, ophthalmic epinephrine with topical miotics, osmotic drugs,* and *topical beta blockers* may cause additive lowering of intraocular pressure. Use with miotics offers the advantage of reducing the ciliary spasm, mydriasis, blurred vision, and increased intraocular pressure that may occur with miotics or epinephrine alone. Use with *cardiac glycosides* and *general anesthetics* (especially *cyclopropane* or *halothane*) may sensitize the myocardium to epinephrine's effects, causing arrhythmias. Use with *ergot alkaloids* or *oxytocics* may cause severe hypertension. Use with *guanethidine* may decrease its hypotensive effects while potentiating epinephrine's effects, resulting in hypertension and arrhythmias. Because *phenothiazines* may cause reversal of its pressor effects, epinephrine shouldn't be used to treat circulatory collapse or hypotension caused by phenothiazines; such use may further lower the blood pressure. Use with other *sympathomimetics* may produce additive effects and toxicity.

ADVERSE REACTIONS
CNS: *nervousness, tremor,* vertigo, *headache,* disorientation, agitation, *drowsiness,* fear, pallor, dizziness, weakness, *cerebral hemorrhage, CVA.* In pa-

tients with Parkinson's disease, drug increases rigidity, tremor; brow ache, headache, light-headedness (with ophthalmic preparation); nervousness, excitation (with nasal solution).
CV: *palpitations;* widened pulse pressure; *hypertension; tachycardia; ventricular fibrillation; shock;* angina; ECG changes, including a decreased T-wave amplitude; palpitations, tachycardia, *arrhythmias,* hypertension (with ophthalmic preparation); *tachycardia* (with nasal solution).
EENT: corneal or conjunctival pigmentation or corneal edema in long-term use, follicular hypertrophy, chemosis, conjunctivitis, iritis, hyperemic conjunctiva, maculopapular rash, eye pain, allergic lid reaction, ocular irritation, eye stinging, burning, and tearing on instillation (with ophthalmic preparation); rebound nasal congestion, slight sting upon application (with nasal solution).
GI: *nausea, vomiting.*
Respiratory: dyspnea.
Skin: urticaria, pain, hemorrhage (at injection site).

▣ KEY CONSIDERATIONS
Besides the recommendations relevant to all adrenergics, consider the following:
● Geriatric patients may be more sensitive to the effects of epinephrine.
● Epinephrine therapy alters blood glucose and serum lactic acid levels (both may be increased), increases BUN levels, and interferes with tests for urine catecholamine levels.
● To hasten drug absorption, massage the site after S.C. or I.M. injection.
● Remember that epinephrine is destroyed by oxidizing agents, alkalies (including sodium bicarbonate), halogens, permanganates, chromates, nitrates, and salts of easily reducible metals such as iron, copper, and zinc.
● To ensure greater accuracy in measurement of parenteral doses, use a tuberculin syringe.
● To avoid hazardous drug errors, check carefully the type of solution prescribed, concentration, dosage, and route before administration. Don't mix with alkali.
● Before withdrawing epinephrine suspension into syringe, shake vial or am-

pule thoroughly to disperse particles; then inject promptly. Don't use if preparation is discolored or contains a precipitate.

• Rotate injection sites and observe for signs of blanching. Repeated injections may cause tissue necrosis from vascular constriction.

• Avoid I.M. injection into buttocks. Epinephrine-induced vasoconstriction favors growth of the anaerobe *Clostridium perfringens*.

• Monitor blood pressure, pulse, respirations, and urine output, and observe patient closely. Epinephrine may widen pulse pressure. If arrhythmias occur, discontinue epinephrine immediately. Watch for changes in intake and output ratio.

• Use a cardiac monitor in patients receiving I.V. epinephrine. Keep resuscitation equipment available.

Patient education

• Urge patient to report diminishing effect. Repeated or prolonged use of epinephrine can cause tolerance to the effects of the drug. Continuing to take epinephrine despite tolerance can be hazardous. Interrupting drug therapy for 12 hours to several days may restore responsiveness to drug.

Inhalation

• Instruct patient in correct use of inhaler.

• Tell patient to avoid contact with eyes and to take no more than 2 inhalations at a time with 1- to 2-minute intervals between them.

• Instruct patient to rinse mouth and throat with water immediately after inhalation to avoid swallowing residual drug (the propellant in the aerosol preparation may cause epigastric pain and systemic effects) and to prevent the oropharyngeal membranes from drying.

• Tell patient to save applicator; refills may be available.

• Advise patient to call immediately if he receives no relief within 20 minutes or if condition worsens.

Nasal

• Tell patient to call if symptoms aren't relieved in 20 minutes or if they become worse and to report bronchial irritation,

nervousness, or sleeplessness, which require dosage reduction.

• Warn patient that intranasal applications may sting slightly and cause rebound congestion or drug-induced rhinitis after prolonged use. Nose drops should be used for only 3 to 4 days. Encourage patient to use drug exactly as prescribed.

• Tell patient to rinse nose dropper or spray tip with hot water after each use to avoid contaminating the solution.

• Instruct patient to gently press finger against nasolacrimal duct for at least 1 to 2 minutes immediately after drug instillation to avoid excessive systemic absorption.

Ophthalmic

• Instruct patient to gently press finger against lacrimal sac during and for 1 to 2 minutes immediately after drug instillation to avoid excessive systemic absorption.

• To prevent contamination, tell patient not to touch applicator tip to any surface and to keep container tightly closed.

• Tell patient not to use if epinephrine solution is discolored or contains a precipitate.

• Advise patient to remove soft contact lenses before instilling eyedrops to avoid staining or damaging them.

• Tell patient to apply a missed dose as soon as possible. If too close to the time for next dose, patient should wait and apply at regularly scheduled time.

• Tell patient to store drug away from heat and light (not in bathroom medicine cabinet, where heat and moisture can cause drug to deteriorate) and out of children's reach.

Overdose & treatment

• Signs and symptoms of epinephrine overdose include a sharp increase in systolic and diastolic blood pressure, a rise in venous pressure, severe anxiety, irregular heartbeat, severe nausea or vomiting, severe respiratory distress, unusually large pupils, unusual paleness and coldness of skin, pulmonary edema, renal failure, and metabolic acidosis.

• Treatment is symptomatic and supportive because epinephrine is rapidly inactivated in the body. Monitor vital signs

---

Reactions may be *common*, uncommon, *life-threatening*, or COMMON AND LIFE-THREATENING.

closely. Trimethaphan or phentolamine may be needed for hypotension; beta blockers (such as propranolol), for arrhythmias.

• When drug is administered I.V., check patient's blood pressure repeatedly during first 5 minutes, then every 3 to 5 minutes until patient's condition is stable.

• Intracardiac administration requires external cardiac massage to move drug into coronary circulation.

• Drying effect on bronchial secretions may make mucus plugs more difficult to dislodge. Bronchial hygiene program may be necessary, including postural drainage, breathing exercises, and adequate hydration.

• Epinephrine may increase blood glucose levels. Closely observe patients with diabetes for loss of diabetes control.

• Monitor amount, consistency, and color of sputum.

Inhalation

• Treatment should start with first symptoms of bronchospasm. Patient should use the fewest number of inhalations that provide relief. To prevent overdose, at least 1 to 2 minutes should elapse before taking additional inhalations of epinephrine. Dosage requirements vary. Warn patient that overuse or too-frequent use can cause severe adverse reactions.

Nasal

• To prevent entry of drug into throat, instill nose drops with patient's head in lateral, head-low position.

Ophthalmic

• Ophthalmic preparation may cause mydriasis with blurred vision and sensitivity to light in some patients being treated for glaucoma. To minimize these symptoms, drug is usually administered at bedtime or after prescribed miotic.

• Patients should have regular tonometer readings during continuous therapy.

• When using separate solutions of epinephrine and a topical miotic, instill the miotic 2 to 10 minutes before epinephrine.

epoetin alfa (erythropoietin)
Epogen, Procrit

Glycoprotein, antianemic

Available by prescription only
Injection: 2,000 U; 3,000 U; 4,000 U; 10,000 U; 20,000 U

INDICATIONS & DOSAGE
Anemia associated with chronic renal failure
Adults: Initiate therapy at 50 to 100 U/kg three times weekly. Patients receiving dialysis should receive drug I.V.; patients with chronic renal failure not on dialysis may receive drug S.C. or I.V.
Reduce dosage when target hematocrit is reached or if hematocrit rises more than 4 points within a 2-week period. Increase dosage if hematocrit doesn't rise by 5 to 6 points after 8 weeks of therapy and hematocrit is below target range. Maintenance dosage is highly individualized.
Anemia related to zidovudine therapy in patients with HIV
Adults: Before therapy, determine endogenous serum epoetin alfa levels. Patients with levels of 500 mU/ml or more are unlikely to respond to therapy.
Initial dose for patients with levels less than 500 mU/ml who are receiving 4,200 mg/week or less of zidovudine is 100 U/kg I.V. or S.C. three times weekly for 8 weeks. If response is inadequate after 8 weeks, increase dose by increments of 50 to 100 U/kg three times weekly and reevaluate response q 4 to 8 weeks. Individualize maintenance dose to maintain response, which may be influenced by zidovudine dose or infection or inflammation.
Anemia secondary to cancer chemotherapy
Adults: 150 U/kg S.C. three times weekly for 8 weeks or until target hemoglobin level is reached. If response isn't satisfactory after 8 weeks, increase dose up to 300 U/kg S.C. three times weekly.
Reduction of need for allogeneic blood transfusion in anemic patients scheduled to undergo elective, noncardiac, nonvascular surgery
Adults: 300 U/kg S.C. daily for 10 days

◊ Unlabeled clinical use

before surgery, on day of surgery, and for 4 days after surgery. Alternatively, 600 U/kg S.C. in once-weekly doses (21, 14, and 7 days before surgery) plus a fourth dose on day of surgery. Before initiating treatment, establish that hemoglobin level is between 10 g/dl and 13 g/dl.

PHARMACODYNAMICS

Antianemic action: Epoetin alfa is a glycoprotein consisting of 165 amino acids synthesized using recombinant DNA technology. It mimics naturally occurring erythropoietin, which the kidneys produce. It stimulates the division and differentiation of cells within bone marrow to produce RBCs.

PHARMACOKINETICS

Absorption: Epoetin alfa may be given S.C. or I.V. After S.C. administration, serum levels peak within 5 to 24 hours.
Distribution: Unknown.
Metabolism: Unknown.
Excretion: Unknown.

CONTRAINDICATIONS & PRECAUTIONS

Contraindicated in patients with uncontrolled hypertension and hypersensitivity to mammalian cell–derived products or albumin (human).

INTERACTIONS

None reported.

ADVERSE REACTIONS

CNS: *headache, **seizures,** paresthesia, fatigue,* dizziness, *asthenia.*
CV: *hypertension, edema.*
GI: *nausea, vomiting, diarrhea.*
Musculoskeletal: *arthralgia.*
Respiratory: *cough, shortness of breath.*
Skin: *rash,* urticaria.
Other: increased clotting of arteriovenous grafts, *pyrexia, injection site reactions.*

🔲 KEY CONSIDERATIONS

• Monitor hematocrit at least twice weekly during initiation of therapy and during any dosage adjustment. Close monitoring of blood pressure is also recommended.

• For HIV-infected patients treated with zidovudine, measure hematocrit once weekly until stabilized and then periodically.

• If a patient fails to respond to epoetin alfa therapy, consider the following possible causes: vitamin deficiency, iron deficiency, underlying infection, occult blood loss, underlying hematologic disease, hemolysis, aluminum intoxication, osteitis fibrosa cystica, or increased dosage of zidovudine.

• Most patients eventually require supplemental iron therapy. Before and during therapy, monitor patient's iron stores, including serum ferritin and transferrin saturation.

• Measure hematocrit twice weekly until it has stabilized and during adjustment to a maintenance dosage in patients with chronic renal failure. It may take 2 to 6 weeks for a dosage change to be reflected in the hematocrit level.

• Perform routine monitoring of CBC with differential and platelet counts.

• Moderate increases in BUN, uric acid, creatinine, phosphorus, and potassium levels have been reported.

Patient education

• Explain importance of regularly monitoring blood pressure in light of the potential drug effects.

• Advise patient to adhere to dietary restrictions during therapy. Make sure he understands that drug won't influence the disease process.

Overdose & treatment

• The maximum safe dose hasn't been established. Doses up to 1,500 U/kg have been administered three times weekly for 3 weeks without direct toxic effects. The drug can cause polycythemia.

• Phlebotomy may be used to bring hematocrit within appropriate levels.

---

ergocalciferol (vitamin D₂)
Calciferol, Deltalin, Drisdol, Vitamin D

Vitamin, antihypocalcemic

Available by prescription only

Capsules: 1.25 mg (50,000 U)
Tablets: 1.25 mg (50,000 U)
Injection: 12.5 mg (500,000 U)/ml
Available without a prescription
Liquid: 8,000 U/ml in 60-ml dropper
bottle

INDICATIONS & DOSAGE

Nutritional rickets or osteomalacia
Adults: 25 to 125 mcg P.O. daily if patient has normal GI absorption. With severe malabsorption, 250 mcg to 7.5 mg P.O. or 250 mcg I.M. daily.
Familial hypophosphatemia
Adults: 250 mcg to 1.5 mg P.O. daily with phosphate supplements.
Vitamin D–dependent rickets
Adults: 250 mcg to 1.5 mg P.O. daily.
Anticonvulsant-induced rickets and osteomalacia
Adults: 50 mcg to 1.25 mg P.O. daily.
Hypoparathyroidism and pseudohypoparathyroidism
Adults: 625 mcg to 5 mg P.O. daily with calcium supplements.
◊ **Fanconi's syndrome**
Adults: 1.25 to 5 mg P.O. daily.
◊ **Osteoporosis**
Adults: 25 to 250 mcg P.O. daily or 1.25 mg P.O. weekly with calcium and fluoride supplements.

PHARMACODYNAMICS

Antihypocalcemic action: Once activated, ergocalciferol regulates serum calcium levels by regulating absorption from the GI tract and resorption from bone.

PHARMACOKINETICS

Absorption: Ergocalciferol is absorbed readily from the small intestine. Onset of action is 10 to 24 hours.
Distribution: Drug is distributed widely and bound to proteins stored in the liver.
Metabolism: Drug is metabolized in the liver and kidneys. It has an average half-life of 24 hours and a duration of action up to 6 months.
Excretion: Drug is primarily excreted in bile (feces). A small percentage is excreted in urine.

CONTRAINDICATIONS & PRECAUTIONS

Contraindicated in patients with hypercalcemia, hypervitaminosis A, or renal osteodystrophy with hyperphosphatemia. Use with extreme caution, if at all, in patients with impaired renal function, heart disease, renal calculi, or arteriosclerosis.

INTERACTIONS

Drug-drug. Use with *cardiac glycosides* may result in arrhythmias. *Cholestyramine, colestipol,* and excessive use of *mineral oil* may interfere with the absorption of ergocalciferol. *Corticosteroids* counteract the effects of the drug. With *magnesium-containing antacids,* use may lead to hypermagnesemia. Administration of *phenobarbital* or *phenytoin* may increase metabolism of drug to inactive metabolites. Use with *thiazide diuretics* may cause hypercalcemia in patients with hypoparathyroidism. With *verapamil,* use may induce recurrence of atrial fibrillation when supplemental calcium and calciferol have induced hypercalcemia.

ADVERSE REACTIONS

Adverse reactions listed usually occur only in vitamin D toxicity.
CNS: headache, weakness, somnolence, decreased libido, overt psychosis, irritability.
CV: *calcifications of soft tissues, including the heart;* hypertension; *arrhythmias.*
EENT: rhinorrhea, conjunctivitis (calcific), photophobia.
GI: anorexia, nausea, vomiting, constipation, dry mouth, metallic taste, polydipsia.
GU: polyuria, albuminuria, hypercalciuria, nocturia, *impaired renal function,* reversible azotemia.
Metabolic: weight loss, *hypercalcemia,* hyperthermia.
Musculoskeletal: bone and muscle pain, bone demineralization.
Skin: pruritus.

▣ KEY CONSIDERATIONS

• Use I.M. injection of ergocalciferol dispersed in oil in patients who are unable to absorb the oral form.
• If I.V. route is necessary, use only water-miscible solutions intended for dilution in large-volume parenterals. Use cautiously in cardiac patients, especially if they are receiving cardiotonic glyco-

sides. In such patients, hypercalcemia may precipitate arrhythmias.
• Monitor eating and bowel habits; dry mouth, nausea, vomiting, metallic taste, and constipation can be early signs and symptoms of toxicity.
• To avoid metastatic calcifications and renal calculi, implement dietary phosphate restrictions and administer binding agents in patients with hyperphosphatemia.
• Frequently monitor serum and urine calcium, potassium, and urea levels when high therapeutic doses are used.
• Anticipate the addition of exogenous bile salts in case of malabsorption caused by inadequate bile or hepatic dysfunction
• Remember that doses of 60,000 IU daily can cause hypercalcemia.
• Patients taking ergocalciferol should restrict their intake of magnesium-containing antacids.
• Ergocalciferol may falsely increase serum cholesterol levels and may elevate AST and ALT levels.

Patient education

• Explain the importance of a calcium-rich diet.
• Caution patient not to increase daily dose on his own initiative. Vitamin D is fat-soluble; vitamin-D toxicity is thus more likely to occur.
• Tell patient to avoid magnesium-containing antacids and mineral oil.
• Instruct patient to swallow tablets whole without crushing or chewing.

Overdose & treatment

• Signs and symptoms of overdose include hypercalcemia, hypercalciuria, and hyperphosphatemia.
• To treat overdose, stop therapy, start a low-calcium diet, and increase fluid intake. To increase calcium excretion, give a loop diuretic, such as furosemide, saline I.V. infusion. Also, calcitonin may decrease hypercalcemia. Supportive measures should be provided. In severe cases, death from cardiac or renal failure may occur.

ergotamine tartrate
Cafergot, Ergomar, Ergostat, Gynergen, Medihaler Ergotamine, Wigraine

Ergot alkaloid, vasoconstrictor

Available by prescription only
Tablets (S.L.): 2 mg
Tablets: 1 mg* (with or without caffeine 100 mg)
Aerosol inhaler: 360 mcg/metered spray
Suppositories: 2 mg (with caffeine 100 mg)

INDICATIONS & DOSAGE

To prevent or abort vascular headache, including migraine and cluster headaches
Adults: Initially, 2 mg S.L. or P.O., then 1 to 2 mg S.L. or P.O. q 30 minutes, to maximum of 6 mg per attack or per 24 hours, and 10 mg weekly. Alternatively, initially 1 inhalation; if not relieved in 5 minutes, repeat 1 inhalation. May repeat inhalations at least 5 minutes apart up to maximum of 6 inhalations per 24 hours or 15 inhalations weekly. Patient may also use rectal suppositories. Initially, 2 mg P.R. at onset of attack; repeat in 1 hour, p.r.n. Maximum dosage is 2 suppositories per attack or 5 suppositories weekly.

PHARMACODYNAMICS

Vasoconstrictive action: In therapeutic doses, ergotamine stimulates alpha-adrenergic receptors, causing peripheral vasoconstriction (if vascular tone is low); however, if vascular tone is high, it produces vasodilation. In high doses, it's a competitive alpha-adrenergic blocker. In therapeutic doses, it inhibits the reuptake of norepinephrine, which increases the vasoconstrictive activity of ergotamine. A weaker serotonin antagonist, it reduces the increased rate of platelet aggregation that serotonin causes.

In treating vascular headaches, ergotamine probably causes direct vasoconstriction of dilated carotid artery beds while decreasing the amplitude of pulsations. Its serotoninergic and cate-

---

cholamine effects also seem to be involved.

PHARMACOKINETICS
Absorption: Ergotamine is rapidly absorbed after inhalation and variably absorbed after oral administration. Drug levels peak within ½ to 3 hours. Caffeine may increase the rate and extent of absorption. Drug undergoes first-pass metabolism after oral administration.
Distribution: Drug is widely distributed throughout the body.
Metabolism: Drug is extensively metabolized in the liver.
Excretion: Within 96 hours, 4% of a dose is excreted in urine; remainder of a dose is presumably excreted in feces. Ergotamine is dialyzable. Onset of action depends on how promptly drug is given after onset of headache.

CONTRAINDICATIONS & PRECAUTIONS
Contraindicated in patients with peripheral and occlusive vascular diseases, coronary artery disease, hypertension, hepatic or renal dysfunction, severe pruritus, sepsis, or hypersensitivity to ergot alkaloids.

INTERACTIONS
Drug-drug. Use with *macrolides* may cause acute ergotism, manifested as peripheral ischemia. Use with *beta blockers* or *propranolol* may intensify the vasoconstrictive effects of ergotamine. Use with *troleandomycin* appears to interfere with the detoxification of ergotamine in the liver; use concurrently with caution. Use with *vasodilators* can increase pressor effects, causing dangerous hypertension.
Drug-food. *Caffeine* may increase rate and extent of absorption.
Drug-lifestyle. *Smoking* may increase adverse effects of drug. Avoid use.

ADVERSE REACTIONS
CV: transient tachycardia or bradycardia, precordial distress and pain, increased arterial pressure, angina pectoris, peripheral vasoconstriction.
GI: nausea, vomiting.
Musculoskeletal: weakness in legs, muscle pain in extremities.

Skin: pruritus, localized edema.
Other: numbness and tingling in fingers and toes.

▣ KEY CONSIDERATIONS
Besides the recommendations relevant to all alpha-adrenergic blockers, consider the following:
● Administer ergotamine cautiously to geriatric patients.
● Use drug in prodromal stage of headache or as soon as possible after onset for maximum effectiveness. Provide quiet, low-light environment to relax patient after dose is administered.
● Store drug in light-resistant container.
● Sublingual tablet is best used during early stage of attack because of its rapid absorption.
● To determine possible relation between certain foods and onset of headache, obtain an accurate dietary history.
● Rebound headache or an increase in duration or frequency of headache may occur when drug is stopped.
● If patient experiences severe vasoconstriction with tissue necrosis, administer I.V. sodium nitroprusside or intra-arterial tolazoline. To prevent vascular stasis and thrombosis, I.V. heparin and 10% dextran 40 in D_5W injection also may be administered.
● Drug is ineffective for muscle contraction headaches.

Patient education
● Instruct patient in correct use of inhaler.
● Urge patient to report immediately feelings of numbness or tingling in fingers or toes, red or violet blisters on hands or feet, or muscle, chest, or abdominal pain.
● Caution patient to avoid alcoholic beverages because alcohol may worsen headache, and to avoid smoking because it may increase adverse effects of drug.
● Warn patient to avoid prolonged exposure to very cold temperatures, which may increase adverse effects of drug.
● Tell patient to promptly report illness or infection, which may increase sensitivity to drug effects.
● Inform patient that the body may need time to adjust after discontinuing the

drug, depending on the amount used and length of time involved.

• Advise patient who uses an inhaler to call promptly if mouth, throat, or lung infection occurs or if condition worsens. Cough, hoarseness, or throat irritation may occur; to help prevent hoarseness and irritation, patient should gargle and rinse mouth after each dose.

• Advise patient not to exceed recommended dosage.

• Tell patient not to eat, drink, or smoke while sublingual tablet is dissolving.

Overdose & treatment

• Signs and symptoms of overdose include adverse vasospastic effects, nausea, vomiting, lassitude, impaired mental function, delirium, severe dyspnea, hypotension or hypertension, rapid and/or weak pulse, unconsciousness, spasms of the limbs, seizures, and shock.

• Treatment is supportive and symptomatic, with prolonged and careful monitoring. If patient is conscious and ingestion is recent, empty stomach by inducing vomiting or performing gastric lavage; if patient is comatose, perform gastric lavage after placing an endotracheal tube with cuff inflated. Activated charcoal and a saline (magnesium sulfate) cathartic may be used. Provide respiratory support. Apply warmth (not direct heat) to ischemic extremities if vasospasm occurs. As needed, administer vasodilators (nitroprusside, prazosin, or tolazoline) and, if necessary, I.V. diazepam to treat convulsions. Dialysis may be helpful.

erythromycin (topical)
Akne-Mycin, A/T/S, Del-Mycin, Erycette, EryDerm, Erymax, Ery-Sol, Erythra-Derm, Staticin, T-Stat, Theramycin Z

erythromycin base
E-Base, E-Mycin, ERYC, ERYC Sprinkle*, Ery-Tab, Erythromycin Base/Filmtabs, PCE, Robimycin

erythromycin estolate
Ilosone

erythromycin ethylsuccinate
E.E.S., EryPed, Pediazole

erythromycin gluceptate
Ilotycin Gluceptate

erythromycin lactobionate
Erythrocin Lactobionate

erythromycin stearate
Apo-Erythro-S*, Erythrocin Stearate Filmtab, Novorythro*

Erythromycin, antibiotic

Available by prescription only
erythromycin base
Tablets (enteric-coated): 250 mg, 333 mg, 500 mg
Pellets (enteric-coated): 250 mg
erythromycin estolate
Tablets: 500 mg
Capsules: 250 mg
Suspension: 125 mg/5 ml, 250 mg/5 ml
erythromycin ethylsuccinate
Tablets (chewable): 200 mg
Topical solution: 1.5%, 2%
Topical gel: 2%
Topical ointment: 2%
Oral suspension: 400 mg/5 ml
Powder for oral suspension: 200 mg/5 ml (after reconstitution)
Granules for oral suspension: 400 mg/5 ml (after reconstitution)
Ophthalmic ointment: 5 mg/g
erythromycin gluceptate
Injection: 500-mg and 1-g vials
erythromycin lactobionate
Injection: 500-mg and 1-g vials

Reactions may be *common*, uncommon, **life-threatening**, or COMMON AND LIFE-THREATENING.

erythromycin stearate
Tablets (film-coated): 250 mg, 500 mg

INDICATIONS & DOSAGE

Acute pelvic inflammatory disease caused by Neisseria gonorrhoeae
Adults: 500 mg I.V. (gluceptate, lactobionate) q 6 hours for 3 days, then 250 mg (base, estolate, stearate) or 400 mg (ethylsuccinate) P.O. q 6 hours for 7 days.

Endocarditis prophylaxis for dental procedures in patients allergic to penicillin
Adults: Initially, 800 mg (ethylsuccinate) or 1 g (stearate) P.O. 2 hours before procedure; then 400 mg (ethylsuccinate) or 500 mg (stearate) P.O. 6 hours later.

Treatment of intestinal amebiasis in patients who can't receive metronidazole
Adults: 250 mg (base, estolate, stearate) or 400 mg (ethylsuccinate) P.O. q 6 hours for 10 to 14 days.

Mild to moderately severe respiratory tract, skin, and soft-tissue infections caused by susceptible organisms
Adults: 250 to 500 mg (base, estolate, stearate) P.O. q 6 hours; or 400 to 800 mg (ethylsuccinate) P.O. q 6 hours; or 15 to 20 mg/kg (gluceptate, lactobionate) I.V. daily, in divided doses q 6 hours.

Syphilis
Adults: 500 mg (base, estolate, stearate) P.O. q.i.d. for 14 days.

Legionnaire's disease
Adults: 500 mg to 1 g I.V. or P.O. (base, estolate, stearate) or 800 mg to 1,600 mg (ethylsuccinate) P.O. q 6 hours for 21 days.

Uncomplicated urethral, endocervical, or rectal infections when tetracyclines are contraindicated
Adults: 500 mg (base, estolate, stearate) or 800 mg (ethylsuccinate) P.O. q.i.d. for at least 7 days.

Topical treatment of acne vulgaris
Adults: Apply to the affected area b.i.d.

Acute and chronic conjunctivitis, trachoma, other eye infections
Adults: Apply ⅜" (1-cm) long ribbon of ointment directly into infected eye up to six times daily, depending on severity of infection.

PHARMACODYNAMICS

Antibiotic action: Erythromycin inhibits bacterial protein synthesis by binding to the ribosomal 50S subunit. It's used to treat *Haemophilus influenzae, Entamoeba histolytica, Mycoplasma pneumoniae, Corynebacterium diphtheriae* and *Corynebacterium minutissimum, Legionella pneumophila,* and *Bordetella pertussis.* It may be used as an alternative to penicillins or tetracycline to treat *Streptococcus pneumoniae, Streptococcus viridans, Listeria monocytogenes, Staphylococcus aureus, Chlamydia trachomatis, N. gonorrhoeae,* and *Treponema pallidum.*

PHARMACOKINETICS

Absorption: Because base salt is acid-sensitive, it must be buffered or enterically coated so that gastric acids don't destroy it. Gastric acidity doesn't affect acid salts and esters (estolate, ethylsuccinate, and stearate); therefore, they're well absorbed. Base and stearate preparations should be given on empty stomach. Food may not affect or may enhance absorption of estolate and ethylsuccinate preparations. When administered topically, erythromycin is minimally absorbed .
Distribution: Erythromycin is distributed widely to most body tissues and fluids except CSF, where it appears only in low levels. About 80% of base and 96% of erythromycin estolate bind to protein.
Metabolism: Drug is metabolized partially in the liver to inactive metabolites.
Excretion: Drug is excreted mainly unchanged in bile. Less than 5% of the drug is excreted in urine. In patients with normal renal function, plasma half-life is about 1½ hours. Drug isn't dialyzable.

CONTRAINDICATIONS & PRECAUTIONS

Contraindicated in patients with hypersensitivity to erythromycin or other macrolides. Erythromycin estolate is contraindicated in patients with hepatic disease. Use erythromycin salts cautiously in patients with impaired hepatic function.

INTERACTIONS

Drug-drug. When used with topical desquamating or abrasive *acne preparations*, topical erythromycin has a cumulative irritant effect. Use of erythromycin may inhibit metabolism of *carbamazepine* (possibly causing toxicity), *cyclosporine* (resulting in elevated serum cyclosporine levels and subsequent nephrotoxicity), *theophylline* (possibly leading to elevated serum theophylline levels), and *warfarin* (causing excessive anticoagulant effect).

Drug-food. *Fruit juice* affects absorption. Don't take together. Administer base and stearate preparations on empty stomach.

ADVERSE REACTIONS

CV: *venous irritation, thrombophlebitis* (after I.V. injection).
EENT: bilateral reversible hearing loss (with high systemic or oral doses in patients with renal or hepatic insufficiency); slowed corneal wound healing, blurred vision, itching and burning eyes (with ophthalmic administration).
GI: *abdominal pain, cramping, nausea, vomiting, diarrhea* (with oral or systemic administration).
Hepatic: cholestatic jaundice (with estolate).
Skin: urticaria, rash, eczema (with oral or systemic administration); urticaria, dermatitis (with ophthalmic administration); sensitivity reactions, erythema, burning, *dryness, pruritus,* irritation, peeling, oily skin (with topical application).
Other: overgrowth of nonsusceptible bacteria or fungi; *anaphylaxis;* fever (with oral or systemic administration); overgrowth of nonsusceptible organisms (with long-term use); hypersensitivity reactions (with ophthalmic administration).

◻ KEY CONSIDERATIONS

• Perform culture and sensitivity tests before erythromycin treatment starts and then as needed.
• Administer base and stearate preparations on empty stomach.
• Erythromycin estolate may cause serious hepatotoxicity (reversible cholestatic jaundice). Monitor liver function tests for increased serum bilirubin, AST, and alkaline phosphatase levels. Other erythromycin salts can cause less severe hepatotoxicity. (Patients who develop hepatotoxicity from erythromycin estolate may react similarly to any erythromycin preparation.)
• Monitor serum theophylline levels if patient is receiving erythromycin concomitantly with theophylline.
• Monitor for prolonged PT or INR and abnormal bleeding if patient is receiving erythromycin with warfarin.
• Reconstitute injectable form (lactobionate) based on manufacturer's instructions and dilute every 250 mg in at least 100 ml of normal saline solution. Continuous infusions are preferred, but drug may be given by intermittent infusion at a maximum concentration of 5 mg/ml infused over 20 to 60 minutes.
• Don't administer erythromycin lactobionate with other drugs because of chemical instability. Reconstituted solutions are acidic and should be completely administered within 8 hours of preparation.
• Drug may cause overgrowth of nonsusceptible bacteria or fungi.
• Although drug is bacteriostatic, it may be bactericidal in high levels or against highly susceptible organisms.
• Erythromycin may interfere with fluorometric determination of urine catecholamine levels and, in rare cases, with calorimetric assays, resulting in falsely elevated liver function test results.

Patient education

• For best absorption, instruct patient to take oral form with full glass of water 1 hour before or 2 hours after meals. However, patient receiving enteric-coated tablets may take them with meals. Advise patient not to take drug with fruit juice. If patient is taking chewable tablets, instruct him not to swallow them whole.
• If patient is using topical solution, instruct him to wash, rinse, and dry affected areas before applying it. Warn patient not to apply solution near eyes, nose, mouth, or other mucous membranes.

Reactions may be *common,* uncommon, *life-threatening,* or COMMON AND LIFE-THREATENING.

Caution patient to avoid sharing wash-cloths and towels with family members.
• Instruct patient to wash hands before and after applying ophthalmic ointment. Instruct him to clean eye area of excess exudate before applying ointment. Warn him not to allow tube to touch the eye or surrounding tissue. Instruct him to promptly report symptoms of sensitivity, such as itching eyelids and constant burning.
• Tell patient to take drug exactly as directed and to continue taking it for prescribed period, even after he feels better.
• Instruct patient to report adverse reactions promptly.

estazolam
ProSom

Benzodiazepine, hypnotic
Controlled substance schedule IV

Available by prescription only
Tablets: 1 mg, 2 mg

INDICATIONS & DOSAGE
Short-term management of insomnia characterized by difficulty in falling asleep, frequent nocturnal awakenings, or early morning awakenings
Adults: Initially, 1 mg P.O. h.s.; may increase to 2 mg as needed and tolerated.
Geriatric patients: In small or debilitated patients, initially 0.5 mg P.O. h.s.; may increase with care to 1 mg if needed.

PHARMACODYNAMICS
Hypnotic action: Estazolam depresses the CNS at the limbic and subcortical levels of the brain. It produces a sedative-hypnotic effect by potentiating the effect of the neurotransmitter gamma-aminobutyric acid on its receptor in the ascending reticular activating system, which increases inhibition and blocks both cortical and limbic arousal.

PHARMACOKINETICS
Absorption: Estazolam is rapidly and completely absorbed through the GI tract in 1 to 3 hours. Levels peak within 2 hours (range is ½ to 6 hours).

Distribution: Some 93% binds to protein.
Metabolism: Drug is extensively metabolized in the liver.
Excretion: Metabolites are excreted primarily in the urine. Less than 5% is excreted in urine as unchanged drug; 4% of a 2-mg dose is excreted in feces. Elimination half-life ranges from 10 to 24 hours; clearance is accelerated in smokers.

CONTRAINDICATIONS & PRECAUTIONS
Contraindicated in patients with hypersensitivity to estazolam. Use cautiously in patients with depression, suicidal tendencies, and hepatic, renal, or pulmonary disease.

INTERACTIONS
Drug-drug. Estazolam potentiates CNS depressant effects of *antihistamines, barbiturates, general anesthetics, MAO inhibitors, narcotics, phenothiazines,* and *tricyclic antidepressants.* Use with *cimetidine, disulfiram, isoniazid,* or *oral contraceptives* may diminish hepatic metabolism, resulting in increased plasma estazolam levels and increased CNS depressant effects. Like other benzodiazepines, estazolam increases *digoxin* and *phenytoin* levels, possibly resulting in toxicity. Use with *probenecid* results in more rapid onset and more prolonged benzodiazepine effect. *Rifampin* increases clearance and decreases half-life of estazolam. *Theophylline* antagonizes the pharmacologic effects of estazolam.
Drug-lifestyle. *Alcohol* increases sedation and CNS effects; don't use together. *Heavy smoking* accelerates metabolism of estazolam, reducing the effectiveness of the drug.

ADVERSE REACTIONS
CNS: fatigue, dizziness, *daytime drowsiness, somnolence, asthenia, hypokinesia, abnormal thinking.*
GI: dyspepsia, abdominal pain.
Musculoskeletal: back pain or stiffness.

◙ KEY CONSIDERATIONS

Besides the recommendations relevant to all benzodiazepines, consider the following:

• Geriatric patients may be more susceptible to CNS depressant effects of estazolam. Use with caution. Lower dosage may be required. Patients should be supervised during activities of daily living, especially at the start of treatment and after an increase in dosage, to prevent injury from dizziness and falls.

• Remove all potential safety hazards such as cigarettes from patient's reach.

• Regularly perform blood counts, urinalysis, and blood chemistry analyses.

• Withdraw drug slowly after prolonged use.

• AST levels may be increased.

• Encourage good sleep habits and regular exercise. Advise the patient to avoid caffeine or other stimulants, especially late in the day.

Patient education

• Tell patient to avoid alcohol and other CNS depressants while taking estazolam. After taking drug in the evening, patient should avoid alcohol the next day.

• Advise patient that heavy smoking may decrease effectiveness of drug.

• Tell patient to notify health care provider of other drug therapy and of usual alcohol consumption.

• Warn that drug may cause drowsiness. Advise special caution and avoidance of driving or operating hazardous machinery until adverse CNS effects of the drug are known.

• Inform patient that sleep may be disturbed for 1 or 2 nights after drug is stopped.

• Caution patient not to discontinue drug abruptly after taking it daily for a prolonged period and not to vary dosage or increase dose unless prescribed.

Overdose & treatment

• Benzodiazepine overdose can cause somnolence, confusion with reduced or absent reflexes, respiratory depression, apnea, hypotension, impaired coordination, slurred speech, seizures, or coma. If excitation occurs, don't use barbiturates. Remember that multiple agents may have been ingested.

• Treatment is symptomatic and supportive. Empty the stomach immediately by inducing vomiting or performing gastric lavage. Monitor respirations, pulse rate, and blood pressure. Maintain airway and administer fluids. Flumazenil, a specific benzodiazepine antagonist, may be useful.

esterified estrogens
Estratab, Menest

Estrogen replacement, antineoplastic

Available by prescription only
Tablets: 0.3 mg, 0.625 mg, 1.25 mg, 2.5 mg

INDICATIONS & DOSAGE

Palliative treatment of advanced inoperable prostate cancer
Adults: 1.25 to 2.5 mg P.O. t.i.d.

Breast cancer
Men and postmenopausal women: 10 mg P.O. t.i.d. for 3 or more months.

Female hypogonadism
Adults: 2.5 mg P.O. daily to t.i.d. in cycles of 20 days on, 10 days off.

Castration, primary ovarian failure
Adults: 2.5 mg daily to t.i.d. in cycles of 3 weeks on, 1 week off.

Vasomotor menopausal symptoms
Adults: 0.3 to 1.25 mg P.O. daily in cycles of 3 weeks on, 1 week off; dosage may be increased to 2.5 or 3.75 mg P.O. daily, if necessary.

Atrophic vaginitis and atrophic urethritis
Adults: 0.3 to 1.25 mg P.O. daily in cycles of 3 weeks on, 1 week off.

PHARMACODYNAMICS

Estrogenic action: Esterified estrogen mimics the action of endogenous estrogen in treating female hypogonadism, menopausal symptoms, and atrophic vaginitis.
Antineoplastic action: Drug inhibits growth of hormone-sensitive tissue in advanced, inoperable prostate cancer and in certain carefully selected cases of breast cancer in men and postmenopausal women.

Reactions may be *common,* uncommon, *life-threatening,* or COMMON AND LIFE-THREATENING.

PHARMACOKINETICS
Absorption: After oral administration, esterified estrogens are well absorbed but substantially inactivated by the liver.
Distribution: About 50% to 80% of esterified estrogens bind to plasma proteins, particularly the estradiol-binding globulin. Distribution occurs throughout the body with highest levels in fat.
Metabolism: Esterified estrogens are metabolized primarily in the liver, where they are conjugated with sulfate and glucuronide.
Excretion: Most esterified estrogens are eliminated through the kidneys in the form of sulfate or glucuronide conjugates.

CONTRAINDICATIONS & PRECAUTIONS
Contraindicated in patients with breast cancer (except metastatic disease), estrogen-dependent neoplasia, active thrombophlebitis or thromboembolic disorders, undiagnosed abnormal genital bleeding, hypersensitivity to drug, or history of thromboembolic disease.

Use cautiously in patients with history of hypertension, mental depression, liver impairment, or cardiac or renal dysfunction and in those with bone diseases, migraine, seizures, or diabetes mellitus.

INTERACTIONS
Drug-drug. Use with *adrenocorticosteroids* or *corticotropin* may cause greater risk of fluid and electrolyte accumulation. In patients with diabetes, esterified estrogens may increase blood glucose levels, necessitating dosage adjustment of *insulin* or *oral antidiabetics*. Administration of drugs that induce hepatic metabolism, such as *barbiturates, carbamazepine, phenytoin, primidone,* and *rifampin* may decrease estrogenic effects of a given dose. Use may decrease the effects of *warfarin-type anticoagulants*.

ADVERSE REACTIONS
CNS: headache, dizziness, chorea, depression, *seizures*.
CV: thrombophlebitis; *thromboembolism;* hypertension; *edema; increased risk of CVA, pulmonary embolism, MI.*

EENT: worsening of myopia or astigmatism, intolerance of contact lenses.
GI: nausea, vomiting, abdominal cramps, bloating, anorexia, increased appetite, weight changes, pancreatitis.
GU: in women—breakthrough bleeding, altered menstrual flow, dysmenorrhea, amenorrhea, *increased risk of endometrial cancer, possibly increased risk of breast cancer,* cervical erosion, altered cervical secretions, enlargement of uterine fibromas, vaginal candidiasis; in men—gynecomastia, testicular atrophy, impotence.
Metabolic: hypercalcemia.
Hepatic: gallbladder disease, cholestatic jaundice, *hepatic adenoma.*
Skin: melasma, rash, hirsutism or hair loss, erythema nodosum, dermatitis.
Other: breast changes (tenderness, enlargement, secretion).

KEY CONSIDERATIONS
• Recommendations for administration of esterified estrogens and for care and teaching of the patient during therapy are the same as those for all estrogens.
• Therapy with esterified estrogens increases sulfobromophthalein retention, PT or INR and clotting factors VII to X, and norepinephrine-induced platelet aggregation.
• Because drug may cause thromboembolism, discontinue therapy at least 1 month before procedures that may immobilize the patient for a long time or cause thromboembolism.
• Anticipate increases in the thyroid-binding globulin level, resulting in increased total thyroid levels (measured by protein-bound iodine or total T_4) and decreased uptake of free T_3 resin. Serum folate, pyridoxine, and antithrombin III levels may decrease; triglyceride, glucose, and phospholipid levels may increase. Glucose tolerance may be impaired.

Patient education
• Warn patient to immediately report abdominal pain; pain, numbness, or stiffness in legs or buttocks; pressure or pain in the chest; or signs of hepatic failure.
• Teach patient to perform breast self-examination.

• Inform patient that unusual vaginal bleeding may be a serious sign of other problems.

estradiol
Climara, Estrace, Estrace Vaginal Cream, Estraderm, Vivelle

estradiol cypionate
depGynogen, Depo-Estradiol Cypionate, Depogen, Estro-Cyp, Estrofem

estradiol valerate
Delestrogen*, Dioval 40, Dioval XX, Estra-L 40, Gynogen L.A. 20, Valergen-20

polyestradiol phosphate
Estradurin

Estrogen replacement, antineoplastic

Available by prescription only
estradiol
Tablets: 0.5 mg, 1 mg, 2 mg
Vaginal: 0.1 mg/g cream (in nonliquefying base)
Transdermal: 4 mg/10 cm^2 (delivers 0.05 mg/24 hours); 8 mg/20 cm^2 (delivers 0.1 mg/24 hours)
estradiol cypionate
Injection: 5 mg/ml (in oil)
estradiol valerate
Injection: 10 mg/ml, 20 mg/ml, 40 mg/ml (in oil)
polyestradiol phosphate
Injection: 40 mg/2 ml

INDICATIONS & DOSAGE
Atrophic vaginitis, atrophic dystrophy of the vulva, vasomotor menopausal symptoms, hypogonadism, female castration, primary ovarian failure
estradiol (tablets)
Adults: 1 to 2 mg P.O. daily, in cycles of 21 days on and 7 days off or cycles of 5 days on and 2 days off; or 0.2 to 1 mg I.M. weekly.
estradiol (transdermal)
Adults: Place 1 Estraderm transdermal patch on trunk of the body, preferably the abdomen, twice weekly. Administer

on an intermittent cyclic schedule (3 weeks on and 1 week off).
estradiol valerate
Adults: 10 to 20 mg I.M. once monthly.
Atrophic vaginitis
estradiol (vaginal cream)
Adults: 2 to 4 g daily for 1 to 2 weeks. When vaginal mucosa is restored, begin maintenance dosage of 1 g one to three times weekly.
Female hypogonadism
estradiol cypionate
Adults: 1.5 to 2 mg I.M. at monthly intervals.
Inoperable breast cancer
estradiol (tablets)
Adults: 10 mg P.O. t.i.d. for 3 months.
Inoperable prostate cancer
estradiol (tablets)
Adults: 1 to 2 mg P.O. t.i.d.
estradiol valerate
Adults: 30 mg I.M. q 1 to 2 weeks.
polyestradiol phosphate
Adults: 40 mg I.M. q 2 to 4 weeks.

PHARMACODYNAMICS
Estrogenic action: Estradiol mimics the action of endogenous estrogen in treating female hypogonadism, menopausal symptoms, and atrophic vaginitis.
Antineoplastic action: Drug inhibits growth of hormone-sensitive tissue in advanced, inoperable prostate cancer and in certain carefully selected cases of breast cancer in men and postmenopausal women.

PHARMACOKINETICS
Absorption: After oral administration, estradiol and the other natural unconjugated estrogens are well absorbed but substantially inactivated by the liver. Therefore, unconjugated estrogens are usually administered parenterally.

After I.M. administration, absorption begins rapidly and continues for days. The cypionate and valerate esters administered in oil have prolonged duration of action because they're slowly absorbed. Topically applied estradiol is absorbed readily into the systemic circulation.
Distribution: About 50% to 80% of estradiol and the other natural estrogens bind to plasma proteins, particularly the estradiol-binding globulin. Distribution

---

Reactions may be *common*, uncommon, *life-threatening*, or COMMON AND LIFE-THREATENING.

occurs throughout the body, with the highest levels in fat.

Metabolism: The steroid estrogens, including estradiol, are metabolized primarily in the liver, where they're conjugated with sulfate and glucuronide. Because of the rapid metabolism, nonesterified forms of estrogen, including estradiol, usually must be administered daily.

Excretion: Most estrogen elimination occurs through the kidneys in the form of sulfate or glucuronide conjugates.

CONTRAINDICATIONS & PRECAUTIONS

Contraindicated in patients with thrombophlebitis or thromboembolic disorders, estrogen-dependent neoplasia, breast or reproductive organ cancer (except for palliative treatment), or undiagnosed abnormal genital bleeding. Also contraindicated in patients with history of thrombophlebitis or thromboembolic disorders associated with previous estrogen use (except for palliative treatment of breast and prostate cancer).

Use cautiously in patients with cerebrovascular or coronary artery disease, asthma, bone diseases, migraine, seizures, or cardiac, hepatic, or renal dysfunction and in women with a strong family history of breast cancer or with breast nodules, fibrocystic disease, or abnormal mammographic findings.

INTERACTIONS

Drug-drug. Use with *adrenocorticosteroids* or *corticotropin* increases the risk of fluid and electrolyte accumulation. Administration of *drugs that induce hepatic metabolism*—such as *barbiturates, carbamazepine, phenytoin, primidone,* and *rifampin*—may decrease estrogenic effects from a given dose. Use with *hepatotoxic drugs* (especially *dantrolene*) increases risk of liver damage. In patients with diabetes, estradiol may increase blood glucose levels, necessitating dosage adjustment of *insulin* or *oral antidiabetics.* Use may decrease the effects of *warfarin-type anticoagulants.*

ADVERSE REACTIONS

CNS: headache, dizziness, chorea, depression, *seizures.*

CV: thrombophlebitis, *thromboembolism,* hypertension, edema.

EENT: worsening of myopia or astigmatism, intolerance of contact lenses.

GI: *nausea,* vomiting, abdominal cramps, bloating, increased appetite, weight changes, pancreatitis.

GU: in women—*increased risk of endometrial cancer, possibly increased risk of breast cancer,* cervical erosion, altered cervical secretions, enlargement of uterine fibromas, vaginal candidiasis; in men—*gynecomastia,* testicular atrophy, impotence.

Hepatic: cholestatic jaundice, gallbladder disease, *hepatic adenoma.*

Metabolic: hypercalcemia.

Skin: melasma, urticaria, erythema nodosum, dermatitis, hirsutism or hair loss.

Other: breast changes (tenderness, enlargement, secretion).

▣ KEY CONSIDERATIONS

Besides the recommendations relevant to all estrogens, consider the following:

• Perform frequent physical examinations in postmenopausal women taking estrogen.

• Before injection, make sure drug is well dispersed in solution by rolling the vial with the reconstituted drug between the palms.

• Administer by deep I.M. injection into large muscles.

• Estradiol increases sulfobromophthalein retention, prothrombin and clotting factors VII to X, and norepinephrine-induced platelet aggregation. Increases in thyroid-binding globulin levels may occur, resulting in increased total thyroid levels (measured by protein-bound iodine or total T_4) and decreased uptake of free T_3 resin. Serum folate, pyridoxine, and antithrombin III levels may decrease; triglyceride, glucose, and phospholipid levels may increase. Glucose tolerance may be impaired.

Patient education

• Tell patient not to apply patch to the breast area.

• Remind patient not to use the same skin site for at least 1 week after removing the transdermal system.

estrogenic substances, conjugated
Premarin

Estrogen replacement, antineoplastic, antiosteoporosis drug

Available by prescription only
Tablets: 0.3 mg, 0.625 mg, 0.9 mg, 1.25 mg, 2.5 mg
Injection: 25 mg/5 ml
Vaginal cream: 0.0625%

INDICATIONS & DOSAGE
Abnormal uterine bleeding (hormonal imbalance)
Adults: 25 mg I.V. or I.M. Repeat in 6 to 12 hours.
Castration and primary ovarian failure
Adults: 1.25 mg P.O. daily in cycles of 3 weeks on, 1 week off.
Osteoporosis
Adults: 0.625 mg P.O. daily in cycles of 3 weeks on, 1 week off.
Female hypogonadism
Adults: 2.5 to 7.5 mg P.O. daily in divided doses for 20 consecutive days, followed by 10 days without drug.
Vasomotor menopausal symptoms
Adults: 1.25 mg P.O. daily in cycles of 3 weeks on, 1 week off.
Atrophic vaginitis or kraurosis vulvae
Adults: 0.3 mg to 1.25 mg or more P.O. daily. Alternatively, 2 to 4 g intravaginally or topically once daily in cycles of 3 weeks on, 1 week off.
Palliative treatment of inoperable prostate cancer
Adults: 1.25 to 2.5 mg P.O. t.i.d.
Palliative treatment of breast cancer
Adults: 10 mg P.O. t.i.d. for 3 months or more.

PHARMACODYNAMICS
Estrogenic action: Conjugated estrogenic substances mimic the action of endogenous estrogen in treating female hypogonadism, menopausal symptoms, and atrophic vaginitis.

Antineoplastic action: Drugs inhibit the growth of hormone-sensitive tissue in advanced, inoperable prostate cancer and in certain carefully selected cases of breast cancer in men and postmenopausal women.
Antiosteoporosis action: Drugs retard the progression of osteoporosis by enhancing calcium and phosphate retention and limiting bone decalcification.

PHARMACOKINETICS
Absorption: Unknown. After I.M. administration of conjugated estrogenic substances, absorption begins rapidly and continues for days.
Distribution: About 50% to 80% of conjugated estrogens bind to plasma protein, particularly the estradiol-binding globulin. Distribution occurs throughout the body, with highest levels in fat.
Metabolism: Conjugated estrogens are metabolized primarily in the liver, where they are conjugated with sulfate and glucuronide. Because of the rapid metabolism, nonesterified forms of estrogen usually must be administered daily.
Excretion: Most estrogen elimination occurs through the kidneys, in the form of sulfate or glucuronide conjugates, or both.

CONTRAINDICATIONS & PRECAUTIONS
Contraindicated in patients with thrombophlebitis or thromboembolic disorders, estrogen-dependent neoplasia, breast or reproductive organ cancer (except for palliative treatment), or undiagnosed abnormal genital bleeding.

Use cautiously in patients with cerebrovascular or coronary artery disease, asthma, bone disease, migraine, seizures, or cardiac, hepatic, or renal dysfunction or in women with family history (mother, grandmother, sister) of breast or genitourinary tract cancer or with breast nodules, fibrocystic disease, or abnormal mammographic findings.

INTERACTIONS
Drug-drug. Use with *adrenocorticosteroids* or *corticotropin* increases the risk of fluid and electrolyte accumulation. Administration of *drugs that induce hepatic metabolism*—such as *barbitu-*

rates, carbamazepine, phenytoin, primi-done, and *rifampin*—may decrease estrogenic effects from a given dose. In patients with diabetes, estrogens may cause increases in blood glucose levels, necessitating dosage adjustment of *insulin* or *oral antidiabetics.* Use may decrease the effects of *warfarin-type anticoagulants.*

ADVERSE REACTIONS
CNS: headache, dizziness, chorea, depression, *seizures.*
CV: thrombophlebitis; *thromboembolism;* hypertension; edema; *increased risk of CVA, pulmonary embolism, MI.*
EENT: worsening of myopia or astigmatism, intolerance of contact lenses.
GI: *nausea,* vomiting, abdominal cramps, bloating, anorexia, increased appetite, weight changes, pancreatitis.
GU: in women—breakthrough bleeding, *increased risk of endometrial cancer, possibly increased risk of breast cancer,* cervical erosion, altered cervical secretions, enlargement of uterine fibromas, vaginal candidiasis; in men—gynecomastia, testicular atrophy, impotence.
Hepatic: cholestatic jaundice, *hepatic adenoma,* gallbladder disease.
Metabolic: hypercalcemia.
Skin: melasma, urticaria, flushing (with rapid I.V. administration), hirsutism or hair loss, erythema nodosum, dermatitis.
Other: breast changes (tenderness, enlargement, secretion).

☑ KEY CONSIDERATIONS
Besides the recommendations relevant to all estrogens, consider the following:
• Long-term use for menopausal symptoms may be associated with increased risk of certain types of cancer. Frequent physical examinations are recommended.
• To treat dysfunctional uterine bleeding or reduce surgical bleeding rapidly, administer the drug parenterally.
• Refrigerate before reconstitution. After adding diluent, agitate gently until drug is in solution, then use within a few hours. Reconstituted drug may be safely refrigerated for up to 60 days.
• Therapy with estrogens increases sulfobromophthalein retention, prothrombin and clotting factors VII to X, and

norepinephrine-induced platelet aggregation. Increases in thyroid-binding globulin levels may occur, resulting in increased total thyroid levels (measured by protein-bound iodine or total T_4) and decreased uptake of free T_3 resin. Serum folate, pyridoxine, and antithrombin III levels may decrease; triglyceride, glucose, and phospholipid levels may increase. Glucose tolerance may be impaired.

etanercept
Enbrel

Tumor necrosis factor (TNF) blocker, antirheumatic

Available by prescription only
Injection: 25-mg single-use vial

INDICATIONS & DOSAGE
Reduction in signs and symptoms of moderately to severely active rheumatoid arthritis in patients with demonstrated inadequate response to one or more disease-modifying antirheumatics; in combination with methotrexate in patients who don't respond adequately to methotrexate alone
Adults: 25 mg S.C. two times per week.

PHARMACODYNAMICS
Antirheumatic action: Etanercept binds specifically to TNF and blocks its action with cell-surface TNF receptors, reducing inflammatory and immune responses that come with rheumatoid arthritis.

PHARMACOKINETICS
Absorption: Serum etanercept levels peak in 72 hours.
Distribution: Unknown.
Metabolism: Unknown.
Excretion: Elimination half-life is 115 hours.

CONTRAINDICATIONS & PRECAUTIONS
Contraindicated in patients with sepsis and hypersensitivity to etanercept or any of its components. Don't give live vaccines during drug therapy.

Use cautiously in patients with underlying diseases (such as diabetes, heart failure, and active or chronic infection) that could predispose them to infection.

INTERACTIONS
None reported.

ADVERSE REACTIONS
CNS: asthenia, *headache,* dizziness.
EENT: *rhinitis,* pharyngitis, sinusitis.
GI: abdominal pain, dyspepsia.
Respiratory: *upper respiratory tract infections*, cough, respiratory disorder.
Skin: *injection site reaction,* rash.
Other: *infections,* **malignancies.**

▣ KEY CONSIDERATIONS
• No overall differences in safety and effectiveness were noted between geriatric and younger adults; however, greater sensitivity to drug effects in geriatric population cannot be ruled out.
• Reconstitute aseptically with 1 ml of supplied sterile bacteriostatic water for injection, USP (0.9% benzyl alcohol). Do not filter reconstituted solution during preparation or administration. Inject diluent slowly into vial. Minimize foaming by gently swirling during dissolution rather than shaking. Dissolution takes less than 5 minutes.
• Inspect the solution for particulate matter and discoloration before use. Reconstituted solution should be clear and colorless. Don't use if solution is discolored or cloudy or if particulate matter remains.
• Don't add other drugs or diluents to reconstituted solution.
• Use reconstituted solution as soon as possible; they may be refrigerated in the vial for up to 6 hours at 36° to 46° F (2° to 8° C).
• Make sure that drug is within expiration date before using.
• Use injection sites at least 1″ (2.5 cm) apart; never use areas where skin is tender, bruised, red, or hard. Recommended sites include the thigh, abdomen, and upper arm. Rotate sites regularly.
• Patient may test positive for antinuclear antibodies or anti–double-stranded DNA antibodies, measured by radioimmunoassay and *Crithidia lucilae* assay.
• The needle cover of the diluent syringe contains dry natural rubber (latex) and

shouldn't be handled by anyone sensitive to latex.

Patient education
• Instruct patient who will be self-administering about mixing and injection techniques, including rotation of injection sites.
• Tell patient to use a puncture-resistant container when disposing of needles and syringes.
• Tell patient that injection site reactions generally occur within first month of therapy and decrease thereafter.
• Warn patient to avoid live vaccine administration while receiving drug. Stress importance of alerting other health care providers of drug use.
• Instruct patient to immediately report signs and symptoms of infection.

---

ethacrynate sodium

ethacrynic acid
Edecrin

Loop diuretic

Available by prescription only
Tablets: 25 mg, 50 mg
Injectable: 50 mg (with 62.5 mg of mannitol and 0.1 mg of thimerosal)

INDICATIONS & DOSAGE
Acute pulmonary edema
Adults: 50 mg or 0.5 to 1 mg/kg I.V. to a maximum dose of 100 mg of ethacrynate sodium I.V. slowly over several minutes.
Edema
Adults: 50 to 200 mg P.O. daily. Refractory cases may require up to 200 mg b.i.d.
Hypertension
Adults: Initially, 25 mg P.O. daily. Adjust dose, p.r.n. Maximum maintenance dosage is 200 mg P.O. daily in two divided doses.

PHARMACODYNAMICS
Diuretic action: Ethacrynic acid inhibits sodium and chloride reabsorption in the proximal part of the ascending loop of

---

Henle, promoting the excretion of sodium, water, chloride, and potassium.

PHARMACOKINETICS

Absorption: Ethacrynic acid is absorbed rapidly from the GI tract; diuresis occurs in 30 minutes and peaks in 2 hours. After I.V. administration of ethacrynate sodium, diuresis occurs in 5 minutes and peaks in 15 to 30 minutes.

Distribution: Ethacrynic acid may accumulate in the liver. Drug doesn't enter the CSF.

Metabolism: Drug is metabolized in the liver to a potentially active metabolite.

Excretion: About 30% to 65% of drug is excreted in urine and 35% to 40% is excreted in bile as the metabolite. Duration of action is 6 to 8 hours after oral administration and about 2 hours after I.V. administration.

CONTRAINDICATIONS & PRECAUTIONS

Contraindicated in patients with anuria or hypersensitivity to ethacrynic acid. Use cautiously in patients with electrolyte abnormalities or impaired hepatic function.

INTERACTIONS

Drug-drug. Administration of ethacrynic acid and *aminoglycosides* or other *ototoxic drugs* may increase the incidence of deafness; avoid use of such combinations. Ethacrynic acid may potentiate the hypotensive effect of *antihypertensives*; patients may require dosage reduction. Use of ethacrynic acid with other *diuretics* may enhance the diuretic effect of the other drugs; reduce dosage when adding ethacrynic acid to a diuretic regimen. Diabetic patients may need increased dosages of *insulin* or *oral antidiabetics* when taking ethacrynic acid. Ethacrynic acid may reduce renal clearance of *lithium*, elevating serum lithium levels; monitor lithium levels and adjust dosage. Use of *potassium sparing diuretics*—such as *amiloride*, *spironolactone*, or *triamterene*—may decrease the potassium loss induced by ethacrynic acid and may be a therapeutic advantage; severe potassium loss may occur if ethacrynic acid is administered with other *potassium-depleting drugs*,

such as *amphotericin B* and *corticosteroids*.

ADVERSE REACTIONS

CNS: confusion, fatigue, vertigo, headache, malaise.

CV: volume depletion and dehydration, orthostatic hypotension.

EENT: transient deafness (with too-rapid I.V. injection), blurred vision, tinnitus, hearing loss.

GI: diarrhea, anorexia, nausea, vomiting, GI bleeding, pancreatitis.

GU: oliguria, hematuria, nocturia, polyuria, frequent urination, azotemia.

Hematologic: *agranulocytosis, neutropenia, thrombocytopenia.*

Metabolic: hypokalemia; hypochloremic alkalosis; asymptomatic hyperuricemia; fluid and electrolyte imbalances, including dilutional hyponatremia, hypocalcemia, hypomagnesemia; hyperglycemia; impaired glucose tolerance.

Other: fever, chills.

▣ KEY CONSIDERATIONS

Besides the recommendations relevant to all loop diuretics, consider the following:

● Geriatric patients require close observation because they're more susceptible to drug-induced diuresis. Excessive diuresis promotes rapid dehydration, leading to hypovolemia, hypokalemia, hyponatremia, and circulatory collapse. Reduced dosages may be indicated.

● Don't give drug either I.M. or S.C. because it may cause severe local pain and irritation. When giving I.V., check infusion site frequently for infiltration (edema or skin blanching).

● Drug therapy alters electrolyte balance and liver and renal function tests..

● Infuse drug slowly over 20 to 30 minutes by I.V. infusion or by direct I.V. injection over a period of several minutes; rapid injection may cause hypotension.

● Don't administer drug simultaneously with whole blood or blood products; hemolysis may occur.

● I.V. ethacrynate sodium has been used to treat hypercalcemia and to manage ethylene glycol poisoning and bromide intoxication.

• Assess hearing function periodically in patients receiving high-dose therapy. Ethacrynic acid may potentiate ototoxicity of other drugs.

Patient education
• Advise patient receiving I.V. form of drug to report pain or irritation at I.V. site immediately.
• Notify diabetic patient that antidiabetic dosage may need to be increased.

Overdose & treatment
• Signs and symptoms of overdose include profound electrolyte and volume depletion, which may precipitate circulatory collapse.
• Treatment of ethacrynic acid overdose is primarily supportive; replace fluid and electrolytes as needed.

---

ethambutol hydrochloride
Myambutol

Semisynthetic antituberculotic

Available by prescription only
Tablets: 100 mg, 400 mg

INDICATIONS & DOSAGE
Adjunctive treatment in pulmonary tuberculosis
Adults: Initial treatment for patients who haven't received previous antituberculotic therapy, 15 mg/kg P.O. daily in a single dose. Retreatment: 25 mg/kg P.O. daily single dose for 60 days with at least one other antituberculotic; then decrease to 15 mg/kg P.O. daily single dose.

PHARMACODYNAMICS
Antituberculotic action: Ethambutol is bacteriostatic; it interferes with mycolic acid incorporation into the mycobacterial cell wall. Ethambutol is active against *Mycobacterium tuberculosis, M. bovis,* and *M. marinum;* some strains of *M. kansasii, M. avium, M. fortuitum,* and *M. intracellulare;* and the combined strain of *M. avium* and *M. intracellulare* (MAC). Ethambutol is considered adjunctive therapy in tuberculosis and is combined with other antituberculotics to prevent or delay development of drug resistance by *M. tuberculosis.*

PHARMACOKINETICS
Absorption: Ethambutol is absorbed rapidly from the GI tract; serum levels peak 2 to 4 hours after ingestion.
Distribution: Drug is distributed widely into body tissues and fluids, especially into lungs, erythrocytes, saliva, and kidneys; lesser amounts distribute into brain, ascitic and pleural fluid, and CSF. About 8% to 22% binds to protein.
Metabolism: Drug undergoes partial hepatic metabolism.
Excretion: After 24 hours, about 50% of unchanged ethambutol and 8% to 15% of its metabolites are excreted in urine; 20% to 25% is excreted in feces. Plasma half-life in adults is about 3½ hours; half-life is prolonged with decreased renal or hepatic function. Ethambutol can be removed by peritoneal dialysis and to a lesser extent by hemodialysis.

CONTRAINDICATIONS & PRECAUTIONS
Contraindicated in patients with optic neuritis or hypersensitivity to ethambutol. Use cautiously in patients with impaired renal function, cataracts, recurrent eye inflammation, gout, and diabetic retinopathy.

INTERACTIONS
Drug-drug. Ethambutol may potentiate the adverse effects of *drugs that produce neurotoxicity. Aluminum salts* may delay and reduce the absorption of ethambutol. Separate administration times by several hours.

ADVERSE REACTIONS
CNS: malaise, headache, dizziness, confusion, possible hallucinations, peripheral neuritis (numbness and tingling of extremities).
EENT: optic neuritis (related to dose and duration of treatment).
GI: anorexia, nausea, vomiting, abdominal pain, GI upset.
Hematologic: *thrombocytopenia.*
Hepatic: abnormal liver function tests.
Musculoskeletal: joint pain.
Skin: dermatitis, pruritus, toxic epidermal necrolysis.

Reactions may be *common,* uncommon, *life-threatening,* or COMMON AND LIFE-THREATENING.

Other: *anaphylactoid reactions,* fever, bloody sputum, elevated uric acid levels, precipitation of acute gout.

▣ KEY CONSIDERATIONS

• To prevent gastric irritation, give drug with food if necessary; food doesn't interfere with absorption.
• Obtain specimens for culture and sensitivity testing before first dose, but therapy can begin before test results are complete; repeat periodically to detect drug resistance.
• Assess visual status before therapy; test visual acuity and color discrimination monthly in patients taking more than 15 mg/kg/day. Visual disturbances are dose-related and reversible if detected in time.
• To prevent toxic reaction, monitor blood (including serum uric acid level), renal, and liver function studies before and periodically during therapy.
• Monitor for change in renal function. Dosage may need to be reduced.
• Ethambutol may elevate serum urate levels and liver function test results.

Patient education

• Explain disease and rationale for long-term therapy.
• Teach signs and symptoms of hypersensitivity and other adverse reactions, and emphasize need to notify health care provider if these occur. Urge patient to report any unusual effects, especially blurred vision, red-green color blindness, or changes in urine elimination.
• Assure patient that visual alterations disappear within several weeks or months after drug is discontinued.
• Urge patient to complete entire prescribed regimen, to comply with instructions for daily dosage, to avoid missing doses, and not to discontinue drug without health care provider's approval. Explain importance of keeping follow-up appointments.

ethinyl estradiol
Estinyl

Estrogen replacement, antineoplastic

Available by prescription only
Tablets: 0.02 mg, 0.05 mg, 0.5 mg

INDICATIONS & DOSAGE
Palliative treatment of metastatic breast cancer (at least 5 years after menopause)
Adults: 1 mg P.O. t.i.d. for at least 3 months.
Female hypogonadism
Adults: 0.05 mg daily to t.i.d. for 2 weeks monthly, followed by 2 weeks of progesterone therapy; continue for 3 to 6 monthly dosing cycles, followed by 2 months off.
Vasomotor menopausal symptoms
Adults: 0.02 to 0.05 mg P.O. daily for cycles of 3 weeks on, 1 week off.
Palliative treatment of metastatic, inoperable prostate cancer
Adults: 0.15 to 2 mg P.O. daily.

PHARMACODYNAMICS
Estrogenic action: Ethinyl estradiol mimics the action of endogenous estrogen in treating female hypogonadism and menopausal symptoms.
Antineoplastic action: Drug inhibits growth of hormone-sensitive tissue in advanced, inoperable prostate cancer and in certain carefully selected cases of breast cancer in men and postmenopausal women.

PHARMACOKINETICS
Absorption: After oral administration, estradiol is well absorbed but substantially inactivated by the liver.
Distribution: Some 50% to 80% of estradiol and the other natural estrogens bind to plasma proteins, particularly the estradiol-binding globulin. Distribution occurs throughout the body, with highest levels in fat.
Metabolism: The steroid estrogens, including estradiol, are metabolized primarily in the liver, where they are conjugated with sulfate and glucuronide. Be-

cause of the rapid metabolism, nonesterified forms of estrogen, including estradiol, usually must be administered daily. *Excretion:* Most estrogen elimination occurs through the kidneys in the form of sulfate or glucuronide conjugates.

CONTRAINDICATIONS & PRECAUTIONS
Contraindicated in patients with thrombophlebitis or thromboembolic disorders, estrogen-dependent neoplasia, breast or reproductive organ cancer (except for palliative treatment), or undiagnosed abnormal genital bleeding.

Use cautiously in patients with cerebrovascular or coronary artery disease, asthma, mental depression, bone disease, or cardiac, hepatic, or renal dysfunction and in women with a family history (mother, grandmother, sister) of breast or genital tract cancer or with breast nodules, fibrocystic disease, or abnormal mammographic findings.

INTERACTIONS
Drug-drug. Use with *adrenocorticosteroids* or *corticotropin* increases the risk of fluid and electrolyte accumulation. Use of estrogens with *corticosteroids* may decrease corticosteroid elimination. Administration of *drugs that induce hepatic metabolism*—such as *barbiturates, carbamazepine, phenytoin, primidone,* and *rifampin*—may decrease estrogenic effects from a given dose. These drugs are known to accelerate the rate of metabolism of certain other drugs. In patients with diabetes, ethinyl estradiol may increase blood glucose levels, necessitating dosage adjustment of *insulin* or *oral antidiabetics.* Use may decrease the effects of *warfarin-type anticoagulants.*

ADVERSE REACTIONS
CNS: headache, dizziness, chorea, depression, *seizures.*
CV: thrombophlebitis; ***thromboembolism;*** hypertension; edema, ***increased risk of CVA, pulmonary embolism, MI.***
EENT: worsening of myopia or astigmatism, intolerance to contact lenses.
GI: nausea, vomiting, abdominal cramps, bloating, anorexia, increased appetite, weight changes.

GU: in women—breakthrough bleeding, cervical erosion, ***increased risk of endometrial cancer, possibly increased risk of breast cancer,*** altered cervical secretions, enlargement of uterine fibromas, vaginal candidiasis; in men—gynecomastia, testicular atrophy, impotence.
Hepatic: cholestatic jaundice, gallbladder disease, ***hepatic adenoma.***
Metabolic: hypercalcemia.
Skin: melasma, urticaria, acne, seborrhea, oily skin, hirsutism or hair loss, erythema nodosum, dermatitis.
Other: breast changes (tenderness, enlargement, secretion).

▣ KEY CONSIDERATIONS
Besides the recommendations relevant to all estrogens, consider the following:
● Use with caution in patients whose condition may be aggravated by fluid retention.
● Therapy with ethinyl estradiol increases sulfobromophthalein retention, prothrombin and clotting factors VII to X, and norepinephrine-induced platelet aggregation. Increases in thyroid-binding globulin level may occur, resulting in increased total thyroid level (measured by protein-bound iodine or total T_4) and decreased uptake of free T_3 resin. Serum folate, pyridoxine, and antithrombin III levels may decrease; triglyceride, glucose, and phospholipid levels may increase. Glucose tolerance may be impaired.

ethosuximide
Zarontin

Succinimide derivative, anticonvulsant

Available by prescription only
Capsules: 250 mg
Syrup: 250 mg/5 ml

INDICATIONS & DOSAGE
Absence seizures
Adults: Initially, 250 mg P.O. b.i.d. May increase by 250 mg q 4 to 7 days up to 1.5 g daily.

PHARMACODYNAMICS

Anticonvulsant action: Ethosuximide raises the seizure threshold; it suppresses characteristic spike-and-wave pattern by depressing neuronal transmission in the motor cortex and basal ganglia. It's indicated for absence seizures refractory to other drugs.

PHARMACOKINETICS

Absorption: Ethosuximide is absorbed from the GI tract; steady-state plasma levels occur in 4 to 7 days.
Distribution: Drug is distributed widely throughout the body; protein-binding is minimal.
Metabolism: Drug is metabolized extensively in the liver to several inactive metabolites.
Excretion: Drug is excreted in urine, with small amounts in bile and feces. Plasma half-life is about 60 hours in adults.

CONTRAINDICATIONS & PRECAUTIONS

Contraindicated in patients with hypersensitivity to succinimide derivatives. Use with extreme caution in patients with hepatic or renal disease.

INTERACTIONS

Drug-drug. Use of *other CNS depressants*—such as *antidepressants, antipsychotics, anxiolytics, narcotics,* and *other anticonvulsants*—causes additive CNS depression and sedation. Don't use together.
Drug-lifestyle. Use of *alcohol* causes additive CNS depression and sedation. Don't use together.

ADVERSE REACTIONS

CNS: *drowsiness*, headache, fatigue, dizziness, ataxia, irritability, hiccups, euphoria, lethargy, depression, psychosis.
EENT: myopia, tongue swelling, gingival hyperplasia.
GI: *nausea, vomiting, diarrhea, weight loss, cramps, anorexia, epigastric and abdominal pain.*
GU: vaginal bleeding, urinary frequency.
Hematologic: leukopenia, eosinophilia, *agranulocytosis,* pancytopenia.

Skin: urticaria, pruritic and erythematous rash, hirsutism, ***Stevens-Johnson syndrome.***

▣ KEY CONSIDERATIONS

Besides the recommendations relevant to all succinimide derivatives, consider the following:
• Use with caution in geriatric patients.
• Administer ethosuximide with food to minimize GI distress.
• Avoid abrupt discontinuation of drug, which may precipitate absence seizures.
• Observe patient for dermatologic reactions, joint pain, unexplained fever, or unusual bruising or bleeding (which may signal hematologic or other severe adverse reactions).
• Perform CBC, liver function tests, and urinalysis periodically.
• Ethosuximide may elevate liver enzyme levels and may cause false-positive Coombs' test results. It may also cause abnormal results of renal function tests.

Patient education

• Tell patient to take drug with food or milk to prevent GI distress, to avoid use with alcoholic beverages, and to avoid hazardous tasks that require alertness if drug causes drowsiness, dizziness, or blurred vision.
• Warn patient not to discontinue drug abruptly because doing so may cause seizures.
• Inform patient that drug may color urine pink- to red-brown.
• Encourage patient to wear a medical identification bracelet or necklace.
• Tell patient to report rash, joint pain, fever, sore throat, or unusual bleeding or bruising.

Overdose & treatment

• Signs and symptoms of ethosuximide overdose include CNS depression, ataxia, stupor, and coma.
• Treatment is symptomatic and supportive. Carefully monitor vital signs and fluid and electrolyte balance. Therapeutic plasma levels range from 40 to 100 µg/ml.

etidronate disodium
Didronel

Pyrophosphate analogue, antihypercalcemic

Available by prescription only
Tablets: 200 mg, 400 mg
Injection: 50 mg/ml (300-mg ampule)

INDICATIONS & DOSAGE
Symptomatic Paget's disease
Adults: 5 mg/kg P.O. daily as a single dose 2 hours before a meal with water or juice. Patient shouldn't eat, consume dairy products, or take antacids or vitamins with mineral supplements for 2 hours after dose. May give up to 10 mg/kg/day in severe cases, not to exceed 6 months. Maximum dosage is 20 mg/kg/day, not to exceed 3 months.
Heterotopic ossification in spinal cord injuries
Adults: 20 mg/kg/day P.O. for 2 weeks, then 10 mg/kg/day for 10 weeks. Total treatment period is 12 weeks.
Heterotopic ossification after total hip replacement
Adults: 20 mg/kg/day P.O. for 1 month before total hip replacement and for 3 months afterward.
Hypercalcemia associated with malignancy
Adults: 7.5 mg/kg I.V. daily for 3 days. May repeat up to 7 days. Then wait 7 days before beginning a second course of treatment.

PHARMACODYNAMICS
Bone-metabolism inhibitor action: Although the exact mechanism of action is unknown, etidronate acts on bone by adsorbing to hydroxyapatite crystals in the bone, thereby inhibiting their growth and dissolution. It also decreases the number of osteoclasts in bone, thereby slowing excessive remodeling of pagetic or heterotopic bone.

PHARMACOKINETICS
Absorption: Absorption after an oral dose is variable and is decreased in the presence of food. Absorption may also be dose-related.
Distribution: About half of the dose is distributed to bone.
Metabolism: Etidronate isn't metabolized.
Excretion: About 50% of drug is excreted within 24 hours in urine.

CONTRAINDICATIONS & PRECAUTIONS
Contraindicated in patients with known hypersensitivity to etidronate or in those with osteomalacia. Use cautiously in patients with impaired renal function.

INTERACTIONS
Drug-drug. Use of *antacids* or *vitamins with mineral supplements* affects etidronate absorption. Patient shouldn't take antacids or vitamins with mineral supplements for 2 hours after dose.
Drug-food. Use of *dairy products* affects etidronate absorption. Patient shouldn't consume dairy products for 2 hours after dose.

ADVERSE REACTIONS
CNS: *seizures.*
GI: most common in patients taking 20 mg/kg/day—diarrhea, increased frequency of bowel movements, nausea, constipation, stomatitis.
Hepatic: abnormal hepatic function.
Metabolic: *elevated serum phosphate level,* fluid overload.
Musculoskeletal: increased or recurrent bone pain.
Respiratory: dyspnea.
Other: pain at previously asymptomatic sites, increased risk of fracture, fever, hypersensitivity reactions.

◨ KEY CONSIDERATIONS
• Give drug usually in a single dose. However, if nausea occurs, dosage may be divided.
• Drug may elevate serum phosphate levels.
• Monitor drug effect by serum alkaline phosphate and urine hydroxyproline excretion; both are lowered by effective therapy.

Patient education
• Instruct patient to take drug on an empty stomach with water or juice and to avoid food, dairy, antacids, and vita-

mins with mineral supplements for 2 hours.

• Remind patient that improvement may take at least 3 months and may continue even after the drug is stopped.

Overdose & treatment

• Signs and symptoms of overdose include diarrhea, nausea, and hypocalcemia.

• To treat overdose, induce vomiting or perform gastric lavage. Administer calcium if required.

---

etodolac
Lodine, Lodine XL

NSAID, antarthritic

Available by prescription only
Capsules: 200 mg, 300 mg
Tablets: 400 mg
Tablets (extended-release): 400 mg, 1,000 mg

INDICATIONS & DOSAGE

Acute and long-term management of osteoarthritis, rheumatoid arthritis, and pain

Adults: For acute pain, give 200 to 400 mg P.O. q 6 to 8 hours, p.r.n., not to exceed 1,200 mg daily. For patients weighing 60 kg (132 lb) or less, total daily dose shouldn't exceed 20 mg/kg.

For osteoarthritis or rheumatoid arthritis, give 800 to 1,200 mg P.O. daily in divided doses initially, followed by adjustments of 600 to 1,200 mg in divided doses: 200 mg P.O. t.i.d. or q.i.d.; 300 mg P.O. b.i.d., t.i.d., or q.i.d.; or 400 mg P.O. b.i.d. or t.i.d. Total daily dosage shouldn't exceed 1,200 mg. For patients weighing 60kg or less, total daily dosage shouldn't exceed 20 mg/kg, or 400 to 1,000 mg P.O. daily (extended-release form). Adjust dosage to lowest effective dose based on patient response. Don't exceed the maximum daily dose of 1,000 mg.

PHARMACODYNAMICS

Antarthritic action: Mechanism of action is unknown but is presumed to be associated with inhibition of prostaglandin biosynthesis.

PHARMACOKINETICS

Absorption: Etodolac is well absorbed from the GI tract, with levels peaking in 1 to 2 hours. Onset of analgesic activity occurs within 30 minutes and lasts 4 to 6 hours. Antacids don't appear to affect absorption of etodolac and have no effect when peak levels are reached; however, they can decrease peak levels reached by 15% to 20%.
Distribution: Drug is distributed in liver, lungs, heart, and kidneys.
Metabolism: Drug is extensively metabolized in the liver.
Excretion: Drug is excreted in urine primarily as metabolites; 16% is excreted in feces.

CONTRAINDICATIONS & PRECAUTIONS

Contraindicated in patients with hypersensitivity to etodolac and in those with history of aspirin- or NSAID-induced asthma, rhinitis, urticaria, or other allergic reactions.

Use cautiously in patients with impaired renal or hepatic function, history of peptic ulcer disease, cardiac disease, hypertension, or conditions associated with fluid retention.

INTERACTIONS

Drug-drug. Although the significance is unknown, use with *aspirin* reduces the protein binding of etodolac without altering its clearance. Like other NSAIDs, etodolac may cause changes in elimination of *cyclosporine, digoxin, lithium,* and *methotrexate,* resulting in increased levels of these drugs. It may enhance nephrotoxicity associated with *cyclosporine.* Use with *warfarin* results in decreased protein binding of warfarin but doesn't change its clearance. No dosage adjustment is necessary.

ADVERSE REACTIONS

CNS: *asthenia, malaise, dizziness,* depression, drowsiness, nervousness, insomnia.
CV: hypertension, ***heart failure,*** syncope, flushing, palpitations, edema, fluid retention.

◇ Unlabeled clinical use

EENT: blurred vision, tinnitus, photophobia, dry mouth.
GI: *dyspepsia, flatulence, abdominal pain, diarrhea, nausea,* constipation, gastritis, melena, vomiting, anorexia, peptic ulceration with or without ***GI bleeding*** or perforation, ulcerative stomatitis, thirst.
GU: dysuria, urinary frequency, ***renal failure.***
Hematologic: anemia (rare), leukopenia, ***thrombocytopenia,*** hemolytic anemia, ***agranulocytosis.***
Hepatic: hepatitis.
Metabolic: weight gain.
Respiratory: asthma.
Skin: pruritus, rash, ***Stevens-Johnson syndrome.***
Other: chills, fever.

▣ KEY CONSIDERATIONS

● Drug is well tolerated.
● Minimal GI blood loss has been reported at doses up to 1,200 mg daily; endoscopy scores are comparable to those after placebo at doses up to 1,000 mg daily.
● No apparent interaction occurs when administered with diuretics, phenytoin, or glyburide. Use caution with use of diuretics in patients with cardiac, renal, or hepatic failure.
● Monitor for signs and symptoms of GI ulceration and bleeding.
● Phenolic metabolites may cause a false-positive test for urine bilirubin. Decreased serum uric acid levels and borderline elevations of one or more liver test results may occur.
● A daily dose of 1,200 mg of etodolac causes less GI bleeding than 2,400 mg of ibuprofen daily, 200 mg of indomethacin daily, 750 mg of naproxen daily, or 20 mg of piroxicam daily.
● In patients with chronic conditions, expect a therapeutic response within 2 weeks.

Patient education

● Instruct patient to report GI effects of etodolac.
● Tell patient that drug may be taken with food.

Overdose & treatment

● Signs and symptoms of overdose include lethargy, drowsiness, nausea, vomiting, and epigastric pain. Rare signs include GI bleeding, coma, renal failure, hypertension, and anaphylaxis.
● Treatment is symptomatic and supportive, including stomach decontamination.

Reactions may be *common,* uncommon, *life-threatening,* or COMMON AND LIFE-THREATENING.

famciclovir
Famvir

Synthetic acyclic guanine derivative, antiviral

Available by prescription only
Tablets: 125 mg, 250 mg, 500 mg

INDICATIONS & DOSAGE
Management of acute herpes zoster
Adults: 500 mg P.O. q 8 hours for 7 days
✦ *Dosage adjustment.* For adult patients with reduced renal function, adjust dosage as follows.

Creatinine clearance (ml/min)	Dosage regimen
≥ 60	500 mg q 8 hr
40-59	500 mg q 12 hr
20-39	500 mg q 24 hr
< 20	250 mg q 48 hr

Recurrent genital herpes
Adults: 125 mg P.O. b.i.d. for 5 days.
✦ *Dosage adjustment.* For adult patients with reduced renal function, adjust dosage as follows.

Creatinine clearance (ml/min)	Dosage regimen
≥ 40	125 mg q 12 hr
20-39	125 mg q 24 hr
< 20	125 mg q 48 hr

PHARMACODYNAMICS
Antiviral action: Famciclovir is a pro-drug that undergoes rapid biotransformation to the active antiviral compound penciclovir. It enters viral cells (herpes simplex types 1 and 2, varicella zoster), where it inhibits DNA polymerase, viral DNA synthesis, and, therefore, viral replication.

PHARMACOKINETICS
Absorption: Absolute bioavailability of famciclovir is 77%. Because bioavailability isn't affected by food intake, the drug can be taken without regard to meals.
Distribution: Less than 20% of drug is bound to plasma proteins.
Metabolism: Drug is extensively metabolized in the liver to the active drug penciclovir (98.5%) and other inactive metabolites.
Excretion: Penciclovir is primarily eliminated in the urine.

CONTRAINDICATIONS & PRECAUTIONS
Contraindicated in patients with hypersensitivity to famciclovir. Use cautiously in patients with impaired renal or hepatic function.

INTERACTIONS
Drug-drug. Use with *probenecid* or other drugs that are significantly eliminated by active renal tubular secretion may increase plasma penciclovir levels; monitor patient for increased adverse effects.

ADVERSE REACTIONS
CNS: *headache,* fatigue, dizziness, paresthesia, somnolence.
EENT: pharyngitis, sinusitis.
GI: diarrhea, *nausea,* vomiting, constipation, anorexia, abdominal pain.
Musculoskeletal: back pain, arthralgia.
Skin: pruritus; zoster-related signs, symptoms, and complications.
Other: fever, injury, pain, rigors.

🔲 KEY CONSIDERATIONS
● Information is based on current literature and may change with further experience.

Patient education
● Inform patient that drug may be taken without regard to meals.
● Teach patient to recognize early symptoms of herpes zoster infection, such as tingling, itching, and pain. Explain that treatment is more effective when started within 48 hours of rash onset.

famotidine
Pepcid, Pepcid AC

H_2-receptor antagonist, antiulcerative

Available by prescription only
Tablets: 20 mg, 40 mg
Injection: 10 mg/ml
Injection, premixed: 20 mg/50 ml normal saline solution
Suspension: 40 mg/5 ml
Available without a prescription
Tablets: 10 mg

INDICATIONS & DOSAGE
Duodenal and gastric ulcer
Adults: For acute therapy, 40 mg P.O. h.s. for 4 to 8 weeks; for maintenance therapy, 20 mg P.O. h.s.
Pathologic hypersecretory conditions (such as Zollinger-Ellison syndrome)
Adults: 20 mg P.O. q 6 hours. Up to 160 mg q 6 hours may be administered.
Short-term treatment of gastroesophageal reflux disease (GERD)
Adults: 20 to 40 mg P.O. b.i.d. for up to 12 weeks.
Hospitalized patients with intractable ulcers or hypersecretory conditions or patients who can't take oral drugs; ◇ *patients with GI bleeding;* ◇ *to control gastric pH in critically ill patients*
Adults: 20 mg I.V. q 12 hours.
Prevention or treatment of heartburn
Adults: 10 mg P.O. of Pepcid AC when symptoms occur; or 10 mg P.O. 1 hour before meals for prevention of symptoms. Drug can be used b.i.d. if necessary.
✦ *Dosage adjustment.* In patients with severe renal insufficiency (creatinine clearance less than 10 ml/minute), dosage may be reduced to 20 mg h.s. or the dosing interval may be prolonged to 36 to 48 hours to avoid excess accumulation of drug.

PHARMACODYNAMICS
Antiulcerative action: Famotidine competitively inhibits histamine's action at H_2-receptors in gastric parietal cells. This inhibits basal and nocturnal gastric acid secretion resulting from stimulation by such factors as caffeine, food, and pentagastrin.

PHARMACOKINETICS
Absorption: When administered orally, 40% to 45% of dose is absorbed; onset of action occurs in 1 hour, with peak action in 1 to 3 hours. After parenteral administration, peak action occurs in 30 minutes.
Distribution: Drug is distributed widely to many body tissues.
Metabolism: About 30% to 35% of an administered dose is metabolized by the liver.
Excretion: Most of drug is excreted unchanged in urine. Famotidine has a longer duration of effect than its 2½- to 4-hour half-life suggests.

CONTRAINDICATIONS & PRECAUTIONS
Contraindicated in patients who are hypersensitive to famotidine.

INTERACTIONS
Drug-drug. Famotidine may cause *enteric coatings* to dissolve too rapidly because of increased gastric pH. It may decrease *ketoconazole's* absorption, requiring an increased dose of ketoconazole.

ADVERSE REACTIONS
CNS: *headache,* dizziness, vertigo, malaise, paresthesia.
CV: palpitations.
EENT: tinnitus, taste disorder, orbital edema.
GI: diarrhea, constipation, anorexia, dry mouth.
GU: increased BUN and creatinine levels.
Musculoskeletal: pain.
Skin: acne, dry skin, flushing.
Other: transient irritation (at I.V. site), fever.

🔲 KEY CONSIDERATIONS
Besides the recommendations relevant to all H_2-receptor antagonists, consider the following:
• Use famotidine cautiously in geriatric patients because of increased risk of adverse reactions, particularly those affecting the CNS.

Reactions may be *common,* uncommon, *life-threatening*, or COMMON AND LIFE-THREATENING.

• Don't use drug for longer than 8 weeks in patients with uncomplicated duodenal ulcer.

• After administration via nasogastric tube, flush the tube to clear it and ensure drug's passage to stomach.

• For I.V. push administration, dilute with normal saline solution to total volume of 5 to 10 ml; administer over period exceeding 2 minutes. For I.V. infusion, dilute in 100 ml of D_5W and administer over 15 to 30 minutes. Drug is stable at room temperature for 48 hours. Don't use drug if it's discolored or contains precipitate.

• Administer antacids concurrently if needed.

• Drug may antagonize pentagastrin during gastric acid secretion tests. Famotidine may elevate hepatic enzyme levels. In skin tests using allergen extracts, drug may cause false-negative results.

• Note that drug appears to cause fewer adverse reactions and drug interactions than cimetidine.

Patient education

• Caution patient to take drug only as directed and to continue taking doses even after pain subsides, to ensure adequate healing.

• Instruct patient to take dose at bedtime.

felodipine
Plendil

Calcium channel blocker, antihypertensive

Available by prescription only
Tablets (extended-release): 2.5 mg, 5 mg, 10 mg

INDICATIONS & DOSAGE
Hypertension
Adults: 5 mg P.O. daily. Adjust dosage based on patient response, generally at intervals not less than 2 weeks. Usual dosage is 2.5 to 10 mg daily; doses exceeding 10 mg daily increase rate of peripheral edema and vasodilatory adverse effects.

Geriatric patients: 2.5 mg P.O. daily. Doses above 10 mg shouldn't be considered.

✦ *Dosage adjustment.* Patients with impaired hepatic function should receive a starting dose of 2.5 mg daily.

PHARMACODYNAMICS
Antihypertensive action: A dihydropyridine-derivative calcium channel blocker, felodipine blocks the entry of calcium ions into vascular smooth muscle and cardiac cells. This type of calcium channel blocker shows some selectivity for smooth muscle as compared with cardiac muscle. Effects on vascular smooth muscle are relaxation and vasodilation.

PHARMACOKINETICS
Absorption: Felodipine is almost completely absorbed, but extensive first-pass metabolism reduces absolute bioavailability to about 20%. Plasma levels peak within 2½ to 5 hours after a dose.
Distribution: Drug is more than 99% bound to plasma proteins.
Metabolism: Drug metabolism is probably hepatic; at least six inactive metabolites have been identified.
Excretion: More than 70% of a dose appears in urine, and 10% appears in feces as metabolites.

CONTRAINDICATIONS & PRECAUTIONS
Contraindicated in patients who are hypersensitive to felodipine. Use cautiously in patients with impaired hepatic function or heart failure, especially those receiving beta blockers.

INTERACTIONS
Drug-drug. *Cimetidine* decreases the clearance of felodipine, so lower doses of felodipine should be used. In clinical trials, felodipine decreased peak serum levels of *digoxin*, but total absorbed drug was unchanged; significance is unknown. Felodipine may alter the pharmacokinetics of *metoprolol;* although no dosage adjustment appears necessary, monitor for adverse effects.

ADVERSE REACTIONS
CNS: *headache,* dizziness, paresthesia, asthenia.

CV: *peripheral edema,* chest pain, *flushing,* palpitations.
EENT: rhinorrhea, pharyngitis.
GI: abdominal pain, nausea, constipation, diarrhea, gingival hyperplasia.
Musculoskeletal: muscle cramps, back pain.
Respiratory: upper respiratory tract infection, cough.
Skin: rash.

▣ KEY CONSIDERATIONS

Besides the recommendations relevant to all calcium channel blockers, consider the following:

● Higher blood levels of drug are seen in geriatric patients. Mean clearance of drug from hypertensive geriatric patients (average age 74) was less than half of that observed in young patients (average age 26). Check blood pressures closely during dosage adjustment. Maximum daily dose is 10 mg.
● Note that peripheral edema appears to be both dose- and age-dependent. It's more common in patients taking higher doses, especially those age 60 and older.
● Administer drug without regard to meals.

Patient education

● Tell patient to observe good oral hygiene and to see a dentist regularly because felodipine has been associated with mild gingival hyperplasia.
● Remind patient to swallow tablet whole and not to crush or chew it.
● Inform patient that he should continue taking drug even after he feels better. He should watch his diet and call before taking other drugs, including OTC drugs.

Overdose & treatment

● Expected signs and symptoms are peripheral vasodilation, bradycardia, and hypotension.
● Provide supportive care. I.V. fluids or sympathomimetics may be useful in treating hypotension, and atropine (0.5 to 1 mg I.V.) may be used for bradycardia. It's unknown whether the drug can be removed by dialysis.

fenofibrate (micronized)
Tricor

Fibric acid derivative, antihyperlipidemic

Available by prescription only
Capsules: 67 mg

INDICATIONS & DOSAGE
Adjunct to diet for treatment of patients with very high serum triglyceride levels (type IV and V hyperlipidemia) who are at high risk for pancreatitis and who don't respond adequately to diet alone
Adults: Initiate therapy with 1 (67-mg) capsule P.O. once daily. Based on response, increase dose if necessary after repeat triglyceride levels at 4- to 8-week intervals to maximum dose of three capsules daily (201 mg).
✦ *Dosage adjustment.* Minimize dosage in patients with renal impairment. Initiate therapy at dose of 67 mg/day and increase only after effects on renal function and triglyceride levels have been evaluated at this dose.

PHARMACODYNAMICS
Antihyperlipidemic action: Exact mechanism of action is unknown; fenofibrate is thought to lower triglyceride levels by inhibiting triglyceride synthesis, resulting in a decrease in the amount of very-low-density lipoprotein released into the circulation. Fenofibrate may stimulate the breakdown of triglyceride-rich protein.

PHARMACOKINETICS
Absorption: Fenofibrate is well absorbed. Plasma levels peak within 6 to 8 hours after administration. Food increases the absorption of drug by 35%.
Distribution: Steady-state plasma levels are achieved within 5 days after initiation of therapy. Drug is almost entirely bound to plasma protein.
Metabolism: Drug is rapidly hydrolyzed by esterases to fenofibric acid, an active metabolite. Fenofibric acid is primarily conjugated with glucuronic acid and excreted in urine.

Reactions may be *common*, uncommon, *life-threatening*, or COMMON AND LIFE-THREATENING.

Excretion: Drug is primarily excreted in the urine; 25% is excreted in the feces; elimination half-life is 20 hours.

CONTRAINDICATIONS & PRECAUTIONS

Contraindicated in patients with preexisting gallbladder disease, hepatic dysfunction (including primary biliary cirrhosis), severe renal dysfunction, unexplained persistent liver function abnormalities, or hypersensitivity to drug.

INTERACTIONS

Drug-drug. *Bile acid resins* may bind and inhibit absorption of fenofibrate, so fenofibrate should be taken 1 hour before or 4 to 6 hours after taking these agents. *Cyclosporine*-induced renal dysfunction may compromise the elimination of fenofibrate; therefore, use cautiously. Use extreme caution when administering drug with *coumarin-type anticoagulants* because of protein-binding displacement of the anticoagulant and potentiation of its effects; reduce dose of anticoagulant to maintain PT and INR within desired range. No data are available on use with *HMG-CoA inhibitors* (statins); however, because of risk of myopathy, rhabdomyolysis, and acute renal failure reported with the use of *statins* with *gemfibrozil* (another fibrate derivative), these drugs shouldn't be given together.

ADVERSE REACTIONS

CNS: dizziness, miscellaneous pain, asthenia, fatigue, paresthesia, insomnia, increased appetite, headache, decreased libido.
CV: *arrhythmias.*
EENT: eye irritation, eye floaters, earache, conjunctivitis, blurred vision, rhinitis, sinusitis.
GI: dyspepsia, eructation, flatulence, nausea, vomiting, abdominal pain, constipation, diarrhea.
GU: polyuria, vaginitis.
Musculoskeletal: arthralgia.
Respiratory: cough.
Skin: urticaria, pruritus, rash.
Other: infections, flulike syndrome.

◻ KEY CONSIDERATIONS

• Withdraw therapy in patients who don't achieve an adequate response after 2 months of treatment with the maximum daily dosage.
• Note that fenofibrate lowers serum uric acid levels in normal patients as well as hyperuricemic patients by increasing uric acid excretion.
• Don't use drug for primary or secondary prevention of coronary artery disease.
• If possible, change or discontinue the use of beta blockers, estrogens, and thiazide diuretics because they may increase plasma triglyceride levels.
• Note that drug may cause excretion of cholesterol into the bile, leading to cholelithiasis. If suspected, perform appropriate tests and discontinue drug.
• Note that mild to moderate decreases in hemoglobin, hematocrit, and WBC count may occur on initiation of therapy but should stabilize on long-term administration.
• Pancreatitis may occur in patients receiving fenofibrate; myositis and rhabdomyolysis may occur in those with renal failure. Assess CK levels in patients with myalgia, muscle tenderness, or weakness.
• ALT or AST levels may be increased. Creatinine and BUN levels are increased, and hemoglobin and uric acid levels are decreased.

Patient education

• Advise patient to promptly report symptoms of unexplained muscle weakness, pain, or tenderness, especially if they're accompanied by malaise or fever.
• Instruct patient to follow a triglyceride-lowering diet during treatment.
• Inform patient to take drug with meals to optimize drug absorption.
• Advise patient to continue weight-control measures, including diet and exercise, and to reduce alcohol intake before starting drug therapy.

---

*Canada only   ◊ Unlabeled clinical use

fenoprofen calcium
Nalfon

NSAID, nonnarcotic analgesic, antipyretic

Available by prescription only
Tablets: 600 mg
Capsules: 200 mg, 300 mg

INDICATIONS & DOSAGE
Rheumatoid arthritis and osteoarthritis
Adults: 300 to 600 mg P.O. t.i.d. or q.i.d.
Maximum dosage is 3.2 g daily.
Mild to moderate pain
Adults: 200 mg P.O. q 4 to 6 hours, p.r.n.
◊ *Fever*
Adults: Single oral doses up to 400 mg.
◊ *Acute gouty arthritis*
Adults: 200 mg P.O. q 6 hours; decrease dose based on patient response.

PHARMACODYNAMICS
Analgesic, anti-inflammatory, and antipyretic actions: Mechanism of action is unknown, but fenoprofen is thought to inhibit prostaglandin synthesis. Drug decreases platelet aggregation and may prolong bleeding time.

PHARMACOKINETICS
Absorption: Fenoprofen is absorbed rapidly and completely from the GI tract. The onset of analgesic activity occurs within 15 to 30 minutes, with peak plasma levels achieved in 2 hours. Duration of action is 4 to 6 hours.
Distribution: About 99% of drug is protein-bound.
Metabolism: Drug is metabolized in the liver.
Excretion: Drug is excreted chiefly in urine with a serum half-life of 2½ to 3 hours. A small amount is excreted in feces.

CONTRAINDICATIONS & PRECAUTIONS
Contraindicated in patients with hypersensitivity to fenoprofen, significantly impaired renal function, or history of aspirin- or NSAID-induced asthma, rhinitis, or urticaria.
  Use cautiously in geriatric patients and in patients with history of GI events,
peptic ulcer disease, compromised cardiac function, or hypertension.

INTERACTIONS
Drug-drug. Increased nephrotoxicity may occur with *acetaminophen, gold compounds,* or *other anti-inflammatories.* Use with *anticoagulants* or *thrombolytics*—such as *coumarin derivatives, heparin, streptokinase,* and *urokinase*—may potentiate anticoagulant effects. Fenoprofen may decrease the effectiveness of *antihypertensives* or *diuretics.* Use with *anti-inflammatories, corticotropin, salicylates,* or *steroids* may increase adverse GI reactions, including ulceration and hemorrhage. *Aspirin* may decrease the bioavailability of fenoprofen. Toxicity may occur with *coumarin derivatives, nifedipine, phenytoin,* or *verapamil.* Use with *diuretics* may increase nephrotoxic potential. Bleeding problems may occur if fenoprofen is used with other *drugs that inhibit platelet aggregation*—such as *dextran, dipyridamole, mezlocillin, piperacillin, sulfinpyrazone, ticarcillin,* or *valproic acid*—or with *aspirin, cefamandole, cefoperazone, plicamycin, salicylates,* or *other anti-inflammatories.* Fenoprofen may displace *highly protein-bound drugs* from binding sites. Because of the influence of prostaglandins on glucose metabolism, use with *insulin* or *oral antidiabetics* may potentiate hypoglycemic effects. Fenoprofen may decrease the renal clearance of *lithium* and *methotrexate.*
Drug-lifestyle. *Alcohol* may increase adverse GI reactions, including ulceration and hemorrhage; avoid use.

ADVERSE REACTIONS
CNS: *headache,* dizziness, *somnolence,* fatigue, nervousness, asthenia, tremor, confusion.
CV: peripheral edema, palpitations.
EENT: tinnitus, blurred vision, decreased hearing.
GI: *epigastric distress, nausea,* **GI bleeding,** vomiting, occult blood loss, peptic ulceration, constipation, anorexia, *dyspepsia,* flatulence.
GU: oliguria, interstitial nephritis, proteinuria, reversible renal failure, papillary necrosis, cystitis, hematuria.

Reactions may be *common,* uncommon, *life-threatening,* or COMMON AND LIFE-THREATENING.

Hematologic: prolonged bleeding time, anemia, *aplastic anemia, agranulocytosis, thrombocytopenia, hemorrhage,* bruising, hemolytic anemia.
Hepatic: elevated enzymes, hepatitis.
Respiratory: dyspnea, upper respiratory tract infections, nasopharyngitis.
Skin: *pruritus,* rash, urticaria, increased diaphoresis.
Other: *anaphylaxis, angioedema.*

▣ KEY CONSIDERATIONS

Besides the recommendations relevant to all NSAIDs, consider the following:
• Patients older than 60 years may be more susceptible to the toxic effects of fenoprofen, especially adverse GI reactions. Use with caution.
• Note that the drug's effects on renal prostaglandins may cause fluid retention and edema, a significant drawback for geriatric patients and those with heart failure.
• Note that fenoprofen has been used to treat fever, acute gouty arthritis, and juvenile arthritis.
• Monitor for potential CNS effects. Institute safety measures to prevent injury.
• The physiological effects of drug may increase bleeding time, BUN, serum creatinine, potassium, alkaline phosphatase, LD, and transaminase levels. Drug may also falsely elevate both free and total serum T_3 levels, but thyroid-stimulating hormone and T_4 levels are unaffected.

Patient education

• Tell patient to avoid activities that require alertness or concentration until CNS effects of drug are known.
• Instruct patient in safety measures to prevent injury.
• Advise patient to call for specific instructions before taking OTC analgesics.
• Advise patient to avoid alcohol while taking drug.

Overdose & treatment

• Little is known about the acute toxicity of fenoprofen. Non-oliguric renal failure, tachycardia, and hypotension have been observed. Other signs and symptoms include drowsiness, dizziness, confusion and lethargy, nausea, vomiting, headache, tinnitus, and blurred vision.

Elevations in serum creatinine and BUN levels have been reported.
• To treat an overdose, empty stomach immediately by inducing vomiting with ipecac syrup or by performing gastric lavage. Administer activated charcoal via an NG tube. Provide symptomatic and supportive measures (respiratory support and correction of fluid and electrolyte imbalances). Monitor laboratory parameters and vital signs closely. Dialysis is of little value.
• Monitor renal, hepatic, and auditory function in patients on long-term therapy. Stop drug if abnormalities occur.

fentanyl citrate
Sublimaze

fentanyl transdermal system
Duragesic-25, Duragesic-50, Duragesic-75, Duragesic-100

fentanyl transmucosal
Fentanyl Oralet

Opioid agonist, analgesic, adjunct to anesthesia, anesthetic
Controlled substance schedule II

Available by prescription only
Injection: 50 mcg/ml
Transdermal system: patches designed to release 25 mcg, 50 mcg, 75 mcg, or 100 mcg of fentanyl/hour.
Transmucosal: 200 mcg, 300 mcg, 400 mcg

INDICATIONS & DOSAGE

Preoperatively
Adults: 50 to 100 mcg I.M. 30 to 60 minutes before surgery. Alternatively, 1 oralet unit consisting of 200 mcg, 300 mcg, or 400 mcg P.O. for patient to suck until dissolved, 20 to 40 minutes before surgery.
Adjunct to general anesthesia; low-dose regimen for minor procedures
Adults: 2 mcg/kg I.V.
Moderate-dose regimen for major procedures
Adults: Initial dosage is 2 to 20 mcg/kg I.V.; may give additional doses of 25 to 100 mcg I.V. or I.M., p.r.n.

High-dose regimen for complicated procedures
Adults: Initial dosage is 20 to 50 mcg/kg; additional doses of 25 mcg to one half the initial dose may be administered, p.r.n.
Adjunct to regional anesthesia
Adults: 50 to 100 mcg I.M. or slow I.V. over 1 to 2 minutes.
Postoperative analgesic
Adults: 50 to 100 mcg I.M. q 1 to 2 hours, p.r.n.
Management of chronic pain in patients who have no relief by lesser means
Adults: Apply one transdermal system to the upper torso on skin that isn't irritated and hasn't been irradiated. Initiate therapy with the 25-mcg/hour system; adjust dosage as needed and tolerated. Each system may be worn for 72 hours.

PHARMACODYNAMICS
Analgesic action: Fentanyl binds to the opiate receptors as an agonist to alter the patient's perception of painful stimuli, thus providing analgesia for moderate to severe pain. Its CNS and respiratory depressant effects are similar to those of morphine. Drug has little hypnotic activity and rarely causes histamine release.

PHARMACOKINETICS
Absorption: Onset of action after I.V. administration is immediate; within 7 to 8 minutes of I.M. injection; within 5 to 15 minutes of transmucosal use; onset after transdermal use may take several hours as it's absorbed through the skin. Peak effect after I.V. use occurs in 3 to 5 minutes; after I.M. or transmucosal use, 20 to 30 minutes; after transdermal use, 1 to 3 days.
Distribution: Redistribution has been suggested as the main cause of the brief analgesic effect of fentanyl.
Metabolism: Drug is metabolized in the liver.
Excretion: Drug is excreted in the urine as metabolites and unchanged drug. Elimination half-life is about 7 hours after parenteral use, 5 to 15 hours after transmucosal use, and 18 hours after transdermal use.

CONTRAINDICATIONS & PRECAUTIONS
Contraindicated in patients with known intolerance to fentanyl. Use cautiously in geriatric or debilitated patients and in those with head injuries, increased CSF pressure, COPD, decreased respiratory reserve, compromised respirations, arrhythmias, or hepatic, renal, or cardiac disease.

INTERACTIONS
Drug-drug. Use with *anticholinergics* may cause paralytic ileus. Use with *cimetidine* may also increase respiratory and CNS depression, causing confusion, disorientation, apnea, or seizures; such use requires that dosage of fentanyl be reduced by one-quarter to one-third. Use with other *CNS depressants*—such as *antihistamines, barbiturates, benzodiazepines, general anesthetics, muscle relaxants, narcotic analgesics, phenothiazines, sedative-hypnotics, tricyclic antidepressants*—potentiates drug's respiratory and CNS depression, sedation, and hypotensive effects. When used to supplement *conduction anesthesia,* such as *some peridural anesthetics* and *spinal anesthesia,* fentanyl can alter respiration by blocking intercostal nerves. *Diazepam* may produce CV depression when given with high doses of fentanyl. When used with fentanyl, *droperidol* may cause hypotension and a decrease in pulmonary artery pressure; however, a droperidol-fentanyl combination, Innovar, is available. Drug accumulation and enhanced effects may result from use with other *drugs that are extensively metabolized in the liver*—such as *digitoxin, phenytoin,* and *rifampin.* The manufacturer warns that fentanyl shouldn't be given to a patient who has received *MAO inhibitors* within the past 14 days. Patients who become physically dependent on drug may experience acute withdrawal syndrome if given a *narcotic antagonist.*
Drug-lifestyle. *Alcohol* potentiates drug's respiratory and CNS depression, sedation, and hypotensive effects; discourage alcohol use.

ADVERSE REACTIONS
CNS: *sedation, somnolence, clouded sensorium, euphoria,* dizziness,

---

headache, *confusion, asthenia,* nervousness, hallucinations, anxiety, depression.
CV: *hypotension,* hypertension, ***arrhythmias,*** chest pain.
GI: *nausea, vomiting, constipation,* ileus, abdominal pain, *dry mouth,* anorexia, diarrhea, dyspepsia.
GU: *urine retention.*
Respiratory: *respiratory depression,* hypoventilation, dyspnea, apnea.
Skin: reaction at application site (erythema, papules, edema), *pruritus, diaphoresis.*
Other: physical dependence.

▣ KEY CONSIDERATIONS
Besides the recommendations relevant to all opioid (narcotic) agonists, consider the following:
• Use with caution in geriatric patients because they may be more sensitive to the therapeutic and adverse effects of drug.
• Observe patient for delayed onset of respiratory depression. The high lipid solubility of fentanyl may contribute to this potential adverse effect.
• Monitor patient's heart rate. Fentanyl may cause bradycardia. Pretreatment with an anticholinergic (such as atropine or glycopyrrolate) may minimize this effect.
• Note that high doses can produce muscle rigidity. This effect can be reversed by naloxone.
• Use epidural and intrathecal fentanyl as a potent adjunct to epidural anesthesia.
• Fentanyl increases plasma amylase and lipase levels.
Transdermal form
• Transdermal fentanyl isn't recommended for postoperative pain.
• Use dosage equivalent charts to calculate the transdermal dose of fentanyl based on daily morphine intake—for example, for every 90 mg of oral morphine or 15 mg of I.M. morphine per 24 hours, 25 mcg/hour of transdermal fentanyl is required. Some patients will require alternative means of opiate administration when the dose exceeds 300 mcg/hour.
• Make dosage adjustments gradually in patients using the transdermal system. Reaching steady-state levels of a new

dose may take up to 6 days; delay dose adjustment until after at least 2 applications.
• Monitor patients who develop adverse reactions to the transdermal system for at least 12 hours after removal. Serum levels of fentanyl drop very gradually and may take as long as 17 hours to decline by 50%.
• Most patients experience good control of pain for 3 days while wearing the transdermal system, although a few may need a new application after 48 hours. Because serum fentanyl level rises for the first 24 hours after application, analgesic effect can't be evaluated on the first day. Be sure the patient has adequate supplemental analgesic to prevent breakthrough pain.
• Withdraw the transdermal system gradually when reducing opiate therapy or switching to a different analgesic. Because serum drug level drops gradually after removal, give half of the equianalgesic dose of the new analgesic 12 to 18 hours after removal.

Patient education
• Teach patient proper application of the transdermal patch. Clip hair at the application site, but don't use a razor, which may irritate the skin. Wash area with clear water if necessary, but not with soaps, oils, lotions, alcohol, or other substances that may irritate the skin or prevent adhesion. Dry area completely before applying the patch.
• Tell patient to remove the transdermal system from the package just before applying. Hold in place for 10 to 20 seconds, and be sure the edges of the patch adhere to the skin.
• Teach patient to dispose of the transdermal patch by folding so the adhesive side adheres to itself and then flushing down the toilet.
• If another patch is needed after 72 hours, tell patient to apply to a new site.

Overdose & treatment
• The most common signs and symptoms of fentanyl overdose are an extension of its actions. They include CNS depression, respiratory depression, and miosis (pinpoint pupils). Other acute

toxic effects include hypotension, bradycardia, hypothermia, shock, apnea, cardiopulmonary arrest, circulatory collapse, pulmonary edema, and seizures.

• To treat acute overdose, first establish adequate respiratory exchange via a patent airway and ventilation as needed; administer a narcotic antagonist (naloxone) to reverse respiratory depression. (Because the duration of action of fentanyl is longer than that of naloxone, repeated dosing may be necessary.) Naloxone shouldn't be given unless the patient has significant respiratory or CV depression. Monitor vital signs closely.

• Provide symptomatic and supportive treatment (continued respiratory support, correction of fluid or electrolyte imbalance). Monitor laboratory values, vital signs, and neurologic status closely.

ferrous fumarate
Femiron, Feostat, Fumasorb, Fumerin, Hemocyte, Ircon, Ircon-FA, Neo-Fer*, Nephro-Fer, Novofumar*, Palafer*, Span-FF

Oral iron supplement, hematinic

Available without a prescription. Ferrous fumarate is 33% elemental iron.
Tablets: 63 mg, 195 mg, 200 mg, 324 mg, 325 mg, 350 mg
Tablets (chewable): 100 mg
Capsules (extended-release): 325 mg
Suspension: 100 mg/5 ml
Drops: 45 mg/0.6 ml

INDICATIONS & DOSAGE
Iron-deficiency states
Adults: 50 to 100 mg P.O. of elemental iron t.i.d. Adjust dose gradually, p.r.n., and as tolerated.

PHARMACODYNAMICS
Hematinic action: Ferrous fumarate replaces iron, an essential component in the formation of hemoglobin.

PHARMACOKINETICS
Absorption: Iron is absorbed from the entire length of the GI tract, but primary absorption sites are the duodenum and proximal jejunum. Up to 10% of iron is absorbed by healthy individuals; patients with iron-deficiency anemia may absorb up to 60%. Enteric coating and some extended-release formulas have decreased absorption because they are designed to release iron past the points of highest absorption; food may decrease absorption by 33% to 50%.
Distribution: Iron is transported through GI mucosal cells directly into the blood, where it's immediately bound to a carrier protein, transferrin, and transported to the bone marrow for incorporation into hemoglobin. Iron is highly protein-bound.
Metabolism: Iron is liberated by the destruction of hemoglobin, but is conserved and reused by the body.
Excretion: Healthy individuals lose only small amounts of iron daily. Men and postmenopausal women lose about 1 mg/day, and premenopausal women about 1.5 mg/day. The loss usually occurs in nails, hair, feces, and urine; trace amounts are lost in bile and sweat.

CONTRAINDICATIONS & PRECAUTIONS
Contraindicated in patients with primary hemochromatosis or hemosiderosis, hemolytic anemia unless iron-deficiency anemia is also present, peptic ulcer disease, regional enteritis, or ulcerative colitis, and in those receiving repeated blood transfusions. Use cautiously on long-term basis.

INTERACTIONS
Drug-drug. *Antacids, cholestyramine, pancreatic extracts,* and *vitamin E* decrease ferrous fumarate absorption (separate doses by 1- to 2-hour intervals). *Ascorbic acid* (vitamin C) increases absorption of ferrous fumarate. *Chloramphenicol* delays response to iron therapy. *Doxycycline* may interfere with ferrous fumarate absorption even when doses are separated. Ferrous fumarate decreases *penicillamine* absorption; separate doses by at least 2 hours. Ferrous fumarate may decrease absorption of *quinolones.* Use with *tetracycline* inhibits absorption of both drugs; give tetracycline 3 hours after or 2 hours before ferrous fumarate.

Drug-food. *Citrus products* increase absorption; take together. *Milk* impairs absorption; don't take together.

ADVERSE REACTIONS
GI: *nausea,* epigastric pain, vomiting, *constipation,* diarrhea, black stools, anorexia.
Other: temporary staining of teeth (with suspension and drops).

🔲 KEY CONSIDERATIONS
• Geriatric patients may need higher doses because reduced gastric secretions and achlorhydria may lower capacity for iron absorption.
• Encourage a proper diet in geriatric patients because iron-induced constipation is common.
• Drug may stain teeth.
• Ferrous fumarate blackens feces and may interfere with tests for occult blood in the stool; the guaiac test and ortho-toluidine test may yield false-positive results, but the benzidine test is usually unaffected. Iron overload may decrease uptake of technetium 99m and thus interfere with skeletal imaging.

Patient education
• Instruct patient to take tablets with orange juice or water, but not with milk or antacids.
• Tell patient to take suspension with straw and place drops at back of throat.

Overdose & treatment
• The lethal dose of iron is 200 to 250 mg/kg; fatalities have occurred with lower dosages. Signs and symptoms may follow ingestion of 20 to 60 mg/kg. Signs and symptoms of acute overdose may occur as follows: Between 30 minutes and 8 hours after ingestion, patient may experience lethargy, nausea and vomiting, green then tarry stools, weak and rapid pulse, hypotension, dehydration, acidosis, and coma. If the patient doesn't die immediately, signs and symptoms may clear for about 24 hours. At 12 to 48 hours, signs and symptoms may return, accompanied by diffuse vascular congestion, pulmonary edema, shock, seizures, anuria, and hyperthermia. Death may follow.

• Treatment requires immediate support of airway, respiration, and circulation. In a conscious patient with an intact gag reflex, induce vomiting with ipecac and perform gastric lavage, using a 1% sodium bicarbonate solution, to convert iron to less irritating, poorly absorbed form. (Phosphate solutions have been used, but carry hazard of other adverse effects.) X-ray abdomen to determine continued presence of excess iron; if serum iron levels exceed 350 mg/dl, deferoxamine may be used for systemic chelation.
• Survivors are likely to sustain organ damage, including pyloric or antral stenosis, hepatic cirrhosis, CNS damage, and intestinal obstruction.

ferrous gluconate
Apo-Ferrous Gluconate*, Fergon, Ferralet, Fertinic*, Novoferrogluc*, Simron

Oral iron supplement, hematinic

Available without a prescription. Ferrous gluconate is 11.6% elemental iron.
Tablets: 300 mg (contains 35 mg Fe$^+$), 320 mg (contains 37 mg Fe$^+$), 325 mg (contains 38 mg Fe$^+$)
Capsules: 86 mg (contains 10 mg Fe$^+$), 325 mg (contains 38 mg Fe$^+$)
Elixir: 300 mg/5 ml (contains 35 mg Fe$^+$)

INDICATIONS & DOSAGE
Iron deficiency
Adults: 325 mg P.O. q.i.d., dosage increased, p.r.n., and as tolerated, up to 650 mg q.i.d.

PHARMACODYNAMICS
Hematinic action: Ferrous gluconate replaces iron, an essential component in the formation of hemoglobin.

PHARMACOKINETICS
Absorption: Iron is absorbed from the entire length of the GI tract, but primary absorption sites are the duodenum and proximal jejunum. Healthy individuals absorb up to 10% of iron; patients with iron-deficiency anemia may absorb up to 60%. Food may decrease absorption by 33% to 50%.

Distribution: Iron is transported through GI mucosal cells directly into the blood, where it's immediately bound to a carrier protein, transferrin, and transported to the bone marrow for incorporation into hemoglobin. Iron is highly protein-bound.
Metabolism: Iron is liberated by the destruction of hemoglobin, but is conserved and reused by the body.
Excretion: Healthy individuals lose only small amounts of iron daily. Men and postmenopausal women lose about 1 mg/day, premenopausal women about 1.5 mg/day. Loss usually occurs in nails, hair, feces, and urine; trace amounts are lost in bile and sweat.

CONTRAINDICATIONS & PRECAUTIONS
Contraindicated in patients with peptic ulceration, regional enteritis, ulcerative colitis, hemosiderosis, primary hemochromatosis, hemolytic anemia unless iron-deficiency anemia is also present, and in those receiving repeated blood transfusions. Use cautiously on long-term basis.

INTERACTIONS
Drug-drug. *Antacids, cholestyramine, pancreatic extracts,* and *vitamin E* decrease ferrous gluconate absorption (separate doses by 1- to 2-hour intervals). *Ascorbic acid* (vitamin C) increases absorption of ferrous gluconate. *Chloramphenicol* delays response to iron therapy. *Doxycycline* may interfere with ferrous gluconate absorption even when doses are separated. Ferrous gluconate decreases *penicillamine* absorption; separate doses by at least 2 hours. Drug may decrease absorption of *quinolones*. Use of ferrous gluconate and *tetracycline* inhibits absorption of both drugs; give tetracycline 3 hours after or 2 hours before ferrous gluconate.
Drug-food. *Citrus products* increase absorption; take together. *Milk* impairs absorption; don't take together.

ADVERSE REACTIONS
GI: *nausea,* epigastric pain, vomiting, *constipation,* diarrhea, *black stools,* anorexia.
Other: temporary staining of teeth (with elixir).

▣ KEY CONSIDERATIONS
● Geriatric patients may need higher dosages because reduced gastric secretions and achlorhydria may lower capacity for iron absorption.
● Note that drug can be given between meals or with some food, but absorption may be decreased.
● Stress proper diet in geriatric patients because iron-induced constipation is common.
● Ferrous gluconate blackens feces and may interfere with tests for occult blood in the stools; the guaiac test and ortho-toluidine test may yield false-positive results, but the benzidine test is usually unaffected. Iron overload may decrease uptake of technetium 99m and thus interfere with skeletal imaging.

Patient education
● Instruct patient to take tablets with orange juice or water, but not with milk or antacids.
● Tell patient to take suspension with straw and place drops at back of throat.

Overdose & treatment
● The lethal dosage of iron is 200 to 250 mg/kg; fatalities have occurred with lower doses. Signs and symptoms may follow ingestion of 20 to 60 mg/kg. Signs and symptoms of acute overdose may occur as follows: Between 30 minutes and 8 hours after ingestion, patient may experience lethargy, nausea and vomiting, green then tarry stools, weak and rapid pulse, hypotension, dehydration, acidosis, and coma. If patient doesn't die immediately, signs and symptoms may clear for about 24 hours. At 12 to 48 hours, symptoms may return, accompanied by diffuse vascular congestion, pulmonary edema, shock, seizures, anuria, and hyperthermia. Death may follow.
● Treatment requires immediate support of airway, respiration, and circulation. In a conscious patient with an intact gag reflex, induce vomiting with ipecac and perform gastric lavage, using a 1% sodium bicarbonate solution, to convert iron to less irritating, poorly absorbed form. (Phosphate solutions have been used, but carry hazard of other adverse effects.) Take abdominal X-ray to determine con-

---

Reactions may be *common,* uncommon, *life-threatening,* or COMMON AND LIFE-THREATENING.

tinued presence of excess iron; if serum iron levels exceed 350 mg/dl, deferoxamine may be used for systemic chelation.
• Survivors are likely to sustain organ damage, including pyloric or antral stenosis, hepatic cirrhosis, CNS damage, and intestinal obstruction.

ferrous sulfate
Apo-Ferrous Sulfate*, Feosol, Feratab, Fer-In-Sol, Fer-Iron, Fero-Grad-500*, Fero-Gradumet, Ferospace, Ferralyn Lanacaps, Ferra-TD, Mol-Iron, Novoferrosulfa*, PMS Ferrous Sulfate*, Slow FE

Oral iron supplement, hematinic

Available without a prescription. Ferrous sulfate is 20% elemental iron; dried and powdered (exsiccated), it's about 32% elemental iron.
Tablets: 195 mg, 300 mg, 324 mg, 325 mg; 200 mg (exsiccated); 160 mg (exsiccated, extended-release); 525 mg (timed-release)
Capsules: 150 mg, 190 mg, 250 mg
Capsules (extended-release): 150 mg, 159 mg, 250 mg
Syrup: 90 mg/5 ml
Elixir: 220 mg/5 ml
Liquid: 75 mg/0.6 ml, 125 mg/ml

INDICATIONS & DOSAGE
Iron deficiency
Adults: 300 mg P.O. b.i.d.; dosage gradually increased to 300 mg q.i.d., p.r.n., and as tolerated. For extended-release capsules, 150 to 250 mg P.O. once or twice daily; for extended-release tablets, 160 to 525 mg once or twice daily.

PHARMACODYNAMICS
Hematinic action: Ferrous sulfate replaces iron, an essential component in the formation of hemoglobin.

PHARMACOKINETICS
Absorption: Iron is absorbed from the entire length of the GI tract, but primary absorption sites are the duodenum and proximal jejunum. Up to 10% of iron is absorbed by healthy individuals; patients with iron-deficiency anemia may absorb

up to 60%. Enteric coating and some extended-release formulas have decreased absorption because they are designed to release iron past the points of highest absorption. Food may decrease absorption by 33% to 50%.
Distribution: Iron is transported through GI mucosal cells directly into the blood, where it's immediately bound to a carrier protein, transferrin, and transported to the bone marrow for incorporation into hemoglobin. Iron is highly protein-bound.
Metabolism: Iron is liberated by the destruction of hemoglobin, but is conserved and reused by the body.
Excretion: Healthy individuals lose very little iron each day. Men and postmenopausal women lose about 1 mg/day, and premenopausal women about 1.5 mg/day. The loss usually occurs in nails, hair, feces, and urine; trace amounts are lost in bile and sweat.

CONTRAINDICATIONS & PRECAUTIONS
Contraindicated in patients with hemosiderosis, primary hemochromatosis, hemolytic anemia unless iron-deficiency anemia is also present, peptic ulceration, ulcerative colitis, or regional enteritis, and in those receiving repeated blood transfusions. Use cautiously on long-term basis.

INTERACTIONS
Drug-drug. *Antacids, cholestyramine, pancreatic extracts,* and *vitamin E* decrease ferrous sulfate absorption (separate doses by 1- to 2-hour intervals). *Ascorbic acid* (vitamin C) increases absorption of ferrous sulfate. *Chloramphenicol* delays response to iron therapy. *Doxycycline* may interfere with ferrous sulfate absorption even when doses are separated. Use with *tetracycline* inhibits absorption of both drugs; give tetracycline 3 hours after or 2 hours before ferrous sulfate.
Drug-food. *Citrus products* increase absorption; take together. *Milk* impairs absorption; don't take together.

ADVERSE REACTIONS
GI: *nausea,* epigastric pain, vomiting, *constipation, black stools,* diarrhea, anorexia.

Other: temporary staining of teeth (with liquid forms).

▣ KEY CONSIDERATIONS

• Geriatric patients may need higher doses because reduced gastric secretions and achlorhydria may lower capacity for iron absorption.
• Stress proper diet in geriatric patients because iron-induced constipation is common.
• Note that drug may stain teeth.
• Ferrous sulfate blackens feces and may interfere with tests for occult blood in the stool; the guaiac test and orthotoluidine test may yield false-positive results, but the benzidine test is usually unaffected. Iron overload may decrease uptake of technetium 99m and thus interfere with skeletal imaging.

Patient education

• Instruct patient not to crush or chew extended-release forms.
• Instruct patient to take tablets with orange juice or water, but not with milk or antacids.
• Tell patient to take suspension with a straw and place drops at back of throat.

Overdose & treatment

• The lethal dose of iron is 200 to 250 mg/kg; fatalities have occurred with lower doses. Signs and symptoms may follow ingestion of 20 to 60 mg/kg. Signs and symptoms of acute overdose may occur as follows: Between 30 minutes to 8 hours after ingestion, patient may experience lethargy, nausea and vomiting, green then tarry stools, weak and rapid pulse, hypotension, dehydration, acidosis, and coma. If the patient doesn't die immediately, signs and symptoms may clear for about 24 hours. At 12 to 48 hours, symptoms may return, accompanied by diffuse vascular congestion, pulmonary edema, shock, seizures, anuria, and hyperthermia. Death may follow.
• Treatment requires immediate support of airway, respiration, and circulation. If the patient is conscious and his gag reflex is intact, induce vomiting with ipecac (if the patient is unconscious, perform gastric lavage). After you've in-

duced vomiting, perform gastric lavage using a 1% sodium bicarbonate solution to convert iron to less irritating, poorly absorbed form. (Phosphate solutions have been used, but carry hazard of other adverse effects.) Take abdominal X-ray to detect excess iron; if serum iron levels exceed 350 mg/dl, deferoxamine may be used for systemic chelation.
• Survivors are likely to sustain organ damage, including pyloric or antral stenosis, hepatic cirrhosis, CNS damage, and intestinal obstruction.

---

fexofenadine hydrochloride
Allegra

H_1-receptor antagonist, antihistamine

Available by prescription only
Capsules: 60 mg

INDICATIONS & DOSAGE

Seasonal allergic rhinitis
Adults: 60 mg P.O. b.i.d.
✦ *Dosage adjustment.* In patients with impaired renal function, 60 mg P.O. once daily.

PHARMACODYNAMICS

Antihistamine action: Fexofenadine's principal effects are mediated through selective inhibition of peripheral H_1 receptors.

PHARMACOKINETICS

Absorption: Fexofenadine is rapidly absorbed.
Distribution: Drug is 60% to 70% bound to plasma protein.
Metabolism: About 5% of drug is metabolized.
Excretion: Drug is mainly excreted in feces; less so in urine. Mean elimination half-life of drug is 14.4 hours.

CONTRAINDICATIONS & PRECAUTIONS

Contraindicated in patients with hypersensitivity to fexofenadine or its components. Use cautiously in patients with impaired renal function.

INTERACTIONS
None reported.

ADVERSE REACTIONS
CNS: fatigue, drowsiness.
GI: nausea, dyspepsia.
GU: dysmenorrhea.
Other: viral infection.

▣ KEY CONSIDERATIONS
• Clinical studies show that geriatric and younger adult patients have similar adverse effects.
• There is no information to indicate that abuse or dependency can occur with fexofenadine use.

Patient education
• Caution patient not to perform hazardous activities if drowsiness occurs with drug use.
• Instruct patient not to exceed prescribed dosage and to take drug only when needed.

---

filgrastim (granulocyte colony–stimulating factor, G–CSF)
Neupogen

Biological response modifier, colony-stimulating factor

Available by prescription only
Injection: 300 mcg/ml in 1-ml and 1.6-ml single-dose vials

INDICATIONS & DOSAGE
To decrease incidence of infection after cancer chemotherapy for nonmyeloid malignancies, chronic severe neutropenia, after bone marrow transplantation in cancer patients; to treat ◊ agranulocytosis, ◊ pancytopenia with colchicine overdose, ◊ acute leukemia, ◊ myelodysplastic syndrome, ◊ hematologic toxicity with zidovudine antiviral therapy
Adults: Initially, 5 mcg/kg S.C. or I.V. as a single daily dose; may increase dose incrementally by 5 mcg/kg for each course of chemotherapy according to duration and severity of absolute neutrophil count (ANC) nadir.

Don't administer earlier than 24 hours after or within 24 hours before chemotherapy.

Filgrastim should be given daily for up to 2 weeks until ANC nadir reaches 10,000/mm^3 after the anticipated chemoinduced ANC nadir. Duration of treatment depends on the myelosuppressive potential of the chemotherapy used. Discontinue if ANC nadir surpasses 10,000/mm^3.
◊ AIDS
Adults: 0.3 to 3.6 mcg/kg/day S.C. or I.V.
◊ Aplastic anemia
Adults: 800 to 1,200 mcg/m^2/day S.C. or I.V.
◊ Hairy cell leukemia, myelodysplasia
Adults: 15 to 500 mcg/m^2/day S.C. or I.V.

PHARMACODYNAMICS
Immunostimulant action: Filgrastim is a naturally occurring cytokine glycoprotein that stimulates proliferation, differentiation, and functional activity of neutrophils, causing a rapid rise in WBC counts within 2 to 3 days in patients with normal bone marrow function or 7 to 14 days in patients with bone marrow suppression. Blood counts usually return to pretreatment levels within 1 week after therapy ends.

PHARMACOKINETICS
Absorption: After S.C. bolus dose, blood levels suggest rapid absorption with peak levels in 2 to 8 hours.
Distribution: Unknown.
Metabolism: Unknown.
Excretion: Elimination half-life is about 3½ hours.

CONTRAINDICATIONS & PRECAUTIONS
Contraindicated in patients hypersensitive to proteins derived from *Escherichia coli* or to filgrastim or its components.

INTERACTIONS
None reported.

ADVERSE REACTIONS
CNS: headache, weakness, *fatigue.*
CV: *MI, arrhythmias,* chest pain.

GI: *nausea, vomiting, diarrhea, mucositis,* stomatitis, constipation.
Hematologic: *thrombocytopenia,* leukocytosis.
Musculoskeletal: *skeletal pain.*
Respiratory: dyspnea, cough.
Skin: *alopecia,* rash, cutaneous vasculitis.
Other: *fever, hypersensitivity reactions.*

KEY CONSIDERATIONS

• Store drug in refrigerator; don't freeze. Avoid shaking. Before injection, allow to reach room temperature for a maximum of 24 hours. Discard after 24 hours. Use only 1 dose per vial; don't reenter vial.
• Obtain CBC and platelet counts before and twice weekly during therapy.
• Note that filgrastim is incompatible with normal saline solution.
• Perform regular monitoring of hematocrit and platelet counts.
• Note that adult respiratory distress syndrome may occur in septic patients because of the influx of neutrophils at the site of inflammation.
• Closely monitor patients with preexisting cardiac conditions; MI and arrhythmias have occurred.
• Bone pain is the most frequent adverse reaction and may be controlled with nonnarcotic analgesics if mild to moderate, or may require narcotic analgesics if severe.
• WBC counts may be increased to 100,000/mm^3 or more. Transient increases in neutrophils, as well as reversible elevations in uric acid, LD, and alkaline phosphatase levels have been reported. Transient decreases in blood pressure and increases in serum creatinine and aminotransferase levels were also reported.

Patient education

• Review "Information for Patients" section of package insert with patient. Thorough instruction is essential if home use is prescribed.
• When drug can be self-administered safely and effectively, instruct patient in proper dosage and administration techniques.
• Alert patient that the manufacturer has a hotline to answer questions about insurance reimbursement. It operates Monday through Friday from 9 a.m. to 5 p.m. Eastern Standard Time. The number is 1-800-272-9376; in Washington, D.C., it's (202) 637-6698.

finasteride
Propecia, Proscar

Steroid (synthetic 4-azasteroid) derivative, androgen synthesis inhibitor

Available by prescription only
Tablets: 1 mg, 5 mg

INDICATIONS & DOSAGE

Symptomatic benign prostatic hyperplasia (BPH), ◊ *adjuvant therapy after radical prostatectomy,* ◊ *first-stage prostate cancer,* ◊ *acne,* ◊ *hirsutism*
Adults: 5 mg P.O. daily, usually for 6 to 12 months.
Male-pattern baldness (androgenetic alopecia)
Adults: 1 mg P.O. daily, usually for 3 months or more. Continued use is recommended to sustain benefit. Withdrawal of treatment leads to reversal of effect within 12 months.

PHARMACODYNAMICS

Androgen synthesis inhibition action: Finasteride competitively inhibits steroid 5μ-reductase, an enzyme responsible for formation of the potent androgen 5μ-dihydrotestosterone (DHT) from testosterone. Because DHT influences development of the prostate gland, decreasing levels of this hormone in adult males should relieve the symptoms of BPH. In men with male-pattern baldness, the balding scalp contains miniaturized hair follicles and increased amounts of DHT. Finasteride decreases scalp and serum DHT levels in these men.

PHARMACOKINETICS

Absorption: Average bioavailability was 63% in one study. Plasma levels peak within 2 hours of a dose.
Distribution: Finasteride is about 90% bound to plasma proteins. Drug crosses the blood-brain barrier.

Reactions may be *common,* uncommon, *life-threatening,* or COMMON AND LIFE-THREATENING.

Metabolism: Drug is extensively metabolized by the liver; at least 2 metabolites have been identified. Metabolites are responsible for less than 20% of the drug's total activity.

Excretion: About 39% of an oral dose is excreted in urine as metabolites; 57% in feces. No unchanged drug is found in urine.

CONTRAINDICATIONS & PRECAUTIONS

Contraindicated in patients who are hypersensitive to finasteride.

INTERACTIONS

Drug-drug. Small, insignificant increases in *theophylline* clearance and decreased half-life (10%) have been observed.

ADVERSE REACTIONS

GU: impotence, decreased volume of ejaculate.
Other: decreased libido.

回 KEY CONSIDERATIONS

• Although drug's elimination rate is decreased in geriatric patients, dosage adjustments are unnecessary.
• Closely evaluate patient before therapy for conditions that might mimic BPH, including hypotonic bladder, prostate cancer, infection, stricture, or other neurologic conditions.
• Continue therapy for a minimum of 6 months because it isn't possible to predict which patients will respond to finasteride.
• Carefully monitor patients who have large residual urine volumes or severely diminished urine flow. Not all patients respond to drug, and these patients may not be candidates for finasteride therapy.
• Note that long-term effects of drug on the complications of BPH, including acute urinary obstruction, or the incidence of surgery are unknown.
• Note that dosage adjustments are unnecessary in patients with renal impairment. Decreased excretion of metabolites in urine is associated with increased excretion of metabolites in feces.
• Evaluate carefully any sustained increases in serum prostate-specific antigen (PSA). In patients receiving finas-

teride therapy, this could indicate non-compliance to therapy.
• Note that current investigations aim to determine drug's effectiveness as adjuvant therapy after radical prostatectomy; as adjunctive treatment of prostate cancer; and in acne and hirsutism.
• Finasteride will decrease levels of PSA even in prostate cancer. This doesn't indicate a beneficial effect.

Patient education

• Explain to male patients that drug may decrease the volume of ejaculate but doesn't appear to impair normal sexual function. However, impotence and decreased libido have occurred in less than 4% of patients treated with drug.
• Inform patient that Propecia is indicated for the treatment of male-pattern hair loss in men only. It isn't indicated for use in women.

flecainide acetate
Tambocor

Benzamide derivative local anesthetic (amide), ventricular antiarrhythmic

Available by prescription only
Tablets: 50 mg, 100 mg, 150 mg

INDICATIONS & DOSAGE
Life-threatening ventricular tachycardia and PVCs
Adults: 100 mg P.O. q 12 hours; may increase in increments of 50 mg b.i.d. q 4 days until efficacy is achieved. Maximum dosage is 400 mg daily.
Paroxysmal supraventricular tachycardia, paroxysmal atrial fibrillation or flutter in patients without structural heart disease
Adults: 50 mg P.O. q 12 hours; may increase in increments of 50 mg b.i.d. q 4 days until efficacy is achieved. Maximum dosage is 300 mg/day.
✦ Dosage adjustment. Reduce dosage in patients with renal impairment (creatinine clearance less than 35 ml/minute/ $1.73 m^2$) beginning at 100 mg/day (50 mg b.i.d.); increase dosage cautiously at intervals longer than 4 days. For pa-

tients with less severe renal failure, initial dose is 100 mg q 12 hours, increasing cautiously at intervals longer than 4 days.

PHARMACODYNAMICS

Antiarrhythmic action: A class IC antiarrhythmic agent, flecainide suppresses SA node automaticity and prolongs conduction in the atria, AV node, ventricles, accessory pathways, and His-Purkinje system. It has the most pronounced effect on the His-Purkinje system, as shown by QRS complex widening; this leads to a prolonged QT interval. The drug has relatively little effect on action-potential duration except in Purkinje's fibers, where it shortens it. A proarrhythmic (arrhythmogenic) effect may result from the drug's potent effects on the conduction system. Effects on the sinus node are strongest in patients with sinus node disease (sick sinus syndrome). Flecainide also exerts a moderate negative inotropic effect.

PHARMACOKINETICS

Absorption: Flecainide is rapidly and almost completely absorbed from the GI tract; bioavailability of commercially available tablets is 85% to 90%. Plasma levels usually peak within 2 to 3 hours.
Distribution: Drug is apparently well distributed throughout the body. Only about 40% binds to plasma proteins. Trough serum levels ranging from 0.2 to 1 μg/ml provide the greatest therapeutic benefit. Trough serum levels higher than 0.7 μg/ml have been associated with increased adverse effects.
Metabolism: Drug is metabolized in the liver to inactive metabolites. About 30% of an orally administered dose escapes metabolism and is excreted in the urine unchanged.
Excretion: Elimination half-life averages about 20 hours. Plasma half-life may be prolonged in patients with heart failure and renal disease.

CONTRAINDICATIONS & PRECAUTIONS

Contraindicated in patients with hypersensitivity to flecainide or with cardiogenic shock and in those with preexisting second- or third-degree AV block or right bundle branch block when associated with a left hemiblock (in the absence of an artificial pacemaker).

Use cautiously in patients with heart failure, cardiomyopathy, severe renal or hepatic disease, prolonged QT interval, sick sinus syndrome, or blood dyscrasia.

Tambocor has demonstrated proarrhythmic effects in patients with atrial fibrillation or flutter; it isn't recommended for use in these patients.

INTERACTIONS

Drug-drug. Use with *acidifying and alkalizing drugs* changes urine pH, which in turn alters flecainide elimination; alkalization decreases renal flecainide excretion, and acidification increases it. When drugs that can markedly affect urine acidity (such as *ammonium chloride*) or alkalinity (such as *carbonic anhydrase inhibitors, high-dose antacids, sodium bicarbonate*) are given, monitor for possible subtherapeutic or toxic levels and effects.

Other *antiarrhythmics* may cause additive, synergistic, or antagonistic cardiac effects and may cause additive adverse effects—for example, *amiodarone* may increase serum flecainide levels, *disopyramide* may cause an additive negative inotropic effect, and *verapamil* may have an additive negative inotropic effect and may exacerbate AV nodal dysfunction. Use with *beta blockers* (such as *propranolol*) may cause additive negative inotropic effects. *Cimetidine* may decrease both the renal and nonrenal clearance of flecainide. Use with *digoxin* may cause increased serum digoxin levels.

ADVERSE REACTIONS

CNS: *dizziness, headache,* fatigue, tremor, anxiety, insomnia, depression, malaise, paresthesia, ataxia, vertigo, *light-headedness, syncope,* asthenia.
CV: *new or worsened arrhythmias,* chest pain, flushing, edema, *heart failure, cardiac arrest,* palpitations.
EENT: *blurred vision and other visual disturbances.*
GI: nausea, constipation, abdominal pain, dyspepsia, vomiting, diarrhea, anorexia.
Respiratory: *dyspnea.*

Reactions may be *common*, uncommon, *life-threatening*, or COMMON AND LIFE-THREATENING.

Skin: rash.
Other: fever.

◙ KEY CONSIDERATIONS

• Geriatric patients may be more susceptible to adverse effects. Monitor patient carefully.

• Note that Tambocor has been associated with excessive mortality or nonfatal cardiac arrest in national multicenter trials. Restrict its use to those patients in whom the benefits outweigh the risks.

• Note that Tambocor is a strong negative inotrope and may cause or worsen heart failure, especially in those with cardiomyopathy, preexisting heart failure, or low ejection fraction.

• Note that hypokalemia or hyperkalemia may alter drug effects and should be corrected before drug therapy begins.

• Initiate therapy in the hospital with careful monitoring of patients who have symptomatic heart failure, sinus node dysfunction, sustained ventricular tachycardia, or underlying structural heart disease, and in patients changing from another antiarrhythmic in whom discontinuation of current antiarrhythmic is likely to cause life-threatening arrhythmias.

• Loading doses may exacerbate arrhythmias and aren't recommended. Make dosage adjustments at intervals of at least 4 days because of drug's long half-life.

• Note that most patients need the drug every 12 hours, but some need it every 8 hours.

• Use twice-daily dosing to improve patient compliance.

• Note that full therapeutic effect may take 3 to 5 days. I.V. lidocaine may be administered while awaiting full effect.

• Flecainide is a class IC antiarrhythmic. Incidence of adverse effects increases when trough serum drug levels exceed 0.7 µg/ml. Periodically monitor blood levels, especially in patients with renal failure or heart failure. Therapeutic levels range from 0.2 to 1.0 µg/ml.

• Note that drug may increase short- and long-term endocardial pacing thresholds and may suppress ventricular escape rhythms. Pacing threshold should be determined before drug is administered, after 1 week of therapy, and regularly thereafter. Drug shouldn't be given to patients with preexisting poor thresholds or nonprogrammable artificial pacemakers unless pacing rescue is available.

• In heart failure and myocardial dysfunction, don't exceed initial dosage of 100 mg every 12 hours; common initial dosage is 50 mg every 12 hours.

• Use in hepatic impairment hasn't been fully evaluated; however, because flecainide is metabolized extensively (probably in the liver), it should be used in patients with significant hepatic impairment only when benefits clearly outweigh risks. Dosage reduction may be necessary, and patients should be monitored carefully for signs of toxicity. Serum levels also must be monitored.

Overdose & treatment

• Signs and symptoms of overdose include increased PR and QT intervals, increased QRS complex duration, decreased myocardial contractility, conduction disturbances, and hypotension.

• Treatment generally involves symptomatic and supportive measures along with ECG, blood pressure, and respiratory monitoring. Inotropic agents, including dopamine and dobutamine, may be used. Hemodynamic support, including use of an intra-aortic balloon pump and transvenous pacing, may be needed. Because of drug's long half-life, supportive measures may be needed for extended periods. Hemodialysis is ineffective in reducing serum drug levels.

---

fluconazole
Diflucan

Bis-triazole derivative, antifungal

Available by prescription only
Tablets: 50 mg, 100 mg, 150 mg, 200 mg
Injection: 200 mg/100 ml, 400 mg/200 ml
Suspension: 350 mg/35 ml, 1,400 mg/35 ml

INDICATIONS & DOSAGE

Oropharyngeal and esophageal candidiasis

Adults: 200 mg P.O. or I.V. on day 1 followed by 100 mg P.O. or I.V. once daily. As much as 400 mg/day has been used for esophageal disease. Treatment should continue for at least 2 weeks after resolution of symptoms.

Systemic candidiasis

Adults: Up to 400 mg P.O. or I.V. once daily. Treatment should continue for at least 2 weeks after resolution of symptoms.

Cryptococcal meningitis

Adults: 400 mg I.V. or P.O. on day 1, followed by 200 mg once daily. Continue treatment for 10 to 12 weeks after CSF culture becomes negative. For suppression of relapse in patients with AIDS, give 200 mg once daily.

Vaginal candidiasis

Adults: 150 mg P.O. as a single dose.

Urinary tract infection or peritonitis

Adults: 50 to 200 mg P.O. or I.V. daily.

Prophylaxis in patients undergoing bone marrow transplantation

Adults: 400 mg P.O. or I.V. daily for several days before transplantation and 7 days after neutrophil count rises above $1,000/mm^3$.

◇ *Candidal infection, long-term suppression in patients with HIV infection*
Adults: 100 to 200 mg P.O. or I.V. daily.

◇ *Prophylaxis against mucocutaneous candidiasis, cryptococcosis, coccidioidomycosis, or histoplasmosis in patients with HIV infection*
Adults: 200 to 400 mg P.O. or I.V. daily.

✦ *Dosage adjustment.* Patients receiving hemodialysis should receive one full dose after each session.

Creatinine clearance (ml/min)	Percentage of usual adult dosage
> 50	100
21-49	50
11-20	25

PHARMACODYNAMICS

Antifungal action: Fluconazole exerts its fungistatic effects by inhibiting fungal cytochrome P-450 and interfering with sterols in the fungal cell. The spectrum of activity includes *Cryptococcus neoformans, Candida* sp. (including systemic *C. albicans*), *Aspergillus flavus, A. fumigatus, Coccidioides immitis,* and *Histoplasma capsulatum.*

PHARMACOKINETICS

Absorption: After oral administration, absorption is rapid and complete. After an oral dose, plasma levels peak in 1 to 2 hours.

Distribution: Fluconazole is well distributed to various sites, including CNS, saliva, sputum, blister fluid, urine, normal skin, nails, and blister skin. CNS levels approach 50% to 90% of that of serum. Fluconazole is 12% protein-bound.

Metabolism: Drug is partially metabolized.

Elimination: Drug is primarily excreted via the kidneys. More than 80% of an administered dose is excreted unchanged in the urine. Excretion rate diminishes as renal function decreases.

CONTRAINDICATIONS & PRECAUTIONS

Contraindicated in patients with hypersensitivity to fluconazole and other drugs in the same classification.

INTERACTIONS

Drug-drug. Fluconazole may interact with *cisapride,* causing prolongation of the QT interval and resulting in arrhythmias and serious CV effects. Use with *cimetidine* may reduce serum fluconazole levels. Fluconazole may increase *cyclosporine* levels and may enhance the hypoprothrombinemic effects of *warfarin.* Fluconazole has been shown to increase the hypoglycemic effects of the sulfonylureas *glipizide, glyburide*, and *tolbutamide. Hydrochlorothiazide* decreases clearance of fluconazole, raising serum drug levels. The incidence of elevated hepatic transaminase levels is higher in patients taking *isoniazid, phenytoin, rifampin, sulfonylureas,* or *valproic acid.* Use with *phenytoin* may significantly increase serum phenytoin levels. *Rifampin* can lower fluconazole levels.

Reactions may be *common,* uncommon, *life-threatening,* or COMMON AND LIFE-THREATENING.

ADVERSE REACTIONS

CNS: headache.
GI: *nausea,* vomiting, abdominal pain, diarrhea.
Hepatic: *hepatotoxicity* (rare), elevated liver enzyme levels.
Skin: rash, *Stevens-Johnson syndrome* (rare).
Other: *anaphylaxis.*

▣ KEY CONSIDERATIONS

• Adjust dose in patients with renal dysfunction.
• Increased liver transaminase serum levels may occur with fluconazole.
• Fluconazole is incompatible with other I.V. drugs.
• Bioavailability of oral drug is comparable to I.V. dosing. Administer drug via oral route whenever possible.
• Adverse reactions (including transaminase elevations) are more frequent and more severe in patients with severe underlying illness (including AIDS and malignancies).

flucytosine (5-FC)
Ancobon

Fluorinated pyrimidine, antifungal

Available by prescription only
Capsules: 250 mg, 500 mg

INDICATIONS & DOSAGE

***Severe fungal infections caused by susceptible strains of* Candida *and* Cryptococcus**
Adults weighing more than 50 kg (110 lb): 50 to 150 mg/kg/day P.O., administered in divided doses q 6 hours.
Adults weighing less than 50 kg (110 lb): 1.5 to 4.5 g/m²/day in four divided doses P.O.
◊ ***Chromoblastomycosis***
Adults: 150 mg/kg P.O. daily.
✦ *Dosage adjustment.* For patients with renal failure who have a creatinine clearance of 50 ml/minute or less, reduce dosage by 20% to 80%. For patients with a creatinine clearance of 20 to 40 ml/minute, increase dosage interval to q 12 hours; creatinine clearance of 10 to 20 ml/minute, increase dosage interval

to q 24 hours; and for those with creatinine clearance less than 10 ml/minute, increase dosage interval to q 24 to 48 hours. Serum levels should be monitored. Flucytosine is removed by hemodialysis and peritoneal dialysis.
Dosage of 20 to 50 mg/kg P.O. immediately after hemodialysis q 2 to 3 days ensures therapeutic blood levels.

PHARMACODYNAMICS

Antifungal action: Flucytosine penetrates fungal cells, where it's converted to fluorouracil, which interferes with pyrimidine metabolism; it also may be converted to fluorodeoxyuredylic acid, which interferes with DNA synthesis. Because human cells lack the enzymes needed to convert drug to these toxic metabolites, flucytosine is selectively toxic to fungal, not host cells. It's active against some strains of *Cryptococcus* and *Candida.*

PHARMACOKINETICS

Absorption: About 75% to 90% of an oral dose is absorbed. Plasma levels peak 2 to 6 hours after a dose. Food decreases rate of absorption.
Distribution: Drug is distributed widely into the liver, kidneys, spleen, heart, bronchial secretions, joints, peritoneal fluid, and aqueous humor. CSF levels vary from 60% to 100% of serum levels. Drug is 2% to 4% bound to plasma proteins.
Metabolism: Only small amounts of flucytosine are metabolized.
Excretion: About 75% to 95% of a dose is excreted unchanged in urine; less than 10% is excreted unchanged in feces. Serum half-life is 2½ to 6 hours with normal renal function; as long as 1,160 hours with creatinine clearance less than 2 ml/minute.

CONTRAINDICATIONS & PRECAUTIONS

Contraindicated in patients with hypersensitivity to flucytosine. Use cautiously in patients with impaired renal or hepatic function and bone marrow suppression.

INTERACTIONS

Drug-drug. Flucytosine potentiates the efficacy and toxicity of *amphotericin B.*

Drug-lifestyle. *Photosensitivity* reaction may occur; take precautions.

ADVERSE REACTIONS
CNS: headache, vertigo, sedation, fatigue, weakness, confusion, hallucinations, psychosis, ataxia, hearing loss, paresthesia, parkinsonism, peripheral neuropathy.
CV: chest pain, *cardiac arrest.*
GI: nausea, vomiting, diarrhea, abdominal pain, dry mouth, duodenal ulcer, *hemorrhage,* ulcerative colitis.
GU: azotemia, elevated creatinine and BUN levels, crystalluria, *renal failure.*
Hematologic: anemia, *leukopenia, bone marrow suppression, thrombocytopenia,* eosinophilia, *agranulocytosis, aplastic anemia.*
Hepatic: elevated liver enzyme and serum alkaline phosphatase levels, jaundice.
Metabolic: hypoglycemia, hypokalemia.
Respiratory: *respiratory arrest,* dyspnea.
Skin: occasional rash, pruritus, urticaria, photosensitivity.

▣ KEY CONSIDERATIONS
• Perform hematologic studies and renal and hepatic function studies before therapy and repeat frequently thereafter to evaluate dosage and monitor for adverse effects.
• Give capsules over a 15-minute period to reduce nausea, vomiting, and GI distress.
• Monitor intake and output to ensure adequate renal function.
• Flucytosine causes falsely elevated creatinine values on aminohydrolase enzymatic assay. Drug may increase alkaline phosphatase, AST, ALT, BUN, and serum creatinine levels and may decrease WBC, RBC, and platelet counts.

Patient education
• Teach patient the signs and symptoms of adverse reactions and the need to report them.
• Tell patient to call promptly if urine output decreases or signs of bleeding or bruising occur.
• Advise patient that photosensitivity reaction may occur.

• Explain that an adequate response may require several weeks or months of therapy. Advise patient to follow medical regimen and to return as instructed for follow-up visits.

Overdose & treatment
• Flucytosine overdose may affect CV and pulmonary function.
• Treatment is largely supportive. If within 4 hours after ingestion, induce vomiting or perform gastric lavage. Activated charcoal and osmotic cathartics also may be helpful. Flucytosine is readily removed by either hemodialysis or peritoneal dialysis.
• Flucytosine is usually given with amphotericin B because they're synergistic.
• Protect drug from light.
• Because drug is removed by hemodialysis, adjust dosage in patients undergoing hemodialysis.
• Prolonged serum levels in excess of 100 mcg/ml may be associated with toxicity; monitor serum levels, especially in patients with renal insufficiency.

---

fludarabine phosphate
Fludara

Antimetabolite, antineoplastic

Available by prescription only
Injection: 50 mg as lyophilized powder

INDICATIONS & DOSAGE
Treatment of B-cell chronic lymphocytic leukemia (CLL) in patients who haven't responded or responded inadequately to at least one standard alkylating drug regimen, ◊ ***mycosis fungoides,*** ◊ ***hairy-cell leukemia,*** ◊ ***Hodgkin's and malignant lymphoma***
Adults: Usually, 25 mg/m² I.V. over 30 minutes (◊ rapid I.V. injection or continuous I.V. infusion) for 5 consecutive days q 28 days. Therapy is based on patient response and tolerance.
◊ ***Chronic lymphocytic leukemia***
Adults: Usually, 18 to 30 mg/m² I.V. over 30 minutes (◊ rapid I.V. injection or continuous I.V. infusion) for 5 consecutive days q 28 days. Therapy based on patient response and tolerance.

Reactions may be *common,* uncommon, *life-threatening,* or COMMON AND LIFE-THREATENING.

PHARMACODYNAMICS

Antineoplastic action: After rapid conversion of fludarabine to its active metabolite, the metabolite appears to inhibit DNA synthesis by inhibiting DNA polymerase alpha, ribonucleotide reductase, and DNA primase. The exact mechanism of action isn't fully established.

PHARMACOKINETICS

Absorption: Fludarabine is administered I.V.
Distribution: Drug is widely distributed, with a volume of distribution of 96 to 98 L/m^2 at steady state.
Metabolism: Drug is rapidly dephosphorylated and then phosphorylated intracellularly to its active metabolite.
Excretion: About 23% is excreted in urine as unchanged active metabolite. Half-life is about 10 hours.

CONTRAINDICATIONS & PRECAUTIONS

Contraindicated in patients hypersensitive to fludarabine or its components. Use cautiously in patients with renal insufficiency.

INTERACTIONS

Drug-drug. Use with other *myelosuppressives* may cause additive toxicity.

ADVERSE REACTIONS

CNS: *fatigue, malaise, weakness, paresthesia,* peripheral neuropathy, headache, sleep disorder, depression, cerebellar syndrome, CVA, agitation, *confusion, coma.*
CV: *edema,* angina, transient ischemic attack, phlebitis, *arrhythmias,* **heart failure,** supraventricular tachycardia, deep venous thrombosis, **aneurysm,** hemorrhage.
EENT: *visual disturbances,* hearing loss, delayed blindness (with high doses), sinusitis, pharyngitis, epistaxis.
GI: *nausea, vomiting, diarrhea,* constipation, *anorexia,* stomatitis, **GI bleeding,** esophagitis, mucositis.
GU: *dysuria,* urinary tract infection, urinary hesitancy, proteinuria, hematuria, renal failure.
Hematologic: *myelosuppression.*
Hepatic: liver failure, cholelithiasis.

Metabolic: hypocalcemia, hyperkalemia, hyperglycemia, hyperuricemia, hyperphosphatemia.
Musculoskeletal: *myalgia.*
Respiratory: *cough, pneumonia, dyspnea, upper respiratory tract infection,* allergic pneumonitis, hemoptysis, hypoxia, bronchitis.
Skin: alopecia, rash, pruritus, seborrhea.
Other: *fever, chills, infection, pain,* tumor lysis syndrome, **anaphylaxis, death** (with very high doses), diaphoresis, dehydration.

▣ KEY CONSIDERATIONS

● Advanced age may increase toxicity potential.
● Drug has been used investigationally in the treatment of malignant lymphoma, macroglobulinemic lymphoma, prolymphocytic leukemia or prolymphocytoid variant of CLL, mycosis fungoides, hairy cell leukemia, and Hodgkin's disease.
● Drug should be administered under the direct supervision of a health care provider experienced in antineoplastic therapy.
● Careful hematologic monitoring is required, especially of neutrophil and platelet counts.
● Tumor lysis syndrome (hyperuricemia, hyperphosphatemia, hypocalcemia, metabolic acidosis, hyperkalemia, hematuria, urate crystalluria, and renal failure) has occurred in CLL patients with large tumors.
● Severe neurologic effects, including blindness, are seen when high doses are used to treat acute leukemia.
● Advanced age, renal insufficiency, and bone marrow impairment may predispose patient to severe toxicity; toxic effects are dose-dependent.
● Optimal duration of therapy hasn't been established; three additional cycles after achieving maximal response are recommended before discontinuing drug.
● To prepare, add 2 ml of sterile water for injection to the solid cake of fludarabine. Dissolution should occur within 15 seconds, and each milliliter will contain 25 mg of drug and 25 mg of mannitol. Use within 8 hours of reconstitution.

Fludarabine has been further diluted in 100 ml or 125 ml of D_5W or normal saline solution.
• Follow institutional protocol and guidelines for proper handling and disposal of chemotherapeutic agents.
• Store drug in refrigerator at 35.6° to 46.4° F (2° to 8°C).
• Irreversible CNS toxicity characterized by delayed blindness, coma, and death is associated with high doses. Severe thrombocytopenia and neutropenia secondary to bone marrow suppression also occur. There is no specific antidote, and treatment consists of discontinuing therapy and taking supportive measures.

Patient education
• Tell patient to avoid contact with infected persons and to report signs of infection or unusual bleeding immediately.

fludrocortisone acetate
Florinef

Mineralocorticoid, glucocorticoid, mineralocorticoid replacement

Available by prescription only
Tablets: 0.1 mg

INDICATIONS & DOSAGE
Adrenal insufficiency (partial replacement), salt-losing adrenogenital syndrome
Adults: 0.1 to 0.2 mg P.O. daily.
Postural hypotension in diabetic patients, ◊ orthostatic hypotension
Adults: 0.1 to 0.4 mg P.O. daily.
Postural hypotension due to levodopa therapy
Adults: 0.05 to 0.2 mg P.O. daily.

PHARMACODYNAMICS
Adrenal hormone replacement action: Fludrocortisone, a synthetic glucocorticoid with potent mineralocorticoid activity, is used for partial replacement of steroid hormones in adrenocortical insufficiency and in salt-losing forms of congenital adrenogenital syndrome. In treating adrenocortical insufficiency, an exogenous glucocorticoid must also be administered for adequate control. (Cor-

tisone or hydrocortisone is usually the drug of choice for replacement because they produce both mineralocorticoid and glucocorticoid activity.) Fludrocortisone is administered on a variable schedule ranging from three times weekly to twice daily, depending on individual requirements.

PHARMACOKINETICS
Absorption: Fludrocortisone is absorbed readily from the GI tract.
Distribution: Drug is removed rapidly from blood and distributed to muscle, liver, skin, intestines, and kidneys. It has a plasma half-life of about 30 minutes. It's extensively bound to plasma proteins (transcortin and albumin). Only the unbound portion is active.
Metabolism: Drug is metabolized in the liver to inactive glucuronide and sulfate metabolites.
Excretion: Inactive metabolites and small amounts of unmetabolized drug are excreted by the kidneys. Insignificant quantities of drug are also excreted in feces. Biological half-life is 18 to 36 hours; plasma half-life is 3½ hours or more.

CONTRAINDICATIONS & PRECAUTIONS
Contraindicated in patients with systemic fungal infections or hypersensitivity to drug.

Use cautiously in patients with hypothyroidism, cirrhosis, ocular herpes simplex, emotional instability, psychotic tendencies, nonspecific ulcerative colitis, diverticulitis, fresh intestinal anastomoses, peptic ulcer, renal insufficiency, hypertension, osteoporosis, and myasthenia gravis.

INTERACTIONS
Drug-drug. Fludrocortisone may enhance hypokalemia caused by *amphotericin B* or *diuretic* therapy; the hypokalemia may increase the risk of toxicity in patients concurrently receiving *cardiac glycosides.* Use with *barbiturates, phenytoin,* or *rifampin* may decrease corticosteroid effects because of increased hepatic metabolism. Fludrocortisone may increase the metabolism of *isoniazid* and *salicylates.*

Reactions may be *common*, uncommon, *life-threatening*, or COMMON AND LIFE-THREATENING.

ADVERSE REACTIONS

CV: *sodium and water retention,* hypertension, cardiac hypertrophy, edema, *heart failure.*

Metabolic: hypokalemia.

Skin: bruising, diaphoresis, urticaria, allergic rash.

▣ KEY CONSIDERATIONS

Besides the recommendations relevant to all systemic adrenocorticoids, consider the following:

• Use only with other supplemental measures, such as glucocorticoids, control of electrolytes, and control of infection.

• Anticipate giving supplemental dosages in times of physiological stress from serious illness, trauma, or surgery.

• Monitor patient for significant weight gain, edema, hypertension, or severe headaches.

• Drug therapy increases serum sodium levels and decreases serum potassium levels. Glucose tolerance tests should be performed only if necessary because addisonian patients tend to develop severe hypoglycemia within 3 hours of the test.

Patient education

• Teach patient to recognize the signs of electrolyte imbalance: muscle weakness, paresthesia, numbness, fatigue, anorexia, nausea, altered mental status, increased urination, altered heart rhythm, severe or continuing headaches, unusual weight gain, or swelling of the feet.

• Tell patient to take missed doses as soon as possible unless it's almost time for the next dose and not to double-dose.

Overdose & treatment

• Acute toxicity produces such effects as disturbances in fluid and electrolyte balance, hypokalemia, edema, hypertension, and cardiac insufficiency.

• In acute toxicity, administer symptomatic treatment and correct fluid and electrolyte imbalance.

flumazenil
Romazicon

Benzodiazepine antagonist, antidote

Available by prescription only
Injection: 0.1 mg/ml in 5-ml and 10-ml multiple-dose vials

INDICATIONS & DOSAGE

Complete or partial reversal of the sedative effects of benzodiazepines after anesthesia or short diagnostic procedures (conscious sedation)

Adults: Initially, 0.2 mg I.V. over 15 seconds. If patient doesn't reach desired level of consciousness after 45 seconds, repeat dose. Repeat at 1-minute intervals until a cumulative dose of 1 mg has been given (initial dose plus four additional doses). Most patients respond after 0.6 to 1 mg of drug. If resedation occurs, dosage may be repeated after 20 minutes, but no more than 1 mg should be given at one time, and patient shouldn't receive more than 3 mg/hour.

Management of suspected benzodiazepine overdose

Adults: Initially, 0.2 mg I.V. over 30 seconds. If patient doesn't reach desired level of consciousness after 30 seconds, administer 0.3 mg over 30 seconds. If patient still doesn't respond adequately, give 0.5 mg over 30 seconds; then repeat 0.5-mg doses at 1-minute intervals until a cumulative dose of 3 mg has been given. Most patients with benzodiazepine overdose respond to cumulative doses between 1 and 3 mg; rarely, patients who respond partially after 3 mg may require additional doses. Don't give more than 5 mg over 5 minutes initially; sedation that persists after this dosage is unlikely to be caused by benzodiazepines. If resedation occurs, dosage may be repeated after 20 minutes, but no more than 1 mg should be given at one time, and patient shouldn't receive more than 3 mg/hour.

PHARMACODYNAMICS

Antidote action: Flumazenil competitively inhibits the actions of benzodiazepines on the gamma-aminobutyric acid-benzodiazepine receptor complex.

PHARMACOKINETICS

Absorption: Flumazenil is administered I.V. only.

Distribution: After administration, drug redistributes rapidly (initial distribution half-life is 7 to 15 minutes). It's about 50% bound to plasma proteins.

Metabolism: Drug is rapidly extracted from the blood and metabolized by the liver. Metabolites that have been identified are inactive. Ingestion of food during an I.V. infusion enhances extraction of drug from plasma, probably by increasing hepatic blood flow.

Excretion: About 90% to 95% appears in the urine as metabolites; the rest is excreted in the feces. Plasma half-life is about 54 minutes.

CONTRAINDICATIONS & PRECAUTIONS

Contraindicated in patients who are hypersensitive to flumazenil or benzodiazepines, in patients who show evidence of serious tricyclic antidepressant overdose, and in those who received a benzodiazepine to treat a potentially life-threatening condition (such as status epilepticus).

Use cautiously in alcohol-dependent or psychiatric patients, in those at high risk for developing seizures, or in those with head injuries, signs of seizures, or recent high intake of benzodiazepines (such as patients in the intensive care unit).

INTERACTIONS

Drug-drug. Flumazenil shouldn't be used in an overdose involving several drugs because it can obscure symptoms of poisoning by *drugs that can cause seizures or arrhythmias,* such as *antidepressants.* Seizures or arrhythmias can develop after flumazenil removes the effects of the benzodiazepine overdose.

ADVERSE REACTIONS

CNS: *dizziness, abnormal or blurred vision, headache, seizures,* agitation, emotional lability, tremor, insomnia.
CV: *arrhythmias,* cutaneous vasodilation, palpitations.
GI: nausea, vomiting.
Respiratory: dyspnea, hyperventilation.
Other: *diaphoresis, pain* (at injection site).

🔲 KEY CONSIDERATIONS

● Onset of action is usually evident within 1 to 2 minutes of injection, and peak effect occurs within 6 to 10 minutes. Because duration of action of flumazenil is shorter than that of benzodiazepines, monitor patient carefully and administer additional drug as needed. Duration and degree of effect depend on plasma levels of the sedating benzodiazepine and the dose of flumazenil.

● To minimize pain at injection site, give the drug through a freely flowing I.V. solution running into a large vein. Compatible solutions include D_5W, lactated Ringer's injection, or normal saline solution.

● Resedation may occur after reversal of benzodiazepine effect because flumazenil has a shorter duration of action than that of benzodiazepines. Patients should be monitored for resedation according to duration of drug being reversed. Monitor closely after long-acting benzodiazepines (such as diazepam) or after high doses of shorter-acting benzodiazepines (such as 10 mg of midazolam). Usually, serious resedation is unlikely in patients who fail to show signs of resedation 2 hours after a 1-mg dose of flumazenil.

● Don't expect patients to recall information from the postprocedure period because drug doesn't reverse the amnesiac effects of benzodiazepines. Therefore, give important instructions to the family or caregiver or in writing to the patient.

Patient education

● Because of risk of resedation, advise patient to avoid hazardous activities (such as driving a car), alcohol, CNS depressants, and OTC drugs within 24 hours of the procedure.

Overdose & treatment

● In clinical trials, large doses of flumazenil were administered I.V. to volunteers in the absence of a benzodiazepine agonist. No serious adverse reactions, signs or symptoms, or altered laboratory tests were noted.

● In patients with benzodiazepine overdose, large doses of flumazenil may produce agitation or anxiety, hyperesthesia,

---

Reactions may be *common,* uncommon, *life-threatening,* or COMMON AND LIFE-THREATENING.

increased muscle tone, or seizures. Seizures may be treated with barbiturates, phenytoin, or benzodiazepines.
• Flumazenil can be administered by direct injection or diluted with a compatible solution. Discard within 24 hours unused drug that has been drawn into a syringe or diluted.

fluocinonide
Lidemol*, Lidex, Lidex-E, Lyderm*

Topical adrenocorticoid, anti-inflammatory

Available by prescription only
Cream, gel, ointment, solution: 0.05%

INDICATIONS & DOSAGE
Inflammation of corticosteroid-responsive dermatoses
Adults: Apply sparingly b.i.d. or t.i.d. Occlusive dressings may be used for severe or resistant dermatoses.

PHARMACODYNAMICS
Anti-inflammatory action: Fluocinonide stimulates the synthesis of enzymes needed to decrease the inflammatory response. Fluocinonide is a high-potency fluorinated glucocorticoid categorized as a group II topical steroid.

PHARMACOKINETICS
Absorption: Amount absorbed depends on amount applied and on nature of skin at application site. It ranges from about 1% in areas of thick stratum corneum (such as the palms, soles, elbows, and knees) to as high as 36% in areas of thin stratum corneum (face, eyelids, and genitals). Absorption increases in areas of skin damage, inflammation, or occlusion. Some systemic absorption of steroids occurs, especially through the oral mucosa.
Distribution: After topical application, drug is distributed throughout the local skin. Any drug absorbed into circulation is removed rapidly from the blood and distributed into muscle, liver, skin, intestines, and kidneys.
Metabolism: After topical administration, fluocinonide is metabolized primar-

ily in the skin. The small amount absorbed into the systemic circulation is metabolized primarily in the liver to inactive compounds.
Excretion: Inactive metabolites are excreted by the kidneys, primarily as glucuronides and sulfates, but also as unconjugated products. Small amounts of the metabolites are excreted in feces.

CONTRAINDICATIONS & PRECAUTIONS
Contraindicated in patients hypersensitive to fluocinonide.

INTERACTIONS
None significant.

ADVERSE REACTIONS
GU: glycosuria.
Metabolic: hyperglycemia.
Skin: burning, pruritus, irritation, dryness, erythema, folliculitis, hypertrichosis, hypopigmentation, acneiform eruptions, perioral dermatitis, allergic contact dermatitis; *maceration, secondary infection, atrophy, striae, miliaria* (with occlusive dressings).
Other: *hypothalamic-pituitary-adrenal axis suppression,* Cushing's syndrome.

▣ KEY CONSIDERATIONS
• Recommendations for use of fluocinonide and for care and teaching of patients during therapy are the same as those for all topical adrenocorticoids.

fluorouracil (5-FU)
Adrucil, Efudex

Antimetabolite (cell cycle–phase specific, S phase), antineoplastic

Available by prescription only
Injection: 50 mg/ml in 10-ml, 20-ml, 50-ml, and 100-ml vials
Cream: 1%, 5%
Topical solution: 1%, 2%, 5%

INDICATIONS & DOSAGE
Dosage and indications may vary. Check current literature for recommended protocol.

*Palliative management of colon, rectal,
breast, ◇ ovarian, ◇ cervical, gastric,
◇ bladder, ◇ liver, pancreatic cancers*
Adults: 12 mg/kg I.V. for 4 days; then if
no toxicity occurs, give 6 mg/kg I.V. on
days 6, 8, 10, and 12. Maintenance therapy is a repeated course q 30 days. Don't
exceed 800 mg/day (400 mg/day in severely ill patients).

Actinic or solar keratoses
Adults: Sufficient cream or lotion to cover lesions b.i.d. for 2 to 4 weeks. Usually,
1% preparations are used on head, neck,
and chest; 2% and 5% on hands.

Superficial basal cell carcinomas
Adults: 5% solution or cream in a sufficient amount to cover lesion b.i.d. for 3
to 6 weeks, up to 12 weeks.

PHARMACODYNAMICS
Antineoplastic action: Fluorouracil exerts its cytotoxic activity by acting as an
antimetabolite, competing for the enzyme that is important in the synthesis
of thymidine, an essential substrate for
DNA synthesis. Therefore, DNA synthesis is inhibited. Drug also inhibits RNA
synthesis to a lesser extent.

PHARMACOKINETICS
Absorption: Fluorouracil is given parenterally because it's absorbed poorly after oral administration.
Distribution: Drug distributes widely
into all areas of body water and tissues,
including tumors, bone marrow, liver,
and intestinal mucosa. Fluorouracil
crosses the blood-brain barrier to a significant extent.
Metabolism: A small amount is converted in the tissues to the active metabolite,
with most of drug degraded in the liver.
Excretion: Metabolites of fluorouracil
are primarily excreted through the lungs
as carbon dioxide. A small portion of a
dose is excreted in urine as unchanged
drug.

CONTRAINDICATIONS & PRECAUTIONS
Contraindicated in patients hypersensitive to fluorouracil, patients who are in a
poor nutritional state, patients with bone
marrow suppression (WBC counts of
5,000/mm³ or less or platelet counts of
100,000/mm³ or less), patients with po-

tentially serious infections, and in those
who have had major surgery within the
previous month.
   Use cautiously in patients after high-
dose pelvic radiation therapy or use of
alkylating agents. Also use with caution
in patients with widespread neoplastic
infiltration of bone marrow and impaired renal or hepatic function.

INTERACTIONS
Drug-drug. *Leucovorin calcium* may
enhance the toxicity of fluorouracil.
Drug-lifestyle. Photosensitivity reaction
may occur to *sunlight;* take precautions.

ADVERSE REACTIONS
CNS: acute cerebellar syndrome, confusion, disorientation, euphoria, ataxia,
headache, nystagmus, weakness,
malaise.
CV: myocardial ischemia, angina,
thrombophlebitis.
GI: stomatitis, GI ulcer (may precede
leukopenia), nausea, vomiting, diarrhea,
anorexia, GI bleeding.
Hematologic: leukopenia, thrombocytopenia, agranulocytosis, anemia; WBC
count nadir 9 to 14 days after first dose;
platelet count nadir in 7 to 14 days.
Skin: reversible alopecia, dermatitis;
erythema; scaling; pruritus; nail
changes; pigmented palmar creases; erythematous, contact dermatitis; desqua-
mative rash of hands and feet with long-
term use ("hand-foot syndrome").
Other: pain, burning, soreness, suppura-
tion, swelling (with topical use), *anaphylaxis.*

▣ KEY CONSIDERATIONS
• Drug may be administered I.V. push
over 1 to 2 minutes.
• Drug may be further diluted in D₅W or
normal saline solution for infusions lasting up to 24 hours.
• Use plastic I.V. containers for administering continuous infusions. Solution is
more stable in plastic I.V. bags than in
glass bottles.
• Don't use cloudy solution. If crystals
form, redissolve by warming at a temperature of 140° F (60° C) with vigorous
shaking. Allow solution to cool to body
temperature before using.

- Use new vein site for each dose.
- Fluorouracil may decrease plasma albumin level because of drug-induced protein malabsorption.
- Give antiemetic before administering to decrease nausea.
- If extravasation occurs, treat as a chemical phlebitis with warm compresses.
- Don't refrigerate fluorouracil.
- Drug can be diluted in 120 ml of water and administered orally; however, this isn't an FDA-approved method of administration, and absorption is erratic.
- General photosensitivity occurs for 2 to 3 months after a dose.
- Ingestion and systemic absorption may cause leukopenia, thrombocytopenia, stomatitis, diarrhea or GI ulceration, bleeding, and hemorrhage. A topical local anesthetic may be used to soothe mouth lesions. Encourage good and frequent mouth care.
- Monitor intake and output, CBC, and renal and hepatic function.
- Avoid I.M. injections in patients with low platelet counts.
- Use plastic gloves when applying topical drug. Wash hands immediately after handling drug. Avoid topical use with occlusive dressings.
- Apply topical solution with caution near eyes, nose, and mouth.
- Note that topical application to larger ulcerated areas may cause systemic toxicity.
- For superficial basal cell carcinoma confirmed by biopsy, use 5% strength. Apply 1% concentration on the face. Reserve higher concentrations for thicker-skinned areas or resistant lesions. Occlusion may be required.
- Don't continue to treat lesions resistant to fluorouracil; they should be biopsied.

Patient education
- Warn patient to avoid strong sunlight or ultraviolet light because it will intensify the skin reaction. Encourage use of sunscreens.
- Tell patient to avoid exposure to people with infections. Advise patient to promptly report signs of infection or unusual bleeding.
- Reassure patient that hair should grow back after treatment is discontinued.

- Tell patient to apply topical fluorouracil with gloves and to wash hands thoroughly after application.
- Warn patient that treated area may be unsightly during therapy and for several weeks after therapy is stopped. Complete healing may not occur until 1 to 2 months after treatment is stopped.

Overdose & treatment
- Signs and symptoms of overdose include myelosuppression, diarrhea, alopecia, dermatitis, hyperpigmentation, nausea, and vomiting.
- Treatment is usually supportive and includes transfusion of blood components, antiemetics, and antidiarrheals.

fluoxetine
Prozac, Prozac Pulvules

Selective serotonin reuptake inhibitor (SSRI), antidepressant

Available by prescription only
Capsules: 10 mg, 20 mg
Oral solution: 20 mg/5 ml

INDICATIONS & DOSAGE
Depression, ◇ *panic disorder;* ◇ *bipolar disorder;* ◇ *alcohol dependence;* ◇ *cataplexy;* ◇ *myoclonus*
Adults: 20 mg P.O. daily in the morning. Increase dosage, p.r.n., after several weeks to 40 mg daily with a dose in the morning and midday. Don't exceed 80 mg daily.
Depression in geriatric patients
Geriatric patients: 20 mg P.O. daily in the morning.
Obsessive-compulsive disorder
Adults: Initially, 20 mg P.O. daily. Gradually increase dosage, p.r.n., and as tolerated to 60 to 80 mg daily.
◇ *Obesity*
Adults: 20 to 60 mg P.O. daily.
◇ *Eating disorders*
Adults: 60 to 80 mg P.O. daily.

PHARMACODYNAMICS
Antidepressant action: The antidepressant action of fluoxetine is purportedly related to its inhibition of CNS neuronal uptake of serotonin. Fluoxetine blocks

uptake of serotonin, but not of norepinephrine, into human platelets. Animal studies suggest it's a much more potent uptake inhibitor of serotonin than of norepinephrine.

PHARMACOKINETICS

Absorption: Fluoxetine is well absorbed after oral administration. Food doesn't alter its absorption.
Distribution: Drug is highly protein-bound (about 95%).
Metabolism: Drug is metabolized primarily in the liver to active metabolites.
Excretion: Drug is excreted by the kidneys. Elimination half-life is 2 to 3 days. Norfluoxetine (the primary active metabolite) has an elimination half-life of 7 to 9 days.

CONTRAINDICATIONS & PRECAUTIONS

Contraindicated in patients hypersensitive to fluoxetine and in patients taking MAO inhibitors within 14 days of starting therapy. Use cautiously in patients at high risk of suicide or in those with a history of seizures, diabetes mellitus, or renal, hepatic, or CV disease.

INTERACTIONS

Drug-drug. Use with *diazepam* may prolong half-life of diazepam. Avoid administration with other *highly protein-bound drugs* (such as *warfarin*). Avoid administration with other *psychoactive drugs*—such as *antipsychotics* and *MAO inhibitors*. Use with *tryptophan* may lead to increased adverse CNS effects (agitation, restlessness) and GI distress.
Drug-lifestyle. *Alcohol* increases CNS depression; don't use together.

ADVERSE REACTIONS

CNS: *nervousness, anxiety, insomnia, headache, drowsiness, tremor, dizziness, asthenia,* fatigue.
CV: palpitations, hot flashes.
EENT: nasal congestion, pharyngitis, cough, sinusitis.
GI: *nausea, diarrhea, dry mouth, anorexia, dyspepsia,* constipation, abdominal pain, vomiting, flatulence, increased appetite.
GU: sexual dysfunction.
Metabolic: *weight loss.*

Musculoskeletal: muscle pain.
Respiratory: upper respiratory tract infection, respiratory distress.
Skin: *rash, pruritus,* diaphoresis.
Other: flulike syndrome, *fever.*

▣ KEY CONSIDERATIONS

• Consider the inherent risk of suicide until significant improvement of depressive state occurs. High-risk patients should have close supervision during initial drug therapy. To reduce risk of suicidal overdose, prescribe the smallest quantity of pulvules consistent with good management.
• Note that full antidepressant effect may be delayed until 4 weeks of treatment or longer.
• Note that treatment of acute depression usually requires at least several months of continuous drug therapy; optimal duration of therapy hasn't been established.
• Because of its long elimination half-life, changes in fluoxetine dosage won't be reflected in plasma for several weeks, affecting titration to final dose and withdrawal from treatment.
• Fluoxetine therapy may activate mania or hypomania.
• Use fluoxetine with caution in patients with liver disease. Impaired hepatic function can delay the elimination of fluoxetine and its metabolite norfluoxetine, prolonging the drug's elimination half-life.
• For patients with severely impaired renal function, know that long-term fluoxetine therapy may result in significant accumulation of drug or its metabolites.
• Prescribe lower or less frequent dosages in patients with renal or hepatic impairment. Also consider lower or less frequent dosages in geriatric patients and others with concurrent disease or multidrug therapy.

Patient education

• Inform patient that drug may cause dizziness or drowsiness. Patient should avoid hazardous tasks that require alertness until CNS response to drug is established.
• Caution patient to avoid ingestion of alcohol and to seek medical approval before taking other drugs.

Reactions may be *common,* uncommon, **life-threatening**, or COMMON AND LIFE-THREATENING.

• Tell patient to promptly report rash or hives, anxiety, nervousness, or anorexia (especially in underweight patients).

Overdose & treatment
• Signs and symptoms of overdose include agitation, restlessness, hypomania, and other signs of CNS excitation; and, in patients who take higher doses of fluoxetine, nausea and vomiting. Among 38 reports of acute overdose with fluoxetine, two fatalities involved plasma levels of 4.57 mg/L and 1.93 mg/L. One involved 1.8 g of fluoxetine with an undetermined amount of maprotiline; another death involved combined ingestion of fluoxetine, codeine, and temazepam. One other patient developed two tonic-clonic seizures after taking 3 g of fluoxetine; these seizures remitted spontaneously and didn't require treatment with anticonvulsants.
• To treat fluoxetine overdose, establish and maintain an airway and ensure adequate oxygenation and ventilation. Activated charcoal, which may be used with sorbitol, may be as effective as inducing vomiting or performing gastric lavage.
• Monitor cardiac and vital signs, and provide usual supportive measures. Fluoxetine-induced seizures that don't subside spontaneously may respond to diazepam. Forced diuresis, dialysis, hemoperfusion, and exchange transfusion are unlikely to be of benefit.

fluphenazine decanoate
Modecate Decanoate*, Prolixin Decanoate

fluphenazine enanthate
Moditen Enanthate*, Prolixin Enanthate

fluphenazine hydrochloride
Permitil Hydrochloride, Prolixin Hydrochloride

Phenothiazine (piperazine derivative), antipsychotic

Available by prescription only
fluphenazine decanoate
Depot injection: 25 mg/ml

fluphenazine enanthate
Depot injection: 25 mg/ml
fluphenazine hydrochloride
Tablets: 1 mg, 2.5 mg, 5 mg, 10 mg
Oral concentrate: 5 mg/ml (Prolixin contains 14% alcohol and Permitil contains 1% alcohol)
Elixir: 2.5 mg/5 ml (with 14% alcohol)
I.M. injection: 2.5 mg/ml

INDICATIONS & DOSAGE
Psychotic disorders
Adults: Initially, 0.5 to 10 mg fluphenazine hydrochloride P.O. daily in divided doses q 6 to 8 hours; may increase cautiously to 20 mg. Maintenance dosage is 1 to 5 mg P.O. daily. I.M. doses are one third to one half that of oral doses (starting dose is 1.25 mg I.M.).
Geriatric patients: Use lower doses (1 to 2.5 mg daily).

PHARMACODYNAMICS
Antipsychotic action: Fluphenazine is thought to exert its antipsychotic effects by postsynaptic blockade of CNS dopamine receptors, thereby inhibiting dopamine-mediated effects.

Fluphenazine has many other central and peripheral effects; it produces both alpha and ganglionic blockade and counteracts histamine- and serotonin-mediated activity. Its most prominent adverse reactions are extrapyramidal.

PHARMACOKINETICS
Absorption: Rate and extent of absorption vary with route of administration; oral tablet absorption is erratic and variable. Oral and I.M. dosages have an onset of action within 1 hour. Long-acting decanoate and enanthate salts act within 24 to 72 hours.
Distribution: Fluphenazine is distributed widely into the body. CNS levels are usually higher plasma levels. Drug is 91% to 99% protein-bound. Peak effects of oral dose usually occur at 2 hours; steady-state serum levels are achieved within 4 to 7 days.
Metabolism: Drug is metabolized extensively by the liver, but no active metabolites are formed. Duration of action is about 6 to 8 hours after oral administra-

tion; 1 to 6 weeks (average, 2 weeks) after I.M. depot administration.
Excretion: Drug is mostly excreted in urine via the kidneys; some is excreted in feces via the biliary tract.

CONTRAINDICATIONS & PRECAUTIONS

Contraindicated in patients with hypersensitivity to fluphenazine or in patients experiencing coma, CNS depression, bone marrow suppression or other blood dyscrasia, subcortical damage, or liver damage.

Use cautiously in geriatric or debilitated patients and in those with pheochromocytoma, severe CV disease, peptic ulcer disease, exposure to extreme hot or cold (including antipyretic therapy) or phosphorus insecticides, respiratory or seizure disorders, hypocalcemia, severe reaction to insulin or electroconvulsive therapy, mitral insufficiency, glaucoma, or prostatic hyperplasia. Use parenteral form cautiously in patients with asthma and those allergic to sulfites.

INTERACTIONS

Drug-drug. Additive effects are likely after use with the following drugs: *antiarrhythmics, disopyramide, procainamide,* and *quinidine,* (increased incidence of arrhythmias and conduction defects); *atropine* or other anticholinergics, including *antidepressants, antihistamines, antiparkinsonians, MAO inhibitors, meperidine,* and *phenothiazines* (oversedation, paralytic ileus, visual changes, and severe constipation); *CNS depressants*—including *analgesics, barbiturates, epidural, general, or spinal anesthetics, narcotics,* and *tranquilizers*— or *parenteral magnesium sulfate* (oversedation, respiratory depression, and hypotension); *metrizamide* (increased risk of seizures); and *nitrates* (hypotension).

Pharmacokinetic alterations and subsequent decreased therapeutic response to fluphenazine may follow use with *aluminum-* or *magnesium-containing antacids* or *antidiarrheals* (decreased absorption), *caffeine, heavy smoking* (increased metabolism), or *phenobarbital* (enhanced renal excretion). Use with *appetite suppressants* or *sympatho-*

mimetics—including *ephedrine* (found in many nasal sprays), *epinephrine, phenylephrine,* and *phenylpropanolamine*—may decrease their stimulatory and pressor effects. *Beta blockers* may inhibit fluphenazine metabolism, increasing plasma levels and toxicity. Fluphenazine may antagonize therapeutic effect of *bromocriptine* on prolactin secretion and may inhibit blood pressure response to *centrally acting antihypertensives* such as *clonidine, guanabenz, guanadrel, guanethidine, methyldopa,* and *reserpine.* Fluphenazine may also decrease the vasoconstrictive effects of high-dose *dopamine* and may decrease effectiveness and increase toxicity of *levodopa* (by dopamine blockade). Use with *lithium* may result in severe neurologic toxicity with an encephalitis-like syndrome and a decreased therapeutic response to fluphenazine. Fluphenazine may inhibit metabolism and increase toxicity of *phenytoin* and *tricyclic antidepressants.* Use with *propylthiouracil* increases risk of agranulocytosis.
Drug-lifestyle. *Alcohol* increases CNS depression; don't use together.

ADVERSE REACTIONS

CNS: extrapyramidal reactions, tardive dyskinesia, sedation, pseudoparkinsonism, EEG changes, drowsiness, seizures, dizziness.
CV: orthostatic hypotension, tachycardia, ECG changes.
EENT: ocular changes, blurred vision, nasal congestion.
GI: dry mouth, constipation, increased appetite.
GU: urine retention, dark urine, menstrual irregularities, gynecomastia, inhibited ejaculation.
Hematologic: leukopenia, agranulocytosis, eosinophilia, hemolytic anemia, aplastic anemia, thrombocytopenia.
Hepatic: cholestatic jaundice, abnormal liver function test results.
Metabolic: weight gain.
Skin: mild photosensitivity, allergic reactions.
Other: neuroleptic malignant syndrome (rare).

Reactions may be *common,* uncommon, **life-threatening**, or **COMMON AND LIFE-THREATENING**.

After abrupt withdrawal of long-term therapy: gastritis, nausea, vomiting, dizziness, tremor, feeling of warmth or cold, diaphoresis, tachycardia, headache, insomnia.

▣ KEY CONSIDERATIONS

Besides the recommendations relevant to all phenothiazines, consider the following:
• Note that depot injection (25 mg/ml) and I.M. injection (2.5 mg/ml) aren't interchangeable.
• Depot injection isn't recommended for patients who aren't stabilized on a phenothiazine. This form has a prolonged elimination time; its action can't be terminated in case of adverse reactions.
• Fluphenazine causes false-positive test results for urine porphyrins, urobilinogen, amylase, and 5-hydroxyindoleacetic acid because of darkening of urine by metabolites.
• Fluphenazine elevates test results for liver enzyme levels and protein-bound iodine and causes quinidine-like ECG effects.

Patient education

• Inform patient that drug may cause dizziness or drowsiness. Patient should avoid hazardous tasks that require alertness until CNS response to drug is established.
• Tell patient to avoid ingestion of alcohol and to seek medical approval before taking other drugs.
• Instruct patient to promptly report rash or hives, anxiety, nervousness, or anorexia (especially in underweight patients).

Overdose & treatment

• CNS depression is characterized by deep, unarousable sleep and possible coma, hypotension or hypertension, extrapyramidal symptoms, dystonia, abnormal involuntary muscle movements, agitation, seizures, arrhythmias, ECG changes, hypothermia or hyperthermia, and autonomic nervous system dysfunction.
• Treatment is symptomatic and supportive; maintain vital signs, airway, stable body temperature, and fluid and electrolyte balance.
• Don't induce vomiting: drug inhibits cough reflex, and aspiration may occur. Use gastric lavage, then activated charcoal and saline cathartics; dialysis doesn't help. Regulate body temperature as needed. Treat hypotension with I.V. fluids; don't give epinephrine. Treat seizures with parenteral diazepam or barbiturates; arrhythmias with parenteral phenytoin (1 mg/kg with rate titrated to blood pressure); extrapyramidal reactions with benztropine 1 to 2 mg or parenteral diphenhydramine at 10 to 50 mg.

---

flurazepam hydrochloride
Apo-Flurazepam*, Dalmane, Novoflupam*

Benzodiazepine, sedative-hypnotic
Controlled substance schedule IV

Available by prescription only
Capsules: 15 mg, 30 mg

INDICATIONS & DOSAGE
Insomnia
Adults: 15 to 30 mg P.O. h.s.
Geriatric patients: 15 mg P.O. h.s.

PHARMACODYNAMICS
Sedative-hypnotic action: Flurazepam depresses the CNS at the limbic and subcortical levels of the brain. It produces a sedative effect by potentiating the effect of the neurotransmitter gamma-aminobutyric acid on its receptor in the ascending reticular activating system, which increases inhibition and blocks both cortical and limbic arousal.

PHARMACOKINETICS
Absorption: When administered orally, flurazepam is absorbed rapidly through the GI tract. Onset of action occurs within 20 minutes, with peak action in 1 to 2 hours. Duration of action is 7 to 10 hours.
Distribution: Drug is distributed widely throughout the body. About 97% of an administered dose is bound to plasma protein.

Metabolism: Drug is metabolized in the liver to the active metabolite desalkylflurazepam.

Excretion: Desalkylflurazepam is excreted in urine; half-life is 50 to 100 hours.

CONTRAINDICATIONS & PRECAUTIONS

Contraindicated in patients with hypersensitivity to flurazepam. Use cautiously in patients with impaired renal or hepatic function, chronic pulmonary insufficiency, mental depression, suicidal tendencies, or history of drug abuse.

INTERACTIONS

Drug-drug. Flurazepam potentiates the CNS depressant effects of *antidepressants, antihistamines, barbiturates, general anesthetics, MAO inhibitors, narcotics,* and *phenothiazines.* Use with *cimetidine, disulfiram,* or *ritonavir* diminishes hepatic metabolism of flurazepam, which increases its plasma levels. Flurazepam may decrease plasma *haloperidol* levels and the therapeutic effects of *levodopa.*

Drug-lifestyle. *Alcohol* increases CNS depression; don't use together. *Heavy smoking* accelerates flurazepam's metabolism, thus lowering its effectiveness.

ADVERSE REACTIONS

CNS: *daytime sedation, dizziness, drowsiness, disturbed coordination,* lethargy, confusion, headache, lightheadedness, nervousness, hallucinations, staggering, ataxia, disorientation, *coma.*

GI: nausea, vomiting, heartburn, diarrhea, abdominal pain.

Hepatic: elevated liver enzyme levels.

Other: physical or psychological dependence.

▣ KEY CONSIDERATIONS

Besides the recommendations relevant to all benzodiazepines, consider the following:

• Geriatric patients are more susceptible to CNS depressant effects of flurazepam. They may require assistance and supervision with walking and daily activities during initiation of therapy or after an increase in dose.

• Note that lower doses usually are effective in geriatric patients because of decreased elimination.

• Drug is most effective after 3 or 4 nights of use because of its long half-life. Don't increase dose more frequently than every 5 days.

• Monitor hepatic function and AST, ALT, bilirubin, and alkaline phosphatase levels for changes. Flurazepam therapy may elevate liver function test results. Minor changes in EEG patterns, usually low-voltage, fast activity, may occur during and after flurazepam therapy.

• Drug is useful for patients who have trouble falling asleep and who awaken frequently at night and early in the morning.

• Although prolonged use isn't recommended, this drug has proven effective for up to 4 weeks of continuous use.

• Note that rapid withdrawal after prolonged use can cause withdrawal symptoms.

• Use lower doses in patients with renal or hepatic dysfunction.

• Store in a cool, dry place, away from light.

Patient education

• Warn patient that heavy smoking will decrease the effectiveness of the drug.

• Emphasize the potential for excessive CNS depression if drug is taken with alcohol, even if it's taken the evening before ingestion of alcohol.

• Advise patient that rebound insomnia may occur after stopping drug.

• Warn patient not to discontinue drug abruptly after prolonged therapy.

• Advise patient not to exceed prescribed dosage.

Overdose & treatment

• Signs and symptoms of overdose include somnolence, confusion, hypoactive reflexes, dyspnea, labored breathing, hypotension, bradycardia, slurred speech, unsteady gait or impaired coordination, and, eventually, coma.

• Support blood pressure and respiration until drug effects subside; monitor vital signs. Mechanical ventilatory assistance via endotracheal (ET) tube may be required to maintain a patent airway and

---

Reactions may be *common,* uncommon, *life-threatening,* or COMMON AND LIFE-THREATENING.

support adequate oxygenation. Use I.V. fluids to promote diuresis and vasopressors such as dopamine and phenylephrine to treat hypotension, as needed. Flumazenil, a specific benzodiazepine antagonist, may be useful as an adjunct to supportive therapy.

• If patient is conscious, induce vomiting; use gastric lavage if ingestion was recent, but only if an ET tube is present to prevent aspiration. Then, administer activated charcoal with a cathartic as a single dose. Dialysis is of limited value. Don't use barbiturates if excitation occurs to avoid exacerbation of excitatory state or potentiation of CNS depressant effects.

flurbiprofen
Ansaid

NSAID, phenylalkanoic acid derivative, antiarthritic

Available by prescription only
Tablets: 50 mg, 100 mg

INDICATIONS & DOSAGE
Rheumatoid arthritis and osteoarthritis
Adults: 200 to 300 mg P.O. daily, divided b.i.d., t.i.d., or q.i.d.
✦ **Dosage adjustment.** Patients with end-stage renal disease may exhibit accumulation of flurbiprofen metabolites, but half-life of parent compound is unchanged. Monitor patient closely and adjust dosage accordingly.

PHARMACODYNAMICS
Anti-inflammatory action: Flurbiprofen interferes with the synthesis of prostaglandins.

PHARMACOKINETICS
Absorption: Flurbiprofen is well absorbed after oral administration, with levels peaking in about 1½ hours. Administering with food alters rate, but not extent, of absorption.
Distribution: Drug is highly bound (more than 99%) to plasma proteins.
Metabolism: Drug is metabolized primarily in the liver. The major metabolite shows little anti-inflammatory activity.

Excretion: Drug is excreted primarily in the urine. Average elimination half-life is 6 to 10 hours.

CONTRAINDICATIONS & PRECAUTIONS
Contraindicated in patients with hypersensitivity to flurbiprofen or history of aspirin- or NSAID-induced asthma, urticaria, or other allergic-type reactions. Use cautiously in geriatric or debilitated patients and those with history of peptic ulcer disease, herpes simplex keratitis, impaired renal or hepatic function, cardiac disease, or conditions associated with fluid retention.

INTERACTIONS
Drug-drug. *Antacids* may decrease the rate, but not the extent, of absorption. *Aspirin* may decrease flurbiprofen levels; use isn't recommended. Drug may decrease the effectiveness of *diuretics;* monitor patient closely. Patients taking *oral anticoagulants* may exhibit increased bleeding tendency, so monitor closely.
Drug-food. *Food* may decrease the rate, but not the extent, of absorption.
Drug-lifestyle. Photosensitivity reaction may occur to *sunlight;* take precautions.

ADVERSE REACTIONS
CNS: *headache,* anxiety, insomnia, dizziness, increased reflexes, tremors, amnesia, asthenia, drowsiness, malaise, depression.
CV: *edema,* **heart failure,** hypertension, vasodilation.
EENT: rhinitis, tinnitus, visual changes, epistaxis.
GI: *dyspepsia, diarrhea, abdominal pain, nausea,* constipation, **bleeding,** flatulence, vomiting.
GU: *symptoms suggesting urinary tract infection,* hematuria, interstitial nephritis, **renal failure.**
Hematologic: **thrombocytopenia,** neutropenia, anemia, **aplastic anemia.**
Hepatic: *elevated liver enzyme levels, jaundice.*
Metabolic: weight changes.
Respiratory: asthma.
Skin: rash, photosensitivity, urticaria.
Other: *angioedema.*

▣ KEY CONSIDERATIONS

Besides the recommendations relevant to all NSAIDs, consider the following:

• Closely monitor patients with impaired hepatic or renal function and geriatric or debilitated patients; they may need lower doses. These patients may be at risk for renal toxicity. Periodically monitor renal function.

• Perform periodic liver function studies, ophthalmologic and auditory examinations, and hematocrit determinations in patients receiving long-term therapy.

Patient education

• Teach patient the signs and symptoms of GI bleeding, and tell him to discontinue the drug and call promptly if these occur.

• Tell patient to take drug with food, milk, or antacid to minimize GI upset.

• Advise patient to avoid hazardous activities that require alertness until the adverse CNS effects of the drug are known.

• Tell patient to immediately report edema, substantial weight gain, black stools, rash, itching, or visual disturbances.

• Advise patient that photosensitivity reactions may occur.

Overdose & treatment

• Signs and symptoms of overdose include lethargy, coma, respiratory depression, and epigastric pain and distress.

• Treatment should be supportive. Induce vomiting or perform gastric lavage.

---

fluticasone propionate
Cutivate, Flonase, Flovent

Corticosteroid, topical or inhaled anti-inflammatory

Available by prescription only
Cream: 0.05%
Ointment: 0.005%
Metered nasal spray: 50 mcg/actuation
Inhalation aerosol: 44 mcg/actuation, 110 mcg/actuation, 220 mcg/actuation
Inhalation powder: 50-mcg, 100-mcg, and 250-mcg rotadisk

INDICATIONS & DOSAGE

Relief of inflammation and pruritus of corticosteroid-responsive dermatoses
Adults: Apply sparingly to affected area b.i.d. and rub in gently and completely.
Allergic rhinitis
Adults: 2 sprays in each nostril once daily or 1 spray b.i.d.
Maintenance treatment of asthma as prophylactic therapy
Adults: 88 to 220 mcg inhalation aerosol b.i.d., adjusting to maximum 440 mcg inhalation aerosol b.i.d.
Adults: 100 mcg inhalation powder b.i.d., adjusting to maximum 500 mcg inhalation powder b.i.d.

See also package insert for dosing considerations in combination with oral corticosteroids.

PHARMACODYNAMICS

Anti-inflammatory action: Fluticasone stimulates synthesis of enzymes needed to decrease inflammation.

PHARMACOKINETICS

Absorption: Amount of fluticasone absorbed depends on the amount applied, application site, vehicle used, use of occlusive dressing, and integrity of epidermal barrier. Some systemic absorption does occur.
Distribution: Drug is distributed throughout the local skin.
Metabolism: Drug is metabolized primarily by the skin. Absorbed drug is extensively metabolized by the liver.
Excretion: Less than 5% is excreted in urine as metabolites; the rest is excreted in feces as parent drug and metabolites.

CONTRAINDICATIONS & PRECAUTIONS

Contraindicated in patients hypersensitive to fluticasone or its components and in patients with viral, fungal, herpetic, or tubercular skin lesions.

Flovent inhalation aerosol and powder are contraindicated as the primary treatment in status asthmaticus or other acute episodes of asthma, where intensive measures are required.

Use care when transferring patients from systemically active corticosteroids to Flovent inhalation aerosol or powder because deaths have occurred in asth-

---

Reactions may be *common*, uncommon, *life-threatening*, or COMMON AND LIFE-THREATENING.

matic patients during and after transfer from systemic corticosteroids to less systemically available inhalation corticosteroids. During periods of stress or severe asthma attack, a patient who has been withdrawn from systemic corticosteroids should be instructed to resume oral corticosteroids in large doses immediately and to contact his health care provider for further assistance.

INTERACTIONS
None significant.

ADVERSE REACTIONS
CNS: dizziness, giddiness.
GU: dysmenorrhea, glycosuria.
Metabolic: hyperglycemia.
Musculoskeletal: pain in joints, sprain or strain aches and pains, pain in limbs.
Respiratory: bronchitis, chest congestion.
Skin: stinging, burning, pruritus, irritation, dryness, erythema, folliculitis, skin atrophy, leukoderma, vesicles, numbness of fingers, rash, hypertrichosis, acneiform eruptions, hypopigmentation, perioral dermatitis, allergic contact dermatitis, secondary infection, striae, miliaria.
Other: *hypothalamic-pituitary-adrenal axis suppression,* Cushing's syndrome, fever.

▣ KEY CONSIDERATIONS
• Don't use for treatment of rosacea, perioral dermatitis, or acne.
• Mixing with other bases or vehicles may affect potency far beyond expectations.
• Risk of adverse reactions may be minimized by changing to a less potent agent.
• During withdrawal from oral corticosteroids, some patients may experience symptoms of systemically active corticosteroid withdrawal, such as joint or musculoskeletal pain, malaise, and depression, despite maintenance or improvement of respiratory function.
• Because of the possibility of systemic absorption of inhalation steroids, patients treated with these drugs should be observed carefully for any evidence of systemic corticosteroid effects. Special

care should be taken during periods of stress or postoperatively for adrenal insufficiency.
• Flovent inhalation aerosol and powder aren't indicated for the relief of acute bronchospasm.

Patient education
• Inform patient to apply agent sparingly and to rub in lightly. Washing the area before application may increase drug penetration.
• Instruct patient to report burning, irritation, or persistent or worsened condition.
• Tell patient to avoid prolonged use, contact with eyes, or use around genital area, rectal area, on face, and in skin creases.
• Inform patient to rinse mouth well after steroid inhalation.
• Teach patient taking an inhaled steroid to avoid exposure to chickenpox or measles, and if he is exposed, to consult his health care provider immediately.

---

fluvastatin sodium
Lescol

Hydroxy-methylglutaryl-coenzyme A (HMG-CoA) reductase inhibitor, antilipemic

---

Available by prescription only
Capsules: 20 mg, 40 mg

INDICATIONS & DOSAGE
Reduction of low-density lipoprotein and total cholesterol levels in patients with primary hypercholesterolemia (types IIa and IIb) when response to diet and other nonpharmacologic measures has been inadequate
Adults: Initially, 20 mg P.O. h.s. Increase dosage, p.r.n., to a maximum of 40 mg daily.
✦ *Dosage adjustment.* With a persistent increase in ALT or AST levels of at least 3 times the upper limit of normal, withdrawal of fluvastatin is recommended. Because fluvastatin is cleared hepatically, with less than 5% of the dose excreted into urine, dosage adjustments for mild to moderate renal impairment

aren't necessary. Exercise caution with severe impairment.

PHARMACODYNAMICS

Antilipemic action: Fluvastatin is a competitive inhibitor of HMG-CoA reductase, which is responsible for the conversion of HMG-CoA to mevalonate, a precursor of sterols, including cholesterol. This enzyme is an early (and rate-limiting) step in the synthetic pathway of cholesterol. Fluvastatin increases high-density lipoproteins and decreases low-density lipoproteins, very-low-density lipoproteins, and plasma triglycerides.

PHARMACOKINETICS

Absorption: Fluvastatin is absorbed rapidly and virtually completely (98%) after oral administration on an empty stomach.
Distribution: More than 98% of circulating drug is bound to plasma proteins.
Metabolism: Drug is completely metabolized in the liver. It has no active metabolites.
Excretion: About 5% of drug is excreted in urine and 90% in feces.

CONTRAINDICATIONS & PRECAUTIONS

Contraindicated in patients with hypersensitivity to fluvastatin and in those with active liver disease or conditions associated with unexplained persistent elevations of serum transaminase levels.

Use cautiously in patients with impaired renal function and history of hepatic disease or heavy alcohol consumption.

INTERACTIONS

Drug-drug. *Cholestyramine* or *colestipol* may bind fluvastatin in the GI tract and decrease absorption. Administer fluvastatin at bedtime, at least 2 hours after the resin, to avoid significant interaction from the drug binding to the resin. *Cimetidine, omeprazole,* and *ranitidine* decrease fluvastatin metabolism. The patient should be monitored closely. *Cyclosporine, erythromycin, gemfibrozil, niacin,* and other immunosuppressants increase the risk of polymyositis and rhabdomyolysis when administered with fluvastatin; therefore, use should be

avoided. Fluvastatin may alter *digoxin* pharmacokinetics. Monitor the patient's serum digoxin levels carefully. *Rifampin* enhances fluvastatin metabolism and decreases plasma levels. Monitor the patient closely for lack of effect.

ADVERSE REACTIONS

CNS: headache, fatigue, dizziness, insomnia.
GI: dyspepsia, diarrhea, nausea, vomiting, abdominal pain, constipation, flatulence, tooth disorder.
Hematologic: thrombocytopenia, leukopenia, *hemolytic anemia.*
Hepatic: increased liver enzyme levels.
Musculoskeletal: arthropathy, muscle pain.
Respiratory: sinusitis, *upper respiratory tract infection,* rhinitis, cough, pharyngitis, bronchitis.
Skin: hypersensitivity reactions (rash, pruritus).

▣ KEY CONSIDERATIONS

• Patient should start fluvastatin therapy only after diet and other nonpharmacologic therapies have been ineffective. Patient should maintain a standard low-cholesterol diet during therapy.
• Give drug without regard to meals; however, efficacy is enhanced if drug is taken in the evening.
• Monitor patient closely for signs of myositis.
• Perform liver function tests at the start of therapy, every 4 to 6 weeks during the first 3 months of therapy, every 6 to 12 weeks during the next 12 months, and at 6-month intervals thereafter. Fluvastatin may elevate serum ALT, AST, CK, alkaline phosphatase, and bilirubin levels. Thyroid function test abnormalities also can occur.

Patient education

• Tell patient to take fluvastatin at bedtime to enhance effectiveness.
• Instruct patient about a standard low-cholesterol diet and emphasize the importance of dietary compliance as part of therapy. Also stress importance of weight control and exercise in controlling elevated serum lipid levels.

Reactions may be *common,* uncommon, *life-threatening,* or COMMON AND LIFE-THREATENING.

• Warn patient to restrict alcohol intake because of potentially serious adverse effects.

• Tell patient to report adverse reactions, particularly muscle aches and pains.

---

fluvoxamine maleate
Luvox

Selective serotonin reuptake inhibitor (SSRI), used in the treatment of obsessive-compulsive disorder

---

Available by prescription only
Tablets: 50 mg, 100 mg

INDICATIONS & DOSAGE
Obsessive-compulsive disorder
Adults: Initially, 50 mg P.O. daily h.s. Increase in 50-mg increments q 4 to 7 days until maximum benefit is achieved. Maximum daily dosage is 300 mg. Total daily dosages exceeding 100 mg should be given in 2 divided doses.
✦ *Dosage adjustment.* Because geriatric patients and patients with hepatic impairment have been observed to have decreased clearance of fluvoxamine maleate, dose titration may be appropriate.

PHARMACODYNAMICS
Anticompulsive action: The exact mechanism of action is unknown. Fluvoxamine is a potent selective inhibitor of the neuronal uptake of serotonin, which may improve obsessive-compulsive behavior.

PHARMACOKINETICS
Absorption: Absolute bioavailability of fluvoxamine is 53%.
Distribution: Mean apparent volume of distribution is about 25 L/kg. About 80% of drug is bound to plasma protein (mostly albumin).
Metabolism: Drug is extensively metabolized in the liver, mostly by oxidative demethylation and deamination.
Excretion: Fluvoxamine's metabolites are primarily excreted in urine.

CONTRAINDICATIONS & PRECAUTIONS
Contraindicated in patients with hypersensitivity to fluvoxamine or to other phenylpiperazine antidepressants and within 14 days of MAO inhibitor therapy. Use cautiously in patients with hepatic dysfunction, concomitant conditions that may affect hemodynamic responses or metabolism, or history of mania or seizures.

INTERACTIONS
Drug-drug. Because fluvoxamine causes reduced clearance of *benzodiazepines, theophylline,* and *warfarin,* they should be used cautiously; however, *diazepam* shouldn't be administered with fluvoxamine, so diazepam dosage may need to be adjusted. Fluvoxamine may cause elevated serum levels of *carbamazepine, clozapine, methadone, metoprolol, propranolol,* and *tricyclic antidepressants;* use with caution and monitor patient closely for adverse reactions (dosage adjustments may be necessary). *Diltiazem* may cause bradycardia; therefore, monitor patient's heart rate. Because *lithium* and *tryptophan* may enhance the effects of fluvoxamine, use cautiously. *MAO inhibitors* may cause severe excitation, hyperpyrexia, myoclonus, delirium, and coma; avoid use.
Drug-lifestyle. *Alcohol* may enhance the effects of the drug; don't use together.

ADVERSE REACTIONS
CNS: headache, asthenia, somnolence, insomnia, nervousness, dizziness, tremor, anxiety, vasodilation, hypertonia, agitation, depression, CNS stimulation, taste perversion.
CV: palpitations, vasodilation.
EENT: amblyopia.
GI: *nausea, diarrhea, constipation, dyspepsia,* anorexia, *vomiting,* flatulence, tooth disorder, dysphagia, *dry mouth.*
GU: decreased libido, abnormal ejaculation, urinary frequency, impotence, anorgasmia, urine retention.
Respiratory: upper respiratory tract infection, dyspnea, yawning.
Skin: sweating.
Other: flulike syndrome, chills.

◙ KEY CONSIDERATIONS

• Drug clearance is decreased by about 50% in geriatric patients compared with younger patients, so administer drug cautiously and adjust dosage slowly during initiation of therapy.
• At least 14 days should be allowed after stopping fluvoxamine before patient is started on an MAO inhibitor. Also, at least 14 days should be allowed before patient may start fluvoxamine after MAO inhibitor therapy has been discontinued.
• Record mood changes. Monitor patient for suicidal tendencies, and allow a minimum supply of drug.

Patient education

• Warn patient not to engage in hazardous activity until CNS effects are known.
• Advise patient to avoid alcoholic beverages while taking fluvoxamine.
• Alert patient that smoking may decrease the effectiveness of drug.
• Tell patient to report rash, hives, or a related allergic reaction.
• Inform patient that several weeks of therapy may be required to obtain the full antidepressant effect. Once improvement is seen, advise patient not to discontinue the drug until directed by health care provider.
• Advise patient to call before taking OTC drugs because of possible drug interactions.

Overdose & treatment

• Common signs and symptoms of fluvoxamine overdose include drowsiness, vomiting, diarrhea, and dizziness; coma, tachycardia, bradycardia, hypotension, ECG abnormalities, liver function abnormalities, and seizures may also occur. Symptoms such as aspiration pneumonitis, respiratory difficulties, or hypokalemia may occur because of loss of consciousness or vomiting.
• Treatment is supportive. Besides maintaining an open airway and monitoring vital signs and ECG, administering activated charcoal may be as effective as inducing vomiting or performing gastric lavage. Because absorption with overdose may be delayed, measures to minimize absorption may be necessary for up to 24 hours after ingestion. Dialysis isn't believed to be beneficial.

folic acid
Folvite

Folic acid derivative, vitamin supplement

Available by prescription only
Tablets: 1 mg
Injection: 10-ml vials (folic acid 5 mg/ml contains 1.5% benzyl alcohol and EDTA; Folvite 5 mg/ml contains 1.5% benzyl alcohol)
Available without a prescription
Tablets: 0.4 mg, 0.8 mg

INDICATIONS & DOSAGE
Megaloblastic or macrocytic anemia secondary to folic acid deficiency, hepatic disease, alcoholism, intestinal obstruction, excessive hemolysis
Adults: 0.4 mg P.O., S.C., or I.M. daily for 4 to 5 days. After anemia secondary to folic acid deficiency is corrected, proper diet and RDA supplements are necessary to prevent recurrence.
Nutritional supplement
Adults: Give 0.15 to 0.2 mg P.O., S.C., or I.M. daily for males; 0.15 to 0.18 mg P.O., S.C., or I.M. daily for females.
Tropical sprue
Adults: 3 to 15 mg P.O. daily.

PHARMACODYNAMICS
Nutritional action: Exogenous folate is required to maintain normal erythropoiesis and to perform nucleoprotein synthesis. Folic acid stimulates production of RBCs, WBCs, and platelets in certain megaloblastic anemias.

Dietary folic acid is present in foods, primarily as reduced folate polyglutamate. This vitamin is absorbed only after hydrolysis, reduction, and methylation occur in the GI tract. Conversion to active tetrahydrofolate may require vitamin B_{12}.

The oral synthetic form of folic acid is a monoglutamate and is absorbed completely after administration, even in malabsorption syndromes.

Reactions may be *common*, uncommon, *life-threatening*, or COMMON AND LIFE-THREATENING.

PHARMACOKINETICS

Absorption: Folic acid is absorbed rapidly from the GI tract, mainly from the proximal part of the small intestine. Peak folate activity in blood occurs within 30 to 60 minutes after oral administration. Normal serum folate levels range from 0.005 to 0.015 µg/ml. Usually, serum levels less than 0.005 µg/ml indicate folate deficiency; those below 0.002 µg/ml usually result in megaloblastic anemia.
Distribution: The active tetrahydrofolic acid and its derivatives are distributed into all body tissues; the liver contains about half of the total body folate stores. Folate is actively concentrated in the CSF.
Metabolism: Folic acid is metabolized in the liver to N-methyltetrahydrofolic acid, the main form of folate storage and transport.
Excretion: A single 0.1- to 0.2-mg dose of folic acid usually results in only a trace amount of drug in the urine. After large doses, excess folate is excreted unchanged in urine. Small amounts of folic acid have been recovered in feces. About 0.05 mg/day of normal body folate is lost in urine and feces and through oxidative cleavage of the molecule.

CONTRAINDICATIONS & PRECAUTIONS

Contraindicated in patients with undiagnosed anemia because it may mask pernicious anemia, and in those with vitamin B_{12} deficiency.

INTERACTIONS

Drug-drug. *Folic acid antagonists, pyrimethamine, triamterene,* or *trimethoprim* may cause dihydrofolate reductase deficiency, which may interfere with folic acid use. *Para-aminosalicylic acid* and *sulfasalazine* may cause a similar deficiency. Conversely, *phenytoin* and *primidone* may decrease serum folate levels and produce symptoms of folic acid deficiency in long-term therapy. Also, use with folic acid (15 to 20 mg/day) decreases serum *phenytoin* levels to subtherapeutic levels, possibly with increased frequency of seizures. Folic acid appears to increase the metabolic clearance of phenytoin and cause redistribution of phenytoin in the CSF and brain. Folic acid may interfere with the antimicrobial actions of *pyrimethamine* against toxoplasmosis.

ADVERSE REACTIONS

CNS: general malaise.
Respiratory: *bronchospasm.*
Skin: allergic reactions (rash, pruritus, erythema).

▣ KEY CONSIDERATIONS

- The RDA for folic acid is 180 to 200 mcg in adults; 100 mcg/day is considered an adequate oral supplement.
- The preferred route of administration for folic acid is P.O. The manufacturer recommends deep I.M., S.C., or I.V. administration only when P.O. treatment isn't feasible or when malabsorption is suspected.
- Alcohol can cause folate deficiencies.
- Ensure that patients don't also have vitamin B_{12} deficiency; folic acid can improve hematologic measurements while allowing progression of neurologic damage. Don't use as sole treatment of pernicious anemia.
- Note that patients undergoing renal dialysis are at risk for folate deficiency.
- Monitor CBC to measure effectiveness of drug treatment. Folic acid therapy alters serum and erythrocyte folate levels; falsely low serum and erythrocyte folate levels may occur with the *Lactobacillus casei* assay in patients receiving antiinfectives, such as tetracycline, which suppress the growth of this organism.
- Protect folic acid injections from light.

Patient education

- Teach patient about dietary sources of folic acid, such as yeast, whole grains, leafy vegetables, beans, nuts, and fruit.
- Tell patient that folate is destroyed by overcooking and canning.
- Stress importance of administering folic acid only under medical supervision.

foscarnet sodium
(phosphonoformic acid)
Foscavir

Pyrophosphate analogue, antiviral

Available by prescription only
Injection: 24 mg/ml in 250-ml and
500-ml vials

INDICATIONS & DOSAGE
Cytomegalovirus (CMV) retinitis in patients with AIDS
Adults: Initially, 60 mg/kg I.V. as an induction treatment in patients with normal renal function. Administer as an I.V. infusion over 1 hour q 8 hours for 2 to 3 weeks, depending on response. Follow with a maintenance infusion of 90 mg/kg daily administered over 2 hours; increase as needed and tolerated to 120 mg/kg daily if disease shows signs of progression.
Mucocutaneous acyclovir-resistant herpes simplex virus (HSV) infection
Adults: 40 mg/kg I.V. Administer as an I.V. infusion over 1 hour q 8 to 12 hours for 2 or 3 weeks, depending on response.
◊ *Varicella zoster infection*
Adults: 40 mg/kg I.V. q 8 hours for 10 to 21 days or until complete healing occurs.
✦ *Dosage adjustment.* For adults with renal failure, calculate weight-adjusted creatinine clearance (ml/minute/kg) from this equation.
For men:

$$\frac{\text{creatinine}}{\text{clearance}} = \frac{(140 - \text{age})}{(\text{serum creatinine} \times 72)}$$

For women: Multiply the above value by 0.85.

Administer according to the following tables.

Induction dosage

Creatinine clearance (ml/min/kg)	Dose to be administered q 8 hr (mg/kg)
≥ 1.6	60
1.5	57
1.4	53
1.3	49
1.2	46
1.1	42
1	39
0.9	35
0.8	32
0.7	28
0.6	25
0.5	21
0.4	18

Maintenance dosage

Creatinine clearance (ml/min/kg)	Equivalent to 90 mg/kg/day	Equivalent to 120 mg/kg/day
≥ 1.4	90	120
1.2-1.4	78	104
1-1.2	75	100
0.8-1	71	94
0.6-0.8	63	84
0.4-0.6	57	76

PHARMACODYNAMICS
Antiviral action: An organic analogue of pyrophosphate, a compound used in many enzymatic reactions, foscarnet inhibits all known herpes viruses in vitro by blocking the pyrophosphate binding site on DNA polymerases and reverse transcriptases.

PHARMACOKINETICS
Absorption: Unknown.
Distribution: Foscarnet is about 14% to 17% bound to plasma proteins. Animal studies indicate that the drug is deposited in bone.
Metabolism: Unknown.
Excretion: About 80% to 90% of drug appears in the urine unchanged. Drug clearance is dependent on renal function. Plasma half-life is about 3 hours.

CONTRAINDICATIONS & PRECAUTIONS

Contraindicated in patients with hypersensitivity to foscarnet. Use with extreme caution in patients with impaired renal function.

INTERACTIONS

Drug-drug. *Nephrotoxic drugs,* such as *aminoglycosides* and *amphotericin B,* may increase risk of nephrotoxicity; avoid use. *Pentamidine* may increase the risk of nephrotoxicity and severe hypocalcemia; don't use together. *Zidovudine* may increase the incidence or severity of anemia; monitor blood counts.

ADVERSE REACTIONS

CNS: *headache, seizures,* fatigue, malaise, pain, asthenia, paresthesia, dizziness, hypoesthesia, neuropathy, tremor, ataxia, generalized spasms, dementia, stupor, sensory disturbances, meningitis, aphasia, abnormal coordination, EEG abnormalities, depression, confusion, anxiety, insomnia, somnolence, nervousness, amnesia, agitation, aggressive reaction, hallucinations.
CV: *hypertension, palpitations, ECG abnormalities, sinus tachycardia,* cerebrovascular disorder, *first-degree AV block, hypotension, flushing,* chest pain, edema.
EENT: visual disturbances, taste perversion, eye pain, conjunctivitis.
GI: *nausea, diarrhea, vomiting, abdominal pain, anorexia,* constipation, dysphagia, rectal hemorrhage, dry mouth, dyspepsia, melena, flatulence, ulcerative stomatitis, ***pancreatitis.***
GU: *abnormal renal function, decreased creatinine clearance and increased serum creatinine levels, albuminuria, dysuria, polyuria, urethral disorder, urine retention, urinary tract infections,* **acute renal failure,** candidiasis.
Hematologic: **anemia, granulocytopenia, leukopenia, bone marrow suppression, thrombocytopenia,** platelet count abnormalities, thrombocytosis, WBC count abnormalities, lymphadenopathy.
Hepatic: abnormal hepatic function, increased liver enzyme levels.
Metabolic: hypokalemia, hypomagnesemia, hypophosphatemia or hyperphosphatemia, hypocalcemia.

Musculoskeletal: leg cramps, back pain, arthralgia, myalgia.
Respiratory: *cough, dyspnea,* pneumonitis, sinusitis, pharyngitis, rhinitis, respiratory insufficiency, pulmonary infiltration, stridor, pneumothorax, *bronchospasm,* hemoptysis.
Skin: pruritus, skin ulceration, erythematous rash, seborrhea, skin discoloration, facial edema, *rash, increased sweating.*
Other: ***death,*** *fever,* flulike syndrome, sepsis, rigors, inflammation and pain at infusion site, lymphoma-like disorder, sarcoma, bacterial or fungal infections, abscess.

KEY CONSIDERATIONS

● It's unknown whether age alters drug response. However, geriatric patients are likely to have preexisting renal function impairment, which requires alterations in dosage.
● Anemia is common (up to 33% of patients treated with drug) and may be severe enough to require transfusions.
● Don't exceed the recommended dosage, infusion rate, or frequency of administration. All doses must be individualized according to patient's renal function.
● An infusion pump must be used to administer foscarnet.
● Unlike ganciclovir, foscarnet doesn't require cellular activation by thymidine kinase or other kinases. Foscarnet may be active against certain CMV strains resistant to ganciclovir.

Patient education

● Make sure patient understands that adverse reactions to drug are common and that he should report for all laboratory studies and follow-up appointments to check his progress.
● Advise patient to report perioral tingling, numbness in the extremities, and paresthesia.

---

fosinopril sodium
Monopril

ACE inhibitor, antihypertensive

Available by prescription only
Tablets: 10 mg, 20 mg, 40 mg

INDICATIONS & DOSAGE
Treatment of hypertension
Adults: Initially, 10 mg P.O. daily; adjust dose based on blood pressure response at peak and trough levels. Usual dose: 20 to 40 mg daily; maximum up to 80 mg daily. Dose may be divided.
Treatment of heart failure
Adults: Initially, 10 mg P.O. daily; maximum dose up to 40 mg daily. Doses may be divided.

PHARMACODYNAMICS
Antihypertensive action: Fosinopril is believed to lower blood pressure primarily by suppressing the renin-angiotensin-aldosterone system, although it has also been effective in patients with low-renin hypertension.

PHARMACOKINETICS
Absorption: Fosinopril is absorbed slowly through the GI tract, primarily via the proximal small intestine.
Distribution: More than 95% is protein-bound; levels peak in about 3 hours.
Metabolism: Drug is hydrolyzed primarily in the liver and gut wall by esterases.
Excretion: About 50% of drug is excreted in urine; the remainder in feces.

CONTRAINDICATIONS & PRECAUTIONS
Contraindicated in patients with hypersensitivity to fosinopril or other ACE inhibitors. Use cautiously in patients with impaired renal or hepatic function.

INTERACTIONS
Drug-drug. *Antacids* may impair absorption of fosinopril; separate administration by at least 2 hours. Excessive hypotension may occur with use of *diuretics,* especially if patient is volume depleted; effect may be minimized by stopping diuretic. When used with *lithium,* increased serum lithium levels and symptoms of lithium toxicity may occur; monitor lithium levels frequently (risk is increased if diuretic is also used.). Use of *potassium sparing diuretics* or *potassium supplements* may result in hyperkalemia; monitor potassium levels.
Drug-lifestyle. Photosensitivity reaction may occur to *sunlight;* take precautions.

ADVERSE REACTIONS
CNS: headache, dizziness, fatigue, syncope, paresthesia, sleep disturbance, *CVA.*
CV: chest pain, angina, *MI, hypertensive crisis,* rhythm disturbances, palpitations, hypotension, orthostatic hypotension.
EENT: tinnitus, sinusitis.
GI: nausea, vomiting, diarrhea, pancreatitis, hepatitis, dry mouth, abdominal distention, abdominal pain, constipation.
GU: sexual dysfunction, renal insufficiency.
Metabolic: hyperkalemia.
Musculoskeletal: arthralgia, pain, myalgia.
Respiratory: *dry, persistent, tickling, nonproductive cough; bronchospasm.*
Skin: urticaria, rash, photosensitivity, pruritus.
Other: *angioedema,* gout, decreased libido.

▣ KEY CONSIDERATIONS
• Diuretic therapy is usually discontinued 2 to 3 days before start of ACE inhibitor therapy to reduce risk of hypotension. If fosinopril doesn't adequately control blood pressure, diuretic may be reinstituted with care. Monitor potassium levels.
• Perform CBC with differential counts before therapy, then every 2 weeks for 3 months, and periodically thereafter.
• The incidence of postural hypotension is low.
• Remember that blood pressure is lowered within 1 hour of a single dose of 10 to 40 mg, with peak reductions occurring 2 to 6 hours after dose. The antihypertensive effect lasts 24 hours.
• Falsely low measurements of digoxin levels may result with the DIGI TAB radioimmunoassay kit for digoxin; other kits may be used. Transient elevations of

---

Reactions may be *common,* uncommon, *life-threatening,* or COMMON AND LIFE-THREATENING.

BUN, serum creatinine levels, and liver function tests and decreases in hematocrit or hemoglobin may also occur.

• Effectiveness of fosinopril is unaffected by age, sex, or weight.

Patient education

• Tell patient to take dose 1 hour before or 2 hours after food or antacids.

• Tell patient to report light-headedness in the first few days of therapy and signs of infection, such as fever or sore throat. He should also call if he experiences swelling of tongue, face, mucous membranes, eyes, lips, or extremities; difficulty swallowing or breathing; or hoarseness. He should discontinue the drug immediately.

• Advise patient to maintain the same salt intake as before therapy because salt restriction can lead to a precipitous drop in blood pressure with initial doses of this drug. Large reductions in blood pressure may also occur with excessive perspiration and dehydration.

• Warn patient to avoid sudden position changes until effect of drug is known; however, postural hypotension is infrequent.

• Advise patient of potential photosensitivity reactions.

fosphenytoin sodium
Cerebyx

Hydantoin derivative, anticonvulsant

Available by prescription only
Injection: 2 ml (150 mg fosphenytoin sodium equivalent to 100 mg phenytoin sodium), 10 ml (750 mg fosphenytoin sodium equivalent to 500 mg phenytoin sodium)

INDICATIONS & DOSAGE
Status epilepticus
Adults: Give 15 to 20 mg phenytoin sodium equivalent (PE)/kg I.V. at 100 to 150 PE/minute as a loading dose, then 4 to 6 mg PE/kg/day I.V. as a maintenance dose. (Phenytoin may be used instead of fosphenytoin as maintenance using the appropriate dose.)

Prevention and treatment of seizures during neurosurgery
Adults: Administer 10 to 20 mg PE/kg I.M. or I.V. at an I.V. infusion rate not exceeding 150 mg PE/minute as a loading dose. Maintenance dose is 4 to 6 mg PE/kg/day I.V.
Short-term substitution for oral phenytoin therapy
Adults: Same total daily dosage as oral phenytoin sodium therapy given as a single daily dose I.M. or I.V. at an I.V. infusion rate not exceeding 150 mg PE/minute. (Some patients may require more frequent dosing.)

PHARMACODYNAMICS
Anticonvulsant action: Fosphenytoin is a prodrug of phenytoin; therefore, its anticonvulsant action is that of phenytoin. Phenytoin stabilizes neuronal membranes and limits seizure activity by modulation of voltage-dependent sodium channels of neurons, inhibition of calcium flux across neuronal membranes, modulation of voltage-dependent calcium channels of neurons, and enhancement of sodium-potassium adenosine triphosphatase activity of neurons and glial cells.

PHARMACOKINETICS
Absorption: Plasma fosphenytoin levels peak about 30 minutes after I.M. administration or at end of the I.V. infusion.
Distribution: About 95% to 99% is bound to plasma proteins, primarily albumin. Volume of distribution increases with dose and rate and ranges from 4.3 to 10.8 L.
Metabolism: Conversion half-life of fosphenytoin to phenytoin is about 15 minutes. Phosphatases are believed to play a major role in conversion.
Excretion: Unknown, although drug isn't excreted in urine.

CONTRAINDICATIONS & PRECAUTIONS
Contraindicated in patients with hypersensitivity to fosphenytoin or its components, phenytoin, or other hydantoins. Also contraindicated in patients with sinus bradycardia, SA block, second- and third-degree AV block, and Adams-Stokes syndrome because of the effect of

parenteral phenytoin on ventricular automaticity.

Use cautiously in patients with hypotension, severe myocardial insufficiency, impaired renal or hepatic function, hypoalbuminemia, porphyria, diabetes mellitus, and history of hypersensitivity to similarly structured drugs, such as barbiturates and succinimides.

INTERACTIONS

Drug-drug. Most significant drug interactions are those that are commonly seen with phenytoin.

Drugs that may decrease plasma phenytoin levels include *carbamazepine* and *reserpine. Drugs that may increase plasma phenytoin levels* (and thus its therapeutic effects) include *amiodarone, chloramphenicol, chlordiazepoxide, cimetidine, diazepam, dicumarol, disulfiram, estrogens, ethosuximide, fluoxetine, H_2-antagonists, halothane, isoniazid, methylphenidate, phenothiazines, phenylbutazone, salicylates, succinimides, sulfonamides, tolbutamide,* and *trazodone. Drugs that may increase or decrease plasma phenytoin levels* include *phenobarbital, sodium valproate,* and *valproic acid;* similarly, the effects of phenytoin on the levels of these drugs are unpredictable. *Drugs whose efficacy may be decreased by phenytoin because of increased hepatic metabolism* include *coumarin, digitoxin, doxycycline, estrogens, furosemide, oral contraceptives, quinidine, rifampin, theophylline,* and *vitamin D. Tricyclic antidepressants* may lower seizure threshold and may require adjustments in phenytoin dosage.

Drug-lifestyle. Plasma phenytoin levels may be decreased by *long-term alcohol abuse* and increased by *acute alcohol intake.*

ADVERSE REACTIONS

CNS: increased reflexes, speech disorder, dysarthria, intracranial hypertension, thinking abnormality, nervousness, hypesthesia, confusion, twitching, positive Babinski's sign, circumoral paresthesia, hemiplegia, hypotonia, seizure, extrapyramidal syndrome, insomnia, meningitis, depersonalization, CNS depression, hypokinesia, hyperkinesia, brain edema, paralysis, psychosis, aphasia, emotional lability, ***coma,*** hyperesthesia, myoclonus, personality disorder, acute brain syndrome, encephalitis, subdural hematoma, encephalopathy, hostility, akathisia, amnesia, neurosis, migraine, syncope, cerebral infarct, asthenia, headache, nystagmus, dizziness, somnolence, ataxia, stupor, incoordination, paresthesia, tremor, agitation, vertigo.

CV: hypertension, ***cardiac arrest, cerebral hemorrhage,*** palpitation, sinus bradycardia, atrial flutter, ***bundle branch block,*** cardiomegaly, orthostatic hypotension, ***pulmonary embolus,*** QT interval prolongation, thrombophlebitis, ventricular extrasystoles, ***heart failure,*** vasodilation, tachycardia, hypotension.

EENT: taste perversion, deafness, visual field defect, eye pain, conjunctivitis, photophobia, hyperacusis, mydriasis, parosmia, ear pain, taste loss, tinnitus, diplopia, amblyopia, pharyngitis, sinusitis, rhinitis, epistaxis.

GI: constipation, dyspepsia, diarrhea, anorexia, GI hemorrhage, increased salivation, abnormal liver function tests, tenesmus, tongue edema, dysphagia, flatulence, gastritis, ileus, nausea, dry mouth, vomiting.

GU: urine retention, oliguria, dysuria, vaginitis, albuminuria, genital edema, kidney failure, polyuria, urethral pain, urinary incontinence, vaginal candidiasis.

Hematologic: ***thrombocytopenia,*** anemia, leukocytosis, hypochromic anemia, leukopenia, ecchymosis.

Metabolic: hypokalemia, hyperglycemia, hypophosphatemia, alkalosis, acidosis, hyperkalemia.

Musculoskeletal: myasthenia, myopathy, leg cramps, arthralgia, myalgia, pelvic pain, back pain.

Respiratory: cyanosis, pneumonia, hyperventilation, ***apnea,*** aspiration pneumonia, asthma, dyspnea, atelectasis, increased cough, increased sputum, hypoxia, pneumothorax, hemoptysis, bronchitis.

Skin: petechia, rash, maculopapular rash, urticaria, sweating, skin discoloration, contact dermatitis, pustular rash, skin nodule, *pruritus.*

Other: diabetes insipidus, lymphadenopathy, dehydration, ketosis.

Reactions may be *common,* uncommon, *life-threatening,* or COMMON AND LIFE-THREATENING.

▣ KEY CONSIDERATIONS

• Geriatric patients metabolize and excrete phenytoin slowly; therefore, fosphenytoin should be administered cautiously to older adults.

• Fosphenytoin should always be prescribed and dispensed in phenytoin sodium equivalent units (PE). Don't make adjustments in the recommended doses when substituting fosphenytoin for phenytoin and vice versa.

• Before I.V. infusion, dilute fosphenytoin in D_5W or normal saline solution for injection to a concentration ranging from 1.5 to 25 mg PE/ml. Don't administer at a rate exceeding 150 mg PE/minute.

• Dose of I.V. fosphenytoin used to treat status epilepticus should be administered at a maximum rate of 150 mg PE/minute. The typical infusion of drug administered to a 50-kg patient takes 5 to 7 minutes, whereas that of an identical molar dose of phenytoin can't be accomplished in less than 15 to 20 minutes because of the untoward CV effects that accompany the direct I.V. administration of phenytoin at rates above 50 mg/minute. Don't use I.M. fosphenytoin because therapeutic phenytoin levels may not be reached as rapidly as with I.V. administration.

• If rapid phenytoin loading is a primary goal, I.V. administration of fosphenytoin is preferred because the time to achieve therapeutic plasma phenytoin levels is greater after I.M. than after I.V. administration.

• Monitor patient's ECG, blood pressure, and respiration continuously throughout the period when maximal serum phenytoin levels occur, about 10 to 20 minutes after the end of fosphenytoin infusions. Severe CV complications are most common in geriatric or gravely ill patients. Reduce rate of administration or discontinue dosing if needed.

• Patients receiving fosphenytoin at doses of 20 mg PE/kg at 150 mg PE/minute are expected to experience some sensory discomfort, with the groin being the most common location. The occurrence and intensity of the discomfort can be lessened by slowing or temporarily stopping the infusion.

• The phosphate load provided by fosphenytoin (0.0037 mmol phosphate/mg PE fosphenytoin) must be taken into consideration when treating patients who require phosphate restriction, such as those with severe renal impairment.

• Discontinue drug if rash appears. If rash is exfoliative, purpuric, or bullous or if lupus erythematosus, Stevens-Johnson syndrome, or toxic epidermal necrolysis is suspected, discontinue drug and seek alternative therapy. If the rash is mild (measleslike or scarlatiniform), therapy may be resumed after it has completely disappeared. If the rash recurs on reinstitution of therapy, further fosphenytoin or phenytoin administration is contraindicated.

• Discontinue drug in patients with acute hepatotoxicity and don't readminister to these patients.

• I.M. drug administration generates systemic phenytoin levels that are similar enough to oral phenytoin sodium to allow essentially interchangeable use.

• A dose of 15 to 20 mg PE/kg of fosphenytoin infused I.V. at 100 to 150 mg PE/minute yields plasma-free phenytoin levels over time that approximate those achieved when an equivalent dose of phenytoin sodium (such as parenteral dilantin) is administered at 50 mg/minute I.V.

• After drug administration, don't monitor phenytoin levels until conversion to phenytoin is essentially complete: about 2 hours after the end of an I.V. infusion or 4 hours after I.M. administration.

• Interpretation of total plasma phenytoin levels should be made cautiously in patients with renal or hepatic disease or hypoalbuminemia because of an increased fraction of unbound phenytoin. Unbound phenytoin levels may be more useful in these patients. Also, these patients are at increased risk for both the frequency and severity of adverse reactions when fosphenytoin is administered I.V.

• Abrupt withdrawal of drug may precipitate status epilepticus.

• Fosphenytoin may decrease serum T_4 levels. It may also produce artificially low results on dexamethasone or metyrapone tests. Phenytoin may also cause increased serum levels of glucose, alkaline phosphatase, and gamma glutamyl transpeptidase.

Patient education
• Warn patient that sensory disturbances may occur with I.V. drug administration.
• Tell patient to report adverse reactions, especially rash, immediately.

Overdose & treatment
• There are no reports of fosphenytoin overdose. However, because it's a prodrug of phenytoin, overdosage may be similar. Early signs and symptoms of phenytoin overdose may include drowsiness, nausea, vomiting, nystagmus, ataxia, dysarthria, tremor, and slurred speech; hypotension, respiratory depression, and coma may follow. Death is caused by respiratory and circulatory depression. The estimated lethal dose of phenytoin in adults is 2 to 5 g.
• Formate and phosphate are metabolites of fosphenytoin and therefore may contribute to signs and symptoms of toxicity after overdose. Signs and symptoms of formate toxicity are similar to those of methanol toxicity and are associated with severe anion-gap metabolic acidosis. Large amounts of phosphate, delivered rapidly, could cause hypocalcemia with paresthesia, muscle spasms, and seizures. Ionized free calcium levels can be measured and, if low, used to guide treatment.
• First, induce vomiting or perform gastric lavage; then, provide supportive treatment. Monitor vital signs and fluid and electrolyte balance. Forced diuresis is of little or no value. Hemodialysis or peritoneal dialysis may be helpful.

---

furosemide
Apo-Furosemide*, Lasix, Lasix Special*, Novosemide*, Uritol*

Loop diuretic, diuretic, antihypertensive

Available by prescription only
Tablets: 20 mg, 40 mg, 80 mg
Solution: 10 mg/ml, 40 mg/5 ml
Injection: 10 mg/ml

INDICATIONS & DOSAGE
Acute pulmonary edema
Adults: 40 mg I.V. injected slowly; then 80 mg I.V. within 1 hour, p.r.n.
Edema
Adults: 20 to 80 mg P.O. daily in the morning, with second dose given in 6 to 8 hours, carefully titrated up to 600 mg daily p.r.n.; or 20 to 40 mg I.M. or I.V. Increase by 20 mg q 2 hours until desired response is achieved. I.V. dose should be given slowly over 1 to 2 minutes.
Hypertension
Adults: 40 mg P.O. b.i.d. Adjust dosage according to response.
◊ *Hypercalcemia*
Adults: 80 to 100 mg I.V. q 1 to 2 hours; or 120 mg P.O. daily.
✦ *Dosage adjustment.* Reduced dosages may be indicated in geriatric patients.

PHARMACODYNAMICS
Diuretic action: Loop diuretics inhibit sodium and chloride reabsorption in the proximal part of the ascending loop of Henle, promoting the excretion of sodium, water, chloride, and potassium.
Antihypertensive action: This drug effect may be the result of renal and peripheral vasodilation and a temporary increase in glomerular filtration rate, and a decrease in peripheral vascular resistance.

PHARMACOKINETICS
Absorption: About 60% of a given furosemide dose is absorbed from the GI tract after oral administration. Food delays oral absorption but doesn't alter diuretic response. Diuresis begins in 30 to 60 minutes; peak diuresis occurs 1 to 2 hours after oral administration. Diuresis follows I.V. administration within 5 minutes and peaks in 20 to 60 minutes.
Distribution: About 95% of drug is plasma protein-bound.
Metabolism: Drug is metabolized minimally by the liver.
Excretion: About 50% to 80% of a dose is excreted in urine; plasma half-life is about 30 minutes. Duration of action is 6 to 8 hours after oral administration and about 2 hours after I.V. administration.

Reactions may be *common*, uncommon, *life-threatening*, or COMMON AND LIFE-THREATENING.

CONTRAINDICATIONS & PRECAUTIONS
Contraindicated in patients with anuria or hypersensitivity to furosemide. Use cautiously in patients with hepatic cirrhosis.

INTERACTIONS
Drug-drug. Furosemide potentiates the hypotensive effect of most other *antihypertensives* and of other *diuretics;* both actions are used to therapeutic advantage. Patients receiving I.V. furosemide within 24 hours of a dose of *chloral hydrate* have experienced sweating, flushing, and blood pressure fluctuations; if possible, use an alternative sedative in patients receiving I.V. furosemide. *Indomethacin* and *probenecid* may reduce furosemide's diuretic effect; combined use isn't recommended, but if no therapeutic alternative exists, the furosemide dosage may need to be increased. Furosemide may reduce renal clearance of *lithium* and increase lithium levels; lithium dosage may require adjustment. Furosemide could prolong neuromuscular blockade by *muscle relaxants.* Administration of furosemide with *nephrotoxic* or *ototoxic drugs* may enhance toxicity. Use with other *potassium-depleting drugs,* such as *amphotericin B* and *corticosteroids,* may cause severe potassium loss; use with *potassium sparing diuretics*—such as *amiloride, spironolactone,* and *triamterene*—may decrease furosemide-induced potassium loss.

ADVERSE REACTIONS
CNS: vertigo, headache, dizziness, paresthesia, restlessness, weakness, transient pain (at I.M. injection site).
CV: volume depletion and dehydration, orthostatic hypotension, thrombophlebitis (with I.V. administration).
EENT: transient deafness with too rapid I.V. injection, blurred vision.
GI: abdominal discomfort and pain, diarrhea, anorexia, nausea, vomiting, constipation, pancreatitis.
GU: nocturia, polyuria, frequent urination, oliguria.
Hematologic: *agranulocytosis,* leukopenia, *thrombocytopenia,* azotemia, anemia, *aplastic anemia.*

Metabolic: hypokalemia; hypochloremic alkalosis; asymptomatic hyperuricemia; fluid and electrolyte imbalances, including dilutional hyponatremia, hypocalcemia, and hypomagnesemia; hyperglycemia and impaired glucose tolerance.
Musculoskeletal: muscle spasm.
Skin: dermatitis, purpura.
Other: fever.

◉ KEY CONSIDERATIONS
Besides the recommendations relevant to all loop diuretics, consider the following:
● Geriatric and debilitated patients require close observation because they are more susceptible to drug-induced diuresis. Excessive diuresis promotes rapid dehydration, leading to hypovolemia, hypokalemia, hyponatremia, and circulatory collapse.
● Give I.V. furosemide slowly, over 1 to 2 minutes. For I.V. infusion, dilute furosemide in D_5W, normal saline solution, or lactated Ringer's solution, and use within 24 hours. If high-dose furosemide therapy is needed, administer as a controlled infusion not exceeding 4 mg/minute.
● Drug therapy alters electrolyte balance and liver and renal function tests.

Patient education
● Warn patient that photosensitivity reaction may occur. Explain that reaction is a photoallergy in which ultraviolet radiation alters drug structure, causing allergic reactions in some individuals.
● Tell patient that photosensitivity reactions occur 10 days to 2 weeks after initial sun exposure.

Overdose & treatment
● Signs and symptoms of overdose include profound electrolyte and volume depletion, which may precipitate circulatory collapse.
● Treatment is chiefly supportive; replace fluids and electrolytes.

G

gabapentin
Neurontin

1-amino-methyl cyclohexoneacetic acid, anticonvulsant

Available by prescription only
Capsules: 100 mg, 300 mg, 400 mg

INDICATIONS & DOSAGE
Adjunctive treatment of partial seizures with and without secondary generalization
Adults: 300 mg P.O. on day 1, 300 mg P.O. b.i.d. on day 2, and 300 mg P.O. t.i.d. on day 3. Increase dosage as needed and tolerated to 1,800 mg daily, in 3 divided doses. Usual dosage is 300 to 600 mg P.O. t.i.d., but dosages up to 3,600 mg/day have been well tolerated.
✦ ***Dosage adjustment.*** In adult patients with renal failure, if creatinine clearance is greater than 60 ml/minute, give 400 mg P.O. t.i.d.; if creatinine clearance is between 30 and 60 ml/minute, give 300 mg P.O. b.i.d.; if creatinine clearance is between 15 and 30 ml/minute, give 300 mg P.O. daily; and if creatinine clearance is less than 15 ml/minute, give 300 mg P.O. every other day. Patients on hemodialysis should receive a loading dose of 300 to 400 mg P.O.; then 200 mg to 300 mg P.O. q 4 hours after hemodialysis.

PHARMACODYNAMICS
Anticonvulsant action: Gabapentin's mechanism of action is unknown. Although it's structurally related to gamma-aminobutyric acid (GABA), the drug doesn't interact with GABA receptors, isn't converted metabolically into GABA or a GABA agonist, and doesn't inhibit GABA uptake or degradation. Gabapentin doesn't exhibit affinity for other common receptor sites.

PHARMACOKINETICS
Absorption: Gabapentin bioavailability isn't dose related. A 400-mg dose, for example, is about 25% less bioavailable

than a 100-mg dose. Over the recommended dose range of 300 to 600 mg t.i.d., however, differences in bioavailability aren't large and bioavailability is about 60%. Food has no effect on the rate or extent of absorption.
Distribution: Gabapentin circulates largely unbound (less than 3%) to plasma protein. Drug crosses the blood-brain barrier with about 20% of the corresponding plasma levels found in CSF.
Metabolism: Drug isn't appreciably metabolized in humans.
Excretion: Drug is eliminated from the systemic circulation by renal excretion as unchanged drug. Its elimination half-life is 5 to 7 hours. Drug can be removed from plasma by hemodialysis.

CONTRAINDICATIONS & PRECAUTIONS
Contraindicated in patients hypersensitive to gabapentin.

INTERACTIONS
Drug-drug. *Antacids* decrease the absorption of gabapentin; administration of the two drugs should be separated by at least 2 hours.

ADVERSE REACTIONS
CNS: *fatigue, somnolence, dizziness, ataxia, nystagmus, tremor,* nervousness, dysarthria, amnesia, depression, abnormal thinking, twitching, incoordination.
CV: peripheral edema, vasodilation.
EENT: *diplopia, rhinitis,* pharyngitis, dry throat, coughing, *amblyopia.*
GI: dental abnormalities, increased appetite, nausea, vomiting, dyspepsia, dry mouth, constipation.
GU: impotence.
Hematologic: leukopenia, decreased WBC count.
Metabolic: weight gain.
Musculoskeletal: back pain, myalgia, fractures.
Skin: pruritus, abrasion.

🔲 KEY CONSIDERATIONS
• Discontinue drug therapy or substitute alternative drug gradually over at least 1 week to minimize risk of seizures. Don't

---

suddenly withdraw other anticonvulsant drugs in patients starting gabapentin therapy.

• Routine monitoring of plasma drug levels is unnecessary. Drug doesn't appear to alter plasma levels of other anticonvulsants.

• Don't use Ames N-Multistix SG dipstick to test for urine protein; false-positive results can occur when gabapentin is added to other antiepileptic drugs. The more specific sulfosalicylic acid precipitation procedure is recommended to determine the presence of urine protein.

Patient education

• Warn patient to avoid driving or operating heavy machinery until adverse CNS effects of drug are known.

• Instruct patient to take first dose at bedtime to minimize drowsiness, dizziness, fatigue, and ataxia.

• Inform patient that drug can be taken without regard to meals.

Overdose & treatment

• Acute overdose of gabapentin may cause double vision, slurred speech, drowsiness, lethargy, and diarrhea.

• Supportive care is recommended. In addition, gabapentin can be removed by hemodialysis; this may be indicated by the patient's clinical state or in patients with significant renal impairment.

ganciclovir (DHPG)
Cytovene

Synthetic nucleoside, antiviral

Available by prescription only
Injection: 500-mg vial
Capsules: 250 mg

INDICATIONS & DOSAGE
Treatment of cytomegalovirus (CMV) retinitis
Adults: Initially, 5 mg/kg I.V. (given at a constant rate over 1 hour) q 12 hours for 14 to 21 days; followed by a maintenance dose of 5 mg/kg I.V. once daily for 7 days weekly; or 6 mg/kg I.V. once daily for 5 days weekly. These I.V. infusions should be given at a constant rate over 1

hour. Alternately, a maintenance dose of 1,000 mg P.O. t.i.d. or 500 mg P.O. q 3 hours while awake (six times daily) may be used.

Prevention of CMV in transplant recipients
Adults: 5 mg/kg I.V. over 1 hour q 12 hours for 7 to 14 days, followed by a maintenance dose of 5 mg/kg once daily for 7 days weekly or 6 mg/kg once daily for 5 days weekly.

◊ **Other CMV infections**
Adults: 5 mg/kg I.V. over 1 hour q 12 hours for 14 to 21 days; or 2.5 mg/kg I.V. q 8 hours for 14 to 21 days.

✦ **Dosage adjustment.** Adjust dosage for patients with renal failure. Consider reducing dosage for patients with neutropenia, anemia, or thrombocytopenia.

Creatinine clearance (ml/min)	Dosage
I.V. induction dosage	
≥ 70	5 mg/kg I.V. q 12 hr
50-69	2.5 mg/kg I.V. q 12 hr
25-49	2.5 mg/kg I.V. q 24 hr
10-24	1.25 mg/kg I.V. q 12 hr
< 10	1.25 mg/kg I.V. three times weekly after hemodialysis
P.O. dosage	
≥ 70	1,000 mg P.O. t.i.d. or 500 mg q 3 hr six times daily
50-69	1,500 mg P.O. daily or 500 mg P.O. t.i.d.
25-49	1,000 mg P.O. daily or 500 mg P.O. b.i.d.
10-24	500 mg P.O. daily
< 10	500 mg P.O. three times weekly after hemodialysis

PHARMACODYNAMICS
Antiviral action: Ganciclovir is a synthetic nucleoside analogue of 2′-deoxyguanosine. It competitively inhibits viral DNA polymerase and may be incorporated within viral DNA to cause early termination of DNA replication. It has shown activity against CMV, herpes simplex virus type 1 and type 2 (HSV-1

and HSV-2), varicella zoster virus, Epstein-Barr virus, and hepatitis B virus.

PHARMACOKINETICS

Absorption: Ganciclovir is administered I.V. because less than 7% is absorbed after oral administration.

Distribution: Drug is only 2% to 3% protein-bound. It preferentially concentrates within CMV-infected cells because of action of cellular kinases that convert it to ganciclovir triphosphate.

Metabolism: Most drug (more than 90%) is excreted unchanged.

Excretion: Elimination half-life is about 3 hours in patients with normal renal function; it can be as long as 30 hours in patients with severe renal failure. The primary route of excretion is through the kidneys by glomerular filtration and some renal tubular secretion.

CONTRAINDICATIONS & PRECAUTIONS

Contraindicated in patients with hypersensitivity to ganciclovir and with an absolute neutrophil count less than 500/mm^3 or a platelet count less than 25,000/mm^3. Use cautiously in patients with impaired renal function.

INTERACTIONS

Drug-drug. Use with *cytotoxic drugs* may result in additive toxicity, including bone marrow depression, stomatitis, and alopecia. Use of *imipenem-cilastatin* may increase the risk of seizures. Use with *probenecid* may decrease the renal clearance of ganciclovir. There may be a higher incidence of neutropenia in patients also receiving *zidovudine*.

ADVERSE REACTIONS

CNS: altered dreams, confusion, ataxia, headache, *seizures, coma,* dizziness, somnolence, tremor, abnormal thinking, agitation, amnesia, anxiety, neuropathy, paresthesia, asthenia, pain (at injection site).

EENT: retinal detachment (in CMV retinitis patients).

GI: *nausea, vomiting, diarrhea, anorexia, abdominal pain,* flatulence, dyspepsia, dry mouth.

Hematologic: *granulocytopenia, **thrombocytopenia,** leukopenia, anemia.*

Hepatic: abnormal liver function tests, increased serum creatinine levels.

Respiratory: pneumonia.

Skin: *rash; sweating;* pruritus, inflammation (at injection site).

Other: phlebitis, chills, sepsis, *fever,* infection.

▣ KEY CONSIDERATIONS

● Use cautiously in geriatric patients with compromised renal function.

● Administer drug over 1 hour; don't administer as a rapid I.V. bolus. Don't give I.M. or S.C.

● Reconstitute with sterile water for injection. Don't reconstitute with bacteriostatic water for injection because this may lead to the formation of a precipitate.

● Note that reconstituted solutions are stable for 12 hours. Don't refrigerate.

● Monitor CBC to detect neutropenia, which may occur in as many as 40% of patients. It usually appears after about 10 days of therapy and may be associated with a higher dosage (15 mg/kg/day). Neutropenia is reversible but may necessitate discontinuation of therapy. Patients may resume drug therapy when blood counts return to normal.

Patient education

● Tell patient that maintenance infusions are necessary to prevent recurrence of disease.

● Instruct patients to have regular ophthalmic examinations to monitor retinitis.

● Advise patient to immediately report signs or symptoms of infection (fever, sore throat) or easy bruising or bleeding.

● Inform patient to take oral dose with food.

Overdose & treatment

● Overdose may result in vomiting, neutropenia, or GI disturbances.

● Treatment should be symptomatic and supportive. Hemodialysis may be useful. Hydrate the patient to reduce plasma levels.

Reactions may be *common*, uncommon, **life-threatening**, or COMMON AND LIFE-THREATENING.

gemfibrozil
Lopid

Fibric acid derivative, antilipemic

Available by prescription only
Tablets: 600 mg

INDICATIONS & DOSAGE
Type IV hyperlipidemia (hypertriglyc-eridemia) and severe hypercholestero-lemia unresponsive to diet and other drugs; reducing risk of cardiac disease, only in type IIb patients without history of disease
Adults: 1,200 mg P.O. administered in 2 divided doses 30 minutes before morning and evening meals.

PHARMACODYNAMICS
Antilipemic action: Gemfibrozil decreases serum triglyceride levels and very-low-density lipoprotein (VLDL) cholesterol while increasing serum high-density lipoprotein cholesterol, inhibits lipolysis in adipose tissue, and reduces hepatic triglyceride synthesis; drug is closely related to clofibrate pharmacologically.

PHARMACOKINETICS
Absorption: Gemfibrozil is well absorbed from the GI tract; plasma levels peak 1 to 2 hours after an oral dose. Plasma levels of VLDL decrease in 2 to 5 days; peak effect occurs in 4 weeks. Further decreases in plasma VLDL levels occur over several months.
Distribution: Drug is 95% protein-bound.
Metabolism: Drug is metabolized by the liver.
Excretion: Drug is eliminated mostly in urine, but some is excreted in feces. After a single dose, half-life is 1½ hours; after multiple doses, half-life decreases to about 1¼ hours.

CONTRAINDICATIONS & PRECAUTIONS
Contraindicated in patients with hypersensitivity to gemfibrozil, hepatic or severe renal dysfunction (including primary biliary cirrhosis), and preexisting gallbladder disease.

INTERACTIONS
Drug-drug. Myopathy with rhabdomyolysis can occur with use of gemfibrozil and *lovastatin,* as well as with similar *antilipemics* (such as *pravastatin* and *simvastatin*); avoid concomitant use. Gemfibrozil enhances the effect of *oral anticoagulants,* increasing the risk of hemorrhage; adjust anticoagulant dose to maintain the desired PT and INR and monitor frequently.

ADVERSE REACTIONS
CNS: headache, fatigue, vertigo.
CV: atrial fibrillation.
GI: abdominal and epigastric pain, diarrhea, nausea, vomiting, *dyspepsia,* constipation, acute appendicitis.
Hematologic: anemia, leukopenia, eosinophilia, *thrombocytopenia.*
Hepatic: bile duct obstruction, elevated liver enzyme levels.
Skin: rash, dermatitis, pruritus, eczema.

▣ KEY CONSIDERATIONS
● Because drug is pharmacologically related to clofibrate, adverse reactions associated with clofibrate may also occur with gemfibrozil. Some studies suggest that clofibrate increases risk of death from cancer, postcholecystectomy complications, and pancreatitis. These hazards haven't been studied in gemfibrozil but should be kept in mind.
● Drug therapy may elevate serum levels of CK, ALT, AST, alkaline phosphatase, and LD; it may also decrease serum potassium and hemoglobin levels, hematocrit, and WBC counts.

Patient education
● Stress importance of close medical supervision and tell patient to report adverse reactions promptly; encourage him to comply with prescribed regimen, diet, and exercise.
● Warn patient not to exceed prescribed dose.
● Advise patient to take drug with food to minimize GI discomfort.

gentamicin sulfate
Cidomycin*, Garamycin, Genoptic, Genoptic S.O.P., Gentacidin, Gentak, Jenamicin

Aminoglycoside, antibiotic

Available by prescription only
Injection: 40 mg/ml (adult), 2 mg/ml (intrathecal)
Ophthalmic ointment: 3 mg/g
Ophthalmic solution: 3 mg/ml
Topical cream or ointment: 0.1%

INDICATIONS & DOSAGE
Serious infections caused by susceptible organisms
Adults with normal renal function:
3 mg/kg/day I.M. or I.V. infusion (in 50 to 100 ml of normal saline solution or D_5W infused over 30 minutes to 2 hours) daily in divided doses q 8 hours. May be given by direct I.V. push if necessary. For life-threatening infections, patient may receive up to 5 mg/kg/day in 3 to 4 divided doses.
Meningitis
Adults: Systemic therapy as above; may also use 4 to 8 mg intrathecally daily.
Endocarditis prophylaxis for GI or GU procedure or surgery
Adults: 1.5 mg/kg I.M. or I.V. 30 minutes before procedure or surgery. Maximum dosage is 80 mg given with ampicillin (vancomycin in penicillin-allergic patients).
External ocular infections caused by susceptible organisms
Adults: Instill 1 or 2 gtt in eye q 4 hours. In severe infections, may use up to 2 drops q hour. Apply ointment to lower conjunctival sac b.i.d. or t.i.d.
Primary and secondary bacterial infections; superficial burns; skin ulcers; and infected lacerations, abrasions, insect bites, or minor surgical wounds
Adults: Rub in small amount gently t.i.d. or q.i.d. with or without gauze dressing.
Pelvic inflammatory disease
Adults: Initially 2 mg/kg I.M. or I.V; then 1.5 mg/kg q 8 hours.
✦ Dosage adjustment. In patients with renal failure, initial dose is same as for those with normal renal function. Subse-

quent doses and frequency determined by renal function studies and blood levels; keep peak serum levels between 4 and 10 µg/ml and trough serum levels between 1 and 2 µg/ml. One method is to administer 1-mg/kg doses and adjust the dosing interval based on steady-state serum creatinine level, using this formula:

$$\frac{\text{creatinine}}{\text{(mg/100 ml)}} \times 8 = \frac{\text{dosing interval}}{\text{(hours)}}.$$

Posthemodialysis to maintain therapeutic blood levels
Adults: 1 to 1.7 mg/kg I.M. or I.V. after each dialysis.

PHARMACODYNAMICS
Antibiotic action: Gentamicin is bactericidal; it binds directly to the 30S ribosomal subunit, thus inhibiting bacterial protein synthesis. Its spectrum of activity includes many aerobic gram-negative organisms (including most strains of *Pseudomonas aeruginosa*) and some aerobic gram-positive organisms. Gentamicin may act against some bacterial strains resistant to other aminoglycosides; bacterial strains resistant to gentamicin may be susceptible to tobramycin, netilmicin, or amikacin.

PHARMACOKINETICS
Absorption: Gentamicin is absorbed poorly after oral administration and is given parenterally; after I.M. administration, serum levels peak at 30 to 90 minutes.
Distribution: Drug is distributed widely after parenteral administration; intraocular penetration is poor. CSF penetration is low even in patients with inflamed meninges. Intraventricular administration produces high levels throughout the CNS. Protein-binding is minimal.
Metabolism: Not metabolized.
Excretion: Drug is excreted primarily in urine by glomerular filtration; a small amount may be excreted in bile. Elimination half-life in adults is 2 to 3 hours. In patients with severe renal damage, half-life may extend to 24 to 60 hours.

Reactions may be *common*, uncommon, *life-threatening*, or COMMON AND LIFE-THREATENING.

CONTRAINDICATIONS & PRECAUTIONS

Contraindicated in patients hypersensitive to gentamicin or in those who may exhibit cross-sensitivity with other aminoglycosides, such as neomycin. Use systemic treatment cautiously in geriatric patients or in those with renal or neuromuscular disorders.

INTERACTIONS

Drug-drug. Use with the following drugs may increase the risk of nephrotoxicity, ototoxicity, or neurotoxicity: other *aminoglycosides, amphotericin B, capreomycin, cephalosporins, cisplatin, methoxyflurane, polymyxin B,* and *vancomycin.* Risk of ototoxicity is also increased during use with *bumetanide, ethacrynic acid, furosemide, mannitol,* or *urea. Dimenhydrinate* and other *antiemetic* and *antivertigo drugs* may mask gentamicin-induced ototoxicity. Gentamicin may potentiate neuromuscular blockade produced by *general anesthetics* or *neuromuscular blockers* such as *succinylcholine* and *tubocurarine.* Use with a *penicillin* results in synergistic bactericidal effect against *P. aeruginosa, Escherichia coli, Klebsiella, Citrobacter, Enterobacter, Serratia,* and *Proteus mirabilis;* however, the drugs are physically and chemically incompatible and are inactivated when mixed or given together.

ADVERSE REACTIONS

CNS: headache, lethargy, encephalopathy, confusion, pain at the injection site, dizziness, *seizures,* numbness, peripheral neuropathy (with injected form).
CV: hypotension (with injected form).
EENT: *ototoxicity,* blurred vision (with injected form); burning, stinging, blurred vision (with ophthalmic ointment); transient irritation (with ophthalmic solution); conjunctival hyperemia (with ophthalmic form).
GI: vomiting, nausea (with injected form).
GU: *nephrotoxicity* (with injected form).
Hematologic: anemia, eosinophilia, *leukopenia, thrombocytopenia, granulocytopenia* (with injected form).

Musculoskeletal: muscle twitching, myasthenia gravis-like syndrome (with injected form).
Respiratory: *apnea (*with injected form).
Skin: rash, urticaria, pruritus, tingling (with injected form); minor skin irritation, possible photosensitivity, allergic contact dermatitis (with topical administration).
Other: fever, *anaphylaxis* (with injected form); hypersensitivity reactions, overgrowth of nonsusceptible organisms (with ophthalmic form and long-term use).

▣ KEY CONSIDERATIONS

Besides the recommendations relevant to all aminoglycosides, consider the following:
● Risk of toxicity is increased with prolonged peak serum level greater than 10 µg/ml and trough serum level greater than 2 µg/ml.
● For local application to skin infections, remove crusts by gently soaking with warm water and soap or wet compresses before applying ointment or cream; cover with protective gauze. Systemic absorption from excessive use may cause systemic toxicities.
● Because drug is dialyzable, patients undergoing hemodialysis may need dosage adjustments.
● Gentamicin-induced nephrotoxicity may elevate BUN, nonprotein nitrogen, and serum creatinine levels, and increase urine excretion of casts.

Patient education

● Teach patient proper topical application of drug; emphasize need to call promptly if lesions worsen or skin irritation occurs.

Overdose & treatment

● Signs and symptoms of overdose include ototoxicity, nephrotoxicity, and neuromuscular toxicity.
● Drug can be removed by hemodialysis or peritoneal dialysis. Treatment with calcium salts or anticholinesterases reverses neuromuscular blockade.

glimepiride
Amaryl

Sulfonylurea, antidiabetic

Available by prescription only
Tablets: 1 mg, 2 mg, 4 mg

INDICATIONS & DOSAGE
***Adjunct to diet and exercise to lower
blood glucose in patients with type 2 diabetes mellitus whose hyperglycemia
can't be managed by diet and exercise
alone***
Adults: Initially, 1 to 2 mg P.O. once daily with first main meal of the day; usual
maintenance dosage is 1 to 4 mg P.O.
once daily. Maximum recommended
dosage is 8 mg once daily. After dose of
2 mg is reached, increases in dosage
should be made in increments not exceeding 2 mg at 1- to 2-week intervals,
based on patient's blood glucose response.
***Adjunct to insulin therapy in patients
with type 2 diabetes mellitus whose hyperglycemia can't be managed by diet
and exercise in conjunction with an
oral antidiabetic***
Adults: 8 mg P.O. once daily with first
main meal of the day in combination
with low-dose insulin. Insulin should be
adjusted upward weekly as needed and
guided by patient's blood glucose response.
✦ ***Dosage adjustment.*** Patients with renal impairment require cautious dosing.
Give 1 mg P.O. once daily with first
main meal of the day, followed by appropriate dose titration, p.r.n.

PHARMACODYNAMICS
Antidiabetic action: Exact mechanism of
glimepiride to lower blood glucose appears to depend on stimulating the release of insulin from functioning pancreatic beta cells. Also, drug can lead to increased sensitivity of peripheral tissues
to insulin.

PHARMACOKINETICS
Absorption: Glimepiride is completely
absorbed from the GI tract. Significant
absorption occurs within 1 hour after ad-

ministration, and peak drug levels occur
at 2 to 3 hours.
Distribution: Drug's protein-binding is
greater than 99.5%.
Metabolism: Drug is completely metabolized by oxidative biotransformation.
Excretion: Glimepiride's metabolites are
excreted in urine (about 60%) and feces
(about 40%).

CONTRAINDICATIONS & PRECAUTIONS
Contraindicated in patients with hypersensitivity to glimepiride and in those
with diabetic ketoacidosis (with or without coma) because this condition should
be treated with insulin. Use cautiously in
debilitated or malnourished patients and
in those with adrenal, pituitary, hepatic,
or renal insufficiency because these patients are more susceptible to the hypoglycemic action of glucose-lowering
drugs.

INTERACTIONS
Drug-drug. Use with *beta blockers* may
mask symptoms of hypoglycemia. Use
of *drugs that tend to produce hyperglycemia*—such as *corticosteroids, estrogens, isoniazid, nicotinic acid, oral contraceptives, phenothiazines, phenytoin,
sympathomimetics, thiazides* and *other
diuretics,* and *thyroid drugs*—may require dosage adjustments. *NSAIDs* and
other *drugs that are highly protein-
bound* (such as *beta blockers, chloramphenicol, coumarins MAO inhibitors,
probenecid, salicylates,* and *sulfonamides*) may potentiate the hypoglycemic action of sulfonylureas such as
glimepiride.

ADVERSE REACTIONS
CNS: dizziness, asthenia, headache.
EENT: changes in accommodation,
blurred vision.
GI: vomiting, abdominal pain, nausea,
diarrhea.
Hematologic: *leukopenia,* hemolytic
anemia, *agranulocytosis, thrombocy-
topenia, aplastic anemia, pancytopenia.*
Hepatic: cholestatic jaundice, elevated
transaminase levels.
Metabolic: hypoglycemia.

Reactions may be *common*, uncommon, *life-threatening*, or COMMON AND LIFE-THREATENING.

Skin: allergic skin reactions (pruritus, erythema, urticaria, morbilliform or maculopapular eruptions).

▣ KEY CONSIDERATIONS

Besides the recommendations relevant to all sulfonylureas, consider the following:
• In geriatric, debilitated, or malnourished patients or in patients with renal or hepatic insufficiency, the initial dosing, dose increments, and maintenance dosage should be conservative to avoid hypoglycemic reactions.
• During maintenance therapy, glimepiride should be discontinued if satisfactory lowering of blood glucose is no longer achieved. Secondary failures to glimepiride monotherapy can be treated with glimepiride-insulin combination therapy.
• Fasting blood glucose should be monitored periodically to determine therapeutic response. Glycosylated hemoglobin should also be monitored, usually every 3 to 6 months, to assess more precisely long-term glycemic control.
• Oral hypoglycemic agents have been associated with an increased risk of CV mortality compared with diet or diet and insulin therapy.

Patient education

• Instruct patient to take drug with first meal of the day.
• Make sure patient understands that therapy relieves symptoms but doesn't cure disease.
• Stress importance of adhering to specific diet, weight reduction, exercise, and personal hygiene programs. Explain how and when he should check his blood glucose level.
• Teach patient how to recognize and manage the signs and symptoms of hyperglycemia and hypoglycemia.
• Advise patient to carry medical identification regarding diabetic status.

Overdose & treatment

• Overdose of sulfonylureas can produce hypoglycemia.
• Mild hypoglycemic symptoms without loss of consciousness or neurologic findings should be treated aggressively with oral glucose and adjustments in drug

dosage and meal patterns. Monitor patient closely until out of danger. Severe hypoglycemic reactions with coma, seizure, or other neurologic impairment occur infrequently but constitute medical emergencies requiring immediate hospitalization. If hypoglycemic coma occurs or is suspected, give a rapid I.V. injection of concentrated (50%) glucose solution, followed by continuous infusion of a more dilute (10%) glucose solution at a rate that will maintain the blood glucose at a level above 100 mg/dl. Patient should be closely monitored for at least 24 to 48 hours because hypoglycemia may recur after apparent recovery.

---

glipizide
Glucotrol, Glucotrol XL

Sulfonylurea, antidiabetic

Available by prescription only
Tablets: 5 mg, 10 mg
Tablets (extended-release): 5 mg, 10 mg

INDICATIONS & DOSAGE

Adjunct to diet to lower blood glucose levels in patients with type 2 diabetes mellitus
Adults: Initially, 5 mg P.O. daily 30 minutes before breakfast; dose should be adjusted in increments of 2.5 to 5 mg. Usual maintenance dosage is 10 to 15 mg. Maximum recommended daily dose is 40 mg. Total daily doses greater than 15 mg should be divided except when using extended-release tablets.
Geriatric patients: Initial dosage may be 2.5 mg.
✦ ***Dosage adjustment.*** Initial dosage in patients with hepatic disease may be 2.5 mg.
Extended-release tablets
Adults: Initially, 5 mg P.O. daily, adjust dosage in 5-mg increments q 3 months based on level of glycemic control. Maximum daily dose is 20 mg.
To replace insulin therapy
Adults: If insulin dosage is more than 20 U daily, patient may be started at usual dosage of glipizide besides 50% of insulin dosage. If insulin dosage is less than 20 U, insulin may be discontinued.

PHARMACODYNAMICS
Antidiabetic action: Glipizide lowers blood glucose levels by stimulating insulin release from functioning beta cells in the pancreas. After prolonged administration, the drug's hypoglycemic effects appear to reflect extrapancreatic effects, possibly including reduction of basal hepatic glucose production and enhanced peripheral sensitivity to insulin. The latter may result either from an increase in the number of insulin receptors or from changes in events subsequent to insulin binding.

PHARMACOKINETICS
Absorption: Glipizide is absorbed rapidly and completely from the GI tract. Onset of action occurs within 15 to 30 minutes, with maximum hypoglycemic effects within 2 to 3 hours.
Distribution: Drug is probably distributed within the extracellular fluid. It's 92% to 99% protein-bound.
Metabolism: Drug is metabolized almost completely by the liver to inactive metabolites.
Excretion: Drug and its metabolites are excreted primarily in urine; small amounts in feces. Renal clearance of unchanged glipizide increases with increasing urine pH. Duration of action is 10 to 24 hours; half-life is 2 to 4 hours.

CONTRAINDICATIONS & PRECAUTIONS
Contraindicated in patients with hypersensitivity to glipizide or with diabetic ketoacidosis with or without coma. Use cautiously in patients with impaired renal or hepatic function and in geriatric, malnourished, or debilitated patients.

INTERACTIONS
Drug-drug. Use with *anticoagulants* may increase plasma levels of both drugs and, after continued therapy, may reduce plasma levels and effectiveness of the anticoagulant. Use with *beta blockers* (including *ophthalmics*) may mask symptoms of hypoglycemia, such as rising pulse rate and blood pressure, and may prolong hypoglycemia by blocking gluconeogenesis. Use with *chloramphenicol, guanethidine, insulin, MAO inhibitors, probenecid, salicylates,* or *sulfonamides* may enhance the hypoglycemic effect by displacing glipizide from its protein-binding sites. *Cimetidine* may potentiate the hypoglycemic effects by preventing hepatic metabolism. Use with *drugs that may increase blood glucose levels (adrenocorticoids, amphetamines, baclofen, corticotropin, epinephrine, estrogens, ethacrynic acid, furosemide, glucocorticoids, oral contraceptives, phenytoin, thiazide diuretics, thyroid hormones,* and *triamterene*) may require dosage adjustments.
Drug-lifestyle. Use of glipizide with *alcohol* may produce a disulfiram-like reaction consisting of nausea, vomiting, abdominal cramps, and headaches. Because *smoking* increases corticosteroid release, patients who smoke may require higher dosages of glipizide; monitor closely.

ADVERSE REACTIONS
CNS: dizziness, drowsiness, headache.
GI: nausea, constipation, diarrhea.
Hematologic: *leukopenia,* hemolytic anemia, *agranulocytosis, thrombocytopenia, aplastic anemia.*
Hepatic: cholestatic jaundice.
Metabolic: *hypoglycemia.*
Skin: rash, pruritus.

▣ KEY CONSIDERATIONS
Besides the recommendations relevant to all sulfonylureas, consider the following:
● Geriatric patients may be more sensitive to the effects of glipizide.
● Patients who may be more sensitive to drug, such as debilitated or malnourished individuals, should begin therapy with a lower dosage (2.5 mg once daily).
● Hypoglycemia causes more neurologic symptoms in geriatric patients.
● To improve glucose control in patients who receive 15 mg/day or more, give divided doses, usually 30 minutes before the morning and evening meals.
● Some patients taking glipizide can be controlled effectively on a once-daily regimen; others show better response with divided dosing.
● Glipizide is a second-generation sulfonylurea oral hypoglycemic. It appears to cause fewer adverse reactions than first-generation sulfonylureas.

Reactions may be *common,* uncommon, *life-threatening*, or COMMON AND LIFE-THREATENING.

• Drug has a mild diuretic effect that may be useful in patients with heart failure or cirrhosis.
• When substituting glipizide for chlorpropamide, monitor patient carefully during the first week because of the prolonged retention of chlorpropamide.
• Glipizide therapy alters cholesterol, alkaline phosphatase, AST, LD, and BUN levels.
• Oral antidiabetics have been associated with an increased risk of CV mortality as compared with diet or diet and insulin therapy.

Patient education
• Emphasize importance of following prescribed diet, exercise, and medical regimen.
• Instruct patient to take the drug at the same time each day.
• Tell patient that if he misses a dose, he should take it immediately unless it's almost time to take the next dose. Patient shouldn't double-dose.
• Advise patient to avoid alcohol when taking glipizide. Remind him that many foods and OTC drugs contain alcohol.
• Encourage patient to wear a medical identification bracelet or necklace.
• Tell patient to take glipizide with food to minimize GI upset.
• Teach patient how to monitor blood glucose, urine glucose, and ketone levels, as prescribed.
• Teach patient how to recognize and manage the signs and symptoms of hyperglycemia and hypoglycemia.

Overdose & treatment
• Signs and symptoms of overdose include low blood glucose levels, tingling of lips and tongue, hunger, nausea, decreased cerebral function (lethargy, yawning, confusion, agitation, and nervousness), increased sympathetic activity (tachycardia, sweating, and tremor), and ultimately seizures, stupor, and coma.
• Mild hypoglycemia (without loss of consciousness or neurologic findings) responds to treatment with oral glucose and dosage adjustments. If the patient looses consciousness or experiences other neurologic changes, he should receive a rapid injection of $D_{50}W$, followed by

continuous infusion of $D_{10}W$ at a rate to maintain blood glucose levels of more than 100 mg/dl. Monitor for 24 to 48 hours.

glucagon

Antidiabetic, diagnostic

Available by prescription only
Powder for injection: 1 mg (1 U)/vial, 10 mg (10 U)/vial

INDICATIONS & DOSAGE
Coma of insulin-shock therapy
Adults: 0.5 to 1 mg S.C., I.M., or I.V. 1 hour after coma develops; may repeat within 25 minutes, if necessary. In deep coma, give glucose 10% to 50% I.V. for faster response. When patient responds, give additional carbohydrate immediately.
Severe insulin-induced hypoglycemia during diabetic therapy
Adults: 0.5 to 1 mg S.C., I.M., or I.V.; may repeat q 20 minutes for 2 doses, if necessary.
Diagnostic aid for radiologic examination
Adults: 0.25 to 2 mg I.V. or I.M. before initiation of radiologic procedure.

PHARMACODYNAMICS
Antidiabetic action: Glucagon increases plasma glucose levels and causes smooth-muscle relaxation and an inotropic myocardial effect because adenylate cyclase is stimulated to produce cAMP. Then cAMP initiates a series of reactions that leads to the degradation of glycogen to glucose. Hepatic stores of glycogen are necessary for glucagon to exert an antihypoglycemic effect.
Diagnostic action: The mechanism by which glucagon relaxes the smooth muscles of the stomach, esophagus, duodenum, small bowel, and colon hasn't been fully defined.

PHARMACOKINETICS
Absorption: Glucagon is destroyed in the GI tract; therefore, it must be given parenterally. After I.V. administration, hyperglycemic activity peaks within 30 minutes; relaxation of the GI smooth

muscle occurs within 1 minute. After I.M. administration, relaxation of the GI smooth muscle occurs within 10 minutes. Administration to comatose hypoglycemic patients (with normal liver glycogen stores) usually produces a return to consciousness within 20 minutes.
Distribution: Distribution isn't fully understood.
Metabolism: Glucagon is degraded extensively by the liver, in the kidneys and plasma, and at its tissue receptor sites in plasma membranes.
Excretion: Metabolic products are excreted by the kidneys. Half-life is about 3 to 10 minutes. Duration after I.M. administration is up to 32 minutes; after I.V. administration, up to 25 minutes.

CONTRAINDICATIONS & PRECAUTIONS
Contraindicated in patients with pheochromocytoma or hypersensitivity to glucagon. Use cautiously in patients with insulinoma and as a diagnostic agent in patients with diabetes mellitus.

INTERACTIONS
Drug-drug. Use of glucagon with *epinephrine* increases and prolongs the hyperglycemic effect. *Phenytoin* appears to inhibit glucagon-induced insulin release.

ADVERSE REACTIONS
CV: hypotension.
GI: nausea, vomiting.
Respiratory: respiratory distress.
Other: hypersensitivity reactions (***bronchospasm,*** rash, dizziness, lightheadedness).

◙ KEY CONSIDERATIONS
• Glucagon should be used only under direct medical supervision.
• If patient experiences nausea and vomiting from glucagon administration and can't retain some form of sugar for 1 hour, consider administration of I.V. dextrose.
• For I.V. drip infusion, glucagon is compatible with dextrose solution but forms a precipitate in chloride solutions.
• Glucagon has a positive inotropic and chronotropic action on the heart and may be used to treat overdose of beta blockers.

• Glucagon may be used as a diagnostic aid in radiologic examination of the stomach, duodenum, small intestine, and colon when a hypotonic state is desirable.
• Mixed solutions with diluent are stable for 48 hours when stored at 41° F (5° C). After reconstitution with sterile water, use immediately.
• Glucagon lowers serum potassium levels.

Patient education
• Teach patient how to mix and inject the drug properly, using an appropriate-sized syringe and injecting at a 90-degree angle.
• Tell patient to mix doses of 2 mg or less using manufacturer's diluent; to mix doses over 2 mg using sterile water for injection.
• Instruct patient and family members how to administer glucagon and how to recognize hypoglycemia. Urge them to call immediately in emergencies.
• Tell patient to expect response usually within 20 minutes after injection; injection may be repeated if no response occurs. Patient should seek medical assistance if second injection is needed.

glyburide
DiaBeta, Glynase PresTab, Micronase

Sulfonylurea, antidiabetic

Available by prescription only
Tablets: 1.25 mg, 2.5 mg, 5 mg
Tablets (micronized): 1.5 mg, 3 mg, 6 mg

INDICATIONS & DOSAGE
Adjunct to diet to lower blood glucose levels in patients with type 2 diabetes mellitus
Adults: Initially, 2.5 to 5 mg P.O. daily with breakfast. Patients who are more sensitive to antidiabetics should be started at 1.25 mg daily. Usual maintenance dosage is 1.25 to 20 mg daily, either as a single dose or in divided doses.
   For micronized tablets, initially give 1.5 to 3 mg P.O. with breakfast. Usual

maintenance dosage is 0.75 to 12 mg P.O. daily.

Geriatric patients: Start therapy with 1.25 mg P.O. once daily.

◆ *Dosage adjustment.* In debilitated or malnourished patients or those with renal or liver dysfunction, start therapy with 1.25 mg once daily.

To replace insulin therapy

Adults: If insulin dosage is more than 40 U/day, patient may be started on 5 mg of glyburide daily besides 50% of the insulin dose. Patients maintained on less than 20 U/day should receive 2.5 to 5 mg/day; those maintained on 20 to 40 U/day should receive 5 mg/day. In all patients, glyburide is substituted and insulin is discontinued abruptly.

For micronized tablets, if insulin dosage is more than 40 U/day, give 3 mg P.O. with a 50% reduction in insulin. Patients maintained on 20 to 40 U/day should receive 3 mg P.O. as a single daily dose; those maintained on less than 20 U/day should receive 1.5 to 3 mg/day as a single dose.

PHARMACODYNAMICS

Antidiabetic action: Glyburide lowers blood glucose levels by stimulating insulin release from functioning beta cells in the pancreas. After prolonged administration, the drug's hypoglycemic effects appear to be related to extrapancreatic effects, possibly including reduction of basal hepatic glucose production and enhanced peripheral sensitivity to insulin. The latter may result either from an increase in the number of insulin receptors or from changes in events subsequent to insulin binding.

PHARMACOKINETICS

Absorption: Glyburide is almost completely absorbed from the GI tract. Onset of action occurs within 2 hours; hypoglycemic effects peak within 3 to 4 hours. A micronized tablet results in significant absorption; a 3-mg micronized tablet provides blood levels similar to a 5-mg conventional tablet.

Distribution: Drug is 99% protein-bound. Its distribution isn't fully understood.

Metabolism: Drug is metabolized completely by the liver to inactive metabolites.

Excretion: Drug is excreted as metabolites in urine and feces in equal proportions. Its duration of action is 24 hours; its half-life is 10 hours.

CONTRAINDICATIONS & PRECAUTIONS

Contraindicated in patients with hypersensitivity to glyburide or with diabetic ketoacidosis with or without coma. Use cautiously in patients with impaired renal or hepatic function and in geriatric, malnourished, or debilitated patients.

INTERACTIONS

Drug-drug. Use with *anticoagulants* may increase plasma levels of both drugs and, after continued therapy, may reduce plasma levels and anticoagulant effect. Use of glyburide with *beta blockers* (including *ophthalmics*) may increase the risk of hypoglycemia, mask its symptoms (increased pulse rate and blood pressure), and prolong its effects by blocking gluconeogenesis. Use with *chloramphenicol, guanethidine, insulin, MAO inhibitors, probenecid, salicylates,* or *sulfonamides* may enhance the hypoglycemic effect by displacing glyburide from its protein-binding sites. Use with *drugs that may increase blood glucose levels*—including *adrenocorticoids, amphetamines, baclofen, corticotropin, diazoxide, epinephrine, ethacrynic acid, furosemide, glucocorticoids, phenytoin, thiazide diuretics, thyroid hormones,* and *triamterene*) may require dosage adjustments.

Drug-lifestyle. Use of glyburide with *alcohol* may produce a disulfiram-like reaction consisting of nausea, vomiting, abdominal cramps, and headaches; don't use together. Because *smoking* increases corticosteroid release, smokers may require higher dosages of glyburide; monitor closely.

ADVERSE REACTIONS

EENT: changes in accommodation or blurred vision.

GI: nausea, epigastric fullness, heartburn.

Hematologic: *leukopenia*, hemolytic anemia, *agranulocytosis, thrombocytopenia, aplastic anemia.*
Hepatic: cholestatic jaundice, hepatitis, abnormal liver function.
Metabolic: *hypoglycemia.*
Musculoskeletal: arthralgia, myalgia.
Skin: rash, pruritus, other allergic reactions.
Other: *angioedema.*

◙ KEY CONSIDERATIONS
Besides the recommendations relevant to all sulfonylureas, consider the following:
• Geriatric patients may be more sensitive to drug's effects because of reduced metabolism and elimination.
• Hypoglycemia causes more neurologic symptoms in geriatric patients.
• To improve control in patients receiving 10 mg/day or more, give divided doses before the morning and evening meals.
• Some patients taking glyburide may be controlled effectively on a once-daily regimen, whereas others show better response with divided dosing.
• Glyburide is a second-generation sulfonylurea oral antidiabetic. It appears to cause fewer adverse reactions than first-generation drugs.
• Drug has a mild diuretic effect that may be useful in patients who have heart failure or cirrhosis.
• When substituting glyburide for chlorpropamide, monitor patient closely during the first week because of the prolonged retention of chlorpropamide in the body.
• Oral antidiabetics have been associated with an increased risk of CV mortality compared with diet or diet and insulin therapy.
• Glyburide therapy alters cholesterol, alkaline phosphatase, and BUN levels.

Patient education
• Emphasize importance of following prescribed diet, exercise, and medical regimen.
• Tell patient to take drug at the same time each day. If a dose is missed, it should be taken immediately, unless it's almost time to take the next dose. Instruct patient not to double-dose.

• Advise patient to avoid alcohol while taking glyburide. Remind him that many foods and OTC drugs contain alcohol.
• Encourage patient to wear a medical identification bracelet or necklace.
• Suggest that drug be taken with food if GI upset occurs.
• Teach patient how to monitor blood glucose and urine glucose and ketone levels as prescribed.
• Teach patient how to recognize the signs and symptoms of hyperglycemia and hypoglycemia and what to do if they occur.

Overdose & treatment
• Signs and symptoms of overdose include low blood glucose levels, tingling of lips and tongue, hunger, nausea, decreased cerebral function (lethargy, yawning, confusion, agitation, and nervousness), increased sympathetic activity (tachycardia, sweating, and tremor), and ultimately seizures, stupor, and coma.
• Mild hypoglycemia, without loss of consciousness or neurological findings, responds to treatment with oral glucose and dosage adjustments. The patient with severe hypoglycemia should be hospitalized immediately. If hypoglycemic coma is suspected, the patient should receive rapid injection of $D_{50}W$, followed by a continuous infusion of $D_{10}W$ at a rate to maintain blood glucose levels greater than 100 mg/dl. Monitor for 24 to 48 hours.

glycerin (glycerol)
Ophthalgan, Osmoglyn, Sani-Supp

Trihydric alcohol, ophthalmic osmotic vehicle, laxative (osmotic), adjunct in treating glaucoma, lubricant

Available by prescription only
Ophthalmic solution: 7.5-ml containers
Oral solution: 50% (0.6 g/ml), 75% (0.94 g/ml)
Available without a prescription
Suppository: 3 g (adults)
Rectal solution: 4 ml/applicator

Reactions may be *common*, uncommon, *life-threatening*, or COMMON AND LIFE-THREATENING.

INDICATIONS & DOSAGE
Constipation
Adults: 3 g as a suppository or 5 to 15 ml as an enema.
Reduction of intraocular pressure
Adults: 1 to 2 g/kg P.O. 60 to 90 minutes preoperatively.

Drug is useful in acute angle-closure glaucoma; before iridectomy (with carbonic anhydrase inhibitors or topical miotics); in trauma or disease, such as congenital glaucoma and some secondary glaucoma forms; and before or after surgery, such as retinal detachment surgery, cataract extraction, or keratoplasty.
Reduction of corneal edema
Adults: 1 or 2 gtt of ophthalmic solution topically before eye examination; 1 or 2 gtt q 3 to 4 hours for corneal edema.

Drug is used to facilitate ophthalmoscopic and gonioscopic examination and to differentiate superficial edema and deep corneal edema.
To act as an osmotic diuretic
Adults: 1 to 2 g/kg P.O. 1 to 1½ hours before surgery.

PHARMACODYNAMICS
Laxative action: Glycerin suppositories produce laxative action by causing rectal distention, thereby stimulating the urge to defecate; by causing local rectal irritation; and by triggering a hyperosmolar mechanism that draws water into the colon.

Antiglaucoma action: Orally administered glycerin helps reduce intraocular pressure by increasing plasma osmotic pressure, thereby drawing water into the blood from extravascular spaces. It also reduces intraocular fluid volume independently of routine flow mechanisms, decreasing intraocular pressure; it may cause tissue dehydration and decreased CSF pressure.

Lubricant action: Topically applied glycerin produces a hygroscopic (moisture-retaining) effect that reduces edema and improves visualization in ophthalmoscopy or gonioscopy. Glycerin reduces fluid in the cornea via its osmotic action and clears corneal haze.

PHARMACOKINETICS
Rectal form
Absorption: Glycerin suppositories are absorbed poorly; after rectal administration, laxative effect occurs in 15 to 30 minutes.

Distribution: When administered by suppository, glycerin is distributed locally.

Metabolism: Unknown.

Excretion: Drug is excreted in the feces.
Oral form
Absorption: Drug is absorbed rapidly from the GI tract, with peak serum levels occurring in 60 to 90 minutes with oral administration; intraocular pressure decreases in 10 to 30 minutes. Peak action occurs in 30 minutes to 2 hours, with effects persisting for 4 to 8 hours. Intracranial pressure (ICP) decreases in 10 to 60 minutes; this effect persists for 2 to 3 hours.

Distribution: Drug is distributed throughout the blood but doesn't enter ocular fluid.

Metabolism: After oral administration, about 80% of dose is metabolized in the liver, 10% to 20% in the kidneys.

Excretion: Drug is excreted in feces and urine.

CONTRAINDICATIONS & PRECAUTIONS
Contraindicated in patients hypersensitive to glycerin. Rectal administration of drug is contraindicated in those with intestinal obstruction, undiagnosed abdominal pain, vomiting or other signs of appendicitis, fecal impaction, or acute surgical abdomen.

Use oral form cautiously in geriatric or dehydrated patients and in those with diabetes or cardiac, renal, or hepatic disease.

INTERACTIONS
Drug-drug. Use with *diuretics* may result in additive effects.

ADVERSE REACTIONS
CNS: mild headache, dizziness (with oral administration).
EENT: eye pain, irritation.
GI: cramping pain, thirst, nausea, vomiting, diarrhea (with oral administration); rectal discomfort, hyperemia of rectal mucosa (with rectal administration).

GU: mild glycosuria.
Metabolic: mild hyperglycemia.

⊡ KEY CONSIDERATIONS

• Dehydrated geriatric patients may experience seizures and disorientation.
• When administering glycerin orally, don't give hypotonic fluids to relieve thirst and headache from glycerin-induced dehydration because these will counteract drug's osmotic effects.
• Use topical tetracaine hydrochloride or proparacaine before ophthalmic instillation to prevent discomfort.
• Don't touch tip of dropper to eye, surrounding tissues, or tear-film; glycerin will absorb moisture.
• To prevent or relieve headache, have patient remain supine during and after oral administration.
• Monitor diabetic patients for possible alteration of serum and urine glucose levels; dosage adjustment may be necessary.
• Drug should be discontinued if symptoms of hypersensitivity occur.
• Commercially available solutions may be poured over ice and sipped through a straw.
• Hyperosmolar laxatives are used most commonly to help laxative-dependent patients reestablish normal bowel habits.
• Other uses include reducing ICP in patients with CVA, meningitis, encephalitis, Reye's syndrome, or CNS trauma or tumors; and reducing brain volume during neurosurgical procedures through oral or I.V. administration, or both.
• Store drug in tightly closed original container.

Patient education

• Instruct patient to call if he experiences severe headache from oral dose.
• Teach patient correct way to instill drops and warn him not to touch eye with the dropper.
• Tell patient to lie down during and after administration of glycerin to prevent or relieve headache.

glycopyrrolate
Robinul, Robinul Forte

Anticholinergic, antimuscarinic, GI antispasmodic

Available by prescription only
Tablets: 1 mg, 2 mg
Injection: 0.2 mg/ml in 1-ml, 2-ml, 5-ml, and 20-ml vials

INDICATIONS & DOSAGE
Blockade of cholinergic effects of anticholinesterases used to reverse neuromuscular blockade
Adults: 0.2 mg I.V. for each 1 mg of neostigmine or 5 mg of pyridostigmine. May be given I.V. without dilution or may be added to dextrose injection and given by infusion.
Preoperatively to diminish secretions and block cardiac vagal reflexes
Adults: 0.0044 mg/kg of body weight given I.M. 30 to 60 minutes before anesthesia.
Adjunctive therapy in peptic ulcers and other GI disorders
Adults: 1 to 2 mg P.O. t.i.d. or 0.1 mg I.M. t.i.d. or q.i.d. Dosage should be individualized.

PHARMACODYNAMICS
Anticholinergic action: Glycopyrrolate inhibits acetylcholine's muscarinic actions on autonomic effectors innervated by postganglionic cholinergic nerves. That action blocks adverse muscarinic effects associated with anticholinesterases used to reverse curariform-induced neuromuscular blockade. Glycopyrrolate decreases secretions and GI motility by the same mechanism. Glycopyrrolate blocks cardiac vagal reflexes by blocking vagal inhibition of the SA node.

PHARMACOKINETICS
Absorption: Glycopyrrolate is poorly absorbed from the GI tract (10% to 25%) after oral administration. Glycopyrrolate is rapidly absorbed when given I.M.; serum levels peak in 30 to 45 minutes. Action begins in 1 minute after I.V. and 15 to 30 minutes after I.M. or S.C. administration.

Reactions may be *common*, uncommon, *life-threatening*, or COMMON AND LIFE-THREATENING.

Distribution: Drug is rapidly distributed. Because it's a quaternary amine, it doesn't cross the blood-brain barrier or enter the CNS.

Metabolism: Exact metabolic fate is unknown. Duration of effect is up to 7 hours when given parenterally and up to 12 hours when given orally.

Excretion: A small amount of drug is eliminated in the urine as unchanged drug and metabolites. Drug is mostly excreted unchanged in feces or bile.

CONTRAINDICATIONS & PRECAUTIONS

Contraindicated in patients with hypersensitivity to glycopyrrolate and in those with glaucoma, obstructive uropathy, obstructive disease of the GI tract, myasthenia gravis, paralytic ileus, intestinal atony, unstable CV status in acute hemorrhage, severe ulcerative colitis, or toxic megacolon.

Use cautiously in patients with autonomic neuropathy, hyperthyroidism, coronary artery disease, arrhythmias, heart failure, hypertension, hiatal hernia, hepatic or renal disease, and ulcerative colitis. Also use with caution in hot or humid conditions when drug-induced heat stroke may occur.

INTERACTIONS

Drug-drug. Administration of *antacids* decreases oral absorption of anticholinergics; administer glycopyrrolate at least 1 hour before antacids. Decreased GI absorption of many drugs has been reported after the use of *anticholinergics* (for example, *ketoconazole* and *levodopa*); conversely, *slowly dissolving digoxin tablets* may yield higher serum digoxin levels when administered with anticholinergics. Administration of *drugs with anticholinergic effects* may cause additive toxicity. Use cautiously with *oral potassium supplements* (especially wax-matrix formulations) because the incidence of potassium-induced GI ulcerations may be increased.

ADVERSE REACTIONS

CNS: weakness; nervousness; insomnia; drowsiness; dizziness; headache; may cause confusion or excitement in geriatric patients.

CV: palpitations, tachycardia.
EENT: *dilated pupils, blurred vision,* photophobia, increased intraocular pressure.
GI: *constipation, dry mouth,* nausea, loss of taste, abdominal distention, vomiting, epigastric distress.
GU: *urinary hesitancy, urine retention,* impotence.
Skin: urticaria, decreased sweating or anhidrosis, other dermal signs and symptoms.
Other: allergic reactions *(anaphylaxis),* fever.

▣ KEY CONSIDERATIONS

Besides the recommendations relevant to all anticholinergics, consider the following:

• Administer glycopyrrolate cautiously to geriatric patients. However, glycopyrrolate may be the preferred anticholinergic in geriatric patients.
• Check all dosages carefully. Even a slight overdose can lead to toxic effects.
• For immediate treatment of bradycardia, some clinicians prefer atropine over glycopyrrolate.
• Don't mix glycopyrrolate with I.V. solutions containing sodium chloride or bicarbonate.
• Drug may be administered with neostigmine or physostigmine in same syringe.
• Note that drug is incompatible with thiopental, methohexital, secobarbital, pentobarbital, chloramphenicol, dimenhydrinate, and diazepam.

Patient education

• Instruct patient to take oral drug 30 to 60 minutes before meals.
• Warn patient to avoid activities that require alertness until drug's CNS effects are known.
• Advise patient to report signs of urinary hesitancy or urine retention.

Overdose & treatment

• Signs and symptoms of overdose include peripheral effects such as dilated, nonreactive pupils; blurred vision; flushed, hot, dry skin; dryness of mucous membranes; dysphagia; decreased or absent bowel sounds; urine retention;

hyperthermia; tachycardia; hypertension; and increased respiration.
• Treatment is primarily symptomatic and supportive, as needed. If patient is alert, induce vomiting (or perform gastric lavage) and follow with a saline cathartic and activated charcoal to prevent further drug absorption. In severe life-threatening cases, physostigmine may be administered to block the antimuscarinic effects of glycopyrrolate. Give fluids, as needed, to treat shock. If urine retention occurs, catheterization may be necessary.

granisetron hydrochloride
Kytril

Selective 5-hydroxytryptamine (5-HT$_3$) receptor antagonist, antiemetic, antinauseant

Available by prescription only
Tablets: 1 mg
Injection: 1 mg/ml

INDICATIONS & DOSAGE
Prevention of nausea and vomiting associated with emetogenic cancer chemotherapy
Adults: 10 mcg/kg I.V. infused over 5 minutes. Begin infusion within 30 minutes before administration of chemotherapy.
Oral form
Adults: 1 mg P.O. b.i.d. Give the first 1-mg tablet 1 hour before chemotherapy administration and the second tablet 12 hours after the first. Give only on days when chemotherapy is given. Continued treatment without chemotherapy hasn't been found to be useful.

PHARMACODYNAMICS
Antiemetic action: Granisetron, a selective 5-HT$_3$ receptor antagonist, is thought to bind to serotonin receptors of the 5-HT$_3$ type located peripherally on vagal nerve terminals and centrally in the chemoreceptor trigger zone of the area postrema. This binding blocks serotonin stimulation and subsequent vomiting after emetogenic stimuli, such as cisplatin.

PHARMACOKINETICS
Absorption: Unknown.
Distribution: Granisetron is distributed freely between plasma and RBCs. Plasma protein-binding is about 65%.
Metabolism: Drug is metabolized by the liver, possibly mediated by the cytochrome P-450 3A subfamily.
Excretion: About 12% of drug is eliminated unchanged in the urine in 48 hours; the rest is excreted as metabolites, 48% in urine and 38% in feces.

CONTRAINDICATIONS & PRECAUTIONS
Contraindicated in patients hypersensitive to granisetron.

INTERACTIONS
None significant.

ADVERSE REACTIONS
CNS: *headache, asthenia,* somnolence, dizziness, anxiety.
CV: hypertension.
GI: diarrhea, *constipation,* abdominal pain, *nausea,* vomiting, decreased appetite.
Hematologic: *leukopenia,* anemia, ***thrombocytopenia.***
Hepatic: elevated liver function tests.
Skin: alopecia.
Other: fever.

▣ KEY CONSIDERATIONS
• Dilute drug with normal saline injection or D$_5$W to a volume of 20 to 50 ml. Infuse I.V. over 5 minutes. Diluted solutions are stable for 24 hours at room temperature.
• Don't mix with other drugs; information about compatibility is limited.
• Although clearance is slower and half-life is prolonged in geriatric patients and in patients with hepatic disease, dosage adjustments aren't necessary.
• No dosage adjustment is recommended in patients with renal impairment.

Patient education
• Tell patient to watch for signs of an anaphylactoid reaction—local or generalized hives, chest tightness, wheezing, and dizziness or weakness—and to report them immediately.

Reactions may be *common,* uncommon, *life-threatening,* or COMMON AND LIFE-THREATENING.

griseofulvin microsize
Fulvicin-U/F, Grifulvin V, Grisactin

griseofulvin ultramicrosize
Fulvicin P/G, Grisactin Ultra, Gris-PEG

Penicillium antibiotic, antifungal

Available by prescription only
Microsize
Capsules: 250 mg
Tablets: 250 mg, 500 mg
Oral suspension: 125 mg/5 ml
Ultramicrosize
Tablets: 125 mg, 165 mg, 250 mg, 330 mg
Tablets (film-coated): 125 mg, 250 mg

INDICATIONS & DOSAGE
Tinea corporis, tinea capitis, tinea barbae, or tinea cruris infections
Adults: 330 mg ultramicrosize P.O. daily, or 500 mg microsize P.O. daily.
Tinea pedis or tinea unguium infections
Adults: 660 mg ultramicrosize P.O. daily or 1 g microsize P.O. daily.

PHARMACODYNAMICS
Antifungal action: Griseofulvin disrupts the fungal cell's mitotic spindle, interfering with cell division; it also may inhibit DNA replication. Drug is also deposited in keratin precursor cells, inhibiting fungal invasion. It's active against *Trichophyton, Microsporum,* and *Epidermophyton.*

PHARMACOKINETICS
Absorption: Absorption of griseofulvin is primarily in the duodenum and varies among individuals. Ultramicrosize preparations are absorbed almost completely; microsize absorption ranges from 25% to 70% and may be increased by giving with a high-fat meal. Levels peak at 4 to 8 hours.
Distribution: Drug concentrates in skin, hair, nails, fat, liver, and skeletal muscle; it's tightly bound to new keratin.
Metabolism: Drug is oxidatively demethylated and conjugated with glucuronic acid to inactive metabolites in the liver.

Excretion: About 50% of drug and its metabolites is excreted in urine and 33% in feces within 5 days. Less than 1% of a dose appears unchanged in urine. Griseofulvin is also excreted in perspiration. Elimination half-life is 9 to 24 hours.

CONTRAINDICATIONS & PRECAUTIONS
Contraindicated in patients with hypersensitivity to griseofulvin and in those with porphyria or hepatocellular failure. Use cautiously in penicillin-sensitive patients.

INTERACTIONS
Drug-drug. Use with *barbiturates* may impair absorption of griseofulvin and increase dosage requirements. Griseofulvin may decrease PT and INR in patients taking *warfarin,* by enzyme induction.
Drug-lifestyle. Drug may potentiate *alcohol* effects, producing tachycardia and flushing; advise patient to avoid alcohol during therapy. Photosensitivity reactions may occur to *sunlight;* take precautions.

ADVERSE REACTIONS
CNS: headache (in early stages of treatment), transient decrease in hearing, fatigue with large doses, occasional mental confusion, impaired performance of routine activities, psychotic symptoms, dizziness, insomnia, paresthesia of the hands and feet after extended therapy.
GI: oral thrush, nausea, vomiting, flatulence, diarrhea, epigastric distress, *bleeding.*
GU: proteinuria.
Hematologic: *leukopenia, granulocytopenia* (requires discontinuation of drug), porphyria.
Hepatic: *hepatic toxicity.*
Skin: *rash, urticaria,* photosensitivity, angioneurotic edema.
Other: hypersensitivity reactions (rash), lupus erythematosus.

▣ KEY CONSIDERATIONS
• Commercial formulation of drug has changed, decreasing the dosage required for an equivalent therapeutic effect. Dosages equivalent to the original formulation (before 1971) for 1 g of griseofulvin are 250 mg ultramicrosize or

500 mg microsize. Dosages may vary slightly depending on the manufacturer.
• Identify organism before therapy begins.
• Give drug with or after meals consisting of a high fat content (if allowed) to minimize GI distress.
• Assess nutrition and monitor food intake; drug may alter taste sensation, suppressing appetite.
• Check CBCs regularly for possible adverse effects; monitor renal and liver function studies periodically. Griseofulvin can cause proteinuria; it also may decrease granulocyte counts.
• Anticipate treating tinea pedis with combined oral and topical therapy.
• Ultramicrosize griseofulvin is absorbed more rapidly and completely than microsize and is effective at one half to two thirds the usual dose.

Patient education
• Encourage patient to maintain adequate nutritional intake; offer suggestions to improve taste of food.
• Stress importance of completing prescribed regimen to prevent relapse, even though symptoms may abate quickly.
• Teach signs and symptoms of adverse effects and hypersensitivity, and tell patient to report them immediately.
• Advise patient to avoid exposure to intense indoor light and sunlight to reduce the risk of photosensitivity reactions.
• Explain that drug may potentiate alcohol's effects, and advise patient to avoid alcohol during therapy.
• Teach correct personal hygiene and skin care.

Overdose & treatment
• Signs and symptoms of overdose include headache, lethargy, confusion, vertigo, blurred vision, nausea, vomiting, and diarrhea.
• Treatment is supportive. After recent ingestion (within 4 hours), induce vomiting or perform gastric lavage. Follow with activated charcoal to decrease absorption. A cathartic may also be helpful.

guaifenesin
Amonidrin, Anti-Tuss, Balminil Expectorant*, Breonesin, Fenesin, Gee-Gee, Genatuss, GG-CEN, Glyate, Glycotuss, Glytuss, Guiatuss, Halotussin, Humibid L.A., Humibid Sprinkle, Hytuss, Hytuss 2X, Malotuss, Mytussin, Naldecon Senior EX, Neo-Spec*, Organidin NR, Resyl*, Robitussin, Scot-Tussin, Uni-Tussin

Propanediol derivative, expectorant

Available without a prescription
Tablets: 100 mg, 200 mg
Tablets (extended-release): 600 mg
Capsules: 200 mg
Capsules (extended-release): 300 mg
Syrup: 100 mg/5 ml, 200 mg/5 ml

INDICATIONS & DOSAGE
As expectorant
Adults: 100 to 400 mg q 4 hours; maximum dosage is 2.4 g/day.
Extended-release
Adults: 600 to 1,200 mg q 12 hours, not to exceed 2,400 mg in 24 hours. For self-medication, recommended dosage is half the usual dosage.

PHARMACODYNAMICS
Expectorant action: Guaifenesin increases respiratory tract fluid by reducing adhesiveness and surface tension, decreasing viscosity of the secretions and thereby facilitating their removal.

PHARMACOKINETICS
Absorption: Unknown.
Distribution: Unknown.
Metabolism: Unknown.
Excretion: Unknown.

CONTRAINDICATIONS & PRECAUTIONS
Contraindicated in patients hypersensitive to guaifenesin.

INTERACTIONS
None significant.

ADVERSE REACTIONS
CNS: dizziness, headache.
GI: vomiting and nausea.

Reactions may be *common*, uncommon, *life-threatening*, or COMMON AND LIFE-THREATENING.

Skin: rash.

◙ KEY CONSIDERATIONS
• Efficacy of guaifenesin as an expectorant hasn't been clearly established because of conflicting results of clinical studies.
• Drug should be taken with a glass of water to help loosen mucus in lungs.
• Drug may cause color interference with tests for 5-hydroxyindoleacetic acid and vanillylmandelic acid.

Patient education
• Instruct patient to call if cough persists for more than 1 week, if cough recurs, or if cough is accompanied by fever, rash, or persistent headache.
• Advise patient to use sugarless throat lozenges to decrease throat irritation and associated cough and to report cough that persists longer than 7 days.
• Recommend that patient use a humidifier to filter out dust, smoke, and air pollutants.
• Encourage patient to perform deep-breathing exercises.

---

guanabenz acetate
Wytensin

Centrally acting antiadrenergic, antihypertensive

Available by prescription only
Tablets: 4 mg, 8 mg

INDICATIONS & DOSAGE
Hypertension (generally considered a step 2 agent)
Adults: Initially, 2 to 4 mg P.O. b.i.d. Dosage may be increased in increments of 4 to 8 mg/day q 1 to 2 weeks. The usual maintenance dosage ranges from 8 to 16 mg daily. Maximum dosage is 32 mg b.i.d.
◊ *Management of opiate withdrawal*
Adults: 4 mg P.O. b.i.d. to q.i.d.

PHARMACODYNAMICS
Antihypertensive action: Guanabenz lowers blood pressure by stimulating central alpha$_2$-adrenergic receptors, decreasing cerebral sympathetic outflow and thus decreasing peripheral vascular resistance. Guanabenz may also antagonize ADH secretion and ADH activity in the kidney.

PHARMACOKINETICS
Absorption: After oral administration, 70% to 80% of guanabenz is absorbed from the GI tract; antihypertensive effect occurs within 60 minutes, peaking at 2 to 4 hours.
Distribution: Drug appears to be distributed widely into the body; drug is about 90% protein-bound.
Metabolism: Drug is metabolized extensively in the liver; several metabolites are formed.
Excretion: Drug and its metabolites are excreted primarily in urine; remaining drug is excreted in feces. Duration of antihypertensive effect varies from 6 to 12 hours.

CONTRAINDICATIONS & PRECAUTIONS
Contraindicated in patients with hypersensitivity to guanabenz. Use cautiously in geriatric patients and in patients with impaired renal or hepatic function, severe coronary insufficiency, recent MI, and cerebrovascular disease.

INTERACTIONS
Drug-drug. Guanabenz may increase the CNS depressant effects of *barbiturates, benzodiazepines, phenothiazines,* and other *sedatives; tricyclic antidepressants* may inhibit antihypertensive effects of guanabenz.
Drug-lifestyle. *Alcohol* may increase CNS depressant effects; avoid use.

ADVERSE REACTIONS
CNS: *drowsiness, sedation, dizziness, weakness,* headache.
CV: *rebound hypertension.*
GI: *dry mouth.*

◙ KEY CONSIDERATIONS
• Geriatric patients may be more sensitive to the antihypertensive and sedative effects of guanabenz.
• Give last dose at bedtime to ensure overnight blood pressure control and minimize daytime drowsiness.

• Investigational uses include managing opiate withdrawal and adjunctive therapy in patients with chronic pain.
• Reduce guanabenz gradually over 2 to 4 days; abrupt discontinuation will cause severe rebound hypertension.
• Reduced dosages may be required in patients with hepatic impairment.
• Guanabenz may reduce serum cholesterol and total triglyceride levels slightly, but it doesn't alter the high-density lipoprotein fraction; drug may cause nonprogressive elevations in liver enzyme levels. Long-term use of guanabenz decreases plasma norepinephrine, dopamine, beta-hydroxylase, and plasma renin activity.

Patient education
• Explain signs and symptoms of adverse effects and the importance of reporting them.
• Warn patient to avoid hazardous activities that require mental alertness and to avoid alcohol and other CNS depressants.
• Suggest taking drug at bedtime until tolerance develops to sedation, drowsiness, and other CNS effects.
• Advise patient to avoid sudden position changes to minimize orthostatic hypotension, and to relieve dry mouth with ice chips or sugarless gum.
• Warn patient to seek medical approval before taking OTC cold preparations.
• Advise patient not to discontinue drug suddenly; severe rebound hypertension may occur.

Overdose & treatment
• Signs and symptoms of overdose include bradycardia, CNS depression, respiratory depression, hypothermia, apnea, seizures, lethargy, agitation, irritability, diarrhea, and hypotension.
• Don't induce vomiting; CNS depression occurs rapidly. After adequate respiration is assured, empty stomach by gastric lavage; then give activated charcoal and a saline cathartic to decrease absorption. Follow with symptomatic and supportive care.

guanadrel sulfate
Hylorel

Adrenergic neuron blocker, antihypertensive

Available by prescription only
Tablets: 10 mg, 25 mg

INDICATIONS & DOSAGE
Hypertension
Adults: Initially, 5 mg P.O. b.i.d.; adjust dosage until blood pressure is controlled. Most patients require 20 to 75 mg daily, usually given b.i.d. (400 mg daily is rarely used).
✦ *Dosage adjustment.* For patients with renal impairment whose creatinine clearance is 30 to 60 ml/minute, reduce dose to 5 mg q 24 hours; if creatinine clearance is less than 30 ml/minute, increase dosing interval to q 48 hours.

PHARMACODYNAMICS
Antihypertensive action: Guanadrel reduces blood pressure by peripheral inhibition of norepinephrine release in adrenergic nerve endings, thus decreasing arteriolar vasoconstriction.

PHARMACOKINETICS
Absorption: Guanadrel is absorbed rapidly and almost completely from the GI tract. Antihypertensive effect usually occurs at ½ to 2 hours; peak effect occurs at 4 to 6 hours.
Distribution: Drug is distributed widely into the body and is about 20% protein-bound; it doesn't enter the CNS.
Metabolism: About 40% to 50% of a given dose is metabolized by the liver.
Excretion: Drug and its metabolites are eliminated primarily in urine. Antihypertensive activity persists for 4 to 14 hours. Plasma half-life is about 10 hours, but varies considerably among individuals.

CONTRAINDICATIONS & PRECAUTIONS
Contraindicated in patients with hypersensitivity to guanadrel, known or suspected pheochromocytoma, or frank heart failure. Also contraindicated in patients receiving MAO inhibitors or with-

---

Reactions may be *common*, uncommon, *life-threatening*, or COMMON AND LIFE-THREATENING.

in 1 week of discontinuing MAO inhibitor therapy.

Use cautiously in patients with regional vascular disease, bronchial asthma, or peptic ulcer disease.

INTERACTIONS
Drug-drug. Guanadrel may potentiate the antihypertensive effects of other *antihypertensives* and the pressor effects of such agents as *metaraminol* and *norepinephrine*. *Amphetamines, ephedrine, MAO inhibitors, methylphenidate, norepinephrine, phenothiazines,* or *tricyclic antidepressants* may antagonize the antihypertensive effects of guanadrel. Use of other *antihypertensives* or *diuretics* increases the antihypertensive effects of guanadrel.
Drug-lifestyle. Use of *alcohol* may increase the risk of guanadrel-induced orthostatic hypotension. Avoid use.

ADVERSE REACTIONS
CNS: *fatigue, drowsiness, faintness, headache, confusion, paresthesia.*
CV: *palpitations, chest pain, peripheral edema, orthostatic hypotension.*
EENT: *glossitis, visual disturbances.*
GI: *diarrhea,* dry mouth, *indigestion,* constipation, anorexia, nausea, vomiting, abdominal pain.
GU: impotence, *ejaculation disturbances, nocturia, urinary frequency.*
Metabolic: *weight gain.*
Musculoskeletal: *aching limbs, leg cramps.*
Respiratory: *shortness of breath, cough.*

▣ KEY CONSIDERATIONS
• Geriatric patients may be more susceptible to orthostatic hypotension.
• Monitor supine and standing blood pressure, especially during periods of dosage adjustment.
• Assess for signs and symptoms of edema.
• Discontinue guanadrel 48 to 72 hours before surgery to minimize the risk of vascular collapse during anesthesia.
• Separate use of guanadrel and MAO inhibitors by at least 1 week.

Patient education
• Teach patient signs and symptoms of adverse effects and importance of reporting them; patient should also report excessive weight gain (more than 2.25 kg [5 lb] weekly).
• Explain that orthostatic hypotension can be minimized by rising slowly from a supine position and avoiding sudden position changes; it may be aggravated by fever, hot weather, hot showers, prolonged standing, exercise, and alcohol.
• Warn patient to avoid hazardous activities that require mental alertness and to take drug at bedtime until tolerance develops to sedation, drowsiness, and other CNS effects.
• Advise patient to avoid alcohol while taking drug.
• Advise patient to use ice chips or sugarless hard candy or gum to relieve dry mouth.
• Warn patient to seek medical approval before taking OTC cold preparations.

Overdose & treatment
• Signs and symptoms of overdose include hypotension, dizziness, blurred vision, and syncope.
• After acute ingestion, induce vomiting or perform gastric lavage. The effect of activated charcoal in absorbing guanadrel hasn't been determined. Further treatment is usually symptomatic and supportive.

guanethidine monosulfate
Ismelin

Adrenergic neuron blocker, antihypertensive

Available by prescription only
Tablets: 10 mg, 25 mg

INDICATIONS & DOSAGE
Moderate to severe hypertension,
◇ signs and symptoms of thyrotoxicosis
Adults: Initially, 10 mg P.O. once daily; increase by 10 mg at weekly to monthly intervals, p.r.n. Usual dosage is 25 to 50 mg once daily; some patients may require up to 300 mg.

PHARMACODYNAMICS

Antihypertensive action: Guanethidine acts peripherally; it decreases arteriolar vasoconstriction and reduces blood pressure by inhibiting norepinephrine release and depleting norepinephrine stores in adrenergic nerve endings.

PHARMACOKINETICS

Absorption: Guanethidine is absorbed incompletely from the GI tract. Maximal antihypertensive effects usually aren't evident for 1 to 3 weeks.
Distribution: Drug is distributed throughout the body; it isn't protein-bound but demonstrates extensive tissue binding.
Metabolism: Drug undergoes partial hepatic metabolism to pharmacologically less-active metabolites.
Excretion: Drug and metabolites are excreted primarily in urine; small amounts are excreted in feces. Elimination half-life after long-term administration is biphasic.

CONTRAINDICATIONS & PRECAUTIONS

Contraindicated in patients with pheochromocytoma, frank heart failure, or hypersensitivity to guanethidine, and in those receiving MAO inhibitors. Use cautiously in patients with severe cardiac disease, recent MI, cerebrovascular disease, peptic ulcer, impaired renal function, or bronchial asthma, and in those taking other antihypertensives.

INTERACTIONS

Drug-drug. Use with *cardiac glycosides* may result in additive bradycardia. Use with *diuretics, levodopa,* or *other antihypertensives* may potentiate the antihypertensive effect of guanethidine. Administration with *MAO inhibitors, oral contraceptives,* or *tricyclic antidepressants* may antagonize the antihypertensive effect of guanethidine. Guanethidine potentiates pressor effects of such drugs as *metaraminol, norepinephrine,* and *oral sympathomimetic nasal decongestants.* Use with *rauwolfia alkaloids* may cause excessive postural hypotension, bradycardia, and mental depression.

Drug-lifestyle. *Alcohol* may potentiate the antihypertensive effect of guanethidine; avoid use.

ADVERSE REACTIONS

CNS: *syncope, fatigue, headache, drowsiness, paresthesia, confusion.*
CV: *palpitations, chest pain, orthostatic hypotension, peripheral edema.*
EENT: *visual disturbances,* glossitis.
GI: *diarrhea, indigestion, constipation, anorexia,* nausea, vomiting.
GU: *nocturia, urinary frequency, ejaculation disturbances,* impotence.
Musculoskeletal: *aching limbs, leg cramps.*
Respiratory: shortness of breath, cough.
Other: *weight gain.*

◻ KEY CONSIDERATIONS

• Geriatric patients may be more sensitive to drug's antihypertensive effects.
• Dosage requirements may be reduced in the presence of fever.
• If diarrhea develops, atropine or paregoric may be prescribed.
• Discontinue drug 2 to 3 weeks before elective surgery to reduce risk of CV collapse during anesthesia.
• When drug is replacing MAO inhibitors, wait at least 1 week before initiating guanethidine; if replacing ganglionic blockers, withdraw them slowly to prevent a spiking blood pressure response during the transfer period.
• Guanethidine has been used topically as a 5% ophthalmic solution to treat chronic open-angle glaucoma or endocrine ophthalmopathy.

Patient education

• Teach patient signs and symptoms of adverse effects and importance of reporting them; tell patient to report persistent diarrhea and excessive weight gain (2.25 kg [5 lb] weekly). Advise him not to discontinue the drug but to call for further instructions if adverse reactions occur.
• Warn patient to avoid hazardous activities that require mental alertness and to take drug at bedtime until tolerance develops to sedation, drowsiness, and other CNS effects.

Reactions may be *common,* uncommon, *life-threatening,* or COMMON AND LIFE-THREATENING.

- Advise patient to avoid sudden position changes, strenuous exercise, heat, and hot showers to minimize orthostatic hypotension. Tell him to relieve dry mouth with ice chips, hard candy, or gum.
- Tell patient not to double next scheduled dose if he misses one; he should take only the next scheduled dose.
- Advise patient to seek medical approval before taking OTC cold preparations.
- Advise patient to avoid alcohol while taking drug.

Overdose & treatment

- Signs and symptoms of overdose include hypotension, blurred vision, syncope, bradycardia, and severe diarrhea.
- After acute ingestion, induce vomiting or perform gastric lavage and give activated charcoal to reduce absorption. Further treatment is usually symptomatic and supportive.

guanfacine hydrochloride
Tenex

Centrally acting antiadrenergic, antihypertensive

Available by prescription only
Tablets: 1 mg, 2 mg

INDICATIONS & DOSAGE
Mild to moderate hypertension
Adults: Initially, 0.5 to 1 mg P.O. daily h.s. Average dose is 1 to 3 mg daily.
◇ **Heroin withdrawal**
Adults: 0.03 to 1.5 mg P.O. daily.
◇ **Migraine**
Adults: 1 mg P.O. daily for 12 weeks.

PHARMACODYNAMICS
Antihypertensive action: Guanfacine is a centrally acting alpha$_2$-adrenoreceptor agonist with a mechanism of action that isn't clearly understood. It appears to stimulate central alpha$_2$-adrenergic receptors that decrease peripheral release of norepinephrine, thus decreasing peripheral vascular resistance and lowering blood pressure. Drug reduces heart rate by reducing sympathetic nerve impulses from the vasomotor center to the heart. Systolic and diastolic blood pressure are both decreased; cardiac output is unaltered.

Elevated plasma renin activity and plasma catecholamine levels are lowered; however, there is no correlation with individual blood pressure. Single doses of guanfacine stimulate growth hormone secretion, but long-term use has no effect on growth hormone levels.

PHARMACOKINETICS
Absorption: Guanfacine is absorbed well and completely after oral administration and is about 80% bioavailable. Plasma levels peak in 1 to 4 hours.
Distribution: About 70% is protein-bound; high distribution to tissues is suggested.
Metabolism: Drug is metabolized in the liver.
Excretion: About 50% is eliminated in urine as unchanged drug, the rest as conjugates of metabolites.

CONTRAINDICATIONS & PRECAUTIONS
Contraindicated in patients with hypersensitivity to guanfacine. Use cautiously in patients with renal or hepatic insufficiency, severe coronary insufficiency, recent MI, or cerebrovascular disease.

INTERACTIONS
Drug-drug. Use with other *antihypertensives* or *diuretic* combinations may potentiate the antihypertensive effects; this often is used to therapeutic advantage. Guanfacine may enhance the depressant effects of *CNS depressants*, such as *barbiturates, benzodiazepines,* and *phenothiazines.* Blood pressure may be increased by *estrogen*-induced fluid retention; monitor patient carefully. *Estrogens, NSAIDs* (especially *indomethacin),* and *sympathomimetics* may reduce the antihypertensive effects of guanfacine. *Indomethacin* and other *NSAIDs* may inhibit renal prostaglandin synthesis or cause sodium and fluid retention, thus antagonizing the antihypertensive activity of guanfacine.
Drug-lifestyle. Guanfacine may enhance the depressant effects of *alcohol.* Discourage alcohol use.

ADVERSE REACTIONS

CNS: *dizziness,* fatigue, headache, insomnia, *somnolence,* asthenia.
CV: bradycardia.
GI: *constipation,* diarrhea, nausea, *dry mouth.*
Skin: dermatitis, pruritus.

▣ KEY CONSIDERATIONS

• Dizziness, drowsiness, hypotension, or faintness occur more frequently in geriatric patients, who may be more sensitive to the effects of guanfacine.
• Give drug at bedtime to reduce daytime drowsiness.
• Withdrawal syndrome may occur if guanfacine is stopped abruptly or discontinued before surgery; therefore, the anesthesiologist must be informed if drug was withdrawn more than 2 days before surgery, or if drug hasn't been withdrawn.
• Dry mouth may contribute to development of dental caries, periodontal disease, oral candidiasis, and discomfort.
• Monitor blood pressure at regular intervals.
• Drug therapy alters urine catecholamine levels and urine vanillylmandelic acid excretion (may be decreased during therapy but may increase on abrupt withdrawal). Plasma growth hormone levels may be increased after a single dose; continuous elevation doesn't follow long-term use.

Patient education

• Stress importance of diet and the possible need for sodium restriction and weight reduction.
• Tell patient to take drug as directed even if feeling well and to take daily dose at bedtime to minimize daytime drowsiness.
• Advise patient that drug may cause drowsiness or dizziness. Urge patient to avoid use of alcohol and other CNS depressants, which may add to this effect. Tell patient to avoid driving or performing other tasks that require alertness until effects of drug are known.
• Inform patient to take a missed dose as soon as possible; if taking more than one dose per day and it's almost time for next dose, skip the missed dose and return to regular schedule.
• Store drug away from heat and light, and out of children's reach.
• Tell patient to advise new health care provider that he is taking this drug before having surgery, including dental surgery, or emergency treatment.
• Advise chewing sugarless gum, candy, ice, or saliva substitute for treatment of dry mouth. If condition continues longer than 2 weeks, patient should call for further recommendations.
• Instruct patient not to take other drugs unless they have been prescribed. This is particularly important with drugs for cough, cold, asthma, hay fever, or sinus.
• Tell patient not to stop taking drug abruptly; rebound hypertension may occur.

Overdose & treatment

• Signs and symptoms of overdose include difficulty breathing, extreme dizziness, faintness, slow heartbeat, and severe or unusual tiredness or weakness.
• Treat symptomatically, with careful cardiac monitoring. Perform gastric lavage and infuse isoproterenol as appropriate. Guanfacine is dialyzed poorly.

halobetasol propionate
Ultravate

Corticosteroid, topical anti-inflammatory

Available by prescription only
Cream: 0.05%
Ointment: 0.05%

INDICATIONS & DOSAGE
Relief of inflammation and pruritus of corticosteroid-responsive dermatoses
Adults: Apply sparingly to affected areas daily to b.i.d. and rub in gently and completely. Treatment beyond 2 consecutive weeks isn't recommended; total dosage shouldn't exceed 50 g weekly. Don't use an occlusive dressing.

PHARMACODYNAMICS
Anti-inflammatory action: Halobetasol is classified as a "super high-potency" (group I) corticosteroid. Its anti-inflammatory response results from stimulation of the synthesis of enzymes needed to decrease inflammation.

PHARMACOKINETICS
Absorption: Amount of halobetasol absorbed depends on amount applied, application site, vehicle, use of occlusive dressing, and integrity of skin. Some systemic absorption occurs.
Distribution: Drug is distributed throughout the local skin.
Metabolism: Drug is metabolized primarily by the skin.
Excretion: Unknown.

CONTRAINDICATIONS & PRECAUTIONS
Contraindicated in patients hypersensitive to halobetasol or its components; not for use as monotherapy in primary bacterial infections or for ophthalmic indications.

INTERACTIONS
None significant.

ADVERSE REACTIONS
CV: fluid retention.
GU: glycosuria.
Metabolic: hyperglycemia.
Skin: stinging, burning, pruritus, irritation, dryness, erythema, folliculitis, skin atrophy, leukoderma, vesicles, rash, hypertrichosis, acneiform eruptions, hypopigmentation, perioral dermatitis, allergic contact dermatitis, secondary infection, striae, miliaria.
Other: *hypothalamic-pituitary-adrenal (HPA) axis suppression,* Cushing's syndrome.

▣ KEY CONSIDERATIONS
● The corticotropin-stimulation test, morning plasma cortisol, and urine cortisol levels are useful in determining the extent of HPA axis suppression.
● Limit treatment to 2 weeks in a dosage less than 50 g weekly.
● Don't use occlusive dressings.
● Don't use to treat rosacea or perioral dermatitis. Discontinue drug if infection occurs.
● If HPA axis suppression occurs, discontinue drug, reduce frequency of application, or substitute a less potent corticosteroid.
● Don't use on face, groin, or axillae.

Patient education
● Warn patient to use externally and only as directed and to avoid contact with eyes.
● Tell patient not to cover, bandage, or wrap treated area unless instructed.
● Tell patient to report signs of stinging, burning, or irritation.
● Caution patient to use drug exactly as prescribed.

---

haloperidol
Apo-Haloperidol*, Haldol, Novo-
Peridol*, Peridol*

haloperidol decanoate
Haldol Decanoate, Haldol
Decanoate 100, Haldol LA*

haloperidol lactate
Haldol, Haldol Concentrate,
Haloperidol Intensol

Butyrophenone, antipsychotic

Available by prescription only
haloperidol
Tablets: 0.5 mg, 1 mg, 2 mg, 5 mg,
10 mg, 20 mg
haloperidol decanoate
Injection: 50 mg/ml, 100 mg/ml
haloperidol lactate
Oral concentrate: 2 mg/ml
Injection: 5 mg/ml

INDICATIONS & DOSAGE
*Psychotic disorders, ◊ alcohol depen-
dence*
Adults: Dosage varies for each patient
and symptomatology. Initial dosage
range is 0.5 to 5 mg P.O. b.i.d. or t.i.d.;
or 2 to 5 mg I.M. q 4 to 8 hours, increased rapidly if necessary for prompt
control. Maximum dosage is 100 mg
P.O. daily. Doses over 100 mg have been
used for patients with severely resistant
conditions.
*Patients with chronic psychosis who re-
quire long-term therapy*
Adults: 100 mg I.M. of haloperidol decanoate q 4 weeks. Experience with doses over 450 mg monthly is limited.
*Control of tics, vocal utterances in
Tourette syndrome*
Adults: 0.5 to 5 mg P.O. b.i.d. or t.i.d.,
increased, p.r.n.

PHARMACODYNAMICS
Antipsychotic action: Haloperidol is
thought to exert its antipsychotic effects
by strong postsynaptic blockade of CNS
dopamine receptors, thereby inhibiting
dopamine-mediated effects; its pharmacologic effects are most similar to those
of piperazine antipsychotics. Its mecha-

nism of action in Tourette syndrome is
unknown.
  Haloperidol has many other central
and peripheral effects; it has weak peripheral anticholinergic effects and
antiemetic effects, produces both alpha
and ganglionic blockade, and counteracts histamine- and serotonin-mediated
activity. Its most prominent adverse reactions are extrapyramidal.

PHARMACOKINETICS
Absorption: Rate and extent of absorption vary with route of administration.
Oral tablet absorption yields 60% to
70% bioavailability. I.M. dose is 70%
absorbed within 30 minutes. After oral
administration plasma levels peak at 2 to
6 hours; after I.M. administration, 30 to
45 minutes; and after long-acting I.M.
(decanoate) administration, 6 to 7 days.
Distribution: Haloperidol is distributed
widely into the body, with high levels in
adipose tissue. Drug is 90% to 92% protein-bound.
Metabolism: Drug is metabolized extensively by the liver; there may be only one
active metabolite that is less active than
parent drug.
Excretion: About 40% of a given dose is
excreted in urine within 5 days; about
15% is excreted in feces via the biliary
tract.

CONTRAINDICATIONS & PRECAUTIONS
Contraindicated in patients with hypersensitivity or in those experiencing
parkinsonism, coma, or CNS depression.
  Use cautiously in geriatric or debilitated patients; in patients with history of
seizures, EEG abnormalities, CV disorders, allergies, angle-closure glaucoma,
or urine retention; and in those receiving
anticoagulants, anticonvulsants, antiparkinsonians, or lithium.

INTERACTIONS
Drug-drug. Pharmacokinetic alterations
and subsequent decreased therapeutic response to haloperidol may follow use
with *aluminum- or magnesium-containing antacids* and *antidiarrheals* (decreased absorption) or *phenobarbital*
(enhanced renal excretion). Additive effects are likely after use with the follow-

---

Reactions may be *common*, uncommon, *life-threatening*, or COMMON AND LIFE-THREATENING.

ing drugs: *antiarrhythmics, disopyramide, procainamide,* or *quinidine* (increased incidence of arrhythmias and conduction defects); *atropine* or *other anticholinergics,* including *antidepressants, antihistamines, antiparkinsonians, MAO inhibitors, meperidine,* and *phenothiazines* (oversedation, paralytic ileus, visual changes, and severe constipation); *CNS depressants,* including *analgesics; barbiturates; epidural, general,* or *spinal anesthetics; narcotics;* and *parenteral magnesium sulfate* or *tranquilizers* (oversedation, respiratory depression, and hypotension); *metrizamide* (increased risk of seizures); and *nitrates* (hypotension).

Use with *appetite suppressants* or *sympathomimetics*—including *ephedrine* (found in many nasal sprays), *epinephrine, phenylephrine,* and *phenylpropanolamine*—may decrease their stimulatory and pressor effects. *Beta blockers* may inhibit haloperidol metabolism, increasing plasma levels and toxicity. Haloperidol may antagonize the therapeutic effect of *bromocriptine* on prolactin secretion, decrease the vasoconstrictive effects of high-dose *dopamine,* decrease effectiveness and increase toxicity of *levodopa* (by dopamine blockade), and inhibit metabolism and increase toxicity of *phenytoin.* Haloperidol may inhibit blood pressure response to *centrally acting antihypertensives,* such as *clonidine, guanabenz, guanadrel, guanethidine, methyldopa,* and *reserpine.* Use with *lithium* may result in severe neurologic toxicity with an encephalitis-like syndrome, and a decreased therapeutic response to haloperidol. Use with *propylthiouracil* increases risk of agranulocytosis.

Drug-lifestyle. Additive effects—such as oversedation, respiratory depression, and hypotension—are likely after use with *alcohol;* don't use together. *Heavy smoking* may increase metabolism of haloperidol.

ADVERSE REACTIONS

CNS: *severe extrapyramidal reactions, tardive dyskinesia,* sedation, drowsiness, lethargy, headache, insomnia, confusion, vertigo, *seizures.*

CV: tachycardia, hypotension, hypertension, ECG changes.
EENT: *blurred vision.*
GI: dry mouth, anorexia, constipation, diarrhea, nausea, vomiting, dyspepsia.
GU: urine retention, menstrual irregularities, gynecomastia, priapism.
Hematologic: *leukopenia,* leukocytosis.
Hepatic: altered liver function tests, jaundice.
Skin: rash, other skin reactions, diaphoresis.
Other: *neuroleptic malignant syndrome* (rare).

▣ KEY CONSIDERATIONS

• Haloperidol is especially useful for agitation associated with senile dementia.
• Geriatric patients usually require lower initial doses and a more gradual dosage titration.
• Drug has few adverse CV effects and may be preferred in patients with cardiac disease.
• Assess patient periodically for abnormal body movement.
• Tardive dyskinesia may occur after prolonged use. It may not appear until months or years later and may disappear spontaneously or persist for life.
• Protect drug from light. Slight yellowing of injection or concentrate is common and doesn't affect potency. Discard markedly discolored solutions.
• Don't withdraw drug abruptly unless required by severe adverse reactions.
• Note that a dose of 2 mg is therapeutic equivalent of 100 mg chlorpromazine.
• When changing from tablets to decanoate injection, give patient initially 10 to 20 times the oral dose once monthly (maximum, 100 mg).
• Administer drug by deep I.M. injection. Don't administer decanoate form I.V.

Patient education

• Warn patient against activities that require alertness and good psychomotor coordination until CNS response to drug is determined. Drowsiness and dizziness usually subside after a few weeks.
• Tell patient to report adverse effects, such as extrapyramidal reactions.

• Instruct patient to avoid combining with alcohol or other depressants.

Overdose & treatment

• CNS depression is characterized by deep, unarousable sleep and possible coma, hypotension or hypertension, extrapyramidal symptoms, dystonia, abnormal involuntary muscle movements, agitation, seizures, arrhythmias, ECG changes (may show QT prolongation and torsades de pointes), hypothermia or hyperthermia, and autonomic nervous system dysfunction. Overdose with long-acting decanoate requires prolonged recovery time.

• Treatment is symptomatic and supportive; maintain vital signs, airway, stable body temperature, and fluid and electrolyte balance. Ipecac may be used to induce vomiting, with due regard for haloperidol's antiemetic properties and hazard of aspiration. Gastric lavage also may be used, followed by activated charcoal and saline cathartics; dialysis doesn't help.

• Regulate body temperature as needed. Treat hypotension with I.V. fluids; don't give epinephrine. Treat seizures with parenteral diazepam or barbiturates; arrhythmias with parenteral phenytoin (1 mg/kg I.V. with rate titrated to blood pressure, not to exceed 50 mg/minute with ECG monitoring; may repeat every 5 minutes up to 10 mg/kg); and extrapyramidal reactions with benztropine at 1 to 2 mg or parenteral diphenhydramine at 10 to 50 mg.

heparin sodium
Heparin Lock Flush, Hep-Lock, Hep-Lock U/P, Liquaemin

Anticoagulant

Available products are derived from bovine lung or porcine intestinal mucosa. All are injectable and available by prescription only.
heparin sodium
Vials: 1,000 U/ml, 5,000 U/ml, 10,000 U/ml, 20,000 U/ml, 40,000 U/ml
Unit-dose ampules: 1,000 U/ml, 5,000 U/ml, 10,000 U/ml

Disposable syringes: 1,000 U/ml, 2,500 U/ml, 5,000 U/ml, 7,500 U/ml, 10,000 U/ml, 20,000 U/ml
Carpuject: 5,000 U/ml
Premixed I.V. solutions: 1,000 U in 500 ml normal saline solution; 2,000 U in 1,000 ml normal saline solution; 12,500 U in 250 ml half-normal saline solution; 25,000 U in 250 ml half-normal saline solution; 25,000 U in 500 ml half-normal saline solution; 10,000 U in 100 ml D_5W; 12,500 U in 250 ml D_5W; 25,000 U in 250 ml D_5W; 25,000 U in 500 ml D_5W
heparin sodium flush
Vials: 10 U/ml, 100 U/ml
Disposable syringes: 10 U/ml, 25 U/2.5 ml, 2,500 U/2.5 ml

INDICATIONS & DOSAGE

Deep vein thrombosis, pulmonary embolism
Adults: Initially, 5,000 to 10,000 U I.V. push, then adjust dose according to PTT results and give dose I.V. q 4 hours (usually 4,000 to 5,000 U); or 5,000 U I.V. bolus, then 20,000 to 40,000 U in 24 hours by I.V. infusion pump. Wait 4 to 6 hours after bolus dose, and adjust hourly rate based on PTT.
Embolism prophylaxis, ◊post MI, ◊cerebral thrombosis in evolving stroke, ◊left ventricular thrombi
Adults: 5,000 U S.C. q 8 to 12 hours.
Open-heart surgery
Adults: (total body perfusion) 150 to 400 U/kg continuous I.V infusion.
DIC
Adults: 50 to 100 U/kg I.V. q 4 hours as a single injection or constant infusion. Discontinue if no improvement in 4 to 8 hours.
To maintain patency of I.V. indwelling catheters
Adults: 10 to 100 U as an I.V. flush (not intended for therapeutic use).
◊ Unstable angina
Adults: Keep PTT 1.5 to 2 times control during first week of anginal pain.
◊ Anticoagulation in blood transfusion and samples
Transfusions and samples: Mix 7,500 U and 100 ml of normal saline and add 6 to 8 ml of mixture to each 100 ml of

whole blood or 70 to 150 U to each 10 to 20 ml of blood sample.

Note: Heparin dosing is highly individualized, depending on disease state, age, and renal and hepatic status.

PHARMACODYNAMICS

Anticoagulant action: Heparin accelerates formation of antithrombin III-thrombin complex; it inactivates thrombin and prevents conversion of fibrinogen to fibrin.

PHARMACOKINETICS

Absorption: Heparin isn't absorbed from the GI tract and must be given parenterally. After I.V. use, onset of action is almost immediate; after S.C. injection, onset of action occurs in 20 to 60 minutes.
Distribution: Drug is extensively bound to lipoprotein, globulins, and fibrinogen.
Metabolism: Although metabolism isn't completely described, drug is thought to be removed by the reticuloendothelial system, with some metabolism occurring in the liver.
Excretion: Little known; a small fraction is excreted in urine as unchanged drug. Plasma half-life is 1 to 2 hours.

CONTRAINDICATIONS & PRECAUTIONS

Contraindicated in patients with hypersensitivity to heparin. Conditionally contraindicated in patients with active bleeding; blood dyscrasia; or bleeding tendencies, such as hemophilia, thrombocytopenia, or hepatic disease with hypoprothrombinemia; suspected intracranial hemorrhage; suppurative thrombophlebitis; inaccessible ulcerative lesions (especially of GI tract) and open ulcerative wounds; extensive denudation of skin; ascorbic acid deficiency and other conditions that increase capillary permeability; during or after brain, eye, or spinal cord surgery; during spinal tap or spinal anesthesia; during continuous tube drainage of stomach or small intestine; in subacute bacterial endocarditis; shock; advanced renal disease; threatened abortion; or severe hypertension. Although heparin use is clearly hazardous in these conditions, its risks and benefits must be evaluated.

Use cautiously in patients with mild hepatic or renal disease, alcoholism, or history of asthma, allergies, or GI ulcer; or in those with occupations that have a high incidence of accidents.

INTERACTIONS

Drug-drug. *Antihistamines, cardiac glycosides, nicotine,* or *tetracyclines* may partially counteract the anticoagulant action of heparin. Use with *oral anticoagulants* and *platelet inhibitors* increases anticoagulant effect; if it isn't possible to avoid using these together, monitor INR, PT, and PTT.

ADVERSE REACTIONS

CNS: mild pain.
GI: ulceration.
Hematologic: *hemorrhage* (with excessive dosage), *overly prolonged clotting time, thrombocytopenia.*
Other: irritation, hematoma, cutaneous or subcutaneous necrosis, "white clot" syndrome, hypersensitivity reactions (including chills, fever, pruritus, rhinitis, urticaria, *anaphylactoid reactions*).

▣ KEY CONSIDERATIONS

• Women older than age 60 may have the greatest risk of hemorrhage.
• Obtain pretherapy baseline INR, PT, and PTT; measure PTT regularly. Anticoagulation is present when PTT values are 1.5 to 2 times control values; draw blood for PTT 4 to 6 hours after an I.V. bolus dose and 12 to 24 hours after an S.C. dose. Blood may be drawn at any time after 4 to 6 hours of constant I.V. infusion; if I.V. therapy is intermittent, draw blood 30 minutes before next scheduled dose to avoid falsely prolonged PTT. Never draw blood for PTT from the I.V. tubing of the heparin infusion, or from vein of infusion; falsely prolonged PTT will result. Always draw blood from opposite arm.
• Heparin therapy prolongs PT, may falsely elevate AST and ALT levels, and may cause false elevations in some tests for serum thyroxine levels.
• I.V. administration is preferred because S.C. and I.M. injections are irregularly absorbed. When possible, administer I.V.

heparin by infusion pump for maximum safety.

• When using heparin flush solution, keep intermittent I.V. line patent by flushing it with saline solution before and after heparin; many drugs are incompatible with heparin and may form precipitates if they come in contact with heparin.

• For S.C. injection, use one needle to withdraw solution from vial and another to inject drug. Give low-dose S.C. injections sequentially between iliac crests in lower abdomen; give slowly and deep into subcutaneous fat. After inserting needle into skin, don't withdraw plunger to check for blood, to reduce risk of tissue injury and hematoma; leave needle in place for 10 seconds after S.C. injection. Alternate site every 12 hours: right for morning, left for evening. Don't massage after S.C. injection; watch for local bleeding, hematoma, or inflammation. Rotate site.

• Check patient regularly for bleeding gums, bruises on arms or legs, petechiae, nosebleeds, melena, tarry stools, hematuria, or hematemesis. Monitor platelet counts regularly.

• Check I.V. infusions regularly, even when pumps are in good working order, to prevent overdose or underdose; don't piggyback other drugs into line while heparin infusion is running because many antibiotics and other drugs inactivate heparin. Never mix any drug with heparin in syringe when bolus therapy is used.

• Avoid excessive I.M. injection of other drugs to prevent or minimize hematomas. If possible, don't give any I.M. injections.

• Abrupt withdrawal may increase coagulability; heparin is usually followed by prophylactic oral anticoagulant therapy.

Patient education
• Teach injection technique and methods of record-keeping if patient or family will be giving drug.

• Encourage compliance with drug schedule, follow-up appointments, and need for routine monitoring of blood studies; teach patient and family signs of bleeding and stress importance of calling immediately at first sign of excess bleeding.

• Caution patient not to double-dose if he misses a dose; tell him to call for instructions instead.

• Warn patient against use of aspirin and other OTC drugs; stress need to seek medical approval before taking new drugs, and to inform health care provider and dentist about heparin use.

Overdose & treatment
• The major sign of overdose is hemorrhage. Immediate withdrawal of drug usually allows the hemorrhage to resolve; however, severe hemorrhage may require treatment with protamine sulfate. Usually, 1 mg protamine sulfate will neutralize 90 U of bovine heparin or 115 U of porcine heparin.

• Heparin administered I.V. disappears rapidly from the blood, so the protamine dose depends on when heparin was administered. Protamine should be given slowly by I.V. injection (over 3 minutes), and not more than 50 mg should be given in any 10-minute period.

• Heparin administered by S.C. route is slowly absorbed. Protamine should be given as a 25- to 50-mg loading dose, followed by constant infusion of the remainder of the calculated dose over 8 to 16 hours. For severe bleeding, transfusions may be required.

hepatitis A vaccine, inactivated
Havrix

Viral vaccine

Available by prescription only
Injection: 360 ELISA U (ELU)/0.5 ml, 1,440 ELU/1 ml

INDICATIONS & DOSAGE
Immunization against disease caused by hepatitis A virus
Adults: 1,440 ELU/1 ml I.M. as a single dose. Give booster dose of 1,440 ELU/ 1 ml I.M. any time between 6 and 12 months after initial dosage to ensure highest antibody titers.

PHARMACODYNAMICS

Immunostimulant action: Hepatitis A vaccine, inactivated, promotes active immunity to hepatitis A virus. Immunity isn't permanent or predictable.

PHARMACOKINETICS

Absorption: Unknown.
Distribution: Unknown.
Metabolism: Unknown.
Excretion: Unknown.

CONTRAINDICATIONS & PRECAUTIONS

Contraindicated in patients with hypersensitivity to any component of vaccine. Use cautiously in patients with thrombocytopenia or bleeding disorders or in those taking anticoagulants because bleeding may occur after I.M. injection in these individuals.

INTERACTIONS

None significant.

ADVERSE REACTIONS

CNS: *fatigue, malaise,* headache, hypertonic episode, insomnia, photophobia, vertigo.
GI: *anorexia, nausea,* abdominal pain, diarrhea, dysgeusia, vomiting.
Hepatic: jaundice, hepatitis.
Musculoskeletal: arthralgia, elevated CK level, myalgia.
Respiratory: pharyngitis, other upper respiratory tract infections.
Skin: pruritus, *rash,* urticaria, *induration, redness, swelling,* hematoma.
Other: *fever,* lymphadenopathy.

▣ KEY CONSIDERATIONS

• As with any vaccine, administration of hepatitis A vaccine should be delayed, if possible, in patients with febrile illness.
• Although anaphylaxis is rare, keep epinephrine readily available to treat an anaphylactoid reaction.
• If vaccine is administered to immunosuppressed patients or those receiving immunosuppressive therapy, the expected immune response may not be obtained.
• Use the vaccine in people traveling to or living in areas endemic for hepatitis A (Africa, Asia [except Japan], the Mediterranean basin, Eastern Europe, the Middle East, Central and South America, Mexico, and parts of the Caribbean), military personnel, native people of Alaska and the Americas, persons engaging in high-risk sexual activity, and users of illicit injectable drugs. Also, certain institutional workers, employees of child day-care centers, laboratory workers who handle live hepatitis A virus, and handlers of primate animals may benefit from immunization.
• Shake vial or syringe well before withdrawal and use. With thorough agitation, the vaccine is an opaque white suspension. Discard if it appears otherwise. No dilution or reconstitution is necessary.
• Administer as I.M. injection into the deltoid region in adults. Don't administer in the gluteal region; such injections may result in suboptimal response. Never inject I.V., S.C., or intradermally.
• Note that hepatitis A vaccine won't prevent infection in persons with unrecognized hepatitis A infection at the time of vaccination.

Patient education

• Inform patient that vaccine won't prevent hepatitis caused by other agents such as hepatitis B virus, hepatitis C virus, hepatitis E virus, or other pathogens known to infect the liver.

hepatitis B immune globulin, human (HBIG)

H-BIG, Hep-B-Gammagee, HyperHep

Immune serum, hepatitis B prophylaxis

Available by prescription only
Injection: 1-ml, 4-ml, and 5-ml vials
Prefilled syringe: 0.5 ml

INDICATIONS & DOSAGE

Hepatitis B exposure

Adults: 0.06 ml/kg I.M. within 7 days after exposure. Repeat 28 days after exposure.

PHARMACODYNAMICS

Postexposure prophylaxis of hepatitis B: HBIG provides passive immunity to hepatitis B.

PHARMACOKINETICS

Absorption: HBIG is absorbed slowly after I.M. injection. Antibodies to hepatitis B surface antigen (HBsAg) appear in serum within 1 to 6 days, peak within 3 to 11 days, and persist for about 2 to 6 months.
Distribution: Unknown.
Metabolism: Unknown.
Excretion: Serum half-life for antibodies to HBsAg is reportedly 21 days.

CONTRAINDICATIONS & PRECAUTIONS

Contraindicated in patients with history of anaphylactic reactions to immune serum or thimerosal allergy.

INTERACTIONS

Drug-drug. HBIG may interfere with immune response to vaccination with *live virus vaccines,* such as *measles, mumps,* and *rubella;* such vaccines should be administered 2 weeks before or 3 months after HBIG whenever possible.

ADVERSE REACTIONS

Other: *anaphylaxis,* urticaria, *angioedema,* pain or tenderness (at injection site).

▣ KEY CONSIDERATIONS

• Obtain a thorough history of allergies and reactions to immunizations.
• Epinephrine solution 1:1,000 should be available to treat allergic reactions.
• Administer drug I.M. only. Severe, even fatal, reactions may occur if it's administered I.V.
• Gluteal or deltoid areas are the preferred injection sites.
• HBIG may be given simultaneously, but at different sites, with hepatitis B vaccine.
• Store between 36° and 46° F (2° and 8° C). Don't freeze.
• Hospital staff should receive immunization if exposed to hepatitis B (for example, from a needle stick or direct contact).

• HBIG hasn't been associated with a higher incidence of AIDS. The immune globulin is devoid of HIV. Immune globulin recipients don't develop antibodies to HIV.

Patient education

• Explain that patient's chances of getting AIDS after receiving HBIG are very small.
• Inform patient that HBIG provides temporary protection against hepatitis B only.
• Tell patient what to expect after vaccination: local pain, swelling, and tenderness at the injection site. Recommend acetaminophen to relieve minor discomfort.
• Encourage patient to promptly report headache, skin changes, or difficulty breathing.

hepatitis B vaccine, recombinant
Engerix-B, Recombivax HB, Recombivax HB Dialysis Formulation

Viral vaccine

Available by prescription only
Injection: 10 mcg HBsAg/ml (Recombivax HB); 20 mcg HBsAg/ml (Engerix-B); 40 mcg HBsAg/ml (Recombivax HB Dialysis Formulation)

INDICATIONS & DOSAGE

Immunization against infection from all known subtypes of hepatitis B; primary preexposure prophylaxis against hepatitis B; postexposure prophylaxis (when given with hepatitis B immune globulin)
Engerix-B
Adults: Initially, give 20 mcg I.M., followed by a second dose of 20 mcg I.M. 30 days later. Give a third dose of 20 mcg I.M. 6 months after the initial dose.
Adults undergoing dialysis or receiving immunosuppressant therapy: Initially, give 40 mcg I.M. (divided into two 20-mcg doses and administered at different sites). Follow with a second dose of 40 mcg I.M. in 30 days, a third dose

after 2 months, and a final dose of 40 mcg I.M. 6 months after the initial dose.

Note: Alternative dosing schedule in certain populations (patients recently exposed to the virus and travelers to high-risk areas) who may receive the initial vaccine dose (20 mcg for adults) followed by a second dose in 1 month and the third dose after 2 months. For prolonged maintenance of protective antibody titers, a booster dose is recommended 12 months after the initial dose.

Recombivax HB
Adults: Initially, give 10 mcg I.M., followed by a second dose of 10 mcg I.M. 30 days later. Give a third dose of 10 mcg I.M. 6 months after the initial dose.
Adults undergoing dialysis or receiving immunosuppressant therapy: Initially, give 40 mcg I.M. (1-ml dialysis formulation). Follow with a second dose of 40 mcg I.M. in 30 days, and give a final dose of 40 mcg I.M. 6 months after the initial dose.

PHARMACODYNAMICS
Hepatitis B prophylaxis: Hepatitis B vaccine promotes active immunity to hepatitis B.

PHARMACOKINETICS
Absorption: After I.M. administration, antibody to HBsAg appears in serum within about 2 weeks, peaks after 6 months, and persists for at least 3 years.
Distribution: Unknown.
Metabolism: Unknown.
Excretion: Unknown.

CONTRAINDICATIONS & PRECAUTIONS
Contraindicated in patients hypersensitive to yeast; recombinant vaccines are derived from yeast cultures. Use cautiously in patients with active infections or compromised cardiac and pulmonary status or in those in whom a febrile or systemic reaction could pose a risk.

INTERACTIONS
Drug-drug. *Corticosteroids* or *immunosuppressants* may impair the immune response to hepatitis B vaccine; larger-than-usual doses of vaccine may be nec-

essary to develop adequate circulating antibody levels.

ADVERSE REACTIONS
CNS: headache, dizziness, insomnia, transient malaise.
EENT: pharyngitis.
GI: nausea, anorexia, diarrhea, vomiting.
Musculoskeletal: paresthesia, neuropathy, arthralgia, myalgia.
Other: slight fever, flulike syndrome, local inflammation, *soreness* (at injection site).

▣ KEY CONSIDERATIONS
• Obtain a thorough history of allergies and reactions to immunizations.
• Have epinephrine solution 1:1,000 available.
• The Centers for Disease Control and Prevention reports that response to hepatitis B vaccine is significantly better after injection into the deltoid rather than the gluteal muscle.
• Hepatitis B vaccine may be administered S.C., but only to persons who are at risk of hemorrhage from I.M. injection, such as hemophiliacs and patients with thrombocytopenia. Don't administer I.V.
• Hepatitis B vaccine may be given simultaneously, but at different sites, with hepatitis B immune globulin, influenza virus vaccine, Haemophilus influenzae type B conjugate vaccine, polyvalent pneumococcal vaccine, or DTP.
• Although unnecessary for most patients, serologic testing (to confirm immunity to hepatitis B after the 3-dose regimen) is recommended for persons older than age 50, those at high risk of needle-stick injury (who might require postexposure prophylaxis), hemodialysis patients, immunocompromised patients, and those who inadvertently received one or more injections into the gluteal muscle.
• Thoroughly agitate vial just before administration to restore a uniform suspension (white and slightly opaque).
• Store opened and unopened vial in the refrigerator. Don't freeze.

Patient education
• Tell patient that there is no risk of contracting HIV infection or AIDS from hepatitis B vaccine because it's synthetically derived.
• Explain that hepatitis B vaccine provides protection against hepatitis B only, not against hepatitis A or hepatitis C.
• Tell patient to expect some discomfort at injection site and possible fever, headache, or upset stomach. Recommend acetaminophen to relieve such effects. Encourage patient to report distressing adverse reactions.

hetastarch (HES, hydroxyethyl starch)
Hespan

Amylopectin derivative, plasma volume expander

Available by prescription only
Injection: 500 ml (6 g/100 ml in normal saline solution)

INDICATIONS & DOSAGE
Plasma expander in shock and cardiopulmonary bypass surgery
Adults: 500 to 1,000 ml I.V. depending on amount of blood lost and resultant hemoconcentration. Total dosage usually shouldn't exceed 20 ml/kg, up to 1,500 ml/day. Up to 20 ml/kg (1.2 g/kg)/hour may be used in hemorrhagic shock; in burns or septic shock, rate should be reduced.
Leukapheresis adjunct
Hetastarch is an adjunct in leukapheresis to improve harvesting and increase the yield of granulocytes.
Adults: Hetastarch 250 to 700 ml is infused at a constant fixed ratio, usually 1:8 to venous whole blood during continuous flow centrifugation (CFC) procedures. Up to 2 CFC procedures weekly, with total number of 7 to 10 procedures using hetastarch, have been found safe and effective. Safety of more procedures is unknown.

Note: Hetastarch can be used as a priming fluid in pump oxygenators for perfusion during extracorporeal circulation or as a cryoprotective agent for long-term storage of whole blood.

PHARMACODYNAMICS
Plasma volume expanding action: Hetastarch has an average molecular weight of 450,000 and exhibits colloidal properties similar to human albumin. After an I.V. infusion of hetastarch 6%, the plasma volume expands slightly in excess of the volume infused because of the colloidal osmotic effect. Maximum plasma volume expansion occurs in a few minutes and decreases over 24 to 36 hours. Hemodynamic status may improve for 24 hours or longer.
    As a leukapheresis adjunct, hetastarch enhances the yield of granulocytes by centrifugal means.

PHARMACOKINETICS
Absorption: After I.V. administration, plasma volume expands within a few minutes.
Distribution: Drug is distributed in the blood plasma.
Metabolism: Hetastarch molecules larger than 50,000 molecular weight are slowly degraded enzymatically to molecules that can be excreted.
Excretion: About 40% of hetastarch molecules smaller than 50,000 molecular weight are excreted in urine within 24 hours. Hetastarch molecules that aren't hydroxyethylated are slowly degraded to glucose. About 90% of dose is eliminated from the body with an average half-life of 17 days; remainder has a half-life of 48 days.

CONTRAINDICATIONS & PRECAUTIONS
Contraindicated in patients with severe bleeding disorders, severe heart failure, or renal failure with oliguria and anuria.

INTERACTIONS
None reported.

ADVERSE REACTIONS
CNS: headache.
CV: peripheral edema of lower extremities.
EENT: periorbital edema.
GI: nausea, vomiting.
Musculoskeletal: muscle pain.

Reactions may be *common*, uncommon, *life-threatening*, or COMMON AND LIFE-THREATENING.

Respiratory: wheezing.
Skin: urticaria.
Other: mild fever, chills.

🔲 KEY CONSIDERATIONS

• Use hetastarch with caution in geriatric patients, who are more prone to fluid overload; a lower dosage may be sufficient to produce desired plasma volume expansion.
• To avoid circulatory overload, carefully monitor patients with impaired renal function and those at high risk of pulmonary edema or heart failure. Hetastarch 6% in normal saline contains 77 mEq sodium and chloride per 500 ml.
• Don't administer as a substitute for blood or plasma.
• Discard partially used bottle because it doesn't contain a preservative.
• Monitor CBC; total leukocyte, platelet, and leukocyte differential counts; hematocrit; and hemoglobin, PT, INR, PTT, electrolyte, BUN, and creatinine levels.
• When added to whole blood, hetastarch increases the erythrocyte sedimentation rate.
• Assess vital signs and cardiopulmonary status to obtain baseline at start of infusion to prevent fluid overload.
• Monitor I.V. site for signs of infiltration and phlebitis.
• Observe patient for edema.

Patient education
• Explain use and administration of drug to patient and family.
• Instruct patient to report adverse reactions promptly.

Overdose & treatment
• Signs and symptoms of overdose include those listed under adverse reactions.
• Stop infusion if an overdose occurs and treat supportively.

---

hydralazine hydrochloride
Apresoline, Novo-Hylazin*

Peripheral vasodilator, antihypertensive

Available by prescription only

Tablets: 10 mg, 25 mg, 50 mg, 100 mg
Injection: 20 mg/ml

INDICATIONS & DOSAGE
Moderate to severe hypertension
Adults: Initially, 10 mg P.O. q.i.d. for 2 to 4 days, then increased to 25 mg q.i.d. for remainder of week. If necessary, increase dosage to 50 mg q.i.d. Maximum recommended dosage is 200 mg daily, but some patients may require 300 to 400 mg daily.
  For severe hypertension, give 10 to 50 mg I.M. or 10 to 20 mg I.V. repeated p.r.n. Switch to oral antihypertensives as soon as possible.
◊*Management of severe heart failure*
Adults: Initially, 50 to 75 mg P.O., then adjusted according to patient response. Most patients respond to 200 to 600 mg daily, divided q 6 to 12 hours, but dosages as high as 3 g daily have been used.

PHARMACODYNAMICS
Antihypertensive action: Hydralazine has a direct vasodilating effect on vascular smooth muscle, thus lowering blood pressure. Hydralazine's effect on resistance vessels (arterioles and arteries) is greater than that on capacitance vessels (venules and veins).

PHARMACOKINETICS
Absorption: Hydralazine is absorbed rapidly from GI tract after oral administration; peak plasma levels occur in 1 hour; bioavailability is 30% to 50%. Antihypertensive effect occurs 20 to 30 minutes after oral dose, 5 to 20 minutes after I.V. administration, and 10 to 30 minutes after I.M. administration. Food enhances absorption.
Distribution: Distributed widely throughout the body; drug is 88% to 90% protein-bound.
Metabolism: Hydralazine is metabolized extensively in the GI mucosa and the liver. Hydralazine is subject to polymorphic acetylation. Slow acetylators have higher plasma levels, generally requiring lower doses.
Excretion: Drug is mostly excreted in urine, primarily as metabolites; about 10% of an oral dose is excreted in feces.

Antihypertensive effect persists 2 to 4 hours after an oral dose and 2 to 6 hours after I.V. or I.M. administration.

CONTRAINDICATIONS & PRECAUTIONS
Contraindicated in patients with hypersensitivity to hydralazine, coronary artery disease, or mitral valvular rheumatic heart disease. Use cautiously in patients with suspected cardiac disease, CVA, or severe renal impairment, and in those receiving other antihypertensive drugs.

INTERACTIONS
Drug-drug. Hydralazine may potentiate the effects of *diuretics* and *other antihypertensives*; profound hypotension may occur if drug is given with *diazoxide*. Hydralazine may decrease the pressor response to *epinephrine;* administration with *MAO inhibitors* may synergistically decrease blood pressure.

ADVERSE REACTIONS
CNS: peripheral neuritis, *headache,* dizziness.
CV: orthostatic hypotension, *tachycardia,* edema, *angina, palpitations.*
GI: *nausea, vomiting, diarrhea, anorexia,* constipation.
Hematologic: *neutropenia, leukopenia, agranulocytosis.*
Skin: rash.
Other: *lupus-like syndrome* (especially with high doses).

▣ KEY CONSIDERATIONS
• Geriatric patients may be more sensitive to antihypertensive effects. Use with special caution in patients with history of stroke or impaired renal function; patients with renal impairment may respond to lower maintenance dosages.
• CBC, lupus erythematosus (LE) cell preparation, and antinuclear antibody (ANA) titer determinations should be performed before therapy and at regular intervals during long-term therapy.
• Incidence of drug-induced systemic lupus erythematosus (SLE) syndrome is greatest in patients receiving more than 200 mg/day for prolonged periods.

• Headache and palpitations may occur 2 to 4 hours after first oral dose but should subside spontaneously.
• Advise precautions for postural hypotension.
• Hydralazine may cause positive ANA titer; positive LE cell preparation; blood dyscrasias, including leukopenia, agranulocytosis, and purpura; and hematologic abnormalities, including decreased hemoglobin and RBC count.
• Food enhances oral absorption and helps minimize gastric irritation; adhere to consistent schedule.
• Some preparations contain tartrazine, which may precipitate allergic reactions, especially in aspirin-sensitive patients.
• For I.V. use: Monitor blood pressure every 5 minutes until stable, then every 15 minutes; put patient in Trendelenburg's position if he is faint or dizzy. Too-rapid reduction in blood pressure can cause mental changes from cerebral ischemia.
• Inject drug as soon as possible after draining through needle into syringe; drug changes color after contact with metal.
• Sodium retention can occur with long-term use; monitor patient for signs of weight gain and edema.

Patient education
• Teach patient about disease and therapy, and explain why drug should be taken exactly as prescribed, even when he feels well; advise him never to discontinue drug suddenly because severe rebound hypertension may occur.
• Explain adverse effects and advise patient to report unusual effects, especially symptoms of SLE (sore throat, fever, rash, and muscle and joint pain).
• Explain how to minimize impact of adverse effects: avoid operation of hazardous equipment until tolerance develops to sedation, drowsiness, and other CNS effects; avoid sudden position changes, to minimize orthostatic hypotension; avoid alcohol; and take drug with meals to enhance absorption and minimize gastric irritation.
• Reassure patient that headaches and palpitations occurring 2 to 4 hours after

---

Reactions may be *common,* uncommon, ***life-threatening****,* or COMMON AND LIFE-THREATENING.

initial dose usually subside spontaneously; if not, he should report such effects.
• Instruct patient to weigh himself at least weekly. Advise him to report weight gain that exceeds 2.3 kg (5 lb) weekly.
• Warn patient to seek medical approval before taking OTC cold preparations.

Overdose & treatment
• Signs and symptoms of overdose include hypotension, tachycardia, headache, and skin flushing; arrhythmias and shock may occur.
• After acute ingestion, induce vomiting or perform gastric lavage and give activated charcoal to reduce absorption. Follow with symptomatic and supportive care.

hydrochlorothiazide
Apo-Hydro*, Aquazide-H, Diuchlor H*, Esidrix, Hydro-chlor, Hydro-D, HydroDIURIL, Mictrin, Neo-Codema*, Novo-Hydrazide*, Oretic, Urozide*

Thiazide diuretic, antihypertensive

Available by prescription only
Tablets: 25 mg, 50 mg, 100 mg
Solution: 50 mg/5 ml, 100 mg/ml

INDICATIONS & DOSAGE
Edema
Adults: Initially, 25 to 200 mg P.O. daily for several days or until dry weight is attained. Maintenance dose is 25 to 100 mg P.O. daily or intermittently. A few refractory patients may require up to 200 mg daily.
Hypertension
Adults: 25 to 50 mg P.O. once daily or in divided doses. Daily dosage is increased or decreased based on blood pressure.

PHARMACODYNAMICS
Diuretic action: Hydrochlorothiazide increases urine excretion of sodium and water by inhibiting sodium reabsorption in the cortical diluting tubule of the nephron, thus relieving edema.
Antihypertensive action: Exact mechanism of drug's antihypertensive effect is unknown. It may result partially from direct arteriolar vasodilation and a decrease in total peripheral resistance.

PHARMACOKINETICS
Absorption: Hydrochlorothiazide is absorbed from the GI tract; the rate and extent of absorption vary with different formulations.
Distribution: Unknown.
Metabolism: None.
Excretion: Excreted unchanged in urine, usually within 24 hours; half-life is 5.6 to 14.8 hours.

CONTRAINDICATIONS & PRECAUTIONS
Contraindicated in patients with anuria or hypersensitivity to other thiazides or other sulfonamide derivatives. Use cautiously in patients with severely impaired renal or hepatic function or progressive hepatic disease.

INTERACTIONS
Drug-drug. Hydrochlorothiazide potentiates the hypotensive effects of most other *antihypertensives*; this may be used to therapeutic advantage. *Cholestyramine* and *colestipol* may bind hydrochlorothiazide, preventing its absorption; give drugs 1 hour apart. Hydrochlorothiazide may potentiate hyperglycemic, hypotensive, and hyperuricemic effects of *diazoxide*, and its hyperglycemic effect may increase *insulin* or *sulfonylurea* requirements in diabetic patients. Hydrochlorothiazide may reduce renal clearance of *lithium,* elevating serum lithium levels and possibly necessitating reduction in lithium dosage by 50%. Hydrochlorothiazide turns urine slightly more alkaline and may decrease urine excretion of some amines, such as *amphetamine* and *quinidine*; alkaline urine also may decrease therapeutic efficacy of *methenamine compounds* such as *methenamine mandelate.*
Drug-lifestyle. Photosensitivity reactions may occur with *sun exposure;* take precautions.

ADVERSE REACTIONS
CNS: dizziness, vertigo, headache, paresthesia, weakness, restlessness.

CV: volume depletion and dehydration, orthostatic hypotension, allergic myocarditis, vasculitis.
GI: anorexia, nausea, pancreatitis, epigastric distress, vomiting, abdominal pain, diarrhea, constipation.
GU: polyuria, urinary frequency, *renal failure,* interstitial nephritis.
Hematologic: *aplastic anemia, agranulocytosis, leukopenia, thrombocytopenia,* hemolytic anemia.
Hepatic: jaundice.
Metabolic: hypokalemia; asymptomatic hyperuricemia; hyperglycemia and impaired glucose tolerance; fluid and electrolyte imbalances, including dilutional hyponatremia, hypochloremia, metabolic alkalosis, hypercalcemia.
Musculoskeletal: muscle cramps.
Respiratory: respiratory distress, pneumonitis.
Skin: dermatitis, photosensitivity, rash, purpura, alopecia.
Other: hypersensitivity reactions, gout, *anaphylactic reactions.*

▣ **KEY CONSIDERATIONS**
Besides the recommendations relevant to all thiazide diuretics, consider the following:
● Geriatric and debilitated patients require close observation and may require reduced dosages. They are more sensitive to excess diuresis because of age-related changes in CV and renal function. Excess diuresis promotes orthostatic hypotension, dehydration, hypovolemia, hyponatremia, hypomagnesemia, and hypokalemia.
● Drug may cause glucose intolerance in some people. Monitor blood glucose level in diabetic patients. May require dose adjustment of insulin or oral antidiabetic.
● Drug therapy may alter serum electrolyte levels and may increase serum urate, glucose, cholesterol, and triglyceride levels. It also may interfere with tests for parathyroid function and should be discontinued before such tests.

Patient education
● Instruct patient to take drug with food to avoid GI upset.
● Tell patient to take drug in morning or early afternoon to avoid nocturia.

● Advise patient to avoid sudden postural changes.
● Encourage patient to use sunblock to avoid photosensitivity reactions.
● Tell patient to consult health care provider before taking OTC drugs.

Overdose & treatment
● Signs and symptoms of overdose include GI irritation and hypermotility, diuresis, and lethargy, which may progress to coma.
● Treatment is mainly supportive; monitor and assist respiratory, CV, and renal function as indicated. Monitor fluid and electrolyte balance. Induce vomiting with ipecac in conscious patient; otherwise, use gastric lavage to avoid aspiration. Don't give cathartics; these promote additional loss of fluids and electrolytes.

---

hydrocortisone (systemic)
Cortef, Cortenema, Hycort*, Hydrocortone

hydrocortisone acetate
Cortifoam

hydrocortisone cypionate
Cortef

hydrocortisone sodium phosphate
Hydrocortone Phosphate

hydrocortisone sodium succinate
A-hydroCort, Solu-Cortef

Glucocorticoid, mineralocorticoid, adrenocorticoid replacement

---

Available by prescription only
hydrocortisone
Tablets: 5 mg, 10 mg, 20 mg
Injection: 25 mg/ml and 50 mg/ml suspensions
Enema: 100 mg/60 ml
hydrocortisone acetate
Injection: 25 mg/ml and 50 mg/ml suspensions

Reactions may be *common,* uncommon, *life-threatening,* or COMMON AND LIFE-THREATENING.

Enema: 10% aerosol foam (provides 90 mg/application)
hydrocortisone cypionate
Oral suspension: 10 mg/5 ml
hydrocortisone sodium phosphate
Injection: 50 mg/ml solution
hydrocortisone sodium succinate
Injection: 100 mg/vial, 250 mg/vial, 500 mg/vial, 1,000 mg/vial

INDICATIONS & DOSAGE
Severe inflammation, adrenal insufficiency
hydrocortisone
Adults: 5 to 30 mg P.O. b.i.d., t.i.d., or q.i.d. (as much as 80 mg P.O. q.i.d. may be given in acute situations).
hydrocortisone acetate
Adults: 10 to 75 mg into joints or soft tissue at 2- or 3-week intervals. Dose varies with size of joint. In many cases, local anesthetics are injected with dose.
hydrocortisone sodium phosphate
Adults: 15 to 240 mg S.C., I.M., or I.V. daily in divided doses q 12 hours.
hydrocortisone sodium succinate
Adults: Initially, 100 to 500 mg I.M. or I.V., then 50 to 100 mg I.M. as indicated.
Shock (other than adrenal crisis)
hydrocortisone sodium succinate
Adults: 100 to 500 mg I.M. or I.V. q 2 to 6 hours.
Life-threatening shock
hydrocortisone sodium succinate
Adults: 0.5 to 2 g I.V. initially, repeated at 2- to 6-hour intervals, p.r.n. High-dose therapy should be continued only until patient's condition has stabilized. Therapy shouldn't be continued beyond 48 to 72 hours.
Adjunctive treatment of ulcerative colitis and proctitis
hydrocortisone
Adults: One enema (100 mg) nightly for 21 days.
hydrocortisone acetate (rectal foam)
Adults: 90 mg (1 full applicator) once or twice daily for 2 or 3 weeks; decrease frequency to every other day thereafter.

PHARMACODYNAMICS
Adrenocorticoid replacement action:
Hydrocortisone is an adrenocorticoid with both glucocorticoid and mineralocorticoid properties. It's a weak anti-inflammatory agent but a potent mineralocorticoid, having potency similar to that of cortisone and twice that of prednisone. Hydrocortisone (or cortisone) is usually the drug of choice for replacement therapy in patients with adrenal insufficiency. It usually isn't used for immunosuppressant activity because of the extremely large doses necessary and the unwanted mineralocorticoid effects.

Hydrocortisone and hydrocortisone cypionate may be administered orally. Hydrocortisone sodium phosphate may be administered by I.M., S.C., or I.V. injection or by I.V. infusion, usually at 12-hour intervals. Hydrocortisone sodium succinate may be administered by I.M. or I.V. injection or I.V. infusion every 2 to 10 hours, depending on the situation. Hydrocortisone acetate is a suspension that may be administered by intraarticular, intrasynovial, intrabursal, intralesional, or soft-tissue injection. It has a slow onset but a long duration of action. Injectable forms are usually used only when the oral dosage forms can't be used.

PHARMACOKINETICS
Absorption: Hydrocortisone is absorbed readily after oral administration. After oral and I.V. administration, peak effects occur in about 1 to 2 hours. The acetate suspension for injection has a variable absorption over 24 to 48 hours, depending on whether it's injected into an intraarticular space or a muscle, and the blood supply to that muscle.
Distribution: Hydrocortisone is removed rapidly from the blood and distributed to muscle, liver, skin, intestines, and kidneys. Hydrocortisone is bound extensively to plasma proteins (transcortin and albumin). Only the unbound portion is active.
Metabolism: Drug is metabolized in the liver to inactive glucuronide and sulfate metabolites.
Excretion: The inactive metabolites and small amounts of unmetabolized drug are excreted by the kidneys. Insignificant quantities of drug are excreted in feces. The biological half-life of hydrocortisone is 8 to 12 hours.

CONTRAINDICATIONS & PRECAUTIONS

Contraindicated in patients allergic to any component of the formulation, and in those with systemic fungal infections.

Use hydrocortisone sodium phosphate or succinate cautiously in patients with a recent MI, GI ulcer, renal disease, hypertension, osteoporosis, diabetes mellitus, hypothyroidism, cirrhosis, diverticulitis, ulcerative colitis, recent intestinal anastomosis, thromboembolic disorders, seizures, myasthenia gravis, heart failure, tuberculosis, ocular herpes simplex, emotional instability, and psychotic tendencies.

INTERACTIONS

Drug-drug. Hydrocortisone may enhance hypokalemia from *amphotericin B* or *diuretic* therapy; the hypokalemia may increase the risk of toxicity in patients receiving *cardiac glycosides*. *Antacids, cholestyramine,* and *colestipol* decrease corticosteroid effects by adsorbing the corticosteroid, thereby decreasing the amount absorbed. Use of *barbiturates, phenytoin,* or *rifampin* may decrease corticosteroid effects because of increased hepatic metabolism. Use with *estrogens* may reduce the metabolism of corticosteroids by increasing transcortin levels; the half-life of the corticosteroid is then prolonged from increased protein binding. Hydrocortisone increases the metabolism of *isoniazid* and *salicylates.* When used concomitantly, hydrocortisone may, in rare cases, decrease the effects of *oral anticoagulants* by unknown mechanisms. Administration of *ulcerogenic drugs,* such as *NSAIDs,* may increase risk of GI ulceration.

ADVERSE REACTIONS

Most adverse reactions to corticosteroids are dose- or duration-dependent.
CNS: *euphoria, insomnia,* psychotic behavior, pseudotumor cerebri, vertigo, headache, paresthesia, *seizures.*
CV: *heart failure,* hypertension, edema, *arrhythmias,* thrombophlebitis, *thromboembolism.*
EENT: cataracts, glaucoma.

GI: *peptic ulceration,* GI irritation, increased appetite, pancreatitis, nausea, vomiting.
Metabolic: possible hypokalemia, hyperglycemia (requiring dosage adjustment in diabetics), carbohydrate intolerance.
Musculoskeletal: muscle weakness, osteoporosis.
Skin: delayed wound healing, acne, various skin eruptions, easy bruising, hirsutism.
Other: susceptibility to infections, *acute adrenal insufficiency with increased stress (infection, surgery, trauma) or abrupt withdrawal (after long-term therapy),* cushingoid state (moonface, buffalo hump, central obesity).
After abrupt withdrawal: rebound inflammation, fatigue, weakness, arthralgia, fever, dizziness, lethargy, depression, fainting, orthostatic hypotension, dyspnea, anorexia, hypoglycemia. *After prolonged use, sudden withdrawal may be fatal.*

▣ KEY CONSIDERATIONS

Besides the recommendations relevant to all systemic adrenocorticoids, consider the following:
• Hydrocortisone suppresses reactions to skin tests, causes false-negative results in the nitroblue tetrazolium tests for systemic bacterial infections, and decreases ^{131}I uptake and protein-bound iodine levels in thyroid function tests.
• Hydrocortisone may increase glucose and cholesterol levels; may decrease serum potassium, calcium, thyroxine, and triiodothyronine levels; and may increase urine glucose and calcium levels.

Reactions may be *common,* uncommon, *life-threatening,* or COMMON AND LIFE-THREATENING.

hydrocortisone (topical)
Acticort 100, Aeroseb-HC, Ala-Cort, Ala-Scalp, Anusol-HC, Bactine, Barriere-HC*, CaldeCORT, Cetacort, CortaGel, Cortaid, Cortate*, Cort-Dome, Cortizone, Dermacort, DermiCort, Dermolate, Dermtex HC, Emo-Cort*, Hi-Cor, Hydro-Tex, Hytone, LactiCare-HC, Nutracort, Penecort, Rectocort*, S-T Cort, Synacort, Texacort, Unicort*

hydrocortisone acetate
Anusol-HC, CaldeCORT, Cortaid, Cort-Dome, Cortef, Corticaine, Corticreme*, Cortoderm*, Gynecort, Hyderm*, Lanacort, Novohydrocort*, Orabase-HCA, Pharma-Cort, Rhulicort

hydrocortisone buteprate
Pandel

hydrocortisone butyrate
Locoid

hydrocortisone valerate
Westcort

Glucocorticoid, anti-inflammatory

Available by prescription only
hydrocortisone
Cream: 0.5%, 1%, 2.5%
Ointment: 0.5%, 1%, 2.5%
Lotion: 0.25%, 0.5%, 1%, 2%, 2.5%
Gel: 0.5%, 1%
Solution: 0.5%, 1%, 2.5%
Aerosol: 0.5%, 1%
Pledgets (saturated with solution): 0.5%, 1%
hydrocortisone acetate
Cream: 0.5%, 1%
Ointment: 0.5%, 1%
Lotion: 0.5%
Suppositories: 25 mg
Rectal foam: 10%
Paste: 0.5%
Solution: 1%
hydrocortisone buteprate
Cream: 0.1%
hydrocortisone butyrate
Cream, ointment, solution: 0.1%

hydrocortisone valerate
Cream, ointment: 0.2%

INDICATIONS & DOSAGE
Inflammation of corticosteroid-responsive dermatoses, including those on face, groin, armpits, and under breasts; seborrheic dermatitis of scalp
Adults: Apply cream, lotion, ointment, foam, or aerosol sparingly once daily to q.i.d.
Aerosol
Shake can well. Direct spray onto affected area from a distance of 6" (15 cm). Apply for only 3 seconds (to avoid freezing tissues). Apply to dry scalp after shampooing; no need to massage or rub drug into scalp after spraying. Apply daily until acute phase is controlled, then reduce dosage to 1 to 3 times weekly, p.r.n., to maintain control.
Rectal administration
Shake can well. Apply once daily or b.i.d. for 2 to 3 weeks, then every other day, p.r.n.
Dental lesions
Adults: Apply paste b.i.d. or t.i.d. and h.s.

PHARMACODYNAMICS
Anti-inflammatory action: Hydrocortisone stimulates the synthesis of enzymes needed to decrease the inflammatory response. Hydrocortisone, a corticosteroid secreted by the adrenal cortex, is about 1.25 times more potent an anti-inflammatory agent than equivalent doses of cortisone, but both have twice the mineralocorticoid activity of the other glucocorticoids.

Hydrocortisone 0.5%, 1%, and hydrocortisone acetate 0.5% are available without a prescription for the temporary relief of minor skin irritation, itching, and rashes caused by eczema, insect bites, soaps, and detergents.

Hydrocortisone is also administered rectally as a retention enema for the temporary treatment of acute ulcerative colitis. Hydrocortisone acetate suspension is also available as a rectal suppository or aerosol foam suspension for the temporary treatment of inflammatory conditions of the rectum such as hemorrhoids, cryptitis, proctitis, and pruritus ani.

PHARMACOKINETICS

Absorption: Absorption depends on potency of preparation, amount applied, and nature of skin at application site. It ranges from about 1% in areas with a thick stratum corneum (such as the palms, soles, elbows, and knees) to as high as 36% in areas where the stratum corneum is thinnest (face, eyelids, and genitals). Absorption increases with skin damage, inflammation, or occlusion. Some systemic absorption occurs, especially through the oral mucosa.
Distribution: After topical application, hydrocortisone is distributed throughout the local skin layers. Any drug absorbed into the circulation is removed rapidly from the blood and distributed into muscle, liver, skin, intestines, and kidneys.
Metabolism: After topical administration, hydrocortisone is metabolized primarily in the skin. The small amount absorbed into the systemic circulation is metabolized primarily in the liver to inactive compounds.
Excretion: Inactive metabolites are excreted by the kidneys, primarily as glucuronides and sulfates, but also as unconjugated products. Small amounts of the metabolites are excreted in feces.

CONTRAINDICATIONS & PRECAUTIONS

Contraindicated in patients hypersensitive to hydrocortisone.

INTERACTIONS

None significant.

ADVERSE REACTIONS

Metabolic: hyperglycemia, glycosuria.
Skin: burning, pruritus, irritation, dryness, erythema, folliculitis, hypertrichosis, hypopigmentation, acneiform eruptions, allergic contact dermatitis; *maceration, secondary infection, atrophy, striae, miliaria* (with occlusive dressings).
Other: *hypothalamic-pituitary-adrenal axis suppression,* Cushing's syndrome.

▣ KEY CONSIDERATIONS

Besides the recommendations relevant to all topical adrenocorticoids, consider the following:
• To prevent skin damage, gently rub in drug, leaving a thin coat.

• Stop drug if skin infection, striae, or atrophy occurs.
• If antifungals or antibiotics are used, stop corticosteroid until infection is controlled, as indicated.

PATIENT EDUCATION

• Teach patient or family member how to apply drug.
• If occlusive dressing is indicated, advise patient not to leave it in place longer than 12 hours each day and not to use occlusive dressing on infected or exudative lesions.

hydromorphone hydrochloride
Dilaudid, Dilaudid-HP, Hydrostat IR

Opioid, analgesic, antitussive
Controlled substance schedule II

Available by prescription only
Tablets: 1 mg, 2 mg, 3 mg, 4 mg, 8 mg
Oral liquid: 5 mg/5 ml
Injection: 1 mg/ml, 2 mg/ml, 3 mg/ml, 4 mg/ml, 10 mg/ml
Suppository: 3 mg

INDICATIONS & DOSAGE
Moderate to severe pain
Adults: 2 to 10 mg P.O. q 3 to 6 hours, p.r.n., or around the clock; or 2 to 4 mg I.M., S.C., or I.V. q 4 to 6 hours, p.r.n., or around the clock (I.V. dose should be given over 3 to 5 minutes); or 3-mg rectal suppository q 6 to 8 hours, p.r.n., or around the clock. (Give 1 to 14 mg Dilaudid-HP S.C. or I.M. q 4 to 6 hours.)
Note: Hydromorphone hydrochloride should be given in the smallest effective dose and as infrequently as possible to minimize the development of tolerance and physical dependence. Dose must be individually adjusted based on patient's severity of pain, age, and size.
Cough
Adults: 1 mg P.O. q 3 to 4 hours, p.r.n.

PHARMACODYNAMICS
Analgesic action: Hydromorphone has analgesic properties related to opiate receptor affinity and is recommended for

---

Reactions may be *common*, uncommon, *life-threatening*, or COMMON AND LIFE-THREATENING.

moderate to severe pain. There is no intrinsic limit to the analgesic effect of hydromorphone, unlike the other opioids.
Antitussive action: Hydromorphone acts directly on the cough center in the medulla, producing an antitussive effect.

PHARMACOKINETICS
Absorption: Hydromorphone is well absorbed after oral, rectal, or parenteral administration. Onset of action occurs in 15 to 30 minutes, with peak effect at ½ to 1 hour after dosing.
Distribution: Unknown.
Metabolism: Drug is metabolized primarily in the liver, where it undergoes conjugation with glucuronic acid.
Excretion: Drug is excreted primarily in the urine as the glucuronide conjugate. Duration of action is 4 to 5 hours.

CONTRAINDICATIONS & PRECAUTIONS
Contraindicated in patients with hypersensitivity to hydromorphone, intracranial lesions associated with increased intracranial pressure, and whenever ventilator function is depressed, such as in status asthmaticus, COPD, cor pulmonale, emphysema, and kyphoscoliosis.
   Use cautiously in geriatric or debilitated patients and in those with hepatic or renal disease, Addison's disease, hypothyroidism, prostatic hyperplasia, or urethral strictures.

INTERACTIONS
Drug-drug. Use with *cimetidine* may also increase respiratory and CNS depression, causing confusion, disorientation, apnea, or seizures; such use usually requires reduced dosage of hydromorphone. Use with other *CNS depressants*—including *antihistamines, barbiturates, benzodiazepines, general anesthetics, muscle relaxants, narcotic analgesics, phenothiazines, sedative-hypnotics,* and *tricyclic antidepressants*—potentiates the respiratory and CNS depression, sedation, and hypotensive effects of the drug. Drug accumulation and enhanced effects may result from use with other *drugs that are extensively metabolized in the liver*—such as *rifampin, phenytoin,* and *digitoxin;* use with *anticholinergics* may cause paralytic ileus. Severe CV depres-

sion may result from use with *general anesthetics.* Patients who become physically dependent on drug may experience acute withdrawal syndrome if given a *narcotic antagonist.*
Drug-lifestyle. *Alcohol* potentiates drug's respiratory and CNS depression, sedation, and hypotensive effects; discourage use.

ADVERSE REACTIONS
CNS: *sedation, somnolence, clouded sensorium,* dizziness, *euphoria.*
CV: *hypotension,* bradycardia.
EENT: blurred vision, diplopia, nystagmus.
GI: *nausea, vomiting, constipation,* ileus.
GU: *urine retention.*
Respiratory: *respiratory depression, bronchospasm.*
Other: induration (with repeated S.C. injections), physical dependence.

▣ KEY CONSIDERATIONS
Besides the recommendations relevant to all opioids, consider the following:
● Lower doses are usually indicated for geriatric patients because they may be more sensitive to the therapeutic and adverse effects of drug.
● Before administration, visually inspect all parenteral products for particulate matter and yellow discoloration.
● Oral dosage form is particularly convenient for patients with chronic pain because tablets are available in several strengths, enabling patient to adjust dosage precisely.
● Dilaudid-HP, a highly concentrated form (10 mg/ml), may be administered in smaller volumes, preventing discomfort associated with large-volume injections.
● Drug increases plasma amylase and lipase levels. It may also delay gastric emptying; increased biliary tract pressure resulting from contraction of the sphincter of Oddi may interfere with hepatobiliary imaging studies.

Patient education
● Instruct patient to take or ask for drug before pain becomes intense.

---

*Canada only   ◊ Unlabeled clinical use

• Tell patient to store suppositories in the refrigerator.
• Encourage coughing or deep breathing to avoid atelectasis (postoperatively).
• Instruct patient to avoid hazardous activities that require mental alertness.
• Advise patient to avoid alcohol.

Overdose & treatment

• The most common signs and symptoms of hydromorphone overdose are CNS depression, respiratory depression, and miosis. Other acute toxic effects include hypotension, bradycardia, hypothermia, shock, apnea, cardiopulmonary arrest, circulatory collapse, pulmonary edema, and seizures.
• To treat an acute overdose, first establish adequate respiratory exchange via a patent airway and ventilation as needed; administer naloxone to reverse respiratory depression. (Because the duration of action of hydromorphone is longer than that of naloxone, repeated dosing is necessary.) Don't give naloxone unless patient has significant respiratory or CV depression. Monitor vital signs closely.
• If patient presents within 2 hours of ingestion of an oral overdose, immediately induce vomiting with ipecac syrup or perform gastric lavage. Use caution to avoid risk of aspiration. Administer activated charcoal via an NG tube to further remove drug.
• Provide symptomatic and supportive treatment (continued respiratory support, correction of fluid or electrolyte imbalance). Monitor laboratory values, vital signs, and neurologic status closely.
• Contact the local or regional poison control center for further information.

hydroxychloroquine sulfate
Plaquenil Sulfate

4-aminoquinoline, antimalarial, anti-inflammatory

Available by prescription only
Tablets: 200 mg (155-mg base)

INDICATIONS & DOSAGE
Suppressive prophylaxis of malarial attacks
Adults: 400 mg of sulfate (310-mg base) P.O. weekly on exactly the same day each week. (Begin 2 weeks before entering and continue for 8 weeks after leaving the endemic area.)
Treatment of acute attack of malaria
Adults: 800 mg (620-mg base) followed by 400 mg (310-mg base) in 6 to 8 hours and 400 mg (310-mg base) on each of 2 consecutive days.
Lupus erythematosus (chronic discoid and systemic)
Adults: 400 mg P.O. daily or b.i.d., continued for several weeks or months, based on response. Prolonged maintenance is 200 to 400 mg P.O. daily.
◊ **Rheumatoid arthritis**
Adults: Initially, 400 to 600 mg P.O. daily. When good response occurs (usually in 4 to 12 weeks), reduce dosage by half.

PHARMACODYNAMICS
Antimalarial action: Hydroxychloroquine binds to DNA, interfering with protein synthesis. It also inhibits DNA and RNA polymerases. It's active against asexual erythrocytic forms of *Plasmodium malariae, P. ovale, P. vivax,* and many strains of *P. falciparum.*
Anti-inflammatory action: Mechanism of action is unknown. Drug may antagonize histamine and serotonin and inhibit prostaglandin effects by inhibiting conversion of arachidonic acid to prostaglandin F_2; it may also inhibit chemotaxis of polymorphonuclear leukocytes, macrophages, and eosinophils.

PHARMACOKINETICS
Absorption: Hydroxychloroquine is absorbed readily and almost completely, with peak plasma levels at 1 to 2 hours.
Distribution: Drug is bound to plasma proteins. It concentrates in the liver, spleen, kidneys, heart, and brain, and is strongly bound in melanin-containing cells.
Metabolism: Drug is metabolized by the liver to desethylchloroquine and desethylhydroxychloroquine.
Excretion: Most of an administered dose is excreted unchanged in urine. Drug and its metabolites are excreted slowly in urine; unabsorbed drug is excreted in feces. Small amounts of drug may be

---

Reactions may be *common,* uncommon, *life-threatening,* or COMMON AND LIFE-THREATENING.

present in urine for months after it's discontinued.

CONTRAINDICATIONS & PRECAUTIONS
Contraindicated in patients with hypersensitivity to hydroxychloroquine and in patients with retinal or visual field changes or porphyria. Use cautiously in patients with severe GI, neurologic, or blood disorders.

INTERACTIONS
Drug-drug. Use with *digoxin* may increase serum digoxin levels. Administration of *kaolin* or *magnesium trisilicate* may decrease absorption of hydroxychloroquine.

ADVERSE REACTIONS
CNS: irritability, nightmares, ataxia, *seizures,* psychosis, vertigo, nystagmus, dizziness, ataxia, lassitude, headache.
EENT: visual disturbances (blurred vision; difficulty in focusing; reversible corneal changes; typically irreversible, sometimes progressive or delayed retinal changes, such as narrowing of arterioles; macular lesions; pallor of optic disk; optic atrophy; visual field defects; patchy retinal pigmentation, commonly leading to blindness; ototoxicity (irreversible nerve deafness, tinnitus, labyrinthitis).
GI: anorexia, abdominal cramps, diarrhea, nausea, vomiting.
Hematologic: *agranulocytosis, leukopenia, thrombocytopenia, hemolysis (in patients with G6PD deficiency), aplastic anemia.*
Metabolic: weight loss.
Musculoskeletal: hypoactive deep tendon reflexes, skeletal muscle weakness.
Skin: pruritus, lichen planus eruptions, skin and mucosal pigmentary changes, pleomorphic skin eruptions, alopecia, bleaching of hair.

▣ KEY CONSIDERATIONS
• Baseline and periodic ophthalmologic examinations are necessary in prolonged or high-dosage therapy.
• Monitor for blurred vision, increased sensitivity to light, hearing loss, pronounced GI disturbances, or muscle weakness.

• Give drug immediately before or after meals on the same day each week to minimize gastric distress.
• Drug is ineffective for chloroquine-resistant strains of *P. falciparum.*
• Drug may cause inversion or depression of the T wave or widening of the QRS complex on ECG.

Patient education
• To prevent drug-induced dermatoses, warn patient to avoid excessive exposure to the sun.

Overdose & treatment
• Signs and symptoms of drug overdose may appear within 30 minutes after ingestion and may include headache, drowsiness, visual changes, CV collapse, and seizures, followed by respiratory and cardiac arrest.
• Treatment is symptomatic. Induce vomiting or perform gastric lavage. Then, if given within 30 minutes of drug ingestion, activated charcoal in an amount at least five times the estimated amount of drug ingested may be helpful.
• Ultra-short-acting barbiturates may help control seizures. Intubation may become necessary. Peritoneal dialysis and exchange transfusions may also be useful. Forced fluids and acidification of the urine are helpful after the acute phase.

hydroxyurea
Hydrea

Antimetabolite (cell cycle–phase specific, S phase), antineoplastic

Available by prescription only
Capsules: 500 mg

INDICATIONS & DOSAGE
Dosage and indications may vary. Check current literature for recommended protocol.
Solid tumors
Adults: 80 mg/kg P.O. as a single dose q 3 days; or 20 to 30 mg/kg P.O. as a single daily dose.
Head and neck cancer
Adults: 80 mg/kg P.O. as a single dose q 3 days.

Resistant chronic myelocytic leukemia
Adults: 20 to 30 mg/kg P.O. as a single
daily dose.

PHARMACODYNAMICS

Antineoplastic action: Exact mechanism
of hydroxyurea's cytotoxic action is unclear. Hydroxyurea inhibits DNA synthesis without interfering with RNA or
protein synthesis. Drug may act as an
antimetabolite, inhibiting the incorporation of thymidine into DNA, and may
also damage DNA directly.

PHARMACOKINETICS

Absorption: Hydroxyurea is well absorbed after oral administration, with
peak serum levels occurring 2 hours after a dose. Higher serum levels are
achieved if drug is given as a large, single dose rather than in divided doses.
Distribution: Drug crosses the blood-
brain barrier.
Metabolism: About 50% of an oral dose
is degraded in the liver.
Excretion: The remaining 50% is excreted in urine as unchanged drug. The
metabolites are excreted through the
lungs as carbon dioxide and in urine as
urea.

CONTRAINDICATIONS & PRECAUTIONS

Contraindicated in patients hypersensitive to hydroxyurea and with marked
bone marrow depression (leukopenia
[less than 2,500 WBCs/mm³], thrombocytopenia [less than 100,000 platelets/
mm³], or severe anemia).
    Use cautiously in patients with im-
paired renal function.

INTERACTIONS

Drug-drug. Use of hydroxyurea may
decrease the activity of *fluorouracil;* hydroxyurea appears to inhibit the conversion of fluorouracil to its active metabolite. (Neurotoxicity may occur when administered together.)

ADVERSE REACTIONS

CNS: hallucinations, headache, dizziness, disorientation, *seizures,* malaise.
GI: *anorexia, nausea, vomiting, diarrhea,* stomatitis, constipation.

GU: increased BUN and serum creatinine levels.
Hematologic: *leukopenia, thrombocytopenia,* anemia, *megaloblastosis, bone
marrow suppression,* with rapid recovery (dose-limiting and dose-related).
Skin: rash, alopecia, erythema.
Other: fever, chills.

◙ KEY CONSIDERATIONS

• Geriatric patients may be more sensitive to drug's effects, requiring a lower
dosage.
• Dose modification may be required after other chemotherapy or radiation therapy.
• Monitor intake and output levels; keep
patient hydrated.
• Obtain BUN, uric acid, and serum creatinine levels routinely.
• Note that drug may exacerbate postir-
radiation erythema.
• Note that auditory and visual hallucinations and blood toxicity increase when
renal function is decreased.
• Avoid all I.M. injections when platelet
counts are less than 100,000/mm³.
• Store capsules in tight container at
room temperature. Avoid exposure to excessive heat.
• Drug is now under investigation for the
treatment of sickle cell anemia. Widespread use of drug for this disease isn't
recommended because of the potential
for toxicity. Hydroxyurea therapy elevates BUN, serum creatinine, and serum
uric acid levels.

Patient education

• Instruct patient to empty contents of
capsule in water and drink immediately
if capsule can't be swallowed.
• Emphasize importance of continuing
drug therapy despite nausea and vomiting.
• Tell patient to call immediately if vomiting occurs shortly after taking a dose.
• Encourage daily fluid intake of 10 to
12 (8-oz [240-ml]) glasses to increase
urine output and facilitate excretion of
uric acid.
• Tell patient to report unusual bruising
or bleeding.

Reactions may be *common,* uncommon, *life-threatening,* or COMMON AND LIFE-THREATENING.

• Advise patient to avoid exposure to people with infections and to report signs of infection immediately.

Overdose & treatment
• Signs and symptoms of overdose include myelosuppression, ulceration of buccal and GI mucosa, facial erythema, maculopapular rash, disorientation, hallucinations, and impairment of renal tubular function.
• Treatment is usually supportive and includes transfusion of blood components.

---

hydroxyzine hydrochloride
Anxanil, Apo-Hydroxyzine*, Atarax, Hydroxacen, Hyzine-50, Multipax*, Novo-Hydroxyzin*, Quiess, Vistacon-50, Vistazine-50

hydroxyzine pamoate
Vistaril

Antihistamine (piperazine derivative), anxiolytic, sedative, antipruritic, antiemetic, antispasmodic

---

Available by prescription only
hydroxyzine hydrochloride
Capsules: 10 mg, 25 mg, 50 mg
Tablets: 10 mg, 25 mg, 50 mg, 100 mg
Syrup: 10 mg/5 ml
Injection: 25 mg/ml, 50 mg/ml
hydroxyzine pamoate
Capsules: 25 mg, 50 mg, 100 mg
Oral suspension: 25 mg/5 ml

INDICATIONS & DOSAGE
Anxiety, tension, hyperkinesia
Adults: 50 to 100 mg P.O. q.i.d.
Preoperative and postoperative adjunctive sedation; to control vomiting; adjunct to asthma treatment
Adults: 25 to 100 mg I.M. q 4 to 6 hours.

PHARMACODYNAMICS
Anxiolytic and sedative actions: Hydroxyzine produces its sedative and anxiolytic effects through suppression of activity at subcortical levels; analgesia occurs at high doses.
Antipruritic action: Drug is a direct competitor of histamine for binding at cellular receptor sites.

Other actions: Hydroxyzine is used as a preoperative and postoperative adjunct for its sedative, antihistaminic, and anticholinergic activity.

PHARMACOKINETICS
Absorption: Hydroxyzine is absorbed rapidly and completely after oral administration. Serum levels peak within 2 to 4 hours. Sedation and other effects are usually noticed in 15 to 30 minutes.
Distribution: Unknown.
Metabolism: Drug is metabolized almost completely in the liver.
Excretion: Drug metabolites are excreted primarily in urine; small amounts of drug and metabolites are found in feces. Half-life of drug is 3 hours. Sedative effects can last for 4 to 6 hours, and antihistaminic effects can persist for up to 4 days.

CONTRAINDICATIONS & PRECAUTIONS
Contraindicated in patients hypersensitive to hydroxyzine. Use cautiously, with adjustments in dosage, in geriatric or debilitated patients.

INTERACTIONS
Drug-drug. Use with other *anticholinergics* causes additive anticholinergic effects. Hydroxyzine may add to or potentiate the effects of *barbiturates,* other *CNS depressants, opioids,* and *tranquilizers*; the dose of CNS depressants should be reduced by 50%. Hydroxyzine may block the vasopressor action of *epinephrine;* if a vasoconstrictor is needed, use norepinephrine or phenylephrine.
Drug-lifestyle. Hydroxyzine may add to or potentiate the effects of *alcohol;* don't use together.

ADVERSE REACTIONS
CNS: *drowsiness,* involuntary motor activity.
GI: *dry mouth.*
Other: marked discomfort at I.M. injection site, *hypersensitivity reactions* (wheezing, dyspnea, chest tightness).

▣ KEY CONSIDERATIONS
• Geriatric patients may experience greater CNS depression and anticholinergic effects. Lower doses are indicated.

• Observe patients for excessive sedation, especially those receiving other CNS depressants.

• Inject deep I.M. only; drug isn't for I.V., intra-arterial, or S.C. use. Aspirate injection carefully to prevent inadvertent intravascular administration.

• Drug therapy causes falsely elevated urine 17-hydroxycorticosteroid levels. It also may cause false-negative skin allergen tests by attenuating or inhibiting the cutaneous response to histamine.

Patient education

• Tell patient to avoid tasks that require mental alertness or physical coordination until CNS effects of drug are known; advise against use of other CNS depressants with hydroxyzine unless prescribed. Patient should avoid alcohol ingestion.

• Instruct patient to seek medical approval before taking OTC cold or allergy preparations that contain antihistamine, which may potentiate the effects of hydroxyzine.

• Advise patient to use sugarless gum or candy to help relieve dry mouth and to drink plenty of water to help with dry mouth or constipation.

Overdose & treatment

• Signs and symptoms of overdose include excessive sedation and hypotension; seizures may occur.

• Treatment is supportive. For recent oral ingestion, induce vomiting or perform gastric lavage. Correct hypotension with fluids and vasopressors (phenylephrine or metaraminol). Don't give epinephrine because hydroxyzine may counteract its effect.

---

hyoscyamine
Cystospaz

hyoscyamine sulfate
Anaspaz, Cystospaz-M, Levsin, Levsin Drops, Levsinex Timecaps, Neoquess

Belladonna alkaloid, anticholinergic

Available by prescription only
hyoscyamine
Tablets: 0.15 mg

hyoscyamine sulfate
Tablets: 0.125 mg
Capsules (extended-release): 0.375 mg
Oral solution: 0.125 mg/ml
Elixir: 0.125 mg/5 ml
Injection: 0.5 mg/ml

INDICATIONS & DOSAGE
GI tract disorders caused by spasm; adjunctive therapy for peptic ulcers
Adults: 0.125 to 0.25 mg P.O. or S.L. q.i.d. before meals and h.s.; 0.375 to 0.75 mg P.O. (extended-release form) q 12 hours; or 0.25 to 0.5 mg I.M., I.V., or S.C. q 4 hours b.i.d. to q.i.d. (Substitute oral drug when symptoms are controlled.)

PHARMACODYNAMICS
Antispasmodic and antiulcerative action: Hyoscyamine competitively blocks acetylcholine at cholinergic neuroeffector sites, decreasing GI motility and inhibiting gastric acid secretion.

PHARMACOKINETICS
Absorption: Hyoscyamine is well absorbed when taken orally; onset of action usually occurs in 20 to 30 minutes with tablets and 5 to 20 minutes with the elixir. Onset of action with parenteral administration usually occurs in 2 to 3 minutes.
Distribution: Drug is well distributed throughout the body and crosses the blood-brain barrier. About 50% of dose binds to plasma proteins.
Metabolism: Drug is metabolized in the liver. Usual duration of effect is up to 4 hours with standard oral and parenteral administration and up to 12 hours for the extended-release preparation.
Excretion: Drug and metabolites are excreted in the urine.

CONTRAINDICATIONS & PRECAUTIONS
Contraindicated in patients with glaucoma, obstructive uropathy, obstructive disease of the GI tract, severe ulcerative colitis, myasthenia gravis, hypersensitivity to anticholinergics, paralytic ileus, intestinal atony, unstable CV status in acute hemorrhage, or toxic megacolon.

Use cautiously in patients with autonomic neuropathy, hyperthyroidism,

---

coronary artery disease, arrhythmias, heart failure, hypertension, hiatal hernia with reflux esophagitis, hepatic or renal disease, and ulcerative colitis. Also use cautiously in hot or humid environments, where drug-induced heat stroke can occur.

INTERACTIONS
Drug-drug. Use with *amantadine* may increase such adverse anticholinergic effects as confusion and hallucinations. *Antacids* and *antidiarrheals* may decrease absorption of hyoscyamine; administer hyoscyamine 1 hour before these drugs. Use with *haloperidol* or *phenothiazines* may reduce the antipsychotic effectiveness of these drugs, possibly by direct CNS antagonism; *phenothiazines* may also increase adverse anticholinergic effects of hyoscyamine.

ADVERSE REACTIONS
CNS: headache, insomnia, drowsiness, dizziness, nervousness, weakness; *confusion, excitement.*
CV: *palpitations,* tachycardia.
EENT: *blurred vision,* mydriasis, increased intraocular pressure, cycloplegia, photophobia.
GI: *dry mouth, dysphagia, constipation,* heartburn, loss of taste, nausea, vomiting, *paralytic ileus.*
GU: *urinary hesitancy, urine retention,* impotence.
Skin: urticaria, decreased sweating or possible anhidrosis, other dermal signs and symptoms.
Other: fever, allergic reactions.

▣ KEY CONSIDERATIONS
Besides the recommendations relevant to all anticholinergics, consider the following:
• Use drug cautiously in geriatric patients; lower doses are indicated.
• Drug is usually administered P.O. but may be given I.V., I.M., S.C., or S.L. when therapeutic effect is needed or if oral administration is impossible.
• Titrate drug based on patient's response and tolerance.

Patient education
• Advise patient to avoid driving or performing other hazardous activities if he has drowsiness, dizziness, or blurred vision.
• Tell patient to drink fluids to avoid constipation.
• Instruct patient to report rash or other skin eruptions.

Overdose & treatment
• Signs and symptoms of overdose include curare-like symptoms, central stimulation followed by depression, and psychotic symptoms such as disorientation, confusion, hallucinations, delusions, anxiety, agitation, and restlessness. Peripheral effects may include dilated, nonreactive pupils; blurred vision; flushed, hot, dry skin; dryness of mucous membranes; dysphagia; decreased or absent bowel sounds; urine retention; hyperthermia; headache; tachycardia; hypertension; and increased respiration.
• Treatment is primarily symptomatic and supportive, as needed. Maintain patent airway. If patient is alert, induce vomiting (or perform gastric lavage) and follow with a saline cathartic and activated charcoal to prevent further drug absorption. In severe cases, physostigmine may be administered to block antimuscarinic effects. Give fluids as needed to treat shock; diazepam to control psychotic symptoms; and pilocarpine (instilled into the eyes) to relieve mydriasis. If urine retention occurs, catheterization may be necessary.

ibuprofen

Advil, Medipren, Motrin, Motrin IB, Nuprin, Rufen, Trendar

NSAID, nonnarcotic analgesic, antipyretic, anti-inflammatory

Available without a prescription
Tablets: 200 mg
Tablets (chewable): 50 mg, 100 mg
Oral suspension: 100 mg/5 ml
Available by prescription only
Tablets: 100 mg, 300 mg, 400 mg, 600 mg, 800 mg
Oral suspension: 100 mg/5 ml
Oral drops: 40 mg/ml

INDICATIONS & DOSAGE

Arthritis, gout, and postextraction dental pain
Adults: 300 to 800 mg P.O. t.i.d. or q.i.d. Don't exceed 3,200 mg as total daily dose.
Mild to moderate pain
Adults: 400 mg P.O. q 4 to 6 hours.
Fever reduction
Adults: 200 to 400 mg P.O. q 4 to 6 hours, p.r.n. Don't exceed 1,200 mg/day or take for more than 3 days.

PHARMACODYNAMICS

Analgesic, antipyretic, and anti-inflammatory actions: Mechanisms of action are unknown; ibuprofen may inhibit prostaglandin synthesis.

PHARMACOKINETICS

Absorption: About 80% of an oral dose is absorbed from the GI tract.
Distribution: Ibuprofen is highly protein-bound.
Metabolism: Drug undergoes biotransformation in the liver.
Excretion: Excreted mainly in urine, with some biliary excretion. Plasma half-life ranges from 2 to 4 hours.

CONTRAINDICATIONS & PRECAUTIONS

Contraindicated in patients with hypersensitivity to ibuprofen or in those who have the syndrome of nasal polyps, angioedema, and bronchospastic reaction to aspirin or other NSAIDs.

Use cautiously in patients with impaired renal or hepatic function, GI disorders, peptic ulcer disease, cardiac decompensation, hypertension, or known coagulation defects. Because chewable tablets contain aspartame, use cautiously in patients with phenylketonuria.

INTERACTIONS

Drug-drug. Ibuprofen may reduce the blood pressure response to *ACE inhibitors* and may result in an acute reduction in renal function. Increased nephrotoxicity may occur with *acetaminophen, diuretics, gold compounds,* or *other anti-inflammatories. Antacids* may decrease the absorption of ibuprofen. Use of ibuprofen with *anticoagulants* and *thrombolytics (coumarin derivatives, heparin, streptokinase,* and *urokinase)* may potentiate anticoagulant effects. Bleeding problems may occur if ibuprofen is used with other drugs that inhibit platelet aggregation, such as parenteral *aspirin, carbenicillin, cefamandole, cefoperazone, dextran, dipyridamole, mezlocillin, piperacillin, plicamycin, salicylates, sulfinpyrazone, ticarcillin, valproic acid,* or *other anti-inflammatories.* Also, use with *anti-inflammatories, corticotropin, corticosteroids,* and *salicylates* may increase adverse GI effects, including ulceration and hemorrhage, and use with *aspirin* may decrease the bioavailability of ibuprofen. Toxicity may occur with *coumarin derivatives, nifedipine, phenytoin,* or *verapamil.* Use with *furosemide* or *thiazides* may decrease their effectiveness. Ibuprofen may displace *highly protein-bound drugs* from binding sites. Because of the influence of prostaglandins on glucose metabolism, use with *insulin* or *oral antidiabetics* may potentiate hypoglycemic effects. Ibuprofen may decrease the renal clearance of *lithium* and *methotrexate.* Ibuprofen may decrease effectiveness of *antihypertensives* and *diuretics.*

Drug-lifestyle. *Alcohol* may increase the adverse GI effects, including ulceration and hemorrhage; use cautiously.

ADVERSE REACTIONS

CNS: *headache, dizziness,* nervousness, aseptic meningitis.
CV: *peripheral edema,* fluid retention, edema.
EENT: *tinnitus.*
GI: *epigastric distress, nausea, occult blood loss, peptic ulceration,* diarrhea, constipation, dyspepsia, flatulence, heartburn, decreased appetite.
GU: *acute renal failure,* azotemia, cystitis, hematuria.
Hematologic: prolonged bleeding time, anemia, *neutropenia, pancytopenia, thrombocytopenia, aplastic anemia, leukopenia, agranulocytosis.*
Hepatic: elevated liver enzyme levels.
Respiratory: *bronchospasm.*
Skin: pruritus, *rash,* urticaria, *Stevens-Johnson syndrome.*

◨ KEY CONSIDERATIONS

Besides the recommendations relevant to all NSAIDs, consider the following:
• Patients older than age 60 may be more susceptible to the toxic effects of ibuprofen, especially adverse GI reactions. Use lowest possible effective dose.
• The effect of drug on renal prostaglandins may cause fluid retention and edema, a significant drawback for geriatric patients, especially those with heart failure.
• Maximum results in arthritis may require 1 to 2 weeks of continuous therapy with ibuprofen. Improvement may be seen, however, within 7 days.
• Administer drug on an empty stomach, 1 hour before or 2 hours after meals, for maximum absorption. However, it may be administered with meals to lessen GI upset.
• Monitor cardiopulmonary status closely; monitor vital signs, especially heart rate and blood pressure. Observe for possible fluid retention.
• Establish safety measures, including raised side rails and supervised walking, to prevent possible injury from CNS effects.

• Monitor auditory and ophthalmic functions periodically during ibuprofen therapy.
• Ibuprofen's physiological effects may prolong bleeding time; decrease blood glucose levels; increase BUN, serum creatinine, and serum potassium levels; decrease serum uric acid, hemoglobin, and hematocrit levels; prolong PT and INR; and increase serum alkaline phosphatase, serum LD, and serum transaminase levels.

Patient education
• Instruct patient to seek medical approval before taking OTC drugs.
• Advise patient not to self-medicate with ibuprofen for longer than 10 days for analgesic use and not to exceed maximum dosage of 6 tablets (1.2 g) daily for self-medication. Caution patient not to take drug if fever lasts longer than 3 days, unless prescribed.
• Tell patient to report adverse reactions. They are usually dose-related.
• Instruct patient in safety measures to prevent injury. Caution him to avoid hazardous activities that require mental alertness until CNS effects are known.
• Encourage patient to adhere to prescribed drug regimen and stress the importance of medical follow-up.

Overdose & treatment
• Signs and symptoms of overdose include dizziness, drowsiness, paresthesia, vomiting, nausea, abdominal pain, headache, sweating, nystagmus, apnea, and cyanosis.
• To treat drug overdose, immediately induce vomiting with ipecac syrup or perform gastric lavage. Administer activated charcoal via NG tube. Provide symptomatic and supportive measures (respiratory support and correction of fluid and electrolyte imbalances). Monitor laboratory parameters and vital signs closely. Alkaline diuresis may enhance renal excretion. Dialysis is of minimal value because ibuprofen is strongly protein-bound.

imipenem-cilastatin sodium
Primaxin I.M., Primaxin I.V.

Carbapenem (thienamycin class), beta-lactam antibiotic

Available by prescription only
Powder (for I.M. injection): 500-mg and 750-mg vials
Injection: 250-mg and 500-mg vials, ADD-Vantage, and infusion bottles

INDICATIONS & DOSAGE
Mild to moderate lower respiratory tract, skin and skin-structure, or gynecologic infections
Adults weighing at least 70 kg (154 lb): 500 to 750 mg I.M. q 12 hours.
Mild to moderate intra-abdominal infections
Adults weighing at least 70 kg (154 lb): 750 mg I.M. q 12 hours.
Serious respiratory and urinary tract infections; intra-abdominal, gynecologic, bone, joint, or skin infections; bacterial septicemia; endocarditis
Adults weighing at least 70 kg (154 lb): 250 mg to 1 g by I.V. infusion q 6 to 8 hours. Maximum daily dosage is 50 mg/kg/day or 4 g/day, whichever is less.
✦ *Dosage adjustment.* In patients with renal failure and creatinine clearance of 6 to 20 ml/minute/1.73 m^2, 125 to 250 mg I.V. q 12 hours for most pathogens. There may be an increased risk of seizures when doses of 500 mg q 12 hours are administered to these patients. When creatinine clearance is 5 ml/minute/1.73 m^2 or less, drug shouldn't be given unless hemodialysis is instituted within 48 hours.
Note: In patients weighing less than 70 kg or those with impaired renal function, dosages vary. Check current literature for recommended protocol.

PHARMACODYNAMICS
Antibacterial action: A bactericidal drug, imipenem inhibits bacterial cell-wall synthesis. Its spectrum of antimicrobial activity includes many gram-positive, gram-negative, and anaerobic bacteria, including *Staphylococcus* and *Streptococcus* species, *Escherichia coli, Klebsiella, Proteus, Enterobacter* species, *Pseudomonas aeruginosa,* and *Bacteroides* species, including *B. fragilis.* Resistant bacteria include methicillin-resistant *Staphylococci, Clostridium difficile,* and other *Pseudomonas* species.

Cilastatin inhibits imipenem's enzymatic breakdown in the kidneys, making it effective in treating urinary tract infections.

PHARMACOKINETICS
Absorption: After I.M. administration, imipenem blood levels peak within 2 hours; cilastatin levels reach their peak within 1 hour. After I.V. administration, peak levels of both agents appear in about 20 minutes. Imipenem is about 75% bioavailable and cilastatin is about 95% bioavailable after I.M. administration compared with I.V. administration.
Distribution: Imipenem-cilastatin is distributed rapidly and widely. About 20% of imipenem is protein-bound; 40% of cilastatin is protein-bound.
Metabolism: Imipenem is metabolized by kidney dehydropeptidase I, resulting in low urine levels. Cilastatin inhibits this enzyme, thereby reducing imipenem's metabolism.
Excretion: About 70% of an imipenem-cilastatin dose is excreted unchanged by the kidneys (when imipenem is combined with cilastatin) by tubular secretion and glomerular filtration. Imipenem is cleared by hemodialysis; therefore, a supplemental dose is required after this procedure. Half-life of drug is about 1 hour after I.V. administration. The prolonged absorption that occurs after I.M. administration results in a longer half-life (2 to 3 hours).

CONTRAINDICATIONS & PRECAUTIONS
Contraindicated in patients with hypersensitivity to drug. Imipenem and cilastatin sodium reconstituted with lidocaine hydrochloride for I.M. injection is contraindicated in patients with known hypersensitivity to local anesthetics of the amide type and in patients with severe shock or heart block.

Reactions may be *common,* uncommon, ***life-threatening,*** or **COMMON AND LIFE-THREATENING.**

Use cautiously in patients with impaired renal function, seizure disorders, or allergy to penicillins or cephalosporins.

INTERACTIONS
Drug-drug. *Chloramphenicol* may impede the bactericidal effects of imipenem; give chloramphenicol a few hours after imipenem-cilastatin. Generalized seizures have occurred in several patients during combined imipenem-cilastatin and *ganciclovir* therapy. *Probenecid* may prevent tubular secretion of cilastatin (but not imipenem) and thereby prolong plasma cilastatin half-life.

ADVERSE REACTIONS
CNS: *seizures,* dizziness, somnolence.
CV: hypotension.
GI: nausea, vomiting, diarrhea, *pseudomembranous colitis.*
Hematologic: *agranulocytosis,* thrombocytosis.
Skin: rash, urticaria, pruritus.
Other: *hypersensitivity reactions (anaphylaxis), thrombophlebitis, pain at injection site,* fever.

▣ KEY CONSIDERATIONS
• Administer cautiously to geriatric patients because they may also have renal dysfunction.
• Perform culture and sensitivity tests before starting therapy.
• When reconstituting powder, shake until solution is clear. Solution may range from colorless to yellow; color variations within this range don't affect drug potency. After reconstitution, solution remains stable for 10 hours at room temperature and for 48 hours when refrigerated.
• Don't administer drug by direct I.V. bolus injection. Infuse 250- or 500-mg dose over 20 to 30 minutes; infuse 1-g dose over 40 to 60 minutes. If nausea occurs, slow infusion.
• Continue use of anticonvulsants in patients with known seizure disorders. Patients who exhibit CNS toxicity should receive phenytoin or benzodiazepines. Reduce dosage or discontinue drug if CNS toxicity continues.
• This drug has broadest antibacterial spectrum of any available antibiotic. It's most valuable for empiric treatment of unidentified infections and for mixed infections that would otherwise require combination of antibiotics, possibly including an aminoglycoside.
• Prolonged use may result in overgrowth of nonsusceptible organisms. In addition, use of imipenem-cilastatin as a sole course of therapy has resulted in resistance.
• Avoid mixing with aminoglycosides; drug may be physically incompatible.
• Serum levels of AST, ALT, alkaline phosphatase, LD, and bilirubin may be elevated; erythrocyte, platelet, and leukocyte counts may be reduced during drug therapy.

Patient education
• Instruct patient to report adverse reaction promptly.
• Inform patient to notify health care provider if loose stools or diarrhea occur.

Overdose & treatment
• If overdose occurs, discontinue drug, treat symptomatically, and institute supportive measures as required. Drug is hemodialyzable, but use of hemodialysis in treating overdose is questionable.

---

imipramine hydrochloride
Apo-Imipramine*, Impril*, Novopramine*, Tofranil

imipramine pamoate
Tofranil-PM

Dibenzazepine tricyclic antidepressant

Available by prescription only
imipramine hydrochloride
Tablets: 10 mg, 25 mg, 50 mg
Injection: 25 mg/2 ml
imipramine pamoate
Capsules: 75 mg, 100 mg, 125 mg, 150 mg

INDICATIONS & DOSAGE
Depression
Adults: Initially, 75 to 100 mg P.O. or I.M. daily in divided doses, increased in

25- to 50-mg increments, up to 200 mg/day. Alternatively, some patients can start with lower doses (25 mg P.O.) and titrate slowly in 25-mg increments every other day. Maximum dosage is 300 mg daily. Alternatively, entire dosage may be given h.s. I.M. route is rarely used. Maximum dosage is 200 mg/day for outpatients, 300 mg/day for inpatients.

Geriatric patients: Recommended dosage is 25 to 50 mg P.O. daily, not to exceed 100 mg daily. Initiate therapy at low doses (10 mg) and titrate slowly.

PHARMACODYNAMICS

Antidepressant action: Imipramine is thought to exert its antidepressant effects by inhibiting reuptake of norepinephrine and serotonin in CNS nerve terminals (presynaptic neurons), which results in increased levels and enhanced activity of these neurotransmitters in the synaptic cleft.

PHARMACOKINETICS

Absorption: Imipramine is absorbed rapidly from the GI tract and muscle tissue after oral and I.M. administration. *Distribution:* Drug is distributed widely into the body, including the CNS. Drug is 90% protein-bound. Effect peaks in ½ to 2 hours; steady state is achieved within 2 to 5 days. Therapeutic plasma levels (parent drug and metabolite) are thought to range from 150 to 300 ng/ml. *Metabolism:* Metabolized by the liver to the active metabolite desipramine. A significant first-pass effect may explain variability of serum levels in different patients taking the same dosage. *Excretion:* Drug is mostly excreted in urine.

CONTRAINDICATIONS & PRECAUTIONS

Contraindicated during acute recovery phase of MI, in patients with hypersensitivity to imipramine, and in those receiving MAO inhibitors.

Use cautiously in patients at risk for suicide; in those with impaired renal or hepatic function, history of urine retention, angle-closure glaucoma, increased intraocular pressure, CV disease, hyperthyroidism, seizure disorders, or allergy

to sulfites (injectable form only); and in patients receiving thyroid drugs.

INTERACTIONS

Drug-drug. Use with *antiarrhythmics* (*disopyramide, procainamide, quinidine*), *pimozide,* or *thyroid drugs* may increase risk of arrhythmias and conduction defects. Imipramine may decrease the hypotensive effects of centrally acting *antihypertensives,* such as *clonidine, guanabenz, guanadrel, guanethidine, methyldopa,* and *reserpine. Barbiturates* induce imipramine metabolism and decrease therapeutic efficacy. *Beta blockers, cimetidine, methylphenidate,* and *propoxyphene* may inhibit imipramine metabolism, increasing plasma levels and toxicity. Use with *disulfiram* or *etchlorvynol* may cause delirium and tachycardia. *Haloperidol* and *phenothiazines* decrease imipramine metabolism, decreasing therapeutic efficacy. Use of imipramine with *sympathomimetics*—including *ephedrine* (found in many nasal sprays), *epinephrine, phenylephrine,* and *phenylpropanolamine*—may increase blood pressure. Use with *warfarin* may prolong PT and cause bleeding.

Additive effects are likely after use of imipramine with *analgesics, anesthetics, barbiturates, CNS depressants, narcotics,* and *tranquilizers* (oversedation); *atropine* or *other anticholinergics,* including *antihistamines, antiparkinsonians, meperidine,* and *phenothiazines* (oversedation, paralytic ileus, visual changes, and severe constipation); or *metrizamide* (increased risk of seizures). **Drug-lifestyle.** Additive effects are likely after use of imipramine with *CNS depressants,* including *alcohol. Heavy smoking* induces imipramine metabolism and decreases therapeutic efficacy. Don't use together.

ADVERSE REACTIONS

CNS: *drowsiness, dizziness,* excitation, tremor, confusion, hallucinations, anxiety, ataxia, paresthesia, nervousness, EEG changes, **seizures,** extrapyramidal reactions.
CV: *orthostatic hypotension, tachycardia, ECG changes,* hypertension, **MI,**

Reactions may be *common,* uncommon, **life-threatening,** or COMMON AND LIFE-THREATENING.

stroke, arrhythmias, heart block, precipitation of heart failure.
EENT: blurred vision, tinnitus, mydriasis.
Endocrine: gynecomastia (in males), galactorrhea and breast enlargement (in females), altered libido, impotence, testicular swelling, increased or decreased blood glucose levels, inappropriate ADH secretion syndrome.
GI: *dry mouth, constipation,* nausea, vomiting, anorexia, paralytic ileus, abdominal cramps.
GU: *urine retention.*
Skin: rash, urticaria, photosensitivity, pruritus.
Other: *diaphoresis,* **hypersensitivity reaction.**
After abrupt withdrawal of long-term therapy: nausea, headache, malaise (doesn't indicate addiction).

▣ KEY CONSIDERATIONS
Besides the recommendations relevant to all tricyclic antidepressants, consider the following:
• Geriatric patients may be at greater risk for adverse cardiac reactions.
• Check sitting and standing blood pressures after initial dose; imipramine is associated with a high incidence of orthostatic hypotension.
• Don't withdraw drug abruptly, taper gradually over time.
• Tolerance to drug's sedative effects usually develops over several weeks.
• Discontinue drug at least 48 hours before surgical procedures.
• Imipramine may prolong conduction time (elongation of QT and PR intervals, flattened T waves on ECG); it also may elevate liver function test results, decrease WBC counts, and decrease or increase serum glucose levels.

Patient education
• Tell patient to take imipramine exactly as prescribed.
• Explain that full effects of drug may not become apparent for up to 4 to 6 weeks after initiation of therapy.
• Warn patient not to discontinue drug abruptly, not to share drug with others, and not to drink alcoholic beverages while taking drug.

• Advise patient to take drug with food or milk if it causes stomach upset.
• Advise patient that smoking may reduce the effectiveness of the drug.
• Suggest relieving dry mouth with sugarless chewing gum or hard candy. Encourage good dental prophylaxis because persistent dry mouth may lead to increased incidence of dental caries.
• Encourage patient to report unusual or troublesome side effects immediately, including confusion, movement disorders, rapid heartbeat, dizziness, fainting, or difficulty urinating.

Overdose & treatment
• Drug overdose is frequently life-threatening, particularly when drug is combined with alcohol. The first 12 hours after acute ingestion are a stimulatory phase characterized by excessive anticholinergic activity (agitation, irritation, confusion, hallucinations, hyperthermia, parkinsonian symptoms, seizure, urine retention, dry mucous membranes, pupillary dilatation, constipation, and ileus). This phase is followed by CNS depressant effects, including hypothermia, decreased or absent reflexes, sedation, hypotension, cyanosis, and cardiac irregularities, including tachycardia, conduction disturbances, and quinidine-like effects on the ECG.
• Severity of overdose is best indicated by widening of the QRS complex, which usually represents a serum level in excess of 1,000 ng/ml; serum levels usually aren't helpful. Metabolic acidosis may follow hypotension, hypoventilation, and seizures.
• Treatment is symptomatic and supportive; maintain airway, stable body temperature, and fluid or electrolyte balance. Induce vomiting if patient is conscious; follow with gastric lavage and activated charcoal to prevent further absorption. Dialysis is of little use.
• Treat seizures with parenteral diazepam or phenytoin and arrhythmias with parenteral phenytoin or lidocaine. Don't use quinidine, procainamide, or atropine during an overdose. Treat acidosis with sodium bicarbonate. Don't give barbiturates; these may enhance CNS and respiratory depressant effects.

immune globulin (gamma globulin, IG, immune serum globulin, ISG)
immune globulin for I.M. use (IGIM)
Gamastan, Gammar

immune globulin for I.V. use (IGIV)
Gamimune N (5%, 10%), Gammagard S/D, Gammar- P IV, Iveegam, Polygam S/D, Sandoglobulin, Venoglobulin-I, Venoglobulin-S

Immune serum, antibody production stimulator

Available by prescription only
IGIM
Injection: 2-ml and 10-ml vials
IGIV
I.V.: Gamimune N—5% and 10% solution in 10-ml, 50-ml, 100-ml, and 250-ml single-use vials; Gammagard S/D—2.5-g, 5-g, and 10-g single-use vials for reconstitution; Gammar-P IV—1-g, 2.5-g, and 5-g vials with diluent and 10-g vials with administration set and diluent; Iveegam—1-g, 2.5-g, and 5-g vials with diluent; Polygam S/D—2.5-g, 5-g, and 10-g single-use vials with diluent; Sandoglobulin—1-g, 3-g, 6-g, and 12-g vials or kits with diluent or bulk packs without diluent; Venoglobulin-I—2.5-g and 5-g vials with or without reconstitution kits with sterile water, 10-g vials with reconstitution kit and administration set, and 0.5-g vials with reconstitution kit; Venoglobulin-S—5% and 10% in 50-ml, 100-ml, and 200-ml vials.

INDICATIONS & DOSAGE
Agammaglobulinemia, hypogamma-globulinemia, immune deficiency (IGIV)
Adults: For Gamimune N only, 100 to 200 mg/kg or 2 to 4 ml/kg I.V. infusion monthly. Infusion rate is 0.01 to 0.02 ml/kg/minute for 30 minutes. Rate can then be increased to maximum of 0.08 ml/kg/minute for remainder of infusion.

For Gammagard S/D only, initially 200 to 400 mg/kg I.V., followed by 100 mg/kg monthly. Initiate infusion at 0.5 ml/kg/hour, gradually increasing to maximum of 4 ml/kg/hour.

For Gammar-P IV only, 200 to 400 mg/kg q 3 to 4 weeks. Infusion rate is 0.01 ml/kg/minute, increasing to 0.02 ml/kg/minute after 15 to 30 minutes, with gradual increase to 0.06 ml/kg/minute.

For Iveegam only, 200 mg/kg I.V. monthly. If response is inadequate, doses may be increased up to 800 mg/kg or the drug may be administered more frequently. Infuse at 1 to 2 ml/minute.

For Polygam S/D only, 100 mg/kg I.V. monthly. An initial dose of 200 to 400 mg/kg may be administered. Initiate infusion at 0.5 ml/kg/hour, gradually increasing to maximum of 4 ml/kg/hour.

For Sandoglobulin only, 200 mg/kg I.V. monthly. Start with 0.5 to 1 ml/minute of a 3% solution; increase up to 2.5 ml/minute gradually after 15 to 30 minutes.

For Venoglobulin-I only, 200 mg/kg I.V. monthly; may be increased to 300 to 400 mg/kg and may be repeated more frequently than once monthly. Infuse at 0.01 to 0.02 ml/kg/minute for 30 minutes, then increase to 0.04 ml/kg/minute or higher if tolerated.

For Venoglobulin-S only, 200 mg/kg I.V. monthly. Increase dose to 300 to 400 mg/kg monthly or administer more frequently if adequate IgG levels aren't achieved. Initiate infusion at 0.01 to 0.02 ml/kg/minute for 30 minutes, then increase 5% solutions to 0.04 ml/kg/minute and 10% solutions to 0.05 ml/kg/minute if tolerated.

Hepatitis A exposure (IGIM)
Adults: 0.02 to 0.04 ml/kg I.M. as soon as possible after exposure. Up to 0.1 ml/kg may be given after prolonged or intense exposure.

Measles exposure (IGIM)
Adults: 0.25 ml/kg within 6 days after exposure.

Postexposure prophylaxis of measles (IGIM)
Adults: 0.5 ml/kg I.M. within 6 days after exposure.

Reactions may be *common*, uncommon, **life-threatening**, or COMMON AND LIFE-THREATENING.

Chickenpox exposure (IGIM)
Adults: 0.6 to 1.2 ml/kg I.M. as soon as exposed.

Idiopathic thrombocytopenic purpura (IGIV)
Adults: 400 mg/kg Sandoglobulin I.V. for 2 to 5 consecutive days; or 400 mg/kg Gamimune N 5% for 5 days or 1,000 mg/kg Gamimune N 10% for 1 to 2 days. Maintenance dose is 400 to 1,000 mg/kg I.V. of Gamimune N 10% as a single infusion to maintain a platelet count greater than 30,000/mm^3.

Bone marrow transplantation (IGIV)
Adults: Gamimune N 10%, 500 mg/kg on day 7 and day 2 before transplantation; then weekly through 90 days after transplant.

PHARMACODYNAMICS
Immune action: Immune globulin provides passive immunity by increasing antibody titer. The mechanism by which IGIV increases platelet counts in idiopathic thrombocytopenic purpura isn't fully known.

PHARMACOKINETICS
Absorption: After slow I.M. absorption, serum levels peak within 2 days.
Distribution: Drug is distributed evenly between intravascular and extravascular spaces.
Metabolism: Unknown.
Excretion: Serum half-life is reportedly 21 to 24 days in immunocompetent patients.

CONTRAINDICATIONS & PRECAUTIONS
Contraindicated in patients hypersensitive to immune globulin.

INTERACTIONS
Drug-drug. Use of immune globulin may interfere with the immune response to *live virus vaccines* (for example, *measles, mumps, rubella*); don't administer live virus vaccines within 3 months after administration of immune globulin.

ADVERSE REACTIONS
CNS: malaise, headache, faintness.
CV: chest pain.
GI: nausea, vomiting.

Musculoskeletal: joint pain, muscle stiffness (at injection site), hip pain.
Respiratory: dyspnea, shortness of breath.
Skin: erythema, urticaria.
Other: fever, *anaphylaxis,* chills, chest tightness.

▣ KEY CONSIDERATIONS
• Obtain a thorough history of allergies and reactions to immunizations.
• Have epinephrine solution 1:1,000 available to treat allergic reactions.
• Inject I.M. formulation into different sites, preferably into buttocks. Don't inject more than 3 ml per injection site.
• Don't give for hepatitis A exposure if 2 weeks or more have elapsed since exposure, or after onset of clinical illness.
• Closely monitor blood pressure in patients receiving IGIV, especially if it's the patient's first infusion of immune globulin.
• Immune globulin hasn't been associated with an increased frequency of AIDS. It's devoid of HIV. Immune globulin recipients don't develop antibodies to HIV.
• Store Sandoglobulin and Gammagard S/D at room temperature not exceeding 77° F (25° C); Gamimune-N and Iveegam at 36° to 46° F (2° to 8° C) but don't freeze; Gammar-P IV at room temperature below 86° F (30° C) but don't freeze; Venoglobulin-I at room temperature below 86° F.
• Immune globulin has been studied in the treatment of various conditions, including Kawasaki disease, asthma, allergic disorders, autoimmune neutropenia, myasthenia gravis, and platelet transfusion rejection. It also has been used in the prophylaxis of infections in immunocompromised patients.
• Gamimune N can be diluted with D_5W.
• Reconstitute Gammagard S/D with diluent (sterile water for injection) and transfer device provided by manufacturer. Administration set (provided) contains a 15-micron in-line filter that must be used during administration.
• Reconstitute Sandoglobulin with diluent supplied (normal saline).

Patient education
• Explain that patient's chances of getting AIDS or hepatitis after receiving immune globulin are minute.
• Tell patient what to expect after vaccination: some local pain, swelling, and tenderness at the injection site. Recommend acetaminophen to ease minor discomfort.
• Instruct patient to promptly report headache, skin changes, or difficulty breathing.

indapamide
Lozol

Thiazide-like diuretic, antihypertensive

Available by prescription only
Tablets: 1.25 mg, 2.5 mg

INDICATIONS & DOSAGE
Edema of heart failure
Adults: 2.5 mg P.O. as a single daily dose taken in the morning; increase dosage to 5 mg daily after 1 week if response is poor.
Hypertension
Adults: 1.25 mg P.O. as a single daily dose taken in the morning; increase dosage to 2.5 mg daily after 4 weeks if response is poor. Maximum daily dose is 5 mg.

PHARMACODYNAMICS
Diuretic action: Indapamide increases urine excretion of sodium and water by inhibiting sodium reabsorption in the cortical diluting tubule of the nephron, thus relieving edema.
Antihypertensive action: Exact mechanism of the antihypertensive effect is unknown. This effect may result from direct arteriolar vasodilatation via calcium channel blockade. Indapamide also reduces total body sodium.

PHARMACOKINETICS
Absorption: After oral administration, indapamide is absorbed completely from the GI tract; peak serum levels occur at 2 to 2½ hours.
Distribution: Distributes widely into body tissues because of its lipophilicity; drug is 71% to 79% plasma protein-bound.
Metabolism: Drug undergoes significant hepatic metabolism.
Excretion: About 60% of a dose is excreted in urine within 48 hours; 16% to 23% is excreted in feces.

CONTRAINDICATIONS & PRECAUTIONS
Contraindicated in patients with anuria or hypersensitivity to other sulfonamide-derived drugs. Use cautiously in patients with severely impaired renal or hepatic function or progressive hepatic disease.

INTERACTIONS
Drug-drug. Indapamide turns urine slightly more alkaline and may decrease urine excretion of some *amines,* such as *amphetamine* and *quinidine;* alkaline urine may also decrease therapeutic efficacy of *methenamine compounds* such as *methenamine mandelate.* Indapamide potentiates the hypotensive effects of most other *antihypertensives;* this may be used to therapeutic advantage. *Cholestyramine* and *colestipol* may bind indapamide, preventing its absorption; give drugs 1 hour apart. Indapamide may potentiate hyperglycemic, hypotensive, and hyperuricemic effects of *diazoxide,* and its hyperglycemic effect may increase *insulin* or *sulfonylurea* requirements in diabetic patients. Indapamide may reduce renal clearance of *lithium,* elevating serum lithium levels, and may necessitate a reduction in lithium dosage by 50%.

ADVERSE REACTIONS
CNS: headache, nervousness, dizziness, light-headedness, weakness, vertigo, restlessness, drowsiness, fatigue, anxiety, depression, numbness of extremities, irritability, agitation.
CV: volume depletion and dehydration, orthostatic hypotension, palpitations, PVCs, irregular heartbeat, vasculitis.
EENT: rhinorrhea.
GI: anorexia, nausea, epigastric distress, vomiting, abdominal pain, diarrhea, constipation.

Reactions may be *common,* uncommon, *life-threatening*, or COMMON AND LIFE-THREATENING.

GU: nocturia, polyuria, urinary frequency, impotence.

Metabolic: asymptomatic hyperuricemia; fluid and electrolyte imbalances, including dilutional hyponatremia and hypochloremia, metabolic alkalosis, hypokalemia, weight loss.

Musculoskeletal: muscle cramps and spasms.

Skin: rash, pruritus, flushing.

Other: gout.

▣ KEY CONSIDERATIONS

Besides the recommendations relevant for all thiazide and thiazide-like diuretics, consider the following:

• Geriatric and debilitated patients require close observation and may require reduced dosages. They are more sensitive to excess diuresis because of age-related changes in CV and renal function. Excess diuresis promotes orthostatic hypotension, dehydration, hypovolemia, hyponatremia, hypomagnesemia, and hypokalemia.

• Indapamide therapy may alter serum electrolyte levels and may increase serum urate, glucose, cholesterol, and triglyceride levels. It also may interfere with tests for parathyroid function and should be discontinued before such tests.

Overdose & treatment

• Signs and symptoms of overdose include GI irritation and hypermotility, diuresis, and lethargy, which may progress to coma.

• Treatment is mainly supportive; monitor and assist respiratory, CV, and renal function as indicated. Monitor fluid and electrolyte balance. Induce vomiting with ipecac in conscious patient; otherwise, use gastric lavage to avoid aspiration. Don't give cathartics; these promote additional loss of fluids and electrolytes.

indinavir sulfate
Crixivan

HIV protease inhibitor, antiviral

Available by prescription only
Capsules: 200 mg, 400 mg

INDICATIONS & DOSAGE
Treatment of patients with HIV infection when antiretroviral therapy is warranted
Adults: 800 mg P.O. q 8 hours.
✦ *Dosage adjustment.* Reduce dosage to 600 mg P.O. q 8 hours in patients with mild to moderate hepatic insufficiency due to cirrhosis.

PHARMACODYNAMICS
Antiviral action: Indinavir sulfate inhibits HIV protease, an enzyme required for the proteolytic cleavage of the viral polyprotein precursors into the individual functional proteins found in infectious HIV. Indinavir binds to the protease active site and inhibits the activity of the enzyme. This inhibition prevents cleavage of the viral polyproteins, resulting in the formation of immature, noninfectious viral particles.

PHARMACOKINETICS
Absorption: Indinavir is rapidly absorbed in the GI tract when it's administered on an empty stomach. A meal high in calories, fat, and protein significantly interferes with drug absorption, whereas lighter meals don't.
Distribution: About 60% of drug is plasma protein-bound.
Metabolism: Indinavir is metabolized to at least seven metabolites. Cytochrome P-450 3A4 (CYP3A4) is the major enzyme responsible for formation of the oxidative metabolites.
Excretion: Less than 20% of drug is excreted unchanged in urine.

CONTRAINDICATIONS & PRECAUTIONS
Contraindicated in patients with hypersensitivity to any component of indinavir. Use cautiously in patients with hepatic insufficiency due to cirrhosis.

INTERACTIONS
Drug-drug. Indinavir shouldn't be administered with *cisapride, midazolam,* or *triazolam* because competition for CYP3A4 by indinavir could inhibit the metabolism of these drugs and create the potential for serious or life-threatening events, such as arrhythmias or prolonged sedation. If indinavir and *didanosine* are

administered concomitantly, they should be given at least 1 hour apart on an empty stomach; a normal (acidic) gastric pH may be necessary for optimum absorption of indinavir, whereas acid rapidly degrades didanosine, which is formulated with buffering agents to increase pH. *Ketoconazole* increases plasma indinavir levels; a dosage reduction of indinavir should be considered when they are coadministered. Indinavir increases the plasma *rifabutin* levels; a dosage reduction of rifabutin is necessary if administered concomitantly. Because *rifampin* induces CYP3A4, which could markedly diminish plasma indinavir levels, coadministration of indinavir and rifampin isn't recommended.

Drug-food. *Foods high in calories, fat, and protein* reduce the absorption of indinavir, so don't give with these foods; administer on an empty stomach if tolerated.

ADVERSE REACTIONS
CNS: headache, insomnia, dizziness, somnolence, asthenia, fatigue, malaise.
EENT: taste perversion.
GI: abdominal pain, *nausea,* diarrhea, vomiting, acid regurgitation, anorexia, dry mouth.
GU: nephrolithiasis.
Hematologic: decreased hemoglobin level, decreased platelet or neutrophil count.
Hepatic: *hyperbilirubinemia;* elevated ALT, AST, and serum amylase levels.
Musculoskeletal: flank pain, back pain.

▣ KEY CONSIDERATIONS
• Dosage of indinavir is the same whether drug is used alone or in combination with other antiretrovirals. However, antiretroviral activity of indinavir may be increased when used in combination with approved reverse transcriptase inhibitors.
• Drug must be taken at 8-hour intervals.
• When administering rifabutin concomitantly, the dose of rifabutin should be reduced by half. However, when administering ketoconazole concomitantly, the dosage of indinavir should be decreased to 600 mg q 8 hours.

• Drug may cause nephrolithiasis. If signs and symptoms of nephrolithiasis occur, consider stopping drug for 1 to 3 days during the acute phase. To prevent nephrolithiasis, patient should maintain adequate hydration.

Patient education
• Inform patient that indinavir isn't a cure for HIV infection. He may continue to develop opportunistic infections and other complications associated with HIV disease. Drug also hasn't been shown to reduce risk of transmitting HIV to others through sexual contact or blood contamination.
• Caution patient not to adjust dosage or discontinue indinavir therapy without medical approval.
• Advise patient that if he misses a dose of indinavir, he should take the next dose at the regularly scheduled time and shouldn't double-dose.
• Instruct patient to take drug on an empty stomach with water 1 hour before or 2 hours after a meal. Alternatively, he may take it with other liquids (such as skim milk, juice, coffee, or tea) or with a light meal. Inform patient that a meal high in calories, fat, and protein reduces the absorption of indinavir.
• Tell patient to store capsules in the original container and to keep the desiccant in the bottle because the capsules are sensitive to moisture.
• Instruct patient to drink at least 1½ qt (1.5 L) of fluid daily.

indomethacin
Apo-Indomethacin*, Indameth, Indochron E-R, Indocid*, Indocin, Indocin SR, Novomethacin*

indomethacin sodium trihydrate
Indocin I.V.

NSAID, nonnarcotic analgesic, antipyretic, anti-inflammatory

Available by prescription only
Capsules: 25 mg, 50 mg
Capsules (sustained-release): 75 mg
Suspension: 25 mg/5 ml

Reactions may be *common,* uncommon, *life-threatening,* or COMMON AND LIFE-THREATENING.

Injection: 1-mg vials
Suppositories: 50 mg

INDICATIONS & DOSAGE
Moderate to severe arthritis, ankylosing spondylitis
Adults: 25 mg P.O. b.i.d. or t.i.d. with food or antacids; may increase dose by 25 to 50 mg daily q 7 days up to 200 mg daily; or 50 mg P.R. q.i.d. Alternatively, sustained-release capsules may be given at 75 mg to start, in the morning or h.s., followed, if necessary, by 75 mg b.i.d.
Acute gouty arthritis
Adults: 50 mg t.i.d. Reduce dose as soon as possible, then stop it. Don't use sustained-release capsules for this condition.
Acute shoulder pain
Adults: 75 to 150 mg P.O. b.i.d. or t.i.d. with food or antacids; usual treatment is 7 to 14 days.
◇ Bartter's syndrome
Adults: 150 mg/day P.O. with food or antacids.

PHARMACODYNAMICS
Analgesic, antipyretic, and anti-inflammatory actions: Exact mechanisms of action are unknown; indomethacin is thought to produce its analgesic, antipyretic, and anti-inflammatory effects by inhibiting prostaglandin synthesis and possibly by inhibiting phosphodiesterase.

PHARMACOKINETICS
Absorption: Indomethacin is absorbed rapidly and completely from the GI tract.
Distribution: Drug is highly protein-bound.
Metabolism: Drug is metabolized in the liver.
Excretion: Drug is excreted mainly in urine, with some biliary excretion.

CONTRAINDICATIONS & PRECAUTIONS
Contraindicated in patients with hypersensitivity to indomethacin or a history of aspirin- or NSAID-induced asthma, rhinitis, or urticaria. Suppositories are contraindicated in patients with a history of proctitis or recent rectal bleeding.
   Use cautiously in geriatric patients and in those with a history of GI disease, impaired renal or hepatic function, epilepsy, parkinsonism, CV disease, infection, mental illness, or depression.

INTERACTIONS
Drug-drug. Use with *acetaminophen, gold compounds,* or *other anti-inflammatories* may increase nephrotoxicity. Use with *anticoagulants* or *thrombolytics* (such as *coumarin derivatives, heparin, streptokinase, urokinase*) may potentiate anticoagulant effects. Use with *anti-inflammatories, corticotropin, salicylates,* or *steroids* may cause increased adverse GI effects, including ulceration and hemorrhage. Use with *antihypertensives* or *diuretics* may decrease their effectiveness. *Aspirin* may decrease the bioavailability of indomethacin. Toxicity may occur with *coumarin derivatives, nifedipine, phenytoin,* or *verapamil.* Bleeding problems may occur if used with other *drugs that inhibit platelet aggregation,* such as *aspirin, parenteral carbenicillin, cefamandole, cefoperazone, dextran, dipyridamole, mezlocillin, piperacillin, plicamycin, salicylates, sulfinpyrazone, ticarcillin, valproic acid,* or *other anti-inflammatories.* Indomethacin may displace *highly protein-bound drugs* from binding sites. Because of the influence of prostaglandins on glucose metabolism, use with *insulin* or *oral antidiabetics* may potentiate hypoglycemic effects. Indomethacin may decrease the renal clearance of *lithium* and *methotrexate.* Use with *triamterene* isn't recommended because of potential nephrotoxicity; *other diuretics* may also predispose patients to nephrotoxicity.
Drug-lifestyle. Use with *alcohol* may cause increased adverse GI effects, including ulceration and hemorrhage. Discourage alcohol use.

ADVERSE REACTIONS
Oral and rectal forms
CNS: *headache, dizziness,* depression, drowsiness, confusion, somnolence, fatigue, peripheral neuropathy, **seizures,** psychic disturbances, syncope, *vertigo.*
CV: hypertension, *edema,* **heart failure.**
EENT: blurred vision, corneal and retinal damage, hearing loss, tinnitus.

GI: *nausea,* anorexia, *diarrhea, peptic ulceration, GI bleeding,* constipation, dyspepsia, *pancreatitis.*

GU: hematuria, *acute renal failure,* proteinuria, interstitial nephritis.

Hematologic: *hemolytic anemia, aplastic anemia, agranulocytosis, leukopenia, thrombocytopenic purpura,* iron-deficiency anemia.

Skin: pruritus, urticaria, *Stevens-Johnson syndrome.*

Other: hypersensitivity (rash, respiratory distress, *anaphylaxis, angioedema*), hyperkalemia.

I.V. form

GU: *renal failure,* hematuria, proteinuria, interstitial nephritis.

▣ KEY CONSIDERATIONS

Besides the recommendations relevant to all NSAIDs, consider the following:

• Patients older than age 60 may be more susceptible to the toxic effects of indomethacin.

• The effect of drug on renal prostaglandins may cause fluid retention and edema, a significant drawback for geriatric patients and those with heart failure.

• Don't mix oral suspension with liquids or antacids before administering.

• Patient should retain suppository in the rectum for at least 1 hour after insertion to ensure maximum absorption.

• Reconstitute 1-mg vial of I.V. dose with 1 to 2 ml of sterile water for injection or normal saline. Prepare solution immediately before use to prevent deterioration. Don't use solution if it's discolored or contains a precipitate.

• Administer drug by direct I.V. injection over 5 to 10 seconds. Use a large vein to prevent extravasation.

• Monitor I.V. site for complications.

• Monitor cardiopulmonary status for significant changes. Watch for signs and symptoms of fluid overload. Check weight and intake and output daily.

• Monitor renal function studies before start of therapy and frequently during therapy to prevent adverse effects.

• Severe headache may occur. If headache persists, decrease dose.

• Monitor carefully for bleeding and for reduced urine output.

• Drug therapy may interfere with dexamethasone suppression test results and urine 5-hydroxyindoleacetic acid determinations.

Patient education

• Instruct patient in proper administration of dosage form prescribed, such as suppository, sustained-release capsule, or suspension.

• Advise patient to seek medical approval before taking OTC drugs.

• Caution patient to avoid hazardous activities that require alertness or concentration. Instruct him in safety measures to prevent injury.

• Tell patient to report signs and symptoms of adverse reactions. Encourage patient to adhere to prescribed drug regimen and recommended follow-up.

Overdose & treatment

• Signs and symptoms of overdose include dizziness, nausea, vomiting, intense headache, mental confusion, drowsiness, tinnitus, sweating, blurred vision, paresthesia, and seizures.

• To treat indomethacin overdose, empty stomach immediately: Induce vomiting with ipecac syrup or perform gastric lavage. Administer activated charcoal via NG tube. Provide symptomatic and supportive measures (respiratory support and correction of fluid and electrolyte imbalances). Monitor laboratory parameters and vital signs closely. Dialysis may have little value because indomethacin is strongly protein-bound.

Reactions may be *common,* uncommon, *life-threatening,* or COMMON AND LIFE-THREATENING.

influenza virus vaccine, 1999-2000 trivalent types A & B (purified surface antigen)
Fluvirin

influenza virus vaccine, 1999-2000 trivalent types A & B (subvirion or purified subvirion)
Fluogen, FluShield, Fluzone

influenza virus vaccine, 1999-2000 trivalent types A & B (whole virion)
Fluzone

Viral vaccine

Available by prescription only
Injection: 0.5-ml prefilled syringe; 5-ml vials

INDICATIONS & DOSAGE
Annual influenza prophylaxis in high-risk patients
Adults: 0.5 ml I.M.

PHARMACODYNAMICS
Influenza prophylaxis: Vaccine promotes active immunity to influenza by inducing antibody production. Protection is provided only against those strains of virus from which the vaccine is prepared (or closely related strains).

PHARMACOKINETICS
Absorption: Duration of immunity varies widely, but usually lasts about 1 year.
Distribution: Unknown.
Metabolism: Unknown.
Excretion: Unknown.

CONTRAINDICATIONS & PRECAUTIONS
Contraindicated in patients with hypersensitivity to chicken eggs or any component of the vaccine, such as thimerosal. Defer vaccination in patients with acute respiratory or other active infection, and delay immunization in those with an active neurologic disorder.

INTERACTIONS
Drug-drug. Influenza vaccine may decrease serum *aminopyrine* and *phenytoin* levels and increase serum *theophylline* levels. Use with *corticosteroids* or *immunosuppressants* may impair the immune response to the vaccine. Rarely, patients receiving *warfarin* with influenza vaccine have shown prolonged PT and INR, GI bleeding, transient gross hematuria, and epistaxis.

ADVERSE REACTIONS
Other: *anaphylaxis,* fever and malaise (most commonly in those not exposed to influenza viruses), myalgia, erythema, induration, and *soreness at injection site.* Severe reactions in adults are rare.

▣ KEY CONSIDERATIONS
• Annual vaccination is highly recommended for patients older than age 65.
• Annual influenza prophylaxis also is recommended for adults with chronic CV, pulmonary, or renal disorders; metabolic disease; severe anemia; or compromised immune function. Vaccine is recommended for medical personnel who have extensive contact with high-risk patients, and residents of nursing homes or other long-term care facilities. Also, vaccine should be given to persons who wish to reduce their risk of acquiring an influenza infection.
• Obtain a thorough history of allergies, especially to eggs or chicken feathers, and of reactions to previous immunizations.
• Patients with known or suspected hypersensitivity to egg protein should have a skin test to assess sensitivity to vaccine. Administer a scratch test with 0.05 to 0.1 ml of a 1:100 dilution in normal saline solution for injection. Patients with positive skin test reactions shouldn't receive the influenza virus vaccine.
• Epinephrine solution 1:1,000 should be available to treat allergic reactions.
• Influenza vaccine shouldn't be administered to patients with active influenza infection. Such infection should be treated with amantadine.
• The preferred I.M. injection site is the deltoid muscle in adults.

• Pneumococcal vaccine, DTP, or live attenuated measles virus vaccine may be given simultaneously, but at a different injection site.

• Store vaccine between 36° and 46° F (2° and 8° C). Don't freeze.

Patient education

• Tell patient that he may experience discomfort at the injection site after immunization; he also may develop fever, malaise, and muscle aches 6 to 12 hours after vaccination that may persist for several days. Recommend acetaminophen to alleviate these effects.

• Encourage patient to report distressing adverse reactions promptly.

• Warn patient that many cases of Guillain-Barré syndrome were reported after vaccination for the swine flu in 1976. This condition usually causes reversible paralysis and muscle weakness, but it can be fatal in some individuals. Influenza vaccines made after 1976 haven't been associated with as high an incidence of Guillain-Barré syndrome, but the condition still occurs rarely. Patients with a history of Guillain-Barré syndrome have a greater risk for repeat episodes.

• Tell patient that he will need to be vaccinated annually.

insulin (regular)

Humulin-R, Novolin R, Novolin R PenFill, Pork Regular Iletin II, Regular (Concentrated) Iletin II, Regular Insulin, Regular Purified Pork Insulin, Velosulin Human

insulin (lispro)

Humalog

Prompt insulin zinc suspension (semilente)

Iletin Semilente*

isophane insulin suspension (NPH)

Humulin N, NPH Iletin*, NPH Insulin*, NPH-N, Novolin N, Novolin N PenFill, Pork NPH Iletin II

insulin zinc suspension (lente)

Humulin L, Lente Iletin II, Lente L, Novolin L

extended zinc insulin suspension (ultralente)

Humulin U Ultralente, Ultralente*

isophane insulin suspension and insulin injection (70% isophane insulin and 30% insulin injection)

Humulin 70/30, Novolin 70/30, Novolin 70/30 PenFill

isophane insulin suspension and insulin injection (50% isophane insulin and 50% insulin injection)

Humulin 50/50

Pancreatic hormone, antidiabetic

Available without a prescription
insulin (regular)
Injection (pork): 100 U/ml, 500 U/ml
Injection (human): 100 U/ml
insulin (lispro)
Injection (human): 100 U/ml
Cartridge (human): 1.5 ml
Prompt insulin zinc suspension (semilente)
Injection(pork): 100 U/ml
isophane insulin suspension (NPH)
Injection (pork): 100 U/ml
Injection (human): 100 U/ml
insulin zinc suspension (lente)
Injection (pork): 100 U/ml
Injection (human): 100 U/ml
extended zinc insulin suspension (ultralente)
Injection (pork): 100 U/ml
Injection (human): 100 U/ml
Available by prescription only
regular (concentrated) Iletin II insulin
Injection (pork): 500 U/ml

INDICATIONS & DOSAGE

Diabetic ketoacidosis (regular insulin)
Adults: Administer loading dose of 0.15 U/kg I.V. followed by 0.1 U/kg/hour

as a continuous infusion. Rate of insulin infusion should be decreased when plasma glucose level reaches 300 mg/dl. Infusion of D_5W should be started separately from the insulin infusion when plasma glucose reaches 250 mg/dl. Thirty minutes before discontinuing insulin infusion, a dose of insulin should be administered S.C.; intermediate-acting insulin is recommended.

Alternative dosage schedule is 50 to 100 U I.V. and 50 to 100 U S.C. immediately; subsequent doses should be based on therapeutic response and glucose, acetone, or ketone levels monitored at 1- to 2-hour intervals, or 2.4 to 7.2 U I.V. loading dose followed by 2.4 to 7.2 U/hour.

Type 1 diabetes mellitus, diabetes mellitus inadequately controlled by diet and oral antidiabetics
Adults: Dosage is individualized based on patient's blood and urine glucose levels.

Hyperkalemia
Adults: 5 to 10 U of regular insulin with 50 ml of D_5W over 5 minutes. Alternatively, 25 U of regular insulin given S.C. and an infusion of 1,000 ml $D_{10}W$ with 90 mEq sodium bicarbonate; infuse 330 ml over 30 minutes and the balance over 3 hours.

Provocative test for growth hormone secretion
Adults: Rapid I.V. injection of regular insulin 0.05 to 0.15 U/kg.

PHARMACODYNAMICS
Antidiabetic action: Insulin is used as a replacement for the physiological production of endogenous insulin in patients with type 1 diabetes mellitus and diabetes mellitus inadequately controlled by diet and oral antidiabetics. Insulin increases glucose transport across muscle and fat-cell membranes to reduce blood glucose levels. It also promotes conversion of glucose to its storage form, glycogen; triggers amino acid uptake and conversion to protein in muscle cells and inhibits protein degradation; stimulates triglyceride formation and inhibits release of free fatty acids from adipose tissue; and stimulates lipoprotein lipase activity, which converts circulating lipoproteins to fatty acids. Insulin is available in various forms, which differ mainly in onset, peak, and duration of action. Characteristics of the various insulin preparations are compared in the following chart.

PHARMACOKINETICS
Absorption: Insulin must be given parenterally because it's destroyed in the GI tract. Commercially available preparations are formulated to differ in onset, peak, and duration after S.C. administration. They are classified as rapid-acting (½- to 1-hour onset), intermediate-acting (1- to 2-hour onset), and long-acting (4- to 8-hour onset). The chart summarizes major pharmacokinetic differences.
Distribution: Insulin is distributed widely throughout the body.
Metabolism: Some insulin is bound and inactivated by peripheral tissues, but the majority appears to be degraded in the liver and kidneys.
Excretion: Insulin is filtered by the renal glomeruli and undergoes some tubular reabsorption. Plasma half-life is about 9 minutes after I.V. administration.

CONTRAINDICATIONS & PRECAUTIONS
No known contraindications.

INTERACTIONS
Drug-drug. *Anabolic steroids, beta blockers, clofibrate, fenfluramine, MAO inhibitors, salicylates,* and *tetracycline* can cause a prolonged hypoglycemic effect; monitor blood glucose levels carefully. *Corticosteroids, dextrothyroxine sodium, epinephrine,* and *thiazide diuretics* can diminish insulin response; monitor for hyperglycemia.
Drug-lifestyle. *Alcohol* can prolong the hypoglycemic effect; monitor blood glucose levels carefully. Use of *marijuana* may increase insulin requirements; monitor closely. *Smoking* decreases absorption of insulin administered S.C.; advise patient not to smoke within 30 minutes after insulin injection.

ADVERSE REACTIONS
Metabolic: *hypoglycemia,* hyperglycemia (rebound, or Somogyi, effect).
Skin: urticaria, pruritus, swelling, redness, stinging, warmth at injection site.

COMPARING INSULIN PREPARATIONS

This table lists the various forms of insulin and times of onset, peak, and duration. Individual responses can vary. Purified insulins contain < 10 ppm of proinsulin.

Preparation	Purified	Onset (hr)	Peak (hr)	Duration (hr)
Rapid-acting insulins				
insulin injection (regular, crystalline zinc)				
Regular Insulin	No	½	2½-5	8
Pork Regular Iletin II	Yes	½	2-4	6-8
Velosulin BR Human	Yes	½	1-3	8
Regular Purified Pork Insulin	Yes	½	2½-5	8
Humulin R	NA	½	2-4	6-8
Novolin R/Novolin R PenFill	NA	½	2½-5	8
Iletin Regular	No	½ to 1	2-4	5-7
insulin injection (lispro)				
Humalog	Yes	< ½	½-1½	< 6
prompt insulin zinc suspension (semilente)				
Iletin Semilente	No	1-3	2-8	12-16
Intermediate-acting insulins				
isophane insulin suspension (NPH)				
NPH Iletin I	No	1-2	6-12	18-24
NPH	No	1½	4-12	24
Pork NPH Iletin II	Yes	1-2	6-12	18-24
Humulin N	NA	1-2	6-12	18-24
Novolin N/Novolin N PenFill	NA	1½	4-12	24
insulin zinc suspension (lente)				
Lente Iletin I	No	1-3	6-12	18-24
Lente Iletin II	Yes	1-3	6-12	18-24
Lente L	Yes	2½	7-15	22
Humulin L	NA	1-3	6-12	18-24
Novolin L	NA	2½	7-15	22
isophane (NPH) 70%, regular insulin 30%				
Humulin 70/30	NA	½	4-8	24
Novolin 70/30/Novolin 70/30 PenFill	NA	½	2-12	24
isophane (NPH) 50%, regular insulin 50%				
Humulin 50/50	NA	½	4-8	24
Long-acting insulins				
extended insulin zinc suspension (ultralente)				
Iletin Ultralente	No	4-8	18-24	28-36
Ultralente	No	4	10-30	36
Humulin U Ultralente	Yes	4-6	8-20	24-28

NA means not applicable.

Reactions may be *common*, uncommon, *life-threatening*, or COMMON AND LIFE-THREATENING.

Other: *lipoatrophy, lipohypertrophy,* hypersensitivity reactions *(anaphylaxis,* rash).

▣ KEY CONSIDERATIONS

• Accuracy of measurement is very important, especially with regular insulin concentrated. Aids, such as a magnifying sleeve or dose magnifier, may help improve accuracy.
• With regular insulin concentrated, a secondary hypoglycemic reaction may occur 18 to 24 hours after injection. This may be caused by a repository effect of drug and the high concentration of insulin in the preparation (500 U/ml).
• Dosage is always expressed in USP U.
• Human insulin may be advantageous for patients who are allergic to pork or beef forms, for non-insulin-dependent patients requiring intermittent or short-term therapy (such as for surgery, infection, or total parenteral nutrition therapy), for patients with insulin resistance, or for those who develop lipoatrophy.
• Don't interchange single-source beef or pork insulins without considering the need for dosage adjustment.
• Lente, semilente, and ultralente insulins may be mixed in any proportion.
• Regular insulin may be mixed with NPH or lente insulins in any proportion. However, in vitro binding will occur over time until an equilibrium is reached. These mixtures should be administered either immediately after preparation or after stability occurs (15 minutes for NPH regular, 24 hours for lente regular) to minimize variability in patient response. Note that switching from separate injections to a prepared mixture also may alter the patient's response. When mixing two insulins, always draw regular insulin into the syringe first.
• Lispro insulin may be mixed with Humulin N or Humulin U and should be given within 15 minutes before a meal to prevent a hypoglycemic reaction. The effects of mixing lispro insulin with insulins of animal source or insulin preparations produced by other manufacturers haven't been studied; such use may require a change in dosage.

• Store insulin in cool area. Refrigeration is desirable but not essential, except with regular insulin concentrated.
• Don't use insulin that has changed color or becomes clumped or granular in appearance.
• Check expiration date on vial before using contents.
• Administration route is S.C. because it allows slower absorption and causes less pain than I.M. injections. Patients who are severely ill or who have type 1 or newly diagnosed diabetes and who also have very high blood glucose levels may require hospitalization and I.V. treatment with regular fast-acting insulin. Patients with type 2 diabetes may be treated as outpatients with intermediate-acting insulin after they have received instructions on how to alter dosage according to self-performed urine or blood glucose determinations. Some patients, brittle diabetics, may use a dextrometer to perform fingerstick blood glucose tests at home.
• Press but don't rub site after injection. Rotate injection sites. Record sites to avoid overuse of one area. However, unstable diabetics may achieve better control if injection site is rotated within same anatomic region.
• To mix insulin suspension, swirl vial gently or rotate between palms or between palm and thigh. Don't shake vigorously; this causes bubbling and air in syringe.
• Some patients may develop insulin resistance and require large insulin doses to control symptoms of diabetes. U-500 insulin is available for such patients as Purified Pork Iletin Regular Insulin, U-500. Although not every pharmacy may normally stock it, it's readily available. Patient should notify pharmacist several days before prescription refill is needed. Give hospital pharmacy sufficient notice before refill of in-house prescription. Never store U-500 insulin in same area as other insulin preparations because of danger of severe overdose if given accidentally to other patients. U-500 insulin must be administered with a U-100 syringe because no syringes are made for this drug.

• Human insulin may help patients who are allergic to pork or beef forms. Humulin is synthesized by a genetically altered strain of *Escherichia coli*. Novolin brands are derived by enzymatic alteration of pork insulin.

• The physiological effects of insulin may decrease serum magnesium, potassium, or inorganic phosphate levels.

Patient education

• Be sure patient knows that insulin therapy relieves symptoms but doesn't cure the disease.

• Tell patient about nature of disease, importance of following therapeutic regimen, specific diet, weight reduction, exercise, personal hygiene, avoidance of infection, and timing of injection and eating.

• Tell patient to adhere strictly to manufacturer's instructions regarding assembly, administration, and care of specialized delivery systems, such as insulin pumps.

• Emphasize importance of eating meals at regular times and not omitting meals.

• Teach patient that blood glucose monitoring is an essential guide to correct dosage and to therapeutic success.

• Emphasize importance of recognizing hypoglycemic symptoms because insulin-induced hypoglycemia is hazardous and may cause brain damage if prolonged.

• Advise patient to always wear a medical identification bracelet or pendant, to carry ample insulin supply and syringes on trips, to have carbohydrates (sugar or candy) on hand for emergency, and to note time-zone changes for dose schedule when traveling.

• Instruct patient not to change the order of mixing insulins or change the model or brand of syringe or needle. Be sure he knows that when mixing two insulins, he should always draw regular insulin into the syringe first.

• Inform patient that use of marijuana may increase insulin requirements.

• Inform patient that cigarette smoking decreases absorption of insulin administered S.C. Advise him not to smoke within 30 minutes after insulin injection.

Overdose & treatment

• Insulin overdose may produce signs and symptoms of hypoglycemia (tachycardia, palpitations, anxiety, hunger, nausea, diaphoresis, tremors, pallor, restlessness, headache, and speech and motor dysfunction).

• Treat the hypoglycemia based on patient's symptoms. If patient is responsive, give 10 to 15 g of a fast-acting oral carbohydrate. If patient's signs and symptoms persist after 15 minutes, give an additional 10 g carbohydrate. If patient is unresponsive, an I.V. bolus $D_{50}W$ solution should immediately increase blood glucose. Some prefer to use $D_{25}W$ because it's less irritating should extravasation occur. A common infusion rate is based on glucose content: 10 to 20 mg/kg/minute. Parenteral glucagon or epinephrine S.C. may also be given; both drugs raise blood glucose levels in a few minutes by stimulating glycogenolysis. Fluid and electrolyte imbalance may require I.V. fluids and electrolyte (such as potassium) replacement.

interferon beta-1b
Betaseron

Biological response modifier, antiviral, immunoregulator

Available by prescription only
Powder for injection, lyophilized: 9.6 million IU (0.3 mg)

INDICATIONS & DOSAGE
Reduction of the frequency of exacerbations in relapsing-remitting multiple sclerosis
Adults: 8 million IU (0.25 mg) S.C. every other day.

PHARMACODYNAMICS
Antiviral/immunoregulator actions: The mechanisms by which interferon beta-1b exerts its actions in multiple sclerosis aren't clearly understood. However, it's known that the biological response-modifying properties of interferon beta-1b are mediated through its interactions with specific cell receptors found on the surface of human cells. The binding to

---

Reactions may be *common*, uncommon, ***life-threatening**, or COMMON AND LIFE-THREATENING.

these receptors induces the expression of a number of interferon-induced gene products that are believed to mediate the biological actions of interferon beta-1b.

PHARMACOKINETICS

Absorption: Serum levels of interferon beta-1b are undetectable after the recommended dose; after higher doses, serum levels peak within 1 to 8 hours after S.C. administration.
Distribution: Unknown.
Metabolism: Unknown.
Excretion: Unknown for patients with multiple sclerosis; however, elimination half-life for healthy patients ranges from 8 minutes to 4 hours.

CONTRAINDICATIONS & PRECAUTIONS

Contraindicated in patients hypersensitive to interferon beta or human albumin.

INTERACTIONS

Drug-lifestyle. Photosensitivity may occur to *sunlight;* take precautions.

ADVERSE REACTIONS

CNS: depression, anxiety, emotional lability, depersonalization, *suicidal tendencies,* confusion, somnolence, *hypertonia, asthenia, migraine, seizures, headache, dizziness.*
CV: palpitations, hypertension, tachycardia, peripheral vascular disorder, *hemorrhage.*
EENT: laryngitis, *sinusitis, conjunctivitis,* abnormal vision.
GI: diarrhea, constipation, *abdominal pain, vomiting.*
Hematologic: *decreased WBC and absolute neutrophil counts.*
Hepatic: *elevated ALT levels, elevated bilirubin levels.*
Metabolic: diabetes insipidus, diabetes mellitus, hypothyroidism, SIADH secretion.
Musculoskeletal: *myasthenia.*
Respiratory: dyspnea.
Skin: diaphoresis; alopecia; inflammation, pain, and necrosis at injection site.
Other: Cushing's syndrome, *flulike signs and symptoms (fever, chills, malaise, myalgia, diaphoresis),* breast pain, *pelvic pain, lymphadenopathy,* generalized edema.

🔲 KEY CONSIDERATIONS

• Drug is being investigated in the treatment of AIDS, AIDS-related Kaposi's sarcoma, metastatic renal-cell carcinoma, malignant melanoma, cutaneous T-cell lymphoma, and acute hepatitis C as unlabeled uses.
• Safety and efficacy in chronic progressive multiple sclerosis haven't been evaluated.
• Drug use may cause depression and suicidal ideation. Other mental disorders can include anxiety, emotional lability, depersonalization, and confusion. It isn't known whether these symptoms may be related to the underlying neurologic basis of multiple sclerosis, to interferon beta-1b treatment, or to a combination of both. Closely monitor patient with these symptoms and consider stopping therapy.
• Before initiating therapy and at periodic intervals thereafter, perform hemoglobin levels, complete and differential WBC counts, platelet counts, and blood chemistries, including liver function tests.
• Have patient take drug at bedtime to minimize mild flulike signs and symptoms that commonly occur.
• To reconstitute, inject 1.2 ml of supplied diluent (half-normal saline injection) into vial and gently swirl to dissolve drug. Don't shake. Reconstituted solution will contain 8 million IU (0.25 mg)/ml. Discard vial containing particulate material or discolored solution.
• Inject drug immediately after preparation.
• Refrigerate drug or reconstituted product (up to 3 hours) at 36° to 46° F (2° to 8° C). Don't freeze.

Patient education
• Caution patient to take protective measures against photosensitization (for example, sunscreens, protective clothing, avoidance of exposure to ultraviolet light or sunlight) until tolerance is determined.
• Teach patient how to self-administer S.C. injections, including solution preparation, use of aseptic technique, rotation of injection sites, and equipment disposal. Periodically reevaluate patient's technique.

• Instruct patient to rotate injection sites to minimize local reactions.
• Inform patient that flulike symptoms are common after initiation of therapy. Recommend taking drug at bedtime to help minimize the symptoms.
• Caution patient not to change dosage or schedule of administration without medical consultation.
• Advise patient to report depression or suicidal ideation.

ipecac syrup

Alkaloid emetic

Available with and without a prescription
Syrup: 70 mg powdered ipecac/ml

INDICATIONS & DOSAGE
To induce vomiting in poisoning
Adults: 15 to 30 ml P.O., followed by 200 to 300 ml of water. Dose may be repeated once after 20 minutes, if necessary.

PHARMACODYNAMICS
Emetic action: Ipecac syrup directly irritates the GI mucosa and directly stimulates the chemoreceptor trigger zone through the effects of emetine and cephalin, its two alkaloids.

PHARMACOKINETICS
Absorption: Ipecac syrup is absorbed in significant amounts mainly when it doesn't produce vomiting. Onset of action usually occurs in 20 minutes.
Distribution: Unknown.
Metabolism: Unknown.
Excretion: Emetine is excreted in urine slowly, over a period lasting up to 60 days. Duration of effect is 20 to 25 minutes.

CONTRAINDICATIONS & PRECAUTIONS
Contraindicated in semicomatose or unconscious patients or those with severe inebriation, seizures, shock, or loss of gag reflex. Don't give after ingestion of gasoline, kerosene, volatile oils, or caustic substances (lye).

INTERACTIONS
Drug-drug. *Activated charcoal* may inactivate ipecac; use with *antiemetics* may decrease therapeutic effectiveness of ipecac.
Drug-food. Use with *carbonated beverages* may cause abdominal distention. Use with *dairy products* may decrease therapeutic effectiveness of ipecac. *Vegetable oil* delays absorption. Avoid administering with any of the above.

ADVERSE REACTIONS
CNS: depression, *drowsiness.*
CV: *arrhythmias,* bradycardia, hypotension; atrial fibrillation, *fatal myocarditis* (with excessive doses).
GI: diarrhea.

▣ KEY CONSIDERATIONS
• Administer ipecac syrup before giving activated charcoal, not after. Follow dose with 1 or 2 glasses of water. If vomiting doesn't occur after second dose, give activated charcoal to adsorb both ipecac syrup and ingested poison. Follow with gastric lavage.
• Inspect vomitus for ingested substances, such as tablets or capsules.
• Ipecac syrup usually empties the stomach completely within 30 minutes (in more than 90% of patients); average emptying time is 20 minutes.
• Be careful not to confuse ipecac syrup with ipecac fluid extract, which is rarely used but 14 times more potent. Never store these two drugs together; the wrong drug could cause death.
• In antiemetic toxicity, ipecac syrup is usually effective if less than 1 hour has passed since ingestion of antiemetic.
• Little if any systemic toxicity occurs with doses of 30 ml or less.
• Patients with an eating disorder (such as bulimia or anorexia nervosa) may abuse the drug.
• Ipecac syrup also may be used in small amounts as an expectorant in cough preparations; however, this use has doubtful therapeutic benefit.

Patient education
• Advise patient to seek medical attention immediately when poisoning is suspected.

Reactions may be *common,* uncommon, *life-threatening,* or COMMON AND LIFE-THREATENING.

• Caution patient to call poison information center before taking ipecac syrup.
• Warn patient to avoid drinking milk or carbonated beverages with ipecac syrup because they may decrease drug's effectiveness; instead, instruct him to take syrup with 1 or 2 glasses of water.
• Advise patient to take activated charcoal only after vomiting has stopped.

Overdose & treatment
• Signs and symptoms of overdose include diarrhea, persistent nausea or vomiting (longer than 30 minutes), stomach cramps or pain, arrhythmias, hypotension, myocarditis, difficulty breathing, and unusual fatigue or weakness.
• Toxicity from ipecac overdose usually involves use of the concentrated fluid extract in dosage appropriate for the syrup. Signs and symptoms of cardiotoxicity include tachycardia, T-wave depression, atrial fibrillation, depressed myocardial contractility, heart failure, and myocarditis. Other toxic effects include bloody stools and vomitus, hypotension, shock, seizures, and coma. Heart failure is the usual cause of death.
• Treatment requires discontinuation of drug followed by symptomatic and supportive care, which may include digitalis and pacemaker therapy to treat cardiotoxic effects. However, no antidote exists for the cardiotoxic effects of ipecac, which may be fatal despite intensive treatment.

ipratropium bromide
Atrovent

Anticholinergic, bronchodilator

Available by prescription only
Inhaler: each metered-dose supplies 18 mcg
Inhalation solution: 2.5 ml
Nasal spray: 0.03%, 0.06%

INDICATIONS & DOSAGE
Bronchospasm in chronic bronchitis and emphysema
Adults: Usually, 2 inhalations (36 mcg) q.i.d.; patient may take additional inhalations p.r.n., but shouldn't exceed 12 inhalations in 24 hours or 500 mcg q 6 to 8 hours via oral nebulizer.
Rhinorrhea associated with allergic and nonallergic perennial rhinitis
0.03% nasal spray
Adults: 2 sprays (42 mcg)/nostril b.i.d. or t.i.d.
Rhinorrhea associated with the common cold
0.06% nasal spray
Adults: 2 sprays (84 mcg)/nostril t.i.d. or q.i.d.

PHARMACODYNAMICS
Anticholinergic action: Ipratropium appears to inhibit vagally mediated reflexes by antagonizing the action of acetylcholine. Anticholinergics prevent the increases in intracellular levels of cyclic guanosine monophosphate (cyclic GMP) that result from interaction of acetylcholine with the muscarinic receptor on bronchial smooth muscle.
Brochodilator action: The bronchodilation after inhalation is primarily a local, site-specific effect, not a systemic one.

PHARMACOKINETICS
Absorption: Ipratropium isn't readily absorbed into the systemic circulation either from the surface of the lung or from the GI tract, as confirmed by blood levels and renal excretion studies. Much of an inhaled dose is swallowed, as shown by fecal excretion studies.
Distribution: None.
Metabolism: Hepatic; elimination half-life is about 2 hours.
Excretion: Most of an administered dose is excreted unchanged in feces. Absorbed drug is excreted in urine and bile.

CONTRAINDICATIONS & PRECAUTIONS
Contraindicated in patients with hypersensitivity to ipratropium or atropine or its derivatives and in those with a history of hypersensitivity to soya lecithin or related food products, such as soybeans and peanuts. Use cautiously in patients with angle-closure glaucoma, prostatic hyperplasia, and bladder-neck obstruction.

INTERACTIONS

Drug-drug. Use of ipratropium with *antimuscarinics*, including *ophthalmic preparations,* may produce additive effects. Increased risk of fluorocarbon toxicity may result from too-closely timed administration of ipratropium and other *fluorocarbon propellant–containing oral inhalants,* such as *adrenocorticoids, cromolyn, glucocorticoids,* or *sympathomimetics;* a 5-minute interval between such drugs is recommended.

ADVERSE REACTIONS

CNS: dizziness, headache, nervousness, pain.
CV: palpitations, chest pain.
EENT: cough, blurred vision, rhinitis, sinusitis.
GI: nausea, GI distress, dry mouth.
Musculoskeletal: back pain.
Respiratory: *upper respiratory tract infection, bronchitis,* cough, dyspnea, pharyngitis, **bronchospasm,** increased sputum.
Skin: rash.
Other: flulike syndrome.

⊡ KEY CONSIDERATIONS

• Because of delayed onset of bronchodilation, drug isn't recommended to treat acute respiratory distress.

Patient education

• Tell patient to shake drug well before using.
• Initial nasal spray pump requires priming with 7 actuations of the pump. If used regularly as recommended, no further priming is needed. If not used for over 24 hours, the pump will require 2 actuations. If not used for over 7 days, the pump will require 7 actuations to reprime.
• Instruct patient to store drug away from heat and direct sunlight and to protect it from freezing.
• Tell patient that temporary blurred vision may result if aerosol is sprayed into eyes.
• Advise patient to allow 1 minute between inhalations.
• Instruct patient to take a missed dose as soon as possible, unless it's almost time for the next scheduled dose, in which case he should skip the missed dose. Warn him to never double-dose.
• Suggest sugarless hard candy, gum, ice, or saliva substitute to relieve dry mouth. Tell patient to report dry mouth if it persists longer than 2 weeks.
• Instruct patient to call if he experiences no benefits within 30 minutes after administration, or if condition worsens.

---

irbesartan
Avapro

Angiotensin II receptor antagonist, antihypertensive

Available by prescription only
Tablets: 75 mg, 150 mg, 300 mg

INDICATIONS & DOSAGE

Treatment of hypertension—alone or in combination with other antihypertensives
Adults: initially 150 mg P.O. once daily, increased to maximum of 300 mg once daily if necessary, without regard to food.
✦ *Dosage adjustment.* In volume- and salt-depleted patients, give 75 mg P.O. initially.

PHARMACODYNAMICS

Antihypertensive action: Drug blocks the vasoconstrictor and aldosterone-secreting effects of angiotensin II by selectively blocking the binding of angiotensin II to its receptor sites.

PHARMACOKINETICS

Absorption: Irbesartan is absorbed rapidly and completely. The average absolute bioavailability is 60% to 80% and isn't affected by food. Plasma levels peak 1½ to 2 hours after ingestion.
Distribution: Drug is 90% bound to plasma proteins. It may cross the blood-brain barrier. Steady state is achieved within 3 days. Drug is widely distributed.
Metabolism: Drug is metabolized by conjugation and oxidation. Cytochrome P-450 2C9 is the major enzyme responsible for formation of the oxidative metabolites. Metabolites don't appear to

---

add appreciably to the pharmacologic activity.

Excretion: Drug is excreted in the bile and urine; 20% is excreted in urine and the rest in feces. Elimination half-life is 11 to 15 hours.

CONTRAINDICATIONS & PRECAUTIONS

Contraindicated in patients who are hypersensitive to irbesartan or its components.

Use cautiously in volume- or salt-depleted patients, in patients whose renal function may depend on the activity of the renin-angiotensin-aldosterone system (for example, patients with severe heart failure), and in those with unilateral or bilateral renal artery stenosis.

INTERACTIONS

None reported.

ADVERSE REACTIONS

CNS: fatigue, anxiety, dizziness, headache.
CV: chest pain, edema, tachycardia.
EENT: pharyngitis, rhinitis, sinus abnormality.
GI: diarrhea, dyspepsia, abdominal pain, nausea, vomiting.
GU: urinary tract infection.
Musculoskeletal: musculoskeletal trauma or pain.
Respiratory: cough, upper respiratory tract infection.
Skin: rash.

▣ KEY CONSIDERATIONS

• Pharmacokinetics of drug aren't altered in patients with renal impairment or in patients on hemodialysis. Irbesartan isn't removed by hemodialysis. Dosage adjustment isn't necessary in patients with mild to severe renal impairment unless patient with renal impairment is also volume depleted.
• Dosage adjustment isn't necessary in patients with hepatic insufficiency.
• Patients not adequately treated by the maximum 300-mg once-daily dose are unlikely to derive additional benefit from a higher dose or twice-daily dosing.
• Monitor blood pressure regularly. A transient hypotensive response isn't a

contraindication to further treatment. Therapy can usually be continued once blood pressure has stabilized.
• Drug therapy may cause a minor increase in BUN or serum creatinine levels.

Patient education

• Tell patient that drug may be taken once daily with or without food.
• Advise patient that if a dose is missed to take it as soon as possible, but not to double-dose.
• Warn patient about symptoms of hypotension and what to do.
• Caution patient not to discontinue drug without medical approval.

iron dextran
DexFerrum, InFeD

Parenteral iron supplement, hematinic

Available by prescription only
Injection: 50 mg elemental iron/ml in 2-ml single-dose vials

INDICATIONS & DOSAGE
Iron-deficiency anemia
Adults: Dosage is highly individualized and is based on patient's weight and hemoglobin level. Drug is usually given I.M.; preservative-free solution can be given I.V. Check current literature for recommended protocol.

PHARMACODYNAMICS
Hematinic action: Iron dextran is a complex of ferric hydroxide and dextran in a colloidal solution. After I.M. injection, 10% to 50% remains in the muscle for several months; remainder enters the bloodstream, increasing plasma iron levels for up to 2 weeks. Iron is an essential component of hemoglobin.

PHARMACOKINETICS
Absorption: I.M. doses are absorbed in two stages: 60% after 3 days and up to 90% by 3 weeks. Remainder is absorbed over several months or longer.
Distribution: During first 3 days, local inflammation facilitates passage of drug

into the lymphatic system; drug is then ingested by macrophages, which enter lymph and blood.

Metabolism: After I.M. or I.V. administration, iron dextran is cleared from plasma by reticuloendothelial cells of the liver, spleen, and bone marrow.

Excretion: In doses of 500 mg or less, half-life is 6 hours. Traces are excreted in urine, bile, and feces. Drug can't be removed by hemodialysis.

CONTRAINDICATIONS & PRECAUTIONS

Contraindicated in patients with hypersensitivity to iron dextran, in those with all anemias except iron-deficiency anemia, and in those with acute infectious renal disease. Use cautiously in patients with impaired hepatic function, rheumatoid arthritis, and other inflammatory diseases.

INTERACTIONS

None significant.

ADVERSE REACTIONS

CNS: headache, transitory paresthesia, arthralgia, myalgia, dizziness, malaise.
CV: *hypotensive reaction, peripheral vascular flushing (with overly rapid I.V. administration).*
GI: nausea, anorexia.
Respiratory: *bronchospasm,* dyspnea.
Skin: rash, urticaria, purpura.
Other: *soreness, inflammation, brown skin discoloration (at I.M. injection site); local phlebitis (at I.V. injection site);* sterile abscess; necrosis; atrophy; fibrosis; *anaphylaxis;* delayed sensitivity reactions; fever; chills.

🔲 KEY CONSIDERATIONS

• Discontinue oral iron before giving iron dextran.
• Use 10-ml multidose vial only for I.M. injections because it contains phenol as a preservative; use only 2- or 5-ml ampule without preservative for I.V. administration.
• Administer test dose of 0.5 ml iron dextran I.M. or I.V. Be alert for anaphylaxis on test dose; monitor vital signs for drug reaction. Keep epinephrine (0.5 ml of a 1:1,000 solution) readily available for such an emergency.

• Inject I.M. preparation deeply into upper outer quadrant of buttocks (never an arm or other exposed area) using a 2- to 3-inch (5- to 8-cm), 19G or 20G needle. Use Z-track technique to avoid leakage into S.C. tissue and skin stains, and minimize staining by using a separate needle to withdraw drug from its container.
• Note that I.V. use is controversial, and some health care facilities don't allow it.
• Give drug I.V. if patient has insufficient muscle mass for deep injection, impaired absorption from muscle because of stasis or edema, a risk of uncontrolled I.M. bleeding from trauma (as in hemophilia), or need for massive and prolonged parenteral therapy (as in chronic substantial blood loss). Don't administer more than 50 mg of iron/minute (1 ml/minute) if using drug undiluted.
• After I.V. iron dextran administration, flush vein with 10 ml of normal saline injection to minimize local irritation. Have patient rest for 15 to 30 minutes because orthostatic hypotension may occur.
• Monitor hemoglobin level, hematocrit, and reticulocyte count during therapy. An increase of about 1 g/dl weekly in hemoglobin level is usual.
• Large doses (over 250 mg iron) may color the serum brown.
• Iron dextran may cause false elevations in serum bilirubin level and false reductions in serum calcium level.
• Iron dextran prevents meaningful measurement of serum iron level and total iron binding capacity for up to 3 weeks; I.M. injection may cause dense areas of activity on bone scans using technetium 99m diphosphonate, for 1 to 6 days.

Patient education

• Warn patient of possibility of skin staining with I.M. injections.

Reactions may be *common*, uncommon, *life-threatening*, or COMMON AND LIFE-THREATENING.

isoniazid (INH)
Isotamine*, Laniazid, Laniazid C.T., Nydrazid, PMS Isoniazid*, Rimifon*

Isonicotinic acid hydrazine, antituberculotic

Available by prescription only
Tablets: 50 mg, 100 mg, 300 mg
Oral solution: 50 mg/5 ml
Injection: 100 mg/ml

INDICATIONS & DOSAGE
Primary treatment against actively growing tubercle bacilli
Adults: 5 mg/kg P.O. or I.M. daily in a single dose, up to 300 mg/day, continued for 9 months to 2 years.
Prophylaxis against tubercle bacilli of those closely exposed or with positive skin test
Adults: 300 mg P.O. daily as a single dose, continued for 6 months to 1 year.

PHARMACODYNAMICS
Antituberculotic action: INH interferes with lipid and DNA synthesis, thus inhibiting bacterial cell wall synthesis. Its action is bacteriostatic or bactericidal, depending on organism susceptibility and drug level at infection site. INH is active against *Mycobacterium tuberculosis, M. bovis,* and some strains of *M. kansasii.*

Resistance by *M. tuberculosis* develops rapidly when INH is used to treat tuberculosis, and it's usually combined with another antituberculotic to prevent or delay resistance. During prophylaxis, however, resistance isn't a problem and isoniazid can be used alone.

PHARMACOKINETICS
Absorption: INH is rapidly and completely absorbed from the GI tract after oral administration; serum levels peak 1 to 2 hours after ingestion. INH also is absorbed readily after I.M. injection.
Distribution: Drug is distributed widely into body tissues and fluids, including ascitic, synovial, pleural, and cerebrospinal fluids; lungs and other organs; and sputum and saliva.

Metabolism: Drug is inactivated primarily in the liver by genetically controlled acetylation. Rate of metabolism varies individually; fast acetylators metabolize drug five times as rapidly as others. About 50% of blacks and whites are slow acetylators of INH, whereas more than 80% of Chinese, Japanese, and Inuits are fast acetylators.
Excretion: About 75% of a dose is excreted in urine as unchanged drug and metabolites in 24 hours; some drug is excreted in saliva, sputum, and feces. Plasma half-life in adults is 1 to 4 hours, depending on metabolic rate. Drug is removed by peritoneal dialysis or hemodialysis.

CONTRAINDICATIONS & PRECAUTIONS
Contraindicated in patients with acute hepatic disease or drug-associated hepatic damage. Use cautiously in geriatric patients and in those with severe, non-INH-associated hepatic disease, seizure disorders (especially those taking phenytoin), severe renal impairment, or chronic alcoholism.

INTERACTIONS
Drug-drug. Use with *antacids* decreases oral absorption of INH. Use with *anticoagulants* may increase anticoagulant activity. Use with *benzodiazepines* (such as *diazepam*), *carbamazepine,* or *phenytoin* inhibits metabolism of these drugs, thus elevating their serum levels and increasing the risk of toxicity. Use with *corticosteroids* may decrease INH efficacy. Use with *cycloserine* increases hazard of CNS toxicity, drowsiness, and dizziness from cycloserine. Use with *disulfiram* may cause coordination difficulties and psychotic episodes. Use with *rifampin* may accelerate INH metabolism to hepatotoxic metabolites because of rifampin-induced enzyme production.
Drug-lifestyle. Daily use of *alcohol* may increase the incidence of INH-induced hepatitis and seizures; don't use together.

ADVERSE REACTIONS
CNS: peripheral neuropathy (dose-related and especially in patients who are malnourished, alcoholic, diabetic, or slow acetylators), usually preceded by

paresthesia of hands and feet, *seizures,* toxic encephalopathy, memory impairment, toxic psychosis.
EENT: optic neuritis, atrophy.
GI: nausea, vomiting, epigastric distress.
GU: gynecomastia.
Hematologic: *agranulocytosis,* hemolytic anemia, *aplastic anemia,* eosinophilia, *thrombocytopenia,* sideroblastic anemia.
Hepatic: *hepatitis* (occasionally severe and sometimes fatal, especially in geriatric patients), jaundice, *elevated serum transaminase levels,* bilirubinemia.
Metabolic: hyperglycemia, metabolic acidosis, hypocalcemia, hypophosphatemia.
Other: rheumatic and lupuslike syndromes, hypersensitivity reactions (fever, rash, lymphadenopathy, vasculitis), pyridoxine deficiency, irritation at I.M. injection site.

▣ KEY CONSIDERATIONS

• Use with caution in geriatric patients; incidence of hepatic effects is increased after age 35. Drug prophylaxis in older patients with a positive purified protein derivative (PPD) test may not be indicated because of risk of hepatotoxicity.
• At least 12 months of preventive therapy is recommended for persons with past tuberculosis and HIV-infected individuals.
• If compliance is a problem, twice-weekly supervised drug administration may be effective. Recommended twice-weekly dose for adults is 15 mg/kg P.O., not to exceed 900 mg.
• Oral doses should be taken on empty stomach for maximum absorption, or with food if gastric irritation occurs.
• Aluminum-containing antacids or laxatives should be taken 1 hour after oral dose of INH.
• Obtain specimens for culture and sensitivity testing before first dose, but therapy may begin before test results are complete; repeat periodically to detect drug resistance.
• Monitor blood, renal, and hepatic function studies before and periodically during therapy to minimize toxicity; assess visual function periodically.

• Observe patient for adverse effects, especially hepatic dysfunction, CNS toxicity, and optic neuritis. Establish safety measures in case of postural hypotension.
• Drug may hinder stabilization of serum glucose level in patients with diabetes mellitus.
• Improvement is usually evident after 2 to 3 weeks of therapy.
• Some recommend pyridoxine 50 mg P.O. daily to prevent peripheral neuropathy from large doses of INH. It may also be useful in patients at risk of developing peripheral neuropathy (malnourished patients, diabetics, and alcohol abusers). Pyridoxine (50 to 200 mg daily) has been used to treat drug-induced neuropathy.
• Because drug is dialyzable, patients undergoing hemodialysis or peritoneal dialysis may need dosage adjustments.
• Hepatotoxicity appears to be age-related and may limit use for prophylaxis. Alcohol consumption or history of alcohol-related liver disease also increases risk of hepatotoxicity.
• INH alters the results of urine glucose tests that use the cupric sulfate method (Benedict's reagent, Diastix, or Chemstrip uG).
• Elevated liver function study results occur in about 15%; most abnormalities are mild and transient, but some persist throughout treatment.

Patient education
• Explain disease process and rationale for long-term therapy.
• Teach signs and symptoms of hypersensitivity and other adverse reactions, particularly visual disturbances, and emphasize need to report these; urge patient to report any unusual effects.
• Warn patient not to use alcohol; explain hazard of serious CNS toxicity and increased hazard of hepatitis.
• Teach patient how and when to take drug; instruct patient to take INH on an empty stomach, at least 1 hour before or 2 hours after meals. If GI irritation occurs, drug may be taken with food.
• Urge patient to comply with and complete prescribed regimen. Advise patient not to discontinue drug without medical

---

Reactions may be *common,* uncommon, *life-threatening,* or COMMON AND LIFE-THREATENING.

approval; explain importance of follow-up appointments.
• Inform patient that drug therapy is usually continued for 18 months to 2 years for treatment of active tuberculosis; 12 months for prophylaxis; 9 months if INH and rifampin therapy are combined.
• Emphasize importance of uninterrupted therapy to prevent relapse and spread of infection.

Overdose & treatment
• Early signs and symptoms of overdose include nausea, vomiting, slurred speech, dizziness, blurred vision, and visual hallucinations, occurring 30 minutes to 3 hours after ingestion; gross overdose causes CNS depression progressing from stupor to coma, with respiratory distress, intractable seizures, and death.
• To treat, establish ventilation; control seizures with diazepam. Pyridoxine is administered to equal dose of INH. Initial dose is 1 to 4 g pyridoxine I.V., followed by 1 g every 30 minutes thereafter, until the entire dose is given. Clear drug with gastric lavage after seizure control and correct acidosis with parenteral sodium bicarbonate; force diuresis with I.V. fluids and osmotic diuretics, and, if necessary, enhance clearance of the drug with hemodialysis or peritoneal dialysis.

---

isoproterenol
Isuprel

isoproterenol hydrochloride
Isuprel, Isuprel Glossets, Isuprel Mistometer, Norisodrine

isoproterenol sulfate
Medihaler-Iso

Adrenergic, bronchodilator, cardiac stimulant

Available by prescription only
isoproterenol
Nebulizer inhaler: 0.25%, 0.5%, 1%
isoproterenol hydrochloride
Tablets (S.L.): 10 mg, 15 mg

Aerosol inhaler: 120 mcg/metered spray, 131 mcg/metered spray
Injection: 200 mcg/ml
isoproterenol sulfate
Aerosol inhaler: 80 mcg/metered spray

INDICATIONS & DOSAGE
Complete heart block after closure of ventricular septal defect
Adults: I.V. bolus, 0.02 to 0.06 mg (1 to 3 ml of a 1:50,000 dilution).
To prevent heart block
Adults: 10 to 30 mg S.L. 4 to 6 times daily.
Maintenance therapy of AV block
Adults: Initially, 10 mg S.L., followed by 5 to 50 mg, p.r.n. Alternatively, 5 mg (half of a 10-mg tablet) administered P.R., followed by 5 to 15 mg, p.r.n.
Bronchospasm during mild acute asthma attacks
isoproterenol hydrochloride
Adults: One aerosol inhalation initially, repeated, p.r.n., after 1 to 5 minutes, to maximum six inhalations daily. Maintenance dose is one or two inhalations four to six times daily at 3- to 4-hour intervals. Via hand-bulb nebulizer, 5 to 15 deep inhalations of a 0.5% solution; if needed, may be repeated in 5 to 10 minutes. May be repeated up to five times daily.
Alternatively, three to seven deep inhalations of a 1% solution, repeated once in 5 to 10 minutes if needed. May be repeated up to five times daily.
isoproterenol sulfate
Adults: For acute dyspneic episodes, one inhalation initially; repeated if needed after 2 to 5 minutes. Maximum six inhalations daily. Maintenance dosage is one or two inhalations up to six times daily.
Bronchospasm in COPD
isoproterenol hydrochloride
Adults: Via hand-bulb nebulizer: 5 to 15 deep inhalations of a 0.5% solution, or 3 to 7 deep inhalations of a 1% solution no more frequently than q 3 to 4 hours.
Bronchospasm during mild acute asthma attacks or in COPD
isoproterenol hydrochloride
Adults: Oral inhalation of 2 ml of 0.125% solution or 2.5 ml of 0.1% solution up to 5 times daily.

Acute asthma attacks unresponsive to inhalation therapy or control of bronchospasm during anesthesia
isoproterenol hydrochloride
Adults: 0.01 to 0.02 mg (0.5 to 1 ml of a 1:50,000 dilution) I.V. Repeat if needed.
For bronchodilation
isoproterenol hydrochloride
Adults: 10 to 20 mg S.L., not to exceed 60 mg daily.
Emergency treatment of arrhythmias
isoproterenol hydrochloride
Adults: Initially, 0.02 to 0.06 mg I.V. bolus. Subsequent doses at 0.01 to 0.2 mg I.V. Alternatively, 5 mcg/minute titrated to patient's response. Range, 2 to 20 mcg/minute. Alternatively, 0.2 mg I.M. or S.C.; subsequent doses at 0.02 to 1 mg I.M. or 0.15 to 0.2 mg S.C. In extreme cases, 0.02 mg (0.1 ml of 1:5,000) intracardiac injection.
Immediate temporary control of atropine-resistant, hemodynamically significant bradycardia
isoproterenol hydrochloride
Adults: 2 to 10 mcg/minute I.V. infusion, titrated to patient's response.
Heart block, Stokes-Adams attacks, and shock
isoproterenol hydrochloride
Adults: 0.5 to 5 mcg/minute by continuous I.V. infusion titrated to patient's response; or 0.02 to 0.06 mg I.V. boluses with 0.01 to 0.2 mg additional doses; or 0.2 mg I.M. or S.C. with 0.02 to 1 mg I.M. or 0.15 to 0.2 mg S.C. additional doses.

PHARMACODYNAMICS

Bronchodilator action: Isoproterenol relaxes bronchial smooth muscle by direct action on beta$_2$-adrenergic receptors, relieving bronchospasm, increasing vital capacity, decreasing residual volume in lungs, and facilitating passage of pulmonary secretions. It also produces relaxation of GI and uterine smooth muscle via stimulation of beta$_2$ receptors. Peripheral vasodilation, cardiac stimulation, and relaxation of bronchial smooth muscle are the main therapeutic effects.
Cardiac stimulant action: Isoproterenol acts on beta$_1$-adrenergic receptors in the heart, producing a positive chronotropic and inotropic effect; it usually increases cardiac output. In patients with AV block, isoproterenol shortens conduction time and the refractory period of the AV node and increases the rate and strength of ventricular contractions.

PHARMACOKINETICS

Absorption: After injection or oral inhalation, isoproterenol is absorbed rapidly; after sublingual or rectal administration, absorption is variable and often unreliable. Onset of action is prompt after oral inhalation and persists up to 1 hour. Effects persist for a few minutes after I.V. injection, up to 2 hours after S.C. or sublingual administration, and up to 4 hours after rectal administration of sublingual tablet.
Distribution: Drug is distributed widely throughout the body.
Metabolism: Drug is metabolized by conjugation in the GI tract and by enzymatic reduction in the liver, lungs, and other tissues.
Excretion: Excreted primarily in urine as unchanged drug and its metabolites.

CONTRAINDICATIONS & PRECAUTIONS

Contraindicated in patients with tachycardia caused by digitalis intoxication, in patients with preexisting arrhythmias (other than those who may respond to treatment with isoproterenol), and in those with angina pectoris. Use cautiously in geriatric patients and in those with impaired renal function, CV disease, coronary insufficiency, diabetes, hyperthyroidism, or sensitivity to sympathomimetic amines.

INTERACTIONS

Drug-drug. Use with *beta blockers* antagonizes isoproterenol's cardiac-stimulating, bronchodilating, and vasodilating effects. Arrhythmias may occur more readily when drug is used with *cardiac glycosides, potassium-depleting drugs,* or *other drugs that affect cardiac rhythm.* Isoproterenol should be used with caution in patients receiving *cyclopropane* or *halogenated hydrocarbon general anesthetics.* Use of isoproterenol with *epinephrine* and other *sympathomimetics* may cause additive CV reactions. However, these drugs may be used together if at least 4 hours elapse between administration times. Use with *ergot alkaloids* may increase blood pressure.

ADVERSE REACTIONS
CNS: *headache, mild tremor,* weakness, dizziness, *nervousness,* insomnia, ***Stokes-Adams seizures.***
CV: palpitations, *tachycardia, anginal pain,* **arrhythmias, cardiac arrest,** *rapid rise and fall in blood pressure.*
GI: *nausea, vomiting, heartburn.*
Metabolic: hyperglycemia.
Respiratory: ***bronchospasm,*** bronchitis, sputum increase, pulmonary edema.
Other: diaphoresis, swelling of parotid glands (with prolonged use).

🔲 KEY CONSIDERATIONS
Besides the recommendations relevant to all adrenergics, consider the following:
• Geriatric patients may be more sensitive to the therapeutic and adverse effects of isoproterenol.
• Drug doesn't replace administration of blood, plasma, fluids, or electrolytes in patients with blood volume depletion.
• Severe paradoxical airway resistance may follow oral inhalations.
• Hypotension must be corrected before isoproterenol is administered.
• If three to five treatments within 6 to 12 hours provide minimal or no relief, reevaluate therapy.
• Continuously monitor ECG during I.V. administration.
• Carefully monitor response to therapy by frequent determinations of heart rate, ECG pattern, blood pressure, and central venous pressure, as well as (for patients in shock) urine volume, blood pH, and Pco_2 levels.
• Prescribed I.V. infusion rate should include specific guidelines for regulating flow or terminating infusion in relation to heart rate, premature beats, ECG changes, precordial distress, blood pressure, and urine flow. Because of danger of precipitating arrhythmias, rate of infusion is usually decreased or infusion may be temporarily discontinued if heart rate exceeds 110 beats/minute.

• A constant-infusion pump prevents sudden infusion of excessive amounts of drug.
• Sublingual doses shouldn't be given more frequently than every 3 to 4 hours or more than 3 times daily.
• Sublingual tablet may be administered rectally, if indicated.
• Monitor patient for rebound bronchospasm when drug's effects end.
• Isoproterenol has also been used to aid diagnosis of coronary artery disease and mitral regurgitation.
• Don't inject solutions intended for oral inhalation.
• Isoproterenol may reduce the sensitivity of spirometry in the diagnosis of asthma.

Patient education
• Remind patient to save applicator; refills may be available.
• Urge patient to call if no relief is gained or if condition worsens.
• Advise patient to store oral forms away from heat and light (not in bathroom medicine cabinet, where heat and moisture will cause deterioration of the drug). Keep drug out of the reach of children.
Inhalation
• Give patient instructions on proper use of inhaler.
• Tell patient that saliva and sputum may appear red or pink after oral inhalation because isoproterenol turns red on exposure to air.
• Advise patient to rinse mouth with water after drug is absorbed completely and between doses.
Sublingual
• Tell patient to allow sublingual tablet to dissolve under tongue, without sucking, and not to swallow saliva (may cause epigastric pain) until drug has been absorbed completely.
• Warn patient that frequent use of sublingual tablets may damage teeth because of drug acidity.

Overdose & treatment
• Signs and symptoms of overdose include exaggeration of common adverse reactions, particularly arrhythmias, extreme tremors, nausea, vomiting, and profound hypotension.

• Treatment includes symptomatic and supportive measures. Monitor vital signs closely. Sedatives (barbiturates) may be used to treat CNS stimulation. Use a cardioselective beta blocker to treat tachycardia and arrhythmias. These agents should be used with caution; they may induce asthmatic attack.

isosorbide dinitrate
Apo-ISDN*, Coronex*, Dilatrate-SR, Iso-Bid, Isonate, Isordil, Isordil Tembids, Isordil Titradose, Isotrate, Novosorbide*, Sorbitrate, Sorbitrate SA

Nitrate, antianginal, vasodilator

Available by prescription only
Tablets: 5 mg, 10 mg, 20 mg, 30 mg, 40 mg
Tablets (S.L.): 2.5 mg, 5 mg, 10 mg
Tablets (extended-release): 40 mg
Tablets (chewable): 5 mg, 10 mg
Capsules (extended-release): 40 mg

INDICATIONS & DOSAGE
Treatment or prophylaxis of acute anginal attacks; treatment of chronic ischemic heart disease (by preload reduction)
Adults: **S.L. form**—2.5 to 10 mg S.L. for prompt relief of angina pain, repeated q 2 to 3 hours during acute phase, or q 4 to 6 hours for prophylaxis.

Chewable form—2.5 to 10 mg, p.r.n., for acute attack or q 2 to 3 hours for prophylaxis, but only after initial test dose of 5 mg to determine risk of severe hypotension.

Oral form—10 to 20 mg P.O. t.i.d. or q.i.d. for prophylaxis only (use smallest effective dose).

Extended-release forms—20 to 40 mg P.O. q 8 to 12 hours.
◊ *Adjunctive treatment of heart failure*
Adults: 5 to 10 mg S.L. q 3 to 4 hours. Alternatively, give 20 to 40 mg P.O. (or chewable tablets) q 4 hours. Usually administered with vasodilators.
◊ *Diffuse esophageal spasm without gastroesophageal reflux*
Adults: 10 to 30 mg P.O. q 4 hours.

PHARMACODYNAMICS
Antianginal action: Isosorbide dinitrate reduces myocardial oxygen demand through peripheral vasodilation, resulting in decreased venous filling pressure (preload) and, to a lesser extent, decreased arterial impedance (afterload). These combined effects result in decreased cardiac work and, consequently, reduced myocardial oxygen demands. Drug also redistributes coronary blood flow from epicardial to subendocardial regions.
Vasodilating action: Drug dilates peripheral vessels (primarily venous), helping to manage pulmonary edema and heart failure caused by decreased venous return to the heart (preload). Arterial vasodilatory effects also decrease arterial impedance (afterload) and thus left ventricular work, benefiting the failing heart. These combined effects may help some patients with acute MI. (Use of isosorbide dinitrate in patients with heart failure and acute MI is currently unapproved.)

PHARMACOKINETICS
Absorption: Oral form is well absorbed from the GI tract but undergoes first-pass metabolism, resulting in bioavailability of about 50% (depending on dosage form used). With S.L. and chewable forms, onset of action is 3 minutes; with other oral forms, 30 minutes; with extended-release forms, 1 hour.
Distribution: Limited information is available on drug's plasma protein-binding and distribution. Like nitroglycerin, it's distributed widely throughout the body.
Metabolism: Drug is metabolized in the liver to active metabolites.
Excretion: Metabolites are excreted in the urine; elimination half-life is about 5 to 6 hours with oral administration; 2 hours with S.L. administration. About 80% to 100% of absorbed dose is excreted in the urine within 24 hours. Duration of effect is longer than that of S.L. preparations. With S.L. and chewable forms, duration of effect is 30 minutes to 2 hours; with other oral forms, 5 to 6 hours.

Reactions may be *common*, uncommon, *life-threatening*, or COMMON AND LIFE-THREATENING.

CONTRAINDICATIONS & PRECAUTIONS

Contraindicated in patients with hypersensitivity or idiosyncratic reaction to nitrates, severe hypotension, shock, or acute MI with low left ventricular filling pressure. Use cautiously in patients with hypotension or blood volume depletion (such as from diuretic therapy).

INTERACTIONS

Drug-drug. Use of isosorbide with *antihypertensives, calcium channel blockers, phenothiazines,* or *vasodilators* may cause additive hypotensive effects; monitor closely.

Drug-lifestyle. Use of isosorbide with *alcohol* may cause additive hypotensive effects; discourage use.

ADVERSE REACTIONS

CNS: *headache* (sometimes with throbbing), dizziness, weakness.
CV: *orthostatic hypotension, tachycardia, palpitations, ankle edema, flushing,* fainting.
GI: nausea, vomiting, sublingual burning.
Skin: cutaneous vasodilation, rash.
Other: hypersensitivity reactions.

▣ KEY CONSIDERATIONS

• Drug may cause headache, especially at first. Dose may need to be reduced temporarily, but tolerance usually develops to this effect. In the interim, patient may relieve headache with aspirin or acetaminophen.
• Additional dose may be given before anticipated stress or at bedtime if angina is nocturnal.
• Monitor blood pressure and intensity and duration of patient's response to drug.
• Drug may cause orthostatic hypotension. To minimize this, have patient stand up slowly, walk up and down stairs carefully, and lie down at first sign of dizziness.
• Don't discontinue drug abruptly because this may cause coronary vasospasm.
• Store drug in cool place, in tightly closed container away from light.
• Maintenance of continuous 24-hour plasma levels may result in refractory

tolerance. Dosing regimens should include dose-free intervals, which vary based on form of drug used.
• Isosorbide dinitrate may interfere with serum cholesterol tests using the Zlatkis-Zak color reaction, causing a falsely decreased value.

Patient education

• Instruct patient to take drug as prescribed, and to keep it easily accessible at all times. Drug is physiologically necessary but not addictive.
• Warn patient that headache may occur initially, but may respond to usual headache remedies or dosage reduction. Assure patient that headache usually subsides gradually with continued treatment.
• If patient is taking oral tablet, tell him to take it on empty stomach, either 30 minutes before or 1 to 2 hours after meals; to swallow oral tablets whole; and to chew chewable tablets thoroughly before swallowing.
• Advise patient to sit when self-administering S.L. tablets. He should lubricate tablet with saliva or place a few milliliters of fluid under tongue with tablet. If patient experiences tingling sensation with drug placed sublingually, he may try to hold tablet in buccal pouch. Dose may be repeated every 10 to 15 minutes for maximum of 3 doses. If no relief occurs, he should call or go to hospital emergency room.
• Warn patient to change position gradually to avoid excessive dizziness.
• Instruct patient to avoid alcohol while taking drug because severe hypotension and CV collapse may occur.
• Advise patient to report blurred vision, dry mouth, or persistent headache.
• Caution patient not to stop long-term therapy abruptly.

Overdose & treatment

• Signs and symptoms of overdose result primarily from vasodilation and methemoglobinemia and include hypotension, persistent throbbing headache, palpitations, visual disturbance, flushing of the skin and sweating (with skin later becoming cold and cyanotic), nausea and vomiting, colic and bloody diarrhea, orthostatism, initial hyperpnea, dyspnea, slow respiratory rate, bradycardia, heart block, increased intracranial pressure with confusion, fever, paralysis, and tissue hypoxia, which can lead to cyanosis, metabolic acidosis, coma, clonic seizures, and circulatory collapse. Death may result from circulatory collapse or asphyxia.

• Treatment includes gastric lavage followed by administration of activated charcoal to remove remaining gastric contents. Blood gases and methemoglobin levels should be monitored, as indicated. Supportive care includes respiratory support and oxygen administration, passive movement of extremities to aid venous return, recumbent positioning (Trendelenburg position, if necessary), maintenance of adequate body temperature, and administration of I.V. fluids.

• An I.V. adrenergic agonist (such as phenylephrine) may be considered if further treatment is required. For methemoglobinemia, methylene blue (1 to 2 mg/kg I.V.) may be given. (Epinephrine and related compounds are contraindicated in isosorbide dinitrate overdose.)

isosorbide mononitrate
IMDUR, ISMO, Monoket

Nitrate, antianginal

Available by prescription only
Tablets: 10 mg, 20 mg
Tablets (extended-release): 30 mg, 60 mg, 120 mg

INDICATIONS & DOSAGE
Prevention of angina pectoris due to coronary artery disease (but not to abort acute anginal attacks)
Adults: 20 mg P.O. b.i.d., with doses 7 hours apart and first dose on awakening. For extended-release tablets, 30 to 60 mg P.O. once daily, on arising; after several days, dosage may be increased to 120 mg once daily; rarely, 240 mg may be required.

PHARMACODYNAMICS
Antianginal action: Isosorbide mononitrate is the major active metabolite of isosorbide dinitrate. It relaxes vascular smooth muscle and consequently dilates peripheral arteries and veins. Dilation of the veins promotes peripheral pooling of blood and decreases venous return to the heart, thereby reducing left ventricular end-diastolic pressure and pulmonary capillary wedge pressure (preload). Arteriolar relaxation reduces systemic vascular resistance, systolic arterial pressure, and mean arterial pressure (afterload). Dilation of the coronary arteries also occurs.

PHARMACOKINETICS
Absorption: Absolute bioavailability of isosorbide mononitrate is almost 100%. Serum levels peak 30 to 60 minutes after ingestion.
Distribution: Drug volume of distribution is about 0.6 L/kg. Less than 4% is bound to plasma proteins.
Metabolism: Drug isn't subject to first-pass metabolism in the liver.
Excretion: Less than 1% of isosorbide mononitrate is eliminated in urine. Overall elimination half-life of drug is about 5 hours.

CONTRAINDICATIONS & PRECAUTIONS
Contraindicated in patients with hypersensitivity or idiosyncratic reaction to nitrates, severe hypotension, shock, or acute MI with low left ventricular filling pressure. Use cautiously in patients with hypotension or blood volume depletion (such as from diuretic therapy).

INTERACTIONS
Drug-drug. Use with *calcium channel blockers* or *organic nitrates* can cause marked symptomatic orthostatic hypotension; dose adjustments of either class of drugs may be necessary. Use with *vasodilators* may cause additive vasodilating effects; monitor closely.
Drug-lifestyle. Use with *alcohol* may cause additive vasodilating effects; discourage use.

ADVERSE REACTIONS
CNS: headache (sometimes with throbbing), dizziness, weakness.

Reactions may be *common*, uncommon, *life-threatening*, or **COMMON AND LIFE-THREATENING**.

CV: *orthostatic hypotension, tachycardia, palpitations, ankle edema, flushing,* fainting.
GI: nausea, vomiting, sublingual burning.
Musculoskeletal: arthralgia.
Respiratory: bronchitis, pneumonia, upper respiratory tract infection.
Skin: cutaneous vasodilation, rash.
Other: hypersensitivity reactions.

▣ KEY CONSIDERATIONS

• Monitor geriatric patients closely for dizziness and other signs of hypotension.
• Drug-free interval sufficient to avoid tolerance to drug isn't completely defined. The recommended regimen involves two daily doses given 7 hours apart, with a gap of 17 hours between the second dose of 1 day and the first dose of the next day. Considering the relatively long half-life of drug, this result is consistent with those obtained for other organic nitrates.
• The asymmetric twice-daily regimen successfully avoids significant rebound or withdrawal effects. In studies of other nitrates, the incidence and magnitude of such phenomena appear to be highly dependent on the schedule of nitrate administration.
• Onset of action of oral drug isn't fast enough to be useful in aborting an acute anginal episode.
• Benefits of drug in patients with acute MI or heart failure haven't been established. Because drug's effects are difficult to terminate rapidly, its use isn't recommended in such patients. If it's used, however, careful clinical or hemodynamic monitoring must be performed to avoid the hazards of hypotension and tachycardia.
• Methemoglobinemia has occurred in patients receiving other organic nitrates and probably could occur as an adverse reaction. Significant methemoglobinemia has occurred in association with moderate overdoses of organic nitrates. Suspect methemoglobinemia in patients who exhibit signs of impaired oxygen delivery despite adequate cardiac output and adequate PaO_2. Classically, methemoglobinemic blood is chocolate brown, without color change on exposure to air.

Treatment of choice for methemoglobinemia is methylene blue, 1 to 2 mg/kg I.V.

Patient education

• Tell patient to follow prescribed dosing schedule carefully (two doses taken 7 hours apart) to maintain antianginal effect and to prevent tolerance.
• Warn patient that daily headaches sometimes accompany treatment with nitrates, including isosorbide mononitrate, and are a marker of drug activity. Patient shouldn't alter treatment schedule because loss of headache may be associated with simultaneous loss of antianginal efficacy. Tell patient to treat headaches with aspirin or acetaminophen.
• Warn patient to avoid alcohol while taking drug because of increased risk of light-headedness.
• Tell patient to rise slowly from recumbent or seated position to avoid light-headedness caused by sudden drop in blood pressure.
• Advise patient that extended-release tablets shouldn't be crushed or chewed.

Overdose & treatment

• Signs and symptoms of overdose may include increased intracranial pressure; persistent, throbbing headache; confusion; moderate fever; vertigo; palpitations; visual disturbances; nausea and vomiting (possibly with colic and even bloody diarrhea); syncope (especially with upright position); air hunger and dyspnea (later followed by reduced ventilatory effort); diaphoresis, with skin either flushed or cold and clammy; heart block and bradycardia; paralysis; coma; seizures; and death.
• No specific antagonist to drug's vasodilator effects is known. However, drug is significantly removed from the blood during hemodialysis.
• If drug is ingested, induce vomiting or perform gastric lavage, followed by activated charcoal administration. Because drug is rapidly and completely absorbed, however, gastric lavage may be effective only with recent ingestion. Treat severe hypotension and reflex tachycardia by elevating the legs and administering I.V.

fluids. Epinephrine is ineffective in reversing severe hypotension associated with overdose, and epinephrine and related compounds are contraindicated. Administer oxygen and artificial ventilation if necessary. Monitor methemoglobin levels as indicated.

---

isradipine
DynaCirc

Calcium channel blocker, antihypertensive

Available by prescription only
Capsules: 2.5 mg, 5 mg

INDICATIONS & DOSAGE
Management of hypertension
Adults: Individualize dosage. Initially, 2.5 mg P.O. b.i.d. alone or with thiazide diuretic. Maximal response may require 2 to 4 weeks; therefore, dosage adjustments of 5 mg daily should be made at 2- to 4-week intervals up to maximum of 20 mg daily. Doses of 10 mg or more per day haven't been shown to be more effective but increase the incidence of adverse reactions.

PHARMACODYNAMICS
Antihypertensive action: A dihydropyridine calcium channel blocker, isradipine binds to calcium channels and inhibits calcium flux into cardiac and smooth muscle, which results in dilation of arterioles. This dilation reduces systemic resistance and lowers blood pressure while producing small increases in resting heart rate.

PHARMACOKINETICS
Absorption: About 90% to 95% of isradipine is absorbed after oral administration; levels peak in 1½ hours.
Distribution: About 95% is bound to plasma protein.
Metabolism: Drug is completely metabolized before elimination, with extensive first-pass metabolism.
Excretion: About 60% to 65% of drug is excreted in urine; 25% to 30% in feces.

CONTRAINDICATIONS & PRECAUTIONS
Contraindicated in patients with hypersensitivity to isradipine. Use cautiously in patients with heart failure, especially if combined with a beta blocker.

INTERACTIONS
Drug-drug. Severe hypotension has been reported with use of a *beta blocker* and a *calcium channel blocker* during *fentanyl anesthesia* but hasn't been seen with isradipine. Additive negative inotropic effects are possible when used with a *beta blocker* in patients with some degree of heart failure.

ADVERSE REACTIONS
CNS: dizziness, *headache,* fatigue.
CV: edema, flushing, syncope, angina, tachycardia.
GI: nausea, diarrhea, abdominal discomfort, vomiting.
Respiratory: dyspnea.
Skin: rash.

▣ KEY CONSIDERATIONS
• Drug has no significant effect on heart rate and no adverse effects on cardiac contractility, conduction or digitalis clearance, or lipid or renal function.
• Administration with food increases the time to reach peak levels by about 1 hour. However, food has no effect on total bioavailability of drug.
• Elevated liver function test results have been reported in some patients.
• Individualize dosage. Allow 2 to 4 weeks between dosage adjustments.

Patient education
• Instruct patient to report irregular heartbeat, shortness of breath, swelling of hands or feet, pronounced dizziness, constipation, nausea, or hypotension.

Overdose & treatment
• No well-documented cases of overdose have been reported; however, this would presumably cause excessive peripheral vasodilation with marked and prolonged systemic hypotension.
• Symptomatic and supportive treatment should be provided, including active CV support, monitoring of input and output and cardiac and respiratory function, el-

---

Reactions may be *common*, uncommon, *life-threatening*, or COMMON AND LIFE-THREATENING.

evation of lower extremities, and fluid replacement as needed. Vasoconstrictors should be used only when not specifically contraindicated.

itraconazole
Sporanox

Synthetic triazole, antifungal

Available by prescription only
Capsules: 100 mg

INDICATIONS & DOSAGE
Treatment of blastomycosis (pulmonary and extrapulmonary), histoplasmosis (including chronic cavitary pulmonary disease and disseminated nonmeningeal histoplasmosis)
Adults: 200 mg P.O. once daily. If condition doesn't improve or shows evidence of progressive fungal disease, increase dose in 100-mg increments to maximum of 400 mg daily. Give doses over 200 mg/day in 2 divided doses.
Aspergillosis (pulmonary and extrapulmonary) in patients who are intolerant of or refractory to amphotericin B therapy
Adults: 200 to 400 mg P.O. daily.
◊ *Treatment of superficial mycoses (dermatophytoses, pityriasis versicolor, sebopsoriasis, candidiasis [vaginal, oral, or chronic mucocutaneous], onychomycosis),* ◊ *systemic mycoses (candidiasis, cryptococcal infections [meningitis, disseminated],* ◊ *dimorphic infections [paracoccidioidomycosis, coccidioidomycosis]),* ◊ *subcutaneous mycoses (sporotrichosis, chromomycosis),* ◊ *cutaneous leishmaniasis,* ◊ *fungal keratitis,* ◊ *alternariatoxicosis, and* ◊ *zygomycosis*
Adults: 50 to 400 mg P.O. daily. Duration of therapy varies from 1 day to greater than 6 months, depending on the condition and mycologic response.

PHARMACODYNAMICS
Antifungal action: Itraconazole is a synthetic triazole antifungal agent. In vitro, itraconazole inhibits the cytochrome P-450-dependent synthesis of ergosterol,

a vital component of fungal cell membranes.

PHARMACOKINETICS
Absorption: Oral bioavailability of itraconazole is maximal when taken with food; absolute oral bioavailability is 55%.
Distribution: Plasma protein-binding of drug is 99.8%; 99.5% for its metabolite, hydroxyitraconazole.
Metabolism: Drug is extensively metabolized by the liver into a large number of metabolites, including hydroxyitraconazole, the major metabolite.
Excretion: Fecal excretion of parent drug varies between 3% and 18% of the dose. Renal excretion of parent drug is less than 0.03% of dose. About 40% of dose is excreted as inactive metabolites in the urine. Drug isn't removed by hemodialysis.

CONTRAINDICATIONS & PRECAUTIONS
Contraindicated in patients with hypersensitivity to itraconazole. Coadministration with cisapride is contraindicated because serious CV events (prolonged QT interval), including death, have occurred in patients taking itraconazole with cisapride.

Use cautiously in patients with hypochlorhydria or HIV infection and in those receiving drugs that are highly protein-bound.

INTERACTIONS
Drug-drug. Itraconazole may increase plasma *cyclosporine* levels; reduce cyclosporine dosage by 50% when using itraconazole doses greater than 100 mg/day, and monitor cyclosporine levels. Itraconazole may increase *digoxin* levels, so these levels should be monitored. *H_2 antagonists, isoniazid, phenytoin,* and *rifampin* may reduce plasma itraconazole levels. Itraconazole can increase plasma levels of the *nonsedating antihistamines,* resulting in rare instances of life-threatening arrhythmias and death; avoid use. Itraconazole can increase levels of *cisapride,* causing prolongation of the QT interval and, rarely, serious ventricular arrhythmias; avoid use. Itraconazole may alter *phenytoin* metabolism; moni-

tor phenytoin levels. Use with *sulfonyl-ureas* may cause hypoglycemia; monitor blood glucose levels. Itraconazole may enhance the anticoagulant effect of *warfarin;* monitor PT and INR.

Drug-food. *Food* enhances absorption; take together.

ADVERSE REACTIONS

CNS: headache, dizziness, somnolence, fatigue, malaise.
CV: hypertension, edema.
GI: *nausea,* vomiting, diarrhea, abdominal pain, anorexia.
GU: albuminuria, decreased libido, impotence.
Hepatic: impaired hepatic function.
Metabolic: hypokalemia.
Skin: rash, pruritus.
Other: fever.

◎ KEY CONSIDERATIONS

● In life-threatening situations, the recommended loading dose is 200 mg 3 times daily (600 mg/day) for first 3 days. Continue treatment for minimum of 3 months and until clinical parameters and laboratory tests indicate that the active fungal infection has subsided. An inadequate period of treatment may lead to recurrence of active infection.
● Obtain specimens for fungal cultures and other relevant laboratory studies (wet mount, histopathology, serology) before therapy to isolate and identify causative organisms. Therapy may be instituted before results of cultures and other laboratory studies are known; once results become available, adjust anti-infective therapy accordingly.
● The course of histoplasmosis in HIV-infected patients is more severe and usually requires maintenance therapy to prevent relapse. Because hypochlorhydria has occurred in HIV-infected patients, absorption of itraconazole may be decreased.
● Monitor hepatic enzymes in patients with preexisting hepatic function abnormalities. Discontinue drug if patient develops signs and symptoms consistent with liver disease that may be attributable to itraconazole.

Patient education
● Instruct patient to take drug with food to enhance absorption.
● Tell patient to report signs and symptoms that may suggest liver dysfunction (jaundice, unusual fatigue, anorexia, nausea, vomiting, dark urine, pale stool) so that appropriate laboratory testing can be performed.

Overdose & treatment
● Signs and symptoms of overdose are similar to those reported in Adverse reactions.
● In the event of accidental overdose, use supportive measures, including gastric lavage with sodium bicarbonate. Itraconazole isn't removed by dialysis.

Reactions may be *common*, uncommon, *life-threatening*, or COMMON AND LIFE-THREATENING.

Handbook of Geriatric Drug Therapy
Photoguide to tablets and capsules

This photoguide provides full-color photographs of some of the most commonly prescribed tablets and capsules in the United States. Shown in actual size, the drugs are organized alphabetically by trade or generic name for quick reference.

Accupril

10 mg   20 mg

Adalat CC

30 mg
(extended-release)

Allegra

60 mg

Altace

2.5 mg   5 mg

Ambien

5 mg   10 mg

---

amitriptyline hydrochloride

25 mg   50 mg   75 mg

100 mg

---

amoxicillin trihydrate

250 mg   500 mg

Amoxil

125 mg
(chewable)

250 mg
(chewable)

250 mg

500 mg

atenolol

25 mg

Ativan

0.5 mg

1 mg

Augmentin

250 mg/125 mg

500 mg/125 mg

125 mg/31.25 mg
(chewable)

250 mg/62.5 mg
(chewable)

Axid

150 mg

300 mg

Biaxin

250 mg

500 mg

Bumex

0.5 mg

1 mg

2 mg

BuSpar

5 mg

10 mg

15 mg

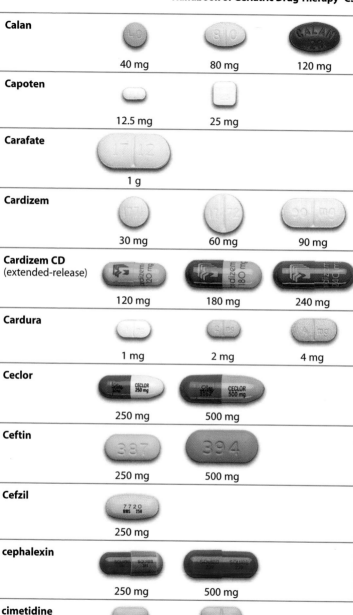

Calan			
	40 mg	80 mg	120 mg

Capoten		
	12.5 mg	25 mg

Carafate	
	1 g

Cardizem			
	30 mg	60 mg	90 mg

Cardizem CD (extended-release)			
	120 mg	180 mg	240 mg

Cardura			
	1 mg	2 mg	4 mg

Ceclor		
	250 mg	500 mg

Ceftin		
	250 mg	500 mg

Cefzil	
	250 mg

cephalexin		
	250 mg	500 mg

cimetidine		
	300 mg	400 mg

Cipro			
	250 mg	500 mg	750 mg

Claritin	
	10 mg

Compazine	
	5 mg	10 mg

Cordarone	
	200 mg

Coreg		
	3.125 mg	6.25 mg	12.5 mg
	25 mg		

Coumadin		
	1 mg	2 mg	2.5 mg
	5 mg	7.5 mg	10 mg

Cozaar	
	25 mg	50 mg

cyclobenzaprine hydrochloride	
	10 mg

Darvocet-N 100	
	100 mg/650 mg

Daypro

600 mg

Deltasone

2.5 mg   5 mg   10 mg

20 mg

Depakote
(delayed-release)

125 mg   250 mg   500 mg

Depakote Sprinkle

125 mg

DiaBeta

1.25 mg   2.5 mg   5 mg

Diflucan

100 mg   150 mg   200 mg

Dilacor XR

180 mg   240 mg

Dilantin Infatabs

50 mg

Dilantin Kapseals

     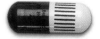

30 mg   100 mg

doxepin hydrochloride

75 mg

Duricef

500 mg

E.E.S.

400 mg

Effexor

25 mg 37.5 mg 50 mg

75 mg 100 mg

Ery-Tab
(delayed-release)

250 mg 333 mg

Erythrocin Stearate Filmtab

250 mg

Erythromycin Base Filmtab

250 mg 500 mg

Estrace

1 mg 2 mg

Fiorinal with Codeine

 325 mg aspirin, 50 mg butalbital, 40 mg caffeine, 30 mg codeine phosphate

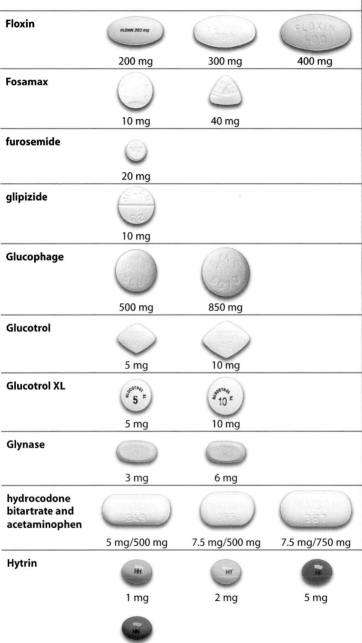

Floxin

200 mg   300 mg   400 mg

Fosamax

10 mg   40 mg

furosemide

20 mg

glipizide

10 mg

Glucophage

500 mg   850 mg

Glucotrol

5 mg   10 mg

Glucotrol XL

5 mg   10 mg

Glynase

3 mg   6 mg

hydrocodone bitartrate and acetaminophen

5 mg/500 mg   7.5 mg/500 mg   7.5 mg/750 mg

Hytrin

1 mg   2 mg   5 mg

10 mg

Inderal

10 mg	20 mg	40 mg

60 mg

K-Dur

10 mEq	20 mEq

Klonopin

0.5 mg	1 mg	2 mg

Lanoxin

0.125 mg	0.25 mg

Lasix

20 mg	40 mg

Levoxyl

0.025 mg	0.05 mg	0.075 mg

0.088 mg	0.1 mg	0.112 mg

0.125 mg	0.137 mg	0.15 mg

0.175 mg	0.2 mg	0.3 mg

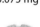

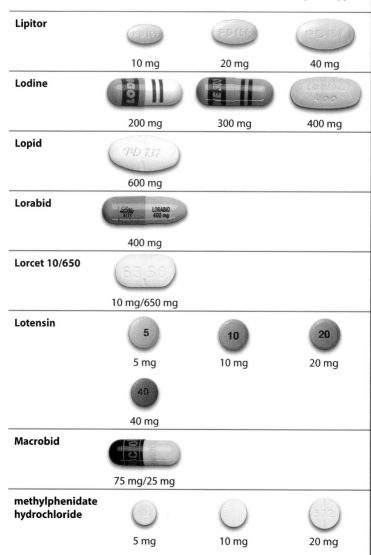

Lipitor

10 mg   20 mg   40 mg

Lodine

200 mg   300 mg   400 mg

Lopid

600 mg

Lorabid

400 mg

Lorcet 10/650

10 mg/650 mg

Lotensin

5 mg   10 mg   20 mg

40 mg

Macrobid

75 mg/25 mg

methylphenidate hydrochloride

5 mg   10 mg   20 mg

20 mg
(extended-release)

Mevacor

| 10 mg | 20 mg | 40 mg |

Micro-K Extencaps
(controlled-release)

10 mEq (750 mg)

Micronase

| 2.5 mg | 5 mg |

Motrin

| 400 mg | 600 mg | 800 mg |

Naprosyn

| 250 mg | 375 mg | 500 mg |

naproxen

| 375 mg | 500 mg |

Nitrostat

| 0.3 mg | 0.4 mg | 0.6 mg |

Nolvadex

10 mg

**nortriptyline
hydrochloride**

| 10 mg | 25 mg | 50 mg |

Norvasc

| 5 mg | 10 mg |

Oruvail

 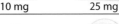

| 100 mg | 150 mg | 200 mg |

Pamelor

10 mg   25 mg   50 mg

75 mg

Paxil

20 mg   30 mg

PCE

333 mg   500 mg

Pepcid

20 mg   40 mg

Percocet

5 mg/325 mg

potassium chloride

10 mEq
(extended-release)

Pravachol

10 mg   20 mg   40 mg

Premarin

0.3 mg
0.625 mg   0.9 mg

1.25 mg
2.5 mg

Prevacid

15 mg   30 mg

Prilosec

10 mg   20 mg

Prinivil

5 mg   10 mg   20 mg

Procardia XL
(extended-release)

30 mg   60 mg   90 mg

propoxyphene napsylate with acetaminophen

100 mg/650 mg

Propulsid

10 mg

Provera

2.5 mg   5 mg   10 mg

Prozac

10 mg   20 mg

Relafen

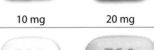
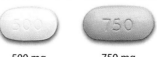

500 mg   750 mg

Risperdal

1 mg

2 mg

3 mg

4 mg

Roxicet

5 mg/325 mg

Sinemet

10 mg/100 mg

25 mg/250 mg

Sinemet CR

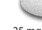
25 mg/100 mg
(extended-release)

Slo-bid Gyrocaps
(extended-release)

50 mg

75 mg

100 mg

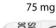
200 mg

300 mg

Sumycin

250 mg

Tagamet

200 mg

300 mg

Tenormin

| 25 mg | 50 mg | 100 mg |

Theo-Dur
(extended-release)

| 100 mg | 200 mg | 300 mg |

450 mg

Ticlid

250 mg

Toprol XL

| 50 mg | 100 mg | 200 mg |

Toradol

10 mg

Trental

400 mg

Trimox

| 250 mg | 500 mg |

Tylenol with Codeine No. 3

300 mg/30 mg

Ultram

50 mg

Valium

2 mg   5 mg   10 mg

Vasotec

2.5 mg   5 mg   10 mg

20 mg

Veetids

250 mg   500 mg

verapamil hydrochloride

180 mg
(sustained-release)

Verelan
(sustained-release)

120 mg   240 mg

Xanax

0.25 mg   0.5 mg   1 mg

Zantac

150 mg   300 mg

Zantac EFFERdose

150 mg

Zestril

5 mg

10 mg

20 mg

40 mg

Zithromax

250 mg

Zocor

5 mg

10 mg

20 mg

Zoloft

50 mg

100 mg

Zovirax

200 mg

400 mg

800 mg

Zyrtec

5 mg

10 mg

ketoconazole
Nizoral

Imidazole derivative, antifungal

Available by prescription only
Tablets: 200 mg
Cream: 2%
Shampoo: 2%

INDICATIONS & DOSAGE
Severe fungal infections caused by susceptible organisms
Adults: Initially, 200 mg P.O. daily as a single dose. Dosage may be increased to 400 mg once daily in patients who don't respond to lower dosage.
Topical treatment of tinea corporis, tinea cruris, tinea versicolor, and tinea pedis
Adults: Apply once daily or b.i.d. for about 2 weeks; for tinea pedis, apply for 6 weeks.
Seborrheic dermatitis
Adults: Apply b.i.d. for about 4 weeks.
Dandruff
Adults: Apply for 1 minute, rinse, then reapply for 3 minutes. Shampoo twice weekly for 4 weeks with at least 3 days between shampoos.
◊***Prostate cancer***
Adults: 400 mg P.O. q 8 hours.

PHARMACODYNAMICS
Antifungal action: Ketoconazole is fungicidal and fungistatic, depending on concentrations. It inhibits demethylation of lanosterol, thereby altering membrane permeability and inhibiting purine transport. The in vitro spectrum of activity includes most pathogenic fungi. However, CSF levels after oral administration are unpredictable. Drug shouldn't be used to treat fungal meningitis, and specimens should be obtained for susceptibility testing before therapy. Currently available tests may not accurately reflect in vivo activity, so interpret results with caution.

Drug is used orally to treat disseminated or pulmonary coccidiomycosis, para-

coccidiomycosis, or histoplasmosis; oral candidiasis; and candiduria (but low renal clearance may limit its usefulness).

It's also useful in some dermatophytoses, including tinea capitis, tinea cruris, tinea pedis, tinea manus, and tinea unguium (onychomycosis) caused by *Epidermophyton, Microsporum,* or *Trichophyton.*

PHARMACOKINETICS
Absorption: Ketoconazole is converted to the hydrochloride salt before absorption. Absorption is erratic; it's decreased by raised gastric pH and may be increased in extent and consistency by food. Plasma levels peak at 1 to 4 hours.
Distribution: Drug is distributed into bile, saliva, cerumen, synovial fluid, and sebum; CSF penetration is erratic and considered minimal. Drug is 84% to 99% bound to plasma proteins.
Metabolism: Drug is converted into several inactive metabolites in the liver.
Excretion: More than 50% of a dose is excreted in feces within 4 days; drug and metabolites are secreted in bile. About 13% is excreted unchanged in urine. Half-life is biphasic, initially 2 hours, with a terminal half-life of 8 hours.

CONTRAINDICATIONS & PRECAUTIONS
Contraindicated in patients with hypersensitivity to ketoconazole and in those taking cisapride because of potential for serious CV adverse events. Use oral form cautiously in patients with hepatic disease. Because CSF levels of ketoconazole are unpredictable after oral administration, don't use drug alone to treat fungal meningitis.

INTERACTIONS
Drug-drug. Use with *corticosteroids* may result in increased plasma corticosteroid levels. Ketoconazole may interfere with the metabolism of *cyclosporine* and thus raise serum cyclosporine levels. Use of ketoconazole with *drugs that raise gastric pH*—such as *antacids, antimuscarinics, cimetidine, famotidine,* and *ranitidine*—decreases absorption of

ketoconazole. Ketoconazole may enhance the toxicity of other *hepatotoxic drugs*. Ketoconazole may intensify the effects of *oral sulfonylureas*. Use with *phenytoin* may alter serum levels of both drugs. *Rifampin* may decrease serum ketoconazole levels, making the drug ineffective. Ketoconazole may enhance the anticoagulant effects of *warfarin*.

Drug-food. *Citrus juice* increases absorption; encourage patient to take oral forms with citrus juice.

Drug-lifestyle. Ketoconazole may interact with *alcohol* to cause a disulfiram-like reaction. Discourage alcohol use.

ADVERSE REACTIONS

CNS: headache, nervousness, dizziness, somnolence, photophobia, *suicidal tendencies,* severe depression (with oral administration).

GI: *nausea, vomiting,* abdominal pain, diarrhea (with oral administration).

GU: gynecomastia with tenderness, fever, chills, impotence (with oral administration).

Hematologic: *thrombocytopenia,* hemolytic anemia, *leukopenia* (with oral administration).

Hepatic: elevated liver enzyme levels, *fatal hepatotoxicity* (with oral administration).

Skin: pruritus; severe irritation, stinging (with topical administration).

☒ KEY CONSIDERATIONS

● Identify organism, but don't delay therapy for results of laboratory tests.
● Give drug with citrus juice.
● Monitor for signs of hepatotoxicity: persistent nausea, unusual fatigue, jaundice, dark urine, and pale stools.
● Drug requires acidity for absorption and is ineffective in patients with achlorhydria.
● Drug has been reported to cause transient elevations of AST, ALT, and alkaline phosphatase levels; it has also been reported to cause transient alterations of serum cholesterol and triglyceride levels.

Patient education

● Teach achlorhydric patients how to take ketoconazole: dissolve each tablet in 4 ml of 0.2N hydrochloric acid solution or take with 200 ml of 0.1N hydrochloric acid, and administer through a glass or plastic straw to avoid damaging tooth enamel. Tell patient to drink a glass of water after each dose.
● Tell patient to avoid driving or performing other hazardous activities if dizziness or drowsiness occur; these often occur early in treatment but abate as treatment continues.
● Caution patient not to alter dose or dosage interval or to discontinue drug without medical approval. Explain that therapy must continue until active fungal infection is completely eradicated to prevent recurrence.
● Reassure patient that nausea will subside; to minimize reaction, patient may take drug with food or may divide dosage into two doses.
● Advise patient to avoid self-prescribed preparations for GI distress (for example, antacids); some may alter gastric pH and interfere with drug action.
● Encourage patient to get medical approval before taking other drugs with ketoconazole.

Overdose & treatment

● Overdose may cause dizziness, tinnitus, headache, nausea, vomiting, or diarrhea; patients with adrenal hypofunction or patients on long-term corticosteroid therapy may show signs of adrenal crisis.
● To treat overdose, induce vomiting and perform sodium bicarbonate lavage, followed by activated charcoal and a cathartic, and supportive measures as needed.

---

ketoprofen
Actron, Orudis, Orudis KT, Oruvail

NSAID, nonnarcotic analgesic, antipyretic, anti-inflammatory

Available by prescription only
Capsules: 25 mg, 50 mg, 75 mg
Capsules (extended-release): 100 mg, 150 mg, 200 mg
Available without a prescription
Tablets: 12.5 mg

Reactions may be *common*, uncommon, *life-threatening*, or **COMMON AND LIFE-THREATENING**.

INDICATIONS & DOSAGE

Rheumatoid arthritis and osteoarthritis
Adults: Usual dose is 75 mg t.i.d. or 50 mg q.i.d. P.O. Maximum dosage is 300 mg/day; or 200 mg (extended-release capsules) P.O. daily.
Mild to moderate pain; dysmenorrhea
Adults: 25 to 50 mg P.O. q 6 to 8 hours, p.r.n.
Temporary relief of mild aches and pain, fever (self-medication)
Adults: 12.5 mg q 4 to 6 hours. Don't exceed 75 mg in a 24-hour period.

PHARMACODYNAMICS

Analgesic, antipyretic, and anti-inflammatory actions: Mechanisms of action are unknown; ketoprofen is thought to inhibit prostaglandin synthesis.

PHARMACOKINETICS

Absorption: Ketoprofen is absorbed rapidly and completely from the GI tract.
Distribution: Drug is highly protein-bound. Extent of body-tissue fluid distribution is unknown, but therapeutic levels range from 0.4 to 6 µg/ml.
Metabolism: Drug is metabolized in the liver.
Excretion: Drug is excreted in urine as parent drug and its metabolites.

CONTRAINDICATIONS & PRECAUTIONS

Contraindicated in patients with hypersensitivity to ketoprofen or history of aspirin- or NSAID-induced asthma, urticaria, or other allergic-type reactions. Use cautiously in patients with impaired renal or hepatic function, peptic ulcer disease, heart failure, hypertension, or fluid retention.

INTERACTIONS

Drug-drug. Use with *acetaminophen, gold compounds,* or *other anti-inflammatories* may increase nephrotoxicity Use of ketoprofen with *anticoagulants* or *thrombolytics* (such as *coumarin derivatives, heparin, streptokinase,* and *urokinase*) may potentiate anticoagulant effects. Ketoprofen may decrease the effectiveness of *antihypertensives* and *diuretics;* use with diuretics may increase nephrotoxic potential. Use with *anti-inflammatories, corticotropin, salicy-*lates, or *steroids* may cause increased GI adverse effects, including ulceration and hemorrhage. *Aspirin* may decrease the bioavailability of ketoprofen. Toxicity may occur with *coumarin derivatives, nifedipine, phenytoin,* or *verapamil.* Bleeding problems may occur if ketoprofen is used with other *drugs that inhibit platelet aggregation,* such as *anti-inflammatories, aspirin, parenteral carbenicillin, cefamandole, cefoperazone, dextran, dipyridamole, mezlocillin, piperacillin, plicamycin, salicylates, sulfinpyrazone, ticarcillin,* or *valproic acid.* Ketoprofen may displace *highly protein-bound drugs* from binding sites. Because of the influence of prostaglandins on glucose metabolism, use with *insulin* or *oral antidiabetics* may potentiate hypoglycemic effects. Ketoprofen may decrease renal clearance of *lithium* and *methotrexate.*

Drug-lifestyle. *Alcohol* may increase risk for bleeding; advise patient to avoid alcoholic beverages during therapy. *Sun exposure* increases the risk of photosensitivity reactions; take precautions.

ADVERSE REACTIONS

CNS: *headache, dizziness, CNS excitation* or depression.
EENT: tinnitus, visual disturbances.
GI: *nausea, abdominal pain, diarrhea, constipation, flatulence, **peptic ulceration,*** dyspepsia, anorexia, vomiting, stomatitis.
GU: *nephrotoxicity,* elevated BUN levels.
Hematologic: prolonged bleeding time, ***thrombocytopenia, agranulocytosis.***
Hepatic: elevated liver enzyme levels.
Respiratory: dyspnea, ***bronchospasm, laryngeal edema.***
Skin: rash, photosensitivity, ***exfoliative dermatitis.***
Other: peripheral edema.

▣ KEY CONSIDERATIONS

Besides the recommendations relevant to all NSAIDs, consider the following:
• Patients older than age 60 may be more susceptible to the toxic effects of ketoprofen. Plasma and renal clearance are reduced and plasma half-life is pro-

longed in geriatric patients. Use with caution.

• The effects of drug on renal prostaglandins may cause fluid retention and edema, a significant drawback for geriatric patients and those with heart failure. The manufacturer recommends that initial dose be reduced by 33% to 50% in geriatric patients.

• Administer tablets on an empty stomach either 30 minutes before or 2 hours after meals to ensure adequate absorption.

• Capsules may be taken with food or antacids to minimize GI distress.

• Store suppositories in refrigerator.

• Monitor CNS effects of drug. Institute safety measures, such as assisted walking, raised side rails, and gradual position changes, to prevent injury.

• Watch for possible photosensitivity reactions.

• Monitor laboratory test results for abnormalities.

Patient education

• Instruct patient in prescribed drug regimen and proper drug administration.

• Tell patient to seek medical approval before taking OTC drugs (especially aspirin and aspirin-containing products).

• Caution patient to avoid activities that require alertness or concentration. Instruct him in safety measures to prevent injury.

• Advise patient of potential photosensitivity reactions. Recommend use of sunscreen.

• Instruct patient to report adverse reactions.

• Advise patient to avoid alcoholic beverages during therapy.

Overdose & treatment

• Signs and symptoms of overdose include nausea and drowsiness.

• To treat drug overdose, immediately induce vomiting with ipecac syrup or perform gastric lavage. Administer activated charcoal via NG tube. Provide symptomatic and supportive measures (respiratory support and correction of fluid and electrolyte imbalances). Monitor laboratory parameters and vital signs closely. Hemodialysis may be useful in removing ketoprofen and assisting in care of renal failure.

ketorolac tromethamine
Toradol

NSAID, analgesic

Available by prescription only
Tablets: 10 mg
Injection: 15 mg/ml (1-ml cartridge), 30 mg/ml (1-ml and 2-ml cartridges)

INDICATIONS & DOSAGE
Short-term management of pain
Adults: Dosage should be based on patient response. Initially, 60 mg I.M. or 30 mg I.V. as a single dose, or multiple doses of 30 mg I.M. or I.V. q 6 hours. Maximum daily dose shouldn't exceed 120 mg.
Geriatric patients: In adults age 65 or older, 30 mg I.M. or 15 mg I.V. initially as a single dose, or multiple doses of 15 mg I.M. or I.V. q 6 hours. Maximum daily dose shouldn't exceed 60 mg.
✦ *Dosage adjustment.* In patients with renal impairment or those who weigh less than 50 kg (110 lb), 30 mg I.M. or 15 mg I.V. initially as a single dose, or multiple doses of 15 mg I.M. or I.V. q 6 hours. Maximum daily dose shouldn't exceed 60 mg.
Short-term management of moderately severe, acute pain when switching from parenteral to oral administration
Adults younger than age 65: 20 mg P.O. as a single dose followed by 10 mg P.O. q 4 to 6 hours, not to exceed 40 mg/day.
Geriatric patients: 10 mg P.O. as a single dose, followed by 10 mg P.O. q 4 to 6 hours, not to exceed 40 mg/day.
✦ *Dosage adjustment.* In patients with renal impairment or those who weigh less than 50 kg (110 lb), 10 mg P.O. as a single dose, followed by 10 mg P.O. q 4 to 6 hours, not to exceed 40 mg/day.

PHARMACODYNAMICS
Analgesic action: Ketorolac is an NSAID that acts by inhibiting the synthesis of prostaglandins.

Reactions may be *common,* uncommon, *life-threatening,* or COMMON AND LIFE-THREATENING.

PHARMACOKINETICS

Absorption: Ketorolac is completely absorbed after I.M. administration. After oral administration, food delays absorption but doesn't decrease total amount of drug absorbed.

Distribution: Mean plasma levels peak about 30 minutes after a 50-mg dose and range from 2.2 to 3 mcg/ml. More than 99% of drug is protein-bound.

Metabolism: Primarily hepatic; a para-hydroxy metabolite and conjugates have been identified; less than 50% of a dose is metabolized. Liver impairment doesn't substantially alter drug clearance.

Excretion: Primary excretion is in the urine (more than 90%); the rest in feces. Terminal plasma half-life is 3.8 to 6.3 hours (average 4.5 hours); it's substantially prolonged in patients with renal failure.

CONTRAINDICATIONS & PRECAUTIONS

Contraindicated in patients with hypersensitivity to ketorolac, active peptic ulcer disease, recent GI bleeding or perforation, advanced renal impairment, risk for renal impairment due to volume depletion, suspected or confirmed cerebrovascular bleeding, hemorrhagic diathesis, incomplete hemostasis, or high risk of bleeding.

Also contraindicated in patients with history of peptic ulcer disease or GI bleeding, or past allergic reactions to aspirin or other NSAIDs. In addition, drug is contraindicated as a prophylactic analgesic before major surgery or intraoperatively when hemostasis is critical; in patients receiving aspirin, an NSAID, or probenecid; and in those requiring analgesics to be administered epidurally or intrathecally.

Use cautiously in patients with impaired renal or hepatic function.

INTERACTIONS

Drug-drug. Use with *diuretics* may decrease efficacy of diuretic and enhance nephrotoxicity. Ketorolac increases *lithium* levels, decreases *methotrexate* clearance and increase its toxicity, and increases blood levels of free (unbound) *salicylates* or *warfarin* (significance is unknown).

Drug-lifestyle. *Alcohol* may increase risk of bleeding; advise patient to avoid alcoholic beverages during therapy.

ADVERSE REACTIONS

CNS: *drowsiness, sedation,* dizziness, *headache.*
CV: edema, hypertension, palpitations, *arrhythmias.*
GI: *nausea, dyspepsia, GI pain,* diarrhea, peptic ulceration, vomiting, constipation, flatulence, stomatitis.
GU: *renal failure.*
Hematologic: decreased platelet adhesion, purpura, *thrombocytopenia.*
Skin: pruritus, rash.
Other: pain (at injection site), diaphoresis.

▣ KEY CONSIDERATIONS

• In clinical trials, terminal half-life of drug was longer in geriatric patients than in patients younger than age 65 (average was 7 hours in geriatric patients).
• Like other NSAIDs, ketorolac has been associated with borderline elevations of one or more liver function test results. Meaningful elevations of AST or ALT—three times the upper normal limit—occur in less than 1% of patients. Because drug inhibits platelet aggregation, it can prolong bleeding time.
• Drug is intended for short-term management of pain. The rate and severity of adverse reactions should be less than those observed in patients taking NSAIDs on a regular basis.
• I.M. injections in patients with coagulopathies or those receiving anticoagulants may cause bleeding and hematoma at the site of injection.
• The combined duration of ketorolac I.M., I.V., or P.O. shouldn't exceed 5 days. Oral use is only for continuation of I.V. or I.M. therapy.
• Hypovolemia should be corrected before initiating therapy with ketorolac.

Patient education

• Warn patient that GI ulceration, bleeding, and perforation can occur at any time, with or without warning, in anyone taking NSAIDs on a long-term basis. Teach patient how to recognize the signs and symptoms of GI bleeding.

---

*Canada only   ◊ Unlabeled clinical use

• Instruct patient to avoid aspirin, aspirin-containing products, and alcoholic beverages during therapy.

Overdose & treatment

• Doses greater than 100 mg/kg may decrease motor activity and cause diarrhea, pallor, crackles, labored breathing, and vomiting.
• Withhold drug and provide supportive treatment.

L

labetalol hydrochloride
Normodyne, Trandate

Alpha-adrenergic blocker and beta blocker, antihypertensive

Available by prescription only
Tablets: 100 mg, 200 mg, 300 mg
Injection: 5 mg/ml in 20-ml, 40-ml, and 60-ml vials and 4-ml and 8-ml disposable syringes

INDICATIONS & DOSAGE
Hypertension
Adults: 100 mg P.O. b.i.d. with or without a diuretic. Dosage may be increased by 100 mg b.i.d. q 2 or 4 days until optimum response is reached. Usual maintenance dosage is 200 to 400 mg b.i.d.; maximum daily dose is 2,400 mg.
Severe hypertension and hypertensive emergencies; ◇pheochromocytoma; ◇clonidine withdrawal hypertension
Adults: Initially, 20-mg I.V. bolus slowly over 2 minutes; may repeat injections of 40 to 80 mg q 10 minutes to maximum dose of 300 mg.
   Alternatively, may be given as continuous I.V. infusion at an initial rate of 2 mg/minute until satisfactory response is obtained. Usual cumulative dose is 50 to 200 mg.
◇Intraoperative hypertension
Adults: Initially, 10 to 30 mg I.V. bolus slowly; may repeat injections of 5 to 10 mg I.V., p.r.n.

PHARMACODYNAMICS
Antihypertensive action: Labetalol inhibits catecholamine access to both beta and postsynaptic alpha-adrenergic receptor sites. Drug may also have a vasodilating effect.

PHARMACOKINETICS
Absorption: Oral absorption is high (90% to 100%); however, labetalol undergoes extensive first-pass metabolism in the liver, and only about 25% of an oral dose reaches the systemic circulation unchanged. Antihypertensive effect

occurs in 20 minutes to 2 hours, peaking in 1 to 4 hours. After direct I.V. administration, antihypertensive effect occurs in 2 to 5 minutes; maximal effect occurs in 5 to 15 minutes.
Distribution: Drug is distributed widely throughout the body; it's about 50% protein-bound.
Metabolism: Orally administered drug is metabolized extensively in the liver and possibly in GI mucosa.
Excretion: About 5% of a dose is excreted unchanged in urine; the rest is excreted as metabolites in urine and feces (biliary elimination). Antihypertensive effect of an oral dose persists for about 8 to 24 hours; after I.V. administration, it lasts 2 to 4 hours. Plasma half-life is about 5½ hours after I.V. administration or 6 to 8 hours after oral administration.

CONTRAINDICATIONS & PRECAUTIONS
Contraindicated in patients with bronchial asthma, overt cardiac failure, greater than first-degree heart block, cardiogenic shock, severe bradycardia, other conditions associated with severe and prolonged hypotension, and hypersensitivity to labetalol.
   Use cautiously in patients with heart failure, hepatic failure, chronic bronchitis, emphysema, preexisting peripheral vascular disease, and pheochromocytoma.

INTERACTIONS
Drug-drug. Labetalol may antagonize bronchodilation produced by *beta agonists*. Oral *cimetidine* may increase bioavailability of oral labetalol, so labetalol dosage should be adjusted. Labetalol may potentiate the antihypertensive effects of *diuretics* and *other antihypertensives;* use of *I.V. labetalol* may result in synergistic antihypertensive effect. *Glutethimide* may decrease bioavailability of oral labetalol, requiring adjustment in labetalol dosage. *Halothane* at concentrations of 3% or more may cause myocardial depression; avoid use. Labetalol blunts the reflex tachycardia produced by *nitroglycerin* without preventing its

hypotensive effect; if used with nitroglycerin in patients with angina, additional antihypertensive effects may occur. Use with *tricyclic antidepressants* may increase incidence of labetalol-induced tremor.

ADVERSE REACTIONS

CNS: vivid dreams, fatigue, headache, paresthesia, syncope, transient scalp tingling.
CV: *orthostatic hypotension, dizziness, ventricular arrhythmias.*
EENT: nasal stuffiness.
GI: nausea, vomiting, diarrhea.
GU: sexual dysfunction, urine retention.
Musculoskeletal: muscle spasm, toxic myopathy.
Respiratory: dyspnea, *bronchospasm.*
Skin: rash.

▣ KEY CONSIDERATIONS

Besides the recommendations relevant to all beta blockers, consider the following:
• Geriatric patients may require lower maintenance dosages of labetalol because of increased bioavailability or delayed metabolism; they also may experience enhanced adverse effects. Use drug with caution in geriatric patients.
• Unlike other beta blockers, labetalol doesn't decrease resting heart rate or cardiac output.
• Dosage reduction may be needed in patients with hepatic insufficiency.
• Dizziness is the most troublesome adverse effect; it tends to occur in early stages of treatment and in patients taking diuretics or receiving higher doses.
• Transient scalp tingling occurs occasionally at beginning of drug therapy. This usually subsides quickly.
• Investigational uses include managing chronic stable angina pectoris, excessive sympathetic activity associated with tetanus, and uncontrolled hypertension before and during anesthesia.
• Don't mix labetalol with 5% sodium bicarbonate injection because of incompatibility.
• When changing hospitalized patients from parenteral to oral labetalol, begin with 200 mg, then give 200 to 400 mg P.O. after 6 to 12 hours. Oral dosage may then be increased in usual increments at 1-day intervals, if necessary, to achieve the desired blood pressure control. Dose may be given 2 or 3 times daily.
• Drug therapy may cause a false-positive increase of urine free and total catecholamine levels when measured by fluorometric or photometric methods. Use specific radioenzyme or HPLC assay techniques.

Patient education
• Advise patient that transient scalp tingling may occur during initiation of therapy.

Overdose & treatment
• Signs and symptoms of overdose include severe hypotension, bradycardia, heart failure, and bronchospasm.
• After acute ingestion, empty stomach by inducing vomiting or performing gastric lavage, and give activated charcoal to reduce absorption. Subsequent treatment is usually symptomatic and supportive.

---

lactulose
Cephulac, Cholac, Chronulac, Constilac, Constulose, Duphalac, Enulose

Disaccharide, laxative

Available by prescription only
Syrup: 10 g/15 ml, bulk bottles, 30-ml unit dose cups
Rectal solution: 3.33 g/5 ml

INDICATIONS & DOSAGE
Constipation
Adults: 15 to 30 ml P.O. daily (may increase to 60 ml if needed).
To prevent and treat portal-systemic encephalopathy, including hepatic precoma and coma in patients with severe hepatic disease
Adults: Initially, 20 to 30 g (30 to 45 ml) P.O. t.i.d. or q.i.d., until 2 or 3 soft stools are produced daily. Usual dosage is 60 to 100 g daily in divided doses; can also be given by retention enema. Mix 300 ml of lactulose with 700 ml of water or normal saline solution and retain for 60 minutes. May repeat q 4 to 6 hours.

Reactions may be *common,* uncommon, *life-threatening,* or COMMON AND LIFE-THREATENING.

◇ *After barium meal examination*
Adults: 5 to 10 ml P.O. b.i.d. for 1 to 4 weeks.
◇ *To restore bowel movements after hemorrhoidectomy*
Adults: 15 ml P.O. twice during day before surgery and for 5 days postoperatively.

PHARMACODYNAMICS

Laxative action: Because lactulose is indigestible, it passes through the GI tract to the colon unchanged; there, it's digested by normally occurring bacteria. The weak acids produced in this manner increase the stool's fluid content and cause distention, thus promoting peristalsis and bowel evacuation.

Lactulose also is used to reduce serum ammonia levels in patients with hepatic disease. Lactulose breakdown acidifies the colon; this, in turn, converts ammonia (NH_3) to ammonium (NH_4^+), which isn't absorbed and is excreted in the stool. Furthermore, this "ion trapping" effect causes ammonia to diffuse from the blood into the colon, where it's excreted as well.

PHARMACOKINETICS

Absorption: Lactulose is absorbed minimally.
Distribution: Drug is distributed locally, primarily in the colon.
Metabolism: Drug is metabolized by colonic bacteria (absorbed portion isn't metabolized).
Excretion: Mostly excreted in feces; absorbed portion is excreted in urine.

CONTRAINDICATIONS & PRECAUTIONS

Contraindicated in patients on a low-galactose diet. Use cautiously in patients with diabetes mellitus.

INTERACTIONS

Drug-drug. *Neomycin* and *other antibiotics* theoretically may decrease lactulose effectiveness by eliminating the bacteria needed to digest it into the active form. *Nonabsorbable antacids* may decrease lactulose effectiveness by preventing a decrease in the pH of the colon.

ADVERSE REACTIONS

GI: *abdominal cramps, belching, diarrhea, gaseous distention, flatulence,* nausea, vomiting, diarrhea (with excessive dosage).

🔲 KEY CONSIDERATIONS

• Monitor patient's serum electrolyte levels; geriatric patients are more sensitive to possible hypernatremia.
• After administration of drug via nasogastric tube, flush the tube with water to clear it and to ensure drug's passage to stomach.
• Dilute drug with water or fruit juice to minimize its sweet taste.
• For administration by retention enema, patient should retain drug for 30 to 60 minutes. If retained less than 30 minutes, dose should be repeated immediately. Begin oral therapy before discontinuing retention enemas.
• Monitor frequency and consistency of stools.
• Don't administer drug with other laxatives because the loose stools produced may be falsely interpreted as an indication that an adequate dosage of lactulose has been achieved.

Patient education

• Advise patient to take drug with juice to improve taste.

---

lamivudine (3TC)
Epivir, Epivir-HBV

Synthetic nucleoside analogue, antiviral

Available by prescription only
Tablets: 100 mg, 150 mg
Oral solution: 5 mg/ml, 10 mg/ml

INDICATIONS & DOSAGE

Treatment of patients with HIV infection concomitantly with zidovudine
Adults weighing 50 kg (110 lb) or more: 150 mg P.O. b.i.d.
Adults weighing less than 50 kg (110 lb): 2 mg/kg P.O. b.i.d.
✦ *Dosage adjustment.* For patients with renal failure, refer to table.

Treatment of chronic hepatitis B
Adults: 100 mg P.O. daily
✦ *Dosage adjustment.* For patients with renal failure, refer to table.

Creatinine clearance (ml/min)	Recommended dosage
≥ 50	100 mg b.i.d.
30-49	150 mg once daily
15-29	150 mg first dose; then 100 mg once daily
5-14	150 mg first dose; then 50 mg once daily
< 5	50 mg first dose; then 25 mg once daily

PHARMACODYNAMICS
Antiviral action: Lamivudine inhibits HIV reverse transcription via viral DNA chain termination. RNA- and DNA-dependent DNA polymerase activities are also inhibited.

PHARMACOKINETICS
Absorption: Lamivudine is rapidly absorbed after oral administration in HIV-infected patients.
Distribution: Drug is believed to distribute into extravascular spaces. Volume of distribution is independent of dose and doesn't correlate with body weight. Less than 36% is bound to plasma proteins.
Metabolism: Metabolism of lamivudine is a minor route of elimination. The only known metabolite is the trans-sulfoxide metabolite.
Excretion: Drug is primarily eliminated unchanged in urine. Mean elimination half-life ranges from 5 to 7 hours.

CONTRAINDICATIONS & PRECAUTIONS
Contraindicated in patients with hypersensitivity to lamivudine. In patients with history of pancreatitis or other significant risk factors for developing pancreatitis, drug should be used with extreme caution—and only if there's no satisfactory alternative therapy. Treatment with lamivudine should be stopped immediately if signs, symptoms, or laboratory abnormalities suggesting pancreatitis occur.

Use cautiously in patients with impaired renal function; dosage reduction in these patients is necessary.

INTERACTIONS
Drug-drug. Use with *trimethoprim/ sulfamethoxazole* may increase blood lamivudine levels because of decreased drug clearance, but the significance of this interaction is unknown; monitor patient closely.

ADVERSE REACTIONS
Adverse reactions are related to the combination therapy of lamivudine and zidovudine.
CNS: *malaise, headache, fatigue, neuropathy, dizziness, insomnia and other sleep disorders, depressive disorders.*
EENT: *nasal symptoms, sore throat.*
GI: *nausea, diarrhea, vomiting, anorexia,* abdominal pain, abdominal cramps, dyspepsia.
Hematologic: *neutropenia,* anemia, ***thrombocytopenia.***
Hepatic: elevated liver enzyme and bilirubin levels.
Musculoskeletal: *musculoskeletal pain,* myalgia, arthralgia.
Respiratory: *cough.*
Skin: rash.
Other: *fever, chills.*

▣ KEY CONSIDERATIONS
● Drug must be administered concomitantly with zidovudine when treating HIV. It isn't intended for use as monotherapy.
● Safety of drug for greater than 1 year and in patients with liver disease or transplantation hasn't been established when treating for hepatitis B.
● Test for HIV before treating with hepatitis B dosage. Resistance for HIV treatment may occur with the lower dosage.
● Monitor patient's CBC, platelet count, and liver function studies throughout therapy because abnormalities may occur.

Patient education
● Inform patient that long-term effects of lamivudine are unknown.

• Inform the patient about testing for HIV before and during hepatitis treatment. Dosage isn't protective for HIV.
• Tell patient that tablets and oral solution are for oral ingestion only.
• Stress importance of taking drug exactly as prescribed.

lamotrigine
Lamictal

Phenyltriazine, anticonvulsant

Available by prescription only
Tablets: 25 mg, 100 mg, 150 mg, 200 mg
Chewable tablets: 5 mg, 25 mg

INDICATIONS & DOSAGE
Adjunct therapy in treatment of partial seizures caused by epilepsy
Adults: 50 mg P.O. daily for 2 weeks, followed by 100 mg daily in two divided doses for 2 weeks. Thereafter, usual maintenance dose is 300 to 500 mg P.O. daily given in two divided doses. For patients also taking valproic acid, give 25 mg P.O. every other day for 2 weeks, followed by 25 mg P.O. daily for 2 weeks. Thereafter, maximum dosage is 150 mg P.O. daily in two divided doses.

PHARMACODYNAMICS
Anticonvulsant action: Unknown. It's believed to involve inhibition of the release of glutamate and aspartate in the brain. This may occur by action on voltage-sensitive sodium channels.

PHARMACOKINETICS
Absorption: Lamotrigine is rapidly and completely absorbed from the GI tract, with negligible first-pass metabolism. Absolute bioavailability is 98%.
Distribution: About 55% is bound to plasma proteins.
Metabolism: Drug is metabolized predominantly by glucuronic acid conjugation; the major metabolite is an inactive 2-N-glucuronide conjugate.
Excretion: Drug is excreted primarily in urine, with only a small portion excreted in feces.

CONTRAINDICATIONS & PRECAUTIONS
Contraindicated in patients with hypersensitivity to lamotrigine. Use cautiously in patients with impaired renal, hepatic, or cardiac function.

INTERACTIONS
Drug-drug. *Carbamazepine, phenobarbital, phenytoin,* and *primidone* decrease steady-state lamotrigine levels; monitor patient closely. Lamotrigine may not affect *folate inhibitors* (such as *co-trimoxazole* and *methotrexate*) because it inhibits dihydrofolate reductase, an enzyme involved in the synthesis of folic acid; monitor patient closely because drug may have an additive effect. *Valproic acid* decreases clearance of lamotrigine, which increases steady-state drug levels; monitor patient closely for toxicity.
Drug-lifestyle. Photosensitivity reaction may occur to *sunlight;* take precautions.

ADVERSE REACTIONS
CNS: *dizziness, headache, ataxia, somnolence,* incoordination, insomnia, tremor, depression, anxiety, seizures, irritability, speech disorder, decreased memory, concentration disturbance, malaise, sleep disorder, emotional lability, vertigo, mind racing, **suicide attempts.**
CV: palpitations.
EENT: *diplopia, blurred vision,* vision abnormality, nystagmus.
GI: *nausea, vomiting,* diarrhea, dyspepsia, abdominal pain, constipation, tooth disorder, anorexia, dry mouth.
GU: vaginitis.
Musculoskeletal: dysarthria, muscle spasm, neck pain.
Respiratory: rhinitis, pharyngitis, cough, dyspnea.
Skin: *Stevens-Johnson syndrome, rash,* pruritus, hot flashes, alopecia, acne, photosensitivity.
Other: flulike syndrome, fever, infection, chills.

▣ KEY CONSIDERATIONS
• Safety and effectiveness in patients older than age 65 haven't been established.
• Don't discontinue drug abruptly because of risk of increasing seizure fre-

quency. Instead, taper drug over at least 2 weeks.

• Stop drug immediately if drug-induced rash occurs.

• If lamotrigine is added to a multidrug regimen that includes valproate, reduce dose of lamotrigine. Use a lower maintenance dosage in patients with severe renal impairment.

• Evaluate patient for reduction in the frequency and duration of seizures. Periodically evaluate serum levels of the adjunct anticonvulsant.

Patient education

• Inform patient that rash may occur, especially during first 6 weeks of therapy. Combination therapy with valproic acid and lamotrigine is likely to precipitate a serious rash. Although it may resolve with continued therapy, tell patient to report it immediately in case drug needs to be discontinued.

• Warn patient not to perform hazardous activities until CNS effects are known.

• Advise patient to take protective measures against photosensitivity reactions until tolerance is known.

lansoprazole
Prevacid

Proton pump inhibitor, antiulcerative

Available by prescription only
Capsules (delayed-release): 15 mg, 30 mg

INDICATIONS & DOSAGE
Short-term treatment of gastric ulcer
Adults: 30 mg P.O. daily before meals for 8 weeks.
Short-term treatment of duodenal ulcer
Adults: 15 mg P.O. daily before meals for 4 weeks.
Maintenance of healed duodenal ulcers
Adults: 15 mg P.O. daily before meals.
Short-term treatment of symptomatic gastroesophageal reflux disease
Adults: 15 mg P.O. daily before meals for up to 8 weeks.
Long-term treatment of pathological hypersecretory conditions, including Zollinger-Ellison syndrome

Adults: Initially, 60 mg P.O. once daily. Increase dosage, p.r.n., to 180 mg/day. Daily dosages exceeding 120 mg should be administered in divided doses.
Short-term treatment of erosive esophagitis
Adults: 30 mg P.O. daily before meals for 8 weeks. If healing doesn't occur, an additional 8 weeks of therapy may be needed.
Maintenance of healing of erosive esophagitis
Adults: 15 mg P.O. daily before meals.
Eradication of Helicobacter pylori to reduce the risk of duodenal ulcer recurrence
Adults: Triple therapy with lansoprazole 30 mg, amoxicillin 1 g, and clarithromycin 500 mg all given P.O. b.i.d. for 10 or 14 days. Alternatively, dual therapy with lansoprazole 30 mg and amoxicillin 1 g, P.O. t.i.d. for 14 days.

PHARMACODYNAMICS
Antiulcer action: Lansoprazole inhibits activity of the acid (proton) pump and binds to hydrogen-potassium adenosine triphosphatase, located at the secretory surface of the gastric parietal cells, to block the formation of gastric acid.

PHARMACOKINETICS
Absorption: Lansoprazole is rapidly absorbed, with absolute bioavailability of greater than 80%.
Distribution: Drug is 97% bound to plasma proteins.
Metabolism: Drug is extensively metabolized in the liver.
Excretion: About two-thirds of dose is excreted in feces; one third in urine.

CONTRAINDICATIONS & PRECAUTIONS
Contraindicated in patients with hypersensitivity to lansoprazole.

INTERACTIONS
Drug-drug. Lansoprazole may interfere with the absorption of *ampicillin esters, iron salts,* and *ketoconazole.* Monitor patient closely. *Sucralfate* delays lansoprazole absorption. Give lansoprazole at least 30 minutes before sucralfate. Lansoprazole may cause a mild increase in *theophylline* excretion; use cautiously.

Reactions may be *common,* uncommon, *life-threatening,* or COMMON AND LIFE-THREATENING.

(Theophylline dosage may need to be adjusted when lansoprazole is started or stopped.)

ADVERSE REACTIONS
GI: diarrhea, nausea, abdominal pain.

🔲 KEY CONSIDERATIONS
• Dosage adjustment is unnecessary in geriatric patients or in those with renal insufficiency; however, it may be required for patients with severe liver disease.
• Although initial dosing regimen need not be altered for geriatric patients, subsequent doses over 30 mg/day shouldn't be administered unless additional gastric acid suppression is necessary.
• For patients with an NG tube in place, capsules can be opened and the intact granules mixed in 1 oz (30 ml) of apple juice and administered through the tube into the stomach. Then, clear the tube by flushing it with more juice.
• A symptomatic response to lansoprazole doesn't rule out the possbility of gastric malignancy.
• Drug shouldn't be used as maintenance therapy for patients with duodenal ulcer disease or erosive esophagitis.

Patient education
• Instruct patient to take drug before meals.
• Caution patient not to chew or crush capsules; capsules should be swallowed whole.
• Tell patient who has trouble swallowing to open the capsule, sprinkle contents over 1 tbs of applesauce, and swallow immediately.

latanoprost
Xalatan

Prostaglandin analogue, antiglaucoma drug, ocular antihypertensive

Available by prescription only
Ophthalmic solution: 0.005%

INDICATIONS & DOSAGE
Treatment of increased intraocular pressure (IOP) in patients with ocular hypertension or open-angle glaucoma who are intolerant of other IOP-lowering drugs or insufficiently responsive to another IOP-lowering drug
Adults: Instill 1 drop in the conjunctival sac of the affected eye once daily in the evening.

PHARMACODYNAMICS
Antiglaucoma and ocular antihypertensive actions: Although exact mechanism of action is unknown, latanoprost is believed to increase the outflow of aqueous humor, thus lowering IOP.

PHARMACOKINETICS
Absorption: Latanoprost is absorbed through the cornea. Drug levels in the aqueous humor peak about 2 hours after topical administration.
Distribution: Drug distribution volume is about 0.16 L/kg. The acid of latanoprost can be measured in aqueous humor during first 4 hours and in plasma only during first hour after local administration.
Metabolism: Drug is hydrolyzed by esterases in the cornea to the biologically active acid. The active acid of drug reaching the systemic circulation is primarily metabolized by the liver.
Excretion: Metabolites are mainly eliminated in urine.

CONTRAINDICATIONS & PRECAUTIONS
Contraindicated in patients with hypersensitivity to latanoprost, benzalkonium chloride, or other ingredients in the product. Use cautiously in patients with impaired renal or hepatic function.

INTERACTIONS
Drug-drug. Precipitation occurs when eyedrops containing *thimerosal* are mixed with latanoprost; they should be administered at least 5 minutes apart.

ADVERSE REACTIONS
CV: angina pectoris.
EENT: *blurred vision; burning; stinging;* itching; conjunctival hyperemia; foreign body sensation; increased pigmentation of iris; punctate epithelial keratopathy; dry eye; excessive tearing; photophobia; conjunctivitis; diplopia;

eye pain or discharge; retinal artery embolus (rare); retinal detachment (rare); vitreous hemorrhage from diabetic retinopathy (rare); lid crusting, edema, erythema, discomfort, or pain.

Musculoskeletal: muscle, joint, back, or chest pain.

Respiratory: upper respiratory tract infection, cold.

Skin: rash; allergic skin reaction.

Other: flu.

◙ KEY CONSIDERATIONS

• Latanoprost may gradually change eye color, increasing the amount of brown pigment in the iris. The change in iris color occurs slowly, may not be noticeable for several months to years, and may be permanent.

Patient education

• Inform patient about potential change in iris color. Patients who are receiving treatment in only one eye should be told about the potential for increased brown pigmentation in the treated eye and thus, heterochromia between the eyes.

• Teach patient how to instill drops. Advise him to wash hands before and after instilling solution, and warn him not to touch dropper or tip to eye or surrounding tissue.

• Advise patient to apply light finger pressure on lacrimal sac for 1 minute after instillation to minimize systemic absorption of drug.

• Instruct patient to report ocular reactions, especially conjunctivitis and lid reactions.

• Tell patient using contact lenses to remove them before administration of the solution and not to reinsert them until 15 minutes have elapsed after administration.

• Advise patient that if more than one topical ophthalmic drug is being used, the drugs should be administered at least 5 minutes apart.

• Stress importance of compliance with recommended therapy.

• Teach patient to protect bottle from light. Refrigerate unopened bottle. Once open, the bottle should be stored at room temperature for up to 6 weeks.

leucovorin calcium (citrovorum factor or folinic acid)
Wellcovorin

Formyl derivative (active reduced form of folic acid), vitamin, antidote

Available by prescription only
Tablets: 5 mg, 15 mg, 25 mg
Injection: 1-ml ampule (3 mg/ml with 0.9% benzyl alcohol, 5 mg/ml with methyl and propyl parabens); 50-mg, 100-mg, and 350-mg vials for reconstitution (contain no preservatives)

INDICATIONS & DOSAGE

Overdose of folic acid antagonist
Adults: P.O., I.M., or I.V. dose equivalent to weight of antagonist given as soon as possible after the overdose.

Leucovorin rescue after large methotrexate dose in treatment of cancer
Adults: Administer 24 hours after last dose of methotrexate according to protocol. Give 15 mg I.M., I.V., or P.O. q 6 hours until methotrexate serum level is less than 5×10^{-8} M.

Toxic effects of methotrexate used to treat severe psoriasis
Adults: 4 to 8 mg I.M. 2 hours after methotrexate dose.

Hematologic toxicity from pyrimethamine or trimethoprim therapy
Adults: 5 to 15 mg P.O. or I.M. daily.

Advanced colorectal cancer
Adults: 200 mg /m^2 by slow I.V. injection over 3 minutes followed by 5-fluorouracil (5-FU), or 20 mg/m^2 by slow I.V. injection over 3 minutes followed by 5-FU. Repeat treatment for 5 days. May repeat course at 4-week intervals for 2 courses and then at 4- to 5-week intervals provided the patient has recovered from toxic effects of previous treatment. Dosage of 5-FU should be individualized.

Megaloblastic anemia from congenital enzyme deficiency
Adults: 3 to 6 mg I.M. daily, then 1 mg P.O. daily for life.

Folate-deficient megaloblastic anemias
Adults: Up to 1 mg of leucovorin P.O. or
I.M. daily. Duration of treatment de-
pends on hematologic response.

PHARMACODYNAMICS
Reversal of folic acid antagonism: Leucovorin is a derivative of tetrahydrofolic
acid, the reduced form of folic acid. Leucovorin performs as a cofactor in 1-
carbon transfer reactions in the biosynthesis of purines and pyrimidines of nucleic acids. Impairment of thymidylate
synthesis in patients with folic acid deficiency may account for defective DNA
synthesis, megaloblast formation, and
megaloblastic and macrocytic anemias.
Antidote action: Leucovorin is a potent
antidote for the hematopoietic and reticuloendothelial toxic effects of folic acid
antagonists (trimethoprim,
pyrimethamine, and methotrexate). Leucovorin rescue is used to prevent or decrease toxicity of massive methotrexate
doses. Folinic acid rescues normal cells
without reversing the oncolytic effect of
methotrexate.

PHARMACOKINETICS
Absorption: After oral administration,
leucovorin is absorbed rapidly; serum
folate levels peak less than 2 hours after
a 15-mg dose. The increase in plasma
and serum folate activity after oral administration is mainly from 5-methylte-
trahydrofolate (the major transport and
storage form of folate in the body).
Distribution: Tetrahydrofolic acid and its
derivatives are distributed throughout the
body; the liver contains about half of the
total body folate stores.
Metabolism: Leucovorin is metabolized
in the liver.
Excretion: Drug is excreted by the kidneys as 10-formyl tetrahydrofolate and
5,10-methenyl tetrahydrofolate. Duration of action is 3 to 6 hours.

CONTRAINDICATIONS & PRECAUTIONS
Contraindicated in patients with pernicious anemia and other megaloblastic
anemias secondary to lack of vitamin B_{12}.

INTERACTIONS
Drug-drug. Leucovorin increases toxicity of *fluorouracil*; lower doses of fluorouracil should be used.

Use with *phenytoin* decreases serum
phenytoin levels and increases frequency
of seizures. Although this interaction has
occurred solely in patients receiving
folic acid, it should be considered when
leucovorin is administered. The mechanism by which this occurs appears to be
an increased metabolic clearance of
phenytoin or a redistribution of phenytoin in the CSF and brain. *Phenytoin* and
primidone may decrease serum folate
levels, producing symptoms of folate deficiency. After chemotherapy with *folic
acid antagonists*, parenteral administration is preferable to oral dosing because
vomiting may cause loss of the leucovorin; to treat an overdose of folic acid
antagonists, leucovorin should be administered within 1 hour if possible, because
it's usually ineffective after a 4-hour delay. Leucovorin has no effect on other
methotrexate toxicities.

ADVERSE REACTIONS
Skin: hypersensitivity reactions (urticaria, ***anaphylactoid reactions***).

▣ KEY CONSIDERATIONS
• Continue drug administration until
plasma methotrexate levels are below
5×10^{-8} M.
• To prepare drug for parenteral use, add
5 ml of bacteriostatic water for injection
to vial containing 50 mg of base drug.
• Maximum rate of leucovorin infusion
shouldn't exceed 160 mg/minute because of calcium concentration of solution.
• Don't use as sole treatment of pernicious anemia or vitamin B_{12} deficiency.
• To treat overdose of folic acid antagonists, use the drug within 1 hour; it's ineffective after a 4-hour delay.
• Monitor patient for signs of drug allergy, such as rash, wheezing, pruritus, and
urticaria.
• Monitor serum creatinine levels daily
to detect possible renal function impairment.
• Administer drug parenterally if giving
more than 25 mg.

• Store at room temperature in a light-resistant container, not in high-moisture areas.
• Leucovorin may mask the diagnosis of pernicious anemia.

Patient education
• Emphasize importance of taking leucovorin only under medical supervision.

---

levobunolol hydrochloride
AKBeta, Betagan

Beta blocker, antiglaucoma drug

Available by prescription only
Ophthalmic solution: 0.25%, 0.5%

INDICATIONS & DOSAGE
Chronic open-angle glaucoma and ocular hypertension
Adults: Instill 1 or 2 gtt (0.5% solution) daily or 1 or 2 gtt (0.25% solution) b.i.d. in eye(s).

PHARMACODYNAMICS
Antiglaucoma action: Levobunolol is a nonselective beta blocker that reduces intraocular pressure. Exact mechanisms are unknown, but the drug appears to reduce formation of aqueous humor.

PHARMACOKINETICS
Absorption: Onset of activity usually occurs within 60 minutes; peak effect in 2 to 6 hours.
Distribution: Unknown.
Metabolism: Unknown.
Excretion: Duration of effect is 24 hours.

CONTRAINDICATIONS & PRECAUTIONS
Contraindicated in patients with hypersensitivity to levobunolol or with bronchial asthma, history of bronchial asthma or severe COPD, sinus bradycardia, second- or third-degree AV block, cardiac failure, and cardiogenic shock. Use cautiously in patients with chronic bronchitis, emphysema, diabetes mellitus, hyperthyroidism, and myasthenia gravis.

INTERACTIONS
Drug-drug. Levobunolol may increase the systemic effect of *oral beta blockers*, further reduce intraocular pressure induced by *carbonic anhydrase inhibitors, epinephrine,* or *pilocarpine,* and enhance the hypotensive and bradycardiac effects of *catecholamine-depleting drugs* and *reserpine.*

ADVERSE REACTIONS
CNS: headache, depression, insomnia.
CV: slight reduction in resting heart rate.
EENT: *transient eye stinging and burning,* tearing, erythema, itching, keratitis, corneal punctate staining, photophobia; decreased corneal sensitivity (with long-term use).
GI: nausea.
Skin: urticaria.
Other: evidence of beta blockade and systemic absorption *(hypotension, bradycardia, syncope, asthma attacks in patients with history of asthma, heart failure).*

▣ KEY CONSIDERATIONS
• Drug should be used with caution in geriatric patients with cardiac or pulmonary disease, who may experience exacerbation of symptoms, depending on extent of systemic absorption.
• Cardiac output is reduced in both healthy patients and those with heart disease. Drug may decrease heart rate and blood pressure and produces beta blockade in bronchi and bronchioles. No effect on pupil size or accommodation has been noted.
• In some patients, a few weeks' treatment may be required to stabilize pressure-lowering response; determine intraocular pressure after 4 weeks of treatment.
• Although oral beta blockers have been reported to decrease serum glucose levels from blockage of normal glycogen release after hypoglycemia, such instances haven't been reported with the use of ophthalmic beta blockers.

Patient education
• Warn patient not to touch dropper to eye or surrounding tissue.

Reactions may be common, *uncommon,* **life-threatening,** *or* **COMMON AND LIFE-THREATENING.**

• Show patient how to instill drug. Teach him to press lacrimal sac lightly for 1 minute after drug administration to decrease chance of systemic absorption.

• Remind patient not to blink more than usual or to close eyes tightly during treatment.

• Although transient stinging and discomfort are common, tell patient to call if reaction is severe.

Overdose & treatment

• Overdose is extremely rare with ophthalmic use. However, usual signs and symptoms include bradycardia, hypotension, bronchospasm, heart block, and cardiac failure.

• Within 30 minutes of ingestion, induce vomiting, providing the patient isn't obtunded, comatose, or having seizures. Follow with activated charcoal. Treat bradycardia, conduction defects, and hypotension with I.V. fluids, glucagon, atropine, or isoproterenol. Treat bronchoconstriction with I.V. aminophylline and seizures with I.V. diazepam.

• Levobunolol is faster-acting than timolol.

levodopa
Dopar, Larodopa

Dopamine precursor, antiparkinsonian

Available by prescription only
Tablets: 100 mg, 250 mg, 500 mg
Capsules: 100 mg, 250 mg, 500 mg

INDICATIONS & DOSAGE
Parkinsonism

Levodopa is indicated in treating idiopathic, postencephalitic, arteriosclerotic parkinsonism and symptomatic parkinsonism that may follow injury to the nervous system by carbon monoxide intoxication and manganese intoxication.
Adults: Initially, 0.5 to 1 g P.O. daily, given b.i.d., t.i.d., or q.i.d. with food; increase by no more than 0.75 g daily q 3 to 7 days, as tolerated. The usual optimal dose is 3 to 6 g daily divided into 3 doses. Don't exceed 8 g daily, except in unusual cases. A significant therapeutic re-

sponse may not be obtained for 6 months. Larger dose requires close supervision.

PHARMACODYNAMICS
Antiparkinsonian action: Precise mechanism of levodopa hasn't been established. A small percentage of each dose crossing the blood-brain barrier is decarboxylated. The dopamine then stimulates dopaminergic receptors in the basal ganglia to enhance the balance between cholinergic and dopaminergic activity, resulting in improved modulation of voluntary nerve impulses transmitted to the motor cortex.

PHARMACOKINETICS
Absorption: Levodopa is absorbed rapidly from the small intestine by an active amino acid transport system, with 30% to 50% reaching the general circulation.
Distribution: Drug is distributed widely to most body tissues but not to the CNS, which receives less than 1% of dose because of extensive metabolism in the periphery.
Metabolism: About 95% of levodopa is converted to dopamine by l-aromatic amino acid decarboxylase enzyme in the lumen of the stomach and intestines and on the first pass through the liver.
Excretion: Excreted primarily in urine; 80% of dose is excreted within 24 hours as dopamine metabolites. Half-life is 1 to 3 hours.

CONTRAINDICATIONS & PRECAUTIONS
Contraindicated in patients receiving concurrent therapy with MAO inhibitors within 14 days and in those with hypersensitivity to levodopa, acute angle-closure glaucoma, melanoma, or undiagnosed skin lesions.

Use cautiously in patients with severe renal, CV, hepatic, and pulmonary disorders; peptic ulcer; psychiatric illness; MI with residual arrhythmias; bronchial asthma; emphysema; and endocrine disorders.

INTERACTIONS
Drug-drug. Use with *amantadine, benztropine, procyclidine,* or *trihexyphenidyl* may increase the efficacy of

levodopa. *Anesthetics* or *hydrocarbon inhalation* may cause arrhythmias because of increased endogenous dopamine level; levodopa should be discontinued 6 to 8 hours before administration of anesthetics such as halothane. *Antacids containing calcium, magnesium, or sodium bicarbonate* may increase absorption of levodopa. *Anticholinergics* used with levodopa may produce a mild synergy and increased efficacy (gradual reduction in anticholinergic dosage is necessary). Use of *anticonvulsants* (such as *hydantoins* and *phenytoin*), *benzodiazepines, haloperidol, papaverine, phenothiazines, rauwolfia alkaloids*, or *thioxanthenes* may decrease therapeutic effects of levodopa. *Antihypertensives* used concurrently with levodopa may increase the hypotensive effect. *Bromocriptine* may produce additive effects, allowing reduced levodopa dosage. Use with *MAO inhibitors* may cause hypertensive crisis; MAO inhibitors should be discontinued 2 to 4 weeks before starting levodopa. *Methyldopa* may alter the antiparkinsonian effects of levodopa and may produce additive toxic CNS effects. *Pyridoxine* in a 10-mg dose reverses the antiparkinsonian effects of levodopa. *Sympathomimetics* may increase the risk of arrhythmias (dosage reduction of the sympathomimetic is recommended; the administration of *carbidopa* with levodopa reduces the tendency of sympathomimetics to cause dopamine-induced arrhythmias); decrease levodopa dose.

Drug-food. *Foods high in protein* appear to interfere with transport of drug; avoid such foods before and after administration. Drug should be given between meals and with *low-protein snack* to maximize drug absorption and minimize GI upset.

ADVERSE REACTIONS

CNS: *aggressive behavior; choreiform, dystonic, and dyskinetic movements; involuntary grimacing, head movements, myoclonic body jerks, seizures,* ataxia, tremor, muscle twitching; bradykinetic episodes; psychiatric disturbances; mood changes, nervousness, anxiety, disturbing dreams, euphoria, malaise, fatigue;

severe depression, *suicidal tendencies,* dementia, delirium, hallucinations (may require reduction or withdrawal of drug).
CV: *orthostatic hypotension,* cardiac irregularities, phlebitis.
EENT: blepharospasm, blurred vision, diplopia, mydriasis or miosis, activation of latent Horner's syndrome, oculogyric crises, excessive salivation.
GI: dry mouth, bitter taste, *nausea, vomiting, anorexia,* weight loss (at start of therapy), constipation, flatulence, diarrhea, abdominal pain.
GU: urinary frequency, urine retention, incontinence, darkened urine, priapism.
Hematologic: *hemolytic anemia, leukopenia, agranulocytosis.*
Hepatic: elevated liver enzyme levels, *hepatotoxicity.*
Respiratory: hiccups.
Other: dark perspiration, hyperventilation.

▣ KEY CONSIDERATIONS

- Smaller doses may be required in geriatric patients because of reduced tolerance to drug's effects.
- Geriatric patients, especially those with osteoporosis, should resume normal activity gradually because increased mobility may increase risk of fractures.
- Geriatric patients are more likely to develop psychological adverse effects, such as anxiety, confusion, or nervousness; those with preexisting heart disease are more susceptible to levodopa's cardiac effects.
- Drug should be given between meals and with low-protein snack to maximize drug absorption and minimize GI upset. Foods high in protein appear to interfere with transport of drug.
- Maximum effectiveness of drug may not occur for several weeks or months after therapy begins.
- Monitor patient also receiving an antihypertensive for possible drug interactions. Discontinue MAO inhibitors at least 2 weeks before levodopa therapy begins.
- Adjust dosage based on patient's response and tolerance. Observe and monitor vital signs, especially while adjusting dose.

- Monitor patient for muscle twitching and blepharospasm (twitching of eyelids), which may be an early sign of drug overdose.
- Test patients on long-term therapy regularly for diabetes and acromegaly; check blood tests and liver and kidney function studies periodically for adverse effects. Leukopenia may require cessation of therapy.
- Because of risk of precipitating a symptom complex resembling neuroleptic malignant syndrome, observe patient closely if levodopa dosage is reduced abruptly or discontinued.
- If restarting therapy after a long period of interruption, adjust drug dosage gradually to previous level.
- Patients undergoing surgery should continue levodopa as long as oral intake is permitted, usually 6 to 24 hours before surgery. Drug should be resumed as soon as patient is able to take oral drug.
- Protect drug from heat, light, and moisture. If preparation darkens, it has lost potency and should be discarded.
- Monitor serum laboratory tests periodically. Coombs' test occasionally becomes positive during extended use. Colorimetric test for uric acid has shown false elevations. False-positive results have been noted on tests for urine glucose using the copper-reduction method; false-negative results have occurred with the glucose oxidase method. Levodopa also may interfere with tests for urine ketones, urine norepinephrine, and urine protein determinations.
- Alkaline phosphatase, AST, ALT, LD, bilirubin, BUN, and protein-bound iodine levels show transient elevations in patients receiving levodopa; WBC, hemoglobin, and hematocrit levels show occasional reduction.
- Although controversial, a medically supervised period of drug discontinuance (drug holiday) may reestablish the effectiveness of a lower dose regimen.
- Combination of levodopa-carbidopa usually reduces the amount of levodopa needed, thus reducing incidence of adverse reactions.
- Levodopa has also been used to relieve pain of herpes zoster.

- Tablets and capsules may be crushed and mixed with applesauce or baby-food fruits for patients who have difficulty swallowing pills.

Patient education
- Warn patient and family not to increase drug dose without specific instruction. (They may be tempted to do this as disease symptoms of parkinsonism progress.)
- Explain that therapeutic response may not occur for up to 6 months.
- Advise patient and family that multivitamin preparations, fortified cereals, and certain OTC products may contain pyridoxine (vitamin B_6), which can reverse the effects of levodopa.
- Warn patient of possible dizziness and orthostatic hypotension, especially at start of therapy. Tell patient to change position slowly and dangle legs before getting out of bed. Instruct patient in use of elastic stockings to control this adverse reaction if appropriate.
- Inform patient of signs and symptoms of adverse reactions and therapeutic effects and the need to report changes.
- Tell patient to take a missed dose as soon as possible but to skip dose if next scheduled dose is within 2 hours; don't take double doses.
- Advise patient not to take drug with food, but that eating something about 15 minutes after administration may help reduce GI upset.
- Warn patient of possible darkening of urine, sweat, and other body fluids.

Overdose & treatment
- Signs and symptoms of overdose include spasm or closing of eyelids, irregular heartbeat, or palpitations.
- Treatment includes immediate gastric lavage, maintenance of an adequate airway, and judicious administration of I.V. fluids, and may include antiarrhythmic drugs if necessary. Pyridoxine 10 to 25 mg P.O. has been reported to reverse toxic and therapeutic effects of levodopa. (Its usefulness hasn't been established in acute overdose.)

levodopa-carbidopa
Sinemet, Sinemet CR

Decarboxylase inhibitor-dopamine precursor combination, antiparkinsonian

Available by prescription only
Tablets: 10 mg carbidopa with 100 mg levodopa (Sinemet 10-100), 25 mg carbidopa with 100 mg levodopa (Sinemet 25-100), 25 mg carbidopa with 250 mg levodopa (Sinemet 25-250)
Tablets (sustained-release): 50 mg carbidopa with 200 mg levodopa (Sinemet CR 50-200), 25 mg carbidopa with 100 mg levodopa (Sinemet CR 25-100)

INDICATIONS & DOSAGE
Parkinsonism
Adults: Most patients respond to a 25-mg/100-mg combination (1 tablet t.i.d.). Dose may be increased q 1 or 2 days; or 1 tablet of 10 mg/100 mg t.i.d. or q.i.d. up to 2 tablets q.i.d.; or 1 sustained-release tablet b.i.d. at intervals at least 6 hours apart. Intervals may be adjusted based on patient response. Usual dose is 2 to 8 tablets daily in divided doses of 4 to 8 hours while awake.

Maintenance therapy must be adjusted carefully based on patient tolerance and desired therapeutic response.

Usual maintenance dosage is 3 to 6 tablets of 25 mg carbidopa/250 mg levodopa daily in divided doses. Don't exceed 8 tablets of 25 mg carbidopa/ 250 mg levodopa daily. Optimum daily dosage must be determined by careful titration for each patient.

Daily dosage of carbidopa should be 70 mg or more to suppress the peripheral metabolism of levodopa but shouldn't exceed 200 mg.

PHARMACODYNAMICS
Decarboxylase inhibiting action: Carbidopa inhibits the peripheral decarboxylation of levodopa, thus slowing its conversion to dopamine in extracerebral tissues. This increases the availability of levodopa for transport to the brain, where it undergoes decarboxylation to dopamine.

PHARMACOKINETICS
Absorption: About 40% to 70% of dose is absorbed after oral administration. Plasma levodopa levels are increased when carbidopa and levodopa are administered concomitantly because carbidopa inhibits the peripheral metabolism of levodopa.
Distribution: Carbidopa is distributed widely in body tissues except the CNS.
Metabolism: Carbidopa isn't metabolized extensively. It inhibits metabolism of levodopa in the GI tract, thus increasing its absorption from the GI tract and its level in plasma.
Excretion: About 30% of dose is excreted unchanged in urine within 24 hours. When given with carbidopa, the amount of levodopa excreted unchanged in urine is increased by about 6%. Half-life is 1 to 2 hours.

CONTRAINDICATIONS & PRECAUTIONS
Contraindicated in patients with hypersensitivity to levodopa-carbidopa or with acute angle-closure glaucoma, melanoma, or undiagnosed skin lesions, and within 14 days of MAO inhibitor therapy.

Use cautiously in patients with severe CV, endocrine, pulmonary, renal, or hepatic disorders; peptic ulcer; psychiatric illness; MI with residual arrhythmias; bronchial asthma; emphysema; and well-controlled, chronic, open-angle glaucoma.

INTERACTIONS
Drug-drug. Use with *amantadine, benztropine, procyclidine,* or *trihexyphenidyl* may increase the efficacy of levodopa. *Anesthetics* or *hydrocarbon inhalation* may cause arrhythmias because of increased endogenous dopamine level; levodopa-carbidopa should be stopped 6 to 8 hours before administration of anesthetics such as *halothane. Antacids containing calcium, magnesium,* or *sodium bicarbonate* may increase absorption of levodopa. Use of *anticonvulsants (hydantoin), benzodiazepines, droperidol, haloperidol, loxapine, metyrosine, papaverine, phenothiazines, rauwolfia alkaloids,* and *thioxanthines* may decrease therapeutic

---

Reactions may be *common*, uncommon, *life-threatening*, or **COMMON AND LIFE-THREATENING**.

effects of levodopa. Use with *antihypertensives* may increase the hypotensive effect. *Bromocriptine* may produce additive effects, allowing reduced levodopa dosage. Use of *MAO inhibitors* may cause hypertensive crisis; discontinue MAO inhibitors 2 to 4 weeks before starting levodopa-carbidopa. *Methyldopa* may alter the antiparkinsonian effects of levodopa and may produce additive toxic CNS effects. *Molindone* may inhibit antiparkinsonian effects of levodopa by blocking dopamine receptors in the brain. *Sympathomimetics* may increase risk of arrhythmias (reduced dosage of the sympathomimetic is recommended; however, administration of carbidopa with levodopa reduces the tendency of sympathomimetics to cause dopamine-induced arrhythmias).

ADVERSE REACTIONS
CNS: *choreiform, dystonic, dyskinetic movements; involuntary grimacing, head movements, myoclonic body jerks, ataxia,* tremor, muscle twitching; bradykinetic episodes; psychiatric disturbances, anxiety, disturbing dreams, euphoria, malaise, fatigue; severe depression, *suicidal tendencies,* dementia, delirium, hallucinations (may necessitate reduction or withdrawal of drug); confusion; insomnia; agitation.
CV: *orthostatic hypotension, cardiac irregularities,* phlebitis.
EENT: blepharospasm, blurred vision, diplopia, mydriasis or miosis, oculogyric crises, excessive salivation.
GI: *dry mouth,* bitter taste, *nausea, vomiting, anorexia,* weight loss at start of therapy; constipation; flatulence; diarrhea; abdominal pain.
GU: urinary frequency, urine retention, urinary incontinence, darkened urine, priapism.
Hematologic: *hemolytic anemia, thrombocytopenia, leukopenia, agranulocytosis.*
Hepatic: *hepatotoxicity.*
Respiratory: hiccups.
Other: dark perspiration, hyperventilation.

▣ KEY CONSIDERATIONS
• In geriatric patients, smaller doses may be required because of reduced tolerance to the effects of levodopa-carbidopa. Geriatric patients, especially those with osteoporosis, should resume normal activity gradually because increased mobility may increase the risk of fractures.
• Geriatric patients are especially vulnerable to CNS adverse effects, such as anxiety, confusion, or nervousness; those with preexisting heart disease are more susceptible to cardiac effects.
• Carefully monitor patient who is also receiving antihypertensive or hypoglycemic agents. Discontinue MAO inhibitors at least 2 weeks before therapy begins.
• Adjust dosage based on patient's response and tolerance to drug. Therapeutic and adverse reactions occur more rapidly with levodopa-carbidopa combination than with levodopa alone. Observe and monitor vital signs, especially while dosage is being adjusted.
• Muscle twitching and blepharospasm (twitching of eyelids) may be an early sign of overdose.
• Test patients on long-term therapy regularly for diabetes and acromegaly; periodically repeat blood test and liver and kidney function studies.
• If patient is being treated with levodopa, discontinue at least 8 hours before starting levodopa-carbidopa.
• The combination drug usually reduces the amount of levodopa needed by 75%, thereby reducing the incidence of adverse reactions.
• Pyridoxine (vitamin B_6) doesn't reverse the beneficial effects of levodopa-carbidopa. Multivitamins can be taken without fear of losing control of symptoms.
• If therapy is interrupted temporarily, usual daily dosage may be given as soon as patient resumes oral drugs.
• Maximum effectiveness of drug may not occur for several weeks or months after therapy begins.
• Sustained-release tablets may be split, but never crushed or chewed.
• Antiglobulin determinations (Coombs' test) are occasionally positive after long-term use. Thyroid function determina-

tions may inhibit thyroid-stimulating hormone response to protirelin.

• Levodopa-carbidopa therapy may elevate serum gonadotropin levels. Serum and uric acid determinations may show false elevations.

• Urine glucose determinations using copper reduction method may show false-positive results; with the glucose oxidase method, false-negative results. Urine ketone determination using dipstick method, urine norepinephrine determinations, and urine protein determinations using Lowery test may show false-positive results.

• Systemic effects of drug may elevate levels of BUN, ALT, AST, alkaline phosphatase, serum bilirubin, LD, and serum protein-bound iodine.

Patient education

• Instruct patient to report adverse reactions and therapeutic effects.

• Warn patient of possible dizziness or orthostatic hypotension, especially at start of therapy. Tell patient to change position slowly and dangle legs before getting out of bed. Elastic stockings may be helpful in some patients.

• Tell patient to take food shortly after taking drug to relieve gastric irritation.

• Inform patient that drug may cause urine or sweat to darken.

• Tell patient to take a missed dose as soon as possible, to skip a missed dose if next scheduled dose is within 2 hours, and never to double-dose.

Overdose & treatment

• Overdose with carbidopa is unknown. Signs and symptoms of levodopa overdose are irregular heartbeat and palpitations, severe continuous nausea and vomiting, and spasm or closing of eyelids.

• Treatment of overdose includes immediate gastric lavage and an antiarrhythmic if necessary. Pyridoxine is ineffective in reversing the actions of carbidopa and levodopa combinations.

levofloxacin
Levaquin

Fluorinated carboxyquinolone, broad-spectrum antibacterial

Available by prescription only
Tablets: 250, 500 mg
Single-use vials: 500 mg
Infusion (premixed): 250 mg in 50 ml D_5W, 500 mg in 100 ml D_5W

INDICATIONS & DOSAGE

***Acute maxillary sinusitis caused by susceptible strains of* Streptococcus pneumoniae, Moraxella catarrhalis, *or* Haemophilus influenzae**
Adults: 500 mg P.O. or I.V. daily for 10 to 14 days.

***Acute bacterial exacerbation of chronic bronchitis caused by* Staphylococcus aureus, S. pneumoniae, M. catarrhalis, H. influenzae, *or* H. parainfluenzae**
Adults: 500 mg P.O. or I.V. daily for 7 days.

***Community-acquired pneumonia caused by* S. aureus, S. pneumoniae, M. catarrhalis, H. influenzae, H. parainfluenzae, Klebsiella pneumoniae, Chlamydia pneumoniae, Legionella pneumophila, *or* Mycoplasma pneumoniae**
Adults: 500 mg P.O. or I.V. daily for 7 to 14 days.

***Uncomplicated skin and soft-tissue infections (mild to moderate) caused by* S. aureus *or* S. pyogenes**
Adults: 500 mg P.O. or I.V. daily for 7 to 10 days.

✦ *Dosage adjustment.* If creatinine clearance is 20 to 49 ml/minute, subsequent dosages are half the initial dose. If creatinine clearance is 10 to 19 ml/minute, subsequent dosages are half the initial dose and the interval is prolonged to q 48 hours.

***Complicated urinary tract infections (mild to moderate) caused by* Enterococcus faecalis, Enterobacter cloacae, Escherichia coli, K. pneumoniae, Proteus mirabilis, *or* Pseudomonas aeruginosa**
Adults: 250 mg P.O. or I.V. daily for 10 days.

Reactions may be *common*, uncommon, ***life-threatening***, or **COMMON AND LIFE-THREATENING**.

Acute pyelonephritis (mild to moderate) caused by E. coli
Adults: 250 mg P.O. or I.V. daily for 10 days.
✦ *Dosage adjustment.* If creatinine clearance is 10 to 19 ml/minute, dosage interval is increased to q 48 hours.

PHARMACODYNAMICS
Antibacterial action: Drug inhibits bacterial DNA gyrase, an enzyme required for DNA replication, transcription, repair, and recombination in susceptible bacteria.

PHARMACOKINETICS
Absorption: The plasma level after I.V. administration is comparable with that observed for equivalent oral doses (on a mg/mg basis). Therefore, oral and I.V. routes can be considered interchangeable. Plasma levels peak within 1 to 2 hours after oral dosing. Steady-state levels are reached within 48 hours on a 500-mg/day regimen.
Distribution: Mean volume of distribution ranges from 89 to 112 L after single and multiple 500-mg doses, indicating widespread distribution into body tissues. Drug also penetrates well into lung tissues; lung tissue levels are generally twofold to fivefold higher than plasma levels.
Metabolism: Drug undergoes limited metabolism in humans. The only identified metabolites are the desmethyl and N-oxide metabolites, which have little relevant pharmacologic activity.
Excretion: Primarily excreted unchanged in the urine. Mean terminal half-life is 6 to 8 hours.

CONTRAINDICATIONS & PRECAUTIONS
Contraindicated in patients with hypersensitivity to levofloxacin, its components, or quinolone antimicrobials.
Use cautiously in patients with history of seizure disorders or other CNS diseases, such as cerebral arteriosclerosis, because quinolones can cause CNS stimulation and increased intracranial pressure. This may lead to seizures (lowered seizure threshold), toxic psychoses, tremors, restlessness, anxiety, lightheadedness, confusion, hallucinations,

paranoia, depression, nightmares, insomnia, and, rarely, suicidal thoughts or acts. These can occur after the first dose.

INTERACTIONS
Drug-drug. *Antacids containing aluminum or magnesium, iron salts, products containing zinc,* and *sucralfate* may interfere with GI absorption of levofloxacin; administer at least 2 hours apart. *Antidiabetics* may alter blood glucose levels; monitor glucose levels closely. *NSAIDs* may increase CNS stimulation; monitor for seizure activity. Coadministration with *theophylline* may result in decreased clearance of theophylline; monitor theophylline levels. *Warfarin* and derivatives may cause increased effect of oral anticoagulant with some fluoroquinolones; monitor PT and INR.
Drug-lifestyle. Photosensitivity reaction may occur to *sunlight;* take precautions.

ADVERSE REACTIONS
CNS: headache, pain, insomnia, dizziness, encephalopathy, paresthesia, *seizures.*
CV: chest pain, palpitations, vasodilation.
GI: nausea, diarrhea, constipation, vomiting, abdominal pain, dyspepsia, flatulence, *pseudomembranous colitis.*
GU: vaginitis.
Hematologic: eosinophilia, hemolytic anemia.
Musculoskeletal: back pain, tendon rupture.
Respiratory: allergic pneumonitis.
Skin: rash, photosensitivity, pruritus, erythema multiforme, *Stevens-Johnson syndrome.*
Other: *hypersensitivity reactions,* injection site reaction, *anaphylaxis, multisystem organ failure.*

🔲 KEY CONSIDERATIONS
• If patient experiences symptoms of excessive CNS stimulation (restlessness, tremor, confusion, hallucinations), discontinue drug. Institute seizure precautions.
• Ruptures of tendons and tendonitis have occurred with quinolone therapy. Discontinue drug if pain, inflammation,

or rupture of a tendon occurs. These ruptures can occur after therapy has been stopped.

• Because rapid or bolus administration may result in hypotension, I.V. levofloxacin should be administered only by slow infusion over 60 minutes.

• Avoid excessive exposure to sunlight.

• Levofloxacin may cause abnormal EEG and a decreased glucose level and lymphocyte count.

Patient education

• Tell patient to take drug as prescribed, even if symptoms disappear.

• Advise patient to take drug with plenty of fluids and to avoid antacids, sucralfate, and products containing iron or zinc for at least 2 hours before and after each dose.

• Warn patient to avoid hazardous tasks until adverse CNS effects of drug are known.

• Advise patient to use sunblock and wear protective clothing when exposed to excessive sunlight.

• Tell patient to stop drug and call if rash or other signs of hypersensitivity develop.

• Tell patient to report pain or inflammation.

• Tell diabetic patient to monitor blood glucose levels and report if a hypoglycemic reaction occurs.

levothyroxine sodium (T$_4$ or L-thyroxine sodium)
Eltroxin, Levo-T, Levothroid, Levoxine, Levoxyl, Synthroid

Thyroid hormone, thyroid hormone replacement

Available by prescription only
Tablets: 25 mcg, 50 mcg, 75 mcg, 88 mcg, 100 mcg, 112 mcg, 125 mcg, 137 mcg, 150 mcg, 175 mcg, 200 mcg, 300 mcg
Injection: 200 mcg/vial, 500 mcg/vial

INDICATIONS & DOSAGE
Myxedema coma
Adults: 300 to 500 mcg I.V. If no response occurs in 24 hours, give an additional 100 to 300 mcg I.V. in 48 hours. A maintenance dose of 50 to 200 mcg may be given until condition stabilizes and drug can be given orally.

Thyroid hormone replacement for atrophy of gland, surgical removal, excessive radiation or thyroid hormone–depleting drugs, or congenital defect
Adults: For mild hypothyroidism—initially, 50 mcg P.O. daily, increased by 25 to 50 mcg P.O. daily q 2 to 4 weeks until desired response is achieved; may be administered I.V. or I.M. when P.O. ingestion is precluded for long periods.

For severe hypothyroidism—12.5 to 25 mcg daily, increased by 25 to 50 mcg daily q 2 to 4 weeks until desired response is achieved.
Geriatric patients: start at 12.5 to 25 mcg P.O. daily and increase in 12.5- to 25-mcg increments q 2 to 8 weeks.
✦ *Dosage adjustment.* For those with CV disease, start at 12.5 to 25 mcg daily and increase in 12.5- to 25-mcg increments q 2 to 8 weeks.

PHARMACODYNAMICS
Thyroid hormone replacement action: Levothyroxine affects protein and carbohydrate metabolism, promotes gluconeogenesis, increases the use and mobilization of glycogen stores, stimulates protein synthesis, and regulates cell growth and differentiation. Major effect of drug is to increase the metabolic rate of tissue.

PHARMACOKINETICS
Absorption: Absorption varies from 50% to 80% from the GI tract. Full effects don't occur for 1 to 3 weeks after oral therapy begins. After I.M. administration, absorption is variable and poor. After an I.V. dose in patients with myxedema coma, increased responsiveness may occur within 6 to 8 hours, but maximum therapeutic effect may not occur for up to 24 hours.
Distribution: Not fully described; however, drug is distributed into most body tissues and fluids. The highest levels are found in the liver and kidneys; 99% is protein-bound.
Metabolism: Drug is metabolized in peripheral tissues, primarily in the liver, kid-

neys, and intestines. About 85% of levothyroxine metabolized is deiodinated. *Excretion:* Fecal excretion eliminates 20% to 40% of levothyroxine. Half-life is 6 to 7 days.

CONTRAINDICATIONS & PRECAUTIONS

Contraindicated in patients with acute MI and thyrotoxicosis, uncomplicated by hypothyroidism, hypersensitivity to levothyroxine, or uncorrected adrenal insufficiency. Use cautiously in geriatric patients and in those with renal impairment, angina pectoris, hypertension, ischemia, or other CV disorders.

INTERACTIONS

Drug-drug. Use with an *anticoagulant* may alter anticoagulant effect; an increase in levothyroxine dosage may necessitate a decrease in anticoagulant dosage. *Beta blockers* may decrease the conversion of levothyroxine to liothyronine. *Cholestyramine* may delay absorption of levothyroxine. Use with *corticotropin* causes changes in thyroid status; changes in levothyroxine dosages may require dosage changes in corticotropin as well. *Estrogens,* which increase serum thyroxine-binding globulin levels, increase levothyroxine requirements. *Hepatic enzyme inducers* (such as *phenytoin*) may increase hepatic degradation of levothyroxine and raise dosage requirements. Use of levothyroxine with *insulin* or *oral antidiabetics* may affect the dosage requirements of these drugs. Use with *somatrem* may accelerate epiphyseal maturation. Decreased *theophylline* clearance can be expected in hypothyroid patients; clearance returns to normal when euthyroid state is achieved. Use of levothyroxine with *tricyclic antidepressants* or *sympathomimetics* may increase the effects of any or all of these drugs and may lead to coronary insufficiency or arrhythmias.

ADVERSE REACTIONS

CNS: *nervousness, insomnia, tremor,* headache.
CV: *tachycardia, palpitations, **arrhythmias,** angina pectoris, **cardiac arrest.***
GI: diarrhea, vomiting.
Metabolic: weight loss.

Skin: allergic skin reactions, diaphoresis.
Other: heat intolerance, fever.

🔲 KEY CONSIDERATIONS

Besides the recommendations relevant to all thyroid hormones, consider the following:
● Geriatric patients are more sensitive to effects of drug. In patients older than age 60, initial dosage should be 25% lower than usual recommended dosage.
● Administer as a single dose before breakfast.
● Carefully observe patient for adverse effects during initial titration phase.
● Monitor for aggravation of concurrent diseases, such as Addison's disease or diabetes mellitus.
● Patients with history of lactose intolerance may be sensitive to Levothroid, which contains lactose.
● Synthroid 100- and 300-mcg tablets contain tartrazine, a dye that causes allergic reactions in susceptible individuals.
● When switching from levothyroxine to liothyronine, levothyroxine dosage should be stopped when liothyronine treatment begins. After residual effects of levothyroxine have disappeared, liothyronine dosage can be increased in small increments. When switching from liothyronine to levothyroxine, levothyroxine therapy should begin several days before withdrawing liothyronine to avoid relapse.
● A patient taking levothyroxine who requires ^{131}I uptake studies must discontinue drug 4 weeks before test. Levothyroxine therapy alters radioactive iodine (^{131}I) thyroid uptake, protein-bound iodine levels, and liothyronine uptake.
● Protect drug from moisture and light. Prepare I.V. dose immediately before injection. Don't mix with other I.V. solutions.
● Levothyroxine has predictable effects because of standard hormone content; therefore, it's the usual drug of choice for thyroid hormone replacement.

Patient education

● Instruct patient to take drug at same time each day; encourage morning dosing to avoid insomnia.

• Tell patient to report headache, diarrhea, nervousness, excessive sweating, heat intolerance, chest pain, increased pulse rate, or palpitations.
• Encourage patient to use the same product consistently because all brands don't have equal bioavailability.
• Advise patient not to store drug in warm, humid areas, such as the bathroom, to prevent deterioration of product.
• Tell patient that replacement therapy must be taken essentially for life, except in cases of transient hypothyroidism.

Overdose & treatment
• Signs and symptoms of overdose include evidence of hyperthyroidism, including weight loss, increased appetite, palpitations, nervousness, diarrhea, abdominal cramps, sweating, tachycardia, increased blood pressure, widened pulse pressure, angina, arrhythmias, tremor, headache, insomnia, heat intolerance, fever, and menstrual irregularities.
• Treatment of overdose requires reduction of GI absorption and efforts to counteract central and peripheral effects, primarily sympathetic activity. Perform gastric lavage or induce vomiting, followed by activated charcoal up to 4 hours after ingestion. If the patient is comatose or is having seizures, inflate cuff on endotracheal tube to prevent aspiration. Treatment may include oxygen and artificial ventilation as needed to support respiration. It also should include appropriate measures to treat heart failure and to control fever, hypoglycemia, and fluid loss. Propranolol (or another beta blocker) may be used to combat many of the effects of increased sympathetic activity. Levothyroxine should be gradually withdrawn over 2 to 6 days, then resumed at a lower dose.

lidocaine (lignocaine)
Xylocaine

lidocaine hydrochloride
Anestacon, Dilocaine, L-Caine, Lidoject, LidoPen Auto-Injector, Nervocaine, Xylocaine, Xylocaine 10% Oral, Xylocaine Viscous, Zilactin-L

Amide derivative, ventricular antiarrhythmic, local anesthetic

Available without a prescription
Ointment: 2.5%
Liquid: 2.5%
Cream: 0.5%
Spray: 0.5%
Gel: 0.5%, 2.5%
Available by prescription only
Injection: 5 mg/ml, 10 mg/ml, 15 mg/ml, 20 mg/ml, 40 mg/ml, 100 mg/ml, 200 mg/ml
Premixed solutions: 2 mg/ml, 4 mg/ml, 8 mg/ml in D_5W
Ointment: 5%
Topical solution: 2%, 4%
Jelly: 2%
Spray: 10%

INDICATIONS & DOSAGE
Ventricular arrhythmias from MI, cardiac manipulation, or cardiac glycosides
Adults: 50 to 100 mg (1 to 1.5 mg/kg) I.V. bolus at 25 to 50 mg/minute. Repeat bolus q 3 to 5 minutes until arrhythmias subside or adverse effects develop. Don't exceed 300-mg total bolus during a 1-hour period. Simultaneously, begin constant infusion of 1 to 4 mg/minute. If single bolus has been given, repeat smaller bolus (usually half the initial bolus) 5 to 10 minutes after start of infusion to maintain therapeutic serum level. After 24 hours of continuous infusion, decrease rate by half.
Geriatric patients: Give half the bolus amount and use slower infusion rates.
♦ *Dosage adjustment.* Give half the bolus amount to lightweight patients and to those with heart failure or hepatic disease. Use slower infusion rate in those with heart failure or hepatic disease, or

patients weighing less than 50 kg (110 lb).

For I.M. administration: 300 mg (4.3 mg/kg) in deltoid muscle has been used in early stages of acute MI.

◊ *Status epilepticus*
Adults: 1 mg/kg I.V. bolus; then, if seizure continues, administer 0.5 mg/kg 2 minutes after first dose; infusion at 30 mcg/kg/minute may be used.

Local anesthesia of skin or mucous membranes, pain from dental extractions, stomatitis
Adults: Apply 2% to 5% solution or ointment or 15 ml of Xylocaine Viscous q 3 to 4 hours to oral or nasal mucosa.

Local anesthesia in procedures involving the male or female urethra
Adults: Instill about 15 ml (male) or 3 to 5 ml (female) into urethra.

Pain, burning, or itching caused by burns, sunburn, or skin irritation
Adults: Apply liberally.

PHARMACODYNAMICS

Ventricular antiarrhythmic action: One of the oldest antiarrhythmics, lidocaine remains among the most widely used drugs for treating acute ventricular arrhythmias. According to the Advanced Cardiac Life Support guidelines (American Heart Association, 1994), lidocaine is the drug of choice to treat ventricular tachycardia and fibrillation.

As a class IB antiarrhythmic, it suppresses automaticity and shortens the effective refractory period and action potential duration of His-Purkinje fibers and suppresses spontaneous ventricular depolarization during diastole. Therapeutic levels don't significantly affect conductive atrial tissue and AV conduction. Unlike quinidine and procainamide, lidocaine doesn't significantly alter hemodynamics when given in usual doses. Drug seems to act preferentially on diseased or ischemic myocardial tissue; exerting its effects on the conduction system, it inhibits reentry mechanisms and halts ventricular arrhythmias.

Local anesthetic action: As a local anesthetic, lidocaine blocks initiation and conduction of nerve impulses by decreasing the permeability of the nerve cell membrane to sodium ions.

PHARMACOKINETICS

Absorption: Lidocaine is absorbed after oral administration; however, a significant first-pass effect occurs in the liver and only about 35% of drug reaches the systemic circulation. Oral doses high enough to achieve therapeutic blood levels result in unacceptable toxicity, probably from high levels of lidocaine.

Distribution: Drug is distributed widely throughout the body and has a high affinity for adipose tissue. After I.V. bolus administration, plasma levels decline rapidly; this decline is associated mainly with distribution into highly perfused tissues (such as the kidneys, lungs, liver, and heart), followed by a slower elimination phase in which metabolism and redistribution into skeletal muscle and adipose tissue occur. The first (early) distribution phase occurs rapidly, calling for initiation of a constant infusion after an initial bolus dose. Distribution volume declines in patients with liver or hepatic disease, resulting in toxic levels with usual doses. About 60% to 80% of circulating drug is bound to plasma proteins. Usual therapeutic drug level is 1.5 to 5 μg/ml. Although toxicity may occur within this range, levels greater than 5 μg/ml are considered toxic and warrant dosage reduction.

Metabolism: Lidocaine is metabolized in the liver to two active metabolites. Less than 10% of a parenteral dose escapes metabolism and reaches the kidneys unchanged. Metabolism is affected by hepatic blood flow, which may decrease after MI and with heart failure. Liver disease also may limit metabolism.

Excretion: Drug's half-life undergoes a biphasic process, with an initial phase of 7 to 30 minutes followed by a terminal half-life of 1.5 to 2 hours. Elimination half-life may be prolonged in patients with heart failure or liver disease. Continuous infusions longer than 24 hours also may cause an apparent half-life increase.

CONTRAINDICATIONS & PRECAUTIONS

Contraindicated in patients with hypersensitivity to amide-type local anesthetics, Stokes-Adams syndrome, Wolff-Parkinson-White syndrome, and severe degrees of SA, AV, or intraventricular block in the absence of an artificial pacemaker. Also contraindicated in patients with inflammation or infection in puncture region, septicemia, severe hypertension, spinal deformities, and neurologic disorders.

Use cautiously in geriatric patients and in those with renal or hepatic disease, complete or second-degree heart block, sinus bradycardia, or heart failure; and in those weighing less than 50 kg (110 lb).

INTERACTIONS

Drug-drug. Use with other *antiarrhythmics*—including *phenytoin, procainamide, propranolol,* and *quinidine*—may cause additive or antagonist effects as well as additive toxicity. Use of lidocaine with *beta blockers* or *cimetidine* may cause lidocaine toxicity from reduced hepatic clearance. Use of high-dose lidocaine with *succinylcholine* may increase neuromuscular effects of succinylcholine.

ADVERSE REACTIONS

CNS: anxiety, nervousness, lethargy, somnolence, paresthesia, muscle twitching; *confusion, tremor, stupor, restlessness, light-headedness,* hallucinations, *seizures* (with systemic form); apprehension, seizures followed by drowsiness, unconsciousness, *respiratory arrest,* confusion, tremors, stupor, restlessness, slurred speech, euphoria, depression, light-headedness, *seizures* (with topical use).
CV: bradycardia, CARDIAC ARREST; *hypotension, new or worsened arrhythmias* (with systemic form); hypotension, myocardial depression, *arrhythmias* (with topical use).
EENT: *tinnitus, blurred or double vision* (with systemic form); tinnitus, blurred or double vision (with topical use).
GI: nausea, vomiting (with topical use).
Skin: dermatologic reactions, sensitization, rash (with topical use).
Other: *anaphylaxis;* soreness at injection site, sensation of cold (with systemic form); edema, *status asthmaticus,* diaphoresis (with topical use).

▣ KEY CONSIDERATIONS

● Use drug with caution in geriatric patients, those weighing less than 50 kg (110 lb), and those with heart failure or renal or hepatic disease. Such patients will need dosage reduction.
● Because of prevalence of concurrent diseases and declining organ system function in geriatric patients, conservative lidocaine doses should be used.
● Monitor patient receiving I.V. lidocaine infusion on cardiac monitor at all times. Use infusion pump or microdrip system and timer to monitor infusion precisely. Never exceed infusion rate of 4 mg/minute. A faster rate greatly increases risk of toxicity.
● Don't administer lidocaine with epinephrine (for local anesthesia) to treat arrhythmias. Use solutions with epinephrine cautiously in patients with CV disorders and in body areas with limited blood supply (ears, nose, fingers, toes).
● Monitor vital signs and serum electrolyte, BUN, and creatinine levels.
● Monitor ECG constantly if administering drug I.V., especially in patients with liver disease, heart failure, hypoxia, respiratory depression, hypovolemia, or shock because these conditions may affect drug metabolism, excretion, or distribution volume, predisposing patient to drug toxicity.
● Monitor for signs of excessive depression of cardiac conductivity (such as sinus node dysfunction, PR-interval prolongation, QRS-interval widening, and appearance or exacerbation of arrhythmias). If they occur, reduce dosage or discontinue drug.
● In severely ill patients, seizures may be the first sign of toxicity. However, severe reactions are usually preceded by somnolence, confusion, and paresthesias. Regard all signs and symptoms of toxicity as serious, and promptly reduce dosage or discontinue therapy. Continued infusion could lead to seizures and coma. Give oxygen via nasal cannula, if not contraindicated. Keep oxygen and CPR equipment handy.
● Doses of up to 400 mg I.M. have been advocated in prehospital phase of acute MI.

Reactions may be *common,* uncommon, ***life-threatening***, OR COMMON AND **LIFE-THREATENING**.

• Patients receiving lidocaine I.M. will show a 7-fold increase in serum CK level. Such CK originates in skeletal muscle, not the heart. Test isoenzyme levels to confirm MI if using I.M. route.

• Don't use solutions containing preservatives for spinal, epidural, or caudal block.

• With epidural use, inject a 2- to 5-ml test dose at least 5 minutes before giving total dose to check for intravascular or subarachnoid injection. Motor paralysis and extensive sensory anesthesia indicate subarachnoid injection.

• Therapeutic serum levels range from 2 to 5 µg/ml.

• Discard partially used vials containing no preservatives.

• Drug has been used investigationally to treat refractory status epilepticus.

Overdose & treatment

• Signs and symptoms of overdose include evidence of CNS toxicity, such as seizures or respiratory depression, and CV toxicity (as indicated by hypotension).

• Treatment includes general supportive measures and drug discontinuation. A patent airway should be maintained and other respiratory support measures carried out immediately. Diazepam or thiopental may be given to treat seizures. To treat significant hypotension, vasopressors (including dopamine and norepinephrine) may be administered.

lindane (gamma benzene hexachloride)
G-well, Kwell, Scabene

Chlorinated hydrocarbon insecticide, scabicide, pediculicide

Available by prescription only
Cream: 1%
Lotion: 1%
Shampoo: 1%

INDICATIONS & DOSAGE
Note: Maximum dosage is 2 oz/application.
Scabies
Adults: After bathing with soap and water, apply a thin layer of cream or lotion

and gently massage it on all skin surfaces, moving from the neck to the toes. After 8 to 12 hours, remove drug by bathing and scrubbing well. Treatment may be repeated after 1 week if needed.
Pediculosis
Adults: Apply shampoo to dry, affected area and wait 4 minutes. Then add a small amount of water and lather for 4 to 5 minutes; rinse thoroughly. Comb hair to remove nits. Treatment may be repeated after 1 week if needed.

PHARMACODYNAMICS
Scabicide and pediculicide actions: Lindane is toxic to the parasitic arthropod *Sarcoptes scabiei* and its eggs, and to *Pediculus capitis, Pediculus corporis,* and *Phthirus pubis.* Drug is absorbed through the organism's exoskeleton and causes its death.

PHARMACOKINETICS
Absorption: About 10% of topical dose may be absorbed in 24 hours.
Distribution: Lindane is stored in body fat.
Metabolism: Metabolism occurs in the liver.
Excretion: Lindane is excreted in urine and feces.

CONTRAINDICATIONS & PRECAUTIONS
Contraindicated in patients hypersensitive to lindane, when skin is raw or inflamed, or in patients with seizure disorders.

INTERACTIONS
None reported.

ADVERSE REACTIONS
CNS: *dizziness,* **seizures.**
Skin: *irritation* (with repeated use).

▣ KEY CONSIDERATIONS
• Make sure patient's body is clean (scrubbed well) and dry before application.
• Avoid applying drug to acutely inflamed skin or raw, weeping surfaces.
• Place hospitalized patient in isolation with linen-handling precautions.

Patient education
• Explain correct use of drug.

• Warn patient that itching may continue for several weeks, even if treatment is effective, especially in scabies infestation.
• If drug accidentally contacts eyes, tell patient to flush with water and call for further instructions. He should avoid inhaling vapor.
• Explain that reapplication usually is unnecessary unless live mites are found; advise reapplication if drug is accidentally washed off, but caution against overuse.
• Tell patient he may use drug to clean combs and brushes, and to wash them thoroughly afterward; advise patient that all clothing and bed linen that may have been contaminated within the past 2 days should be machine washed in hot water and dried in hot dryer, or dry-cleaned, to avoid reinfestation or transmission of organism.
• Discourage repeated use of drug, which may irritate skin and cause systemic toxicity.
• Caution patient to avoid use of other oils or ointments.
• Advise patient that family and close contacts, including sexual contacts, should be treated concurrently.
• Warn patient not to use if open wounds, cuts, or sores are present on scalp or groin, unless directed by health care provider.

Overdose & treatment
• Accidental ingestion may cause extreme CNS toxicity; reported signs and symptoms include CNS stimulation, dizziness, and seizures.
• To treat lindane ingestion, induce vomiting or perform gastric lavage; follow with saline cathartic (don't use oil laxative). Treat seizures with pentobarbital, phenobarbital, or diazepam, as needed.

---

liothyronine sodium (T_3)
Cytomel, Triostat

Thyroid hormone, thyroid hormone replacement

Available by prescription only
Tablets: 5 mcg, 25 mcg, 50 mcg
Injection: 10 mcg/ml

INDICATIONS & DOSAGE
Myxedema
Adults: Initially, 5 mcg daily, increased by 5 to 10 mcg q 1 to 2 weeks. Maintenance dosage is 50 to 100 mcg daily.
Myxedema coma, precoma
Adults: Initially, 25 to 50 mcg I.V.; reassess after 4 to 12 hours, then switch to P.O. as soon as possible. Patients with known or suspected cardiac disease should receive 10 to 20 mcg I.V.
Nontoxic goiter
Adults: Initially, 5 mcg P.O. daily; may be increased by 5 to 10 mcg daily at intervals of 1 to 2 weeks until dosage of 25 mcg daily is reached. Thereafter, dosage may be increased by 12.5 to 25 mcg daily at intervals of 1 to 2 weeks until desired response is noted. Usual maintenance dosage is 75 mcg daily.
Geriatric patients: Initially, 5 mcg P.O. daily, increased by 5-mcg increments q 1 to 2 weeks until dosage of 25 mcg is reached. Thereafter, dosage may be increased by 12.5 to 25 mcg daily q 1 to 2 weeks.
Thyroid hormone replacement
Adults: Initially, 25 mcg P.O. daily, increased by 12.5 to 25 mcg q 1 to 2 weeks until satisfactory response is achieved. Usual maintenance dosage is 25 to 75 mcg daily.
Liothyronine suppression test to differentiate hyperthyroidism from euthyroidism
Adults: 75 to 100 mcg daily for 7 days.

PHARMACODYNAMICS
Thyroid hormone replacement action: Liothyronine is usually a second-line drug in the treatment of hypothyroidism, myxedema, and cretinism. This component of thyroid hormone affects protein and carbohydrate metabolism, promotes gluconeogenesis, increases the utilization and mobilization of glycogen stores, stimulates protein synthesis, and regulates cell growth and differentiation. The major effect of liothyronine is to increase the metabolic rate of tissue. It may be most useful in syndromes of thyroid hormone resistance.

PHARMACOKINETICS

Absorption: Liothyronine is 95% absorbed from the GI tract. Peak effect occurs within 24 to 72 hours.
Distribution: Drug is highly protein-bound. Its distribution hasn't been fully described.
Metabolism: Unknown
Excretion: Half-life is 1 to 2 days.

CONTRAINDICATIONS & PRECAUTIONS

Contraindicated in patients with hypersensitivity to liothyronine, acute MI uncomplicated by hypothyroidism, untreated thyrotoxicosis, or uncorrected adrenal insufficiency. Use cautiously in geriatric patients and in those with angina pectoris, hypertension, ischemia, other CV disorders, renal insufficiency, diabetes, or myxedema.

INTERACTIONS

Drug-drug. Use of liothyronine with *adrenocorticoids* or *corticotropin* alters thyroid status; changes in liothyronine dosages may require dosage changes in the adrenocorticoid or corticotropin as well. Use with *anticoagulants* may impair the latter's effects; an increase in liothyronine dosage may require a lower dosage of the anticoagulant. *Estrogens,* which increase serum thyroxine-binding globulin levels, increase liothyronine requirements. Use with *insulin* or *oral antidiabetics* may affect dosage requirements of these agents. Use with *sympathomimetics* or *tricyclic antidepressants* may increase the effects of any or all of these drugs, causing coronary insufficiency or arrhythmias.

ADVERSE REACTIONS

CNS: *nervousness, insomnia, tremor,* headache.
CV: *tachycardia,* **arrhythmias,** angina pectoris, **cardiac decompensation and collapse.**
GI: diarrhea, vomiting.
Metabolic: weight loss.
Skin: diaphoresis, skin reactions.
Other: heat intolerance.

▣ KEY CONSIDERATIONS

Besides the recommendations relevant to all thyroid hormones, consider the following:

● Geriatric patients are more sensitive to drug's effects. In patients older than age 60, initial dosage should be 25% lower than usual recommended dosage.

● Liothyronine may be preferred when rapid effect is desired or when GI absorption or peripheral conversion of levothyroxine to liothyronine is impaired.

● Oral absorption may be reduced in patients with heart failure.

● When switching from levothyroxine to liothyronine, discontinue levothyroxine and start liothyronine at low dosage, increasing in small increments after residual effects of levothyroxine have disappeared. When switching from liothyronine to levothyroxine, start levothyroxine several days before withdrawing liothyronine to avoid relapse.

● Discontinue drug 7 to 10 days before patient undergoes radioactive iodine uptake studies. Liothyronine therapy alters radioactive iodine (^{131}I) uptake and protein-bound iodine levels.

Patient education

● Tell patient to report headache, diarrhea, nervousness, excessive sweating, heat intolerance, chest pain, increased pulse rate, or palpitations.

● Advise patient not to store drug in warm, humid areas, such as the bathroom, to prevent deterioration of drug.

● Encourage patient to take drug at the same time each day, preferably in the morning to avoid insomnia.

Overdose & treatment

● Signs and symptoms of overdose include evidence of hyperthyroidism, including weight loss, increased appetite, palpitations, diarrhea, nervousness, abdominal cramps, sweating, headache, tachycardia, increased blood pressure, widened pulse pressure, angina, arrhythmias, tremor, insomnia, heat intolerance, fever, and menstrual irregularities.

● Treatment of overdose reduces GI absorption and counteracts central and peripheral effects, primarily sympathetic activity. Perform gastric lavage or induce vomiting, followed by activated charcoal up to 4 hours after ingestion. If patient is comatose or having seizures, inflate the cuff on an endotracheal tube to prevent aspiration. Treatment may include oxygen and ventilation to maintain respiration. It also should include appropriate measures to treat heart failure and to control fever, hypoglycemia, and fluid loss. Propranolol (or another beta blocker) may be used to counteract many of the effects of increased sympathetic activity. Liothyronine should be withdrawn gradually over 2 to 6 days, then resumed at a lower dose.

liotrix
Euthroid, Thyrolar

Thyroid hormone, thyroid hormone replacement

Available by prescription only
Tablets: Euthroid-1/2—levothyroxine sodium 30 mcg and liothyronine sodium 7.5 mcg
Euthroid-1—levothyroxine sodium 60 mcg and liothyronine sodium 15 mcg
Euthroid-2—levothyroxine sodium 120 mcg and liothyronine sodium 30 mcg
Euthroid-3—levothyroxine sodium 180 mcg and liothyronine sodium 45 mcg
Thyrolar-1/4—levothyroxine sodium 12.5 mcg and liothyronine sodium 3.1 mcg
Thyrolar-1/2—levothyroxine sodium 25 mcg and liothyronine sodium 6.25 mcg
Thyrolar-1—levothyroxine sodium 50 mcg and liothyronine sodium 12.5 mcg
Thyrolar-2—levothyroxine sodium 100 mcg and liothyronine sodium 25 mcg
Thyrolar-3—levothyroxine sodium 150 mcg and liothyronine sodium 37.5 mcg

INDICATIONS & DOSAGE
Hypothyroidism
Dosages must be individualized to approximate deficit in patient's thyroid secretion.

Adults: Initially, 15 to 30 mg thyroid equivalent P.O. daily, increased by 15 to 30 mg thyroid equivalent q 1 to 2 weeks until desired response is achieved.

PHARMACODYNAMICS
Thyroid hormone replacement action: Liotrix affects protein and carbohydrate metabolism, promotes gluconeogenesis, increases the use and mobilization of glycogen stores, stimulates protein synthesis, and regulates cell growth and differentiation. The major effect of liotrix is to increase the metabolic rate of tissue. It's used to treat hypothyroidism (myxedema, cretinism, and thyroid hormone deficiency).

Liotrix is a synthetic preparation combining levothyroxine sodium and liothyronine sodium. Such combination products were developed because circulating T_3 was assumed to result from direct release from the thyroid gland. About 80% of T_3 is now known to be derived from deiodination of T_4 in peripheral tissues, and patients receiving only T_4 have normal serum T_3 and T_4 levels. Therefore, combining thyroid drugs isn't advantageous; actually, it could result in excessive T_3 levels.

PHARMACOKINETICS
Absorption: About 50% to 95% is absorbed from the GI tract.
Distribution: Distribution isn't fully understood.
Metabolism: Liotrix is metabolized partially in peripheral tissues (liver, kidneys, and intestines).
Excretion: Drug is excreted partially in feces.

CONTRAINDICATIONS & PRECAUTIONS
Contraindicated in patients with hypersensitivity to liotrix, acute MI uncomplicated by hypothyroidism, untreated thyrotoxicosis, or uncorrected adrenal insufficiency.

Use cautiously in geriatric patients and in those with impaired renal function, ischemia, angina pectoris, hypertension, other CV disorders, myxedema, and diabetes mellitus or insipidus.

Reactions may be *common,* uncommon, *life-threatening,* or COMMON AND LIFE-THREATENING.

INTERACTIONS

Drug-drug. Use of liotrix with an *adrenocorticoid* or *corticotropin* alters thyroid status; changes in liotrix dosage may require adrenocorticoid or corticotropin dosage changes as well. Use with *anticoagulants* may alter anticoagulant effect; an increase in liotrix dosage may require a lower anticoagulant dose. *Beta blockers* may decrease the conversion of T_4 to T_3. *Cholestyramine* may delay absorption of T_4. *Estrogens*, which increase serum thyroxine-binding globulin levels, increase liotrix dosage requirements. *Hepatic enzyme inducers* (such as *phenytoin*) may increase hepatic degradation of T_4, resulting in increased requirement for T_4. Use with *insulin* or *oral antidiabetics* may affect dosage requirements of these drugs. Use with *somatrem* may accelerate epiphyseal maturation. Use with *sympathomimetics* or *tricyclic antidepressants* may increase the effects of any or all of these drugs and may lead to coronary insufficiency or arrhythmias.

ADVERSE REACTIONS

CNS: *nervousness, insomnia, tremor,* headache.
CV: *tachycardia, arrhythmias,* angina pectoris, ***cardiac decompensation and collapse.***
GI: diarrhea, vomiting.
Metabolic: weight loss.
Skin: diaphoresis, allergic skin reactions.
Other: heat intolerance.

▣ KEY CONSIDERATIONS

Besides the recommendations relevant to all thyroid hormones, consider the following:
• Geriatric patients are more sensitive to drug's effects and may require a lower dosage.
• Note that T_4 is the drug of choice for hypothyroidism. Hepatic conversion of T_4 to T_3 is usually adequate. Excessive exogenous supplementation of T_3 usually causes toxicity.
• Liotrix therapy alters radioactive iodine (^{131}I) thyroid uptake, protein-bound iodine levels, and T_3 uptake.
• The two commercially prepared liotrix brands contain different amounts of each ingredient; don't change from one brand to the other without considering the differences in potency.
• Monitor patient's pulse rate and blood pressure.
• Protect drug from heat and moisture.

Patient education

• Tell patient to report headache, diarrhea, nervousness, excessive sweating, heat intolerance, chest pain, increased pulse rate, or palpitations.
• Advise patient not to store liotrix in warm and humid areas, such as the bathroom.
• Encourage patient to take single daily dose in the morning to avoid insomnia.

Overdose & treatment

• Signs and symptoms of overdose include evidence of hyperthyroidism, including weight loss, increased appetite, palpitations, nervousness, diarrhea, abdominal cramps, sweating, tachycardia, increased pulse rate and blood pressure, angina, arrhythmias, tremor, headache, insomnia, heat intolerance, fever, and menstrual irregularities.
• Treatment requires reduction of GI absorption and efforts to counteract central and peripheral effects, primarily sympathetic activity. Perform gastric lavage or induce vomiting, then follow with activated charcoal if less than 4 hours since ingestion. If patient is comatose or having seizures, inflate the cuff on an endotracheal tube to prevent aspiration. Treatment may include oxygen and artificial ventilation as needed to maintain respiration. It should also include appropriate measures to treat heart failure and to control fever, hypoglycemia, and fluid loss. Propranolol (or atenolol, metoprolol, acebutolol, nadolol, or timolol) may be used to combat many of the effects of increased sympathetic activity. Thyroid therapy should be withdrawn gradually over 2 to 6 days, then resumed at a lower dosage.

lisinopril
Prinivil, Zestril

ACE inhibitor, antihypertensive

Available by prescription only
Tablets: 2.5 mg, 5 mg, 10 mg, 20 mg,
40 mg

INDICATIONS & DOSAGE
Mild to severe hypertension
Adults: Initially, 10 mg P.O. daily. Most
patients are well controlled on 20 to
40 mg daily as a single dose. Doses up
to 80 mg have been used.
Heart failure
Adults: Initially, 5 mg P.O. daily. Most
patients are well controlled on 5 to
20 mg daily as a single dose.
Acute MI
Adults: Initially, 5 mg P.O.; then give
5 mg after 24 hours, 10 mg after 48
hours, and 10 mg daily for 6 weeks.
    In patients with an acute MI and low
systolic blood pressure (less than
120 mm Hg), give 2.5 mg P.O. when
treatment is started or during the first 3
days after an infarct. If hypotension occurs, a daily maintenance dose of 5 mg
may be given with temporary reductions
to 2.5 mg if needed.
◆ *Dosage adjustment.* In adults with renal failure, initially, 5 mg/day P.O. if creatinine clearance is between 10 and
30 ml/minute, and 2.5 mg/day P.O. if it's
less than 10 ml/minute. Dosage may be
adjusted upward until blood pressure is
controlled or to maximum of 40 mg daily. Dosage for patients with heart failure
who have a creatinine clearance less than
30 ml/minute is 2.5 mg/day P.O.

PHARMACODYNAMICS
Antihypertensive action: Lisinopril inhibits ACE, preventing the conversion of
angiotensin I to angiotensin II, a potent
vasoconstrictor. Reduced formation of
angiotensin II decreases peripheral arterial resistance and aldosterone secretion,
thereby reducing sodium and water retention and blood pressure.

PHARMACOKINETICS
Absorption: Variable absorption occurs
after oral administration; an average of
about 25% of an oral dose has been absorbed by test subjects. Peak serum levels occur in about 7 hours. Onset of antihypertensive activity occurs in about 1
hour and peaks in about 6 hours.
Distribution: Lisinopril is distributed
widely in tissues. Plasma protein-
binding appears insignificant. Minimal
amounts enter the brain.
Metabolism: Drug isn't metabolized.
Excretion: Drug is excreted unchanged
in the urine.

CONTRAINDICATIONS & PRECAUTIONS
Contraindicated in patients with hypersensitivity to ACE inhibitors or history
of angioedema related to previous treatment with an ACE inhibitor. Use cautiously in patients at risk for hyperkalemia or in those with impaired renal
function.

INTERACTIONS
Drug-drug. Use with *diuretics* may
cause excessive hypotension. *Indomethacin* may attenuate the hypotensive effect of lisinopril. Use with *lithium* may
increase plasma lithium levels. Use with
potassium sparing diuretics or *potassium supplements* may lead to hyperkalemia.
Drug-food. *Potassium-containing salt
substitutes* increase the likelihood of hyperkalemia; avoid use.

ADVERSE REACTIONS
CNS: *dizziness, headache, fatigue,
paresthesia.*
CV: hypotension, *orthostatic hypoten-
sion,* chest pain.
EENT: *nasal congestion.*
GI: *diarrhea,* nausea, dyspepsia.
GU: impotence.
Hematologic: *neutropenia, bone mar-
row suppression, thrombocytopenia.*
Metabolic: hyperkalemia.
Respiratory: *dry, persistent, tickling,
nonproductive cough;* dyspnea.
Skin: rash.
Other: *angioedema, anaphylaxis.*

Reactions may be *common*, uncommon, *life-threatening*, or COMMON AND LIFE-THREATENING.

⊡ KEY CONSIDERATIONS

Besides the recommendations relevant to all ACE inhibitors, consider the following:

• Geriatric patients may require lower doses because of impaired drug clearance. They may also be more sensitive to drug's hypotensive effects.

• Drug absorption is unaffected by food.

• Lisinopril attenuates potassium loss of thiazide diuretics.

• If patient is taking a diuretic, discontinue diuretic 2 to 3 days before lisinopril therapy, or reduce lisinopril dosage to 5 mg once daily to reduce the likelihood of hypotension..

• Drug's physiologic effects may elevate serum potassium, serum creatinine, BUN, and serum bilirubin levels; slightly reduce hemoglobin level and hematocrit; and change liver enzyme levels.

• If drug doesn't adequately control blood pressure, diuretics may be added.

• Review WBC and differential counts before treatment, every 2 weeks for 3 months, and periodically thereafter.

• Lower the dosage in patients with impaired renal function.

• Be aware that the beneficial effects of lisinopril may require several weeks of therapy.

Patient education

• Tell patient to report light-headedness, especially in first few days of treatment, so dose can be adjusted; signs of infection such as sore throat or fever because drug may decrease WBC count; facial swelling or difficulty breathing because drug may cause angioedema; and loss of taste, which may necessitate discontinuation of drug.

• Tell patient that a dry, persistent, tickling, nonproductive cough may occur. If it becomes bothersome, he should notify the health care provider; the drug may need to be stopped.

• Advise patient to avoid sudden postural changes to minimize orthostatic hypotension.

• Warn patient to seek medical approval before taking OTC cold preparations.

• Instruct patient to avoid potassium-containing salt substitutes.

lithium carbonate
Carbolith*, Duralith*, Eskalith, Eskalith CR, Lithane, Lithizine*, Lithobid, Lithonate, Lithotabs

lithium citrate
Cibalith-S

Alkali metal, antimanic, antipsychotic

Available by prescription only
lithium carbonate
Capsules: 150 mg, 300 mg, 600 mg
Tablets: 300 mg
Tablets (sustained-release): 300 mg, 450 mg
lithium citrate
Syrup (sugarless): 300 mg/5 ml (with 0.3% alcohol)

INDICATIONS & DOSAGE

Prevention or control of mania; prevention of depression in patients with bipolar illness
Adults: Acute and maintenance dosage, 900 mg (sustained-release tablet) P.O. in morning and h.s., or 600 mg (tablet or capsule) in the morning, noon, and h.s.
◊ *Major depression,* ◊ *schizoaffective disorder,* ◊ *schizophrenic disorder,* ◊ *alcohol dependence*
Adults: 300 mg lithium carbonate P.O. t.i.d. or q.i.d.
◊ *Chemotherapy-induced neutropenia in patients with AIDS receiving zidovudine*
Adults: 300 to 1,000 mg P.O. daily.

PHARMACODYNAMICS

Antimanic and antipsychotic actions: Lithium is thought to exert its antipsychotic and antimanic effects by competing with other cations for exchange at the sodium-potassium ion pump, thus altering cation exchange at the tissue level. It also inhibits adenyl cyclase, reducing intracellular levels of cAMP and, to a lesser extent, cyclic guanosine monophosphate (cGMP).

PHARMACOKINETICS

Absorption: Rate and extent of absorption vary with dosage form; absorption is complete within 6 hours of oral administration of conventional tablets and capsules.

Distribution: Distributed widely into the body; levels in thyroid gland, bone, and brain tissue exceed serum levels. Peak effects occur at 30 minutes to 3 hours; liquid form peaks at 15 minutes to 1 hour. Steady-state serum level is achieved in 12 hours; therapeutic effect begins in 5 to 10 days and is maximal within 3 weeks. Therapeutic and toxic serum levels and therapeutic effects show good correlation. Therapeutic range is 0.6 to 1.2 mEq/L; adverse reactions increase as level reaches 1.5 to 2 mEq/L—such levels may be necessary in acute mania. Toxicity usually occurs at levels above 2 mEq/L.

Metabolism: Lithium isn't metabolized.

Excretion: Excreted 95% unchanged in urine; about 50% to 80% of a given dose is excreted within 24 hours. Level of renal function determines elimination rate.

CONTRAINDICATIONS & PRECAUTIONS

Contraindicated if therapy can't be closely monitored. Use cautiously in geriatric patients; patients with thyroid disease, seizure disorders, renal or CV disease, severe dehydration or debilitation, or sodium depletion; and in those receiving neuroleptics, neuromuscular blockers, and diuretics.

INTERACTIONS

Drug-drug. *Antacids* and *other drugs containing aminophylline, caffeine, calcium, sodium,* or *theophylline* may increase lithium excretion by renal competition for elimination, thus decreasing lithium's therapeutic effect. *Carbamazepine, mazindol, methyldopa, phenytoin,* and *tetracyclines* may increase lithium toxicity. Lithium may decrease the effects of *chlorpromazine.* Acute neurotoxicity with delirium has occurred in patients receiving lithium and *electroconvulsive therapy* (ECT); lithium dosage should be reduced or withdrawn before ECT. *Fluoxetine* increases lithium serum levels. Use with *haloperidol* may result in severe encephalopathy characterized by confusion, tremors, extrapyramidal effects, and weakness; use this combination with caution. *Indomethacin, phenyl-*

butazone, piroxicam, and *other NSAIDs* also decrease renal excretion of lithium and may require a 30% reduction in lithium dosage. Use of lithium with *thiazide diuretics* may decrease renal excretion and enhance lithium toxicity; diuretic dosage may need to be reduced by 30%. Lithium also may potentiate the effects of *neuromuscular blockers* (such as *atracurium, pancuronium,* and *succinylcholine*) and interfere with the pressor effects of *sympathomimetics,* especially *norepinephrine.*

Drug-food. *Caffeine* and *calcium* may increase lithium excretion by renal competition for elimination, thus decreasing lithium's therapeutic effect. *Dietary sodium* may alter the renal elimination of lithium. Increased sodium intake may increase elimination of drug; decreased intake may decrease elimination.

ADVERSE REACTIONS

CNS: tremors, drowsiness, headache, confusion, restlessness, dizziness, psychomotor retardation, lethargy, **coma,** blackouts, **epileptiform seizures,** EEG changes, worsened organic mental syndrome, impaired speech, ataxia, muscle weakness, incoordination.

CV: *reversible ECG changes,* **arrhythmias,** hypotension, bradycardia, **peripheral vascular collapse** (rare).

EENT: tinnitus, blurred vision.

GI: dry mouth, metallic taste, nausea, vomiting, anorexia, diarrhea, *thirst,* abdominal pain, flatulence, indigestion.

GU: *polyuria,* glycosuria, renal toxicity with long-term use, decreased creatinine clearance, albuminuria.

Hematologic: *leukocytosis with WBC count of 14,000 to 18,000/mm^3* (reversible).

Metabolic: transient hyperglycemia, goiter, hypothyroidism (lowered T_3, T_4, and protein-bound iodine, but elevated ^{131}I uptake), hyponatremia.

Skin: pruritus, rash, diminished or absent sensation, drying and thinning of hair, psoriasis, acne, alopecia.

Other: ankle and wrist edema.

▣ KEY CONSIDERATIONS

• Geriatric patients are more susceptible to chronic overdose and toxic effects, es-

---

Reactions may be *common,* uncommon, *life-threatening*, or COMMON AND LIFE-THREATENING.

pecially dyskinesias. These patients usually respond to a lower dosage.

• Shake syrup formulation before administration.

• Discontinue drug before ECT therapy.

• Administer drug with food or milk to reduce GI upset.

• Monitor baseline ECG, thyroid and renal studies, and electrolyte levels. Monitor lithium blood levels 8 to 12 hours after first dose, usually before morning dose, 2 or 3 times weekly for the first month, then weekly to monthly on maintenance therapy.

• Note that determination of serum drug levels is crucial for safe use of drug. Don't use drug in patients who can't have regular serum drug level checks. Be sure patient or responsible family member can comply with instructions.

• When lithium blood levels are less than 1.5 mEq/L, adverse reactions usually are mild.

• Monitor fluid intake and output, especially when surgery is scheduled.

• Expect lag of 1 to 3 weeks before drug's beneficial effects are noticed. Other psychotropic drugs (for example, chlorpromazine) may be necessary during interim.

• Drug causes false-positive test results on thyroid function tests; it also elevates neutrophil count.

• Monitor for signs of edema or sudden weight gain.

• Adjust fluid and salt ingestion to compensate if excessive loss occurs through protracted sweating or diarrhea. Patient should have fluid intake of 2,500 to 3,000 ml daily and a balanced diet with adequate salt intake.

• Arrange for outpatient follow-up of thyroid and renal function every 6 to 12 months. Thyroid should be palpated to check for enlargement.

• Check urine for specific gravity less than 1.015, which may indicate diabetes insipidus.

• Drug may alter glucose tolerance in diabetic patients. Monitor blood glucose levels closely.

• Lithium is used investigationally to increase WBC count in patients undergoing cancer chemotherapy. It has also been used investigationally to treat clus-ter headaches, aggression, organic brain syndrome, and tardive dyskinesia. Drug has been used to treat SIADH.

• Monitor serum levels and signs of impending toxicity.

• Lithane tablets contain tartrazine, a dye that may precipitate an allergic reaction in certain individuals, particularly asthmatic patients sensitive to aspirin.

• Monitor drug dosing carefully when patient's initial manic symptoms begin to subside because the ability to tolerate high serum lithium levels decreases as symptoms resolve.

• EEG changes include diffuse slowing, widening of frequency spectrum, potentiation, and disorganization of background rhythm. Vomiting and diarrhea occur within 1 hour of acute ingestion (induce vomiting in noncomatose patients if it isn't spontaneous). Death has occurred in patients ingesting 10 to 60 g of lithium; patients have ingested 6 g with minimal toxic effects. Serum lithium levels above 3.4 mEq/L are potentially fatal.

Patient education

• Explain that lithium has a narrow therapeutic margin of safety. A serum drug level that is even slightly high can be dangerous.

• Warn patient and family to watch for signs of toxicity (diarrhea, vomiting, dehydration, drowsiness, muscle weakness, tremor, fever, and ataxia) and to expect transient nausea, polyuria, thirst, and discomfort during first few days. If toxic symptoms occur, tell patient to withhold one dose and call promptly.

• Warn ambulatory patient to avoid activities that require alertness and good psychomotor coordination until CNS response to drug is determined.

• Advise patient to maintain adequate water intake and adequate—but not excessive—salt in diet.

• Explain importance of regular follow-up visits to measure lithium serum levels.

• Tell patient to avoid large amounts of caffeine, which will interfere with drug's effectiveness.

• Advise patient to seek medical approval before initiating weight-loss program.

• Tell patient not to switch brands of lithium or take other prescription or OTC drugs without medical approval. Different brands may not provide equivalent effect.

• Tell patient to take drug with food.

• Warn patient against stopping drug abruptly.

• Tell patient to explain to close friends or family members the signs of lithium overdose in case emergency aid is needed.

• Instruct patient to carry identification and instruction card with toxicity and emergency information.

Overdose & treatment

• Overdose with chronic lithium ingestion may follow altered pharmacokinetics, drug interactions, or volume or sodium depletion; sedation, confusion, hand tremors, joint pain, ataxia, muscle stiffness, increased deep tendon reflexes, visual changes, and nystagmus may occur. Symptoms may progress to coma, movement abnormalities, tremors, seizures, and CV collapse.

• Treatment is symptomatic and supportive; closely monitor vital signs. Induce vomiting or perform gastric lavage. Monitor fluid and electrolyte balance; correct sodium depletion with normal saline solution. Institute hemodialysis if serum level is above 3 mEq/L, in severely symptomatic patients unresponsive to fluid and electrolyte correction, or if urine output decreases significantly. Serum rebound of tissue lithium stores (from high volume distribution) commonly occurs after dialysis and may necessitate prolonged or repeated hemodialysis. Peritoneal dialysis may help but is less effective.

loperamide hydrochloride
Imodium, Imodium A-D, Kaopectate II, Maalox Anti-Diarrheal, Pepto Diarrhea Control

Piperidine derivative, antidiarrheal

Available by prescription only
Capsules: 2 mg
Available without a prescription

Tablets: 2 mg
Solution: 1 mg/5 ml

INDICATIONS & DOSAGE
Acute, nonspecific diarrhea
Adults: Initially, 4 mg P.O., then 2 mg after each unformed stool. Maximum dosage, 16 mg daily.
Chronic diarrhea
Adults: Initially, 4 mg P.O., then 2 mg after each unformed stool until diarrhea subsides. Adjust dose to individual response.
Relief of diarrhea (self-medication)
Adults: 4 tsp or 2 tablets after the first loose bowel movement, followed by 2 tsp or 1 tablet after each subsequent loose bowel movement. Don't exceed 8 mg/day for 2 days.

PHARMACODYNAMICS
Antidiarrheal action: Loperamide reduces intestinal motility by acting directly on intestinal mucosal nerve endings; tolerance to antiperistaltic effect doesn't develop. Drug also may inhibit fluid and electrolyte secretion by an unknown mechanism. Although it's chemically related to opiates, it hasn't shown any physical dependence in humans, and it possesses no analgesic activity.

PHARMACOKINETICS
Absorption: Loperamide is absorbed poorly from the GI tract.
Distribution: Unknown.
Metabolism: Absorbed drug is metabolized in the liver.
Excretion: Drug is excreted primarily in feces; less than 2% is excreted in urine.

CONTRAINDICATIONS & PRECAUTIONS
Contraindicated in patients with hypersensitivity to loperamide or when constipation must be avoided. Also, OTC use is contraindicated in patients with a fever exceeding 101° F (38.3° C) or if blood is present in the stool. Use cautiously in patients with hepatic impairment.

INTERACTIONS
Drug-drug. Use with an *opioid analgesic* may cause severe constipation.

Reactions may be *common*, uncommon, **life-threatening**, or COMMON AND LIFE-THREATENING.

ADVERSE REACTIONS
CNS: drowsiness, fatigue, dizziness.
GI: dry mouth; abdominal pain, distention, or discomfort; *constipation;* nausea; vomiting.
Skin: rash, hypersensitivity reactions.

▣ KEY CONSIDERATIONS
• After administration via nasogastric tube, flush tube to clear it and to ensure drug's passage to stomach.

Patient education
• Warn patient to take drug only as directed and not to exceed recommended dose.
• Caution patient to avoid driving and other tasks requiring alertness because drug may cause drowsiness and dizziness.
• Instruct patient to call if no improvement occurs in 48 hours or if fever develops.

Overdose & treatment
• Signs and symptoms of overdose include constipation, GI irritation, and CNS depression.
• Treat with activated charcoal if ingestion was recent. If patient is vomiting, activated charcoal may be given in a slurry when patient can retain fluids. Alternatively, gastric lavage may be performed, followed by administration of activated charcoal slurry. Monitor for CNS depression; treat respiratory depression with naloxone.

loracarbef
Lorabid

Synthetic beta-lactam antibiotic of carbacephem class, antibiotic

Available by prescription only
Pulvules: 200 mg, 400 mg
Powder for oral suspension:
100 mg/5 ml, 200 mg/5 ml

INDICATIONS & DOSAGE
Secondary bacterial infections of acute bronchitis
Adults: 200 to 400 mg P.O. q 12 hours for 7 days.

Acute bacterial exacerbations of chronic bronchitis
Adults: 400 mg P.O. q 12 hours for 7 days.
Pneumonia
Adults: 400 mg P.O. q 12 hours for 14 days.
Pharyngitis or tonsillitis
Adults: 200 mg P.O. q 12 hours for 10 days.
Sinusitis
Adults: 400 mg P.O. q 12 hours for 10 days.
Uncomplicated skin and skin-structure infections
Adults: 200 mg P.O. q 12 hours for 7 days.
Uncomplicated cystitis
Adults: 200 mg P.O. daily for 7 days.
Uncomplicated pyelonephritis
Adults: 400 mg P.O. q 12 hours for 14 days.
◆ *Dosage adjustment.* Adults with renal failure and creatinine clearance of 50 ml/minute or more don't require dose and interval changes. In patients with creatinine clearance of 10 to 49 ml/minute, use half the usual dose at same interval or normal recommended dose at twice the usual dosage interval; in those with creatinine clearance less than 10 ml/minute, use usual dose q 3 to 5 days. Hemodialysis patients should be given another dose after dialysis.

PHARMACODYNAMICS
Antibiotic action: Loracarbef exerts its bactericidal action by binding to essential target proteins of the bacterial cell wall, leading to inhibition of cell-wall synthesis. Loracarbef is active against gram-positive aerobes, such as *Staphylococcus aureus, S. saprophyticus, Streptococcus pneumoniae,* and *S. pyogenes;* and gram-negative aerobes, such as *Escherichia coli, Haemophilus influenzae,* and *Moraxella (Branhamella) catarrhalis.*

PHARMACOKINETICS
Absorption: After oral administration, loracarbef is about 90% absorbed from the GI tract. When pulvules are taken with food, peak plasma levels are 50% to 60% of those achieved on an empty

stomach. (Effect of food on rate and extent of absorption of suspension form hasn't been studied to date.) Absorption of suspension form is greater than that of pulvule. Average plasma levels of pulvule form peak in about 1.2 hours; those of suspension form peak in about 0.8 hours.

Distribution: About 25% of circulating drug is bound to plasma proteins.

Metabolism: Drug doesn't appear to be metabolized.

Excretion: Drug is eliminated primarily in urine. Elimination half-life in patients with normal renal function averages 1 hour.

CONTRAINDICATIONS & PRECAUTIONS

Contraindicated in patients with hypersensitivity to loracarbef or other cephalosporins and in patients with diarrhea caused by pseudomembranous colitis.

INTERACTIONS

Drug-drug. *Probenecid* decreases the excretion of loracarbef, increasing plasma levels; monitor for toxicity.

Drug-food. *Food* decreases absorption; instruct patient to take drug at least 1 hour before or at least 2 hours after eating.

ADVERSE REACTIONS

CNS: headache, somnolence, nervousness, insomnia, dizziness.

CV: vasodilation.

GI: diarrhea, nausea, vomiting, abdominal pain, anorexia, *pseudomembranous colitis.*

GU: vaginal candidiasis, transient increases in BUN and creatinine levels.

Hematologic: *transient thrombocytopenia, leukopenia,* eosinophilia.

Hepatic: transient elevations in AST, ALT, and alkaline phosphatase levels.

Skin: rash, urticaria, pruritus, *erythema multiforme.*

Other: hypersensitivity reactions, including *anaphylaxis.*

▣ KEY CONSIDERATIONS

• The increased rate of absorption should be considered if oral suspension is to be substituted for pulvule.

• Pseudomembranous colitis has been reported with nearly all antibacterial agents and may range from mild to life-threatening. Therefore, diagnosis must be considered in patients who present with diarrhea after drug administration.

• Obtain specimen for culture and sensitivity tests before giving first dose. Therapy may begin pending test results.

• Drug may cause overgrowth of nonsusceptible bacteria or fungi. Monitor for signs and symptoms of superinfection.

• To reconstitute powder for oral suspension, add 30 ml of water in 2 portions to the 50-ml bottle or 60 ml of water in 2 portions to the 100-ml bottle; shake after each addition.

• After reconstitution, oral suspension is stable for 14 days at room temperature (59° to 86° F [15° to 30° C]).

• Drug can cause prolonged PT and INR, positive direct Coombs' test, elevated LD, pancytopenia, and neutropenia.

Patient education

• Instruct patient to take drug at least 1 hour before or at least 2 hours after eating.

• Tell patient to take drug exactly as prescribed, even after he feels better.

• Inform patient that oral suspension can be stored at room temperature for 14 days. Instruct patient to discard unused portion after 14 days.

Overdose & treatment

• Signs and symptoms of overdose of beta-lactams, such as loracarbef, include nausea, vomiting, epigastric distress, and diarrhea.

• Forced diuresis, peritoneal dialysis, hemodialysis, and hemoperfusion haven't been established as beneficial for an overdose of loracarbef. Hemodialysis is effective in hastening the elimination of loracarbef from plasma in patients with chronic renal failure.

Reactions may be *common*, uncommon, *life-threatening*, or COMMON AND LIFE-THREATENING.

loratadine
Claritin

Tricyclic antihistamine

Available by prescription only
Tablets: 10 mg
Tablets (rapidly disintegrating): 10 mg
Syrup: 1 mg/ml

INDICATIONS & DOSAGE
Symptomatic treatment of seasonal allergic rhinitis and indicated for treatment of idiopathic chronic urticaria
Adults: 10 mg P.O. daily.
✦ *Dosage adjustment.* In patients with liver failure or glomerular filtration rate less than 30 ml/minute, adjust dose to 10 mg every other day.

PHARMACODYNAMICS
Antihistamine action: Loratadine is a long-acting tricyclic antihistamine with selective peripheral H_1-receptor antagonistic activity.

PHARMACOKINETICS
Absorption: Loratadine is readily absorbed, with onset of action beginning within 1 to 3 hours, reaching maximum at 8 to 12 hours, and lasting in excess of 24 hours. Because food may delay plasma levels from peaking by 1 hour, drug should be administered on an empty stomach.
Distribution: About 97% is bound to plasma protein. Drug doesn't readily cross the blood-brain barrier.
Metabolism: Extensively metabolized to an active metabolite (descarboethoxyloratadine). The specific enzyme systems responsible for metabolism haven't been identified.
Excretion: About 80% of total dose administered is equally distributed between urine and feces. Mean elimination half-life is 8.4 hours. Drug isn't eliminated by hemodialysis; it's unknown whether drug is eliminated by peritoneal dialysis.

CONTRAINDICATIONS & PRECAUTIONS
Contraindicated in patients with hypersensitivity to loratadine. Use cautiously in patients with hepatic impairment.

INTERACTIONS
Drug-drug. *Drugs known to inhibit hepatic metabolism* should be coadministered with caution until definitive interaction studies can be completed.
Drug-food. *Food* decreases absorption; instruct patient to take drug at least 1 hour before or at least 2 hours after eating.

ADVERSE REACTIONS
CNS: headache, somnolence, fatigue.
GI: dry mouth.

🔳 KEY CONSIDERATIONS
• No information exists to indicate that drug abuse or dependency occurs.

Patient education
• Instruct patient to take drug on an empty stomach at least 2 hours after a meal and to avoid eating for at least 1 hour after taking drug.
• Tell patient to take drug only once daily. Tell him to call if symptoms persist or worsen.
• Warn patient to stop taking drug 4 days before allergy skin tests to preserve accuracy of tests.

Overdose & treatment
• Somnolence, tachycardia, and headache have been reported with overdoses greater than 10 mg (40 to 180 mg). If overdose occurs, institute symptomatic and supportive measures promptly and maintain for as long as necessary.
• To treat, induce vomiting with ipecac syrup, except in patients with impaired consciousness, followed by administration of activated charcoal to adsorb any remaining drug. If vomiting is unsuccessful or contraindicated, gastric lavage should be performed with normal saline solution. Saline cathartics may be of value for rapid dilution of bowel contents.

*Canada only ◇ Unlabeled clinical use

lorazepam
Apo-Lorazepam*, Ativan, Novo-Lorazem*

Benzodiazepine, anxiolytic, sedative-hypnotic
Controlled substance schedule IV

Available by prescription only
Tablets: 0.5 mg, 1 mg, 2 mg
Tablets (S.L.): 1 mg, 2 mg
Injection: 2 mg/ml, 4 mg/ml

INDICATIONS & DOSAGE
Anxiety, tension, agitation, irritability, especially in anxiety neuroses or organic (especially GI or CV) disorders
Adults: 2 to 6 mg P.O. daily in divided doses; maximum dosage, 10 mg/day.
Insomnia
Adults: 2 to 4 mg P.O. h.s.
Preoperatively
Adults: 0.05 mg/kg I.M. 2 hours before surgery (maximum, 4 mg). Alternatively, 0.044 mg/kg (maximum total dose, 2 mg) I.V. 15 to 20 minutes before surgery; in adults younger than age 50, dosage may be increased to 0.05 mg/kg (maximum, 4 mg) when increased lack of recall of preoperative events is desired.

PHARMACODYNAMICS
Anxiolytic and sedative actions: Lorazepam depresses the CNS at the limbic and subcortical levels of the brain. It produces an antianxiety effect by influencing the effect of the neurotransmitter gamma-aminobutyric acid (GABA) on its receptor in the ascending reticular activating system, which increases inhibition and blocks both cortical and limbic arousal after stimulation of the reticular formation.

PHARMACOKINETICS
Absorption: When administered orally, lorazepam is well absorbed through the GI tract. Peak levels occur in 2 hours.
Distribution: Distributed widely throughout the body. Drug is about 85% protein-bound.
Metabolism: Drug is metabolized in the liver to inactive metabolites.

Excretion: The metabolites of lorazepam are excreted in urine as glucuronide conjugates.

CONTRAINDICATIONS & PRECAUTIONS
Contraindicated in patients with acute angle-closure glaucoma or hypersensitivity to lorazepam, other benzodiazepines, or its vehicle (used in parenteral dosage form).
Use cautiously in patients with pulmonary, renal, or hepatic impairment and in geriatric, acutely ill, or debilitated patients.

INTERACTIONS
Drug-drug. Lorazepam potentiates the CNS depressant effects of *antidepressants, antihistamines, barbiturates, general anesthetics, MAO inhibitors, narcotics,* and *phenothiazines.* Use with *cimetidine* and possibly *disulfiram* causes diminished hepatic metabolism of lorazepam, which increases its plasma level. Use of parenteral lorazepam and *scopolamine* may increase the risk of hallucinations, irrational behavior, and increased sedation.
Drug-lifestyle. Lorazepam potentiates the CNS depressant effects of *alcohol. Heavy smoking* accelerates metabolism of lorazepam, thus lowering effectiveness. Avoid use with either.

ADVERSE REACTIONS
CNS: *drowsiness,* amnesia, insomnia, agitation, *sedation,* dizziness, weakness, unsteadiness, disorientation, depression, headache.
EENT: visual disturbances.
GI: abdominal discomfort, nausea, change in appetite.
Other: *acute withdrawal syndrome* (after sudden discontinuation in physically dependent persons).

▣ KEY CONSIDERATIONS
Besides the recommendations relevant to all benzodiazepines, consider the following:
● Geriatric patients are more sensitive to lorazepam's CNS depressant effects. They may require supervision with ambulation and activities of daily living

---

Reactions may be *common,* uncommon, *life-threatening,* or COMMON AND LIFE-THREATENING.

during initiation of therapy or after an increase in dose.
• Lower doses usually are effective in geriatric patients because of decreased elimination.
• Parenteral administration of drug is more likely to cause apnea, hypotension, bradycardia, and cardiac arrest in geriatric patients.
• Lorazepam is one of the preferred benzodiazepines for patients with hepatic disease.
• Use the lowest possible effective dose to avoid oversedation.
• Parenteral lorazepam appears to possess potent amnestic effects.
• Administer oral drug in divided doses, with the largest dose given before bedtime.
• Arteriospasm may result from intra-arterial injection of lorazepam. Don't administer by this route.
• For I.V. administration, dilute lorazepam with an equal volume of a compatible diluent, such as D_5W, sterile water for injection, or normal saline solution.
• Drug may be injected directly into a vein or into the tubing of a compatible I.V. infusion, such as normal saline solution or D_5W solution. The rate of lorazepam I.V. injection shouldn't exceed 2 mg/minute. Emergency resuscitative equipment should be available when administering I.V.
• Administer diluted lorazepam solutions immediately.
• Don't use drug solutions if they are discolored or contain a precipitate.
• Administer I.M. dose of lorazepam undiluted, deep into a large muscle mass.
• Periodically assess hepatic function studies to prevent cumulative effects and to ensure adequate drug metabolism.
• Drug therapy may elevate liver function test results.

Patient education
• Caution patient not to make changes in drug regimen without specific instructions.
• As appropriate, teach safety measures to protect from injury, such as gradual position changes and supervised walking.
• Advise patient of possible retrograde amnesia after I.V. or I.M. use.

• Tell patient to avoid large amounts of caffeine-containing products, which may interfere with drug's effectiveness.
• Advise patient of potential for physical and psychological dependence with chronic use.
• Tell patient to discontinue drug slowly (over 8 to 12 weeks) after long-term therapy.
• Advise patient that smoking may decrease the effectiveness of the drug.
• Advise patient to avoid alcohol while taking drug.

Overdose & treatment
• Signs and symptoms of overdose include somnolence, confusion, coma, hypoactive reflexes, dyspnea, labored breathing, hypotension, bradycardia, slurred speech, unsteady gait, and impaired coordination.
• Treatment requires support of blood pressure and respiration until drug effects subside; monitor vital signs. Mechanical ventilatory assistance via endotracheal tube may be required to maintain a patent airway and support adequate oxygenation. Flumazenil, a specific benzodiazepine antagonist, may be useful. Use I.V. fluids and vasopressors such as dopamine and phenylephrine to treat hypotension, if necessary. If patient is conscious, induce vomiting; use gastric lavage if ingestion was recent, but only if an endotracheal tube is present to prevent aspiration. Then, administer activated charcoal with a cathartic as a single dose. Dialysis is of limited value.

---

losartan potassium
Cozaar

Angiotensin II receptor antagonist, antihypertensive

Available by prescription only
Tablets: 25 mg, 50 mg

INDICATIONS & DOSAGE
Hypertension
Adults: Initially, 25 to 50 mg P.O. daily. Maintenance dosage is 25 to 100 mg P.O. once daily or b.i.d.

PHARMACODYNAMICS

Antihypertensive action: Losartan is an angiotensin II receptor antagonist. It blocks the vasoconstrictor and aldosterone-secreting effects of angiotensin II by selectively blocking the binding of angiotensin II to its receptor sites found in many tissues, including vascular smooth muscle.

PHARMACOKINETICS

Absorption: Losartan is well absorbed and undergoes substantial first-pass metabolism; systemic bioavailability is about 33%.
Distribution: Both losartan and its active metabolite are highly bound to plasma proteins, primarily albumin.
Metabolism: Cytochrome P-450 2C9 and 3A4 are involved in the biotransformation of drug to its metabolites.
Excretion: Drug and its metabolites are primarily excreted in feces, with a small amount excreted in urine.

CONTRAINDICATIONS & PRECAUTIONS

Contraindicated in patients with hypersensitivity to losartan. Use cautiously in patients with impaired renal or hepatic function.

INTERACTIONS

Drug-drug. Administration of *cimetidine* increases bioavailability without affecting pharmacokinetics of active metabolite. Administration with *phenobarbital* decreases bioavailability of losartan and active metabolite.
Drug-food. *Salt substitutes that contain potassium* can cause hyperkalemia in patients taking losartan; avoid use.

ADVERSE REACTIONS

CNS: dizziness, insomnia.
EENT: nasal congestion, sinus disorder, sinusitis.
GI: diarrhea, dyspepsia.
Musculoskeletal: muscle cramps, myalgia, back or leg pain.
Respiratory: cough, upper respiratory tract infection.

▣ KEY CONSIDERATIONS

• Use lowest dosage (25 mg) initially in patients with impaired hepatic function and in those who have intravascular volume depletion (receiving diuretic therapy).
• Drug can be used alone or in combination with other antihypertensive agents.
• If antihypertensive effect measured at trough (using once-daily dosing) is inadequate, a twice-daily regimen at the same total daily dose or an increased dose may give a more satisfactory response.
• Monitor patient taking diuretics concurrently for treatment of hypertension for symptomatic hypotension.
• Regularly assess patient's renal function (serum creatinine and BUN levels).
• Patients with severe heart failure whose renal function depends on the angiotensin-aldosterone system have experienced acute renal failure during therapy with ACE inhibitors. Manufacturer of losartan states that drug would be expected to do the same. Closely monitor patient, especially during first few weeks of therapy.

Patient education

• Instruct patient not to discontinue drug abruptly.
• Tell patient to avoid sodium substitutes; these products may contain potassium, which can cause hyperkalemia in patients taking losartan.

Overdose & treatment

• The most likely signs are hypotension and tachycardia; bradycardia could occur from parasympathetic stimulation.
• If symptomatic hypotension occurs, initiate supportive treatment. Neither losartan nor its active metabolite can be removed by hemodialysis.

lovastatin
Mevacor

Lactone, 3-hydroxy 3-methylglutaryl coenzyme A (HMG-CoA) reductase inhibitor, antilipemic

Available by prescription only
Tablets: 10 mg, 20 mg, 40 mg

Reactions may be *common*, uncommon, *life-threatening*, or COMMON AND LIFE-THREATENING.

INDICATIONS & DOSAGE
Reduction of low-density lipoprotein and total cholesterol levels in patients with primary hypercholesterolemia (types IIa and IIb), atherosclerosis
Adults: Initially, 20 mg once daily with evening meal. For patients with severely elevated cholesterol levels (for example, more than 300 mg/dl), initial dose should be 40 mg. Recommended range is 20 to 80 mg in single or divided doses.

PHARMACODYNAMICS
Antilipemic action: Lovastatin, an inactive lactone, is hydrolyzed to the beta-hydroxy acid, which specifically inhibits HMG-CoA reductase. This enzyme is an early (and rate-limiting) step in the synthetic pathway of cholesterol. At therapeutic doses, the enzyme isn't blocked, and biologically necessary amounts of cholesterol can still be synthesized.

PHARMACOKINETICS
Absorption: Animal studies indicate that about 30% of an oral dose is absorbed. Administration of drug with food improves plasma levels of total inhibitors by about 30%. Onset of action is about 3 days, with maximal therapeutic effects seen in 4 to 6 weeks.
Distribution: Less than 5% of an oral dose reaches the systemic circulation because of extensive first-pass hepatic extraction; the liver is the drug's principal site of action. Both the parent compound and its principal metabolite are highly bound (more than 95%) to plasma proteins. Animal studies indicate that lovastatin can cross the blood-brain barrier.
Metabolism: Drug is converted to the active beta-hydroxy acid form in the liver. Other metabolites include the 6' hydroxy derivative and two unidentified compounds.
Excretion: About 80% of lovastatin is excreted primarily in feces, about 10% in urine.

CONTRAINDICATIONS & PRECAUTIONS
Contraindicated in patients with hypersensitivity to lovastatin and in those with active liver disease or conditions associated with unexplained persistent elevations of serum transaminase levels.

Use cautiously in patients who consume excessive amounts of alcohol or have a history of liver disease.

INTERACTIONS
Drug-drug. Administration with *cholestyramine* or *colestipol* may enhance lipid-reducing effects but may decrease bioavailability of lovastatin. Administration of *cyclosporine, erythromycin, gemfibrozil,* or *niacin* may increase risk of severe myopathy or rhabdomyolysis. *Isradipine* may increase clearance of lovastatin and its metabolites. Administration of *itraconazole* increases HMG-CoA reductase inhibitor levels. Therapy with lovastatin should be temporarily interrupted if *systemic azole antifungal treatment* is required. Lovastatin may increase the anticoagulant effects of *warfarin.*
Drug-lifestyle. Photosensitivity reaction may occur to *sunlight;* take precautions.

ADVERSE REACTIONS
CNS: headache, dizziness, peripheral neuropathy, insomnia.
CV: chest pain.
EENT: blurred vision.
GI: constipation, diarrhea, dyspepsia, flatulence, abdominal pain or cramps, heartburn, nausea, vomiting.
Hepatic: elevated serum transaminase levels, abnormal liver test results.
Musculoskeletal: muscle cramps, myalgia, myositis, *rhabdomyolysis.*
Skin: rash, pruritus, alopecia, photosensitivity.

▣ KEY CONSIDERATIONS
• Initiate drug therapy only after diet and other nonpharmacologic therapies have proven ineffective. Patient should be on a standard cholesterol-lowering diet and continue on this diet during therapy.
• Administer drug with evening meal; absorption is enhanced and cholesterol biosynthesis is greater in the evening.
• Therapeutic response occurs in about 2 weeks, with maximum effects in 4 to 6 weeks.
• Monitor for signs of myositis; have patient report muscle aches and pains.

• Perform liver function tests frequently during initiation of therapy and periodically thereafter.
• Store tablets at room temperature in a light-resistant container.
• Don't exceed 20 mg/day if patient is receiving immunosuppressive drugs.
• Lovastatin may elevate serum CK or serum transaminase levels.

Patient education
• Stress importance of lowering cholesterol.
• Advise patient to restrict alcohol intake.
• Instruct patient to take drug with evening meal.
• Tell patient to report adverse reactions, particularly muscle aches and pains, and to take precautions with exposure to sun and other ultraviolet light until tolerance is determined.

loxapine hydrochloride
Loxitane C, Loxitane IM

loxapine succinate
Loxapac*, Loxitane

Dibenzoxazepine, antipsychotic

Available by prescription only
Capsules: 5 mg, 10 mg, 25 mg, 50 mg
Oral concentrate: 25 mg/ml
Injection: 50 mg/ml

INDICATIONS & DOSAGE
Psychotic disorders
Adults: 10 mg P.O. b.i.d. to q.i.d., rapidly increasing to 60 to 100 mg P.O. daily for most patients (dose varies from patient to patient), or 12.5 to 50 mg I.M. q 4 to 6 hours. Maximum daily dose, 250 mg. Don't administer drug I.V.

PHARMACODYNAMICS
Antipsychotic action: Loxapine is the only tricyclic antipsychotic; it's structurally similar to amoxapine. Loxapine is thought to exert its antipsychotic effects by postsynaptic blockade of CNS dopamine receptors, thus inhibiting dopamine-mediated effects. Loxapine has many other central and peripheral ef-

fects; its most prominent adverse reactions are extrapyramidal.

PHARMACOKINETICS
Absorption: Loxapine is absorbed rapidly and completely from the GI tract. Sedation occurs in 30 minutes.
Distribution: Distributed widely into the body. Peak effect occurs at 1½ to 3 hours; steady-state serum level is achieved within 3 to 4 days. Drug is 91% to 99% protein-bound.
Metabolism: Drug is metabolized extensively by the liver, forming a few active metabolites; duration of action is 12 hours.
Excretion: Mostly excreted as metabolites in urine; some is excreted in feces via the biliary tract. About 50% of drug is excreted in urine and feces within 24 hours.

CONTRAINDICATIONS & PRECAUTIONS
Contraindicated in patients with hypersensitivity to dibenzoxazepines and in patients experiencing coma, severe CNS depression, or drug-induced depressed states. Use cautiously in patients with seizure or CV disorders, glaucoma, or history of urine retention.

INTERACTIONS
Drug-drug. *Aluminum- and magnesium-containing antacids* and *antidiarrheals* decrease loxapine absorption and, thus, its therapeutic effects. Use of loxapine with *appetite suppressants* or *sympathomimetics*—including *ephedrine* (found in many nasal sprays), *epinephrine*, *phenylephrine,* and *phenylpropanolamine*—may decrease their stimulatory and pressor effects; loxapine may inhibit the vasopressor effect of epinephrine by causing epinephrine reversal. *Beta blockers* may inhibit loxapine metabolism, increasing plasma levels and toxicity. Loxapine may inhibit blood pressure response to *centrally acting antihypertensives,* such as *clonidine, guanabenz, guanadrel, guanethidine, methyldopa,* and *reserpine.* Loxapine may antagonize the therapeutic effect of *bromocriptine* on prolactin secretion; it may also decrease the vasoconstrictive effects of high-dose *dopamine,* and may decrease

---

effectiveness and increase toxicity of *levodopa* (by dopamine blockade). Use with *lithium* may result in severe neurologic toxicity with an encephalitis-like syndrome and in decreased therapeutic response to loxapine.

Additive effects are likely after use with the following drugs: *antiarrhythmics, disopyramide, procainamide,* and *quinidine* (increased incidence of arrhythmias and conduction defects); *atropine* and *other anticholinergics,* including *antidepressants, antihistamines, antiparkinsonians, MAO inhibitors, meperidine, phenothiazines* (oversedation, paralytic ileus, visual changes, and severe constipation); *CNS depressants,* including *analgesics, anesthetics (general, epidural,* and *spinal), barbiturates, parenteral magnesium sulfate,* and *narcotics, tranquilizers* (oversedation, respiratory depression, and hypotension); and *nitrates* (hypotension).

Drug-lifestyle. Additive effects are likely after use with *alcohol;* discourage use. Photosensitivity reaction may occur to *sunlight;* take precautions.

ADVERSE REACTIONS

CNS: *extrapyramidal reactions, sedation, drowsiness, seizures,* numbness, confusion, syncope, *tardive dyskinesia,* pseudoparkinsonism, EEG changes, dizziness.
CV: *orthostatic hypotension, tachycardia,* ECG changes, hypertension.
EENT: *blurred vision,* nasal congestion.
GI: *dry mouth, constipation,* nausea, vomiting, paralytic ileus.
GU: *urine retention,* menstrual irregularities, gynecomastia.
Hematologic: *leukopenia, agranulocytosis, thrombocytopenia.*
Skin: *mild photosensitivity,* allergic reactions, rash, pruritus.
Other: weight gain, *neuroleptic malignant syndrome,* jaundice.

▣ KEY CONSIDERATIONS

• Geriatric patients are highly sensitive to antimuscarinic, hypotensive, and sedative effects of drug and have a higher risk of developing extrapyramidal adverse reactions, such as parkinsonism and tardive dyskinesia. These patients

develop higher plasma levels and therefore require a lower initial dosage and more gradual titration.
• Assess patient periodically for abnormal body movement.
• Tardive dyskinesia may occur, usually after prolonged use. It may not appear until months or years after treatment and may disappear spontaneously or persist for life.
• Avoid combining drug with alcohol or other depressants.
• Obtain baseline blood pressure measurements before starting therapy and monitor regularly.
• Dilute liquid concentrate with orange or grapefruit juice just before giving.
• Periodic ophthalmic tests are recommended.
• Dose of 10 mg is therapeutic equivalent of 100 mg chlorpromazine.
• Photosensitivity warnings may apply with loxapine.
• Drug causes false-positive test results for urine porphyrin, urobilinogen, amylase, and 5-hydroxyindoleacetic acid (5-HIAA) levels because of darkening of urine by metabolites.
• Loxapine elevates test results for liver enzyme and protein-bound iodine levels, and causes quinidine-like effects on the ECG.

Patient education

• Warn against activities that require alertness and good psychomotor coordination until CNS response to drug is determined. Drowsiness and dizziness usually subside after first few weeks.
• Recommend sugarless gum or candy, mouthwash, ice chips, or artificial saliva to help alleviate dry mouth.
• Advise patient to get up slowly to avoid orthostatic hypotension.
• Advise patient to avoid alcohol while taking drug.
• Advise patient to take precautions when exposed to the sun to prevent photosensitivity reactions.

Overdose & treatment

• CNS depression is characterized by deep, unarousable sleep and possible coma, hypotension or hypertension, extrapyramidal symptoms, abnormal involuntary muscle movements, agitation, seizures, arrhythmias, ECG changes, hypothermia or hyperthermia, and autonomic nervous system dysfunction.

• Treatment is symptomatic and supportive; maintain vital signs, airway, stable body temperature, and fluid and electrolyte balance.

• Don't induce vomiting; drug inhibits cough reflex, and aspiration may occur. Use gastric lavage, then activated charcoal and saline cathartics; hemodialysis may be helpful. Regulate body temperature as needed. Treat hypotension with I.V. fluids; don't give epinephrine. Treat seizures with parenteral diazepam or barbiturates; arrhythmias with parenteral phenytoin (1 mg/kg with rate titrated to blood pressure); and extrapyramidal reactions with benztropine at 1 to 2 mg or parenteral diphenhydramine at 10 to 50 mg.

magnesium hydroxide (milk of magnesia)

Concentrated Phillips' Milk of Magnesia, Milk of Magnesia, Phillips' Milk of Magnesia

Magnesium salt, antacid, antiulcerative, laxative

Available without prescription
Tablets: 300 mg, 600 mg
Tablets (chewable): 311 mg
Liquid: 400 mg/5 ml, 800 mg/5 ml
Suspension (concentrated): 10 ml
(equivalent to 30 ml milk of magnesia)
Suspension: 77.5 mg/g

INDICATIONS & DOSAGE

Constipation, bowel evacuation before surgery
Adults: 10 to 20 ml concentrated milk of magnesia P.O.; 15 to 60 ml milk of magnesia P.O.
Laxative
Adults: 30 to 60 ml P.O., usually h.s.
Antacid
Adults: 5 to 15 ml (liquid) P.O., p.r.n., up to q.i.d.; 2.5 to 7.5 ml (liquid concentrate) P.O., p.r.n., up to q.i.d.; 2 to 4 tablets P.O., p.r.n., up to q.i.d.

PHARMACODYNAMICS

Antacid action: Magnesium hydroxide reacts rapidly with hydrochloric acid in the stomach to form magnesium chloride and water.
Antiulcerative action: Drug neutralizes gastric acid, decreasing the direct acid irritant effect. This increases pH, which in turn leads to pepsin inactivation. It also enhances mucosal barrier integrity and improves gastric and esophageal sphincter tone.
Laxative action: Drug increases the osmotic gradient in the gut and draws in water, causing distention that stimulates peristalsis and bowel evacuation.

PHARMACOKINETICS

Absorption: About 15% to 30% of magnesium may be absorbed systemically (posing a potential risk to patients with renal failure).
Distribution: None.
Metabolism: None.
Excretion: Unabsorbed drug is excreted in feces; absorbed drug is excreted rapidly in urine.

CONTRAINDICATIONS & PRECAUTIONS

Contraindicated in patients with abdominal pain, nausea, vomiting, or other signs and symptoms of appendicitis or acute surgical abdomen, and patients with myocardial damage, heart block, fecal impaction, rectal fissures, intestinal obstruction or perforation, or renal disease.

Use cautiously in patients with rectal bleeding.

INTERACTIONS

Drug-drug. Use with *aluminum hydroxide* may decrease the absorption rate and extent of *chlordiazepoxide, chlorpromazine, dicumarol, digoxin, iron salts,* and *isoniazid.* Simultaneous administration increases absorption of *buffered* or *enteric-coated aspirin.* Magnesium hydroxide may cause premature release of *enteric-coated drugs* and may decrease absorption of *quinolones* and *tetracyclines.*

ADVERSE REACTIONS

GI: *abdominal cramping, nausea, diarrhea,* laxative dependence (with long-term or excessive use).
Other: fluid and electrolyte disturbances (with daily use).

▣ KEY CONSIDERATIONS

● Give magnesium hydroxide at least 1 hour apart from enteric-coated drugs; shake suspension well.
● After administering drug through an NG tube, flush tube with water to clear it.
● Monitor for signs and symptoms of hypermagnesemia, especially if patient has impaired renal function.

Patient education
- Caution patient to avoid overuse to prevent laxative dependence.
- Instruct patient to shake suspension well or to chew tablets well.

---

magnesium salicylate
Doan's Extra Strength Caplets, Doan's Regular Caplets, Magan, Mobidin

Salicylate, nonnarcotic analgesic, antipyretic, anti-inflammatory

---

Available by prescription only
Tablets: 545 mg, 600 mg
Available without prescription
Tablets: 325 mg, 500 mg

INDICATIONS & DOSAGE
Arthritis
Adults: 545 mg to 1.2 g t.i.d. or q.i.d.
Analgesia and antipyresis
Adults: 300 to 600 mg P.O. q 4 hours, p.r.n.
Analgesia (self-medicated)
Adults: 500 mg to 1 g P.O. initially, then 500 mg q 4 hours, p.r.n., not to exceed 3.5 g in 24 hours. Absorption of buffered or enteric-coated aspirin is increased by simultaneous administration.

PHARMACODYNAMICS
Analgesic action: Magnesium salicylate has an ill-defined effect on the hypothalamus (central action) and blocks generation of pain impulses (peripheral action). The peripheral action may inhibit prostaglandin synthesis.
Antipyretic action: Drug acts on the heat-regulating center in the hypothalamus to produce peripheral vasodilation. This increases peripheral blood supply and promotes sweating, which leads to loss of heat and to cooling by evaporation.
Anti-inflammatory action: Drug is thought to inhibit prostaglandin synthesis; it may also inhibit the synthesis or action of other mediators of inflammation.

PHARMACOKINETICS
Absorption: Magnesium salicylate is absorbed rapidly and completely from the GI tract.
Distribution: Drug is highly protein-bound.
Metabolism: Drug is hydrolyzed in the liver.
Excretion: Metabolites are excreted in urine.

CONTRAINDICATIONS & PRECAUTIONS
Contraindicated in patients with hypersensitivity to magnesium salicylate, other salicylates, or NSAIDs or those with severe chronic renal insufficiency because of risk of magnesium toxicity. Also contraindicated in patients with bleeding disorders. Use cautiously in patients with hypoprothrombinemia or vitamin K deficiency.

INTERACTIONS
Drug-drug. *Ammonium chloride* and other *urine acidifiers* increase magnesium salicylate blood levels; monitor for magnesium salicylate toxicity. *Antacids* delay and decrease absorption of magnesium salicylate. *Antacids in high doses* and other *urine alkalizers* decrease drug blood levels; monitor for decreased salicylate effect. *Anticoagulants* and *thrombolytics* may to some degree potentiate the platelet-inhibiting effects of magnesium salicylate. *Corticosteroids* enhance magnesium salicylate. Monitor therapy closely for both drugs. Use of drug with *highly protein-bound drugs* (such as *phenytoin, sulfonylureas,* and *warfarin*) may cause displacement of either drug and adverse effects; monitor therapy closely for both drugs. Use with other *GI irritants* (such as *antibiotics,* other *NSAIDs,* and *corticosteroids*) may potentiate the adverse GI effects of magnesium salicylate; use together with caution.

ADVERSE REACTIONS
EENT: tinnitus, hearing loss.
GI: nausea, vomiting, GI distress.
Hepatic: increased serum levels of AST, ALT, alkaline phosphatase, and bilirubin; hepatitis.
Skin: rash, bruising.
Other: hypersensitivity reactions (**anaphylaxis**, asthma), Reye's syndrome.

Reactions may be *common*, uncommon, *life-threatening*, or COMMON AND LIFE-THREATENING.

⊡ KEY CONSIDERATIONS

Besides the recommendations relevant to all salicylates, consider the following:

• Patients older than age 60 may be more susceptible to the toxic effects of magnesium salicylate. Use with caution.

• The effects of salicylates on renal prostaglandins may cause fluid retention and edema, a significant drawback for geriatric patients and those with heart failure.

• GI disturbances are less common with this drug than with other anti-inflammatories.

• High doses of drug may cause false-positive urine glucose test results using copper sulfate method; it may cause false-negative urine glucose test results using glucose enzymatic method.

• False increases or decreases have occurred in urine vanillylmandelic acid tests. Drug may interfere with the Gerhardt test for urine acetic acid.

• Drug has a less profound effect on inhibiting platelet aggregation than other salicylates.

• Obtain hemoglobin levels and PT periodically.

• To prevent toxicity, especially in patients with renal insufficiency, monitor serum magnesium levels.

• Discontinue use if patient experiences dizziness, tinnitus, or impaired hearing.

Patient education

• Instruct patient to follow prescribed regimen and report problems.

• Advise patient not to take magnesium salicylate longer than 10 days without medical supervision.

• Caution patient to keep drug out of children's reach.

Overdose & treatment

• Signs and symptoms of overdose include metabolic acidosis with respiratory alkalosis, hyperpnea, and tachypnea from increased carbon dioxide production and direct stimulation of the respiratory center.

• To treat overdose, empty stomach immediately: Induce vomiting with ipecac syrup if patient is conscious or perform gastric lavage if he isn't. Administer activated charcoal via an NG tube. Provide symptomatic and supportive measures, such as respiratory support and correction of fluid and electrolyte imbalances. Monitor laboratory values and vital signs closely. Alkaline diuresis may enhance renal excretion.

magnesium sulfate

Mineral/electrolyte, anticonvulsant

Available by prescription only
Injectable solutions: 10%, 12.5%, 20%, and 50% in 2-ml, 5-ml, 8-ml, 10-ml, 20-ml, 30-ml, and 50-ml ampules, vials, and prefilled syringes

INDICATIONS & DOSAGE

Hypomagnesemic seizures

Adults: 1 to 2 g (as 10% solution) I.V. over 15 minutes, then 1 g I.M. q 4 to 6 hours, based on patient's response and magnesium blood levels.

Seizures secondary to hypomagnesemia in acute nephritis, life-threatening arrhythmias

Adults: For patient with sustained ventricular tachycardia or torsades de pointes, give 2 to 6 g I.V. over several minutes, followed by 3 to 20 mg/minute I.V. infusion for 5 to 48 hours, depending on patient response and serum magnesium levels. For patients with paroxysmal atrial tachycardia, give 3 to 4 g I.V. over 30 seconds.

Barium poisoning, ◊ asthma

Adults: 1 to 2 g I.V.

Mild hypomagnesemia

Adults: 1 g I.M. q 4 to 6 hours; or 5 g in 1 L D_5W or dextrose 5% in normal saline solution I.V. over 3 hours.

PHARMACODYNAMICS

Anticonvulsant action: Magnesium sulfate has CNS and respiratory depressant effects. It acts peripherally, causing vasodilation; moderate doses cause flushing and sweating, whereas high doses cause hypotension. It prevents or controls seizures by blocking neuromuscular transmission.

Drug is used to treat hypomagnesemic seizures in adults.

PHARMACOKINETICS

Absorption: I.V. magnesium sulfate acts immediately; effects last about 30 minutes. After I.M. injection, it acts within 60 minutes and lasts for 3 to 4 hours. Effective serum levels are 2.5 to 7.5 mEq/L.

Distribution: Drug is distributed widely throughout the body.

Metabolism: None.

Excretion: Drug is excreted unchanged in urine.

CONTRAINDICATIONS & PRECAUTIONS

Parenteral administration of magnesium sulfate is contraindicated in patients with heart block or myocardial damage. Use cautiously in patients with impaired renal function.

INTERACTIONS

Drug-drug. Use with *antidepressants, antipsychotics, anxiolytics, barbiturates, general anesthetics, hypnotics,* or *narcotics* may increase CNS depressant effects; reduced dosages may be required. Give with *cardiac glycosides* with extreme caution; changes in cardiac conduction in patients receiving *digoxin* may lead to heart block if *I.V. calcium* is administered. Use with *succinylcholine* or *tubocurarine* potentiates and prolongs neuromuscular blocking action of these drugs; use with caution.

Drug-lifestyle. *Alcohol* increases CNS depressant effects.

ADVERSE REACTIONS

CNS: drowsiness, *depressed reflexes,* flaccid paralysis, hypothermia.

CV: *hypotension, flushing,* **circulatory collapse,** depressed cardiac function.

Metabolic: hypocalcemia.

Respiratory: *respiratory paralysis.*

Other: diaphoresis.

▣ KEY CONSIDERATIONS

• Inject I.V. bolus slowly (to avoid respiratory or cardiac arrest).

• Administer by constant infusion pump, if available; maximum infusion rate is 150 mg/minute. Rapid drip causes feeling of heat.

• Discontinue magnesium sulfate as soon as needed effect is achieved.

• Concentration of drug for I.V. administration shouldn't exceed 20% at a rate no greater than 150 mg/minute (1.5 ml of 10% concentration or equivalent). For I.M. administration in adults, a concentration of 25% or 50% is generally used.

• When giving repeated doses, test knee-jerk reflex before each dose; if absent, discontinue drug. Use of drug beyond this point risks respiratory center failure.

• Respiratory rate must be 16 breaths/minute or more before each dose. Keep I.V. calcium salts on hand.

• To calculate grams of magnesium in a percentage of solution: $x\% = x$ g/100 ml (for example, $25\% = 25$ g/100 ml = 250 mg/ml).

• To avoid overdose, monitor serum magnesium load and clinical status.

Overdose & treatment

• Signs and symptoms of overdose include a sharp decrease in blood pressure and respiratory paralysis, ECG changes (increased PR interval, QRS complex, and QT interval), heart block, and asystole.

• Treatment requires artificial ventilation and I.V. calcium salts to reverse depression and heart block. Usual dose is 5 to 10 mEq of calcium (10 to 20 ml of 10% calcium gluconate sodium).

---

mannitol
Osmitrol, Resectisol

Osmotic diuretic, prevention and management of acute renal failure or oliguria, reduction of intracranial or intraocular pressure, treatment of drug intoxication

---

Available by prescription only

Injection: 5%, 10%, 15%, 20%, 25%

Urogenital solution: 5 g/100 ml distilled water

INDICATIONS & DOSAGE

Test dose for marked oliguria or suspected inadequate renal function

Adults: 200 mg/kg or 12.5 g as a 15% or 20% solution I.V. over 3 to 5 minutes. Response is adequate if 30 to 50 ml of urine/hour is excreted over 2 to 3 hours.

Treatment of oliguria
Adults: 50 to 100 g as a 15% to 20% solution I.V. over 90 minutes to several hours.

Prevention of oliguria or acute renal failure
Adults: 50 to 100 g followed by a 5% to 10% solution I.V. Exact concentration is determined by fluid requirements.

Treatment of edema and ascites
Adults: 100 g as a 10% to 20% solution I.V. over 2 to 6 hours.

To reduce intraocular pressure (IOP) or intracranial pressure (ICP)
Adults: 1.5 to 2 g/kg as a 15% to 25% solution I.V. over 30 to 60 minutes administered 60 to 90 minutes before surgery.

To promote diuresis in drug intoxication
Adults: 25-g loading dose, followed by an infusion maintaining urine output of 100 to 500 ml/hour and positive fluid balance. For patients with barbiturate poisoning, give 0.5 g/kg, followed by a 5% to 10% solution.

Urologic irrigation
Adults: 2.5% solution.

PHARMACODYNAMICS
Diuretic action: Mannitol increases the osmotic pressure of glomerular filtrate, inhibiting tubular reabsorption of water and electrolytes, thus promoting diuresis. This action also promotes urine excretion of certain drugs, which is useful for preventing or managing acute renal failure or oliguria. This action is also useful for reducing IOP or ICP because mannitol elevates plasma osmolality, enhancing flow of water into extracellular fluid.

PHARMACOKINETICS
Absorption: Mannitol isn't absorbed from the GI tract. I.V. mannitol lowers IOP in 30 to 60 minutes and ICP in 15 minutes; it produces diuresis in 1 to 3 hours.
Distribution: Drug remains in the extracellular compartment. It doesn't cross the blood-brain barrier.
Metabolism: Drug is metabolized minimally to glycogen in the liver.
Excretion: Drug is filtered by the glomeruli; half-life in adults with normal renal function is about 100 minutes.

CONTRAINDICATIONS & PRECAUTIONS
Contraindicated in patients with hypersensitivity to mannitol and in those with anuria, severe pulmonary congestion, frank pulmonary edema, severe heart failure, severe dehydration, metabolic edema, progressive renal disease or dysfunction, or active intracranial bleeding, except during craniotomy.

INTERACTIONS
Drug-drug. Use with *cardiac glycosides* may enhance the possibility of digitalis toxicity. Drug may increase the effects of other *diuretics,* including *carbonic anhydrase inhibitors.* Mannitol may enhance renal excretion of *lithium* and lower serum lithium levels.

ADVERSE REACTIONS
CNS: *seizures,* dizziness, headache.
CV: edema, thrombophlebitis, hypotension, hypertension, **heart failure,** tachycardia, angina-like chest pain.
EENT: blurred vision, rhinitis, dry mouth.
GI: thirst, nausea, vomiting, *diarrhea.*
GU: urine retention.
Other: fluid and electrolyte imbalance, dehydration, local pain, fever, chills, urticaria.

▣ KEY CONSIDERATIONS
Besides the recommendations relevant to all osmotic diuretics, consider the following:
• Geriatric patients require close observation and may require lower dosages. Excessive diuresis promotes rapid dehydration, leading to hypovolemia, hypokalemia, and hyponatremia.
• Mannitol may interfere with tests for inorganic concentration or blood ethylene glycol.
• Use with extreme caution in patients with compromised renal function; monitor vital signs (including central venous pressure) hourly and input and output, weight, renal function, fluid balance, and serum and urine sodium and potassium levels daily.
• For maximum pressure reduction during surgery, give drug 1 to 1¼ hours preoperatively.

• To avoid extravasation, carefully administer drug I.V. via an in-line filter.
• To prevent agglutination, don't administer with whole blood.
• Mannitol solutions commonly crystallize at low temperatures; place crystallized solutions in a hot water bath, shake vigorously to dissolve crystals, and cool to body temperature before use. Don't use solutions with undissolved crystals.

Patient education
• Tell patient he may experience thirst or dry mouth and emphasize importance of drinking only the amount of fluids provided.
• With initial doses, warn patient to change position slowly, especially when rising from lying or sitting position, to prevent dizziness from orthostatic hypotension.
• Instruct patient to immediately report pain in the chest, back, or legs or difficulty breathing.

Overdose & treatment
• Signs and symptoms of overdose include polyuria, cellular dehydration, hypotension, and CV collapse.
• Discontinue infusion and institute supportive measures. Hemodialysis removes mannitol and decreases serum osmolality levels.

mechlorethamine hydrochloride (nitrogen mustard)
Mustargen

Alkylating agent (cell cycle–phase nonspecific), antineoplastic

Available by prescription only
Injection: 10-mg vials

INDICATIONS & DOSAGE
Dosage and indications may vary. Check current literature for recommended protocols.
Hodgkin's disease, bronchogenic cancer, chronic lymphocytic leukemia, chronic myelocytic leukemia, lymphosarcoma, polycythemia vera
Adults: 0.4 mg/kg I.V. per course of therapy as a single dose or 0.1 to 0.2 mg/kg on 2 to 4 successive days q 3 to 6 weeks. Give through running I.V. infusion. Don't give a subsequent course until the patient has recovered hematologically from the previous course. Dose is based on ideal or actual body weight, whichever is less.
Intracavitary doses for neoplastic effusions
Adults: 0.2 to 0.4 mg/kg.

PHARMACODYNAMICS
Antineoplastic action: Mechlorethamine exerts its cytotoxic activity through alkylation. Drug causes cross-linking of DNA strands, single-strand breakage of DNA, abnormal base pairing, and interruption of other intracellular processes, resulting in cell death.

PHARMACOKINETICS
Absorption: Mechlorethamine is well absorbed after oral administration; however, because drug is very irritating to tissue, it must be administered I.V. After intracavitary administration, drug is absorbed incompletely, probably from deactivation by body fluids in the cavity.
Distribution: Drug doesn't cross the blood-brain barrier.
Metabolism: Drug undergoes rapid chemical transformation and reacts quickly with various cellular components before being deactivated.
Excretion: Metabolites are excreted in urine. Less than 0.01% of an I.V. dose is excreted unchanged in urine.

CONTRAINDICATIONS & PRECAUTIONS
Contraindicated in patients with hypersensitivity to mechlorethamine and with known infectious diseases. Use cautiously in patients with severe anemia or depressed neutrophil or platelet count and in those who have recently undergone chemotherapy or radiation therapy.

INTERACTIONS
None reported.

ADVERSE REACTIONS
CNS: weakness, vertigo.

Reactions may be *common*, uncommon, *life-threatening*, or **COMMON AND LIFE-THREATENING**.

EENT: tinnitus, deafness (with high doses).

GI: *nausea, vomiting, anorexia (beginning within minutes, lasting 8 to 24 hours).*

Hematologic: *thrombocytopenia,* lymphocytopenia, *agranulocytosis,* nadir of myelosuppression occurs by days 4 to 10 and lasts 10 to 21 days; mild anemia begins in 2 to 3 weeks.

Skin: rash, sloughing, severe irritation (if drug extravasates or touches skin).

Other: *alopecia,* ANAPHYLAXIS, precipitation of herpes zoster, hyperuricemia, *thrombophlebitis,* amyloidosis, jaundice, impaired spermatogenesis.

◻ KEY CONSIDERATIONS

- Mechlorethamine may increase blood and urine uric acid levels.
- To reconstitute powder, use 10 ml sterile water for injection or normal saline solution to give a concentration of 1 mg/ml.
- When reconstituted, drug is a clear colorless solution. Don't use if solution is discolored or if droplets of water are visible within vial before reconstitution.
- Solution is very unstable. Prepare immediately before infusion and use within 15 minutes. Discard unused solution.
- Drug may be administered I.V. push over a few minutes into the tubing of a freely flowing I.V. infusion.
- Dilution of drug into a large volume of I.V. solution isn't recommended because it may react with the diluent and isn't stable for a prolonged period.
- Treatment of extravasation includes local injections of a 1/6-M sodium thiosulfate solution. Prepare solution by mixing 4 ml sodium thiosulfate 10% with 6 ml sterile water for injection. Also, apply ice packs for 6 to 12 hours to minimize local reactions.
- During intracavitary administration, patient should be turned from side to side every 15 minutes for 1 hour to distribute drug.
- Avoid contact with skin or mucous membranes. To prevent accidental skin contact, wear gloves when preparing solution and during administration. If contact occurs, wash with copious amounts of water.

- Monitor uric acid levels, CBC, and liver function tests.
- To prevent hyperuricemia with resulting uric acid nephropathy, allopurinol may be given; keep patient well hydrated.
- Anticoagulants should be used cautiously. Watch closely for signs of bleeding.
- Avoid all I.M. injections when platelet count is low.
- Drug has been used topically to treat mycosis fungoides.

Patient education

- Tell patient to avoid exposure to people with infections.
- Instruct patient that adequate fluid intake facilitates excretion of uric acid.
- Reassure patient that hair should grow back after treatment has ended.
- Tell patient to promptly report signs or symptoms of bleeding or infection

Overdose & treatment

- Signs and symptoms of overdose include severe leukopenia, anemia, thrombocytopenia, and a hemorrhagic diathesis with subsequent delayed bleeding. Death may follow.
- Treatment is usually supportive and includes transfusion of blood components and antibiotic treatment of complicating infections.

---

meclizine hydrochloride
Antivert, Antivert/25, Antrizine, Bonine, Dizmiss, Meclizine, Meni-D, Ru-Vert-M

Piperazine-derivative antihistamine, antiemetic, antivertigo drug

---

Available with or without prescription
Tablets: 12.5 mg, 25 mg, 50 mg
Tablets (chewable): 25 mg
Capsules: 25 mg, 30 mg

INDICATIONS & DOSAGE
Dizziness
Adults: 25 to 100 mg P.O. daily in divided doses; dosage varies with patient response.

Motion sickness
Adults: 25 to 50 mg P.O. 1 hour before travel; may repeat dose daily for duration of journey.
Vertigo
Adults: 25 to 100 mg daily in divided doses.

PHARMACODYNAMICS
Antiemetic action: Meclizine hydrochloride probably inhibits nausea and vomiting by centrally decreasing sensitivity of labyrinth apparatus that relays stimuli to the chemoreceptor trigger zone and stimulates the vomiting center in the brain.
Antivertigo action: Drug decreases labyrinth excitability and conduction in vestibular-cerebellar pathways.

PHARMACOKINETICS
Absorption: Onset of action about 60 minutes.
Distribution: Meclizine is well distributed throughout the body.
Metabolism: Drug is probably metabolized in the liver.
Excretion: Half-life is about 6 hours; action persists for 8 to 24 hours. Drug is excreted unchanged in feces; metabolites are found in urine.

CONTRAINDICATIONS & PRECAUTIONS
Contraindicated in patients hypersensitive to meclizine hydrochloride. Use cautiously in patients with asthma, glaucoma, or prostatic hyperplasia.

INTERACTIONS
Drug-drug. Additive sedative and CNS depressant effects may occur when meclizine is used with other *CNS depressants*, such as *anxiolytics, barbiturates, sleeping agents,* and *tranquilizers.* Drug shouldn't be given to patients taking *ototoxic drugs*—such as *aminoglycosides, cisplatin, loop diuretics, salicylates,* and *vancomycin*—because it may mask signs of ototoxicity.
Drug-lifestyle. Use with *alcohol* may increase the sedative effect.

ADVERSE REACTIONS
CNS: *drowsiness,* restlessness, excitation, nervousness, auditory and visual hallucinations.
CV: hypotension, palpitations, tachycardia.
EENT: blurred vision, diplopia, tinnitus, dry nose and throat.
GI: dry mouth, constipation, anorexia, nausea, vomiting, diarrhea.
GU: urine retention, urinary frequency.
Skin: urticaria, rash.

▣ KEY CONSIDERATIONS
Besides the recommendations relevant to all antihistamines, consider the following:
• Meclizine should be discontinued 4 days before diagnostic skin tests to avoid preventing, reducing, or masking test response.
• Geriatric patients are usually more sensitive to adverse effects of antihistamines and are likely to experience a greater degree of dizziness, sedation, hyperexcitability, dry mouth, and urine retention than younger patients.
• Tablets may be placed in mouth and allowed to dissolve without water, or they may be chewed or swallowed whole.
• Abrupt withdrawal of drug after long-term use may cause paradoxical reactions or sudden reversal of improved state.

Patient education
• Instruct patient to avoid activities that require mental alertness and physical coordination, such as driving and operating dangerous machinery.

Overdose & treatment
• Signs and symptoms of moderate overdose include hyperexcitability alternating with drowsiness. Seizures, hallucinations, and respiratory paralysis may occur in profound overdose. Anticholinergic signs and symptoms, such as dry mouth, flushed skin, fixed and dilated pupils, and GI symptoms, are common.
• Treat overdose by performing gastric lavage to empty stomach; inducing vomiting with ipecac syrup may be ineffective. Treat hypotension with vasopres-

---

Reactions may be *common,* uncommon, *life-threatening,* or COMMON AND LIFE-THREATENING.

sors, and control seizures with diazepam or phenytoin. Don't give stimulants.

---

medroxyprogesterone acetate
Amen, Curretab, Cycrin, Depo-Provera, Depot, Provera

Progestin, antineoplastic

Available by prescription only
Tablets: 2.5 mg, 5 mg, 10 mg
Injection: 150 mg/ml, 400 mg/ml

INDICATIONS & DOSAGE
Abnormal uterine bleeding from hormonal imbalance
Adults: 5 to 10 mg P.O. daily for 5 to 10 days beginning on day 16 or 21 of menstrual cycle. If patient has received estrogen, then 10 mg P.O. daily for 10 days beginning on day 16 of cycle.
Endometrial or renal carcinoma
Adults: 400 to 1,000 mg I.M. weekly.
◊ ***Paraphilia in males***
Adults: Initially, 200 mg I.M. b.i.d. or t.i.d. or 500 mg I.M. weekly. Adjust dosage based on response.

PHARMACODYNAMICS
Progestational action: Parenteral medroxyprogesterone suppresses ovulation, causes thickening of cervical mucous membrane, and induces sloughing of the endometrium.
Antineoplastic action: Drug may inhibit growth progression of progestin-sensitive endometrial or renal cancer tissue by an unknown mechanism.

PHARMACOKINETICS
Absorption: Medroxyprogesterone is slowly absorbed after I.M. administration.
Distribution: Unknown.
Metabolism: Drug is primarily metabolized in the liver.
Excretion: Drug is primarily excreted from the kidneys.

CONTRAINDICATIONS & PRECAUTIONS
Contraindicated in patients with hypersensitivity to medroxyprogesterone, active thromboembolic disorders, or past history of thromboembolic disorders, cerebral vascular disease, apoplexy, breast cancer, undiagnosed abnormal vaginal bleeding, or hepatic dysfunction. Tablets are also contraindicated in patients with liver dysfunction or known or suspected malignant disease of the genital organs.
    Use cautiously in patients with diabetes mellitus, seizures, migraines, cardiac or renal disease, asthma, or mental depression.

INTERACTIONS
Drug-drug. *Aminoglutethimide* may increase the hepatic metabolism of medroxyprogesterone, possibly decreasing its therapeutic effect. In patients receiving *bromocriptine,* progestins may cause amenorrhea or galactorrhea, thus interfering with the action of bromocriptine; use of these drugs isn't recommended.

ADVERSE REACTIONS
CNS: depression.
CV: thrombophlebitis, *pulmonary embolism,* edema, *thromboembolism, CVA.*
EENT: exophthalmos, diplopia.
GU: cervical erosion, abnormal secretions.
Hepatic: cholestatic jaundice.
Skin: rash, pain, induration, sterile abscesses, acne, pruritus, melasma, alopecia, hirsutism.
Other: breast tenderness, enlargement, or secretion; changes in weight.

▣ KEY CONSIDERATIONS
Besides the recommendations relevant to all progestins, consider the following:
• Use cautiously in patients with diabetes mellitus, seizures, migraine, cardiac or renal disease, asthma, and mental depression.
• Parenteral form is for I.M. administration only. Inject deep into large muscle mass, preferably the gluteal muscle. Monitor for development of sterile abscesses. To ensure complete suspension of drug, it must be shaken vigorously immediately before each use.
• I.M. injection may be painful. Monitor sites for evidence of sterile abscess. To

---

prevent muscle atrophy, rotate injection sites.

• Medroxyprogesterone has been used to treat obstructive sleep apnea and to manage paraphilia.

Patient teaching

• Make sure patient reads package insert explaining possible adverse effects of progestins before he receives the first dose. Also, give him a verbal explanation.

• Tell patient to report unusual symptoms immediately and to stop drug and call health care provider if visual disturbances or migraine occur.

• Teach patient how to perform routine monthly breast self-examination.

megestrol acetate
Megace

Progestin, antineoplastic

Available by prescription only
Tablets: 20 mg, 40 mg
Suspension: 200 mg/5 ml

INDICATIONS & DOSAGE

Dosage and indications may vary. Check current literature for recommended protocol.

Palliative treatment of breast cancer
Adults: 40 mg (tablets) P.O. q.i.d.

Palliative treatment of endometrial cancer
Adults: 10 to 80 mg (tablets) P.O. q.i.d.

Anorexia, cachexia, or weight loss in patients with AIDS
Adults: 800 mg (suspension) P.O. daily; 100 to 400 mg for AIDS-related cachexia.

PHARMACODYNAMICS

Antineoplastic action: Megestrol inhibits growth and causes regression of progestin-sensitive breast and endometrial cancer tissue by an unknown mechanism.

Treatment of anorexia, cachexia, or weight loss: Mechanism of action is unknown. It may stimulate appetite by interfering with the production of such mediators as cachectin.

PHARMACOKINETICS

Absorption: Megestrol is well absorbed across the GI tract after oral administration.

Distribution: Drug appears to be stored in fatty tissue and is highly bound to plasma proteins.

Metabolism: Drug is completely metabolized in the liver.

Excretion: Metabolites are eliminated primarily through the kidneys.

CONTRAINDICATIONS & PRECAUTIONS

Contraindicated in patients hypersensitive to megestrol. Use cautiously in patients with history of thrombophlebitis.

INTERACTIONS

None significant.

ADVERSE REACTIONS

CV: thrombophlebitis, hypertension, edema, chest pain.
GI: nausea, vomiting, diarrhea, flatulence.
GU: impotence, decreased libido.
Hepatic: hepatomegaly.
Metabolic: weight gain, hyperglycemia.
Respiratory: *pulmonary embolism,* dyspnea, pneumonia, cough, pharyngitis.
Skin: rash, pruritus, candidiasis, alopecia.
Other: increased appetite, carpal tunnel syndrome.

▣ KEY CONSIDERATIONS

• Use cautiously in patients with history of thrombophlebitis.

• Blood glucose levels may increase in patients with diabetes.

• Megestrol is a relatively nontoxic drug with a low incidence of adverse effects.

• Two months is an adequate trial when treating patients with cancer.

Patient education

• Inform patient that therapeutic response isn't immediate.

• Tell patient to immediately report shortness of breath or difficulty breathing.

Reactions may be *common,* uncommon, *life-threatening,* OR COMMON AND LIFE-THREATENING.

melphalan (phenylalanine mustard)
Alkeran

Alkylating agent (cell cycle–phase nonspecific), antineoplastic

Available by prescription only
Tablets (scored): 2 mg
Powder for injection: 50 mg

INDICATIONS & DOSAGE
Dosage and indications may vary. Check current literature for recommended protocol.
Multiple myeloma
Adults: 6 mg P.O. daily for 2 to 3 weeks; then stop therapy for 4 weeks. When WBC and platelet count begin to increase, start maintenance dose of 2 mg P.O. daily. Alternatively, give 0.15 mg/kg/day P.O. for 7 days, administered at 2- to 6-week intervals, or 0.25 mg/kg/day P.O. for 4 days at 4- to 6-week intervals; monitor patient's blood counts.

For I.V. administration, give 16 mg/m² over 15 to 20 minutes once at 2-week intervals for four doses. Monitor patient's blood counts and reduce dose as necessary.
Epithelial ovarian cancer
Adults: 200 mcg/kg/day P.O. for 5 days, repeated q 4 to 6 weeks if blood counts return to normal.

PHARMACODYNAMICS
Antineoplastic action: Melphalan forms cross-links of strands of DNA and RNA and inhibits protein synthesis.

PHARMACOKINETICS
Absorption: Absorption from GI tract is incomplete and variable. One study found that absorption ranged from 25% to 89% after an oral dose of 0.6 mg/kg.
Distribution: Melphalan distributes rapidly and widely into total body water. Drug is initially 50% to 60% bound to plasma proteins and eventually increases to 80% to 90% over time.
Metabolism: Drug is extensively deactivated by hydrolysis.
Excretion: Drug elimination has been described as biphasic, with an initial half-

life of 8 minutes and a terminal half-life of 2 hours. Drug and its metabolites are excreted primarily in urine, with 10% of an oral dose excreted as unchanged drug.

CONTRAINDICATIONS & PRECAUTIONS
Contraindicated in patients with hypersensitivity to melphalan and in those whose disease is known to be resistant to the drug. Patients hypersensitive to chlorambucil may have cross-sensitivity to melphalan.

Use cautiously in patients with impaired renal function, severe leukopenia, thrombocytopenia, anemia, or chronic lymphocytic leukemia.

INTERACTIONS
Drug-drug. *Cimetidine* inhibits GI absorption. Because melphalan may increase cyclosporine-induced nephrotoxicity, monitor renal function closely in patients receiving the drug with *cisplatin* or *cyclosporine*. *Interferon-alfa* may decrease serum melphalan levels.
Drug-food. *Food* decreases bioavailability of drug.

ADVERSE REACTIONS
CV: hypotension, tachycardia, edema.
GI: nausea, vomiting, diarrhea, oral ulceration.
Hematologic: *thrombocytopenia, leukopenia, bone marrow suppression,* hemolytic anemia.
Respiratory: *pneumonitis, pulmonary fibrosis,* dyspnea, bronchospasm.
Skin: pruritus, alopecia, urticaria.
Other: *anaphylaxis,* hypersensitivity, *hepatotoxicity,* secondary malignancy.

▣ KEY CONSIDERATIONS
• Use cautiously in geriatric patients because many have decreased hepatic, renal, and cardiac function.
• Oral dose may be taken at one time.
• Administer melphalan on an empty stomach because absorption is decreased by food.
• Drug therapy may increase blood and urine levels of uric acid.
• Fever may enhance elimination of melphalan.
• Frequent hematologic monitoring, including CBC, is necessary for accurate

dosage adjustments and prevention of toxicity.
• Discontinue therapy temporarily or reduce dosage if WBC count falls below 3,000/mm³ or platelet count falls below 100,000/mm³.
• Avoid I.M. injections when platelet count is less than 100,000/mm³.
• Dosage reduction should be considered in patients with renal failure receiving I.V. drug. Increased bone marrow suppression was observed in patients with BUN levels of 30 mg/dl or more.
• Anticoagulants, aspirin, and aspirin-containing products should be used cautiously.

Patient education
• Instruct patient to continue taking drug despite nausea and vomiting.
• Tell patient to call immediately if vomiting occurs shortly after taking dose.
• Explain that adequate fluid intake is important to facilitate excretion of uric acid.
• Instruct patient to avoid exposure to people with infections.
• Reassure patient that hair should grow back after treatment has ended.
• Tell patient to promptly report signs and symptoms of infection or bleeding.

Overdose & treatment
• Signs and symptoms of overdose include myelosuppression, hypocalcemia, severe nausea, vomiting, mouth ulcers, decreased consciousness, seizures, muscular paralysis, and cholinomimetic effects.
• Treatment is usually supportive and includes transfusion of blood components.

meningococcal polysaccharide vaccine
Menomune-A/C/Y/W-135

Bacterial vaccine

Available by prescription only
Injection: a killed bacteria vaccine in single-dose, 10-dose, and 50-dose vials with vial of diluent

INDICATIONS & DOSAGE
Meningococcal meningitis prophylaxis
Adults: 0.5 ml S.C.

PHARMACODYNAMICS
Meningitis prophylaxis: Vaccine promotes active immunity to meningitis caused by *Neisseria meningitidis.*

PHARMACOKINETICS
Absorption: Unknown.
Distribution: Unknown.
Metabolism: Unknown.
Excretion: Unknown.

CONTRAINDICATIONS & PRECAUTIONS
Contraindicated in immunosuppressed patients and patients with hypersensitivity to thimerosal. Vaccination should be deferred in patients with acute illness.

INTERACTIONS
None reported.

ADVERSE REACTIONS
CNS: headache.
Other: *pain, tenderness, erythema, induration* (at injection site); **anaphylaxis,** malaise, chills, fever, muscle cramps.

▣ KEY CONSIDERATIONS
• Obtain a thorough history of allergies and reactions to immunizations.
• Don't give meningitis vaccine I.D., I.M., or I.V., because safety and efficacy haven't been established.
• Epinephrine solution 1:1,000 should be available to treat allergic reactions.
• Reconstitute vaccine with diluent provided. Shake until dissolved. Discard reconstituted solution after 5 days.
• Store vaccine between 36°F and 46°F (2°C and 8°C).
• Protective antibody levels may be achieved within 10 to 14 days after vaccination.

Patient education
• Tell patient that pain and inflammation may occur at injection site. Recommend acetaminophen to alleviate adverse reactions such as fever.
• Encourage patient to report distressing adverse reactions.

- Explain that vaccine will provide immunity only to meningitis caused by one type of bacteria.

meperidine hydrochloride (pethidine hydrochloride)
Demerol

Opioid, analgesic, adjunct to anesthesia
Controlled substance schedule II

Available by prescription only
Tablets: 50 mg, 100 mg
Liquid: 50 mg/5 ml
Injection: 10 mg/ml, 25 mg/ml, 50 mg/ml, 75 mg/ml, 100 mg/ml

INDICATIONS & DOSAGE
Moderate to severe pain
Adults: 50 to 150 mg P.O., I.M., I.V., or S.C. q 3 to 4 hours.
Preoperatively
Adults: 50 to 100 mg I.M., I.V., or S.C. 30 to 90 minutes before surgery.
Support of anesthesia
Adults: Repeated slow I.V. injections of fractional doses (10 mg/ml) or continuous I.V. infusion of 1 mg/ml. Dose should be titrated to meet patient's needs.

PHARMACODYNAMICS
Analgesic action: Meperidine is a narcotic agonist with actions and potency similar to those of morphine, with principle actions at the opiate receptors. It's recommended for the relief of moderate to severe pain.

PHARMACOKINETICS
Absorption: Meperidine given orally is only half as effective as when given parenterally. Onset of analgesia within 10 to 45 minutes. Duration of action is 2 to 4 hours.
Distribution: Drug is distributed widely throughout the body and is 60% to 80% bound to plasma proteins.
Metabolism: Drug is metabolized primarily by hydrolysis in the liver to an active metabolite, normeperidine.
Excretion: About 30% of dose is excreted in the urine as the N-demethylated de-

rivative; about 5% is excreted unchanged. Excretion is enhanced by acidifying the urine. Half-life of parent compound is 3 to 5 hours and the half-life of metabolite is 8 to 21 hours.

CONTRAINDICATIONS & PRECAUTIONS
Contraindicated in patients with hypersensitivity to meperidine and in those who have received MAO inhibitors within the past 14 days.

Use cautiously in geriatric or debilitated patients and in those with increased intracranial pressure, head injury, asthma, other respiratory conditions, supraventricular tachycardia, seizures, acute abdominal conditions, renal or hepatic disease, hypothyroidism, Addison's disease, urethral stricture, and prostatic hyperplasia.

INTERACTIONS
Drug-drug. Use with *anticholinergics* may cause paralytic ileus. Use with *cimetidine* may increase respiratory and CNS depression, causing confusion, disorientation, apnea, or seizures; such use requires reduced dosage. Use with other *CNS depressants*—such as *antihistamines, barbiturates, benzodiazepines, general anesthetics, muscle relaxants, narcotic analgesics, phenothiazines, sedative-hypnotics,* and *tricyclic antidepressants*—potentiates the respiratory and CNS depressant, sedative, and hypotensive effects of meperidine. Severe CV depression may result from use with *general anesthetics*. Meperidine can potentiate the adverse effects of *isoniazid*. Use with *MAO inhibitors* may precipitate unpredictable and occasionally fatal reactions, even in patients who may receive MAO inhibitors within 14 days of receiving meperidine: Some reactions have been characterized by coma, respiratory depression, cyanosis, and hypotension; in others, hyperexcitability, seizures, tachycardia, hyperpyrexia, and hypertension have occurred. Patients who become physically dependent on drug may experience acute withdrawal syndrome if given a *narcotic antagonist*.
Drug-lifestyle. Use with *alcohol* potentiates the respiratory and CNS depres-

sant, sedative, and hypotensive effects of meperidine.

ADVERSE REACTIONS

CNS: *sedation, somnolence, clouded sensorium, euphoria, dizziness,* paradoxical excitement, tremor, *seizures* (with large doses), headache, hallucinations, syncope, *light-headedness.*
CV: *hypotension,* bradycardia, tachycardia, *cardiac arrest, shock.*
GI: *constipation,* ileus, dry mouth, *nausea, vomiting,* biliary tract spasms.
GU: *urine retention.*
Respiratory: *respiratory depression, respiratory arrest.*
Skin: pruritus, urticaria, *diaphoresis.*
Other: physical dependence, muscle twitching, phlebitis (after I.V. delivery), pain (at injection site), local tissue irritation, induration (after S.C. injection).

◙ KEY CONSIDERATIONS

Besides the recommendations relevant to all opioids, consider the following:
● Lower doses are usually indicated for geriatric patients because they may be more sensitive to the therapeutic and adverse effects of meperidine.
● Drug may be administered to some patients who are allergic to morphine.
● Drug and its active metabolite normeperidine accumulate. Monitor the patient for neurotoxic effects, especially in burn patients and those with poor renal function, sickle cell anemia, or cancer.
● Because drug toxicity commonly appears after several days of treatment, this drug isn't recommended for treatment of chronic pain.
● Drug may be given slowly I.V., preferably as a diluted solution. S.C. injection is very painful. During I.V. administration, tachycardia may occur, possibly as a result of drug's atropine-like effects.
● Oral dose is less than half as effective as parenteral dose. Give I.M. if possible. When changing from parenteral to oral route, dosage should be increased.
● Syrup has local anesthetic effect. Give with water.
● Alternating drug with a peripherally active nonnarcotic analgesic (aspirin, acetaminophen, NSAID) may improve pain control while allowing lower narcotic dosages.
● Injectable drug is compatible with sodium chloride and D_5W solutions and their combinations and with lactated Ringer's and sodium lactate solution.
● Question patient carefully regarding possible use of MAO inhibitors—such as isocarboxazid, furazolidone, phenelzine, procarbazine, and tranylcypromine—within the past 14 days.

Patient education

● Caution geriatric patients about getting out of bed or walking. Warn outpatient to avoid driving and other potentially hazardous activities that require mental alertness until drug's CNS effects are known.
● Encourage patient to turn, cough, and breathe deeply and to use an incentive spirometer to prevent atelectasis when drug is used postoperatively.
● Advise patient to avoid alcohol.

Overdose & treatment

● The most common signs and symptoms of meperidine overdose are CNS depression, respiratory depression, skeletal muscle flaccidity, cold and clammy skin, mydriasis, bradycardia, and hypotension. Other acute toxic effects include hypothermia, shock, apnea, cardiopulmonary arrest, circulatory collapse, pulmonary edema, and seizures.
● To treat acute overdose, first establish adequate respiratory exchange via a patent airway and ventilation as needed; administer a narcotic antagonist (naloxone) to reverse respiratory depression. (Because the duration or action of drug is longer than that of naloxone, repeated dosing is necessary.) Naloxone shouldn't be given unless the patient has significant respiratory or CV depression. Monitor vital signs. If patient presents within 2 hours of ingestion of an oral overdose, immediately induce vomiting with ipecac syrup or perform gastric lavage. Use caution to avoid risk of aspiration. Administer activated charcoal via an NG tube to remove more drug. Provide symptomatic and supportive treatment (continued respiratory support, correction of fluid or electrolyte imbalance).

Reactions may be *common,* uncommon, *life-threatening,* or COMMON AND LIFE-THREATENING.

Monitor laboratory values, vital signs, and neurologic status closely.

mephenytoin
Mesantoin

Hydantoin derivative, anticonvulsant

Available by prescription only
Tablets: 100 mg

INDICATIONS & DOSAGE
Generalized tonic-clonic or complex-partial seizures
Adults: 50 to 100 mg P.O. daily; may increase by 50 to 100 mg at weekly intervals, up to 200 mg P.O. q 8 hours. Dosages up to 800 mg/day may be required.

PHARMACODYNAMICS
Anticonvulsant action: Like other hydantoin derivatives, mephenytoin stabilizes the neuronal membranes and limits seizure activity either by increasing efflux or decreasing influx of sodium ions across cell membranes in the motor cortex during generation of nerve impulses. Like phenytoin, drug appears to have antiarrhythmic effects.

Drug is used for prophylaxis of tonic-clonic, psychomotor, focal, and Jacksonian-type partial seizures in patients immune to less toxic agents. It's usually combined with phenytoin, phenobarbital, or primidone; phenytoin is preferred because it causes less sedation than barbiturates. Drug also is used with succinimides to control combined absence and tonic-clonic disorders; use with oxazolidinediones, paramethadione, or trimethadione isn't recommended because of the increased hazard of blood dyscrasias.

PHARMACOKINETICS
Absorption: Mephenytoin is absorbed from the GI tract. Onset of action in 30 minutes, persists for 24 to 48 hours.
Distribution: Drug is distributed widely throughout the body; good seizure control without toxicity occurs with serum levels of drug and major metabolite of 25 to 40 mcg/ml.

Metabolism: Drug is metabolized by the liver.
Excretion: Drug and its metabolites are excreted in urine.

CONTRAINDICATIONS & PRECAUTIONS
Contraindicated in patients with hydantoin hypersensitivity.

INTERACTIONS
Drug-drug. Use with *antihistamines, chloramphenicol, cimetidine, diazepam, diazoxide, disulfiram, isoniazid, oral anticoagulants, phenylbutazone, salicylates, sulfamethizole,* or *valproate* may increase the therapeutic effects of mephenytoin. Drug may decrease the effects of *folic acid* and *oral contraceptives.*
Drug-lifestyle. Use of *alcohol* may decrease the therapeutic effects of drug.

ADVERSE REACTIONS
CNS: ataxia, *drowsiness,* fatigue, irritability, choreiform movements, depression, tremor, insomnia, dizziness.
EENT: conjunctivitis, diplopia, nystagmus, gingival hyperplasia.
GI: nausea and vomiting.
Hematologic: *leukopenia, neutropenia, agranulocytosis, thrombocytopenia,* eosinophilia, leukocytosis.
Respiratory: *pulmonary fibrosis.*
Skin: rash, *exfoliative dermatitis, Stevens-Johnson syndrome, fatal dermatitides.*
Other: edema, lymphadenopathy, polyarthropathy.

▣ KEY CONSIDERATIONS
Besides the recommendations relevant to all hydantoin derivatives, consider the following:
• Mephenytoin may elevate liver function test results.
• Decreased alertness and coordination are most pronounced at the start of treatment. Patient may need help with walking and other activities for first few days.
• Drug shouldn't be discontinued abruptly. Transition from mephenytoin to other anticonvulsant drug should progress over 6 weeks.

• CBC and platelet counts should be performed before therapy, after 2 weeks of initial therapy, and after 2 weeks on maintenance dose; they should be repeated every month for 1 year and subsequently at 3-month intervals.

Patient education
• Tell patient never to discontinue mephenytoin or change dosage except as prescribed and to avoid alcohol, which decreases the effectiveness of the drug and increases sedative effects.
• Explain that follow-up laboratory tests are essential for safe use.
• Instruct patient to report unusual changes immediately (cutaneous reaction, sore throat, glandular swelling, fever, mucous membrane swelling).

Overdose & treatment
• Signs and symptoms of acute mephenytoin toxicity may include restlessness, dizziness, drowsiness, nausea, vomiting, nystagmus, ataxia, dysarthria, tremor, and slurred speech; hypotension, respiratory depression, coma, and death may follow.
• Treat overdose by performing gastric lavage or inducing vomiting and follow with supportive treatment. Carefully monitor vital signs and fluid and electrolyte balance. Forced diuresis is of little or no value. Hemodialysis or peritoneal dialysis may be more helpful.

---

meprobamate
Apo-Meprobamate*, Equanil, Meprospan, Miltown, Neuramate

Carbamate, anxiolytic
Controlled substance schedule IV

Available by prescription only
Tablets: 200 mg, 400 mg, 600 mg
Capsules (sustained-release): 200 mg, 400 mg

INDICATIONS & DOSAGE
Anxiety and tension
Adults: 1.2 to 1.6 g P.O. daily in three or four equally divided doses. Maximum dosage, 2.4 g daily (sustained-release capsules, 400 to 800 mg b.i.d.).

PHARMACODYNAMICS
Anxiolytic action: The cellular mechanism is unknown. Meprobamate causes nonselective CNS depression similar to that seen with barbiturates. Drug acts at multiple sites in the CNS, including the thalamus, hypothalamus, limbic system, and spinal cord, but not the medulla or reticular activating system.

PHARMACOKINETICS
Absorption: Meprobamate is well absorbed after oral administration; serum levels peak in 1 to 3 hours. Sedation usually occurs within 1 hour.
Distribution: Drug is distributed throughout the body; 20% is protein-bound.
Metabolism: Drug is metabolized rapidly in the liver to inactive glucuronide conjugates. Half-life of drug is 6 to 17 hours.
Excretion: Metabolites of drug and 10% to 20% of a single dose as unchanged drug are excreted in urine.

CONTRAINDICATIONS & PRECAUTIONS
Contraindicated in patients hypersensitive to meprobamate or related compounds (such as carisoprodol, mebutamate, tybamate, and carbromal) and in those with porphyria.

Use cautiously in geriatric or debilitated patients and in those with impaired renal or hepatic function, seizure disorders, or suicidal tendencies.

INTERACTIONS
Drug-drug. Meprobamate may add to or potentiate the effects of *antihistamines, barbiturates, narcotics,* other *CNS depressants,* or *tranquilizers.*
Drug-lifestyle. Meprobamate may add to or potentiate the effects of *alcohol.*

ADVERSE REACTIONS
CNS: *drowsiness,* ataxia, dizziness, slurred speech, headache, vertigo, *seizures.*
CV: palpitations, tachycardia, hypotension, *arrhythmias,* syncope.
GI: nausea, vomiting, diarrhea.
Hematologic: *aplastic anemia, thrombocytopenia, agranulocytosis.*

Reactions may be *common,* uncommon, *life-threatening,* or COMMON AND LIFE-THREATENING.

Skin: pruritus, urticaria, erythematous maculopapular rash, *hypersensitivity reactions.*

After abrupt withdrawal of long-term therapy: severe generalized tonic-clonic seizures.

▣ KEY CONSIDERATIONS

• Geriatric patients may have more pronounced CNS effects. Use lowest dose possible.

• Impose safety precautions such as raised bed rails, especially for geriatric patients, when initiating treatment or increasing the dose. Patient may need assistance walking.

• Assess level of consciousness and vital signs frequently.

• Meprobamate may falsely elevate urine 17-ketosteroids, 17-ketogenic steroids (as determined by the Zimmerman reaction), and 17-hydroxycorticosteroid levels (as determined by the Glenn-Nelson technique).

• Periodic evaluation of CBC is recommended during long-term therapy.

• Drug abuse and addiction may occur.

• Withdraw drug gradually; otherwise, withdrawal symptoms may occur if patient has been taking drug for a long time.

Patient education

• Tell patient to avoid alcohol and other CNS depressants—such as antihistamines, narcotics, and tranquilizers—while taking meprobamate, unless prescribed.

• Advise patient not to increase dose or frequency and not to abruptly discontinue or decrease dose unless prescribed.

• Tell patient to avoid tasks requiring mental alertness or physical coordination until drug's CNS effects are known.

• Recommend sugarless candy, gum, or ice chips to relieve dry mouth.

• Advise patient to report sore throat, fever, or unusual bleeding or bruising.

• Inform patient of potential for physical or psychological dependence with long-term use.

Overdose & treatment

• Signs and symptoms of overdose include drowsiness, lethargy, ataxia, coma, hypotension, shock, and respiratory depression.

• Treatment of overdose is supportive and symptomatic, including maintaining adequate ventilation and a patent airway, with mechanical ventilation if needed. Treat hypotension with fluids and vasopressors as needed. Empty gastric contents by inducing vomiting or performing gastric lavage if ingestion was recent, followed by activated charcoal and a cathartic. Treat seizures with parenteral diazepam. Peritoneal dialysis and hemodialysis may effectively remove drug. Serum levels greater than 100 μg/ml may be fatal.

---

mercaptopurine
(6-mercaptopurine, 6-MP)
Purinethol

Antimetabolite (cell cycle–phase specific, S phase), antineoplastic

Available by prescription only
Tablets (scored): 50 mg

INDICATIONS & DOSAGE

Dosage and indications may vary. Check current literature for recommended protocols.

Acute lymphoblastic leukemia, acute myeloblastic leukemia, chronic myelocytic leukemia

Adults: 2.5 mg/kg P.O. daily as a single dose, up to 5 mg/kg daily. Maintenance dosage, 1.5 to 2.5 mg/kg daily.

◊ ***Treatment of regional enteritis (Crohn's disease) and ulcerative colitis***

Adults: Usual dosage is 1.5 mg/kg/day, gradually increased to 2.5 mg/kg/day if tolerated.

PHARMACODYNAMICS

Antineoplastic action: Mercaptopurine is converted intracellularly to its active form, which exerts its cytotoxic antimetabolic effects by competing for an enzyme required for purine synthesis. This results in inhibition of DNA and RNA synthesis. Cross-resistance exists between drug and thioguanine.

PHARMACOKINETICS

Absorption: Mercaptopurine absorption after an oral dose is incomplete and variable; about 50% of a dose is absorbed. Serum levels peak 2 hours after dose.
Distribution: Drug distributes widely into total body water. Drug crosses the blood-brain barrier, but CSF level is too low for treatment of meningeal leukemias.
Metabolism: Drug is extensively metabolized in the liver. It appears to undergo extensive first-pass metabolism, contributing to its low bioavailability.
Excretion: Drug and metabolites are excreted in urine.

CONTRAINDICATIONS & PRECAUTIONS

Contraindicated in patients whose disease has shown resistance to mercaptopurine. Use cautiously after chemotherapy or radiation therapy in patients with depressed neutrophil or platelet counts and in those with impaired renal or hepatic function.

INTERACTIONS

Drug-drug. Use of *allopurinol* at dosages of 300 to 600 mg/day increases the toxic effects of mercaptopurine, especially myelosuppression. This interaction is due to the inhibition of mercaptopurine metabolism by allopurinol. Reduce dosage of mercaptopurine to 25% to 30% when administering with allopurinol.

Drug should be used cautiously with other *hepatotoxic drugs* because of the increased potential for hepatotoxicity. Use with *trimethoprim-sulfamethoxazole* may cause enhanced marrow suppression. Use with mercaptopurine decreases the anticoagulant activity of *warfarin;* the mechanism of this interaction is unknown.

ADVERSE REACTIONS

GI: *nausea, vomiting, anorexia, painful oral ulcers, diarrhea,* **pancreatitis,** *GI ulcers.*
Hematologic: *leukopenia,* **thrombocytopenia,** anemia (all may persist several days after drug is stopped).
Hepatic: *jaundice,* **hepatotoxicity.**
Skin: rash, hyperpigmentation.
Other: hyperuricemia.

▣ KEY CONSIDERATIONS

• This drug may falsely elevate serum glucose and uric acid levels when sequential multiple analyzer is used.
• Monitor weekly blood counts; watch for precipitous decrease.
• Store tablets at room temperature and protect from light.
• After chemotherapy or radiation therapy, in depressed neutrophil or platelet count, and in impaired hepatic or renal function, dosage may need to be modified.
• Monitor intake and output. Encourage patient to drink at least 3 L [3 qt] of fluids daily.
• Monitor hepatic function and hematologic values weekly during therapy.
• Monitor serum uric acid levels. If allopurinol is necessary, use cautiously.
• Observe for signs of bleeding and infection.
• Hepatic dysfunction is reversible when drug is stopped. Watch for jaundice, clay-colored stools, and frothy dark urine. Drug should be stopped if hepatic tenderness occurs.
• Avoid all I.M. injections when platelet count is less than 100,000/mm^3.

Patient education
• Warn patient that improvement may take 2 to 4 weeks or longer.
• Tell patient to continue drug despite nausea and vomiting.
• Instruct patient to call health care provider immediately if vomiting occurs shortly after taking a dose.
• Warn patient to avoid alcoholic beverages while taking drug because of the hepatotoxic effects.
• Urge patient to maintain adequate fluid intake to increase urine output and facilitate the excretion of uric acid.
• Advise patient to avoid exposure to people with infections. Tell patient to call immediately if signs of unusual bleeding or infection occur.

Overdose & treatment
• Signs and symptoms of overdose include myelosuppression, hypocalcemia, severe nausea, vomiting, ulceration of the mouth, decreased consciousness,

---

Reactions may be *common,* uncommon, *life-threatening,* or COMMON AND LIFE-THREATENING.

seizures, muscular paralysis, hepatic necrosis, and cholinomimetic effects.
• Treatment is usually supportive and includes transfusion of blood components and antiemetics. Hemodialysis is thought to be of marginal use because of the rapid intracellular incorporation of mercaptopurine into active metabolites with long persistence.

meropenem
Merrem I.V.

Carbapenem derivative, antibiotic

Available by prescription only
Powder for injection: 500 mg/15 ml, 500 mg/20 ml, 500 mg/100 ml, 1 g/15 ml, 1 g/30 ml, 1 g/100 ml

INDICATIONS & DOSAGE
Complicated appendicitis and peritonitis caused by viridans group streptococci, **Escherichia coli, Klebsiella pneumoniae, Pseudomonas aeruginosa, Bacteroides fragilis, Bacteroides thetaiotaomicron,** *and* **Peptostreptococcus** *species; bacterial meningitis caused by* **Streptococcus pneumoniae, Haemophilus influenzae,** *and* **Neisseria meningitidis**
Adults: Administer 1 g I.V. q 8 hours over 15 to 30 minutes as I.V. infusion or over 3 to 5 minutes as I.V. bolus injection (maximum recommended concentration, 50 mg/ml).
✦ *Dosage adjustment.* In adults with renal failure, give 1 g q 12 hours if creatinine clearance is 26 to 50 ml/minute, 500 mg q 12 hours if it's 10 to 25 ml/minute, and 500 mg q 24 hours if it's less than 10 ml/minute.

PHARMACODYNAMICS
Antibiotic action: Meropenem inhibits cell wall synthesis in bacteria. It readily penetrates the cell wall of most gram-positive and gram-negative bacteria to reach penicillin-binding protein targets.

PHARMACOKINETICS
Absorption: Meropenem is only given I.V.

Distribution: Drug is distributed into most body fluids and tissues, including CSF. It's only about 2% bound to plasma protein.
Metabolism: Drug is thought to undergo minimal metabolism. One inactive metabolite has been identified.
Excretion: Drug is excreted unchanged primarily in urine. Elimination half-life in adults with normal renal function is about 1 hour.

CONTRAINDICATIONS & PRECAUTIONS
Contraindicated in patients with hypersensitivity to any component of meropenem or other drugs in the same class and in those who have demonstrated anaphylactic reactions to beta-lactams. Use cautiously in patients with history of seizure disorders or impaired renal function.

INTERACTIONS
Drug-drug. *Probenecid* competes with meropenem for active tubular secretion and thus inhibits the renal excretion of meropenem. This significantly increases the elimination half-life of meropenem and the extent of systemic exposure; coadministration of probenecid with drug isn't recommended.

ADVERSE REACTIONS
CNS: headache, syncope, insomnia, agitation, delirium, confusion, dizziness, *seizure,* nervousness, paresthesia, hallucinations, somnolence, anxiety, depression.
CV: *heart failure; cardiac arrest; MI; pulmonary embolism;* tachycardia; hypertension; *bradycardia;* hypotension; chest pain; edema, phlebitis, or thrombophlebitis (at injection site).
GI: diarrhea, nausea, vomiting, constipation, abdominal pain or enlargement, oral candidiasis, anorexia.
GU: dysuria, *kidney failure,* increased creatinine clearance or BUN levels, presence of RBCs in urine.
Hematologic: anemia, increased or decreased platelet count, increased eosinophil count, prolonged or shortened PT or PTT, positive direct or indirect Coombs' test, decreased hemoglobin

level or hematocrit, decreased WBC count.

Hepatic: *hepatic failure,* cholestatic jaundice, jaundice, flatulence, ileus, increased levels of ALT, AST, alkaline phosphatase, LD, and bilirubin.

Musculoskeletal: back pain.

Respiratory: *apnea, hypoxia,* respiratory disorder, dyspnea.

Skin: rash, pruritus, urticaria, sweating.

Other: *hypersensitivity and anaphylactic reactions,* inflammation (at injection site), bleeding events, *sepsis, shock,* fever, peripheral edema.

▣ KEY CONSIDERATIONS

• Use cautiously in geriatric patients because of decreased renal function. Adjust dosage in geriatric patients with a creatinine clearance level less than 50 ml/minute.

• Don't use to treat methicillin-resistant staphylococci.

• Obtain specimen for culture and sensitivity tests before giving first dose. Therapy may begin pending test results.

• For I.V. bolus administration, add 10 ml sterile water for injection to 500 mg/20-ml vial size or 20 ml to 1 g/30-ml vial size. Shake to dissolve and let stand until clear. Maximum reconstitution concentration is 50 mg/ml.

• For I.V. infusion, infusion vials (500 mg/100 ml and 1 g/100 ml) may be directly reconstituted with a compatible infusion fluid. Alternatively, an injection vial may be reconstituted, then the resulting solution added to an I.V. container and further diluted with an appropriate infusion fluid. ADD-Vantage vials shouldn't be used.

• For ADD-Vantage vials, reconstitute only with half-normal saline injection, normal saline injection, or D_5W injection in 50-, 100-, or 250-ml Abbott ADD-Vantage flexible diluent containers. Follow manufacturer's guidelines closely when using ADD-Vantage vials.

• Don't mix with or physically add meropenem to solutions containing other drugs.

• Use freshly prepared solutions of drug immediately whenever possible. Stability of drug varies with type of drug used (injection vial, infusion vial, or ADD-Vantage container). Consult manufacturer's literature for details.

• Serious and occasionally fatal hypersensitivity (anaphylactic) reactions have been reported in patients receiving therapy with beta-lactams. Before therapy is initiated, find out if previous hypersensitivity reactions to penicillins, cephalosporins, other beta-lactams, and other allergens have occurred.

• Discontinue drug immediately if an allergic reaction occurs. Serious anaphylactic reactions require immediate emergency treatment with epinephrine, oxygen, I.V. steroids, and airway management. Other therapy may also be required as indicated by the patient's condition.

• Seizures and other CNS adverse reactions associated with drug therapy commonly occur in patients with CNS disorders, bacterial meningitis, and compromised renal function.

• If seizures occur during drug therapy, decrease dosage or discontinue drug.

• Drug may cause overgrowth of nonsusceptible bacteria or fungi. Monitor patient for signs and symptoms of superinfection.

• Periodic assessment of organ system functions, including renal, hepatic, and hematopoietic, is recommended during prolonged therapy.

Overdose & treatment

• Signs and symptoms and treatment of overdosage are unknown.

• If overdose occurs, discontinue drug and give general supportive treatment until renal elimination occurs. Meropenem and its metabolite are readily dialyzable and effectively removed by hemodialysis.

---

mesalamine
Asacol, Pentasa, Rowasa

Salicylate, anti-inflammatory

Available by prescription only
Capsules (controlled-release): 250 mg
Tablets (delayed-release): 400 mg
Suppositories: 500 mg

Rectal suspension: 4 g/60 ml, in units of 7 disposable bottles

INDICATIONS & DOSAGE

Active mild to moderate distal ulcerative colitis, proctosigmoiditis, proctitis

Adults: 800 mg (delayed-release tablets) P.O. t.i.d. for 6 weeks or 1 g (controlled-release capsules) q.i.d. for up to 8 weeks.

Alternatively, use 1 rectal suppository b.i.d. for 3 to 6 weeks. For maximum benefit, the suppository should be retained for 1 to 3 hours or longer. Usual dosage of mesalamine suspension enema in 60-ml U is one rectal instillation (4 g) once daily, preferably h.s., retained for about 8 hours.

Lower doses of suspension enemas of 40 g q 2 to 3 nights or 1 g daily have been effective.

PHARMACODYNAMICS

Anti-inflammatory action: Mechanism of action of mesalamine (and sulfasalazine) is unknown, but appears to be topical rather than systemic. Mucosal production of arachidonic acid metabolites, both through cyclooxygenase pathways (for example, prostaglandins) and through lipoxygenase pathways (for example, leukotrienes and hydroxyeicosatetraenoic acids) is increased in patients with chronic inflammatory bowel disease; drug may possibly diminish inflammation by blocking cyclooxygenase and inhibiting prostaglandin production in the colon.

Sulfasalazine is split by bacterial action in the colon into sulfapyridine (SP) and mesalamine (5-ASA). The mesalamine component is considered therapeutically active in ulcerative colitis. The usual oral dosage of sulfasalazine for active ulcerative colitis in adults is 3 to 4 g/day in divided doses; 4 g sulfasalazine provides 1.6 g free mesalamine to the colon.

PHARMACOKINETICS

Absorption: Mesalamine administered P.R. as a suppository or suspension enema is poorly absorbed from colon. Extent of absorption depends on retention time, with considerable individual variation. Oral tablets coated with an acrylic resin delay the release of drug until tablet is beyond the terminal ileum. About 72% of dose reaches colon; 28% of dose is absorbed. Food doesn't affect absorption. Capsules are formulated to release therapeutic levels throughout the GI tract. About 20% to 30% is absorbed.

Distribution: Maximum plasma levels of oral mesalamine and N-acetyl 5-aminosalicylic acid are about twice as high as those with sulfasalazine therapy. At steady state, 10% to 30% of daily 4-g rectal dose can be recovered in cumulative 24-hour urine collections.

Metabolism: Drug undergoes acetylation, but site is unknown. Most absorbed drug is excreted in urine as the N-acetyl-5-ASA metabolite. Elimination half-life of drug is 0.5 to 1.5 hours; half-life of acetylated metabolite is 5 to 10 hours. Steady-state plasma levels show no accumulation of either free or metabolized drug during repeated daily administrations.

Excretion: After rectal administration, drug is mostly excreted in feces as parent drug and metabolite. After oral administration, drug is mostly excreted in urine as metabolite.

CONTRAINDICATIONS & PRECAUTIONS

Contraindicated in patients hypersensitive to mesalamine, its components (sulfite in rectal preparation), or salicylates. Use cautiously in patients with impaired renal function.

INTERACTIONS

None reported.

ADVERSE REACTIONS

CNS: headache, dizziness, fatigue, malaise, asthenia, chills, anxiety, depression, hyperesthesia, paresthesia, tremor.
CV: chest pain.
GI: abdominal pain, cramps, discomfort, flatulence, diarrhea, rectal pain, bloating, nausea, *pancreatitis,* vomiting, constipation, eructation.
GU: dysuria, hematuria, urinary urgency.
Musculoskeletal: arthralgia, myalgia, back pain, hypertonia.
Respiratory: wheezing.
Skin: itching, rash, urticaria, hair loss.

Other: *anaphylaxis (rare),* fever.

▣ KEY CONSIDERATIONS
• Although the effects of mesalamine may be evident in 3 to 21 days, usual course of therapy is 3 to 6 weeks depending on symptoms and sigmoidoscopic findings. Clinical studies haven't determined if suspension enema modifies relapse rates after the 6-week, short-term treatment.

Patient education
• Tell patient to swallow the tablets whole.
• Instruct patient to retain suppository as long as possible (at least 1 to 3 hours) for maximum effectiveness.
• Instruct patient in correct use of rectal suspension:
– Shake the bottle well to make sure the suspension is homogeneous.
– Remove the protective sheath from the applicator tip. Holding the bottle at the neck won't cause drug to be discharged.
– To administer, lie on the left side to facilitate migration into the sigmoid colon) with the lower leg extended and the right upper leg flexed forward for balance; or use the knee-chest position.
– Gently insert the applicator tip in the rectum, pointing toward the umbilicus.
– Steadily squeeze the bottle to discharge the preparation into the colon.
• Patient instructions are included with every 7-U bottle.

---

mesna
MESNEX

Thiol derivative, uroprotectant

Available by prescription only
Injection: 100 mg/ml in 2-ml and 10-ml ampules

INDICATIONS & DOSAGE
Prevention of ifosfamide-induced hemorrhagic cystitis
Adults: Calculate daily dose as 60% of the ifosfamide dose. Administer in three equally divided bolus doses: Give first dose at time of ifosfamide injection.

Subsequent doses are given at 4 and 8 hours after ifosfamide.
   Protocols that use 1.2 g/m^2 ifosfamide would use 240 mg/m^2 mesna at 0, 4, and 8 hours after ifosfamide.
◇ *Prophylaxis in bone marrow recipients receiving cyclophosphamides*
Adults: 60% to 160% of the cyclophosphamide daily dose given in three to five divided doses or by continuous infusion.

PHARMACODYNAMICS
Uroprotectant action: Mesna disulfide is reduced to mesna in the kidney and reacts with the urotoxic metabolites of ifosfamide to detoxify the drug and protect the urinary system.

PHARMACOKINETICS
Absorption: Mesna is administered I.V.
Distribution: Drug remains in vascular compartment and doesn't distribute through tissues.
Metabolism: Drug is rapidly metabolized to mesna disulfide, its only metabolite.
Excretion: In the kidneys, 33% of dose is eliminated in the urine in 24 hours; half-life of mesna and mesna disulfide are 0.36 and 1.17 hours, respectively.

CONTRAINDICATIONS & PRECAUTIONS
Contraindicated in patients hypersensitive to mesna or thiol-containing compounds.

INTERACTIONS
None reported.

ADVERSE REACTIONS
CNS: headache, fatigue.
CV: hypotension.
GI: soft stools, nausea, vomiting, diarrhea, dysgeusia.
Other: limb pain, allergy.
   Note: Because mesna is used together with ifosfamide and other chemotherapeutic agents, it's difficult to determine adverse reactions attributable solely to mesna.

▣ KEY CONSIDERATIONS
• Instruct patient to report hematuria or allergy immediately.

Reactions may be *common,* uncommon, *life-threatening,* or COMMON AND LIFE-THREATENING.

• MESNEX multidose vials may be stored and used for up to 8 days.
• Discard unused drug from open ampules. It will form an inactive oxidation product (dimesna) on exposure to oxygen.
• Dilute appropriate dose in D_5W injection, normal saline solution injection, or lactated Ringer's injection to a concentration of 20 mg/ml. Once diluted, solution is stable for 24 hours at room temperature.
• Drug is physically incompatible with cisplatin. Don't add mesna to cisplatin infusions.
• Drug may produce a false-positive test result for urine ketones. A red-violet color will return to violet when glacial acetic acid is added.

mesoridazine besylate
Serentil

Phenothiazine (piperidine derivative), antipsychotic

Available by prescription only
Tablets: 10 mg, 25 mg, 50 mg, 100 mg
Oral concentrate: 25 mg/ml (0.6% alcohol)
Injection: 25 mg/ml

INDICATIONS & DOSAGE
Psychoneurotic signs and symptoms (anxiety)
Adults: 10 mg P.O. t.i.d., up to maximum of 150 mg/day.
Schizophrenia
Adults: initially, 50 mg P.O. t.i.d. to maximum of 400 mg/day; or 25 mg I.M. repeated in 30 to 60 minutes, p.r.n., not to exceed 200 mg I.M. daily.
Alcoholism
Adults: 25 mg P.O. b.i.d., up to maximum of 200 mg/day.
Behavioral problems caused by chronic brain syndrome
Adults: 25 mg P.O. t.i.d., up to maximum of 300 mg/day. I.M. dosage form is irritating.

PHARMACODYNAMICS
Antipsychotic action: Mesoridazine, a metabolite of thioridazine, is thought to act by postsynaptic blockade of CNS dopamine receptors, inhibiting dopamine-mediated effects.

Drug has many other central and peripheral effects; it produces both alpha and ganglionic blockade and counteracts histamine-and serotonin-mediated activity. Its most prominent adverse reactions are antimuscarinic and sedative; it causes fewer extrapyramidal effects than other antipsychotics.

PHARMACOKINETICS
Absorption: Mesoridazine appears to be well absorbed from the GI tract following oral administration. I.M. dosage form is absorbed rapidly.
Distribution: Drugs is distributed widely into the body and peaks at 2 to 4 hours; steady-state serum level is achieved within 4 to 7 days. Drug is 91% to 99% protein-bound.
Metabolism: Drug is metabolized extensively by the liver; no active metabolites are formed. Duration of action is 4 to 6 hours.
Excretion: Drug is mostly excreted as metabolites in urine; some is excreted in feces via the biliary tract.

CONTRAINDICATIONS & PRECAUTIONS
Contraindicated in patients with hypersensitivity to mesoridazine or in those experiencing severe CNS depression or comatose states.

INTERACTIONS
Drug-drug. Pharmacokinetic alterations and subsequent decreased therapeutic response to drug may follow use with *aluminum-* or *magnesium-containing antacids* or *antidiarrheals* (decreased absorption) or *phenobarbital* (enhanced renal excretion). Use with *appetite suppressants* or *sympathomimetics*—including *ephedrine* (found in many nasal sprays), *epinephrine, phenylephrine, phenylpropanolamine*—may decrease their stimulatory and pressor effects. *Beta blockers* may inhibit drug metabolism, increasing plasma levels and toxicity. Drug may antagonize therapeutic effect of *bromocriptine* on prolactin secretion; it also may decrease the vasoconstrictive effects of *high-dose*

dopamine and decrease effectiveness and increase toxicity when *levodopa* (by dopamine blockade). Drug may inhibit blood pressure response to *centrally acting antihypertensives*, such as *clonidine, guanabenz, guanadrel, guanethidine, methyldopa,* and *reserpine.* Use with *lithium* may result in severe neurological toxicity with an encephalitis-like syndrome, and a decreased therapeutic response to mesoridazine. *Phenothiazines* can cause epinephrine reversal and produce hypotension when epinephrine is used as a pressor agent. Drug may inhibit metabolism and increase toxicity of *phenytoin.* Use with *propylthiouracil* increases risk for agranulocytosis.

Additive effects are likely after use with the following drugs: *antiarrhythmics, disopyramide, procainamide,* or *quinidine* (increased incidence of arrhythmias and conduction defects); *atropine* or other *anticholinergics,* including *antidepressants, antihistamines, antiparkinsonians, MAO inhibitors, meperidine,* and *phenothiazines* (oversedation, paralytic ileus, visual changes, and severe constipation); *CNS depressants—including analgesics, anesthetics (epidural, general, and spinal), barbiturates, narcotics,* and *tranquilizers—*or *parenteral magnesium sulfate* (oversedation, respiratory depression, and hypotension); *metrizamide* (increased risk for seizures); or *nitrates* (hypotension). **Drug-lifestyle.** Additive effects are likely after use with *alcohol. Caffeine* or *heavy smoking* may increase drug metabolism. *Sun exposure* may cause a photosensitivity reaction. Advise patient to take appropriate precautions.

ADVERSE REACTIONS
CNS: extrapyramidal reactions, *tardive dyskinesia, sedation, drowsiness, tremor, rigidity, weakness, EEG changes, dizziness.*
CV: *hypotension, tachycardia, ECG changes.*
EENT: *ocular changes, blurred vision, retinitis pigmentosa, nasal congestion.*
GI: *dry mouth, constipation, nausea, vomiting.*
GU: *urine retention, gynecomastia, inhibited ejaculation.*

Hematologic: leukopenia, *agranulocytosis, aplastic anemia,* eosinophilia, *thrombocytopenia.*
Hepatic: jaundice, abnormal liver function test results.
Metabolic: weight gain,
Skin: *mild photosensitivity, allergic reactions, pain at I.M. injection site, sterile abscess, rash.*
Other: *neuroleptic malignant syndrome.*
After abrupt withdrawal of long-term therapy: gastritis, nausea, vomiting, dizziness, tremor, feeling of warmth or cold, diaphoresis, tachycardia, headache, insomnia.

▣ KEY CONSIDERATIONS
• Obtain baseline measures of blood pressure before starting therapy and monitor regularly. Watch for orthostatic hypotension, especially with parenteral administration.
• Oral liquid and parenteral forms may cause contact dermatitis. Wear gloves when preparing solutions and prevent contact with skin and clothing.
• Give deep I.M. only in outer upper quadrant of buttocks. Massage slowly afterward to prevent sterile abscess. Injection may sting.
• Monitor patient for tardive dyskinesia, which may occur after prolonged use. It may not appear until months or years later and disappear spontaneously or persist for life, despite discontinuation of drug.
• Monitor therapy with weekly bilirubin tests during first month, periodic blood tests (CBC and liver function), and ophthalmic tests (long-term use), as ordered.
• Assess patient for neuroleptic malignant syndrome (extrapyramidal effects, hyperthermia, autonomic disturbance). It's rare, but in many cases fatal. It isn't necessarily related to length of drug use or type of neuroleptic, but more than 60% of affected patients are men.
• Withhold dose and notify health care provider if patient develops jaundice, signs or symptoms of blood dyscrasia (fever, sore throat, infection, cellulitis, weakness), or persistent extrapyramidal reactions (longer than a few hours).

Reactions may be *common,* uncommon, *life-threatening,* or COMMON AND LIFE-THREATENING.

• Don't withdraw mesoridazine abruptly unless required by severe adverse reactions.
• Protect drug from light. Slight yellowing of injection or concentrate is common and doesn't affect potency. Discard markedly discolored solutions.

Patient teaching
• Warn patient to avoid activities that require alertness and good psychomotor coordination until CNS effects of mesoridazine are known. Drowsiness and dizziness usually subside after a few weeks.
• Advise patient to change position slowly.
• Warn patient to avoid alcohol while taking drug.
• Have patient report urine retention or constipation.
• Tell patient that drug may discolor urine.
• Instruct patient to relieve dry mouth with sugarless gum or hard candy.
• Advise patient to use sunblock and to wear protective clothing to avoid photosensitivity reactions.

Overdose & treatment
• CNS depression is characterized by deep sleep (in which the patient can't be aroused) and possible coma, hypotension or hypertension, extrapyramidal symptoms, abnormal involuntary muscle movements, agitation, seizures, arrhythmias, ECG changes, hypothermia or hyperthermia, and autonomic nervous system dysfunction.
• Treatment is symptomatic and supportive, including maintaining vital signs, airway, stable body temperature, and fluid and electrolyte balance.
• Don't induce vomiting: Drug inhibits cough reflex, and aspiration may occur. Perform gastric lavage, then administer activated charcoal and saline cathartics; dialysis doesn't help. Regulate body temperature as needed. Treat hypotension with I.V. fluids: don't give epinephrine. Treat seizures with parenteral diazepam or barbiturates; arrhythmias, with parenteral phenytoin (15 to 18 mg/kg at a rate not to exceed 50 mcg/minute); extrapyramidal reactions, with benztropine

at 1 to 2 mg or parenteral diphenhydramine at 10 to 50 mg.

metaproterenol sulfate
Alupent, Metaprel

Adrenergic, bronchodilator

Available by prescription only
Tablets: 10 mg, 20 mg
Syrup: 10 mg/5 ml
Aerosol inhaler: 0.65 mg/metered spray
Nebulizer inhaler: 0.4%, 0.6%, and 5% solutions

INDICATIONS & DOSAGE
Bronchial asthma and reversible bronchospasm
Oral
Adults: 20 mg P.O. t.i.d. or q.i.d.
Inhalation
Adults: Administered by metered aerosol, two or three inhalations with at least 2 minutes between inhalations; no more than 12 inhalations in 24 hours. Administered by hand-bulb nebulizer, 10 inhalations of an undiluted 5% solution or alternatively, administered by IPPB, 0.3 ml (range, 0.2 to 0.3 ml of a 5% solution diluted in about 2.5 ml normal saline solution or 2.5 ml of a commercially available 0.4% or 0.6% solution for nebulization).

PHARMACODYNAMICS
Bronchodilator action: Metaproterenol relaxes bronchial smooth muscle and peripheral vasculature by stimulating beta$_2$ receptors, thus decreasing airway resistance via bronchodilation. It has less effect on beta$_1$ receptors and has little or no effect on alpha-adrenergic receptors. In high doses, it may cause CNS and cardiac stimulation, resulting in tachycardia, hypertension, or tremors.

PHARMACOKINETICS
Absorption: Drug is well-absorbed from the GI tract. Onset of action within 1 minute after oral inhalation, 5 to 30 minutes after nebulization, and 15 to 30 minutes after oral administration; effects peak in about 1 hour. Duration of action after oral inhalation is 1 to 4 hours after

single dose, 1 to 2½ hours after multiple doses; after nebulization, 2 to 6 hours after single dose, 4 to 6 hours after repeated doses; after oral administration, 1 to 4 hours.

Distribution: Drug is widely distributed throughout the body.

Metabolism: Drug is extensively metabolized on first pass through the liver.

Excretion: Drug is excreted in urine, mainly as glucuronic acid conjugates.

CONTRAINDICATIONS & PRECAUTIONS
Contraindicated in patients with hypersensitivity to metaproterenol or its ingredients, in use during anesthesia with cyclopropane or halogenated hydrocarbon general anesthetics, and in patients with tachycardia and arrhythmias associated with tachycardia, peripheral or mesenteric vascular thrombosis, profound hypoxia, or hypercapnia.

Use cautiously in patients with hypertension, hyperthyroidism, heart disease, diabetes, or cirrhosis and in those receiving cardiac glycosides.

INTERACTIONS
Drug-drug. *Beta blockers,* especially *propranolol,* antagonize the bronchodilating effects of the drug. Use of metaproterenol with *general anesthetics* (especially *chloroform, cyclopropane, halothane,* and *trichloroethylene*), *cardiac glycosides, levodopa, theophylline derivatives,* other *sympathomimetics,* or *thyroid hormones* may increase the potential for cardiac effects, including severe ventricular tachycardia, arrhythmias, and coronary insufficiency. Use of *MAO inhibitors* or *tricyclic antidepressants* may potentiate the CV actions. Increased CNS stimulation may result from use with other *CNS stimulants,* other *sympathomimetics,* and *xanthines,* and other *sympathomimetics* may also produce additive effects and toxicity.

ADVERSE REACTIONS
CNS: *nervousness, weakness, drowsiness, tremor, vertigo, headache.*
CV: *tachycardia, hypertension, palpitations,* **cardiac arrest** (with excessive use).

GI: *vomiting, nausea, heartburn, dry mouth.*
Respiratory: paradoxical bronchiolar constriction with excessive use, cough, dry and irritated throat.
Skin: rash, hypersensitivity reactions.

◙ KEY CONSIDERATIONS
Besides the recommendations relevant to all adrenergics, consider the following:
• Geriatric patients may be more sensitive to the therapeutic and adverse effects of metaproterenol.
• Adverse reactions are dose-related and characteristic of sympathomimetics and may persist a long time because metaproterenol has a long duration of action.
• Excessive or prolonged use may lead to decreased effectiveness.
• Drug may reduce sensitivity to spirometry in the diagnosis of asthma.
• Avoid simultaneous administration of adrenocorticoid inhalation aerosol. Allow at least 5 minutes to lapse between using the two aerosols.
• Monitor patient for signs and symptoms of toxic effects (nausea and vomiting, tremors, and arrhythmias).
• Aerosol treatments may be used with oral tablet dosing.

Patient education
• Instruct patient to use only as directed and to take no more than two inhalations at one time, with 1- to 2-minute intervals between. Remind patient to save applicator; refills may be available.
• Tell patient to take missed dose if remembered within 1 hour. If beyond 1 hour, patient should skip dose and resume regular schedule. The patient shouldn't double-dose.
• Tell patient to store drug away from heat and light and safely out of children's reach.
• Inform patient to call immediately if no relief occurs or condition worsens.
• Warn patient to avoid simultaneous use of adrenocorticoid aerosol and to allow at least 5 minutes to lapse between using the two aerosols.
• Tell patient that he may experience bad taste in mouth after using oral inhaler.

Reactions may be *common,* uncommon, *life-threatening,* or COMMON AND LIFE-THREATENING.

• Instruct patient to shake container, exhale through nose as completely as possible, then administer aerosol while inhaling deeply through mouth, and hold breath for 10 seconds before exhaling slowly. Patient should wait 1 to 2 minutes before repeating inhalations.

• Tell patient that drug may have shorter duration of action after prolonged use. Advise patient to report failure to respond to usual dose.

• Warn patient not to increase dose or frequency unless prescribed; serious adverse reactions are possible.

Overdose & treatment

• Signs and symptoms of overdose include exaggeration of common adverse reactions, particularly nausea and vomiting, arrhythmias, angina, hypertension, and seizures.

• Treatment includes supportive and symptomatic measures. Monitor vital signs closely. Support CV status. Use cardioselective beta$_1$ blockers (acebutolol, atenolol, metoprolol) to treat symptoms with extreme caution; they may induce severe bronchospasm or asthmatic attack.

metformin hydrochloride
Glucophage

Biguanide, antidiabetic

Available by prescription only
Tablets: 500 mg, 850 mg

INDICATIONS & DOSAGE

Adjunct to diet and exercise to lower blood glucose levels in patients with type 2 diabetes mellitus
Adults: Initially, give 500 mg P.O. b.i.d. with morning and evening meals or 850 mg P.O. once daily with morning meal. When 500-mg dosage used, increase by 500 mg weekly to a maximum of 2,500 mg/day as necessary. When 850-mg dosage used, increase by 850 mg every other week to maximum of 2,550 mg/day as necessary.

PHARMACODYNAMICS

Antidiabetic action: Metformin decreases hepatic glucose production and intestinal absorption of glucose and improves insulin sensitivity (increases peripheral glucose uptake and use).

PHARMACOKINETICS

Absorption: Metformin is absorbed from GI tract with absolute bioavailability of 50% to 60%. Food decreases the extent and slightly delays absorption.
Distribution: Drug is negligibly bound to plasma proteins. It partitions into erythrocytes, most likely as a function of time.
Metabolism: Drug isn't metabolized.
Excretion: About 90% is excreted in urine. Elimination half-life in plasma about 6.2 hours and 17.6 hours in blood.

CONTRAINDICATIONS & PRECAUTIONS

Contraindicated in patients with hypersensitivity to metformin, renal disease, or metabolic acidosis. Drug should be temporarily withheld in patients undergoing radiologic studies involving parenteral administration of iodinated contrast materials because use of such products may result in acute renal dysfunction. Discontinue drug if patient develops a hypoxic state. Avoid use in patients with hepatic disease.

Use cautiously in geriatric, debilitated, or malnourished patients and in those with adrenal or pituitary insufficiency because of increased susceptibility to developing hypoglycemia.

INTERACTIONS

Drug-drug. Cationic drugs such as *amiloride, cimetidine, digoxin, morphine, procainamide, quinidine, quinine, ranitidine, triamterene, trimethoprim,* and *vancomycin* have the potential to compete for common renal tubular transport systems, which may increase metformin plasma levels; monitor patient's blood glucose level. Because *calcium channel blockers, corticosteroids, estrogens, isoniazid, nicotinic acid, oral contraceptives, phenothiazines, phenytoin, sympathomimetics, thiazides* or other *diuretics,* and *thyroid drugs* may produce hyperglycemia, patient's glycemic control should be monitored; metformin dosage may need to be increased. *Nifedipine* increases metformin plasma levels, so monitor patient closely; metformin dosage may need to be decreased.

ADVERSE REACTIONS

GI: diarrhea, nausea, vomiting, abdominal bloating, flatulence, anorexia.
Hematologic: *megaloblastic anemia.*
Skin: rash, dermatitis.
Other: *lactic acidosis,* unpleasant or metallic taste.

▣ KEY CONSIDERATIONS

• Administer cautiously to geriatric patients because of decreased renal function.
• Assess patient's renal function before beginning therapy and then annually thereafter. If renal impairment is detected, give another antidiabetic.
• Administer drug with meals; once-daily dose should be administered with breakfast, twice-daily dose should be administered with breakfast and dinner.
• When changing patients from standard oral antidiabetics other than chlorpropamide to metformin, no transition period is necessary. When changing patients from chlorpropamide, exercise care during the first 2 weeks because of prolonged retention of chlorpropamide in the body, increasing risk for hypoglycemia during this time.
• To evaluate effectiveness, monitor patient's blood glucose level regularly.
• If patient doesn't respond to 4 weeks of maximum dose of metformin, add an oral sulfonylurea while continuing metformin at the maximum dose. If patient still doesn't respond after several months of concomitant therapy at maximum doses, discontinue both drugs and initiate insulin therapy.
• Monitor patient closely during times of increased stress, such as infection, fever, surgery, or trauma. Insulin therapy may be required in these situations.
• Incidence of drug-induced lactic acidosis is very low. Reported cases have occurred primarily in diabetic patients who have had significant renal insufficiency or multiple concomitant medical or sur-

gical problems or who were receiving multidrug therapy. Risk for lactic acidosis increases with advanced age and degree of renal impairment.
• Discontinue drug immediately if patient develops conditions associated with hypoxemia or dehydration because of risk for lactic acidosis associated with these conditions.
• Suspend therapy temporarily for surgical procedures (except minor procedures not associated with restricted intake of food and fluids) or radiologic procedures involving parenteral administration of iodinated contrast, and don't restart until patient's oral intake has resumed and renal function is normal.
• Monitor patient's hematologic status for megaloblastic anemia. Patients with inadequate vitamin B_{12} or calcium intake or absorption appear to be predisposed to developing subnormal vitamin B_{12} levels. These patients should have serum vitamin B_{12} levels checked routinely at 2- to 3-year intervals.
• Instruct patient to discontinue drug immediately and report unexplained hyperventilation, myalgia, malaise, unusual somnolence, or other nonspecific symptoms of early lactic acidosis.
• Warn patient not to consume excessive amounts of alcohol while taking metformin.
• Teach the patient about diabetes as well as the importance of following his therapeutic regimen, specific diet, and personal hygiene program; reducing his weight; exercising; and avoiding infection. Explain how and when to self-monitor blood glucose level, and teach him how to recognize hypoglycemia and hyperglycemia.
• Tell patient not to change drug dosage without medical approval. Encourage him to report abnormal blood glucose levels.
• Advise patient not to take other drugs, including OTC drugs, without calling first.
• Instruct patient to carry medical identification stating that he has diabetes.

Overdose & treatment

• Hypoglycemia hasn't been observed with ingestion of up to 85 g of met-

formin, although lactic acidosis has occurred.
• Hemodialysis may be useful for removing drug.

methadone hydrochloride
Dolophine, Methadose, Physeptone*

Opioid, analgesic, narcotic detoxification adjunct
Controlled substance schedule II

Available by prescription only
Tablets: 5 mg, 10 mg, 40 mg for oral solution (for narcotic abstinence syndrome)
Oral solution: 5 mg/5 ml, 10 mg/5 ml, 10 mg/ml (concentrate)
Injection: 10 mg/ml

INDICATIONS & DOSAGE
Severe pain
Adults: 2.5 to 10 mg P.O., I.M., or S.C. q 3 to 4 hours, p.r.n., or around the clock.
Narcotic abstinence syndrome
Adults: 15 to 20 mg P.O. daily (highly individualized). Maintenance dosage is 20 to 120 mg P.O. daily. Adjust dose, p.r.n. Daily doses exceeding 120 mg require special state and federal approval. If patient feels nauseated, give one-quarter of total P.O. dose in two injections, S.C. or I.M.

PHARMACODYNAMICS
Analgesic action: Methadone is an opiate agonist that has an affinity for the opiate receptors similar to that of morphine. It's recommended for severe, chronic pain and is also used in detoxification and maintenance of patients with opiate abstinence syndrome.

PHARMACOKINETICS
Absorption: Methadone is well absorbed from the GI tract. Oral administration delays onset and prolongs duration of action compared with parenteral administration. Onset of action within 30 to 60 minutes; effect peaks at ¼ to 1 hour.
Distribution: Drug is highly bound to tissue protein, which may explain its cumulative effects and slow elimination.

Metabolism: Drug is metabolized primarily in the liver by N-demethylation.
Excretion: Duration of action is 4 to 6 hours. Half-life is 7 to 11 hours in patients with hepatic dysfunction. Urine excretion, the major route, is dose-dependent. Drug metabolites are also excreted in the feces via the bile.

CONTRAINDICATIONS & PRECAUTIONS
Contraindicated in patients with hypersensitivity to methadone. Use cautiously in geriatric or debilitated patients and in those with severe renal or hepatic impairment, acute abdominal conditions, hypothyroidism, Addison's disease, prostatic hyperplasia, urethral stricture, head injury, increased intracranial pressure, asthma, or other respiratory disorders.

INTERACTIONS
Drug-drug. Use with *cimetidine* may increase respiratory and CNS depression, causing confusion, disorientation, apnea, or seizures; such use usually requires reduced dosage of methadone. Drug accumulation and enhanced effects may result from use with *digitoxin*. Use with other *CNS depressants*—including *antidepressants, antihistamines, barbiturates, benzodiazepines, general anesthetics, muscle relaxants, narcotic analgesics, phenothiazines,* and *sedative-hypnotics*—potentiates the respiratory and CNS depressant, sedative, and hypotensive effects of methadone. *Phenytoin* and *rifampin* decrease serum methadone levels by up to 50%; higher doses may be needed, and withdrawal may occur. Patients who become physically dependent on drug may experience acute withdrawal syndrome if given a *narcotic antagonist;* use with caution, and monitor closely.
Drug-lifestyle. *Alcohol* increases respiratory and CNS depressant, sedative, and hypotensive effects.

ADVERSE REACTIONS
CNS: *sedation, somnolence, clouded sensorium, euphoria, dizziness, choreic movements,* **seizures** *(with large doses), headache, insomnia, agitation, lightheadedness, syncope.*

CV: *hypotension, bradycardia, **shock, cardiac arrest,** palpitations.*
EENT: *visual disturbances.*
GI: *nausea, vomiting, constipation, ileus, dry mouth, anorexia, biliary tract spasm.*
GU: *urine retention, decreased libido.*
Respiratory: *respiratory depression, respiratory arrest.*
Skin: *diaphoresis, pruritus, urticaria, edema.*
Other: physical dependence; pain at injection site; tissue irritation, induration (after S.C. injection).

▣ KEY CONSIDERATIONS
Besides the recommendations relevant to all opioids, consider the following:
• Methadone increases plasma amylase levels.
• Lower doses are usually indicated for geriatric patients because they may be more sensitive to the therapeutic and adverse effects of drug.
• Verify that patient is in a methadone maintenance program to manage narcotic addiction—and, if so, at what dosage—and continue that program appropriately.
• Dispersible tablets may be dissolved in 4 oz (120 ml) of water or fruit juice; oral concentrate must be diluted to at least 3 oz (90 ml) with water before administration.
• Oral liquid form (not tablets) is legally required and is the only form available in drug maintenance programs.
• Regimented scheduling (around the clock) is beneficial for severe, chronic pain. When used for severe, chronic pain, tolerance may develop with long-term use, requiring a higher dose to achieve the same degree of analgesia.
• Patients treated for narcotic abstinence syndrome usually require an additional analgesic if pain control is necessary.
• If used with general anesthetics, tranquilizers, sedatives, hypnotics, alcohol, tricyclic antidepressants, or MAO inhibitors, respiratory depression, hypotension, profound sedation, or coma may occur. Use together with extreme caution. Monitor patient's response.

• Physical and psychological tolerance or dependence may occur. Be aware of potential for abuse.

Patient education
• If appropriate, tell patient that he may experience severe constipation during maintenance with methadone. Instruct him to take a stool softener or other laxative.
• Caution patient to avoid activities that require full alertness, such as driving and operating machinery, because of potential for drowsiness.

Overdose & treatment
• The most common signs and symptoms of overdose are CNS depression, respiratory depression, and miosis (pinpoint pupils). Others include hypotension, bradycardia, hypothermia, shock, apnea, cardiopulmonary arrest, circulatory collapse, pulmonary edema, and seizures. Toxicity may result from accumulation of drug over several weeks.
• To treat acute overdose, first establish adequate respiratory exchange via a patent airway and ventilation as needed. Administer an opioid antagonist (naloxone) to reverse respiratory depression. (Because the duration of action of methadone is longer than that of naloxone, repeated naloxone dosing is necessary.) The antagonist naloxone shouldn't be given unless the patient has significant respiratory or CV depression. Monitor vital signs closely.
• If patient presents within 2 hours of ingestion of an oral overdose, immediately induce vomiting with ipecac syrup or perform gastric lavage. Use caution to avoid risk of aspiration. Administer activated charcoal via NG tube to further remove drug.
• Provide symptomatic and supportive treatment (continued respiratory support, correction of fluid or electrolyte imbalance). Monitor laboratory values, vital signs, and neurologic status closely.

Reactions may be *common,* uncommon, ***life-threatening,*** or **COMMON AND LIFE-THREATENING.**

methimazole
Tapazole

Thyroid hormone antagonist, anti-hyperthyroid drug

Available by prescription only
Tablets: 5 mg, 10 mg

INDICATIONS & DOSAGE
Hyperthyroidism, preparation for thyroidectomy, thyrotoxic crisis
Adults: 15 mg/day P.O. if mild; 30 to
40 mg/day P.O. if moderately severe;
60 mg/day P.O. if severe; all are given in
three equally divided doses q 8 hours.
Continue until patient is euthyroid, then
start maintenance dosage of 5 to
15 mg/day.

PHARMACODYNAMICS
Antithyroid action: Methimazole inhibits
synthesis of thyroid hormone by interfering with the incorporation of iodide into
tyrosyl. Drug also inhibits the formation
of iodothyronine. As preparation for thyroidectomy, drug inhibits synthesis of
the thyroid hormone and causes euthyroid state, reducing surgical problems
during thyroidectomy; as a result, the
mortality for a single-stage thyroidectomy is low. Iodide reduces the vascularity
of the gland, making it less friable. For
treating thyrotoxic crisis (thyrotoxicosis), propylthiouracil theoretically is preferred over methimazole because it inhibits peripheral deiodination of T_4 to T_3.

PHARMACOKINETICS
Absorption: Methimazole is absorbed
rapidly from the GI tract (80% to 95%
bioavailable). Plasma levels peak within
1 hour.
Distribution: Drug is concentrated in the
thyroid. It isn't protein-bound.
Metabolism: Drug undergoes hepatic
metabolism.
Excretion: About 80% of drug and its
metabolites are excreted renally; 7% is
excreted unchanged. Half-life is between
5 and 13 hours.

CONTRAINDICATIONS & PRECAUTIONS
Contraindicated in patients with hypersensitivity to methimazole.

INTERACTIONS
Drug-drug. Use with *adrenocorticoids*
or *corticotropin* and *propylthiouracil*
may require a dosage adjustment of the
steroid when thyroid status changes.
Anti–vitamin K action of drug potentiates the action of *anticoagulants.* Use
with *iodinated glycerol, lithium,* or
potassium iodide may potentiate hypothyroid and goitrogenic effects. Use
with other *bone marrow depressants*
causes an increased risk for agranulocytosis. Use with other *hepatotoxic drugs*
increases the risk of hepatotoxicity.

ADVERSE REACTIONS
CNS: headache, drowsiness, vertigo,
paresthesia, neuritis, neuropathies, CNS
stimulation, depression.
EENT: loss of taste.
GI: diarrhea, nausea, vomiting (may be
dose-related), salivary gland enlargement, epigastric distress.
GU: nephritis.
Hematologic: *agranulocytosis, leukopenia, thrombocytopenia, aplastic anemia.*
Hepatic: jaundice, hepatic dysfunction,
hepatitis.
Musculoskeletal: arthralgia, myalgia.
Skin: rash, urticaria, discoloration, pruritus, erythema nodosum, exfoliative
dermatitis, lupus-like syndrome.
Other: fever, lymphadenopathy, hypothyroidism (mental depression; cold
intolerance; hard, nonpitting edema; hypoprothrombinemia; and bleeding).

▣ KEY CONSIDERATIONS
• Administer dosage around the clock
for best response and give at the same
time each day with respect to meals.
• Methimazole alters selenomethionine
(^{75}Se) uptake by the pancreas and ^{123}I
and ^{131}I uptake by the thyroid.
• Dosages of more than 40 mg/day increase the risk of agranulocytosis.
• A beta blocker, usually propranolol, is
usually given to manage the peripheral
signs of hyperthyroidism, primarily
tachycardia.

• Euthyroid state may take several months to develop.

Patient education
• Tell patient to take methimazole at regular intervals around the clock and to take it at the same time each day with respect to meals.
• If GI upset occurs, tell patient to take drug with meals.
• Tell patient to call promptly if fever, sore throat, malaise, unusual bleeding, yellowing of eyes, nausea, or vomiting occur.
• Advise patient not to store drug in bathroom; heat and humidity cause it to deteriorate.
• Tell patient to inform other health care providers and dentists of drug use.
• Teach patient the signs and symptoms of hyperthyroidism and hypothyroidism and what to do if they occur.

Overdose & treatment
• Signs and symptoms of overdose include nausea, vomiting, epigastric distress, fever, headache, arthralgia, pruritus, edema, and pancytopenia.
• Treatment is supportive. Perform gastric lavage or induce vomiting if possible. If bone marrow depression develops, fresh whole blood, corticosteroids, and anti-infectives may be required.

---

methocarbamol
Robaxin

Carbamate derivative of guaifenesin, skeletal muscle relaxant

---

Available by prescription only
Tablets: 500 mg, 750 mg
Injection: 100 mg/ml

INDICATIONS & DOSAGE
Adjunct in acute, painful musculoskeletal conditions
Adults: 1.5 g P.O. q.i.d. for 2 to 3 days. Maintenance dosage, 4 to 4.5 g P.O. daily in three to six divided doses. Alternatively, 1 g I.M. or I.V. Maximum dosage is 3 g daily I.M. or I.V. for 3 consecutive days.

Supportive therapy in tetanus management
Adults: 1 to 2 g I.V. push (300 mg/minute) and an additional 1 to 2 g may be added to I.V. solution. Total initial I.V. dosage, 3 g. Repeat I.V. infusion of 1 to 2 g q 6 hours until NG tube can be inserted.

PHARMACODYNAMICS
Skeletal muscle relaxant action: Mechanism of action is indirect. The effects of methocarbamol appear to be related to its sedative action. Exact mechanism of action is unknown.

PHARMACOKINETICS
Absorption: Methocarbamol is rapidly and completely absorbed from the GI tract. Onset of action after single oral dose within 30 minutes. Onset of action after single I.V. dose is immediate.
Distribution: Drug is widely distributed throughout the body.
Metabolism: Drug is extensively metabolized in liver via dealkylation and hydroxylation. Half-life is between 0.9 and 1.8 hours.
Excretion: Drug is rapidly and almost completely excreted in urine, mainly as its glucuronide and sulfate metabolites (40% to 50%), as unchanged drug (10% to 15%), and the rest as unidentified metabolites.

CONTRAINDICATIONS & PRECAUTIONS
Contraindicated in patients with hypersensitivity to methocarbamol, impaired renal function (injectable form), or seizure disorder (injectable form).

INTERACTIONS
Drug-drug. Patients with myasthenia gravis who receive an *anticholinesterase* may experience severe weakness if given methocarbamol. Use with other *CNS depressants*—including *anxiolytics, narcotics, psychotics,* and *tricyclic antidepressants*—may cause additive CNS depression. When used with other *depressants,* be careful to avoid overdose.
Drug-lifestyle. Use with *alcohol* may cause additive CNS depression.

Reactions may be *common,* uncommon, *life-threatening*, or COMMON AND LIFE-THREATENING.

ADVERSE REACTIONS

CNS: drowsiness, dizziness, light-headedness, headache, syncope, mild muscular incoordination (with I.M. or I.V. use), *seizures* (with I.V. use only), vertigo.
CV: hypotension, flushing, bradycardia (with I.M. or I.V. use).
EENT: blurred vision, conjunctivitis, nystagmus, diplopia.
GI: nausea, GI upset, metallic taste.
GU: hematuria (with I.V. use only), discoloration of urine.
Respiratory: thrombophlebitis.
Skin: urticaria, pruritus, rash.
Other: extravasation (with I.V. use only), fever, *anaphylactic reactions* (with I.M. or I.V. use).

🔲 KEY CONSIDERATIONS

• Lower doses are indicated for geriatric patients because of increased sensitivity to the effects of the drug.
• Don't administer S.C. Give I.V. undiluted at a rate not exceeding 300 mg/minute. May also be given by I.V. infusion after diluting in D_5W or normal saline solution.
• Patient should be supine during and for at least 10 to 15 minutes after I.V. injection.
• To give via NG tube, crush tablets and suspend in water or normal saline solution.
• When used in tetanus, follow manufacturer's instructions.
• Patient's urine may turn black, blue, brown, or green if left standing.
• Patient needs assistance in walking after parenteral administration.
• Extravasation of I.V. solution may cause thrombophlebitis and sloughing from hypertonic solution.
• Oral administration should replace parenteral use as soon as feasible.
• Adverse reactions after oral administration are usually mild and transient and subside with dosage reduction.
• For I.M. administration, don't give more than 500 mg in each gluteal region.
• Drug therapy alters results of laboratory tests for urine 5-hydroxyindoleacetic acid (5-HIAA) using quantitative method of Udenfriend (false-positive) and for urine vanillylmandelic acid (false-positive when Gitlow screening test used; no problem when quantitative method of Sunderman used).

Patient education

• Tell patient urine may turn black, blue, green, or brown.
• Warn patient drug may cause drowsiness. Patient should avoid hazardous activities that require alertness until degree of CNS depression can be determined.
• Advise patient to make position changes slowly, particularly from recumbent to upright position, and to dangle legs before standing.
• Advise patient to avoid alcoholic beverages and use OTC cold or cough preparations carefully because some contain alcohol.
• Tell patient to store drug away from heat and light (not in bathroom medicine cabinet) and safely out of reach of children.
• Tell patient to take missed dose if remembered within 1 hour. Beyond 1 hour, patient should skip that dose and resume regular schedule. He shouldn't double-dose.

Overdose & treatment

• Signs and symptoms of overdose include extreme drowsiness, nausea and vomiting, and arrhythmias.
• Treatment includes symptomatic and supportive measures. If ingestion is recent, induce vomiting or perform gastric lavage (may reduce absorption). Maintain adequate airway; monitor urine output and vital signs; and administer I.V. fluids if needed.

methotrexate, methotrexate sodium

Folex, Mexate, Mexate-AQ, Rheumatrex Dose Pack

Antimetabolite (cell cycle–phase specific, S phase), antineoplastic

Available by prescription only
Tablets (scored): 2.5 mg
Injection: 20-mg, 25-mg, 50-mg, 100-mg, 250-mg, and 1-g vials of preservative-free lyophilized powder; 25-mg/ml vials of preservative-free solution; 2.5-

mg/ml and 25-mg/ml vials of lyophilized powder, preserved

Dose pack of 2.5-mg tablets, which are given q 12 hours for three doses, once a week

INDICATIONS & DOSAGE

Dosage and indications may vary. Check current literature for recommended protocols.

Trophoblastic tumors (choriocarcinoma, hydatidiform mole)

Adults: 15 to 30 mg P.O. or I.M. daily for 5 days. Repeat after 1 or more weeks, according to response or toxicity.

Acute lymphoblastic leukemia

Adults: 3.3 mg/m² P.O. daily for 4 to 6 weeks or until remission occurs; then 20 to 30 mg/m² P.O. or I.M. twice weekly or 2.5 mg/kg I.V. q 14 days. (Used in combination with prednisone.)

Meningeal leukemia

Adults: 12 mg/m² intrathecally to a maximum dose of 15 mg q 2 to 5 days until CSF is normal. Use only vials of preservative-free powder; dilute using normal saline solution injection without preservatives. Use only new vials of drug and diluent. Use immediately after reconstitution.

Burkitt's lymphoma (stage I or II)

Adults: 10 to 25 mg P.O. daily for 4 to 8 days with 7- to 10-day rest intervals.

Lymphosarcoma (stage III; malignant lymphoma)

Adults: 0.625 to 2.5 mg/kg daily P.O., I.M., or I.V.

Mycosis fungoides (advanced)

Adults: 2.5 to 10 mg P.O. daily, or 50 mg I.M. weekly, or 25 mg I.M. twice weekly.

Psoriasis (severe)

Adults: 10 to 25 mg P.O., I.M., or I.V. as single weekly dose.

Rheumatoid arthritis (severe, refractory)

Adults: 7.5 to 15 mg weekly P.O. in single or divided doses.

Adjunct treatment in osteosarcoma

Adults: Give 12 to 15 g/m² as 4-hour I.V. infusion.

PHARMACODYNAMICS

Antineoplastic action: Methotrexate tightly binds with dihydrofolic acid reductase, an enzyme crucial to purine metabolism, thus inhibiting DNA, RNA, and protein synthesis.

PHARMACOKINETICS

Absorption: Absorption across the GI tract appears to be dose related. Lower doses are essentially completely absorbed; absorption of larger doses is incomplete and variable. I.M. doses are absorbed completely. Serum levels peak 30 minutes to 2 hours after I.M. dose and 1 to 4 hours after P.O. dose.

Distribution: Drug is distributed widely throughout the body, with highest levels in the kidneys, gallbladder, spleen, liver, and skin. Drug crosses the blood-brain barrier but doesn't achieve therapeutic levels in the CSF. About 50% of the drug is bound to plasma protein.

Metabolism: Drug is metabolized only slightly in the liver.

Excretion: Excreted primarily into urine as unchanged drug. Elimination has been described as biphasic, with a first-phase half-life of 45 minutes and a terminal-phase half-life of 4 hours.

CONTRAINDICATIONS & PRECAUTIONS

Contraindicated in patients hypersensitive to drug. Also contraindicated in patients with psoriasis or rheumatoid arthritis who have alcoholism, alcoholic liver, chronic liver disease, immunodeficiency syndromes, or preexisting blood dyscrasia.

Use cautiously in geriatric or debilitated patients and in those with impaired renal or hepatic function, bone marrow suppression, aplasia, leukopenia, thrombocytopenia, anemia, folate deficiency, infection, peptic ulcer, or ulcerative colitis.

Drug exits slowly from third-space compartments (for example, pleural effusions or ascites). This results in a prolonged terminal plasma half-life and unexpected toxicity.

INTERACTIONS

Drug-drug. *Folic acid* may decrease the effectiveness of methotrexate. *Immunizations* may be ineffective when given during drug therapy; because of the risk for disseminated infections, live virus vaccines generally aren't recommended during therapy. *NSAIDs, salicylates, sulfonamides,* and *sulfonylureas* may increase the therapeutic and toxic effects of methotrexate by displacing methotrexate from plasma proteins, increasing the levels of free methotrexate; therefore, use should be avoided if possible. *Oral antibiotics*—such as *nonabsorbable broad-spectrum antibiotics, chloramphenicol,* and *tetracycline*—may decrease absorption of drug. *Phenytoin* serum levels may be decreased by chemotherapeutic regimens that use methotrexate, increasing the risk of seizures. Use with *probenecid* or *salicylates* increases the therapeutic and toxic effects of methotrexate by inhibiting the renal tubular secretion of methotrexate; use of these drugs requires a lower dosage of methotrexate. *Pyrimethamine* shouldn't be given concurrently because of similar pharmacologic action.

ADVERSE REACTIONS
CNS: *arachnoiditis* (within hours of intrathecal use), subacute *neurotoxicity* (may begin a few weeks later), *necrotizing demyelinating leukoencephalopathy* (may occur a few years later), malaise, fatigue, dizziness, headache, drowsiness, *seizures.*
EENT: pharyngitis, gingivitis, blurred vision.
GI: stomatitis, diarrhea, abdominal distress, anorexia, GI ulceration and bleeding, enteritis, *nausea, vomiting.*
GU: nephropathy, *tubular necrosis, renal failure,* hematuria, defective spermatogenesis, cystitis.
Hematologic: WBC and platelet count nadirs occurring on day 7; anemia, *leukopenia, thrombocytopenia* (all dose related).
Hepatic: acute toxicity (elevated transaminase level), *chronic toxicity (cirrhosis, hepatic fibrosis).*
Metabolic: hyperuricemia.
Musculoskeletal: arthralgia, myalgia.
Respiratory: *pulmonary fibrosis; pulmonary interstitial infiltrates;* pneumonitis; dry, nonproductive cough.
Skin: alopecia, *urticaria, pruritus, hyperpigmentation, erythematous rash, ecchymoses, psoriatic lesions (aggravated by exposure to sun), rash, photosensitivity.*

Other: fever, chills, reduced resistance to infection, septicemia, diabetes, *sudden death.*

🔲 KEY CONSIDERATIONS
• Use cautiously in geriatric or debilitated patients and in those with infection, peptic ulcer, ulcerative colitis.
• Dose modification may be required in impaired hepatic or renal function, bone marrow depression, aplasia, leukopenia, thrombocytopenia, or anemia.
• Methotrexate therapy may increase blood and urine levels of uric acid and may alter results of the laboratory assay for folate by inhibiting the organism used in the assay, thus interfering with the detection of folic acid deficiency.
• GI adverse reactions may require drug discontinuation.
• Rash, redness, or ulcerations in mouth or pulmonary adverse reactions may signal serious complications.
• Monitor uric acid levels.
• Monitor intake and output daily. Encourage patient to drink at least 2 to 3 L (2 to 3 qt) daily.
• Alkalinize urine by giving sodium bicarbonate tablets to prevent precipitation of drug, especially with high doses. Maintain urine pH at more than 6.5. Reduce dose if BUN level is 20 to 30 mg/dl or serum creatinine level is 1.2 to 2 mg/dl. Stop drug if BUN level is more than 30 mg/dl or serum creatinine level is more than 2 mg/dl.
• Watch for increases in AST, ALT, and alkaline phosphatase levels, which may signal hepatic dysfunction. Drug shouldn't be used when the potential for third spacing exists.
• Watch for bleeding (especially GI) and infection.
• Monitor temperature daily, and watch for cough, dyspnea, and cyanosis.
• Avoid all I.M. injections in patients with thrombocytopenia.
• Leucovorin rescue is necessary with high-dose protocols (doses greater than 100 mg).
• Drug may be given undiluted by I.V. push injection.
• Drug can be diluted to a higher volume with normal saline solution for I.V. infusion.

---

*Canada only ◇ Unlabeled clinical use

• Use reconstituted solutions of preservative-free drug within 24 hours after mixing.
• For intrathecal administration, use preservative-free formulations only. Dilute with unpreserved normal saline solution.

Patient education
• Emphasize importance of continuing drug despite nausea and vomiting. Advise patient to call immediately if vomiting occurs shortly after taking a dose.
• Emphasize the importance of taking leucovorin exactly as prescribed to avoid potentially serious adverse effects in dosing protocols where leucovorin is used.
• Encourage patient to maintain adequate fluid intake to increase urine output, prevent nephrotoxicity, and facilitate excretion of uric acid.
• Warn patient to avoid alcoholic beverages during therapy.
• Tell patient to avoid prolonged exposure to sunlight and to use a highly protective sunscreen when exposed to sunlight.
• Teach patient good mouth care to prevent superinfection of oral cavity.
• Advise patient that hair should grow back after treatment has ended.
• Recommend salicylate-free analgesics to relieve pain or reduce fever.
• Tell patient to avoid exposure to people with infections and to report signs of infection immediately.
• Advise patient to report unusual bruising or bleeding promptly.

Overdose & treatment
• Signs and symptoms of overdose include myelosuppression, anemia, nausea, vomiting, dermatitis, alopecia, and melena.
• The antidote for diagnosed or anticipated hematopoietic toxicity of methotrexate is calcium leucovorin, started as soon as possible after the administration of methotrexate. Because leucovorin blunts therapeutic response of drug, consult specific disease protocols for details. In many therapeutic protocols, leucovorin is only given if serum methotrexate concentration remains high

(measured by serum assays), or by protocol.

methylcellulose
Citrucel, Methylcellulose Tablets

Adsorbent, bulk-forming laxative

Available without prescription
Powder: 105 mg/g, 364 mg/g
Tablets: 500 mg

INDICATIONS & DOSAGE
Chronic constipation
Adults: Maximum dose is 6 g daily, divided into 0.45 to 3 g/dose.

PHARMACODYNAMICS
Laxative action: Methylcellulose adsorbs intestinal fluid and serves as a source of indigestible fiber, stimulating peristaltic activity.

PHARMACOKINETICS
Absorption: Methylcellulose isn't absorbed. Action begins in 12 to 24 hours, but full effect may not occur for 2 to 3 days.
Distribution: Drug is distributed locally, in the intestine.
Metabolism: None.
Excretion: Drug is excreted in feces.

CONTRAINDICATIONS & PRECAUTIONS
Contraindicated in patients with abdominal pain, nausea, vomiting, or other signs or symptoms of appendicitis or acute surgical abdomen and in those with intestinal obstruction or ulceration, disabling adhesions, or difficulty swallowing.

INTERACTIONS
Drug-drug. When used together, methylcellulose may absorb *oral drugs;* separate administration by at least 1 hour.

ADVERSE REACTIONS
GI: *nausea, vomiting, diarrhea (with excessive use); esophageal, gastric, small intestinal, or colonic strictures (when drug is chewed or taken in dry form);* abdominal cramps, especially in severe

---

Reactions may be *common*, uncommon, *life-threatening*, or COMMON AND LIFE-THREATENING.

constipation; laxative dependence (with long-term or excessive use).

▣ KEY CONSIDERATIONS
• Administer methylcellulose with water or juice (at least 225 ml [8 oz]).
• Drug may absorb oral drugs; schedule at least 1 hour apart from all other drugs.
• Bulk laxatives most closely mimic natural bowel function and don't promote laxative dependence.
• Drug is especially useful in patients who continually abuse laxatives, irritable bowel syndrome, diverticular disease, or colostomies; in debilitated patients; and to empty colon before barium enema examinations.

Patient education
• Instruct patient to take other oral drugs 1 hour before or after methylcellulose.
• Explain that drug's full effect may not occur for 2 to 3 days.

---

methyldopa
Aldomet, Apo-Methyldopa*, Dopamet*, Novomedopa*

Centrally acting antiadrenergic, antihypertensive

Available by prescription only
Tablets: 125 mg, 250 mg, 500 mg
Oral suspension: 250 mg/5 ml
Injection (as methyldopate hydrochloride): 250 mg/5 ml in 5-ml vials

INDICATIONS & DOSAGE
Moderate to severe hypertension
Adults: initially, 250 mg P.O. b.i.d. or t.i.d. in first 48 hours, then increased or decreased, p.r.n., q 2 days. Alternatively, 250 to 500 mg I.V. q 6 hours (maximum dose, 1 g q 6 hours). Adjust dosage if other antihypertensives are added to or deleted from therapy.
   Maintenance dosage is 500 mg to 2 g P.O. daily in two to four divided doses. Maximum recommended daily dose is 3 g. I.V. infusion dosage is 250 to 500 mg given over 30 to 60 minutes q 6 hours. Maximum I.V. dosage, 1 g q 6 hours.

PHARMACODYNAMICS
Antihypertensive action: Exact mechanism is unknown; it's thought to be caused by methyldopa's metabolite, alpha-methylnorepinephrine, which stimulates central inhibitory alpha-adrenergic receptors, decreasing total peripheral resistance; drug may act as a false neurotransmitter. Drug may also reduce plasma renin activity.

PHARMACOKINETICS
Absorption: Methyldopa is absorbed partially from the GI tract. Absorption varies, but usually about 50% of oral dose is absorbed. After oral administration, maximal decline in blood pressure occurs in 3 to 6 hours; full effect isn't evident for 2 to 3 days. No correlation exists between plasma level and antihypertensive effect. After I.V. administration, blood pressure usually begins to fall in 4 to 6 hours.
Distribution: Drug is distributed throughout the body and is bound weakly to plasma proteins.
Metabolism: Drug is metabolized extensively in the liver and intestinal cells.
Excretion: Drug and metabolites are excreted in urine; unabsorbed drug is excreted unchanged in feces. Elimination half-life is about 2 hours. Antihypertensive activity usually persists up to 24 hours after oral administration and 10 to 16 hours after I.V. administration.

CONTRAINDICATIONS & PRECAUTIONS
Contraindicated in patients with hypersensitivity to methyldopa or active hepatic disease (such as acute hepatitis) and active cirrhosis. Also contraindicated if previous methyldopa therapy caused liver disorder. Use cautiously in patients with impaired hepatic function and in those receiving MAO inhibitors.

INTERACTIONS
Drug-drug. Patients undergoing surgery may require reduced dosages of *anesthetics.* *Diuretics* may increase hypotensive effect of drug. Use with *haloperidol* may produce dementia and sedation. Use with *lithium* may increase risk for lithium toxicity. *Oral iron therapy* may decrease hypotensive effects and increase

---

serum methyldopa levels. Methyldopa may potentiate the antihypertensive effects of other *antihypertensives* and the pressor effects of *sympathomimetic amines* such as *phenylpropanolamine*. Use with *phenothiazines* or *tricyclic antidepressants* may reduce the antihypertensive effects of drug. Use with *phenoxybenzamine* may cause reversible urinary incontinence. Drug may impair *tolbutamide* metabolism, enhancing the hypoglycemic effect of drug.

ADVERSE REACTIONS

CNS: *sedation, headache, weakness, dizziness,* decreased mental acuity, paresthesia, parkinsonism, involuntary choreoathetoid movements, psychic disturbances, depression, nightmares.
CV: *bradycardia,* orthostatic hypotension, aggravated angina, *myocarditis,* edema.
EENT: *nasal congestion.*
GI: nausea, vomiting, diarrhea, *pancreatitis,* dry mouth, constipation.
GU: gynecomastia, impotence.
Hematologic: *hemolytic anemia, thrombocytopenia, leukopenia,* bone marrow depression.
Hepatic: *hepatic necrosis,* abnormal liver function test results, *hepatitis.*
Skin: rash.
Other: drug-induced fever, decreased libido.

▣ KEY CONSIDERATIONS

• Patients with impaired renal function may require smaller maintenance dosages of methyldopa.
• Because geriatric patients are more sensitive to sedation and hypotension, dosage may need to be reduced.
• At the initiation of and periodically throughout therapy, monitor hemoglobin level, hematocrit, and RBC count for hemolytic anemia; also monitor liver function tests.
• Drug may falsely elevate urine catecholamine levels, interfering with the diagnosis of pheochromocytoma. A positive direct antiglobulin (Coombs') test may also occur.
• Take blood pressure in supine, sitting, and standing positions during dosage adjustment; take blood pressure at least

every 30 minutes during I.V. infusion until patient's condition is stable.
• Sedation and drowsiness usually disappear with continued therapy; bedtime dosage will minimize this effect. Orthostatic hypotension may indicate a need for dosage reduction. Some patients tolerate receiving the entire daily dose in the evening or at bedtime
• Monitor intake and output and daily weights to detect sodium and water retention; voided urine exposed to air may darken because of the breakdown of drug or its metabolites.
• Tolerance may develop after 2 to 3 weeks. Adding a diuretic or increasing the dosage of drug frequently restores blood pressure control. A thiazide is recommended.
• Signs of hepatotoxicity may occur 2 to 4 weeks after therapy begins.
• Monitor for signs and symptoms of drug-induced depression.
• Drug is administered I.V. I.M. or S.C. administration isn't recommended because of unpredictable absorption.
• Patients receiving drug may become hypertensive after dialysis because drug is dialyzable.

Patient education

• Teach patient signs and symptoms of adverse effects, such as jerky movements, and about the need to report them; he should also report excessive weight gain (2.25 kg [5 lb] weekly), signs of infection, or fever.
• Teach patient to take drug at bedtime until he develops tolerance to sedation, drowsiness, and other CNS effects; avoid sudden position changes to minimize orthostatic hypotension; and to use ice chips, hard candy, or gum to relieve dry mouth.
• Warn patient to avoid hazardous activities that require mental alertness until sedative effects subside.
• Instruct patient to call for instructions before taking OTC cold preparations.

Overdose & treatment

• Signs and symptoms of overdose include sedation, hypotension, impaired AV conduction, and coma.

Reactions may be *common*, uncommon, *life-threatening*, or COMMON AND LIFE-THREATENING.

• Within 4 hours ingestion, induce vomiting or perform gastric lavage. Give activated charcoal to reduce absorption; then treat symptomatically and supportively. In severe cases, hemodialysis may be considered.

methylphenidate hydrochloride
Ritalin, Ritalin-SR

Piperidine CNS stimulant, CNS stimulant (analeptic)
Controlled substance schedule II

Available by prescription only
Tablets: 5 mg, 10 mg, 20 mg
Tablets (sustained-release): 20 mg

INDICATIONS & DOSAGE
Narcolepsy
Adults: 10 mg P.O. b.i.d. or t.i.d., 30 to 45 minutes before meals. Dosage varies with patient needs; average dosage is 40 to 60 mg/day.

When using sustained-release tablets, calculate regular dose in q 8-hour intervals and administer as such.

PHARMACODYNAMICS
Analeptic action: The cerebral cortex and reticular activating system appear to be the primary sites of activity; methylphenidate releases nerve terminal stores of norepinephrine, promoting nerve impulse transmission. At high doses, effects are mediated by dopamine.

PHARMACOKINETICS
Absorption: Methylphenidate is absorbed rapidly and completely after oral administration; plasma levels peak at 1 to 2 hours. Duration of action is usually 4 to 6 hours (with considerable individual variation); sustained-release tablets may act for up to 8 hours.
Distribution: Unknown.
Metabolism: Drug is metabolized by the liver.
Excretion: Drug is excreted in urine.

CONTRAINDICATIONS & PRECAUTIONS
Contraindicated in patients with hypersensitivity to methylphenidate, glaucoma, motor tics, family history of or diagnosis of Tourette syndrome, or history of marked anxiety, tension, or agitation.
Use cautiously in patients with history of seizures, drug abuse, hypertension, or EEG abnormalities.

INTERACTIONS
Drug-drug. Methylphenidate may inhibit metabolism and increase the serum levels of *anticonvulsants (phenobarbital, phenytoin, primidone),* coumarin *anticoagulants, phenylbutazone,* and *tricyclic antidepressants;* it also may decrease the hypotensive effects of *bretylium* and *guanethidine.* Use with *drugs with MAO-inhibiting activity* or *MAO inhibitors* or within 14 days of such therapy may cause severe hypertension.
Drug-lifestyle. Use with *caffeine* may enhance the CNS stimulant effects.

ADVERSE REACTIONS
CNS: *nervousness, insomnia, Tourette syndrome, dizziness, headache, akathisia, dyskinesia,* **seizures,** *drowsiness.*
CV: *palpitations, angina, tachycardia, changes in blood pressure and pulse rate,* **arrhythmias.**
GI: nausea, abdominal pain, anorexia, weight loss.
Hematologic: *thrombocytopenia,* ***thrombocytopenic purpura, leukopenia,*** anemia.
Skin: rash, urticaria, *exfoliative dermatitis, erythema multiforme.*

▣ KEY CONSIDERATIONS
• Monitor initiation of therapy closely; drug may precipitate Tourette syndrome.
• Reduce dosage or discontinue drug if paradoxical aggravation of symptoms occurs during therapy.
• Check vital signs regularly for increased blood pressure or other signs of excessive stimulation. To minimize insomnia, avoid late-day or evening dosing, especially of long-acting dosage forms.

---

*Canada only ◊ Unlabeled clinical use

• Drug may decrease seizure threshold in seizure disorders.

• Monitor CBC, differential, and platelet counts when patient is taking drug long term.

• Intermittent drug-free periods when stress is least evident (weekends) may help prevent development of tolerance and permit decreased dosage when drug is resumed. Sustained-release form allows convenience of single, at-home dosing.

• Drug has abuse potential; discourage use to combat fatigue. Some abusers dissolve tablets and inject drug.

• After high-dose and long-term use, abrupt withdrawal may unmask severe depression. Reduce dosage gradually to prevent acute rebound depression.

• Make sure patient obtains adequate rest; fatigue may result as drug wears off.

• Discourage drug use for analeptic effect; CNS stimulation superimposed on CNS depression may cause neuronal instability and seizures.

Patient education

• Explain rationale for therapy and the risks and benefits that may be anticipated.

• Tell patient to avoid drinks containing caffeine to prevent added CNS stimulation and not to alter dosage unless prescribed.

• Advise narcoleptic patient to take first dose on awakening.

• Tell patient not to chew or crush sustained-release dosage forms.

• Warn patient not to use drug to mask fatigue, to be sure to obtain adequate rest, and to call if excessive CNS stimulation occurs.

• Advise patient to avoid hazardous activities that require mental alertness until degree of sedative effect is determined.

Overdose & treatment

• Signs and symptoms of overdose may include euphoria, confusion, delirium, coma, toxic psychosis, agitation, headache, vomiting, dry mouth, mydriasis, self-injury, fever, diaphoresis, tremors, hyperreflexia, muscle twitching, seizures, flushing, hypertension, tachycardia hyperpyrexia, palpitations, and arrhythmias.

• Treat overdose symptomatically and supportively. Perform gastric lavage or induce vomiting in patients with intact gag reflex. Maintain airway and circulation. Closely monitor vital signs and fluid and electrolyte balance. Maintain in cool room, monitor temperature, minimize external stimulation, and protect patient against self-injury. External cooling blankets may be needed.

methylprednisolone (systemic)
Medrol

methylprednisolone acetate
depMedalone-40, depMedalone-80, Depoject-40, Depoject-80, Depo-Medrol, Depo-Predate-40, Depo-Predate-80, Duralone-40, Duralone-80, Medralone, Rep-Pred-40, Rep-Pred-80

methylprednisolone sodium succinate
A-methaPred, Solu-Medrol

Glucocorticoid, anti-inflammatory, immunosuppressant

Available by prescription only
methylprednisolone
Tablets: 2 mg, 4 mg, 8 mg, 16 mg, 24 mg, 32 mg
methylprednisolone acetate
Injection: 20-mg/ml, 40-mg/ml, and 80-mg/ml suspensions
methylprednisolone sodium succinate
Injection: 40-mg, 125-mg, 500-mg, 1,000-mg, and 2,000-mg vials

INDICATIONS & DOSAGE
Multiple sclerosis
methylprednisolone (systemic)
Adults: 200 mg P.O. daily for 1 week, followed by 80 mg every other day for 1 month.
Inflammation
methylprednisolone
Adults: 2 to 60 mg P.O. daily in four divided doses, depending on disease being treated.

methylprednisolone acetate

Adults: 10 to 80 mg I.M. daily; or 4 to 80 mg into joints and soft tissue, p.r.n., q 1 to 5 weeks; or 20 to 60 mg intralesionally.

methylprednisolone sodium succinate

Adults: 10 to 250 mg I.M. or I.V. q 4 hours.

Shock

methylprednisolone sodium succinate

Adults: 100 to 250 mg I.V. at 2- to 6-hour intervals.

◇ *Severe lupus nephritis*

Adults: 1 g I.V. over 1 hour for 3 days.

◇ *Treatment or minimization of motor and sensory defects caused by acute spinal cord injury*

Adults: Initially, 30 mg/kg I.V. over 15 minutes followed in 45 minutes by I.V. infusion of 5.4 mg/kg/hour for 23 hours.

PHARMACODYNAMICS

Anti-inflammatory action: Methylprednisolone stimulates the synthesis of enzymes needed to decrease the inflammatory response. It suppresses the immune system by reducing activity and volume of the lymphatic system, thus producing lymphocytopenia (primarily T lymphocytes), decreasing immunoglobulin and complement levels, decreasing passage of immune complexes through basement membranes, and possibly depressing reactivity of tissue to antigen-antibody interactions.

Drug is an intermediate-acting glucocorticoid. It has essentially no mineralocorticoid activity but is a potent glucocorticoid, with five times the potency of an equal weight of hydrocortisone. It's used primarily as an anti-inflammatory and immunosuppressant.

Methylprednisolone may be administered orally. Methylprednisolone sodium succinate may be administered by I.M. or I.V. injection or by I.V. infusion, usually at 4- to 6-hour intervals. Methylprednisolone acetate suspension may be administered by intra-articular, intrasynovial, intrabursal, intralesional, or soft-tissue injection. It has a slow onset but a long duration of action. Injectable forms are usually used only when the oral dosage forms can't be used.

PHARMACOKINETICS

Absorption: Methylprednisolone is absorbed readily after oral administration. After oral and I.V. administration, effects peak in about 1 to 2 hours. The acetate suspension for injection has a variable absorption over 24 to 48 hours, depending on whether it's injected into an intra-articular space or a muscle, and on the blood supply to that muscle.

Distribution: Drug is distributed rapidly to muscle, liver, skin, intestines, and kidneys.

Metabolism: Drug is metabolized in the liver to inactive glucuronide and sulfate metabolites.

Excretion: Inactive metabolites and small amounts of unmetabolized drug are excreted in urine. Insignificant quantities of drug are excreted in feces. Biological half-life of drug is 18 to 36 hours.

CONTRAINDICATIONS & PRECAUTIONS

Contraindicated in patients allergic to components of the formulation and in those with systemic fungal infections.

Use cautiously in patients with renal disease, GI ulceration, hypertension, osteoporosis, diabetes mellitus, hypothyroidism, cirrhosis, diverticulitis, nonspecific ulcerative colitis, recent intestinal anastomoses, thromboembolic disorders, seizures, myasthenia gravis, heart failure, tuberculosis, emotional instability, ocular herpes simplex, and psychotic tendencies.

INTERACTIONS

Drug-drug. *Antacids, cholestyramine,* and *colestipol* decrease the corticosteroid effect by adsorbing the corticosteroid, decreasing the amount absorbed. Methylprednisolone may interact with *anticholinesterase,* causing profound weakness. *Barbiturates, phenytoin,* and *rifampin* may cause decreased corticosteroid effects because of increased hepatic metabolism. Use with *cyclosporine* may increase cyclosporine levels. Use with *estrogens* may reduce the metabolism of corticosteroids by increasing transcortin levels; the half-life of the corticosteroid is then prolonged because of increased protein-binding. Use with *isoniazid* and *salicylates* increases metabolism of these drugs; causes hyperglycemia, requiring dosage adjustment of *oral antidiabetics* or *insulin* in diabetic patients; and may enhance hypokalemia caused by *amphotericin B* or *diuretic* therapy—and the hypokalemia may increase the risk of toxicity in patients concurrently receiving *cardiac glycosides.* Adrenocorticoids may decrease the effects of *oral anticoagulants* by unknown mechanisms. Administration of *ulcerogenic drugs* such as *NSAIDs* may increase the risk for GI ulceration. Drug may decrease effectiveness of *vaccines.*

ADVERSE REACTIONS
Most adverse reactions to corticosteroids are dose- or duration-dependent.
CNS: *euphoria, insomnia,* psychotic behavior, pseudotumor cerebri, vertigo, headache, paresthesia, **seizures.**
CV: *heart failure,* hypertension, edema, **arrhythmias,** thrombophlebitis, **thromboembolism, fatal arrest or circulatory collapse** (following rapid administration of large I.V. doses).
EENT: cataracts, glaucoma.
GI: *peptic ulceration,* GI irritation, increased appetite, pancreatitis, nausea, vomiting.
Metabolic: hypokalemia, hyperglycemia, carbohydrate intolerance.
Musculoskeletal: muscle weakness, osteoporosis.
Skin: delayed wound healing, acne, various skin eruptions.
Other: hirsutism, susceptibility to infections, cushingoid state (moonface, buffalo hump, central obesity), **acute adrenal insufficiency may occur with increased stress (infection, surgery, or trauma) or abrupt withdrawal after long-term therapy.**
After abrupt withdrawal: rebound inflammation, fatigue, weakness, arthralgia, fever, dizziness, lethargy, depression, fainting, orthostatic hypotension, dyspnea, anorexia, hypoglycemia. *After prolonged use, sudden withdrawal may be fatal.*

KEY CONSIDERATIONS
• Consider the risk-benefit of corticosteroid use. Consider lower doses because of body changes caused by aging—that is, diminution of muscle mass and plasma volume. Monitor blood pressure and blood glucose and electrolyte levels at least every 6 months.
• Methylprednisolone decreases ^{131}I uptake and protein-bound iodine levels in thyroid function tests.
• Recommendations for use of drug and for care and teaching of patients during therapy are the same as those for all systemic adrenocorticoids.
• Drug suppresses reactions to skin tests; causes false-negative results in the nitroblue tetrazolium test for systemic bacterial infections.

metipranolol hydrochloride
OptiPranolol

Beta blocker, antiglaucoma drug

Available by prescription only
Ophthalmic solution: 0.3% in 5-ml and 10-ml dropper bottles with 0.004% benzalkonium chloride and ethylenediaminetetraacetic acid

INDICATIONS & DOSAGE
Treatment of ocular conditions in which lowering of intraocular pressure (IOP) would be beneficial (ocular hypertension, chronic open-angle glaucoma)
Adults: Instill 1 gtt into affected eye b.i.d. Higher dosage or more frequent administration isn't known to be of benefit. If IOP isn't satisfactory, concomitant therapy to lower IOP may be instituted.

PHARMACODYNAMICS
Antiglaucoma action: Exact mechanism of action isn't known, but metipranolol appears to reduce aqueous humor production. Drug may also slightly increase outflow facility.

Like other noncardioselective beta blockers, drug doesn't have significant local anesthetic (membrane-stabilizing) actions or intrinsic sympathomimetic ac-

---

Reactions may be *common,* uncommon, *life-threatening,* or COMMON AND LIFE-THREATENING.

tivity. It reduces elevated and normal IOP with or without glaucoma with little or no effect on pupil size or accommodation. In patients with IOP more than 24 mm Hg, pressure is reduced an average of 20% to 26%.

PHARMACOKINETICS

Absorption: Metipranolol is intended to act locally, but some systemic absorption may occur. Onset of action in less than 30 minutes.
Distribution: Local.
Metabolism: Unknown.
Excretion: Unknown; maximum effect in about 2 hours; duration of effect is 12 to 24 hours.

CONTRAINDICATIONS & PRECAUTIONS

Contraindicated in patients hypersensitive to metipranolol or its components and in those with bronchial asthma, history of bronchial asthma or severe COPD, sinus bradycardia, second- or third-degree AV block, cardiac failure, and cardiogenic shock.

Use cautiously in patients with nonallergic bronchospasm, chronic bronchitis, emphysema, diabetes mellitus, hyperthyroidism, or cerebrovascular insufficiency.

INTERACTIONS

Drug-drug. Use with caution in patients taking *systemic beta blockers* because of potential for additive effects. The following agents may interact with systemic beta blockers, and thus may interact with ophthalmic beta blockers: *antithyroid agents, calcium channel blockers, catecholamine-depleting drugs, cimetidine, clonidine, digoxin, haloperidol, hydralazine, insulin, lidocaine, morphine, nondepolarizing neuromuscular blockers, NSAIDs, oral contraceptives, phenobarbital, phenothiazines, prazosin, rifampin, salicylates, sympathomimetics, theophylline,* and *thyroid hormones*.
Drug-lifestyle. *Smoking* may also interfere with drug effect.

ADVERSE REACTIONS

CNS: headache, anxiety, dizziness, depression, somnolence, nervousness, asthenia, brow ache.

CV: hypertension, *MI,* atrial fibrillation, angina, palpitations, bradycardia.
EENT: transient local eye discomfort, tearing, conjunctivitis, eyelid dermatitis, blurred vision, blepharitis, abnormal vision, photophobia, eye edema, rhinitis, epistaxis.
GI: nausea.
Musculoskeletal: myalgia.
Respiratory: dyspnea, bronchitis, cough.
Skin: rash.
Other: hypersensitivity reactions.

▣ KEY CONSIDERATIONS

• Pilocarpine and other miotics, dipivefrin, or systemic carbonic anhydrase inhibitors may be administered concomitantly if IOP isn't adequately controlled.
• Proper administration is essential for optimal therapeutic response; instruct patient in correct techniques.
• The normal eye can retain only about 10 µl of fluid; the average dropper delivers 25 to 50 µl/gtt. Thus, the value of more than 1 gtt is questionable. If multidrop therapy is indicated, the best interval between drops is 5 minutes.

Patient education

• Tell patient to wash hands thoroughly before administration and then to follow these directions:
– Tilt head back or lie down and gaze upward.
– Gently grasp lower eyelid below eyelashes and pull eyelid away from eye to form a pouch.
– Place dropper directly over eye, avoiding contact of dropper with eye or any surface.
– Look up just before applying drop; look down for several seconds after applying drop. Slowly release eyelid.
– Close eyes gently for 1 to 2 minutes. Closing eyes tightly after instillation may expel drug from pouch. Apply gentle pressure to inside corner of eye at bridge of nose to retard drainage of solution from intended area.
• Tell patient to avoid rubbing the eye and to minimize blinking.
• Tell patient not to rinse dropper after use.

• Advise patient to check expiration date on bottle before use and not to use eyedrops that have changed color.
• Tell patient who must instill more than one drug to wait at least 5 minutes between instillations.

Overdose & treatment
• Systemic overdose after accidental ingestion may cause bradycardia, hypotension, bronchospasm, or acute cardiac failure.
• For ocular overdose, flush eye with copious amounts of water or normal saline solution. For systemic overdose, discontinue therapy, institute supportive and symptomatic measures, and decrease further absorption, for example, by gastric lavage.

metoclopramide hydrochloride
Apo-Metoclop*, Clopra, Emex*, Maxeran*, Maxolon, Octamide PFS, Reclomide, Reglan

PABA derivative, antiemetic, GI stimulant

Available by prescription only
Tablets: 5 mg, 10 mg
Syrup: 5 mg/5 ml
Injection: 5 mg/ml
Solution: 10 mg/ml

INDICATIONS & DOSAGE
Prevention or reduction of nausea and vomiting induced by highly emetogenic chemotherapy
Adults: 1 to 2 mg/kg I.V. q 2 hours for 2 doses, beginning 30 minutes before emetogenic chemotherapy drug administration, then q 3 hours for 3 doses.
Facilitation of small-bowel intubation and to aid in radiologic examinations
Adults: 10 mg I.V. as a single dose over 1 to 2 minutes.
Delayed gastric emptying secondary to diabetic gastroparesis
Adults: 10 mg P.O. 30 minutes before meals and h.s. for 2 to 8 weeks, depending on response; or 10 mg I.V. over 2 minutes.

Gastroesophageal reflux
Adults: 10 to 15 mg P.O. q.i.d., p.r.n., taken 30 minutes before meals and h.s.
Postoperative nausea and vomiting
Adults: 10 to 20 mg I.M. near end of surgical procedure, repeated q 4 to 6 hours, p.r.n.
◊ **Vomiting**
Adults: 10 mg P.O. taken 30 minutes before meals.

PHARMACODYNAMICS
Antiemetic action: Metoclopramide inhibits dopamine receptors in the brain's chemoreceptor trigger zone to inhibit or reduce nausea and vomiting.
GI stimulant action: Drug relieves esophageal reflux by increasing lower esophageal sphincter tone and reduces gastric stasis by stimulating motility of the upper GI tract, thus reducing gastric emptying time.

PHARMACOKINETICS
Absorption: After oral administration, metoclopramide is absorbed rapidly and thoroughly from the GI tract; action begins in 30 to 60 minutes. After I.M. administration, 74% to 96% of drug is bioavailable; action begins in 10 to 15 minutes. After I.V. administration, onset of action in 1 to 3 minutes.
Distribution: Distributed to most body tissues and fluids, including the brain.
Metabolism: Drug isn't metabolized extensively; a small amount is metabolized in the liver.
Excretion: Drug is mostly excreted in urine and feces. Hemodialysis and renal dialysis remove minimal amounts. Duration of effect is 1 to 2 hours.

CONTRAINDICATIONS & PRECAUTIONS
Contraindicated in patients in whom stimulation of GI motility might be dangerous (for example, those with hemorrhage, obstruction, or perforation) and in those with hypersensitivity to metoclopramide, pheochromocytoma, or seizure disorders.
    Use cautiously in patients with history of depression, Parkinson's disease, and hypertension.

Reactions may be *common*, uncommon, *life-threatening*, or COMMON AND LIFE-THREATENING.

INTERACTIONS

Drug-drug. Metoclopramide may increase or decrease absorption of other drugs, depending on changes in transit time through the intestinal tract; it may increase absorption of *acetaminophen, aspirin, diazepam, levodopa, lithium,* and *tetracycline* and may decrease absorption of *digoxin. Anticholinergics* and *opiates* may antagonize drug effect on GI motility. Use with *antihypertensives* and *CNS depressants* (such as *sedatives* and *tricyclic antidepressants*) may lead to increased CNS depression. Use with *butyrophenone antipsychotics* and *phenothiazine* may potentiate extrapyramidal reactions. A faster gastric emptying time may allow for increased *cyclosporine* absorption, possibly increasing its immunosuppressive and toxic effects. Drug releases catecholamines in patients with essential hypertension; use with caution, if at all, in patients receiving *MAO inhibitors.*

Drug-lifestyle. Use with *alcohol* may increase CNS depression.

ADVERSE REACTIONS

CNS: *restlessness, anxiety, drowsiness, fatigue, lassitude, depression, akathisia, insomnia, confusion, **suicidal ideation, seizures,*** hallucinations, headache, dizziness, extrapyramidal symptoms, tardive dyskinesia, dystonic reactions.
CV: transient hypertension, hypotension, supraventricular tachycardia, bradycardia.
GI: nausea, bowel disturbances, diarrhea.
GU: urinary frequency, incontinence.
Hematologic: *neutropenia, agranulocytosis.*
Respiratory: *bronchospasm.*
Skin: rash, urticaria.
Other: fever, prolactin secretion, loss of libido, porphyria.

◉ KEY CONSIDERATIONS

• Use metoclopramide with caution, especially in patients with impaired renal function; dosage may need to be decreased. Geriatric patients are more likely to experience extrapyramidal symptoms and tardive dyskinesia.

• Don't use drug for more than 12 weeks.
• For I.V. push administration, use undiluted and inject over 1 to 2 minutes. For I.V. infusion, dilute with 50 ml D_5W, dextrose 5% in half-normal saline, normal saline injection, Ringer's injection, or lactated Ringer's injection, and infuse over at least 15 minutes.
• Administer by I.V. infusion 30 minutes before chemotherapy.
• Drug may be used to facilitate nasoduodenal tube placement.
• Diphenhydramine may be used to counteract extrapyramidal effects of high-dose metoclopramide.
• Drug isn't recommended for long-term use.
• Drug has been used investigationally to treat anorexia nervosa, dizziness, migraine, and intractable hiccups; oral dose form is being used investigationally to treat nausea and vomiting.

Patient education
• Warn patient to avoid driving for 2 hours after each dose because metoclopramide may cause drowsiness. Until extent of CNS effect is known, advise patient not to consume alcohol.
• Tell patient to report twitching or involuntary movement.
• Instruct patient to take drug 30 minutes before each meal.

Overdose & treatment
• Signs and symptoms of overdose include drowsiness, dystonia, seizures, and extrapyramidal effects.
• Treatment includes administration of antimuscarinics, antiparkinsonians, or antihistamines with antimuscarinic activity (for example, 50 mg diphenhydramine given I.M.).

---

metolazone
Mykrox, Zaroxolyn

Quinazoline derivative (thiazide-like) diuretic, antihypertensive

---

Available by prescription only
Tablets: 2.5 mg, 5 mg, 10 mg
Tablets (rapid-acting): 0.5 mg (Mykrox)

INDICATIONS & DOSAGE
Tablets
Edema (heart failure)
Adults: 5 to 10 mg P.O. daily.
Edema (renal disease)
Adults: 5 to 20 mg P.O. daily.
Hypertension
Adults: 2.5 to 5 mg P.O. daily; mainte-
nance dosage based on patient's blood
pressure.
Rapid-acting tablets
Hypertension
Adults: 0.5 mg once daily; may be in-
creased to maximum of 1 mg daily.

PHARMACODYNAMICS
Diuretic action: Metolazone increases
urine excretion of sodium and water by
inhibiting sodium reabsorption in the
cortical diluting tubule of the nephron,
thus relieving edema. Drug may be more
effective in edema associated with impaired renal function than thiazide or thiazide-like diuretics.
Antihypertensive action: Exact mechanism of action is unknown; it may result
from direct arteriolar vasodilatation.
Drug also reduces total body sodium
levels and total peripheral resistance.

PHARMACOKINETICS
Absorption: About 65% of a given dose
is absorbed after oral administration to
healthy subjects; in cardiac patients, absorption decreases to 40%. However,
rate and extent of absorption vary
among preparations. Blood levels peak
in 2 to 4 hours with rapid-acting oral
dose (Mykrox) and 8 hours with other
dosage forms.
Distribution: Metolazone is 50% to 70%
erythrocyte-bound and about 33% protein-bound.
Metabolism: Insignificant.
Excretion: Some 70% to 95% of drug is
excreted unchanged in urine. Half-life is
about 14 hours in healthy subjects; it
may be prolonged in patients with decreased creatinine clearance.

CONTRAINDICATIONS & PRECAUTIONS
Contraindicated in patients with anuria,
hepatic coma or precoma, or hypersensitivity to thiazides or other sulfonamide-
derived drugs. Use cautiously in patients
with impaired renal or hepatic function.

INTERACTIONS
Drug-drug. Metolazone turns urine
slightly more alkaline and may decrease
urine excretion of some *amines,* such as
amphetamine and *quinidine;* alkaline
urine may also decrease therapeutic efficacy of *methenamine compounds* such
as *methenamine mandelate.* Drug also
potentiates the hypotensive effects of
most other *antihypertensives;* this may
be used to therapeutic advantage.
Cholestyramine and *colestipol* may bind
drug, preventing its absorption; give
drugs 1 hour apart. Drug may potentiate
hyperglycemic, hypotensive, and hyperuricemic effects of *diazoxide,* and its hyperglycemic effect may increase *insulin*
or *sulfonylurea* requirements in patients
with diabetes. Administration with
furosemide may cause excessive volume
and electrolyte depletion. Drug may reduce renal clearance of *lithium,* elevate
serum lithium levels, and may necessitate a 50% reduction in lithium dosage.

ADVERSE REACTIONS
CNS: *dizziness, headache, fatigue, vertigo, paresthesia, weakness, restlessness,
drowsiness, anxiety, depression, nervousness, blurred vision.*
CV: volume depletion and dehydration,
orthostatic hypotension, palpitations,
vasculitis.
GI: anorexia, nausea, *pancreatitis,* epigastric distress, vomiting, abdominal
pain, diarrhea, constipation, dry mouth.
GU: nocturia, polyuria, frequent urination, impotence.
Hematologic: *aplastic anemia, agranulocytosis,* leukopenia.
Hepatic: jaundice, hepatitis.
Metabolic: hyperglycemia and glucose
tolerance impairment; fluid and electrolyte imbalances, including hypokalemia, dilutional hyponatremia and
hypochloremia, metabolic alkalosis, hypercalcemia.
Musculoskeletal: muscle cramps.
Skin: dermatitis, photosensitivity, rash,
purpura, pruritus, urticaria.

Reactions may be *common*, uncommon, *life-threatening*, or COMMON AND LIFE-THREATENING.

▣ KEY CONSIDERATIONS

Besides the recommendations relevant to all thiazide and thiazide-like diuretics, consider the following:

• Metolazone is effective in patients with decreased renal function.

• Drug is used as an adjunct in furosemide-resistant edema.

• Drug has been used with furosemide to induce diuresis in patients who didn't respond to either diuretic alone.

• Rapid-acting form (Mykrox) isn't interchangeable with other forms of metolazone. Dosage and uses vary. Drug may cause electrolyte disturbance and increase risk for digoxin toxicity. It also may interfere with tests for parathyroid function and should be discontinued before such tests.

Overdose & treatment

• Signs and symptoms of overdose include orthostatic hypotension, dizziness, electrolyte abnormalities, GI irritation and hypermotility, diuresis, and lethargy, which may progress to coma.

• Treatment is mainly supportive; monitor and assist respiratory, CV, and renal function as indicated. Monitor fluid and electrolyte balance. Induce vomiting with ipecac a patient who's conscious; otherwise, use gastric lavage to avoid aspiration. Don't give cathartics; these promote additional loss of fluids and electrolytes.

---

metoprolol tartrate
Lopressor, Toprol XL

Beta blocker, antihypertensive, adjunctive treatment of acute MI

Available by prescription only
Tablets: 50 mg, 100 mg
Tablets (extended-release): 50 mg, 100 mg, 200 mg
Injection: 1 mg/ml in 5-ml ampules or prefilled syringes

INDICATIONS & DOSAGE
Mild to severe hypertension
Adults: initially, 100 mg P.O. daily in single or divided doses; usual maintenance dosage is 100 to 450 mg daily. Alternatively, 50 to 100 mg P.O. extended-release tablets daily (maximum dose, 400 mg daily).
Early intervention in an acute MI
Adults: Three 5-mg I.V. boluses q 2 minutes. Then, beginning 15 minutes after last dose, 50 mg P.O. q 6 hours for 48 hours. Maintenance dose, 100 mg P.O. b.i.d. or 25 to 50 mg P.O. q 6 hours. (Late treatment, 100 mg P.O. b.i.d.)
Angina
Adults: 100 mg in two divided doses. Maintenance dose, 100 to 400 mg daily. Alternatively, 100 mg P.O. extended-release tablets daily (maximum dose, 400 mg daily).

PHARMACODYNAMICS
Antihypertensive action: Metoprolol is classified as a cardioselective beta$_1$ blocker; exact mechanism of effect is unknown. Drug may reduce blood pressure by blocking adrenergic receptors, thus decreasing cardiac output; by decreasing sympathetic outflow from the CNS; or by suppressing renin release.
Action after an acute MI: The exact mechanism by which drug decreases mortality after an MI is unknown. In patients with a MI, drug reduces heart rate, systolic blood pressure, and cardiac output. Drug also appears to decrease the occurrence of ventricular fibrillation in these patients.

PHARMACOKINETICS
Absorption: Orally administered metoprolol is absorbed rapidly and almost completely from the GI tract; food enhances absorption. Plasma levels peak in 90 minutes. After I.V. administration, maximum beta blockade occurs in 20 minutes. Maximum therapeutic effect after 1 week of treatment.
Distribution: Drug is distributed widely throughout the body; about 12% is protein-bound.
Metabolism: Drug is metabolized in the liver.
Excretion: About 95% of a given dose is excreted in urine within 72 hours, largely as metabolite.

CONTRAINDICATIONS & PRECAUTIONS

Contraindicated in patients with hypersensitivity to metoprolol or other beta blockers. Also contraindicated in patients with sinus bradycardia, heart block greater than first degree, cardiogenic shock, or overt cardiac failure when used to treat hypertension or angina. When used to treat an MI, drug also is contraindicated in patients with heart rate less than 45 beats/minute, second- or third-degree heart block, PR interval of 0.24 second or longer with first-degree heart block, systolic blood pressure less than 100 mm Hg, or moderate to severe cardiac failure.

Use cautiously in patients with impaired hepatic or respiratory function, diabetes, or heart failure.

INTERACTIONS

Drug-drug. Drug may enhance bradycardia of *cardiac glycosides*. Metoprolol may potentiate antihypertensive effects of *diuretics* and other *antihypertensives*. Drug may antagonize the beta effects of *sympathomimetics*. *Verapamil* may decrease the bioavailability of metoprolol when administered with antiarrhythmics.

ADVERSE REACTIONS

CNS: *fatigue, dizziness,* depression.
CV: **bradycardia,** *hypotension,* **heart failure.**
GI: nausea, diarrhea.
Hepatic: elevated serum transaminase, alkaline phosphatase, LD, and uric acid levels.
Respiratory: dyspnea, **bronchospasm.**
Skin: rash.

▣ KEY CONSIDERATIONS

Besides the recommendations relevant to all beta blockers, consider the following:
• Geriatric patients may require lower maintenance dosages of metoprolol because of delayed metabolism; they may also experience enhanced adverse effects. Use with caution.
• Drug may be administered daily as a single dose or in divided doses. If a dose is missed, patient should take only the next scheduled dose.
• Administer drug with meals to enhance absorption.

• Reduce dosage in patients with impaired hepatic function.
• Avoid late-evening doses to minimize insomnia.
• Observe patient for signs of mental depression.

Overdose & treatment

• Signs and symptoms of overdose include hypotension, bradycardia, heart failure, and bronchospasm.
• After acute ingestion, induce vomiting or perform gastric lavage, and give activated charcoal to reduce absorption. Subsequent treatment is usually asymptomatic and supportive.

---

metronidazole

Apo-Metronidazole*, Flagyl, Flagyl ER, Metric-21, Novonidazol*, Protostat

metronidazole hydrochloride

Flagyl I.V., Flagyl I.V. RTU, Metro I.V.

Nitroimidazole, antibacterial, antiprotozoal, amebicide

Available by prescription only
Tablets: 250 mg, 500 mg
Tablets (film-coated): 250 mg, 500 mg
Tablets (extended-release, film-coated): 750 mg
Capsules: 375 mg
Powder for injection: 500-mg single-dose vials
Injection (ready to use): 500 mg/dl

INDICATIONS & DOSAGE

Amebic hepatic abscess
Adults: 500 to 750 mg P.O. t.i.d. for 5 to 10 days.
Intestinal amebiasis
Adults: 750 mg P.O. t.i.d. for 5 to 10 days. Centers for Disease Control and Prevention recommends addition of iodoquinol, 650 mg P.O. t.i.d. for 20 days.
Trichomoniasis
Adults (men and women concurrently): 375-mg capsule P.O. b.i.d. for 7 days, or 500-mg tablet P.O. b.i.d. for 7 days, or a

---

single dose of 2 g P.O. or divided into two doses given on same day.

Refractory trichomoniasis

Adults (women): 500 mg P.O. b.i.d. for 7 days.

Bacterial infections caused by anaerobic microorganisms

Adults: Loading dose is 15 mg/kg I.V. infused over 1 hour (about 1 g for a 70-kg [154-lb] adult). Maintenance dosage is 7.5 mg/kg I.V. or P.O. q 6 hours (about 500 mg for a 70-kg adult). First maintenance dose should be administered 6 hours after the loading dose. Maximum dose shouldn't exceed 4 g daily.

◊ *Giardiasis*

Adults: 250 mg P.O. t.i.d. for 5 days, or 2 g once daily for 3 days.

Prevention of postoperative infection in contaminated or potentially contaminated colorectal surgery

Adults: 15 mg/kg infused over 30 to 60 minutes and completed about 1 hour before surgery, then 7.5 mg/kg infused over 30 to 60 minutes at 6 and 12 hours after initial dose.

◊ *Bacterial vaginosis*

Adults: 500 mg P.O. b.i.d. for 7 days; or 2 g P.O. as a single dose.

◊ *Pelvic inflammatory disease*

Adults: 500 mg P.O. b.i.d. for 14 days (given with 400 mg b.i.d. of ofloxacin).

◊ **Clostridium difficile**

Adults: 750 mg to 2 g P.O. daily, in 3 or 4 divided doses for 7 to 14 days.

◊ **Helicobacter pylori** *associated with peptic ulcer disease*

Adults: 250 to 500 mg P.O. t.i.d. (in combination with other drugs).

PHARMACODYNAMICS

Bactericidal, amebicidal, and trichomonacidal actions: The nitro group of metronidazole is reduced inside the infecting organism; this reduction product disrupts DNA and inhibits nucleic acid synthesis. Drug is active in intestinal and extraintestinal sites against most anaerobic bacteria and protozoa, including *Bacteroides fragilis, Bacteroides melaninogenicus, Fusobacterium, Veillonella, Clostridium, Peptococcus, Peptostreptococcus, Entamoeba histolytica, Trichomonas vaginalis, Giardia lamblia,* and *Balantidium coli.*

PHARMACOKINETICS

Absorption: About 80% of an oral dose is absorbed; serum levels peak at about 1 hour. Food delays the rate but not the extent of absorption.

Distribution: Metronidazole is distributed into most body tissues and fluids, including CSF, bone, bile, saliva, pleural and peritoneal fluids, vaginal secretions, seminal fluids, middle-ear fluid, and hepatic and cerebral abscesses. CSF levels approach serum levels in patients with inflamed meninges; they reach about 50% of serum levels in patients with noninflamed meninges. Less than 20% of drug binds to plasma proteins.

Metabolism: Drug is metabolized to an active 2-hydroxymethyl metabolite and also to other metabolites.

Excretion: About 60% to 80% of dose is excreted as parent compound or its metabolites. About 20% of dose is excreted unchanged in urine; 6% to 15% is excreted in feces. Half-life is 6 to 8 hours in adults with normal renal function; half-life may be prolonged in patients with impaired hepatic function.

CONTRAINDICATIONS & PRECAUTIONS

Contraindicated in patients with hypersensitivity to metronidazole or other nitroimidazole derivatives. Use cautiously in patients with history of blood dyscrasia or alcoholism, hepatic disease, retinal or visual field changes, or CNS disorders and in those receiving hepatotoxic drugs.

INTERACTIONS

Drug-drug. Use with *barbiturates* or *phenytoin* may diminish the antimicrobial effectiveness of metronidazole by increasing its metabolism and may require higher doses of metronidazole. Use with *cimetidine* may decrease the clearance of metronidazole, thereby increasing its potential for causing adverse effects. Use with *disulfiram* may precipitate psychosis and confusion and should be avoided. Use with *lithium* may increase lithium levels. Use of metronidazole with *oral anticoagulants* prolongs PT.

Drug-lifestyle. Use with *alcohol* inhibits alcohol dehydrogenase activity, causing a disulfiram-like reaction (nausea, vomiting, headache, abdominal cramps, and flushing) in some patients; it isn't recommended.

ADVERSE REACTIONS

CNS: vertigo, headache, ataxia, dizziness, syncope, incoordination, confusion, irritability, depression, weakness, insomnia, *seizures,* peripheral neuropathy.
CV: ECG change (flattened T wave), edema (with I.V. RTU preparation), flushing, thrombophlebitis (after I.V. infusion).
GI: abdominal cramping; stomatitis; epigastric distress; nausea; vomiting; anorexia; diarrhea; constipation; proctitis; dry mouth; overgrowth of nonsusceptible organisms, especially *Candida* species (glossitis, furry tongue); metallic taste.
GU: darkened urine, polyuria, dysuria, cystitis, decreased libido, dyspareunia, dryness of vagina and vulva, vaginal candidiasis.
Hematologic: *transient leukopenia, neutropenia.*
Musculoskeletal: fleeting joint pain, sometimes resembling serum sickness.
Skin: rash.
Other: fever.

◙ KEY CONSIDERATIONS

• Trichomoniasis should be confirmed by wet smear and amebiasis by culture before giving metronidazole.
• I.V. form should be administered by slow infusion only; if used with a primary I.V. fluid system, discontinue the primary fluid during the infusion; don't give by I.V. push.
• Monitor patient on I.V. drug for candidiasis.
• Drug may interfere with the chemical analyses of aminotransferase and triglyceride, leading to falsely decreased levels.
• When treating amebiasis, monitor number and character of stools. Send fecal specimens to laboratory promptly; infestation is detectable only in warm specimens. Repeat fecal studies at 3-month intervals to ensure elimination of amebae.

• When preparing powder for injection, follow manufacturer's instructions carefully; use solution prepared from powder within 24 hours. I.V. solutions must be prepared in three steps: reconstitution with 4.4 ml normal saline solution injection (with or without bacteriostatic water); dilution with lactated Ringer's injection, D_5W, or normal saline solution; and neutralization with sodium bicarbonate, 5 mEq/500 mg of drug.

Patient education
• Inform patient that metronidazole may cause metallic taste and red-brown urine.
• Tell patient to take tablets with meals to minimize GI distress and that tablets may be crushed to facilitate swallowing.
• Counsel patient on need for medical follow-up after discharge.
• Advise patient to report adverse effects.
• Tell patient to avoid alcohol and alcohol-containing drugs during therapy and for at least 48 hours after the last dose to prevent disulfiram-like reaction.
Amebiasis patients
• Explain that follow-up examinations of stool specimens are necessary for 3 months after treatment is discontinued to ensure elimination of amebae.
• To help prevent reinfection, instruct patient and family members about proper hygiene—including disposing of feces and washing hands after defecation and before handling, preparing, and eating food—and about the risks of eating raw food and the control of contamination by flies.
• Encourage other household members and suspected contacts to be tested and, if necessary, treated.
Trichomoniasis patients
• Teach correct personal hygiene, including perineal care.
• Explain that asymptomatic sexual partners of patients being treated for trichomoniasis should be treated simultaneously to prevent reinfection; patient should refrain from intercourse during therapy or have partner use condom.

Overdose & treatment
- Signs and symptoms of overdose include nausea, vomiting, ataxia, seizures, and peripheral neuropathy.
- No known antidote exists; treatment is supportive. If patient doesn't vomit spontaneously, induce vomiting or perform gastric lavage; activated charcoal and a cathartic may be used. Diazepam or phenytoin may be used to control seizures.

---

metronidazole (topical)
MetroGel, MetroGel-Vaginal, MetroCream, Noritate

Nitroimidazole, antiprotozoal, antibacterial

Available by prescription only
Topical gel: 0.75%
Topical cream: 0.75%, 1%
Vaginal gel: 0.75%

INDICATIONS & DOSAGE
***Topical treatment of acne rosacea,
◇pressure ulcer, inflammatory papules
or pustules***
Adults: Apply a thin film b.i.d. to affected area during the morning and evening (once daily for Noritate). Significant results should be seen within 3 weeks and continue for first 9 weeks of therapy.
Topical treatment of bacterial vaginosis
Adults: One applicator b.i.d. vaginally for 5 days.

PHARMACODYNAMICS
Anti-inflammatory action: Although exact mechanism of action is unknown, topical metronidazole probably exerts effect through its antibacterial and antiprotozoal actions.

PHARMACOKINETICS
Absorption: Under normal conditions, serum metronidazole levels after topical administration are negligible; 20% to 25% is absorbed vaginally, with serum levels peaking in 6 to 12 hours.
Distribution: Drug is less than 20% bound to plasma proteins.
Metabolism: Unknown.

Excretion: Unknown after topical or intravaginal application.

CONTRAINDICATIONS & PRECAUTIONS
Contraindicated in patients hypersensitive to metronidazole or its ingredients (such as parabens) and other nitroimidazole derivatives.

Use cautiously in patients with history of blood dyscrasia. Use vaginal form cautiously in patients with history of CNS disease because risk for seizures or peripheral neuropathy exists.

INTERACTIONS
Drug-drug. Use with *oral anticoagulants* may potentiate the anticoagulant effect. Monitor patient for potential adverse effects.

ADVERSE REACTIONS
CNS: dizziness, light-headedness, headache (with vaginal form).
EENT: lacrimation (if topical gel is applied around the eyes).
GI: cramps, pain, nausea, diarrhea, constipation, metallic or bad taste in mouth, decreased appetite (with vaginal form).
GU: *cervicitis, vaginitis,* urinary frequency (with vaginal form).
Skin: rash, *transient redness, dryness, mild burning, stinging* (with vaginal form).
Other: overgrowth of nonsusceptible organisms (with vaginal form).

▣ KEY CONSIDERATIONS
- Topical metronidazole therapy hasn't been associated with adverse reactions observed with parenteral or oral drug therapy (including disulfiram-like reaction following alcohol ingestion). However, some drug can be absorbed following topical use. Limited clinical experience hasn't shown these adverse effects.

Patient education
- Advise patient to clean area thoroughly before applying metronidazole. Patient may use cosmetics after applying the drug.
- Instruct patient to avoid use of drug on eyelids and to apply cautiously if drug must be used around the eyes.

● If local reactions occur, advise patient to apply drug less frequently or to discontinue use and call for specific instructions.

mexiletine hydrochloride
Mexitil

Lidocaine analogue, sodium channel antagonist, ventricular antiarrhythmic

Available by prescription only
Capsules: 150 mg, 200 mg, 250 mg

INDICATIONS & DOSAGE
Life-threatening documented ventricular arrhythmias, including ventricular tachycardia
Adults: 200 mg P.O. q 8 hours. May increase or decrease dose in increments of 50 to 100 mg q 8 hours if satisfactory control isn't obtained. Alternatively, give loading dose of 400 mg with maintenance dosage of 200 mg P.O. q 8 hours. Some patients may respond well to 450 mg q 12 hours. Maximum daily dose shouldn't exceed 1,200 mg.
◊ *Diabetic neuropathy*
Adults: 150 mg daily for 3 days; then 300 mg daily for 3 days, followed by 10 mg/kg daily.

PHARMACODYNAMICS
Antiarrhythmic action: Mexiletine is structurally similar to lidocaine and exerts similar electrophysiologic and hemodynamic effects. A class IB antiarrhythmic, it suppresses automaticity and shortens the effective refractory period and action potential duration of His-Purkinje fibers and suppresses spontaneous ventricular depolarization during diastole. At therapeutic serum levels, the drug doesn't affect conductive atrial tissue or AV conduction.

Unlike quinidine and procainamide, drug doesn't significantly alter hemodynamics when given in usual doses. Its effects on the conduction system inhibit reentry mechanisms and halt ventricular arrhythmias. Drug doesn't have a significant negative inotropic effect.

PHARMACOKINETICS
Absorption: About 90% of mexiletine is absorbed from the GI tract; serum levels peak in 2 to 3 hours. Absorption rate decreases with conditions that speed gastric emptying.
Distribution: Drug is widely distributed throughout the body. About 50% to 60% of circulating drug binds to plasma proteins. Usual therapeutic drug level is 0.5 to 2 µg/ml. Although toxicity may occur within this range, levels greater than 2 µg/ml are considered toxic and are associated with an increased frequency of adverse CNS effects, warranting dosage reduction.
Metabolism: Drug is metabolized in the liver to relatively inactive metabolites. Less than 10% of a parenteral dose escapes metabolism and reaches the kidneys unchanged. Metabolism is affected by hepatic blood flow, which may be reduced in patients recovering from MI and in those with heart failure. Liver disease also limits metabolism.
Excretion: In healthy patients, drug's half-life is 10 to 12 hours. Elimination half-life may be prolonged in patients with heart failure or liver disease. Urine excretion increases with urine acidification and slows with urine alkalinization.

CONTRAINDICATIONS & PRECAUTIONS
Contraindicated in patients with cardiogenic shock or preexisting second- or third-degree AV block in the absence of an artificial pacemaker.

Use cautiously in patients with hypotension, heart failure, first-degree heart block, ventricular pacemaker, preexisting sinus node dysfunction, or seizure disorders.

INTERACTIONS
Drug-drug. Use with *cimetidine* may decrease mexiletine metabolism, resulting in increased serum levels. Use with *drugs that acidify the urine* (such as *ammonium chloride*) enhances mexiletine excretion; use with *drugs that alkalinize urine* (such as *high-dose antacids, carbonic anhydrase inhibitors,* and *sodium bicarbonate*) decreases mexiletine excretion. Use of mexiletine with *drugs that alter gastric emptying time* (such as

---

Reactions may be *common*, uncommon, *life-threatening*, or COMMON AND LIFE-THREATENING.

antacids containing aluminum-magnesium hydroxide, atropine, and *narcotics*) may delay mexiletine absorption; use with *metoclopramide* may increase absorption. Use with *drugs that alter hepatic enzyme function* (such as *phenobarbital, phenytoin,* and *rifampin*) may induce hepatic metabolism of mexiletine and thus reduce serum drug levels. When used with *theophylline,* drug may increase serum theophylline levels.

ADVERSE REACTIONS

CNS: *tremor, dizziness, confusion,* lightheadedness, incoordination, changes in sleep habits, paresthesia, weakness, fatigue, speech difficulties, depression, *nervousness, headache.*
CV: *new or worsened arrhythmias,* palpitations, chest pain, nonspecific edema, angina.
EENT: *blurred vision, diplopia,* tinnitus.
GI: *nausea, vomiting, upper GI distress, heartburn, diarrhea, constipation, dry mouth, changes in appetite, abdominal pain.*
Skin: rash.

▣ KEY CONSIDERATIONS

• Most geriatric patients require reduced dosages because of reduced hepatic blood flow and decreased metabolism. Geriatric patients also may be more susceptible to CNS adverse effects.
• Mexiletine should be administered with meals, if possible.
• Because of proarrhythmic effects, drug generally isn't recommended for non–life-threatening arrhythmias.
• Avoid administering drug within 1 hour of antacids containing aluminum hydrozide or magnesium hydroxide.
• When changing from lidocaine to mexiletine, stop infusion when first mexiletine dose is given. Keep infusion line open, however, until arrhythmia appears to be satisfactorily controlled.
• Patients who aren't controlled by dosing q 8 hours may respond to dosing q 6 hours.
• Many patients who respond well to drug (300 mg or less q 8 hours) can be maintained on a q 12-hour schedule. The same total daily dose is divided into

twice-daily doses, which improves patient compliance.
• Monitor blood pressure and heart rate and rhythm for significant change.
• Tremor (usually a fine hand tremor) is common in patients taking higher doses of drug.
• Liver function test results may be transiently altered during drug therapy.

Patient education
• Tell patient to take mexiletine with food to reduce risk of nausea.
• Instruct patient to report unusual bleeding or bruising, signs or symptoms of infection (fever, sore throat, stomatitis, or chills), or fatigue.

Overdose & treatment
• Signs and symptoms of overdose are primarily extensions of adverse CNS effects. Seizures are the most serious effect.
• Treatment usually involves symptomatic and supportive measures. In acute overdose, induce emesis or perform gastric lavage. Urine acidification may accelerate drug elimination. If patient has bradycardia and hypotension, atropine may be given.

mezlocillin sodium
Mezlin

Extended-spectrum penicillin, acyclaminopenicillin, antibiotic

Available by prescription only
Injection: 1 g, 2 g, 3 g, 4 g
Infusion: 2 g, 3 g, 4 g

INDICATIONS & DOSAGE
Infections caused by susceptible organisms
Adults: 200 to 300 mg/kg I.V. or I.M. daily given in 4 to 6 divided doses. Usual dose is 3 g q 4 hours or 4 g q 6 hours. For serious infections, up to 24 g daily may be administered.
✦ *Dosage adjustment.* In adult patients with renal failure with creatinine clearance of 10 to 30 ml/minute, give 3 g q 6 to 8 hours for life-threatening or serious infection. For urinary tract infection (UTI), give 1.5 g q 6 to 8 hours. If crea-

tinine clearance is less than 10 ml/minute, give 2 g q 6 to 8 hours for life-threatening or serious infection. For UTI, give 1.5 g q 8 hours.

Patients on hemodialysis should be given 3 to 4 g after each dialysis session, then q 12 hours. Patients on peritoneal dialysis may receive 3 g q 12 hours.

PHARMACODYNAMICS
Antibiotic action: Mezlocillin is bactericidal; it adheres to bacterial penicillin-binding proteins, thereby inhibiting bacterial cell wall synthesis.

Extended-spectrum penicillins are more resistant to inactivation by certain beta-lactamases, especially those produced by gram-negative organisms, but may still be inactivated by certain others.

Drug spectrum of activity includes many gram-negative aerobic and anaerobic bacilli, many gram-positive and gram-negative aerobic cocci, and some gram-positive aerobic and anaerobic bacilli, but many of these organisms are resistant to the drug. It may be effective against some strains of carbenicillin- and ticarcillin-resistant gram-negative bacilli. Drug shouldn't be used as sole therapy because patient will rapidly develop resistance. Some health care providers see no advantage of the drug over ticarcillin or carbenicillin, at least with respect to cure rates. Drug is less active against *Pseudomonas aeruginosa* than other members of this class, such as piperacillin.

PHARMACOKINETICS
Absorption: After an I.M. dose, plasma levels peak at ¾ to 1½ hours.
Distribution: Mezlocillin is distributed widely. It penetrates minimally into CSF with noninflamed meninges and is 16% to 42% protein-bound.
Metabolism: Drug is partially metabolized; about 15% of a dose is metabolized to inactive metabolites.
Excretion: Drug is excreted primarily (39% to 72%) in urine through glomerular filtration and renal tubular secretion; up to 30% of dose is excreted in bile. Elimination half-life in adults is ¾ to 1½ hours; in extensive renal impairment, half-life is extended to 2 to 14 hours. Drug is removed through hemodialysis but not peritoneal dialysis.

CONTRAINDICATIONS & PRECAUTIONS
Contraindicated in patients with hypersensitivity to mezlocillin or other penicillins. Use cautiously in patients with bleeding tendencies, uremia, hypokalemia, or allergy to cephalosporins.

INTERACTIONS
Drug-drug. Use with *aminoglycoside antibiotics* results in a synergistic bactericidal effect against *Pseudomonas aeruginosa; Escherichia coli; Klebsiella, Citrobacter, Enterobacter,* and *Serratia* species; and *Proteus mirabilis.* However, the drugs are physically and chemically incompatible and are inactivated when mixed or given together. Use with *clavulanic acid* also produces a synergistic bactericidal effect against certain beta-lactamase–producing bacteria. Large doses of drug may interfere with renal tubular secretion of *methotrexate*, delaying elimination and elevating serum methotrexate levels. *Probenecid* blocks tubular secretion of penicillins, increasing their serum levels. Drug may prolong neuromuscular blockade in *vecuronium bromide.*

ADVERSE REACTIONS
CNS: neuromuscular irritability, *pain at injection site,* **seizures.**
CV: *phlebitis.*
GI: nausea, diarrhea, vomiting, abnormal taste sensation, pseudomembranous colitis.
GU: interstitial nephritis.
Hematologic: *bleeding* (with high doses), **neutropenia, thrombocytopenia,** eosinophilia, **leukopenia, hemolytic anemia.**
Metabolic: *hypokalemia.*
Other: *hypersensitivity reactions* (**anaphylaxis,** edema, fever, chills, rash, pruritus, urticaria), overgrowth of nonsusceptible organisms, *vein irritation.*

▣ KEY CONSIDERATIONS
Besides the recommendations relevant to all penicillins, consider the following:
• Half-life may be prolonged in geriatric patients because of impaired renal func-

---

tion; monitor for increased adverse effects.

• Mezlocillin may be more suitable than carbenicillin or ticarcillin for patients on salt-free diets; mezlocillin contains only 1.85 mEq/g of sodium.

• Drug alters test results for urine or serum proteins; it interferes with turbidimetric methods that use sulfosalicylic acid, trichloroacetic acid, acetic acid, or nitric acid. Drug doesn't interfere with tests using bromophenol blue (Albustix, Albutest, MultiStix). Positive Coombs' test results have been reported in patients taking carbenicillin disodium

• Monitor serum potassium level and liver function studies.

• Monitor patient with high serum levels for seizures.

• Drug is almost always used with another antibiotic, such as an aminoglycoside, in life-threatening infections.

• Inject I.M. dose slowly over 12 to 15 seconds to minimize pain. Don't exceed 2 g/site.

• If precipitate forms during refrigerated storage, warm to 98.6°F (37°C) in warm water bath and shake well. Solution should be clear.

• Because drug is partially dialyzable, dosage may need adjustment in patients on hemodialysis.

Overdose & treatment

• Signs and symptoms of overdose include neuromuscular sensitivity or seizures.

• A 4- to 6-hour hemodialysis session will remove 20% to 30% of drug.

miconazole nitrate
Femizol-M, Micatin, Monistat 3, Monistat 7, Monistat-Derm

Imidazole derivative, antifungal

Available by prescription only
Vaginal suppositories: 200 mg
Vaginal cream: 2%
Cream: 2%
Available without prescription
Cream: 2%
Powder: 2%
Spray: 2%
Vaginal cream: 2%
Vaginal suppositories: 100 mg, 200 mg

INDICATIONS & DOSAGE
Cutaneous or mucocutaneous fungal infections caused by susceptible organisms
Topical use
Adults: Cover affected area b.i.d. for 2 to 4 weeks.
Vaginal use
Adults: Insert 200-mg suppository h.s. for 3 days, or 100-mg suppository or 1 applicator of vaginal cream h.s. for 7 days.

PHARMACODYNAMICS
Antifungal action: Miconazole is both fungistatic and fungicidal, depending on drug concentration, in *Coccidioides immitis, Candida albicans, Cryptococcus neoformans, Histoplasma capsulatum, Candida tropicalis, Candida parapsilosis, Paracoccidioides brasiliensis, Sporothrix schenckii, Aspergillus flavus, A. ustus, Microsporum canis, Curvularia, Pseudallescheria boydii,* dermatophytes, and some gram-positive bacteria. Drug causes thickening of the fungal cell wall, altering membrane permeability; it also may kill the cell by interference with peroxisomal enzymes, causing accumulation of peroxide within the cell wall. It attacks virtually all pathogenic fungi.

PHARMACOKINETICS
Absorption: About 50% of oral miconazole dose is absorbed; however, no oral dosage form is currently available. A small amount of drug is systemically absorbed after vaginal administration.
Distribution: Drug penetrates well into inflamed joints, vitreous humor, and the peritoneal cavity. Distribution into sputum and saliva is poor, and CSF penetration is unpredictable. More than 90% binds to plasma proteins.
Metabolism: Drug is metabolized in the liver, predominantly to inactive metabolites.
Excretion: Drug elimination is triphasic; terminal half-life is about 24 hours. Between 10% and 14% of oral dose is ex-

creted in urine; 50%, in feces. Up to 1% of vaginal dose is excreted in urine; 14% to 22% of I.V. dose is excreted in urine.

CONTRAINDICATIONS & PRECAUTIONS

Topical form contraindicated in patients with hypersensitivity to miconazole. Use cautiously in patients with hepatic insufficiency.

INTERACTIONS

Drug-drug. Miconazole may antagonize the effects of *amphotericin B*. Drug may increase *phenytoin* levels. Drug enhances the anticoagulant effect of *warfarin*.

ADVERSE REACTIONS

CNS: headache.
GU: vulvovaginal burning, pruritus, or irritation with vaginal cream; pelvic cramps.
Skin: irritation, burning, maceration, allergic contact dermatitis.

▣ KEY CONSIDERATIONS

• Clean affected area before applying cream. After application, massage area gently until cream disappears.
• Continue topical therapy for at least 1 month; improvement should begin in 1 to 2 weeks. If no improvement occurs by 4 weeks, reevaluate diagnosis.
• Insert vaginal applicator high into vagina.

Patient education

• Teach patient the symptoms of fungal infection, and explain treatment rationale.
• Encourage patient to adhere to prescribed regimen and follow-up visits and to report adverse effects.
• Teach patient correct procedure for intravaginal or topical applications.
• To prevent vaginal reinfection, teach correct perineal hygiene and recommend that patient abstain from sexual intercourse during therapy.

midazolam hydrochloride
Versed

Benzodiazepine, preoperative sedative, agent for conscious sedation, adjunct for induction of general anesthesia, amnestic
Controlled substance schedule IV

Available by prescription only
Injection: 1 mg/ml in 2-ml, 5-ml, and 10-ml vials; 5 mg/ml in 1-ml, 2-ml, 5-ml, and 10-ml vials; 5 mg/ml in 2-ml disposable syringe

INDICATIONS & DOSAGE

Preoperative sedation (to induce sleepiness or drowsiness and relieve apprehension)
Adults younger than age 60: 0.07 to 0.08 mg/kg I.M. about 1 hour before surgery. May be administered with atropine or scopolamine and reduced doses of narcotics.
✦ *Dosage adjustment.* Reduce dosage in patients older than age 60, those with COPD, those considered to be high-risk surgical patients, and those who've received concomitant narcotics or other depressants.
Conscious sedation
Adults younger than age 60: initially, 1 to 2.5 mg I.V. administered over at least 2 minutes; repeat in 2 minutes, if needed, in small increments of initial dose over at least 2 minutes to achieve desired effect. Total dose up to 5 mg may be used. Additional doses to maintain desired level of sedation may be given by slow titration in increments of 25% of dose used to reach the sedation end point.
Adults age 60 and older: 1.5 mg or less over at least 2 minutes. If additional titration is needed, give at rate not exceeding 1 mg over 2 minutes. Total doses exceeding 3.5 mg usually aren't necessary.
Induction of general anesthesia
Adults younger than age 55 who haven't been premedicated: 0.3 to 0.35 mg/kg I.V. over 20 to 30 seconds if patient hasn't received preanesthesia drugs, or 0.2 to 0.25 mg/kg I.V. over 20 to 30 seconds

if patient has received preanesthesia drugs. Additional increments of 25% of the initial dose may be needed to complete induction.

Adults age 55 and older who haven't been premedicated: initially, 0.3 mg/kg. For debilitated patients, initial dose is 0.2 to 0.25 mg/kg. For premedicated patients, 0.15 mg/kg may be sufficient.

Continuous infusion for sedation of intubated and mechanically ventilated patients as a component of anesthesia or during treatment in the critical care setting

Adults: If a loading dose is necessary to rapidly initiate sedation, give 0.01 to 0.05 mg/kg slowly or infused over several minutes, with dose repeated at 10- to 15-minute intervals until adequate sedation is achieved. For maintenance of sedation, usual infusion rate is 0.02 to 0.10 mg/kg/hour (1 to 7 mg/hour). Infusion rate should be titrated to the desired amount of sedation. Drug can be titrated up or down by 25% to 50% of the initial infusion rate to achieve optimal sedation without oversedation.

PHARMACODYNAMICS

Sedative and anesthetic action: Although exact mechanism is unknown, midazolam, like other benzodiazepines, is thought to facilitate the action of gamma-aminobutyric acid to provide short-acting CNS depressant action.

Amnesic action: Mechanism of action isn't known.

PHARMACOKINETICS

Absorption: Absorption after I.M. administration appears to be 80% to 100%; serum levels peak in 45 minutes and are about one-half of those after I.V. administration. Sedation begins within 15 minutes after an I.M. dose and within 2 to 5 minutes after I.V. injection. After I.V. administration, anesthesia is induced in 1½ to 2½ minutes.

Distribution: Midazolam has a large volume of distribution and is about 97% protein-bound.

Metabolism: Drug is metabolized in the liver.

Excretion: Metabolites of drug are excreted in urine. Half-life of drug is 1.2 to

12.3 hours. Duration of sedation is usually 1 to 4 hours.

CONTRAINDICATIONS & PRECAUTIONS

Contraindicated in patients with hypersensitivity to midazolam or acute angle-closure glaucoma and in those experiencing shock, coma, or acute alcohol intoxication. Use cautiously in geriatric or debilitated patients and in those with uncompensated acute illnesses.

INTERACTIONS

Drug-drug. Midazolam may add to or potentiate the effects of *antidepressants, antihistamines, barbiturates, narcotics, other CNS and respiratory depressants,* and *tranquilizers. Droperidol, fentanyl,* and *narcotics* used as preoperative drugs potentiate the hypnotic effect of midazolam. *Erythromycin* may decrease plasma clearance of midazolam. Midazolam may decrease the needed dose of *inhaled anesthetics* by depressing respiratory drive. *Isoniazid* may decrease the metabolism of midazolam.

Drug-lifestyle. Drug may add to or potentiate the effects of *alcohol.*

ADVERSE REACTIONS

CNS: headache, oversedation, drowsiness, amnesia, *pain.*
CV: variations in blood pressure (hypotension) and pulse rate, ***cardiac arrest.***
GI: *nausea,* vomiting.
Respiratory: *decreased respiratory rate, hiccups,* ***apnea, respiratory arrest.***
Other: *tenderness (at injection site).*

▣ KEY CONSIDERATIONS

Besides the recommendations relevant to all benzodiazepines, consider the following:

• Midazolam syrup isn't recommended in geriatric patients. Hypoxemia was noted in one geriatric study in 60% of study patients.

• Geriatric or debilitated patients, especially those with COPD, are at significantly increased risk for respiratory depression and hypotension. Lower doses are indicated. Use with caution.

• Individualize dosage; use smallest effective dose possible. Use with extreme caution and reduce dosage in geriatric and debilitated patients.

• Medical personnel who administer midazolam should be familiar with airway management. Close monitoring of cardiopulmonary function is required. Continuously monitor patients who have received drug to detect potentially life-threatening respiratory depression.

• D_5W, normal saline solution, and lactated Ringer's solution are compatible with drug.

• Before I.V. administration, ensure the immediate availability of oxygen and resuscitative equipment. Apnea and death have been reported with rapid I.V. administration. Avoid intra-arterial injection because the hazards of this route are unknown. Avoid extravasation. Administer I.V. dose slowly to prevent respiratory depression.

• Administer I.M. dose deep into a large muscle mass to prevent tissue injury.

• Don't use solution that's discolored or contains a precipitate.

• Hypotension is more common in patients premedicated with narcotics. Monitor vital signs closely.

• Laryngospasm and bronchospasm may occur rarely; countermeasures should be available.

• Drug can be mixed in the same syringe with morphine, meperidine, atropine, and scopolamine.

Patient education

• Advise patient to postpone tasks requiring mental alertness or physical coordination until the effects of midazolam have worn off.

• As necessary, instruct patient in safety measures, such as supervised walking and gradual position changes, to prevent injury.

• Advise patient to call for instructions before taking OTC drugs.

Overdose & treatment

• Signs and symptoms of overdose include confusion, stupor, coma, respiratory depression, and hypotension.

• Treatment is supportive. Maintain patent airway, and ensure adequate ventilation with mechanical support if necessary. Monitor vital signs. Use I.V. flu-

ids or ephedrine to treat hypotension. Flumazenil, a specific benzodiazepine-receptor antagonist, is indicated for complete or partial reversal of the sedative effects.

milrinone lactate
Primacor

Bipyridine phosphodiesterase inhibitor, inotropic vasodilator

Available by prescription only
Solution: 1 mg/ml in 10-ml and 20-ml vials
Cartridge: 5 ml
Injection: premixed 200 mcg/ml in dextrose 5% injection

INDICATIONS & DOSAGE
Short-term I.V. therapy for heart failure
Adults: Initial loading dose of 50 mcg/kg I.V. over 10 minutes, followed by continuous infusion/maintenance dose of 0.375 to 0.75 mcg/kg/minute. Adjust infusion dose based on hemodynamic and clinical response.

✦ **Dosage adjustment.** For patients with renal impairment, refer to the following table.

Note: If hypotension occurs, administration of milrinone should be reduced or temporarily discontinued until patient's condition stabilizes.

Creatinine clearance (ml/min/1.73 m²)	Infusion rate (mcg/kg/min)
5	0.20
10	0.23
20	0.28
30	0.33
40	0.38
50	0.43

PHARMACODYNAMICS
Inotropic vasodilator action: Milrinone is a selective inhibitor of peak III cAMP phosphodiesterase isozyme in cardiac and vascular muscle. This inhibitory action is consistent with cAMP-mediated increases in intracellular ionized calcium and contractile force in cardiac muscle, as well as with cAMP-dependent con-

---

Reactions may be *common,* uncommon, *life-threatening,* or COMMON AND LIFE-THREATENING.

tractile protein phosphorylation and relaxation in vascular muscle. Besides increasing myocardial contractility, drug improves diastolic function, shown by improvements in left ventricular diastolic relaxation.

PHARMACOKINETICS
Absorption: Not applicable.
Distribution: Milrinone is about 70% bound to human plasma protein.
Metabolism: About 12% of dose is metabolized to a glucuronide metabolite.
Excretion: After I.V. administration, about 90% of drug is excreted unchanged in the urine within 8 hours.

CONTRAINDICATIONS & PRECAUTIONS
Contraindicated in patients with hypersensitivity to milrinone, severe aortic or pulmonic valvular disease in place of surgical correction, or during the acute phase of MI. Use cautiously in patients with atrial fibrillation or flutter.

INTERACTIONS
None reported.

ADVERSE REACTIONS
CNS: headache.
CV: *ventricular arrhythmias, ventricular ectopic activity, nonsustained ventricular tachycardia,* SUSTAINED VENTRICULAR TACHYCARDIA, VENTRICULAR FIBRILLATION, hypotension, angina.

▣ KEY CONSIDERATIONS
• Milrinone therapy isn't recommended for patients in acute post-MI phase; clinical studies in this population are lacking.
• Monitor renal function and fluid and electrolyte changes during drug therapy. Correct hypokalemia with potassium supplements before or during use of drug.
• Duration of therapy depends on patient responsiveness. Patients have been maintained on infusions of drug for up to 5 days.
• When furosemide is injected into an I.V. line containing milrinone, an immediate chemical interaction occurs, evidenced by formation of a precipitate.

Furosemide shouldn't be administered in an I.V. line that contains milrinone.

---

mineral oil
Fleet Enema Mineral Oil, Kondremul*, Kondremul Plain, Lansoÿl*, Milkinol, Neo-Cultol, Nujol*, Petrogalar Plain

Lubricant oil, laxative

Available without prescription
Jelly: 180 ml
Emulsion: 2.5 ml/5 ml, 1.4 g/5 ml
Suspension: 1.4 ml/5 ml, 2.75 ml/5 ml, 4.75 ml/5 ml
Rectal oil enema: 120 ml

INDICATIONS & DOSAGE
Constipation, preparation for bowel studies or surgery
Adults: 15 to 45 ml P.O. as single dose or in divided doses, or 120-ml enema.

PHARMACODYNAMICS
Laxative action: Mineral oil acts mainly in the colon, lubricating the intestine and retarding colonic fluid absorption.

PHARMACOKINETICS
Absorption: Mineral oil normally is absorbed minimally; with emulsified drug form, significant absorption occurs. Action begins in 6 to 8 hours.
Distribution: Drug is distributed locally, primarily in the colon.
Metabolism: None.
Excretion: Drug is excreted in feces.

CONTRAINDICATIONS & PRECAUTIONS
Contraindicated in patients with abdominal pain, nausea, vomiting, or other symptoms of appendicitis or acute surgical abdomen and in those with fecal impaction or intestinal obstruction or perforation.
  Contraindicated in patients with colostomy, ileostomy, ulcerative colitis, and diverticulitis. Use cautiously in geriatric or debilitated patients.

INTERACTIONS
Drug-drug. Mineral oil may impair absorption of *fat-soluble vitamins (A, D, E,*

and *K)*, *anticoagulants*, *cardiac glyco-sides*, *oral contraceptives*, and *sulfon-amides*, thus lessening their therapeutic effects. *Stool softeners* such as *docusate* increase mineral oil absorption to poten-tially toxic levels; avoid use, which may cause lipoid pneumonia.

ADVERSE REACTIONS

GI: *nausea; vomiting; diarrhea* (with excessive use); abdominal cramps, espe-cially in severe constipation; decreased absorption of nutrients and fat-soluble vitamins, resulting in deficiency; slowed healing after hemorrhoidectomy; anal pruritus; anal irritation; hemorrhoids; perianal discomfort.
Other: laxative dependence (with long-term or excessive use), **lipid pneumonia.**

▣ KEY CONSIDERATIONS

• Because of increased risk of aspiration, use caution when administering mineral oil to geriatric patients.
• Avoid administering drug to patients lying flat because if drug is aspirated into lungs, pneumonitis may result.
• Don't give drug with food because this may delay gastric emptying, resulting in delayed drug action and increased risk for aspiration. Separate by at least 2 hours.
• To improve taste, give emulsion and suspension with fruit juice or carbonated beverages.
• Prescribe cleansing enema 30 minutes to 1 hour after retention enema.
• Reduce or divide dose or use emulsi-fied drug form to avoid leakage through anal sphincter.
• Drug may impair absorption of fat-soluble vitamins (A, D, E, and K).

Patient education

• Instruct patient not to take mineral oil with stool softeners.
• Warn patient that drug may leak through anal sphincter, especially with repeated use or with enema form. Patient may want undergarment protection.

---

minocycline hydrochloride
Dynacin, Minocin

Tetracycline, antibiotic

Available by prescription only
Capsules: 50 mg, 100 mg
Tablets: 50 mg, 100 mg
Suspension: 50 mg/5 ml
Injection: 100 mg/vial

INDICATIONS & DOSAGE
Infections caused by sensitive organ-isms
Adults: initially, 200 mg P.O., I.V.; then 100 mg q 12 hours or 50 mg P.O. q 6 hours.
Gonorrhea in patients sensitive to peni-cillin
Adults: initially, 200 mg; then 100 mg q 12 hours for 4 days.
Syphilis in patients sensitive to peni-cillin
Adults: initially, 200 mg; then 100 mg q 12 hours for 10 to 15 days.
Meningococcal carrier state
Adults: 100 mg P.O. q 12 hours for 5 days.
Uncomplicated urethral, endocervical, or rectal infection caused by **Chlamy-dia trachomatis** *or* **Ureaplasma ure-alyticum**
Adults: 100 mg P.O. q 12 hours for at least 7 days.
Uncomplicated gonococcal urethritis in men
Adults: 100 mg P.O. q 12 hours for 5 days.
Mycobacterium marinum
Adults: 100 mg P.O. q 12 hours for 6 to 8 weeks.
Cholera
Adults: initially, 200 mg P.O., then 100 mg P.O. q 12 hours for 72 hours.
Acne
Adults: 50 mg P.O. daily, b.i.d. or t.i.d.
◊ *Nocardiosis*
Adults: Usual dose for 12 to 18 months.
◊ *Sclerosing agent for pleural effusions*
Adults: 300 mg mixed in 40 to 50 ml normal saline solution, instilled through a thoracostomy tube.

Reactions may be *common*, uncommon, *life-threatening*, or COMMON AND LIFE-THREATENING.

PHARMACODYNAMICS
Antibacterial action: Minocycline is bacteriostatic; it binds reversibly to ribosomal units, thus inhibiting bacterial protein synthesis.

Drug is active against many gram-negative and gram-positive organisms; *Mycoplasma, Rickettsia,* and *Chlamydia* species; and spirochetes; it may be more active against staphylococci than other tetracyclines.

The potential vestibular toxicity and cost of the drug limit its usefulness. It may be more active than other tetracyclines against *Nocardia asteroides;* it's also effective against *Mycobacterium marinum* infections. It's been used for meningococcal meningitis prophylaxis because of its activity against *Neisseria meningitidis.*

PHARMACOKINETICS
Absorption: About 90% to 100% of drug is absorbed after oral administration; serum levels peak at 2 to 3 hours.
Distribution: Minocycline is widely distributed into body tissues and fluids, including synovial, pleural, prostatic, and seminal fluids; bronchial secretions; saliva; and aqueous humor; CSF penetration is poor. Drug is 55% to 88% protein-bound.
Metabolism: Drug is partially metabolized.
Excretion: Drug is excreted primarily unchanged in urine through glomerular filtration. Plasma half-life is 11 to 22 hours in adults with normal renal function.

CONTRAINDICATIONS & PRECAUTIONS
Contraindicated in patients with hypersensitivity to minocycline or other tetracyclines. Use cautiously in patients with impaired renal or hepatic function.

INTERACTIONS
Drug-drug. Use of minocycline with *antacids containing aluminum, calcium,* or *magnesium* or with *laxatives containing magnesium* decreases oral absorption of minocycline (because of chelation); use with *oral iron products* or *sodium bicarbonate* also decreases absorption. Use of drug necessitates re-duced dosage of *digoxin* because of increased bioavailability and reduced dosage of *oral anticoagulants* because of enhanced effects. Tetracyclines may antagonize bactericidal effects of *penicillin,* inhibiting cell growth through bacteriostatic action; administer penicillin 2 to 3 hours before minocycline.
Drug-food. *Food* and *dairy products* may decrease absorption of drug, but less so than other tetracyclines.

ADVERSE REACTIONS
CNS: headache, *intracranial hypertension (pseudotumor cerebri),* light-headedness, dizziness, vertigo.
CV: pericarditis, *thrombophlebitis.*
EENT: dysphagia, glossitis.
GI: *anorexia, epigastric distress, oral candidiasis, nausea, vomiting, diarrhea,* enterocolitis, inflammatory lesions in anogenital region.
GU: increased BUN level.
Hematologic: *neutropenia,* eosinophilia, *thrombocytopenia,* hemolytic anemia.
Hepatic: elevated liver enzyme levels.
Skin: *maculopapular and erythematous rashes, photosensitivity, increased pigmentation, urticaria.*
Other: hypersensitivity reactions *(anaphylaxis),* superinfection.

▣ KEY CONSIDERATIONS
Besides the recommendations relevant to all tetracyclines, consider the following:
• Reconstitute 100 mg powder with 5 ml sterile water for injection, with further dilution to 500 to 1,000 ml for I.V. infusion.
• Reconstituted solution is stable for 24 hours at room temperature. However, final diluted solution should be used immediately.
• Minocycline causes false-negative results in urine glucose tests using glucose oxidase reagent (Clinistix or glucose enzymatic test strip) and falsely elevates fluorometric test results for urine catecholamines.

Overdose & treatment
• Signs and symptoms of overdose are usually limited to GI tract.

---

*Canada only

◇ Unlabeled clinical use

• If ingestion occurred within preceding 4 hours, perform gastric lavage and give antacids.

minoxidil (systemic)
Loniten

Peripheral vasodilator, antihypertensive

Available by prescription only
Tablets: 2.5 mg, 10 mg

INDICATIONS & DOSAGE
Severe hypertension
Adults: Initially, 5 mg P.O. as a single daily dose. Effective dosage range is usually 10 to 40 mg daily. Maximum dosage is 100 mg/day.

PHARMACODYNAMICS
Antihypertensive action: Minoxidil has a direct vasodilative effect on vascular smooth muscle; the effect on resistance vessels (arterioles and arteries) is greater than that on capacitance vessels (venules and veins).

PHARMACOKINETICS
Absorption: Minoxidil is absorbed rapidly from the GI tract; antihypertensive effects in 30 minutes, peaking at 2 to 3 hours.
Distribution: Drug is distributed widely into body tissues; it isn't bound to plasma proteins.
Metabolism: About 90% of a given dose is metabolized.
Excretion: Drug and metabolites are excreted primarily in urine. Antihypertensive action persists for about 3 days.

CONTRAINDICATIONS & PRECAUTIONS
Contraindicated in patients with pheochromocytoma or hypersensitivity to drug. Use cautiously in patients with impaired renal function or after acute MI.

INTERACTIONS
Drug-drug. Use with *diuretics* or *guanethidine* may cause profound orthostatic hypotension.

ADVERSE REACTIONS
CV: *edema, tachycardia, pericardial effusion and tamponade, **heart failure,*** ECG changes, rebound hypertension.
GI: nausea, vomiting.
Metabolic: *weight gain.*
Skin: rash, ***Stevens-Johnson syndrome.***
Other: *hypertrichosis (elongation, thickening, and enhanced pigmentation of fine body hair), breast tenderness.*

▣ KEY CONSIDERATIONS
• Geriatric patients may be sensitive to the antihypertensive effects of minoxidil. Dosage adjustment may be necessary because of altered drug clearance.
• Drug therapy is usually given concomitantly with other antihypertensives, such as diuretics, beta blockers, or sympathetic nervous system suppressants.
• Monitor blood pressure and pulse after administration, and report significant changes; assess intake, output, and body weight for sodium and water retention.
• Monitor for heart failure, pericardial effusion, and cardiac tamponade; have phenylephrine, dopamine, and vasopressin on hand to treat hypotension.
• Patients with renal failure or on dialysis may require smaller maintenance doses of drug. If dialysis is at 9 a.m., drug should be administered immediately after dialysis because dialysis will remove drug; if dialysis is after 3 p.m., the daily dose is given at 7 a.m. (8 hours before dialysis).
• Drug may alter direction and magnitude of T waves on ECG.

Patient education
• Explain that minoxidil is usually taken with other antihypertensives; emphasize importance of taking drug as prescribed.
• Caution patient to report the following cardiac signs and symptoms promptly: increased heart rate (more than 20 beats/minute over normal), rapid weight gain, shortness of breath, chest pain, severe indigestion, dizziness, light-headedness, or fainting.
• Tell patient to call for instructions before taking OTC cold preparations.
• Advise patient that hypertrichosis will disappear 1 to 6 months after stopping drug.

Reactions may be *common*, uncommon, *life-threatening*, or COMMON AND LIFE-THREATENING.

Overdose & treatment
• Signs and symptoms of overdose include hypotension, tachycardia, headache, and skin flushing.
• After acute ingestion, induce vomiting or perform gastric lavage, and give activated charcoal to reduce absorption. Further treatment is usually symptomatic and supportive. Administer normal saline solution I.V. to maintain blood pressure. Sympathomimetics, such as epinephrine and norepinephrine, should be avoided because of their excessive cardiac stimulating action.

minoxidil (topical)
Rogaine

Direct-acting vasodilator, hair-growth stimulant

Available without a prescription
Topical solution: 2% and 5% in 60-ml bottles

INDICATIONS & DOSAGE
Male pattern baldness (alopecia androgenetica), diffuse hair loss or thinning in women, ◊ ***adjunct to hair transplantation***
Adults: Apply 1 ml to affected area b.i.d. for 4 months or longer.

PHARMACODYNAMICS
Hair-growth stimulation: Exact mechanism is unknown. Minoxidil may alter androgen metabolism in the scalp or exert a local vasodilatation and enhance the microcirculation around the hair follicle. It may also directly stimulate the hair follicle.

PHARMACOKINETICS
Absorption: Minoxidil is poorly absorbed through intact skin. About 0.3% to 4.5% of topically applied dose reaches systemic circulation.
Distribution: Serum levels are generally negligible.
Metabolism: Not fully described.
Excretion: Drug is eliminated primarily from the kidneys. About 95% of topically applied dose is eliminated after 4 days.

CONTRAINDICATIONS & PRECAUTIONS
Contraindicated in patients hypersensitive to minoxidil or a component of the solution. Use cautiously in patients with renal, cardiac, or hepatic disease and in those older than age 50.

INTERACTIONS
Drug-drug. Theoretically, absorbed minoxidil may potentiate orthostatic hypotension in patients taking *diuretics* or *guanethidine*.

ADVERSE REACTIONS
CNS: headache, dizziness, faintness, light-headedness.
CV: edema, chest pain, hypertension, hypotension, palpitations, increased or decreased pulse rate, edema.
EENT: sinusitis.
GI: diarrhea, nausea, vomiting.
GU: urinary tract infection, renal calculi, urethritis.
Metabolic: weight gain.
Musculoskeletal: back pain, tendinitis.
Respiratory: bronchitis, upper respiratory tract infection.
Skin: irritant dermatitis, allergic contact dermatitis, eczema, hypertrichosis, local erythema, pruritus, dry skin or scalp, flaking, alopecia, exacerbation of hair loss.

▣ KEY CONSIDERATIONS
• Don't use with other topical drugs—such as corticosteroids, retinoids, and petroleum jelly—or drugs that enhance percutaneous absorption. Rogaine is for topical use only; each milliliter contains 20 mg or 50 mg minoxidil, and accidental ingestion could cause adverse systemic effects.
• Monitor patient 1 month after starting topical drug therapy and at least every 6 months afterward. Discontinue topical drug if systemic effects occur.
• Alcohol base will burn and irritate the eye and other sensitive surfaces (eye, abraded skin, and mucous membranes). If topical drug contacts sensitive areas, flush with copious amounts of cool water.
• Before starting treatment, check that patient has healthy scalp. Local abrasion

or dermatitis may increase absorption and the risk of adverse effects.

• Before treating a patient with a topical drug, obtain the patient's history, make sure he gets a physical, and advise him of the potential risks of the drug; a risk-benefit decision should be made. Patients with cardiac disease should realize that adverse effects may be especially serious. Alert patient to possibility of tachycardia and fluid retention, and monitor for increased heart rate, weight gain, or other systemic effects.

Patient education

• Tell patient to avoid inhaling the spray.
• Teach patient to apply topical minoxidil as follows: Hair and scalp should be dry before application. One milliliter should be applied to the total affected areas b.i.d. Total daily dose shouldn't exceed 2 ml. If fingertips are used to apply the drug, wash the hands afterward.
• Encourage patient to carefully review patient information leaflet, which is included with each package and in the full product information.
• Inform patient that 4 months of use may be required before results become apparent.

Overdose & treatment

• No overdoses have been reported. However, if topical use produces systemic adverse effects, wash application site thoroughly with soap and water and treat signs and symptoms, as appropriate.
• Signs and symptoms of oral overdose include hypotension, tachycardia, headache, and skin flushing.
• After acute ingestion, induce vomiting or perform gastric lavage, and give activated charcoal to reduce absorption. Further treatment is usually symptomatic and supportive.

mirtazapine
Remeron

Piperazinoazepine derivative, tetracyclic antidepressant

Available by prescription only
Tablets: 15 mg, 30 mg

INDICATIONS & DOSAGE
Depression
Adults: initially, 15 mg P.O. h.s. Maintenance dosage ranges from 15 to 45 mg daily. Dosage adjustments should be made at intervals no less than 1 to 2 weeks apart.

PHARMACODYNAMICS
Antidepressant action: Unknown.

PHARMACOKINETICS
Absorption: Mirtazapine is rapidly and completely absorbed from the GI tract. Absolute bioavailability of drug is about 50%.
Distribution: Drug is about 85% bound to plasma protein.
Metabolism: Drug is extensively metabolized in the liver.
Excretion: Drug is predominantly eliminated in urine (75%), with 15% excreted in feces. Half-life between 20 and 40 hours.

CONTRAINDICATIONS & PRECAUTIONS
Contraindicated in patients with hypersensitivity to mirtazapine. Coadministration with MAO inhibitors is contraindicated.

Use cautiously in patients with CV or cerebrovascular disease, seizure disorders, suicidal ideation, impaired hepatic and renal function, or history of mania or hypomania. Also, use cautiously in patients with conditions that predispose to hypotension, such as dehydration, hypovolemia, or treatment with antihypertensives.

Use cautiously in patients with increased intraocular pressure, history of urine retention, or angle-closure glaucoma because of anticholinergic properties.

INTERACTIONS
Drug-drug. *Diazepam* and other *CNS depressants* may cause additive CNS effects when administered with mirtazapine; avoid use. Drug shouldn't be used with *MAO inhibitors* or within 14 days of initiating or discontinuing therapy with MAO inhibitor because of potential serious and sometimes fatal reactions.

Reactions may be *common,* uncommon, *life-threatening,* or COMMON AND LIFE-THREATENING.

Drug-lifestyle. *Alcohol* may cause additive CNS effects.

ADVERSE REACTIONS
CNS: *somnolence,* dizziness, asthenia, abnormal dreams, abnormal thinking, tremor, confusion.
CV: edema.
GI: nausea, *increased appetite, dry mouth, constipation.*
GU: urinary frequency.
Hematologic: *agranulocytosis* (rare).
Metabolic: *weight gain.*
Musculoskeletal: back pain, myalgia.
Respiratory: dyspnea.
Other: flulike syndrome, peripheral edema.

▣ KEY CONSIDERATIONS
• Administer mirtazapine cautiously in geriatric patients because pharmacokinetic studies reveal a decreased clearance in these patients.
• Use with caution in geriatric patients with increased intraocular pressure, history of urine retention, or history of angle-closure glaucoma because of the anticholinergic properties of the drug.
• Although agranulocytosis is rare, discontinue drug and monitor patient closely if a sore throat, fever, stomatitis, or other signs or signs of infection together with a low WBC count develop.
• Monitor patient closely because it's unknown if drug causes physical or psychological dependence.

Patient education
• Caution patient not to perform hazardous activities if somnolence occurs with mirtazapine use.
• Instruct patient not to use alcohol or other CNS depressants while taking drug because of additive effect.
• Tell patient to report signs and symptoms of infection—such as fever, chills, sore throat, mucous membrane ulceration, or other possible signs or symptoms of infection, including flulike signs and symptoms.
• Stress importance complying with drug therapy.
• Instruct patient not to take other drugs concomitantly without medical approval.

Overdose & treatment
• Overdosage may result in disorientation, drowsiness, impaired memory, and tachycardia.
• Treatment is that for any antidepressant overdosage. If patient is unconscious, establish an airway and provide adequate oxygenation. Gastric lavage, induced vomiting, or both and activated charcoal should be considered. Monitor cardiac and vital signs and provide general symptomatic and supportive measures.

misoprostol
Cytotec

Prostaglandin E¹ analogue, antiulcerative, gastric mucosal protectant

Available by prescription only
Tablets: 100 mcg, 200 mcg

INDICATIONS & DOSAGE
Prevention of gastric ulcer induced by NSAIDs
Adults: 200 mcg P.O. q.i.d with meals and h.s. Reduce dosage to 100 mcg P.O. q.i.d. in patients who can't tolerate this dosage.
◊ **Duodenal or gastric ulcer**
Adults: 100 to 200 mcg P.O. q.i.d. with meals and h.s.
◊ **Prevention of acute graft rejection in renal transplantation**
Adults: 200 mcg P.O. q.i.d. for 12 weeks.

PHARMACODYNAMICS
Antiulcerative action: Misoprostol enhances the production of gastric mucus and bicarbonate and decreases basal, nocturnal, and stimulated gastric acid secretion.

PHARMACOKINETICS
Absorption: Misoprostol is rapidly absorbed after oral administration.
Distribution: Drug is less than 90% bound to plasma proteins. Levels peak in about 12 minutes.
Metabolism: Drug is rapidly de-esterified to misoprostol acid, the biologically active metabolite. The de-ester-

ified metabolite undergoes further oxidation in several body tissues.
Excretion: About 15% of oral dose appears in the feces; the balance is excreted in the urine. Terminal half-life is 20 to 40 minutes.

CONTRAINDICATIONS & PRECAUTIONS
Contraindicated in patients with a known allergy to prostaglandins.

INTERACTIONS
Drug-drug. Misoprostol levels are diminished by administration with *antacids,* and misoprostol diminishes the availability of *aspirin;* however, neither of these effects is significant.

ADVERSE REACTIONS
CNS: headache.
GI: *diarrhea, abdominal pain, nausea, flatulence, dyspepsia, vomiting, constipation.*
GU: cramps.

▣ KEY CONSIDERATIONS
• Diarrhea is usually dose related and develops within the first 2 weeks of therapy. It can be minimized by administering misoprostol after meals and at bedtime and by avoiding magnesium-containing antacids.
• Drug has been used for treatment and prophylaxis of reflux esophagitis, alcohol-induced gastritis, hemorrhagic gastritis, and fat malabsorption in cystic fibrosis.

Patient education
• Instruct patient not to share misoprostol.
• Advise patient to take as prescribed for duration of NSAID therapy.
• Tell patient to take the drug with meals and the last dose at bedtime.

---

moexipril hydrochloride
Univasc

ACE inhibitor, antihypertensive

Available by prescription only
Tablets: 7.5 mg, 15 mg

INDICATIONS & DOSAGE
Hypertension
Adults: initially, 7.5 mg P.O. once daily before meals for patients not receiving diuretics. If control is inadequate, dose can be increased or divided dosing may be attempted. Recommended dosage range is 7.5 to 30 mg daily, administered in one or two divided doses 1 hour before meals. For patients receiving diuretics, give 3.75 mg P.O. once daily before meals. Make subsequent dosage adjustments according to blood pressure response.

PHARMACODYNAMICS
Antihypertensive action: Exact mechanism of action is unknown, but it's thought to result primarily from suppression of the renin-angiotensin-aldosterone system. The active metabolite, moexiprilat, inhibits ACE and thereby inhibits the production of angiotensin II (a potent vasoconstrictor and stimulator of aldosterone secretion). Other mechanisms may also be involved.

PHARMACOKINETICS
Absorption: Moexipril is incompletely absorbed from the GI tract with a bioavailability of about 13%. Food significantly decreases bioavailability of drug.
Distribution: Metabolite is about 50% protein-bound.
Metabolism: Drug is metabolized extensively to the active metabolite, moexiprilat.
Excretion: Drug is excreted primarily in feces, with a small amount excreted in urine. Half-life of drug is 2 to 9 hours.

CONTRAINDICATIONS & PRECAUTIONS
Contraindicated in patients with hypersensitivity to moexipril or history of angioedema related to previous treatment with an ACE inhibitor.
Use cautiously in patients with impaired renal function, heart failure, or renal artery stenosis.

INTERACTIONS
Drug-drug. Because *diuretics* increase the risk of excessive hypotension, they should be discontinued or dose of moex-

---

ipril reduced. Drug increases serum *lithium* levels and lithium toxicity; avoid use. *Potassium sparing diuretics, potassium supplements*, and *sodium substitutes containing potassium* increase the risk of hyperkalemia; monitor serum potassium levels closely.

Drug-food. *Food,* particularly *high-fat foods,* can impair absorption.

ADVERSE REACTIONS
CNS: *dizziness,* headache, fatigue, pain.
CV: peripheral edema, hypotension, orthostatic hypotension, chest pain, flushing.
EENT: *angioedema,* pharyngitis, rhinitis, sinusitis.
GI: diarrhea, dyspepsia, nausea.
GU: urinary frequency.
Hematologic: *neutropenia.*
Metabolic: hyperkalemia.
Musculoskeletal: myalgia.
Respiratory: *dry, persistent, tickling, nonproductive cough;* upper respiratory tract infection.
Skin: rash.
Other: *anaphylactoid reactions, angioedema,* flulike syndrome.

▣ KEY CONSIDERATIONS
• Monitor patient for hypotension. Excessive hypotension can occur when moexipril is given with diuretics. If possible, discontinue diuretic therapy 2 to 3 days before starting moexipril to decrease potential for excessive hypotensive response. If drug doesn't adequately control blood pressure, reinstitute diuretic therapy with care.
• Measure blood pressure at trough (just before a dose) to verify adequate blood pressure control. Be aware that drug is less effective in reducing trough blood pressures in blacks than in nonblacks.
• Assess renal function before treatment and periodically throughout therapy. Monitor serum potassium levels.
• Other ACE inhibitors may cause agranulocytosis and neutropenia. Monitor CBC with differential counts before therapy, especially in patients who have collagen vascular disease with impaired renal function.
• Because angioedema that involves the tongue, glottis, or larynx may cause fatal airway obstruction, have available the appropriate therapy to ensure a patent airway, such as S.C. epinephrine 1:1,000 (0.3 to 0.5 ml) and equipment.
• In patients undergoing major surgery or anesthesia with drugs that produce hypotension, moexipril may block the compensatory renin release. Hypotension can be treated with volume expansion.

Patient education
• Instruct patient to take moexipril on an empty stomach; meals, particularly those high in fat, can impair absorption.
• Tell patient to avoid sodium substitutes; these products may contain potassium, which can cause hyperkalemia in patients taking this drug.
• Inform patient that light-headedness can occur, especially during the first few days of therapy. Tell him to rise slowly to minimize this effect and to report symptoms. If fainting occurs, tell patient to stop drug and call immediately.
• Instruct patient to use caution in hot weather and during exercise. Inadequate fluid intake, vomiting, diarrhea, and excessive perspiration can lead to light-headedness and syncope.
• Advise patient to report signs and symptoms of infection, such as fever and sore throat.
• Tell patient to report easy bruising or bleeding; swelling of tongue, lips, face, eyes, mucous membranes, or extremities; difficulty swallowing or breathing; and hoarseness.

Overdose & treatment
• Although no information is available on overdose of moexipril, it's probably similar to overdose of other ACE inhibitors, with hypotension as the principal adverse reaction.
• Because the hypotensive effect of the drug is achieved through vasodilation and effective hypovolemia, it's reasonable to treat overdose by infusing normal saline solution. In addition, renal function and serum potassium levels should be monitored.

molindone hydrochloride
Moban

Dihydroindolone, antipsychotic

Available by prescription only
Tablets: 5 mg, 10 mg, 25 mg, 50 mg,
100 mg
Oral concentrate: 20 mg/ml

INDICATIONS & DOSAGE
Psychotic disorders
Adults: 50 to 75 mg P.O. daily, increased
100 mg daily in 3 to 4 days to a maximum of 225 mg daily. Maintenance dose
for mild disease is 5 to 15 mg t.i.d. or
q.i.d.; moderate disease, 10 to 25 mg
t.i.d. or q.i.d.; and severe disease,
225 mg daily.

PHARMACODYNAMICS
Antipsychotic action: Molindone is unrelated to other antipsychotics; it's thought
to exert effects by postsynaptic blockade
of CNS dopamine receptors, thereby inhibiting dopamine-mediated effects.

Drug has many other central and peripheral effects; it also produces alpha
and ganglionic blockade. Its most prominent adverse reactions are extrapyramidal.

PHARMACOKINETICS
Absorption: Data are limited, but absorption appears rapid; effects peak
within 1¼ hours.
Distribution: Molindone is distributed
widely into the body.
Metabolism: Drug is metabolized extensively; drug effects persist for 24 to 36
hours.
Excretion: Most of drug is excreted as
metabolites in urine; some is excreted in
feces via the biliary tract. About 90% of
a given dose is excreted within 24 hours.

CONTRAINDICATIONS & PRECAUTIONS
Contraindicated in patients with hypersensitivity to molindone and in those experiencing coma or severe CNS depression. Use cautiously in patients at risk
for seizures or when high physical activity is harmful to patient.

INTERACTIONS
Drug-drug. Use with *appetite suppressants* or *sympathomimetics*—including
ephedrine (found in many nasal sprays),
epinephrine, phenylephrine, and *phenylpropanolamine*—may decrease their
stimulatory and pressor effects; because
of its alpha-blocking potential, molindone may cause *epinephrine* reversal, a
hypotensive response to epinephrine.
Beta blockers may inhibit molindone
metabolism, increasing plasma levels
and toxicity. Drug may antagonize therapeutic effect of *bromocriptine* on prolactin secretion; it may also decrease the
vasoconstrictive effects of *high-dose
dopamine* and may decrease effectiveness and increase toxicity of *levodopa*
via dopamine blockade. Molindone may
inhibit blood pressure response to *centrally acting antihypertensives,* such as
*clonidine, guanabenz, guanadrel,
guanethidine, methyldopa,* and
reserpine. Calcium sulfate in molindone
tablets may inhibit the absorption of
phenytoin. Use with *propylthiouracil* increases risk for agranulocytosis and decreases therapeutic response to molindone.

Additive effects are likely after use
with the following drugs: *antiarrhythmics, disopyramide, quinidine,* or *procainamide* (increased incidence of arrhythmias and conduction defects); atropine or other *anticholinergics,*
including *antidepressants, antihistamines, MAO inhibitors, meperidine, phenothiazines,* and *antiparkinsonians*
(oversedation, paralytic ileus, visual
changes, and severe constipation); *CNS
depressants*—including *analgesics,
anesthetics (epidural, general, or
spinal), barbiturates, narcotics,* and
tranquilizers—or *parenteral magnesium
sulfate* (oversedation, respiratory depression, and hypotension); *metrizamide* (increased risk of seizures); and *nitrates*
(hypotension).
Drug-lifestyle. Additive effects are likely after use with *alcohol.* Caution patient
against *sun exposure* to avoid photosensitivity reaction.

ADVERSE REACTIONS

CNS: *extrapyramidal reactions, tardive dyskinesia, sedation, drowsiness, depression, euphoria, pseudoparkinsonism, EEG changes, dizziness.*
CV: *orthostatic hypotension, tachycardia, ECG changes.*
EENT: *blurred vision.*
GI: *dry mouth, constipation, nausea.*
GU: *urine retention, gynecomastia, inhibited ejaculation.*
Hematologic: *leukopenia,* leukocytosis.
Hepatic: jaundice, abnormal liver function test results.
Skin: *mild photosensitivity, allergic reactions.*
Other: *neuroleptic malignant syndrome* (rare).

▣ KEY CONSIDERATIONS

• Lower doses are recommended for geriatric patients; 30% to 50% of usual dose may be effective. They're at greater risk for tardive dyskinesia and other extrapyramidal effects.
• Molindone may cause GI distress and should be administered with food or fluids.
• Dilute concentrate in 2 to 4 oz of liquid, preferably soup, water, juice, carbonated drinks, milk, or pudding.
• Drug may cause pink to brown discoloration of urine.
• Protect liquid form from light.
• Drug causes additive potential for causing seizures with metrizamide myelography.

Patient education

• Explain risks of dystonic reaction and tardive dyskinesia, and advise patient to report abnormal body movements.
• Warn patient to avoid spilling liquid preparation on the skin; rash and irritation may result.
• Advise patient to avoid temperature extremes (hot or cold baths, sunlamps, or tanning beds) because drug may cause thermoregulatory changes.
• Suggest sugarless gum or candy, ice chips, or artificial saliva to relieve dry mouth.
• Warn patient not to take molindone with antacids or antidiarrheals; not to drink alcoholic beverages or take other

drugs that cause sedation; not to stop taking drug or take other drugs except as instructed; and to take drug exactly as prescribed, without double-dosing after missing a dose.
• Warn patient about sedative effect. Tell patient to report difficult urination, sore throat, dizziness, or fainting.
• Advise patient to get up slowly from a recumbent or seated position to minimize effects of light-headedness.
• Tell patient that drug may contain sodium metabisulfite, which can cause an allergic reaction to those with a sulfite allergy.

Overdose & treatment

• CNS depression is characterized by deep sleep (in which the patient can't be aroused) and possible coma, hypotension or hypertension, extrapyramidal symptoms, abnormal involuntary muscle movements, agitation, seizure, arrhythmia, ECG changes, hypothermia or hyperthermia, and autonomic nervous system dysfunction.
• Treatment is symptomatic and supportive, including maintaining vital signs, airway, stable body temperature, and fluid and electrolyte balance.
• Don't induce vomiting: Drug inhibits cough reflex, and aspiration may occur. Perform gastric lavage, then administer activated charcoal and saline cathartics; dialysis doesn't help. Regulate body temperature as needed. Treat hypotension with I.V. fluids: don't give epinephrine.
• Treat seizures with parenteral diazepam or barbiturates, arrhythmias with 15 to 18 mg/kg of parenteral phenytoin (given at a rate not to exceed 50 mg/minute), and extrapyramidal reactions with 1 to 2 mg of benztropine or 10 to 50 mg of parenteral diphenhydramine.

---

montelukast sodium
Singulair

Leukotriene receptor antagonist, antiasthmatic

Available by prescription only
Tablets: 10 mg
Tablets (chewable): 5 mg

INDICATIONS & DOSAGE
For prophylaxis and long-term treatment of asthma
Adults: 10 mg P.O. once daily in evening.

PHARMACODYNAMICS
Antiasthmatic action: Montelukast causes inhibition of airway cysteinyl leukotriene receptors. Drug binds with high affinity and selectivity to the $CysLT_1$ receptor and inhibits the physiological action of the cysteinyl leukotriene, LTD_4. This receptor inhibition reduces early- and late-phase bronchoconstriction due to antigen challenge.

PHARMACOKINETICS
Absorption: Montelukast is rapidly absorbed after oral administration; mean plasma levels peak in 3 to 4 hours, and mean oral bioavailability is 64%. Food doesn't affect drug absorption. For chewable tablet, levels peak in 2 to 2.5 hours and mean oral bioavailability is 73%.
Distribution: Drug is minimally distributed to the tissues with a steady-state volume of distribution of 8 to 11 L. More than 99% of drug binds to plasma proteins.
Metabolism: Drug is extensively metabolized, but plasma levels of metabolites at therapeutic doses are undetectable. In vitro studies with human liver microsomes demonstrate metabolism involvement by cytochromes P-450 3A4 and 2C9.
Excretion: About 86% of oral dose is metabolized and excreted in the feces, indicating drug and its metabolites are excreted almost exclusively in the bile. Half-life is 2.7 to 5.5 hours.

CONTRAINDICATIONS & PRECAUTIONS
Contraindicated in patients with hypersensitivity to montelukast or its components. Also contraindicated in patients with acute asthma attacks or status asthmaticus. Although airway function is improved in patients with known aspirin hypersensitivity, these patients should avoid aspirin and NSAIDs.

INTERACTIONS
Drug-drug. Use caution when montelukast is used with *drugs known to inhibit 3A4 and 2C9 enzymes*. Patient may need to be monitored if drug is given with *phenobarbital* or *rifampin,* which induce hepatic metabolism.

ADVERSE REACTIONS
CNS: *headache,* dizziness, fatigue, asthenia.
EENT: nasal congestion, dental pain.
GI: dyspepsia, infectious gastroenteritis, abdominal pain.
Respiratory: cough, influenza.
Skin: rash.
Other: fever, trauma.

▣ KEY CONSIDERATIONS
• Montelukast therapy may increase ALT and AST levels.
• Although dose of inhaled corticosteroids may be reduced gradually, montelukast shouldn't be abruptly substituted for inhaled or oral corticosteroids.
• Drug shouldn't be used as monotherapy for management of exercise-induced bronchospasm.
• No added benefit is achieved with doses greater than 10 mg daily.

Patient education
• Advise patient to take montelukast daily, even if asymptomatic, and to contact his health care provider if asthma isn't well controlled.
• Warn patient that drug isn't beneficial in acute asthma attacks or in exercise-induced bronchospasm, and advise him to keep appropriate rescue drugs available.
• Advise patient with known aspirin sensitivity not to take aspirin and NSAIDs.
• Warn patient with phenylketonuria that chewable tablet contains phenylalanine, a component of aspartame.
• Advise patient to seek medical attention if short-acting bronchodilators are needed more often than usual or prescribed.

Reactions may be *common,* uncommon, *life-threatening,* or COMMON AND LIFE-THREATENING.

moricizine hydrochloride
Ethmozine

Sodium channel blocker, anti-arrhythmic

Available by prescription only
Tablets: 200 mg, 250 mg, 300 mg

INDICATIONS & DOSAGE
Treatment of documented, life-threatening ventricular arrhythmias when benefit of treatment outweighs risks
Adults: Dosage must be individualized. Usual range is 600 to 900 mg daily, given q 8 hours in equally divided doses. Dosage may be adjusted within this range in increments of 150 mg daily at 3-day intervals until desired effect is obtained. Hospitalization is recommended for initiation of therapy because patient will be at high risk.
♦ **Dosage adjustment.** For patients with renal or hepatic impairment, initial daily dose is 600 mg or less.

PHARMACODYNAMICS
Antiarrhythmic action: Although moricizine is chemically related to the neuroleptic phenothiazines, it has no demonstrated dopaminergic activities. It has potent local anesthetic activity and myocardial membrane stabilizing effects. A class I antiarrhythmic, it reduces the fast inward current carried by sodium ions. In patients with ventricular tachycardia, drug prolongs AV conduction but has no significant effect on ventricular repolarization. Intra-atrial conduction or atrial effective refractory periods aren't consistently affected, and drug has minimal effect on sinus cycle length and sinus node recovery time. This may be significant in patients with sinus node dysfunction.

In patients with impaired left ventricular function, drug has minimal effects on measurements of cardiac performance: cardiac index, stroke volume, pulmonary capillary wedge pressure, systemic or pulmonary vascular resistance, and ejection fraction either at rest or during exercise. A small but consistent increase in resting blood pressure and heart rate are seen. Drug has no effect on exercise tolerance in patients with ventricular arrhythmias, heart failure, or angina pectoris.

Drug has antiarrhythmic activity similar to that of disopyramide, propranolol, and quinidine. Arrhythmia rebound isn't noted after discontinuation of therapy.

PHARMACOKINETICS
Absorption: Plasma levels usually peak within ½ to 2 hours. Administration within 30 minutes of mealtime delays absorption and lowers peak plasma levels but has no effect on extent of absorption.
Distribution: Moricizine is 95% plasma protein-bound.
Metabolism: Drug undergoes significant first-pass metabolism, resulting in an absolute bioavailability of about 38%. At least 26 metabolites have been identified, with no single one representing at least 1% of the administered dose. It has been shown to induce its own metabolism.
Excretion: About 56% is excreted in feces; 39%, in urine; some is also recycled through enterohepatic circulation.

CONTRAINDICATIONS & PRECAUTIONS
Contraindicated in patients with cardiogenic shock and in those with hypersensitivity to moricizine, preexisting second- or third-degree AV block, or right bundle-branch block when associated with left hemiblock (bifascicular block) unless an artificial pacemaker is present.

Use cautiously in patients with impaired renal, hepatic, or left ventricular function; sick sinus syndrome; or coronary artery disease.

INTERACTIONS
Drug-drug. Use with *cimetidine* decreases moricizine clearance by 49%; no significant changes in efficacy or tolerance were observed, but patients should receive decreased doses of cimetidine (that is, not more than 600 mg/day). Concomitant *digoxin* therapy prolongs the PR interval. Use with *propranolol* may produce a small additive increase in the PR interval. *Theophylline* clearance increases and plasma half-life decreases

with concomitant therapy; monitor when moricizine is added or discontinued.

ADVERSE REACTIONS
CNS: *dizziness, headache, fatigue,* hyperesthesia, anxiety, asthenia, nervousness, paresthesia, sleep disorders.
CV: *proarrhythmic events (ventricular tachycardia, PVCs, supraventricular arrhythmias),* ECG abnormalities (including *conduction defects, sinus pause, junctional rhythm,* or *AV block*), *heart failure,* palpitations, thrombophlebitis, chest pain, *cardiac death,* hypotension, hypertension, vasodilation, cerebrovascular events.
EENT: blurred vision.
GI: *nausea, vomiting, abdominal pain, dyspepsia, diarrhea, dry mouth.*
GU: urine retention, urinary frequency, dysuria.
Musculoskeletal: pain.
Respiratory: dyspnea.
Skin: rash.
Other: drug-induced fever, diaphoresis.

▣ KEY CONSIDERATIONS
• Moricizine may elevate liver function test results.
• When changing from another antiarrhythmic to moricizine, previous therapy should be withdrawn one to two half-lives before initiating moricizine.
• Correct electrolyte imbalances before starting therapy; hypokalemia, hyperkalemia, or hypomagnesemia may alter the effects of the drug.

Overdose & treatment
• Signs and symptoms of overdose include vomiting, lethargy, coma, syncope, hypotension, conduction disturbances, exacerbation of heart failure, MI, sinus arrest, arrhythmias, and respiratory failure. No specific antidote has been identified.
• Treatment should be supportive and include careful monitoring of cardiac, respiratory, and CNS changes. Gastric evacuation, with care to avoid aspiration, may be used as well.

morphine hydrochloride*
Morphitec*, M.O.S.*

morphine sulfate
Astramorph PF, Duramorph, Epimorph*, Infumorph, MS Contin, MSIR, MS/L, MS/S, OMS Concentrate, Oramorph SR, RMS Uniserts, Roxanol, Statex*

Opioid, narcotic analgesic
Controlled substance schedule II

Available by prescription only
morphine hydrochloride*
Tablets: 10 mg, 20 mg, 40 mg, 60 mg
Syrup: 1 mg/ml, 5 mg/ml, 10 mg/ml, 20 mg/ml, 50 mg/ml
Suppositories: 20 mg, 30 mg
morphine sulfate
Tablets: 15 mg, 30 mg
Tablets (extended-release): 15 mg, 30 mg, 60 mg, 100 mg, 200 mg
Tablets (soluble): 10 mg, 15 mg, 30 mg
Oral solution: 4 mg/ml, 10 mg/5 ml, 20 mg/5 ml, 20 mg/ml, 100 mg/5 ml
Injection (with preservative): 1 mg/ml, 2 mg/ml, 3 mg/ml, 4 mg/ml, 5 mg/ml, 8 mg/ml, 10 mg/ml, 15 mg/ml, 25 mg/ml, 50 mg/ml
Injection (without preservative): 500 mcg/ml, 1 mg/ml, 10 mg/ml, 25 mg/ml
Suppositories: 5 mg, 10 mg, 20 mg, 30 mg

INDICATIONS & DOSAGE
Severe pain
Adults: 10 mg q 4 hours S.C. or I.M., or 10 to 30 mg P.O., or 10 to 20 mg P.R. q 4 hours, p.r.n., or around the clock. May be injected by slow I.V. (over 4 to 5 minutes), 2.5 to 15 mg diluted in 4 to 5 ml water for injection. May also administer controlled-release tablets, 30 mg q 8 to 12 hours. As an epidural injection, 5 mg via epidural catheter q 24 hours.
Preoperative sedation and adjunct to anesthesia
Adults: 8 to 10 mg I.M., S.C., or I.V.
Control of pain from an acute MI
Adults: 8 to 15 mg I.M., S.C., or I.V. Additional, smaller doses may be given in 3- to 4-hour intervals, p.r.n.

Reactions may be *common,* uncommon, *life-threatening,* or COMMON AND LIFE-THREATENING.

Adjunctive treatment of acute pulmonary edema
Adults: 10 to 15 mg I.V. at a rate not exceeding 2 mg/minute.

PHARMACODYNAMICS
Analgesic action: Morphine is the principal opium alkaloid, the standard for opiate agonist analgesic activity. Drug is thought to alter the patient's pain perception via the opiate receptors. Morphine is particularly useful in severe, acute pain or severe, chronic pain. Morphine also has a central depressant effect on respiration and on the cough reflex center.

PHARMACOKINETICS
Absorption: Absorption from the GI tract varies. Onset of analgesia is within 15 to 60 minutes. Analgesia peaks ½ to 1 hour after dosing. Morphine 6-glucuronide may accumulate after continuous dosing in patients with renal failure, which may result in enhanced and prolonged opiate activity.
Distribution: Drug is distributed widely through the body.
Metabolism: Drug is metabolized primarily in the liver.
Excretion: Duration of action is 3 to 7 hours. Drug is excreted in urine and bile.

CONTRAINDICATIONS & PRECAUTIONS
Contraindicated in patients with hypersensitivity to morphine or conditions that would preclude administration of opioids by I.V. route (acute bronchial asthma or upper airway obstruction).

Use cautiously in geriatric or debilitated patients and in those with head injury, increased intracranial pressure, seizures, pulmonary disease, prostatic hyperplasia, hepatic or renal disease, acute abdominal conditions, hypothyroidism, Addison's disease, or urethral strictures.

INTERACTIONS
Drug-drug. Use with *anticholinergics* may cause paralytic ileus. Use with *cimetidine* also may increase respiratory and CNS depression, causing confusion, disorientation, apnea, or seizures; dosage of morphine usually needs to be reduced. Use with other *CNS depres-* sants—including *antihistamines, barbiturates, benzodiazepines, general anesthetics, MAO inhibitors, muscle relaxants, narcotic analgesics, phenothiazines, sedative-hypnotics,* and *tricyclic antidepressants*—potentiates the respiratory and CNS depressant, sedative, and hypotensive effects of morphine. Drug accumulation and enhanced effects may result from use with *digitoxin.* Severe CV depression may result from use with *general anesthetics.* Patients who become physically dependent on this drug may experience acute withdrawal syndrome if given a *narcotic antagonist. Phenytoin* and *rifampin* decrease serum morphine levels.
Drug-lifestyle. *Alcohol* potentiates the respiratory and CNS depressant effects of drug.

ADVERSE REACTIONS
CNS: sedation, somnolence, *clouded sensorium, euphoria,* **seizures** (with large doses), *dizziness, nightmares,* light-headedness, hallucinations, nervousness, depression, syncope.
CV: *hypotension, bradycardia,* **shock, cardiac arrest,** tachycardia, hypertension.
GI: *nausea, vomiting, constipation, ileus, dry mouth, biliary tract spasms, anorexia.*
GU: *urine retention, decreased libido.*
Hematologic: **thrombocytopenia.**
Respiratory: **respiratory depression, apnea, respiratory arrest.**
Skin: pruritus, skin flushing; *diaphoresis; edema.*
Other: *physical dependence,* allergic reaction.

▣ KEY CONSIDERATIONS
Besides the recommendations relevant to all opioids, consider the following:
• Morphine increases plasma amylase levels.
• Lower doses are usually indicated for geriatric patients, who may be more sensitive to the therapeutic and adverse effects of drug.
• Morphine is drug of choice in relieving pain from a MI; may cause transient decrease in blood pressure.

• Around-the-clock scheduling is beneficial for severe, chronic pain.

• Oral solutions of various concentrations and a new intensified oral solution are available.

• Note the disparity between oral and parenteral doses.

• Long-term treatment in patients with advanced renal disease may lead to toxicity because of accumulation of the active metabolite morphine 6-glucoronide.

• For S.L. administration, measure oral solution with tuberculin syringe, and administer dose a few drops at a time to allow maximal S.L. absorption and to minimize swallowing.

• Refrigeration of rectal suppositories is unnecessary. Note that in some patients, rectal and oral absorption may not be equivalent.

• Preservative-free preparations are now available for epidural and intrathecal administration. The epidural route is being used more frequently.

• Epidural morphine has proven to be an excellent analgesic for patients with postoperative pain. After epidural administration, monitor closely for respiratory depression up to 24 hours after the injection. Check respiratory rate and depth according to protocol (for example, every 15 minutes for 2 hours, then hourly for 18 hours). Some health care providers advocate a dilute naloxone infusion (5 to 10 mcg/kg/hour) during the first 12 hours to minimize respiratory depression without altering pain relief.

• Drug may worsen or mask gallbladder pain.

• Some commercially available forms of morphine injection contain sulfites, which may cause allergic-type reactions.

Patient education

• Tell patient that oral liquid form of morphine may be mixed with a glass of fruit juice immediately before it's taken, if desired, to improve the taste.

• Tell patient taking long-acting morphine tablets to swallow them whole. Tablets shouldn't be broken, crushed, or chewed before swallowing.

Overdose & treatment

• Rapid I.V. administration may result in overdose because of the delay in maximum CNS effect (30 minutes).

• The most common signs and symptoms of morphine overdose are respiratory depression, with or without CNS depression, and miosis. Other acute toxic effects include hypotension, bradycardia, hypothermia, shock, apnea, cardiopulmonary arrest, circulatory collapse, pulmonary edema, and seizures.

• To treat acute overdose, first establish adequate respiratory exchange via a patent airway and ventilation as needed; administer a narcotic antagonist (naloxone) to reverse respiratory depression. (Because duration of action of morphine is longer than that of naloxone, repeated naloxone dosing is necessary.) Naloxone shouldn't be given if the patient doesn't have significant respiratory or CV depression. Monitor vital signs closely.

• If patient presents within 2 hours of ingestion of an oral overdose, immediately induce vomiting with ipecac syrup or perform gastric lavage, using caution to avoid aspiration. Administer activated charcoal via NG tube to further remove drug.

• Provide symptomatic and supportive treatment (continued respiratory support, correction of fluid or electrolyte imbalance). Monitor laboratory values, vital signs, and neurologic status closely.

Reactions may be *common*, uncommon, *life-threatening*, or COMMON AND LIFE-THREATENING.

nabumetone
Relafen

NSAID, antiarthritic

Available by prescription only
Tablets: 500 mg, 750 mg

INDICATIONS & DOSAGE
***Short- and long-term treatment of
rheumatoid arthritis or osteoarthritis***
Adults: initially, 1,000 mg P.O. daily as a
single dose or in divided doses b.i.d. Adjust dosage based on patient response.
Maximum recommended daily dose is
2,000 mg.

PHARMACODYNAMICS
Anti-inflammatory action: Nabumetone
probably acts by inhibiting the synthesis
of prostaglandins. Drug also has analgesic and antipyretic action.

PHARMACOKINETICS
Absorption: Nabumetone is well absorbed from the GI tract. After absorption, about 35% is rapidly transformed
to 6-methoxy-2-naphthylacetic acid
(6MNA), the principal active metabolite;
the balance is transformed to unidentified metabolites. Administration with
food increases the absorption rate and
peak levels of 6MNA but doesn't change
total drug absorbed. Levels peak in 2½
to 4 hours.
Distribution: 6MNA is more than 99%
bound to plasma proteins.
Metabolism: 6MNA is metabolized to
inactive metabolites in the liver.
Excretion: Metabolites are excreted primarily in urine; about 9% are excreted in
feces. Elimination half-life is about 24
hours; half-life is increased in patients
with renal failure.

CONTRAINDICATIONS & PRECAUTIONS
Contraindicated in patients with hypersensitivity reactions, history of aspirin-
or NSAID-induced asthma, urticaria, or
other allergic-type reactions.

Use cautiously in patients with impaired
renal or hepatic function, heart failure,
hypertension, conditions that predispose
the patient to fluid retention, and history
of peptic ulcer disease.

INTERACTIONS
Drug-drug. Use with *drugs that are
highly bound to plasma proteins* (such as
warfarin) increases the risk of adverse
reactions because nabumetone may displace drug; use together with caution.

ADVERSE REACTIONS
CNS: *dizziness, headache,* fatigue, insomnia, nervousness, somnolence.
CV: vasculitis, edema.
EENT: *tinnitus.*
GI: *diarrhea, dyspepsia, abdominal
pain, constipation, flatulence, nausea,*
dry mouth, gastritis, stomatitis, anorexia,
vomiting, ***bleeding,*** ulceration.
Respiratory: dyspnea, pneumonitis.
Skin: *pruritus, rash,* increased diaphoresis.

▣ KEY CONSIDERATIONS
Besides the recommendations relevant to
all NSAIDs, consider the following:
● Because NSAIDs impair the synthesis
of renal prostaglandins, they can decrease renal blood flow and lead to reversible renal function impairment, especially in geriatric patients; in patients
with preexisting renal failure, liver dysfunction, and heart failure; and in those
taking diuretics. Monitor these patients
closely during therapy.
● During long-term therapy, periodically
monitor renal and liver function, CBC,
and hematocrit.
● Monitor carefully for signs and symptoms of GI bleeding.

Patient education
● Tell patient to take nabumetone with
food, milk, or antacids to enhance drug
absorption.
● Stress importance of follow-up examinations to detect adverse GI effects.

• Teach patient signs and symptoms of GI bleeding, and tell him to report them immediately.
• Advise patient to limit alcohol intake because of risk for additive GI toxicity.

nadolol
Corgard

Beta blocker, antihypertensive, antianginal

Available by prescription only
Tablets: 20 mg, 40 mg, 80 mg, 120 mg, 160 mg

INDICATIONS & DOSAGE
Hypertension
Adults: initially, 20 to 40 mg P.O. once daily. Dosage may be increased in 40- to 80-mg increments daily at 2- to 14-day intervals until optimum response occurs. Usual maintenance dosage is 40 or 80 mg once daily. Dosages up to 240 or 320 mg daily may be necessary.
Long-term prophylaxis for chronic stable angina pectoris
Adults: initially, 40 mg P.O. once daily. Dosage may be increased in 40- to 80-mg increments daily at 3- to 7-day intervals until optimum response occurs. Usual maintenance dosage is 40 or 80 mg once daily. Dosages up to 160 or 240 mg daily may be needed.
◇*Arrhythmias*
Adults: 60 to 160 mg daily.
◇*Prophylaxis of vascular headache*
Adults: 20 to 40 mg once daily; may gradually increase to 120 mg daily if necessary.
✦*Dosage adjustment.* For patients with renal impairment, refer to the following table.

Creatinine clearance (ml/min/1.73m²)	Dosing interval
> 50	q 24 hr
31 to 50	q 24 to 36 hr
10 to 30	q 24 to 48 hr
< 10	q 40 to 60 hr

PHARMACODYNAMICS
Antihypertensive action: Mechanism of action is unknown. Nadolol may reduce blood pressure by blocking adrenergic receptors, thus decreasing cardiac output; by decreasing sympathetic outflow from the CNS; or by suppressing renin release.
Antianginal action: Drug decreases myocardial oxygen consumption, thus relieving angina, by blocking catecholamine-induced increases in heart rate, myocardial contraction, and blood pressure.

PHARMACOKINETICS
Absorption: From 30% to 40% of dose is absorbed from the GI tract; plasma levels peak in 2 to 4 hours. Food doesn't affect absorption.
Distribution: Nadolol is distributed throughout the body; drug is about 30% protein-bound.
Metabolism: None.
Excretion: Most of a given dose is excreted unchanged in urine; the remainder is excreted in feces. Plasma half-life is about 20 hours. Antihypertensive and antianginal effects persist for about 24 hours.

CONTRAINDICATIONS & PRECAUTIONS
Contraindicated in patients with bronchial asthma, sinus bradycardia, greater than first-degree heart block, and cardiogenic shock. Use cautiously in patients with hyperthyroidism, heart failure, diabetes, chronic bronchitis, emphysema, and impaired renal or hepatic function and in those receiving general anesthesia before undergoing surgery.

INTERACTIONS
Drug-drug. *Antimuscarinics* such as *atropine* may antagonize nadolol-induced bradycardia. Nadolol may potentiate antihypertensive effects of *diuretics* and other *antihypertensives* and, at high doses, the neuromuscular blocking effect of *tubocurarine* and related drugs. Use with *epinephrine* may cause a decrease in pulse rate with first- and second-degree heart block and hypertension. Use with other *antiarrhythmics* may have additive or antagonistic cardiac effects and addi-

Reactions may be *common*, uncommon, *life-threatening*, or COMMON AND LIFE-THREATENING.

tive toxic effects. Nadolol may antagonize beta-stimulating effects of *sympathomimetics* such as *isoproterenol.*
Drug-lifestyle. *Cocaine* may inhibit the
therapeutic effects of nadolol.

ADVERSE REACTIONS
CNS: fatigue, dizziness.
CV: *bradycardia, hypotension,* **heart
failure,** peripheral vascular disease,
rhythm and conduction disturbances.
GI: nausea, vomiting, diarrhea, abdomi-
nal pain, constipation, anorexia.
Respiratory: *increased airway resis-
tance.*
Skin: rash.
Other: fever.

▣ KEY CONSIDERATIONS
Besides the recommendations relevant to
all beta blockers, consider the following:
● Geriatric patients may require lower
maintenance dosages of nadolol because
of increased bioavailability or delayed
metabolism; they also may experience
enhanced adverse effects.
● Dosage adjustments may be necessary
in patients with renal impairment.
● Drug has been used as an antiarrhythmic and as prophylaxis for migraine
headaches.
● If long-term therapy is used, gradually
decrease dose over 1 to 2 weeks before
discontinuing drug. Abrupt withdrawal
can exacerbate angina and cause a MI.

Patient education
● Tell patient not to discontinue nadolol
abruptly. Drug dose should be tapered.

Overdose & treatment
● Signs and symptoms of overdose include severe hypotension, bradycardia,
heart failure, and bronchospasm.
● After acute ingestion, induce vomiting
or perform gastric lavage, and give activated charcoal to reduce absorption.
Magnesium sulfate may be given orally
as a cathartic. Subsequent treatment is
usually symptomatic and supportive.

nafcillin sodium
Nallpen, Unipen

*Penicillinase-resistant penicillin, an-
tibiotic*

Available by prescription only
Capsules: 250 mg
Tablets: 500 mg
Injection: 500 mg, 1 g, 2 g

INDICATIONS & DOSAGE
*Systemic infections caused by suscepti-
ble organisms (methicillin-sensitive*
Staphylococcus aureus)
Adults: 2 to 4 g P.O. daily, divided into
doses given q 6 hours; 2 to 12 g I.M. or
I.V. daily, divided into doses given q 4 to
6 hours.

PHARMACODYNAMICS
Antibiotic action: Nafcillin is bactericidal; it adheres to bacterial penicillin-
binding proteins, thus inhibiting bacterial cell wall synthesis.
    Drug resists the effects of penicillin-
ases and is thus active against many
strains of penicillinase-producing bacteria. This activity is most important
against penicillinase-producing staphylococci; some strains may remain resistant. Drug is also active against a few
gram-positive aerobic and anaerobic
bacilli, but has no significant effect on
gram-negative bacilli.

PHARMACOKINETICS
Absorption: Nafcillin is absorbed erratically and poorly from the GI tract; serum
levels peak at ½ to 2 hours after oral
dose and 30 to 60 minutes after I.M.
dose. Food decreases absorption.
Distribution: Drug is widely distributed;
CSF penetration is poor but is enhanced
by meningeal inflammation. Drug is
70% to 90% protein-bound.
Metabolism: Drug is metabolized primarily in the liver; it undergoes enterohepatic circulation. Dosage adjustment
isn't necessary for patients in renal failure.
Excretion: Drug and metabolites are excreted primarily in bile; 25% to 30% is

excreted in urine unchanged. Elimination half-life in adults is ½ to 1½ hours.

CONTRAINDICATIONS & PRECAUTIONS
Contraindicated in patients with hypersensitivity to nafcillin or other penicillins. Use cautiously in patients with GI distress or sensitivity to cephalosporins.

INTERACTIONS
Drug-drug. Use with *aminoglycosides* produces synergistic bactericidal effects against *S. aureus;* however, the drugs are physically and chemically incompatible and are inactivated when mixed or given together. Use with *cyclosporine* may cause subtherapeutic cyclosporine levels, so these levels should be monitored closely, especially in organ transplant recipients. Use with *hepatotoxic drugs* may increase the risk for hepatotoxicity. *Probenecid* blocks renal tubular secretion of penicillins; however, this interaction has only a small effect on the excretion of nafcillin.
Drug-food. Taking drug with *food* decreases absorption.

ADVERSE REACTIONS
CV: thrombophlebitis.
GI: *nausea,* vomiting, diarrhea, ***Pseudomonas colitis.***
Hematologic: transient leukopenia, ***neutropenia, granulocytopenia, thrombocytopenia*** with high doses.
Other: hypersensitivity reactions (chills, fever, rash, pruritus, urticaria, *anaphylaxis*), vein irritation.

▣ KEY CONSIDERATIONS
Besides the recommendations relevant to all penicillins, consider the following:
• Nafcillin alters test results for urine and serum proteins; turbidimetric urine and serum proteins are often falsely positive or elevated in tests using sulfosalicylic acid or trichloroacetic acid.
• Half-life may be prolonged in geriatric patients because of impaired hepatic and renal function.
• Drug should be given with water only; acid in fruit juice or carbonated beverages may inactivate drug.

• Give dose on empty stomach; food decreases absorption.
• Renal, hepatic, and hematologic systems should be evaluated periodically during prolonged drug therapy.

Patient education
• Tell patient to report severe diarrhea or allergic reactions promptly.

---

nalbuphine hydrochloride
Nubain

Narcotic agonist-antagonist; opioid partial agonist, analgesic, adjunct to anesthesia

---

Available by prescription only
Injection: 10 mg/ml, 20 mg/ml

INDICATIONS & DOSAGE
Moderate to severe pain
Adults: 10 to 20 mg S.C., I.M., or I.V. q 3 to 6 hours, p.r.n., or around the clock. Maximum dosage is 160 mg/day.
Supplement to anesthesia
Adults: 0.3 mg/kg to 3 mg/kg I.V. over 10 to 15 minutes; maintenance dose, 0.25 to 0.5 mg/kg I.V.

PHARMACODYNAMICS
Analgesic action: Nalbuphine is believed to relieve moderate to severe pain. The narcotic antagonist effect may result from competitive inhibition at opiate receptors in the CNS. Like other opioids, drug causes respiratory depression, sedation, and miosis. In patients with coronary artery disease or a MI, it appears to produce no substantial changes in heart rate, pulmonary artery or wedge pressure, left ventricular end-diastolic pressure, pulmonary vascular resistance, or cardiac index.

PHARMACOKINETICS
Absorption: Nalbuphine is about one-fifth as effective as an analgesic when administered P.O. as it is when given I.M., apparently because of first-pass metabolism in the GI tract and liver. Onset of action is within 15 minutes; effect peaks at ½ to 1 hour.

Reactions may be *common,* uncommon, ***life-threatening***, or COMMON AND LIFE-THREATENING.

Distribution: Drug isn't appreciably bound to plasma proteins.
Metabolism: Drug is metabolized in the liver; duration of action is 3 to 6 hours.
Excretion: Drug is excreted in urine and to some degree in bile.

CONTRAINDICATIONS & PRECAUTIONS

Contraindicated in patients with hypersensitivity to nalbuphine. Use cautiously in patients with history of drug abuse, emotional instability, head injury, increased intracranial pressure, impaired ventilation, a MI accompanied by nausea and vomiting, upcoming biliary surgery, and hepatic or renal disease.

INTERACTIONS

Drug-drug. If administered within a few hours of *barbiturate anesthetics* such as *thiopental*, nalbuphine may produce additive CNS and respiratory depressant effects and possibly apnea. According to some reports, *cimetidine* may increase narcotic nalbuphine toxicity, causing disorientation, respiratory depression, apnea, and seizures; although this combination isn't contraindicated (data are limited), be prepared to administer a narcotic antagonist if toxicity occurs. Use with *general anesthetics* may cause severe CV depression. Reduced doses of nalbuphine are usually necessary when drug is used with other *CNS depressants*—including *antihistamines, barbiturates, benzodiazepines, muscle relaxants, narcotic analgesics, phenothiazines, sedative-hypnotics,* and *tricyclic antidepressants*—because they may potentiate the respiratory and CNS depressant, sedative, and hypotensive effects of the drug. Drug accumulation and enhanced effects may result if drug is given with other *drugs that are extensively metabolized in the liver,* such as *digitoxin, phenytoin,* and *rifampin.* Patients who become physically dependent on drug may experience acute withdrawal syndrome if given high doses of an *opioid antagonist;* use with caution and monitor closely.
Drug-lifestyle. *Alcohol* may cause additive CNS and respiratory depressant effects.

ADVERSE REACTIONS

CNS: *headache, sedation, dizziness, vertigo,* nervousness, depression, restlessness, crying, euphoria, hostility, unusual dreams, confusion, hallucinations, speech difficulty, delusions.
CV: hypertension, hypotension, tachycardia, bradycardia.
EENT: blurred vision, *dry mouth.*
GI: cramps, dyspepsia, bitter taste, *nausea, vomiting,* constipation, biliary tract spasms.
GU: urinary urgency.
Respiratory: *respiratory depression,* dyspnea, asthma, *pulmonary edema.*
Skin: pruritus, burning, urticaria, *clamminess.*

▣ KEY CONSIDERATIONS

Besides the recommendations relevant to all opioid agonist-antagonists, consider the following:
● Lower doses are usually indicated for geriatric patients, who may be more sensitive to the therapeutic and adverse effects of nalbuphine.
● Drug may obscure the signs and symptoms of an acute abdominal condition or worsen gallbladder pain.
● Drug may cause orthostatic hypotension in ambulatory patients.
● Before administration, inspect all parenteral products for particulate matter and discoloration.
● Parenteral administration of drug provides better analgesia than oral administration. I.V. doses should be given by slow I.V. injection, preferably in diluted solution. Rapid I.V. injection increases the incidence of adverse effects.
● Drug causes respiratory depression, which at 10 mg is equal to the respiratory depression that 10 mg of morphine causes.
● Drug also acts as a narcotic antagonist; it may precipitate abstinence syndrome in narcotic-dependent patients.

Patient education
● Instruct patient to avoid driving or operating machinery because nalbuphine may cause dizziness and fatigue.

Overdose & treatment

● The most common signs and symptoms of overdose are CNS and respiratory depression and miosis (pinpoint pupils). Other acute toxic effects include hypotension, bradycardia, hypothermia, shock, apnea, cardiopulmonary arrest, circulatory collapse, pulmonary edema, and seizures.

● To treat acute overdose, first establish adequate respiratory exchange via a patent airway and ventilation as needed; administer a narcotic antagonist (naloxone) to reverse respiratory depression. Because the duration of action of nalbuphine is longer than that of naloxone, repeated naloxone dosing is necessary. Naloxone shouldn't be given if the patient doesn't have significant respiratory or CV depression. Monitor vital signs closely.

● Provide symptomatic and supportive treatment (continued respiratory support, correction of fluid or electrolyte imbalance). Monitor laboratory values, vital signs, and neurologic status closely.

naloxone hydrochloride
Narcan

Opioid antagonist

Available by prescription only
Injection: 0.4 mg/ml with preservatives, 0.02 mg/ml, 0.4 mg/ml paraben-free

INDICATIONS & DOSAGE
Known or suspected opioid-induced respiratory depression, including that caused by natural and synthetic narcotics, methadone, nalbuphine, pentazocine, and propoxyphene
Adults: 0.4 to 2 mg I.V., S.C., or I.M., repeated q 2 to 3 minutes, p.r.n. If no response is observed after 10 mg has been administered, diagnosis of narcotic-induced toxicity should be questioned.
Postoperative narcotic depression
Adults: 0.1 to 0.2 mg I.V. q 2 to 3 minutes, p.r.n., until desired response is obtained.

Naloxone challenge for diagnosing opiate dependence
Adults: 0.16 mg I.M.; if no signs of withdrawal are apparent after 20 to 30 minutes, give second dose of 0.24 mg I.V.

PHARMACODYNAMICS
Opioid antagonist action: Naloxone is essentially a pure antagonist. In patients who have received an opioid agonist or other analgesic with narcotic-like effects, naloxone antagonizes most of the opioid effects, especially respiratory depression, sedation, and hypotension. Because the duration of action of naloxone in most cases is shorter than that of the opioid, opiate effects may return as those of naloxone dissipate. Drug doesn't produce tolerance or physical or psychological dependence. The precise mechanism of action is unknown but is thought to involve competitive antagonism of more than one opiate receptor in the CNS.

PHARMACOKINETICS
Absorption: Naloxone is rapidly inactivated after oral administration; therefore, it's given parenterally. Onset of action is 1 to 2 minutes after I.V. administration and 2 to 5 minutes after I.M. or S.C. administration. The duration of action is longer after I.M. use and higher doses compared with I.V. use and lower doses.
Distribution: Drug is rapidly distributed into body tissues and fluids.
Metabolism: Drug is rapidly metabolized in the liver, primarily by conjugation.
Excretion: Duration of action is about 45 minutes, depending on route and dose. Drug is excreted in urine. Plasma half-life has been reported to be from 60 to 90 minutes in adults.

CONTRAINDICATIONS & PRECAUTIONS
Contraindicated in patients with hypersensitivity to naloxone. Use cautiously in patients with cardiac irritability and opiate addiction.

INTERACTIONS
Drug-drug. Patients receiving *cardiotoxic drugs* may have serious CV effects with use of naloxone. When given

---

Reactions may be *common,* uncommon, ***life-threatening,*** or COMMON AND LIFE-THREATENING.

to a *narcotic addict,* naloxone may produce an acute abstinence syndrome; use with caution, and monitor closely.

ADVERSE REACTIONS
CNS: *seizures.*
CV: tachycardia, hypertension, hypotension, *ventricular fibrillation, cardiac arrest.*
GI: nausea, vomiting.
Respiratory: pulmonary edema.
Other: tremors, withdrawal symptoms, diaphoresis.

▣ KEY CONSIDERATIONS
Besides the recommendations relevant to all narcotic antagonists, consider the following:
• Lower doses are usually indicated for geriatric patients because they may be more sensitive to the therapeutic and adverse effects of naloxone.
• Before administration, inspect all parenteral products for particulate matter and discoloration.
• Take a careful drug history to rule out possible narcotic addiction, to avoid inducing withdrawal symptoms.
• Because drug's duration of activity is shorter than that of most narcotics, vigilance and repeated doses are usually necessary to manage an acute opioid overdose in a nonaddicted patient.
• Avoid depending on drug too much; give attention to the airway, breathing, and circulation. Maintain adequate respiratory and CV status at all times. Respiratory overshoot may occur; monitor for respiratory rate higher than before respiratory depression. Respiratory rate increases in 1 to 2 minutes, and effect lasts 1 to 4 hours.
• Drug isn't effective in treating respiratory depression caused by nonopioids.
• Drug can be diluted in D_5W or normal saline solution. Use within 24 hours after mixing.
• Naloxone is the safest drug to use when cause of respiratory depression is uncertain.
• Drug may be given via continuous I.V. infusion, which may be necessary to control the adverse effects of epidural morphine. Usual dose is 2 mg/500 ml D_5W or normal saline solution.

naproxen
Naprosyn, EC-Naprosyn

naproxen sodium
Aleve, Anaprox, Naprelan

NSAID, nonnarcotic analgesic, antipyretic, anti-inflammatory

Available by prescription only
naproxen
Tablets: 250 mg, 375 mg, 500 mg
Tablets (delayed-release): 375 mg, 500 mg
Oral suspension: 125 mg/5 ml
naproxen sodium
Tablets (film-coated): 275 mg, 550 mg
Note: 220 mg, 275 mg, 550 mg of naproxen sodium = 200 mg, 250 mg, or 500 mg of naproxen, respectively.
Tablets (controlled-release): 375 mg, 500 mg
Available without prescription
naproxen sodium
Tablets or capsules: 220 mg

INDICATIONS & DOSAGE
Mild to moderately severe musculoskeletal or soft-tissue irritation
naproxen
Adults: 250 to 500 mg P.O. b.i.d. Alternatively, 250 mg in the morning and 500 mg in the evening. *Delayed-release tablets:* 375 to 500 mg P.O. b.i.d.
naproxen sodium
Adults: 275 to 550 mg P.O. b.i.d. Alternatively, 275 mg in the morning and 550 mg in the evening. *Controlled-release tablets:* 750 to 1,000 mg P.O. once daily.
Mild to moderate pain
naproxen
Adults: 500 mg P.O. to start, followed by 250 mg P.O. q 6 to 8 hours, p.r.n. Maximum daily dose shouldn't exceed 1.25 g.
naproxen sodium
Adults: 550 mg P.O. to start, followed by 275 mg P.O. q 6 to 8 hours, p.r.n. Maximum daily dose is 1.375 g.
Controlled-release: 1,000 mg P.O. daily. For patients requiring a greater analgesic benefit, 1,500 mg may be used for a limited period.

Self-medication: 220 mg q 8 to 12 hours. For adults ages 65 and older, maximum daily dose is 440 mg. Drug shouldn't be used for more than 10 days.

Acute gout

naproxen
Adults: 750 mg initially, then 250 mg q 8 hours until episode subsides.

naproxen sodium
Adults: 825 mg initially, then 275 mg q 8 hours until attack subsides.

Controlled-release: 1,000 to 1,500 mg once daily on the first day, followed by 1,000 mg once daily until attack subsides.

PHARMACODYNAMICS

Analgesic, antipyretic, and anti-inflammatory actions: Mechanisms of action are unknown; naproxen is thought to inhibit prostaglandin synthesis.

PHARMACOKINETICS

Absorption: Naproxen is absorbed rapidly and completely from the GI tract. Effect peaks at 2 to 4 hours.
Distribution: Drug is highly protein-bound.
Metabolism: Drug is metabolized in the liver.
Excretion: Drug is excreted in urine; half-life is 10 to 20 hours.

CONTRAINDICATIONS & PRECAUTIONS

Contraindicated in patients with hypersensitivity to naproxen or asthma, rhinitis, or nasal polyps. Use cautiously in geriatric patients and in those with a history of peptic ulcer disease or renal, CV, GI, or hepatic disease.

INTERACTIONS

Drug-drug. Increased nephrotoxicity may occur with *acetaminophen, gold compounds,* or other *anti-inflammatories.* Use of naproxen with *anticoagulants* and *thrombolytics*—including *coumadin derivatives, heparin, streptokinase,* and *urokinase*—may potentiate anticoagulant effects. Naproxen may decrease the effectiveness of *antihypertensives* and *diuretics;* use may increase the risk for nephrotoxicity. Use with *anti-inflammatories, corticotropin, corticosteroids,* or *salicylates,* may cause increased GI adverse reactions, including

ulceration and hemorrhage. *Aspirin* may decrease the bioavailability of naproxen. Toxicity may occur with *coumadin derivatives, nifedipine, phenytoin,* or *verapamil.* Bleeding problems may occur if used with other *drugs that inhibit platelet aggregation,* such as *aspirin, cefamandole, cefoperazone, dextran, dipyridamole, mezlocillin,* other *anti-inflammatories, parenteral carbenicillin, piperacillin, plicamycin, salicylates, sulfinpyrazone, ticarcillin,* or *valproic acid.* Naproxen may displace *highly protein-bound drugs* from binding sites. Because of the influence of prostaglandins on glucose metabolism, use with *insulin* or *oral antidiabetics* may potentiate hypoglycemic effects.
Naproxen may decrease the renal clearance of *lithium* and *methotrexate.*
Drug-lifestyle. Use with *alcohol* may cause increased GI adverse reactions, including ulceration and hemorrhage.

ADVERSE REACTIONS

CNS: *headache, drowsiness, dizziness,* vertigo.
CV: *edema,* palpitations.
EENT: visual disturbances, *tinnitus,* auditory disturbances.
GI: *epigastric distress, occult blood loss, nausea, **peptic ulceration,*** constipation, dyspepsia, heartburn, diarrhea, stomatitis, thirst.
GU: nephrotoxicity, increased BUN and creatinine levels.
Hematologic: ***thrombocytopenia,*** eosinophilia, ***agranulocytosis,*** neutropenia.
Hepatic: elevated liver enzyme levels.
Respiratory: dyspnea.
Skin: *pruritus, rash,* urticaria, ecchymosis, diaphoresis, purpura.

▣ KEY CONSIDERATIONS

Besides the recommendations relevant to all NSAIDs, consider the following:
• Patients older than age 60 are more sensitive to the adverse effects (especially GI toxicity) of naproxen.
• Drug's effect on renal prostaglandins may cause fluid retention and edema. This may be significant in geriatric patients, especially those with heart failure.

• Drug and its metabolites may interfere with urine 5-hydroxyindoleacetic acid and 17-hydroxy-corticosteroid levels.
• Use lowest possible effective dose; 250 mg of naproxen is equivalent to 275 mg of naproxen sodium.
• Relief usually begins within 2 weeks after beginning therapy with naproxen.
• Institute safety measures to prevent injury resulting from possible CNS effects.
• Monitor fluid balance and for signs and symptoms of fluid retention, especially significant weight gain.
• Don't break, crush, or chew sustained-release tablets.

Patient education
• Caution patient to avoid use of OTC drugs.
• Teach patient signs and symptoms of possible adverse reactions and to report them promptly.
• Instruct patient to check his weight every 2 to 3 days and to report a gain of 1.5 kg (3 lb) or more within 1 week.
• Instruct patient in safety measures; advise him to avoid activities that require alertness until CNS effects are known.
• Warn patient against combining naproxen (Naprosyn) with naproxen sodium (Anaprox) because both drugs circulate in the blood as naproxen anion.

Overdose and treatment
• Signs and symptoms of overdose include drowsiness, heartburn, indigestion, nausea, and vomiting.
• To treat overdose of naproxen, immediately induce vomiting with ipecac syrup or perform gastric lavage. Administer activated charcoal via NG tube. Provide symptomatic and supportive measures (respiratory support and correction of fluid and electrolyte imbalances). Monitor laboratory parameters and vital signs closely. Hemodialysis is ineffective in drug removal.

naratriptan hydrochloride
Amerge

Selective 5-hydroxytryptamine$_1$ (5-HT$_1$) receptor subtype agonist, antimigraine drug

Available by prescription only
Tablets: 1 mg, 2.5 mg

INDICATIONS & DOSAGE
Treatment of acute migraine headache attacks with or without aura
Adults: 1 or 2.5 mg P.O. as a single dose. Dose should be individualized, depending on the possible benefit of the 2.5-mg dose and the greater risk for adverse events. If headache returns or if only partial response occurs, may repeat dose after 4 hours for maximum dose of 5 mg within 24 hours.
✦ ***Dosage adjustment.*** In patients with mild to moderate renal or hepatic impairment, consider a lower initial dose; don't exceed maximum dose of 2.5 mg over a 24-hour period. Don't use in patients with severe renal or hepatic impairment.

PHARMACODYNAMICS
Antimigraine action: Naratriptan binds with high affinity to 5-HT$_{1D}$ and 5-HT$_{1B}$ receptors. One theory suggests that activation of 5-HT$_{1D/1B}$ receptors located on intracranial blood vessels leads to vasoconstriction, which helps relieve migraines. Another hypothesis suggests that activation of 5-HT$_{1D/1B}$ receptors on sensory nerve endings in the trigeminal system results in the inhibition of proinflammatory neuropeptide release.

PHARMACOKINETICS
Absorption: Naratriptan is well absorbed, with about 70% oral bioavailability. Plasma levels peak in 2 to 4 hours.
Distribution: Steady-state volume of distribution is 170 L. Plasma protein-binding is 28% to 31%.
Metabolism: In vitro, drug is metabolized by many P-450 cytochrome isoenzymes to inactive metabolites.

Excretion: Drug is predominantly eliminated in urine, with 50% of dose recovered unchanged and 30% as metabolites. Mean elimination half-life is 6 hours.

CONTRAINDICATIONS & PRECAUTIONS

Contraindicated in patients with hypersensitivity to naratriptan or its components and in those with history, symptoms, or signs of ischemic cardiac, cerebrovascular (such as CVA or transient ischemic attack), or peripheral vascular syndromes (such as ischemic bowel disease). Also contraindicated in patients with significant underlying CV diseases, including angina pectoris, MI, and silent myocardial ischemia.

Drug may increase blood pressure and shouldn't be given to patients with uncontrolled hypertension.

Contraindicated in patients with severe renal (creatinine clearance less than 15 ml/minute) or hepatic (Child-Pugh class C) impairment and in those with hemiplegic or basilar migraine.

Drug or other 5-HT₁ agonists are also contraindicated in patients with potential risk factors for coronary artery disease, such as hypertension, hypercholesterolemia, obesity, diabetes, strong family history of coronary artery disease, or smoking.

INTERACTIONS

Drug-drug. *Ergot-containing* or *ergot-type drugs* or *other 5-HT₁ agonists* have been reported to cause prolonged vasospastic reactions because their actions may be additive; use of these drugs within 24 hours of naratriptan is contraindicated. Use with *oral contraceptives* results in slightly higher naratriptan levels. Rarely, *selective serotonin reuptake inhibitors (SSRIs)* (such as *fluoxetine, fluvoxamine, paroxetine,* and *sertraline*) have been reported to cause weakness, hyperreflexia, and incoordination when administered with 5-HT₁ agonists; if therapy with naratriptan and an SSRI is needed, monitor patient.
Drug-lifestyle. *Smoking* increases the clearance of drug by 30%.

ADVERSE REACTIONS

CNS: paresthesia, dizziness, drowsiness, malaise, fatigue, vertigo.
CV: palpitations, increased blood pressure, tachyarrhythmias, *abnormal ECG changes (prolonged PR or QT interval, abnormal ST-T segment, PVCs, atrial flutter, or atrial fibrillation),* syncope.
EENT: ear, nose, and throat infections; photophobia.
GI: nausea, hyposalivation, vomiting.
Other: warm or cold temperature sensations; sensations of pressure, tightness, or heaviness.

▣ KEY CONSIDERATIONS

• Use of naratriptan isn't recommended in geriatric patients because clinical studies didn't include patients older than age 65. Geriatric patients are more likely to have serious adverse effects because of decreased hepatic and renal function. The contraindications alone almost exclusively rule out geriatric patients as an appropriate group to receive this drug.
• Use drug only when a clear diagnosis of migraine has been established. It isn't intended as prophylaxis for migraines or for use in managing hemiplegic or basilar migraine.
• Administer first dose in a medically equipped facility for patients at risk for coronary artery disease but determined to have a satisfactory CV evaluation. Consider ECG monitoring.
• Perform periodic cardiac reevaluation in patients who have or develop risk factors for coronary artery disease.
• Safety and effectiveness haven't been established for cluster headaches.

Patient education

• Tell patient that naratriptan is intended to relieve, not prevent, migraine headaches.
• Teach patient to alert doctor of risk factors for coronary artery disease.
• Tell patient that if more relief is needed after the first tablet, such as when a partial response occurs or if the headache returns, he may take a second tablet but not sooner than 4 hours after the first tablet. Inform patient not to exceed two tablets within 24 hours.

Reactions may be *common*, uncommon, *life-threatening*, or COMMON AND LIFE-THREATENING.

Overdose and treatment
• A significant increase in blood pressure has been observed with overdose, occurring between 30 minutes and 6 hours after ingestion of naratriptan. Blood pressure returned to normal within 8 hours without pharmacologic intervention in some patients, whereas in others, antihypertensive treatment was necessary.
• No specific antidote exists. Monitor ECG for evidence of ischemia. Monitor patient for at least 24 hours after overdose or while symptoms persist. The effect of hemodialysis or peritoneal dialysis is unknown.

---

nedocromil sodium
Tilade

Pyranoquinoline, anti-inflammatory respiratory inhalant

Available by prescription only
Inhalation aerosol: 1.75 mg per actuation in 16.2-g canister (U.S.); 2 mg per actuation in 16.2-g canister (Canada)

INDICATIONS & DOSAGE
Maintenance therapy in mild to moderate bronchial asthma
Adults: 2 inhalations q.i.d., preferably at regular intervals; may gradually decrease dosing interval to b.i.d.

PHARMACODYNAMICS
Anti-inflammatory action: Nedocromil inhibits the activation and release of inflammatory mediators from various cell types in the lumen and mucosa of the bronchial tree. These mediators—which include leukotrienes, histamine, and prostaglandins—are preformed or derived from arachidonic acid metabolism. A range of human cells associated with asthma may be involved. As a result, drug exhibits specific anti-inflammatory properties when administered topically to the bronchial mucosa. It has demonstrated a significant inhibitory effect on allergen-induced early and late asthmatic reactions and on bronchial hyperresponsiveness. Drug also may affect sensory nerves in the lung. The result is inhibition of bradykinin-induced bronchoconstriction.

PHARMACOKINETICS
Absorption: About 2% to 3% of amount swallowed after nedocromil inhalation is absorbed. From 6% to 9% of nedocromil deposited in the lungs is completely absorbed. Onset of action is within 30 minutes. Drug peaks in 5 to 90 minutes, and lasts 6 to 12 hours.
Distribution: Drug is distributed to plasma only. About 89% is reversibly bound to plasma proteins when plasma levels are between 0.5 and 50 mcg/ml.
Metabolism: Drug isn't metabolized.
Excretion: Drug is rapidly excreted unchanged in bile and urine. Half-life is 1.5 to 3.3 hours.

CONTRAINDICATIONS & PRECAUTIONS
Contraindicated in patients hypersensitive to the formulation or in patients experiencing an acute asthma attack or acute bronchospasm.

ADVERSE REACTIONS
CNS: headache, dysphagia, fatigue.
CV: chest pain.
GI: nausea, vomiting, dyspepsia, abdominal pain, dry mouth, *unpleasant taste.*
Respiratory: upper respiratory tract infection, rhinitis, cough, pharyngitis, increased sputum, bronchitis, dyspnea, ***bronchospasm.***

▣ KEY CONSIDERATIONS
• Dosage may be reduced to two inhalations t.i.d. and then b.i.d. after several weeks, when patient's asthma is under control.
• In maintenance therapy, nedocromil must be used regularly, even during symptom-free periods, to achieve benefit.
• A decrease in severity of symptoms or the need for concomitant therapy is a sign of improvement that usually occurs in the first 2 weeks if patient responds to therapy.
• When drug is added to an existing regimen of bronchodilators or inhaled or oral corticosteroids, dosage of the corticosteroid or bronchodilator may be re-

duced in some patients. However, reduction should be gradual and under close medical supervision to avoid exacerbating the asthma.
• Don't exceed 16 mg within 24 hours.
• In some patients, a single dose of drug before activities that precipitate asthma—such as exercise or exposure to cold air, pollutants, or allergens—may prevent bronchospasm.

Patient education
• Warn patient that nedocromil has no direct bronchodilating action and can't replace bronchodilators during an acute asthma attack.
• Tell patient that drug is an adjunct to the regular bronchodilator regimen and may reduce the need for corticosteroids or bronchodilators.
• Emphasize that drug should be taken regularly for best results. Most patients report benefits after 1 week of use; some require longer treatment before improvement occurs.
• Teach patient how to use the inhaler. Instruct him to shake canister immediately before use and to invert it just before actuation. Prime inhaler with three actuations before first use, or if unused for more than 7 days.
• Advise patient to clean inhaler at least twice weekly and to remove canister before rinsing inhaler in hot running water. Allow inhaler to air-dry overnight.

nefazodone hydrochloride
Serzone

Phenylpiperazine, antidepressant

Available by prescription only
Tablets: 100 mg, 150 mg, 200 mg, 250 mg

INDICATIONS & DOSAGE
Depression
Adults: initially, 200 mg/day P.O. divided into two doses. Dosage increased in 100- to 200-mg/day increments at intervals of no less than 1 week, as needed. Usual dosage range is 300 to 600 mg/day.

PHARMACODYNAMICS
Antidepressant action: Action isn't precisely defined. Nefazodone inhibits neuronal uptake of serotonin and norepinephrine. It also occupies central 5-HT$_2$ (serotonin) and alpha$_1$-adrenergic receptors.

PHARMACOKINETICS
Absorption: Nefazodone is rapidly and completely absorbed, but because of extensive metabolism, absolute bioavailability is only about 20%.
Distribution: More than 99% is bound to plasma proteins.
Metabolism: Drug is extensively metabolized by N-dealkylation and aliphatic and aromatic hydroxylation.
Excretion: Drug and its metabolites are excreted in urine; half-life is 2 to 4 hours.

CONTRAINDICATIONS & PRECAUTIONS
Contraindicated in patients with hypersensitivity to nefazodone or other phenylpiperazine antidepressants. Don't use within 14 days of MAO inhibitor therapy, and don't administer with cisapride.
Use cautiously in patients with CV or cerebrovascular disease that could be exacerbated by hypotension (such as history of a MI, angina, or CVA) and conditions that predispose patients to hypotension (such as dehydration, hypovolemia, and antihypertensive therapy). Also use cautiously in patients with history of mania.

INTERACTIONS
Drug-drug. Because administration with *alprazolam* or *triazolam* potentiates the effects of these drugs, don't administer together; however, if necessary, dosage of alprazolam and triazolam may need to be reduced greatly. Use with *cisapride* may decrease metabolism of these drugs, leading to increased levels and cardiotoxicity; avoid use. Use with *CNS-active drugs* may alter CNS activity; use cautiously. Nefazodone may increase *digoxin* level; use cautiously and monitor digoxin levels. Administration with other *highly plasma protein-bound drugs* may increase incidence and severity of adverse reactions; monitor patient

---

Reactions may be *common,* uncommon, *life-threatening,* or COMMON AND LIFE-THREATENING.

closely. Use with *MAO inhibitors* may cause severe excitation, hyperpyrexia, seizures, delirium, or coma; avoid use.

ADVERSE REACTIONS
CNS: *headache, somnolence, dizziness, asthenia,* insomnia, *light-headedness, confusion,* memory impairment, paresthesia, abnormal dreams, decreased concentration, ataxia, incoordination, taste perversion, psychomotor retardation, tremor, hypertonia.
CV: orthostatic hypotension, vasodilation, hypotension, peripheral edema.
EENT: *blurred vision, abnormal vision,* pharyngitis, tinnitus, visual field defect.
GI: *dry mouth, nausea, constipation,* dyspepsia, diarrhea, increased appetite, thirst, vomiting.
GU: urinary frequency, urinary tract infection, urine retention, vaginitis.
Musculoskeletal: neck rigidity, arthralgia.
Respiratory: cough.
Skin: pruritus, rash.
Other: infection, flulike syndrome, chills, fever, breast pain.

▣ KEY CONSIDERATIONS
• Because of increased systemic exposure to nefazodone, initiate treatment at half the usual dose, but adjust dosage upward over the same range as in younger patients. Observe usual precautions in geriatric patients who have other medical illnesses or are receiving concomitant drugs.
• Allow at least 1 week after stopping drug before giving patient an MAO inhibitor. Also, allow at least 14 days before patient is started on nefazodone after MAO inhibitor therapy has been stopped.
• Record mood changes. Monitor patient for suicidal tendencies, and allow a minimum supply of drug.

Patient education
• Warn patient not to engage in hazardous activities until CNS effects are known.
• Tell men that if prolonged or inappropriate erections occur, to stop nefazodone immediately and seek medical attention.

• Instruct patient not to drink alcoholic beverages during therapy.
• Tell patient to report rash, hives, or a related allergic reaction.
• Inform patient that several weeks of therapy may be required to obtain the full antidepressant effect. Once improvement is seen, advise patient not to discontinue drug until directed.

Overdose and treatment
• Signs and symptoms of overdose include nausea, vomiting, and somnolence. Other drug-associated adverse reactions may occur.
• Provide symptomatic and supportive treatment in the case of hypotension or excessive sedation. Use gastric lavage if needed.

---

nelfinavir mesylate
Viracept

HIV protease inhibitor, antiviral

Available by prescription only
Tablets: 250 mg
Powder: 50 mg/g powder

INDICATIONS & DOSAGE
Treatment of HIV infection when antiretroviral therapy is warranted
Adults: 750 mg P.O. t.i.d with meal or light snack; or for powder, 15 level 1-g scoops or 3.75 level tsp.

PHARMACODYNAMICS
Antiviral action: Nelfinavir is an HIV protease inhibitor. Inhibition of the protease enzyme prevents cleavage of the viral polyprotein, resulting in the production of an immature, noninfectious virus.

PHARMACOKINETICS
Absorption: Absolute bioavailability is undetermined. Food increases absorption of nelfinavir. Levels peak 2 to 4 hours after drug is administered with food.
Distribution: Apparent volume of distribution is 2 to 7 L/kg. More than 98% of drug is bound to plasma protein.
Metabolism: Drug is metabolized in the liver by multiple cytochrome P-450 isoforms, including CYP3A.

Excretion: Terminal half-life is 3.5 to 5 hours. Drug is primarily excreted in feces.

CONTRAINDICATIONS & PRECAUTIONS

Contraindicated in patients with hypersensitivity to a component of drug. Use cautiously in patients with hepatic dysfunction or hemophilia types A and B.

INTERACTIONS

Drug-drug. Don't administer nelfinavir with *amiodarone, cisapride, ergot derivatives, midazolam, quinidine,* or *triazolam* because nelfinavir is expected to produce large increases in plasma levels of these drugs, which may increase the risk for serious or life-threatening adverse events. *Anti-HIV protease inhibitors* such as *indinavir* and *ritonavir* may increase plasma nelfinavir levels. *Carbamazepine, phenobarbital,* and *phenytoin* may reduce the effectiveness of nelfinavir by decreasing plasma nelfinavir levels. Coadministration with *drugs primarily metabolized by CYP3A* such as *calcium channel blockers* and *dihydropyridine* may result in increased levels of the other drug and decreased plasma levels of nelfinavir; use cautiously. Use with approved *reverse-transcriptase inhibitors* may increase antiretroviral activity. Nelfinavir dramatically increases plasma *rifabutin* levels; reduce dose of rifabutin to one-half the usual dose. *Rifampin* decreases plasma nelfinavir levels; don't use together.

ADVERSE REACTIONS

CNS: malaise, anxiety, depression, dizziness, emotional lability, hyperkinesia, insomnia, migraine headache, paresthesia, *seizures,* sleep disorders, somnolence, *suicidal ideation.*
EENT: iritis, eye disorders, pharyngitis, rhinitis, sinusitis.
GI: abdominal pain, nausea, *diarrhea,* flatulence, anorexia, dyspepsia, epigastric pain, GI bleeding, pancreatitis, mouth ulceration, vomiting.
GU: sexual dysfunction, kidney calculus, urine abnormality.
Hematologic: anemia, *leukopenia, thrombocytopenia.*
Hepatic: *hepatitis.*

Metabolic: dehydration, diabetes mellitus, hyperlipidemia, hyperuricemia, hypoglycemia.
Musculoskeletal: back pain, arthralgia, arthritis, cramps, myalgia, myasthenia, myopathy.
Respiratory: dyspnea.
Skin: rash, dermatitis, folliculitis, fungal dermatitis, pruritus, sweating, urticaria.
Other: fever.

▣ KEY CONSIDERATIONS

● Decision to use nelfinavir is based on surrogate marker changes in patients who received drug in combination with nucleoside analogues or alone for up to 24 weeks. There are no results from controlled trials evaluating the effect on survival or incidence of opportunistic fungal infections.
● Drug dosage is the same whether used alone or in combination with other antiretrovirals.
● Administer oral powder in patients unable to take tablets; oral powder may be mixed with water, milk, soy milk, or dietary supplements. Tell patient to drink entire contents.
● Don't reconstitute with water in its original container.
● Use reconstituted powder within 6 hours.
● Acidic foods or juice aren't recommended because of bitter taste.
● Monitor CBC with differential (especially neutrophil count) and chemistries; low incidences of laboratory abnormalities were reported in clinical studies. Increases in alkaline phosphatase, amylase, CK, LD, AST, ALT, and GGT levels may occur; monitor closely.

Patient education

● Advise patient to take nelfinavir with food.
● Inform patient that drug doesn't cure HIV infection.
● Tell patient that long-term effects of drug are unknown but that drug reduces the risk of HIV transmission to others.
● Advise patient to take drug daily as prescribed and not to alter the dose or the drug without medical approval.
● If patient misses a dose, tell him to take the dose as soon as possible and re-

---

Reactions may be *common,* uncommon, *life-threatening,* or COMMON AND LIFE-THREATENING.

turn to his normal schedule. If a dose is skipped, advise patient not to double-dose.
• Tell patient that diarrhea is the most common adverse effect and that it can be controlled with loperamide, if necessary.
• Advise patient to report use of other prescribed or OTC drugs.

neostigmine bromide

neostigmine methylsulfate
Prostigmin

Cholinesterase inhibitor, muscle stimulant

Available by prescription only
Tablets: 15 mg
Injection: 0.25 mg/ml, 0.5 mg/ml, 1 mg/ml

INDICATIONS & DOSAGE
Antidote for nondepolarizing neuro-muscular blockers
Adults: 0.5 to 2.5 mg slow I.V. Repeat p.r.n.; maximum total dose, 5 mg. Give 0.6 to 1.2 mg atropine sulfate I.V. before antidote dose if patient is bradycardic.
Postoperative abdominal distention and bladder atony
Adults: 0.5 to 1 mg I.M. or S.C. q 3 hours for five doses after bladder has emptied (treatment); 0.25 mg I.M. or S.C. q 4 to 6 hours for 2 to 3 days (prevention).
Diagnosis of myasthenia gravis
Adults: 0.022 mg/kg I.M. If cholinergic reaction occurs, discontinue test and give 0.4 to 0.6 mg of atropine sulfate I.V.
Symptomatic control of myasthenia gravis
Adults: 0.5 mg S.C. or I.M. Oral dosage can range from 15 to 375 mg/day (average, 150 mg/day). Subsequent dosages must be individualized, based on response and tolerance of adverse effects. Therapy may be required day and night.

PHARMACODYNAMICS
Muscle stimulant action: Neostigmine blocks hydrolysis of acetylcholine by cholinesterase, resulting in acetylcholine accumulation at cholinergic synapses. This leads to increased cholinergic receptor stimulation at the myoneural junction.

PHARMACOKINETICS
Absorption: Neostigmine is poorly absorbed (1% to 2%) from the GI tract after oral administration. Action usually begins 45 to 75 minutes after an oral dose, 20 to 30 minutes after an I.M. dose, and 4 to 8 minutes after an I.V. dose.
Distribution: About 15% to 25% of dose binds to plasma proteins.
Metabolism: Drug is hydrolyzed by cholinesterases and metabolized by microsomal liver enzymes. Duration of effect varies considerably, depending on patient's physical and emotional status and on disease severity.
Excretion: About 80% of dose is excreted in urine as unchanged drug and metabolites in the first 24 hours after administration.

CONTRAINDICATIONS & PRECAUTIONS
Contraindicated in patients with hypersensitivity to cholinergics or to bromide and in those with peritonitis or mechanical obstruction of the intestine or urinary tract. Use cautiously in patients with bronchial asthma, bradycardia, seizure disorders, recent coronary occlusion, vagotonia, hyperthyroidism, arrhythmias, and peptic ulcer.

INTERACTIONS
Drug-drug. *Atropine* antagonizes the muscarinic effects of neostigmine. *Corticosteroids* may decrease cholinergic effects; when corticosteroids are stopped, however, the cholinergic effects of neostigmine may increase, possibly affecting muscle strength. *Magnesium* has a direct depressant effect on skeletal muscle and may antagonize the beneficial effects of neostigmine. Use with *procainamide* or *quinidine* may reverse the cholinergic effect of neostigmine on muscle. Use with *succinylcholine* may result in prolonged respiratory depression from plasma esterase inhibition, causing delayed succinylcholine hydrolysis; use with other *cholinergics* may cause additive toxicity.

ADVERSE REACTIONS

CNS: dizziness, headache, muscle weakness, unconsciousness, drowsiness.
CV: bradycardia, hypotension, tachycardia, AV block, flushing, syncope, *cardiac arrest.*
EENT: blurred vision, lacrimation, miosis.
GI: *nausea, vomiting, diarrhea, abdominal cramps,* excessive salivation, flatulence, increased peristalsis.
GU: urinary frequency.
Musculoskeletal: *muscle cramps,* muscle fasciculations, arthralgia.
Respiratory: *bronchospasm,* dyspnea, respiratory depression, *respiratory arrest,* increased secretions.
Skin: rash, urticaria, diaphoresis.
Other: hypersensitivity reactions *(anaphylaxis).*

◨ KEY CONSIDERATIONS

Besides the recommendations relevant to all cholinesterase inhibitors, consider the following:
• Geriatric patients may be more sensitive to the effects of neostigmine. Use with caution.
• Monitor patient's vital signs, particularly the pulse rate.
• If muscle weakness is severe, determine if this stems from drug toxicity or from exacerbation of myasthenia gravis. A test dose of edrophonium I.V. aggravates drug-induced weakness but temporarily relieves weakness resulting from the disease.
• Hospitalized patients may be able to manage a bedside supply of tablets to take themselves.
• Give drug with food or milk to reduce the chance of GI adverse effects.
• When administering drug to patient with myasthenia gravis, schedule largest dose before anticipated periods of fatigue. For example, if patient has dysphagia, schedule this dose 30 minutes before each meal.
• To prevent additive toxicity, stop all other cholinergics during neostigmine therapy.
• When administering drug to prevent abdominal distention and GI distress, insertion of a rectal tube may be indicated to help passage of gas.

• Administration with atropine can relieve or eliminate adverse reactions; however, these reactions may be signs and symptoms of neostigmine overdose.
• Patients may develop resistance to drug.

Patient education
• Instruct patient to observe and record changes in muscle strength.

Overdose & treatment
• Signs and symptoms of overdose include headache, nausea, vomiting, diarrhea, blurred vision, miosis, excessive tearing, bronchospasm, increased bronchial secretions, hypotension, incoordination, excessive sweating, muscle weakness, cramps, fasciculations, paralysis, bradycardia or tachycardia, excessive salivation, and restlessness or agitation.
• Support respiration; bronchial suctioning may be performed. Discontinue neostigmine immediately. Atropine may be given to block the muscarinic effects of the drug but won't counter paralytic effects of the drug on skeletal muscle. Avoid atropine overdose because it may lead to bronchial plug formation.

---

nevirapine
Viramune

Nonnucleoside reverse transcriptase inhibitor, antiviral

Available by prescription only
Tablets: 200 mg

INDICATIONS & DOSAGE

Adjunct treatment of patients with HIV-1 infection who have experienced clinical or immunologic deterioration
Adults: 200 mg P.O. daily for first 14 days, followed by 200 mg P.O. b.i.d. in combination with nucleoside analogue antiretrovirals.

PHARMACODYNAMICS

Antiviral action: Nevirapine binds directly to reverse transcriptase and blocks the RNA- and DNA-dependent DNA polymerase activities by disrupting the enzyme's catalytic site.

Reactions may be *common,* uncommon, *life-threatening,* or COMMON AND LIFE-THREATENING.

PHARMACOKINETICS

Absorption: Nevirapine is readily absorbed.

Distribution: Drug is widely distributed; about 60% bound to plasma proteins.

Metabolism: Drug is extensively metabolized in the liver.

Excretion: Metabolites are primarily excreted in urine; a small amount is excreted in feces.

CONTRAINDICATIONS & PRECAUTIONS

Contraindicated in patients with hypersensitivity to nevirapine. Use cautiously in patients with impaired renal or hepatic function because the pharmacokinetics of drug haven't been evaluated in these patient groups.

INTERACTIONS

Drug-drug. Nevirapine may reduce the plasma levels of *drugs that are extensively metabolized by P-450 CYP3A;* dosage adjustment of these drugs may be needed. Nevirapine may decrease plasma levels of *oral contraceptives* and *protease inhibitors;* these drugs shouldn't be used with nevirapine.

ADVERSE REACTIONS

CNS: headache, peripheral neuropathy, paresthesia.

GI: nausea, diarrhea, abdominal pain, ulcerative stomatitis.

Hematologic: *decreased neutrophil count,* eosinophilia.

Hepatic: *hepatitis,* abnormal liver function test results, increased ALT, AST, GGT, and total bilirubin levels, *hepatotoxicity.*

Musculoskeletal: myalgia.

Skin: *rash, Stevens-Johnson syndrome, toxic epidermal necrolysis.*

Other: fever.

▣ KEY CONSIDERATIONS

• Pharmacokinetics of nevirapine in HIV-1 infected adults don't appear to change up to age 68; however, the drug hasn't been extensively evaluated in adults older than age 55.

• Perform clinical chemistry tests, including liver function tests, before initiating therapy and regularly throughout therapy.

• Resistant virus emerges rapidly when drug is administered as monotherapy. Always administer in combination with at least one other antiretroviral.

• Discontinue drug if patient develops a severe rash or a rash accompanied by fever, blistering, oral lesions, conjunctivitis, swelling, muscle or joint aches, or general malaise. Use of a 200-mg/day dose as a lead-in period has been shown to decrease the incidence of rash. If rash occurs during the initial 14 days, don't increase dosage until it has resolved. Most rashes occur within the first 6 weeks of therapy.

• Temporarily stop drug in patients with moderate or severe liver function test result abnormalities (excluding GGT) until they have returned to baseline. Restart drug at half the previous dose level. If moderate or severe liver function test abnormalities recur, discontinue drug therapy.

• If therapy is interrupted for more than 7 days, restart therapy as if receiving drug for the first time.

• If disease progresses during therapy, consider altering antiretroviral therapy.

Patient education

• Inform patient that nevirapine isn't a cure for HIV, and the illnesses associated with advanced HIV-1 infection may still occur. Also, tell patient that drug doesn't reduce the risk of transmission of HIV-1 to others through sexual contact or blood contamination.

• Instruct patient to report rash immediately. Therapy may need to be stopped temporarily.

• Stress importance of taking drug exactly as prescribed. If a dose is missed, tell patient to take the next dose as soon as possible. However, if a dose is skipped, he shouldn't double-dose.

• Tell patient not to use other drugs without medical approval.

• Stress that patient should consult health care provider if symptoms of hepatitis occur, and it's important to monitor liver function studies.

---

*Canada only   ◇ Unlabeled clinical use

niacin (vitamin B₃, nicotinic acid)

Niaspan, Nico-400, Nicobid, Nicolar, Nicotinex, Slo-Niacin

B-complex vitamin, vitamin B₃, antilipemic, peripheral vasodilator

---

Available by prescription only
Capsules: 500 mg
Injection: 30-ml vials, 100 mg/ml
Available without prescription
Tablets: 25 mg, 50 mg, 100 mg, 125 mg, 250 mg, 400 mg, 500 mg
Tablets (timed-release): 250 mg, 500 mg, 750 mg
Capsules (timed-release): 125 mg, 250 mg, 300 mg, 400 mg, 500 mg, 750 mg
Tablets (extended-release): 500 mg, 750 mg, 1,000 mg
21-day starter pack: 7 each of 375 mg, 500 mg, and 750 mg
Elixir: 50 mg/5 ml

INDICATIONS & DOSAGE
Pellagra
Adults: 300 to 500 mg in divided doses P.O., S.C., I.M., or I.V. infusion daily, depending on severity of niacin deficiency. Maximum recommended daily dosage is 500 mg, which should be divided into 10 doses, 50 mg each.
Peripheral vascular disease and circulatory disorders
Adults: 100 to 150 mg P.O. three to five times daily.
Adjunctive treatment of hyperlipidemias, especially those associated with hypercholesterolemia
Adults: 1.5 to 3 g daily in three divided doses with or after meals, increased at intervals to 6 g daily to maximum of 9 g daily.
Dietary supplement
Adults: 10 to 20 mg P.O. daily.

PHARMACODYNAMICS
Vitamin replacement action: Niacin functions as a coenzyme essential to tissue respiration, lipid metabolism, and glycogenolysis. Vitamin deficiency causes pellagra, which manifests as dermatitis, diarrhea, and dementia; administration of niacin cures pellagra.
Antilipemic action: Mechanism of action is unknown. Nicotinic acid inhibits lipolysis in adipose tissue, decreases hepatic esterification of triglyceride, and increases lipoprotein lipase activity. It reduces serum cholesterol and triglyceride levels.
Vasodilative action: Niacin acts directly on peripheral vessels, dilating cutaneous vessels and increasing blood flow, predominantly in the face, neck, and chest.

PHARMACOKINETICS
Absorption: Niacin is absorbed rapidly from the GI tract. Plasma levels peak in 45 minutes. Cholesterol and triglyceride levels decrease after several days.
Distribution: Drug coenzymes are distributed widely in body tissues.
Metabolism: Drug is metabolized by the liver to active metabolites.
Excretion: Drug is excreted in urine.

CONTRAINDICATIONS & PRECAUTIONS
Contraindicated in patients with hepatic dysfunction, active peptic ulcer, severe hypotension, arterial hemorrhage, or hypersensitivity to drug. Use cautiously in patients with history of liver disease, peptic ulcer, allergy, gout, gallbladder disease, diabetes mellitus, or coronary artery disease.

INTERACTIONS
Drug-drug. Use with *aspirin* may decrease the metabolic clearance of nicotinic acid. Use with *sympathetic blockers* may cause added vasodilation and hypotension.

ADVERSE REACTIONS
Most reactions are dose-dependent.
CNS: tingling.
CV: *excessive peripheral vasodilation,* hypotension, atrial fibrillation, **flushing, arrhythmias.**
EENT: toxic amblyopia.
GI: *nausea, vomiting, diarrhea,* possible activation of peptic ulceration, epigastric or substernal pain.
Metabolic: hyperglycemia, hyperuricemia.
Hepatic: *hepatic dysfunction.*
Skin: pruritus, dryness.

Reactions may be *common,* uncommon, *life-threatening,* or COMMON AND LIFE-THREATENING.

KEY CONSIDERATIONS

• RDA of niacin in adult males is 19 mg; in adult females, 19 mg.
• For I.V. infusion, use concentration of 10 mg/ml or dilute in 500 ml normal saline solution; give slowly at a rate no faster than 2 mg/minute.
• I.V. administration of drug may cause fibrinolysis, metallic taste in mouth, and anaphylactic shock.
• Megadoses of drug aren't usually recommended.
• Monitor hepatic function and blood glucose levels during initial therapy.
• Aspirin may reduce flushing response.
• Drug therapy alters fluorometric test results for urine catecholamines and urine glucose test results using cupric sulfate (Benedict's reagent).

Patient education

• Explain the patient's disease and the rationale for therapy; stress that niacin isn't simply a vitamin, but a serious drug. Emphasize importance of complying with therapy.
• Instruct patient not to substitute sustained-release (timed) tablets for intermediate-release tablets in equivalent doses. Severe hepatic toxicity, including necrosis, may occur.
• Explain that cutaneous flushing and warmth commonly occur in the first 2 hours; they'll cease with continued therapy.
• Advise patient not to make sudden postural changes to minimize effects of postural hypotension.
• Instruct patient to avoid hot liquids when initially taking drug to reduce flushing response.
• Advise patient to take drug with meals to minimize GI irritation.

nicardipine hydrochloride
Cardene, Cardene SR

Calcium channel blocker, antianginal, antihypertensive

Available by prescription only
Capsules: 20 mg, 30 mg
Capsules (extended-release): 30 mg, 45 mg, 60 mg

Injection: 2.5 mg/ml in 10-ml ampules

INDICATIONS & DOSAGE
Hypertension; management of chronic stable angina
Adults: initially, 20 mg P.O. t.i.d. immediate-release capsules. Titrate dosage based on patient response. Usual dosage range, 20 to 40 mg t.i.d. Extended-release capsules (for hypertension only) can be initiated at 30 mg b.i.d. Usual dose, 30 to 60 mg b.i.d.
Short-term management of hypertension when oral therapy isn't feasible or possible
Adults: initially 5 mg/hour I.V. infusion; titrate infusion by 2.5 mg/hour q 15 minutes up to a maximum of 15 mg/hour, p.r.n.

PHARMACODYNAMICS
Antianginal and antihypertensive actions: Nicardipine inhibits the transmembrane flux of calcium ions into cardiac and smooth-muscle cells. Drug appears to act specifically on vascular muscle and may cause a smaller decrease in cardiac output than other calcium channel blockers because of its vasodilative effect.

PHARMACOKINETICS
Absorption: Nicardipine is completely absorbed after oral administration; absolute bioavailability is 35% because of first-pass metabolism. Plasma levels are detectable within 20 minutes and peak in about 1 hour. Food may decrease absorption. Therapeutic serum levels are 28 to 50 ng/ml.
Distribution: Drug is extensively (more than 95%) bound to plasma proteins.
Metabolism: A substantial first-pass effect reduces absolute bioavailability to about 35%. Drug is extensively metabolized in the liver, and the process is saturable. Increasing dosage yields nonlinear increases in plasma levels.
Excretion: Elimination half-life is about 8.6 hours after steady-state levels are reached.

CONTRAINDICATIONS & PRECAUTIONS
Contraindicated in patients with hypersensitivity to nicardipine and in those

with advanced aortic stenosis. Use cautiously in patients with impaired renal or hepatic function, cardiac conduction disturbances, hypotension, or heart failure.

INTERACTIONS
Drug-drug. Administration of *cimetidine* results in higher plasma nicardipine levels. Coadministration with *cyclosporine* results in increased plasma cyclosporine levels; careful monitoring is recommended. Serum *digoxin* levels should be carefully monitored because some calcium channel blockers may increase plasma levels of *cardiac glycosides*. Severe hypotension has been reported in patients taking calcium channel blockers who undergo *fentanyl* anesthesia.

ADVERSE REACTIONS
CNS: *dizziness, light-headedness, headache, paresthesia, asthenia.*
CV: *peripheral edema, palpitations, flushing,* angina, tachycardia.
GI: nausea, abdominal discomfort, dry mouth.
Skin: rash.

▣ KEY CONSIDERATIONS
Besides the recommendations relevant to all calcium channel blockers, consider the following:
• Allow at least 3 days between oral dosage changes to ensure achievement of steady-state plasma levels.
• When treating patients with chronic stable angina, S.L. nitroglycerin, prophylactic nitrate therapy, and beta blockers may be continued.
• When treating hypertension, monitor blood pressure during plasma level trough (about 8 hours after dose or immediately before subsequent doses). Because of prominent effects that may occur during peak plasma levels, measure blood pressure 1 to 2 hours after dose.
• In patients with hepatic dysfunction, therapy should begin at 20 mg P.O. b.i.d.; carefully titrate subsequent dosage based on patient response.
• Dilute solution in ampule before I.V. infusion; recommended dilution is 0.1 mg/ml in dextrose or saline solution.

• Monitor blood pressure during I.V. administration because nicardipine I.V. decreases peripheral resistance.

nicotine
Habitrol, Nicoderm, Nicotrol, Nicotrol NS, ProStep

Nicotinic cholinergic agonist, smoking cessation aid

Some forms available without prescription
Transdermal system: designed to release nicotine at a fixed rate
Habitrol: 21 mg/day, 14 mg/day, 7 mg/day
Nicoderm: 21 mg/day, 14 mg/day, 7 mg/day
Nicotrol: 15 mg/day, 10 mg/day, 5 mg/day
ProStep: 22 mg/day, 11 mg/day
Nasal spray: metered-spray pump
Nicotrol NS: 10 mg/ml
Available by prescription only
Nicotine inhaler cartridge containing 10 mg nicotine

INDICATIONS & DOSAGE
Relief of nicotine withdrawal symptoms in patients attempting smoking cessation
Adults: One transdermal system applied to nonhairy part of the upper trunk or upper outer arm. Dosage varies slightly from product to product.
Habitrol, Nicoderm
Initially, apply one 21-mg/day system daily for 6 weeks. After 24 hours, the system should be removed and a new system applied to a different site. Then taper dosage to 14 mg/day for 2 to 4 weeks. Finally, taper dosage to 7 mg/day if necessary. Nicotine substitution and gradual withdrawal should take 8 to 12 weeks.
✦ *Dosage adjustment.* Patients who weigh less than 45 kg (100 lb), have CV disease, or smoke less than half a pack of cigarettes daily should start therapy with the 14-mg/day system.
Nicotrol
Initially, apply one 15-mg/day system daily for 12 weeks. The system should

be applied on waking and removed at h.s. Then taper dosage to 10 mg/day for 2 weeks. Finally, taper dosage to 5 mg/day for 2 weeks if necessary. Alternatively, dosage may be reduced in patients who have successfully abstained from smoking q 2 to 4 weeks until 5-mg/day dosage has been used for 2 weeks. Nicotine substitution and gradual withdrawal should take 14 to 20 weeks.

Nicotrol NS
Adults: initially, 1 or 2 doses/hour (1 dose = 2 sprays—one in each nostril). Encourage patient to use at least the recommended minimum of 8 doses/day. Maximum recommended dose is 40 mg or 80 sprays/day. Duration of treatment shouldn't exceed 3 months.

Nicotrol Inhaler
Adults: Initial dose is 6 to 16 cartridges daily. Recommended treatment is up to 3 months and, if needed, gradual reduction over the next 6 to 12 weeks.

ProStep
Initially, apply one 22-mg/day system daily for 4 to 8 weeks. After 24 hours, system should be removed and a new system applied to a different site. In patients weighing less than 45 kg (100 lb), start therapy with the 11-mg/day system; those who have successfully stopped smoking during this period may discontinue drug. If therapy was initiated with the 22-mg/day system, treatment may continue for an additional 2 to 4 weeks at lower dosage (11 mg/day). Nicotine substitution and gradual withdrawal should take 6 to 12 weeks.

PHARMACODYNAMICS
Nicotinic cholinergic action: Nicotine transdermal system and nasal spray provide nicotine, the chief stimulant alkaloid found in tobacco products, which stimulates nicotinic acetylcholine receptors in the CNS, neuromuscular junction, autonomic ganglia, and adrenal medulla.

PHARMACOKINETICS
Absorption: Nicotine is rapidly absorbed.
Distribution: Drug is less than 5% bound by plasma protein.
Metabolism: Drug is metabolized in the liver, kidneys, and lungs. More than 20

metabolites have been identified; primary metabolites are cotinine (15%) and trans-3-hydroxycotinine (45%).
Excretion: Drug is excreted primarily in urine as metabolites; about 10% is excreted unchanged. With high urine flow rates or acidified urine, up to 30% can be excreted unchanged.

CONTRAINDICATIONS & PRECAUTIONS
Contraindicated in patients with hypersensitivity to nicotine or components. Also contraindicated in nonsmokers and in patients with recent MI, life-threatening arrhythmias, and severe or worsening angina pectoris.
Use cautiously in patients with hyperthyroidism, pheochromocytoma, type 1 diabetes mellitus, or peptic ulcer disease.

INTERACTIONS
Drug-drug. Cessation of smoking may decrease induction of hepatic enzymes responsible for metabolizing certain drugs, such as *acetaminophen, caffeine, imipramine, oxazepam, pentazocine, propranolol,* and *theophylline;* dosage reduction of such drugs may be necessary. Cessation of smoking may increase the amount of S.C. *insulin* absorbed and may require reduction of insulin dosage. Cessation of smoking may decrease levels of circulating catecholamines and may require lower doses of *adrenergic antagonists* (such as *labetalol, prazosin*) or higher doses of *adrenergic agonists* (such as *isoproterenol, phenylephrine*).

ADVERSE REACTIONS
CNS: somnolence, dizziness, *headache, insomnia,* paresthesia, abnormal dreams, nervousness.
CV: hypertension.
EENT: pharyngitis, sinusitis, *mouth and throat irritation* (with inhaler use).
Musculoskeletal: back pain, myalgia.
GI: abdominal pain, constipation, dyspepsia, nausea, diarrhea, vomiting, dry mouth.
Respiratory: *increased cough.*
Skin: *local or systemic erythema, pruritus, burning at application site,* cutaneous hypersensitivity, rash.
Other: diaphoresis.

▣ KEY CONSIDERATIONS

• Discourage use of transdermal system for more than 3 months. Long-term nicotine consumption by any route can be dangerous and habit forming.

• Each Nicotrol inhaler cartridge provides about 20 minutes of puffing, or about 80 deep draws or 300 shallow puffs. Best effect is achieved with continuous puffing. Patient must stop smoking completely before using the inhaler.

• Patients who can't stop cigarette smoking during the initial 4 weeks of therapy probably won't benefit from continued use of drug. Patients who are unsuccessful may benefit from counseling to identify factors that led to the unsuccessful attempt. Encourage patient to minimize or eliminate the factors that contributed to treatment failure and to try again, possibly after some interval before the next attempt.

• Health care workers' exposure to the nicotine in the transdermal systems should be minimal; however, avoid unnecessary contact with the system. After contact, wash hands with water alone because soap can enhance absorption.

• Nicotrol NS isn't recommended in patients with chronic nasal disorders or severe reactive airway disease.

Patient education

• Tell patient to discontinue use of patch and to call immediately if a generalized rash or persistent or severe local skin reactions (pruritus, edema, or erythema) occur.

• Make sure patient understands that nicotine can evaporate from the transdermal system once it's removed from its protective packaging. The patch shouldn't be altered (folded or cut) before it's applied. It should be applied promptly after removal of the system's protective packaging. Tell patient not to store patch at temperatures above 86°F (30°C).

• Teach patient how to dispose of transdermal system. After removal, fold the patch in half, bringing the adhesive sides together. If the system comes in a protective pouch, dispose of the used patch in the pouch that contained the new system. Careful disposal is necessary to prevent accidental poisoning of children or pets.

• Make sure that patient reads and understands the patient information that's dispensed with drug when the prescription is filled.

• Instruct patient to refrain from smoking while using the system; he may experience adverse effects from the increased nicotine levels.

• Explain that patient is likely to experience nasal irritation, which may become less bothersome with continued use of Nicotrol NS.

Overdose & treatment

• Signs and symptoms of overdose include those of acute nicotine poisoning, such as nausea, vomiting, diarrhea, weakness, respiratory failure, hypotension, and seizures.

• Treat symptomatically. Barbiturates or benzodiazepines may be used to treat seizures, and atropine may attenuate excessive salivation or diarrhea. Administer fluids to treat hypotension; increase urine flow to enhance elimination of drug.

---

nicotine polacrilex (nicotine resin complex)
Nicorette

Nicotinic agonist, smoking cessation aid

Available with and without prescription
Chewing gum: 2 mg and 4 mg of nicotine resin complex/square

INDICATIONS & DOSAGE

Aid in managing nicotine dependence
Serves as a temporary smoking-cessation aid for a smoker participating in a behavior modification program under medical supervision. Generally, a smoker with physical nicotine dependence is most likely to benefit from use of nicotine chewing gum.
Adults: Chew 1 piece of gum slowly and intermittently for 30 minutes whenever the urge to smoke occurs. Most patients require about 10 pieces of gum daily during 1st month. Patients using the 2-mg strength shouldn't exceed 30 pieces of gum daily; those using the 4-mg strength shouldn't exceed 20 pieces of gum daily.

Reactions may be *common,* uncommon, *life-threatening,* or COMMON AND LIFE-THREATENING.

PHARMACODYNAMICS
Nicotine replacement action: Nicotine is an agonist at the nicotinic receptors in the peripheral nervous system and CNS and produces both behavioral stimulation and depression. It acts on the adrenal medulla to help patients overcome physical dependence on nicotine as they stop smoking.

The CV effects of nicotine are usually dose dependent. Nonsmokers have experienced CNS-mediated signs and symptoms—including hiccuping, nausea, and vomiting—even with a small dose. Most smokers chewing a 2-mg piece of gum every hour don't experience CV adverse effects.

PHARMACOKINETICS
Absorption: Nicotine is bound to ion-exchange resin and is released only during chewing. The blood level depends on the vigor with which the gum is chewed.
Distribution: Distribution into tissues hasn't been fully characterized.
Metabolism: Drug is metabolized mainly in the liver and less so in the kidneys and lungs. The main metabolites are cotinine and nicotine-19-N-oxide.
Excretion: Both drug and its metabolites are excreted in urine, with 10% to 20% excreted unchanged. Acid urine and by high urine output increase excretion of drug.

CONTRAINDICATIONS & PRECAUTIONS
Contraindicated in nonsmokers and in patients with a recent MI, severe or worsening angina pectoris, life-threatening arrhythmias, or active temporomandibular joint disease.

Use cautiously in patients with hyperthyroidism, pheochromocytoma, type 1 diabetes mellitus, peptic ulcer disease, history of esophagitis, oral or pharyngeal inflammation, or dental conditions that might be exacerbated by chewing gum.

INTERACTIONS
Drug-drug. Dosages of *adrenergic agonists* or *adrenergic blockers* may need to be adjusted if used with nicotine polacrilex. Smoking may increase the metabolism of *caffeine, imipramine, penta-*

zocine, and *theophylline;* smoking cessation with nicotine polacrilex may reverse this effect. Nicotine polacrilex can increase circulating levels of *catecholamines* and *cortisol.* Smoking cessation agents may reduce the first-pass metabolism of *propoxyphene.*

ADVERSE REACTIONS
CNS: dizziness, light-headedness, irritability, insomnia, headache, paresthesia.
CV: atrial fibrillation.
EENT: throat soreness, jaw muscle ache (from chewing).
GI: nausea, vomiting, indigestion, eructation, anorexia, excessive salivation.
Respiratory: hiccups.
Other: sweating.

▣ KEY CONSIDERATIONS
• Inform patient that gum is sugar-free and usually doesn't stick to dentures.
• Patients most likely to benefit from drug are smokers with a high physical dependence. Typically, they smoke more than 15 cigarettes daily, prefer brands of cigarettes with high nicotine levels, usually inhale the smoke, smoke the first cigarette within 30 minutes of arising, and find the first morning cigarette the hardest to give up.
• Instruct patient to chew gum slowly and intermittently for about 30 minutes to promote slow and even buccal absorption of nicotine. Fast chewing allows faster absorption and produces more adverse reactions. After about 15 chews, temporarily stop chewing and leave the piece between the cheek and the gums.
• At the initial visit, instruct patient to chew one piece of gum whenever the urge to smoke occurs, instead of having a cigarette. Most patients will require about 10 pieces of gum daily during first month of treatment.
• Tell patient who has successfully abstained to gradually withdraw from gum use after 3 months; he shouldn't use gum for longer than 6 months.

Overdose & treatment
• The risk of overdose is minimized by the early nausea and vomiting that result from excessive nicotine intake. Poisoning manifests as nausea, vomiting, sali-

vation, abdominal pain, diarrhea, cold sweats, headache, dizziness, disturbed hearing and vision, mental confusion, and weakness.
• To treat overdose, induce vomiting with ipecac syrup. A sodium chloride cathartic speeds the gum's passage through the GI tract. Perform gastric lavage followed by activated charcoal in unconscious patients. Provide supportive treatment of respiratory paralysis and CV collapse as needed.

nifedipine
Adalat, Adalat CC, Procardia, Procardia XL

Calcium channel blocker, antianginal

Available by prescription only
Capsules: 10 mg, 20 mg
Tablets (extended-release): 30 mg, 60 mg, 90 mg

INDICATIONS & DOSAGE
Management of Prinzmetal's or variant angina or chronic stable angina pectoris
Adults: Starting dose is 10 mg P.O. t.i.d. Usual effective dosage range is 10 to 20 mg t.i.d. Some patients may require up to 30 mg q.i.d. Maximum daily dose for capsules is 180 mg; for extended-release tablets, 120 mg.
Hypertension
Adults: initially, 30 to 60 mg P.O. once daily (extended-release tablets). Adjust dosage at 7- to 14-day intervals based on patient tolerance and response. Maximum daily dosage is 120 mg.
◊ *Quick reduction of blood pressure*
Adults: 10 to 20 mg q 20 to 30 minutes; capsule should be bitten and then swallowed.

PHARMACODYNAMICS
Antianginal action: Nifedipine dilates systemic arteries, resulting in decreased total peripheral resistance and modestly decreased systemic blood pressure with a slightly increased heart rate, decreased afterload, and increased cardiac index. Reduced afterload and the subsequent

decrease in myocardial oxygen consumption probably account for drug's value in treating chronic stable angina. In Prinzmetal's angina, drug inhibits coronary artery spasm, increasing myocardial oxygen delivery.

PHARMACOKINETICS
Absorption: About 90% of dose is absorbed rapidly from the GI tract after oral administration; however, only 65% to 70% of drug reaches the systemic circulation because of a significant first-pass effect in the liver. Serum levels peak in ½ to 2 hours. Hypotensive effects may occur 5 minutes after S.L. administration. Therapeutic serum levels are 25 to 100 ng/ml.
Distribution: About 92% to 98% of circulating drug binds to plasma proteins.
Metabolism: Drug is metabolized in the liver.
Excretion: Inactive metabolites are excreted in urine and feces. Elimination half-life is 2 to 5 hours. Duration of effect ranges from 4 to 12 hours.

CONTRAINDICATIONS & PRECAUTIONS
Contraindicated in patients with hypersensitivity to nifedipine. Use cautiously in geriatric patients and in those with heart failure or hypotension. Use extended-release form cautiously in patients with GI narrowing. Use cautiously in patients with unstable angina who aren't currently taking a beta blocker because a higher incidence of MI has been reported.

INTERACTIONS
Drug-drug. Use of nifedipine with *beta blockers* may exacerbate angina, heart failure, and hypotension. *Cimetidine* may decrease metabolism of nifedipine and therefore increase nifedipine drug levels; use cautiously. Use with *digoxin* may cause increased serum digoxin levels. Use with *fentanyl* may cause excessive hypotension. Use with other *antihypertensives* may precipitate excessive hypotension. Drug may increase *phenytoin* levels.

Reactions may be *common,* uncommon, *life-threatening,* or COMMON AND LIFE-THREATENING.

ADVERSE REACTIONS

CNS: *dizziness, light-headedness, flushing, headache, weakness,* syncope, nervousness.

CV: *peripheral edema,* hypotension, palpitations, **heart failure, MI, pulmonary edema.**

EENT: nasal congestion.

GI: *nausea,* diarrhea, constipation, abdominal discomfort.

Hepatic: mild to moderate increase in serum levels of alkaline phosphate, LD, AST, and ALT.

Metabolic: hypokalemia.

Musculoskeletal: muscle cramps.

Respiratory: dyspnea, cough.

Skin: rash, pruritus.

Other: fever.

▣ KEY CONSIDERATIONS

• Use nifedipine cautiously in geriatric patients because they may be more sensitive to drug's effects and duration of effect may be prolonged.

• Initial doses or dosage increase may exacerbate angina briefly. Reassure patient that this symptom is temporary.

• Drug isn't available in S.L. form. No advantage has been found in S.L. or intrabuccal use.

• Monitor blood pressure regularly, especially if patient is also taking beta blockers or antihypertensives.

• Although rebound effect hasn't been observed when drug is stopped, reduce dosage slowly.

Patient education

• Instruct patient to swallow capsules whole without breaking, crushing, or chewing them unless instructed otherwise.

• Tell patient that he may experience hypotensive effects during dosage adjustment, and urge compliance with therapy.

Overdose & treatment

• Signs and symptoms of overdose are extensions of the pharmacologic effects of the drug, primarily peripheral vasodilation and hypotension.

• Treatment includes such basic support measures as hemodynamic and respiratory monitoring. If patient requires blood pressure support by a vasoconstrictor, norepinephrine may be administered. Extremities should be elevated and fluid deficit corrected.

---

nimodipine
Nimotop

Calcium channel blocker, cerebral vasodilator

Available by prescription only
Capsules: 30 mg

INDICATIONS & DOSAGE

Improvement of neurologic deficits after subarachnoid hemorrhage from ruptured congenital aneurysms
Adults: 60 mg P.O. q 4 hours for 21 days. Therapy should begin within 96 hours of subarachnoid hemorrhage.

◆ ***Dosage adjustment.*** In adults with hepatic impairment, give 30 mg P.O. q 4 hours.

◇ *Migraine headache*
Adults: 120 mg P.O. daily, 1 hour before or 2 hours after meals.

PHARMACODYNAMICS

Neuronal-sparing action: Nimodipine inhibits calcium ion influx across cardiac and smooth-muscle cells, thus decreasing myocardial contractility and oxygen demand, and dilates coronary arteries and arterioles. Although the action isn't completely known, it's believed that dilation of the small cerebral resistance vessels with increased collateral circulation is possible.

PHARMACOKINETICS

Absorption: Nimodipine is well absorbed after oral administration. However, because of extensive first-pass metabolism, bioavailability is only 3% to 30%.

Distribution: Drug is greater than 95% protein-bound.

Metabolism: Drug is extensively metabolized in the liver. Drug and metabolites undergo enterohepatic recycling.

Excretion: Less than 1% excreted as parent drug. Elimination half-life is 1 to 9 hours.

CONTRAINDICATIONS & PRECAUTIONS
No known contraindications. Use cautiously in patients with hepatic failure.

INTERACTIONS
Drug-drug. Use with *antihypertensives* may enhance the hypotensive effect; use with *calcium channel blockers* may enhance the CV effects of these drugs. Drug may increase *phenytoin* levels.

ADVERSE REACTIONS
CNS: headache, psychic disturbances.
CV: decreased blood pressure, flushing, edema, tachycardia.
GI: nausea, diarrhea, abdominal discomfort.
Musculoskeletal: muscle cramps.
Respiratory: dyspnea.
Skin: dermatitis, rash.

▣ KEY CONSIDERATIONS
Besides the recommendations relevant to all calcium channel blockers, consider the following:
• Unlike other calcium channel blockers, nimodipine isn't used for angina pectoris or hypertension.
• Use lower doses in patients with hepatic failure. Initiate therapy at 30 mg P.O. q 4 hours, and closely monitor blood pressure and heart rate.
• Monitor blood pressure and heart rate in all patients, especially during initiation of therapy.
• If patient can't swallow capsules, puncture the ends of liquid-filled capsule with an 18G needle and draw the contents into a syringe. Instill dose into patient's NG tube and rinse tube with 30 ml normal saline solution.
• When possible, give drug not less than 1 hour before or 2 hours after meals.

Patient education
• Advise patient to rise from supine position slowly to avoid dizziness and hypotension, especially at beginning of therapy.

Overdose & treatment
• Signs and symptoms of overdose include nausea, weakness, drowsiness, confusion, bradycardia, and decreased cardiac output.

• Treatment should be supportive. Administer pressor amines to counter hypotension; use cardiac pacing, atropine, or sympathomimetics to treat bradycardia. Calcium gluconate I.V. has been used to treat calcium channel blocker overdose.

---

nisoldipine
Sular

Calcium channel blocker, antihypertensive

Available by prescription only
Tablets (extended-release): 10 mg, 20 mg, 30 mg, 40 mg

INDICATIONS & DOSAGE
Hypertension
Adults: initially, 20 mg P.O. once daily, then increased by 10 mg/week or at longer intervals, p.r.n. Usual maintenance dosage, 20 to 40 mg once daily. Don't exceed 60 mg daily.
Geriatric patients: Give starting dose of 10 mg P.O. once daily. Monitor blood pressure closely during dosage adjustment.
✦ *Dosage adjustment.* For those with hepatic dysfunction, give starting dose of 10 mg P.O. once daily. Monitor blood pressure closely during dosage adjustment.

PHARMACODYNAMICS
Antihypertensive action: Nisoldipine is a member of the dihydropyridine class of calcium channel blockers. Drug prevents the entry of calcium ions into vascular smooth-muscle cells, thereby causing dilation of the arterioles, which in turn decreases peripheral vascular resistance.

PHARMACOKINETICS
Absorption: Nisoldipine is relatively well absorbed from the GI tract. High-fat foods significantly affect release of drug from the coat-core formulation. Bioavailability is about 5%.
Distribution: Drug is about 99% bound to plasma protein.
Metabolism: Drug is extensively metabolized, with five major metabolites identified.

Reactions may be *common*, uncommon, **life-threatening**, or COMMON AND LIFE-THREATENING.

Excretion: Drug is excreted in urine; half-life is from 7 to 12 hours.

CONTRAINDICATIONS & PRECAUTIONS

Contraindicated in patients with hypersensitivity to dihydropyridine calcium channel blockers. Use cautiously in patients receiving beta blockers or in those who have compromised ventricular or hepatic function and heart failure.

INTERACTIONS

Drug-drug. *Cimetidine* increases bioavailability (rate or extent of absorption) and peak level of nisoldipine. *Quinidine* decreases bioavailability but not peak level of nisoldipine.

Drug-food. *Grapefruit juice* and *high-fat meals* can increase drug levels. Don't give together.

ADVERSE REACTIONS

CNS: *headache,* dizziness.
CV: vasodilation, palpitations, chest pain.
EENT: pharyngitis, sinusitis.
GI: nausea.
Skin: rash.
Other: *peripheral edema.*

▣ KEY CONSIDERATIONS

● Geriatric patients may have twofold to threefold higher plasma levels than younger patients, which requires cautious dosing.

● Monitor patient carefully. Some patients, especially those with severe obstructive coronary artery disease, have developed increased frequency, duration, or severity of angina or even acute MI after initiation of calcium channel blocker therapy or at time of dosage increase.

● Monitor blood pressure regularly, especially during initial administration and adjustment of nisoldipine.

● Patients with cirrhosis should have lower strengths and maintenance doses because plasma levels are higher in patients with cirrhosis.

Patient education

● Tell patient to take nisoldipine exactly as prescribed, even if he feels well.

● Instruct patient to swallow tablet whole and not to chew, divide, or crush tablets.

● Tell patient not to take drug with a high-fat meal or with grapefruit products.

● Advise patient to rise slowly from supine position to avoid dizziness and hypotension, especially at beginning of therapy.

● Tell patient not to stop taking drug abruptly.

---

nitrofurantoin
Furadantin

nitrofurantoin macrocrystals
Macrobid, Macrodantin

Nitrofuran, urinary tract anti-infective

Available by prescription only
Macrocrystals
Capsules: 25 mg, 50 mg, 100 mg
Capsules (dual-release): 100 mg
Microcrystals
Suspension: 25 mg/5 ml

INDICATIONS & DOSAGE

Initial or recurrent urinary tract infections caused by susceptible organisms
Adults: 50 to 100 mg P.O. q.i.d. or 100 mg dual-release capsules q 12 hours.

Long-term suppression therapy
Adults: 50 to 100 mg P.O. daily at h.s. as a single dose.

PHARMACODYNAMICS

Antibacterial action: Nitrofurantoin has bacteriostatic action with low levels and possible bactericidal action with high levels. Although exact mechanism of action is unknown, it may inhibit bacterial enzyme systems, interfering with bacterial carbohydrate metabolism. Drug is most active at an acidic pH.

Drug's spectrum of activity includes many common gram-positive and gram-negative urine pathogens, including *Escherichia coli, Staphylococcus aureus,* enterococci, and certain strains of *Klebsiella* and *Enterobacter.* Organisms that usually resist nitrofurantoin include *Pseudomonas, Acinetobacter, Serratia, Providencia,* and *Proteus* species.

PHARMACOKINETICS

Absorption: When administered orally, nitrofurantoin is well absorbed (mainly by the small intestine) from GI tract. Food aids drug dissolution and speeds absorption. The macrocrystal form exhibits slower dissolution and absorption and causes less GI distress.

Distribution: Drug crosses into bile; 60% binds to plasma proteins. Plasma half-life is about 20 minutes. Urine levels peak in about 30 minutes when drug is given as microcrystals and somewhat later when given as macrocrystals.

Metabolism: Drug is metabolized partially in the liver.

Excretion: About 30% to 50% of dose is eliminated through glomerular filtration and tubular secretion into urine as unchanged drug within 24 hours.

CONTRAINDICATIONS & PRECAUTIONS

Contraindicated in patients with moderate to severe renal impairment, anuria, oliguria, or creatinine clearance less than 60 ml/minute.

Use cautiously in patients with impaired renal function, anemia, diabetes mellitus, electrolyte abnormalities, vitamin B deficiency, debilitating disease, or G6PD deficiency.

INTERACTIONS

Drug-drug. *Anticholinergics* enhance bioavailability of nitrofurantoin by slowing GI motility, thereby increasing the drug dissolution and absorption. Use with *magnesium trisilicate antacids* may decrease nitrofurantoin absorption. *Probenecid* and *sulfinpyrazone* reduce renal excretion of nitrofurantoin, leading to increased serum and decreased urine nitrofurantoin levels: Increased serum levels may lead to increased toxicity; decreased urine levels may reduce the antibacterial effectiveness of the drug. Use with *quinolone derivatives*—including *cinoxacin, ciprofloxacin, nalidixic acid,* and *norfloxacin*—may antagonize the anti-infective effects of the drug.

Drug-food. *Food* enhances bioavailability of drug by slowing GI motility, thereby increasing the drug dissolution and absorption.

ADVERSE REACTIONS

CNS: *peripheral neuropathy,* headache, dizziness, drowsiness, *ascending polyneuropathy* (with high doses or renal impairment).

GI: *anorexia, nausea, vomiting,* abdominal pain, *diarrhea.*

Hematologic: hemolysis in patients with G6PD deficiency (reversed after stopping drug), agranulocytosis, thrombocytopenia.

Hepatic: hepatitis, hepatic necrosis.

Respiratory: pulmonary sensitivity reactions (cough, chest pain, fever, chills, dyspnea, pulmonary infiltration with consolidation or pleural effusion), asthma attacks in patients with history of asthma.

Skin: maculopapular, erythematous, or eczematous eruption; pruritus; urticaria; *exfoliative dermatitis;* Stevens-Johnson syndrome; transient alopecia.

Other: hypersensitivity reactions *(anaphylaxis),* drug fever, overgrowth of nonsusceptible organisms in the urinary tract.

▣ KEY CONSIDERATIONS

- Serum glucose levels may be decreased; bilirubin and alkaline phosphatase levels may be elevated.
- Obtain culture and sensitivity tests before starting therapy; repeat as needed.
- Oral suspension may be mixed with water, milk, fruit juice, and formulas.
- Monitor CBC regularly.
- Monitor fluid intake and output and pulmonary status.
- Nitrofurantoin may turn urine brown or rust yellow.
- Continue treatment for at least 3 days after sterile urine specimens have been obtained.
- Long-term therapy may cause overgrowth of nonsusceptible organisms, especially *Pseudomonas* species.
- Drug may cause false-positive results in urine glucose tests using cupric sulfate reagents (such as Benedict's test, Fehling's test, or Clinitest) because it reacts with these reagents.

Patient education

- Instruct patient to take nitrofurantoin with food or milk to minimize GI distress.

Reactions may be *common,* uncommon, **life-threatening,** or COMMON AND LIFE-THREATENING.

• Caution patient that drug may cause false-positive results in urine glucose tests using cupric sulfate reduction method (Clinitest), but not in glucose oxidase test (glucose enzymatic test strip, Diastix, or Chemstrip uG).
• Emphasize that bedtime dose is important because drug remains in the bladder longer.
• Warn patient that drug may turn urine brown or rust yellow.
• Instruct patient to notify health care provider if fever, chills, cough, chest pain, difficulty breathing, skin rash, numbness or tingling of fingers or toes, or intolerable GI upset occurs.

nitroglycerin (glyceryl trinitrate)
Oral, extended-release
Niong, Nitro-Bid, Nitroglyn, Nitrong, Nitrong SR*, Nitrocine

S.L.
Nitrostat

Translingual
Nitrolingual

I.V.
Nitro-Bid IV, Tridil

Topical
Nitro-Bid, Nitrol

Transdermal
Deponit, Minitran, Nitro-Derm, Nitrodisc, Nitro-Dur, Transderm-Nitro

Transmucosal
Nitrogard

Nitrate, antianginal, vasodilator

Available by prescription only
Tablets (sustained-release): 2.6 mg, 6.5 mg, 9 mg
Tablets (S.L.): 0.15 mg, 0.3 mg, 0.4 mg, 0.6 mg
Tablets (buccal, controlled-release): 1 mg, 2 mg, 3 mg
Capsules (sustained-release): 2.5 mg, 6.5 mg, 9 mg, 13 mg
Aerosol (lingual): 0.4 mg/metered spray

I.V.: 0.5 mg/ml, 0.8 mg/ml, 5 mg/ml
I.V. premixed solutions in dextrose: 100 mcg/ml, 200 mcg/ml, 400 mcg/ml
Topical: 2% ointment
Transdermal: 0.1-mg/hour, 0.2-mg/hour, 0.3-mg/hour, 0.4-mg/hour, 0.6-mg/hour systems

INDICATIONS & DOSAGE
Prophylaxis against chronic angina attacks
Adults: One sustained-release capsule q 8 to 12 hours, or 2% ointment. Start with ½" ointment, increasing by ½" increments until headache occurs, then decreasing to previous dose. Range of dosage with ointment is 2" to 5". Usual dose is 1" to 2". Alternatively, transdermal disc or pad may be applied to hairless site once daily. However, to prevent tolerance, topical forms shouldn't be worn overnight.
Relief of acute angina pectoris, prophylaxis to prevent or minimize angina attacks when taken immediately before stressful events
Adults: one S.L. tablet dissolved under the tongue or in the buccal pouch immediately on indication of angina attack. May repeat q 5 minutes for 15 to 30 minutes, for a maximum of 3 doses. Or use Nitrolingual spray, spray 1 or 2 doses into mouth, preferably onto or under the tongue. May repeat q 3 to 5 minutes to a maximum of 3 doses within a 15-minute period. Or transmucosally, use 1 to 3 mg q 3 to 5 hours during waking hours.
Hypertension, heart failure, angina
Nitroglycerin is indicated to control hypertension from surgery, to treat heart failure from a MI, to relieve angina pectoris in acute situations, and to produce controlled hypotension during surgery (by I.V. infusion).
Adults: Initial infusion rate is 5 mcg/minute. May be increased by 5 mcg/minute q 3 to 5 minutes until a response is noted. If a 20-mcg/minute rate doesn't produce desired response, dosage may be increased by as much as 20 mcg/minute q 3 to 5 minutes.
◊ *Hypertensive crisis*
Adults: Infuse at 5 to 100 mcg/minute.

PHARMACODYNAMICS

Antianginal action: Nitroglycerin relaxes vascular smooth muscle of both the venous and arterial beds, resulting in a net decrease in myocardial oxygen consumption. It also dilates coronary vessels, leading to redistribution of blood flow to ischemic tissue. The systemic and coronary vascular effects of the drug (which may vary slightly with the various nitroglycerin forms) probably account for its value in treating angina.

Vasodilative action: Drug dilates peripheral vessels, making it useful (in I.V. form) in producing controlled hypotension during surgical procedures and in controlling blood pressure in perioperative hypertension. Because peripheral vasodilation decreases venous return to the heart (preload), drug also helps treat pulmonary edema and heart failure. Arterial vasodilation decreases arterial impedance (afterload), thereby decreasing left ventricular work and aiding the failing heart. These combined effects may prove valuable in treating some patients with an acute MI.

PHARMACOKINETICS

Absorption: Nitroglycerin is well absorbed from the GI tract. However, because of first-pass metabolism in the liver, it's incompletely absorbed into the systemic circulation. Onset of action for oral preparations is slow (except for S.L. tablets). After S.L. administration, absorption from the oral mucosa is relatively complete. Drug also is well absorbed after topical administration as an ointment or transdermal system. Onset of action varies as follows: I.V., 1 to 2 minutes; S.L., 1 to 3 minutes; translingual, 2 minutes; transmucosal, 3 minutes; topical, 20 to 60 minutes; P.O. (sustained-release), 40 minutes; transdermal, 40 to 60 minutes.

Distribution: Drug is distributed widely throughout the body; about 60% of circulating drug binds to plasma proteins.

Metabolism: Drug is metabolized in the liver and serum to 1,3 glyceryl dinitrate; 1,2 glyceryl dinitrate; and glyceryl mononitrate. Dinitrate metabolites have a slight vasodilative effect.

Excretion: Metabolites are excreted in urine; elimination half-life is 1 to 4 minutes. Duration of effect varies as follows: I.V., 3 to 5 minutes; S.L., up to 30 minutes; translingual, 30 to 60 minutes; transmucosal, 5 hours; topical, 3 to 6 hours; P.O. (sustained-release), 4 to 8 hours; transdermal, 18 to 24 hours.

CONTRAINDICATIONS & PRECAUTIONS

Contraindicated in patients with hypersensitivity to nitrates and in those with early MI (S.L. form), severe anemia, increased intracranial pressure, angle-closure glaucoma, orthostatic hypotension, and allergy to adhesives (transdermal form). I.V. form is contraindicated in patients with hypersensitivity to I.V. form, cardiac tamponade, restrictive cardiomyopathy, or constrictive pericarditis. Extended-release preparations shouldn't be used in patients with organic or functional GI hypermotility or malabsorption syndrome. Contraindicated in patients taking sildenafil, which potentiates the hypotensive effect of nitrates.

Use cautiously in patients with hypotension or volume depletion.

INTERACTIONS

Drug-drug. Use of nitroglycerin with *antihypertensives, phenothiazines,* or *sildenafil* may cause additive hypotensive effects. Use with *ergot alkaloids* may precipitate angina; oral nitroglycerin may increase the bioavailability of ergot alkaloids.

Drug-lifestyle. Use of nitroglycerin with *alcohol* may cause additive hypotensive effects.

ADVERSE REACTIONS

CNS: headache, sometimes with throbbing; dizziness; weakness.

CV: *orthostatic hypotension, tachycardia,* flushing, *palpitations,* fainting.

GI: nausea, vomiting.

Skin: cutaneous vasodilation, contact dermatitis (patch), rash.

Other: hypersensitivity reactions, S.L. burning.

🔲 KEY CONSIDERATIONS

• Nitroglycerin may interfere with serum cholesterol levels using the Zlatkis-Zak color reaction, resulting in falsely decreased values.

• Verify that patient isn't taking sildenafil to avoid a potentially fatal decrease in blood pressure.

• Use only S.L. and translingual forms to relieve acute angina attack.

• To apply ointment, spread in uniform thin layer to hairless part of skin, except distal parts of arms or legs, because absorption won't be maximal at these sites. Don't rub in. Cover with plastic film to aid absorption and to protect clothing. If using Tape-Surrounded Appli-Ruler (TSAR) system, keep TSAR on skin to protect patient's clothing and make sure ointment remains in place. If serious adverse effects develop in patients using ointment or transdermal system, remove product at once or wipe ointment from skin. Be sure to avoid contact with ointment.

• Administration as I.V. infusion requires special nonabsorbent tubing supplied by manufacturer because regular plastic tubing may absorb up to 80% of drug. Infusion should be prepared in glass bottle or container.

• If drug causes headache (especially likely with initial doses), aspirin or acetaminophen may be indicated. Dosage may need to be reduced temporarily.

• S.L. dose may be administered before anticipated stress or at bedtime if angina is nocturnal.

• Drug may cause orthostatic hypotension. To minimize this, patient should change to upright position slowly, go up and down stairs carefully, and lie down at the first sign of dizziness.

• When administering drug to patient during initial days after an acute MI, monitor hemodynamic and clinical status carefully.

• Monitor blood pressure and intensity and duration of patient's response to drug.

• Remove transdermal patch before defibrillation. Because of patch's aluminum backing, electric current may cause patch to explode.

• When terminating transdermal nitroglycerin treatment for angina, gradually reduce dosage and frequency of application over 4 to 6 weeks.

• To prevent withdrawal symptoms, reduce dosage gradually after long-term use of oral or topical preparations.

• Store drug in cool, dark place in tightly closed container. To ensure freshness, replace supply of S.L. tablets every 3 months. Remove cotton from container because it absorbs drug.

Patient education

• Instruct patient to take the drug regularly, as prescribed, and to keep S.L. form accessible at all times. Nitroglycerin is physiologically necessary but not addictive.

• Teach patient to take oral tablet on empty stomach, either 30 minutes before or 1 to 2 hours after meals; to swallow oral tablets whole; and to chew chewable tablets thoroughly before swallowing.

• Instruct patient to take S.L. tablet at first sign of angina attack. Tell him to wet tablet with saliva, place it under the tongue until completely absorbed, and sit down and rest. If he feels no relief after three tablets, he should call an ambulance and go to the emergency department. If he complains of tingling sensation with drug placed S.L., he may try holding tablet in buccal pouch.

• Advise patient to store S.L. tablets in original container or other container specifically approved for this use away from heat and light. Keep bottle cap tightly closed.

• Instruct patient to place transmucosal tablet under upper lip or in buccal pouch, to let the tablet dissolve slowly, and not to chew or swallow it. Advise him that dissolution rate may increase if he touches tablet with tongue or drinks hot liquids.

• If patient is receiving nitroglycerin lingual aerosol (Nitrolingual), instruct him how to use this device correctly. Remind him not to inhale spray but to release it onto or under the tongue. Also, tell him to wait about 10 seconds before swallowing after administering the spray.

• Caution patient to use care when wearing transdermal patch near microwave oven because leaking radiation may heat the metallic backing of the patch and cause burns.

• Warn patient that headache may follow initial doses, but that this symptom may respond to usual headache remedies or dosage reduction (however, dose should be reduced only with medical approval). Assure patient that headache usually subsides gradually with continued treatment.

• Instruct patient to avoid alcohol while taking drug because severe hypotension and CV collapse may occur.

• Warn patient that drug may cause dizziness or flushing and to move to an upright position slowly.

• Tell patient to report blurred vision, dry mouth, or persistent headache.

Overdose & treatment

• Signs and symptoms of overdose result primarily from vasodilation and methemoglobinemia. They include hypotension, persistent throbbing headache, palpitations, visual disturbances, flushed skin, sweating (with skin later becoming cold and cyanotic), nausea and vomiting, colic, bloody diarrhea, orthostasis, initial hyperpnea, dyspnea, slow respiratory rate, bradycardia, heart block, increased intracranial pressure with confusion, fever, paralysis, tissue hypoxia (from methemoglobinemia) leading to cyanosis, and metabolic acidosis, coma, clonic seizures, and circulatory collapse. Death may result from circulatory collapse or asphyxia.

• Treatment includes gastric lavage followed by administration of activated charcoal to remove remaining gastric contents. ABG measurements and methemoglobin levels should be monitored, as indicated. Supportive care includes respiratory support and oxygen administration, passive movement of the extremities to aid venous return, and recumbent positioning.

---

nitroprusside sodium
Nipride*, Nitropress

Vasodilator, antihypertensive

Available by prescription only

Injection: 50 mg/2-ml and 50 mg/5-ml vials

INDICATIONS & DOSAGE
Hypertensive emergencies
Adults: I.V. infusion titrated to blood pressure, with a range of 0.3 to 10 mcg/kg/minute. Maximum infusion rate is 10 mcg/kg/minute for 10 minutes.
Acute heart failure
Adults: I.V. infusion titrated to cardiac output and systemic blood pressure. Same dosage range as for hypertensive emergencies.

PHARMACODYNAMICS
Antihypertensive action: Nitroprusside acts directly on vascular smooth muscle, causing peripheral vasodilation.

PHARMACOKINETICS
Absorption: Nitroprusside is administered by I.V. route; blood pressure is reduced almost immediately.
Distribution: Unknown.
Metabolism: Drug is metabolized rapidly in erythrocytes and tissues to a cyanide radical and then converted to thiocyanate in the liver.
Excretion: Excreted primarily as metabolites in the urine. Blood pressure returns to pretreatment level 1 to 10 minutes after infusion is completed.

CONTRAINDICATIONS & PRECAUTIONS
Contraindicated in patients with hypersensitivity to drug, compensatory hypertension (such as in arteriovenous shunt or coarctation of the aorta), inadequate cerebral circulation, congenital optic atrophy, or tobacco-induced amblyopia.

Use cautiously in patients with renal or hepatic disease, increased intracranial pressure, hypothyroidism, hyponatremia, or low vitamin B_{12} levels. Contraindicated in patients who recently received sildenafil because of hypotensive effects.

INTERACTIONS
Drug-drug. *General anesthetics,* particularly *enflurane* and *halothane,* may potentiate the antihypertensive effects of the drug. Nitroprusside may potentiate antihypertensive effects of other *antihypertensives. Pressor drugs* such as *epi-*

nephrine may cause an increase in blood pressure during nitroprusside therapy. Patients who have recently taken *sildenafil* have a profound potentiation of hypotensive effects of nitroprusside.

ADVERSE REACTIONS

CNS: *headache, dizziness,* loss of consciousness, apprehension, ***increased intracranial pressure,*** *restlessness.*
CV: ***bradycardia,*** hypotension, tachycardia, palpitations, ECG changes.
GI: *nausea, abdominal pain,* ileus.
GU: possibly increased serum creatinine levels.
Musculoskeletal: *muscle twitching.*
Skin: pink color, flushing, rash, *diaphoresis.*
Other: acidosis, ***thiocyanate toxicity, methemoglobinemia, cyanide toxicity,*** venous streaking, irritation at infusion site, hypothyroidism.

▣ KEY CONSIDERATIONS

● Geriatric patients may be more sensitive to antihypertensive effects of nitroprusside.
● Check blood pressure at least every 5 minutes at start of infusion and every 15 minutes thereafter during infusion.
● Prepare solution using D_5W solution; don't use bacteriostatic water for injection or sterile sodium chloride solution for reconstitution; because of light sensitivity, foil-wrap I.V. solution (but not tubing). Fresh solutions have faint brownish tint; discard after 24 hours.
● Use infusion pump to administer drug.
● Drug is best given piggyback through a peripheral line with no other drugs; don't adjust rate of main I.V. line while drug is running because even small boluses can cause severe hypotension.
● Drug can cause cyanide toxicity; check serum thiocyanate levels every 72 hours. Levels greater than 100 µg/ml are associated with cyanide toxicity, which can produce profound hypotension, metabolic acidosis, dyspnea, ataxia, and vomiting. If such signs and symptoms occur, discontinue infusion and reevaluate therapy.
● Drug may be used to produce controlled hypotension during anesthesia

and to reduce bleeding from surgical procedure.
● Hypertensive patients are more sensitive to drug than normotensive patients. Also, patients taking other antihypertensives are extremely sensitive to nitroprusside. Drug has been used in patients with an acute MI, refractory heart failure, and severe mitral regurgitation.

Patient education
● Instruct patient to report CNS symptoms (such as headache or dizziness) promptly.

Overdose & treatment
● Signs and symptoms of overdose include the adverse reactions previously listed and increased tolerance to antihypertensive effects of nitroprusside.
● Treat overdose by giving nitrites to induce methemoglobin formation. Discontinue drug and administer amyl nitrite inhalations for 15 to 30 seconds each minute until a 3% sodium nitrite solution can be prepared. Administer amyl nitrite cautiously to minimize risk of additional hypotension secondary to vasodilation. Then administer the sodium nitrite solution by I.V. infusion at a rate not exceeding 2.5 to 5 ml/minute, up to a total dose of 10 to 15 ml. Follow with I.V. sodium thiosulfate infusion (12.5 g/ 50 ml of D_5W solution) over 10 minutes. If necessary, repeat infusions of sodium nitrite and sodium thiosulfate at half the initial doses. Further treatment involves symptomatic and supportive care.

nizatidine
Axid, Axid AR

H₂-receptor antagonist, antiulcerative

Available by prescription only
Capsules: 150 mg, 300 mg
Available without prescription
Capsules: 75 mg

INDICATIONS & DOSAGE
Treatment of active duodenal ulcer
Adults: 300 mg P.O. once daily h.s. Alternatively, may give 150 mg P.O. b.i.d.

Maintenance therapy for patients with duodenal ulcer
Adults: 150 mg P.O. once daily h.s.
Gastroesophageal reflux disease
Adults: 150 mg P.O. b.i.d.
Heartburn
Adults: One 75-mg capsule P.O. ½ hour before meals; use up to b.i.d.
✦ *Dosage adjustment.* For adults with renal failure, refer to the table.

Creatinine clearance (ml/min)	Dosage for active duodenal ulcer	Maintenance dosage
20-50	150 mg/day	150 mg q other day
< 20	150 mg q other day	150 mg q 3 days

PHARMACODYNAMICS
Antiulcerative action: Nizatidine is a competitive, reversible inhibitor of H_2 receptors, particularly those in the gastric parietal cells.

PHARMACOKINETICS
Absorption: Nizatidine is well absorbed (more than 90%) after oral administration. Absorption may be slightly enhanced by food and slightly impaired by antacids.
Distribution: About 35% of drug is bound to plasma protein. Plasma levels peak ½ to 3 hours after dose is administered.
Metabolism: Drug probably undergoes hepatic metabolism. About 40% of excreted drug is metabolized; the remainder is excreted unchanged.
Excretion: More than 90% of oral dose is excreted in urine within 12 hours. Renal clearance is about 500 ml/minute, which indicates excretion via active tubular secretion. Less than 6% of administered dose is eliminated in feces. Elimination half-life is 1 to 2 hours. Moderate to severe renal impairment significantly prolongs half-life and decreases clearance of drug. In anephric persons, half-life is 3½ to 11 hours; plasma clearance is 7 to 14 L/hour.

CONTRAINDICATIONS & PRECAUTIONS
Contraindicated in patients hypersensitive to H_2-receptor antagonists. Use cautiously in patients with impaired renal function.

INTERACTIONS
Drug-drug. Because nizatidine doesn't inhibit the cytochrome P-450–linked drug metabolizing enzyme system, drug interactions mediated by inhibition of hepatic metabolism aren't expected. Use of high doses of *aspirin* (3,900 mg/day) with nizatidine (150 mg b.i.d.) increases serum salicylate levels.

ADVERSE REACTIONS
CNS: somnolence.
Hematologic: eosinophilia.
Hepatic: hepatocellular injury, elevated liver function test results.
Skin: *diaphoresis,* rash, urticaria.
Other: hyperuricemia, fever.

▣ KEY CONSIDERATIONS
● False-positive test results for urobilinogen may occur during nizatidine therapy.
● Safety and efficacy in geriatric patients appear similar to those in younger patients; however, consider that geriatric patients have reduced renal function.
● Because drug is excreted primarily from the kidneys, reduce dosage in patients with moderate to severe renal insufficiency.
● Drug is partially metabolized in the liver. In patients with normal renal function and uncomplicated hepatic dysfunction, the disposition of drug is similar to that in patients with normal hepatic function.
● For patients on maintenance therapy, consider that effects of continuous drug therapy for longer than 1 year are unknown.

Patient education
● Advise patient not to smoke because this may increase gastric acid secretion and worsen the disease.

Overdose & treatment
● Signs and symptoms of overdose are cholinergic, including lacrimation, salivation, vomiting, miosis, and diarrhea.
● Treatment may include use of activated charcoal, induced vomiting, or gastric

---

Reactions may be *common,* uncommon, *life-threatening,* or COMMON AND LIFE-THREATENING.

lavage with monitoring and supportive therapy.

norepinephrine bitartrate (formerly levarterenol bitartrate)
Levophed

Direct-acting adrenergic, vasopressor

Available by prescription only
Injection: 1 mg/ml parenteral

INDICATIONS & DOSAGE
To maintain blood pressure in acute hypotensive states
Adults: initially, 8 to 12 mcg/minute I.V. infusion, then titrated to maintain desired blood pressure; maintenance dosage, 2 to 4 mcg/minute.
◇ GI bleeding
Adults: 8 mg/250 ml normal saline solution given intraperitoneally, or 8 mg/100 ml normal saline solution given via NG tube q 1 hour for 6 to 8 hours, then q 2 hours for 4 to 6 hours.

PHARMACODYNAMICS
Vasopressor action: Norepinephrine acts predominantly by direct stimulation of alpha-adrenergic receptors, constricting both capacitance and resistance blood vessels. This results in increased total peripheral resistance; increased systolic and diastolic blood pressure; decreased blood flow to vital organs, skin, and skeletal muscle; and constriction of renal blood vessels, which reduces renal blood flow. It also has a direct stimulating effect on $beta_1$ receptors of the heart, producing a positive inotropic response. Its main therapeutic effects are vasoconstriction and cardiac stimulation.

PHARMACOKINETICS
Absorption: Pressor effect occurs rapidly after infusion, is of short duration, and stops within 1 to 2 minutes after infusion has stopped.
Distribution: Norepinephrine localizes in sympathetic nerve tissues. It doesn't cross the blood-brain barrier.

Metabolism: Drug is metabolized in the liver and other tissues to inactive compounds.
Excretion: Excreted in urine primarily as sulfate and glucuronide conjugates. A small amount is excreted unchanged in urine.

CONTRAINDICATIONS & PRECAUTIONS
Contraindicated in patients with mesenteric or peripheral vascular thrombosis, profound hypoxia, hypercapnia, or hypotension resulting from blood volume deficit and during cyclopropane and halothane anesthesia.

Use cautiously in patients with sulfite allergies or in those receiving MAO inhibitors or triptyline- or imipramine-type antidepressants.

INTERACTIONS
Drug-drug. Use with *atropine* blocks the reflex bradycardia caused by norepinephrine and enhances its pressor effects. Use with *beta blockers* may result in an increased potential for hypertension. (Propranolol may be used to treat arrhythmias occurring during norepinephrine administration.) Use with *furosemide* or other *diuretics* may decrease arterial responsiveness. When used with *general anesthetics,* norepinephrine may cause increased arrhythmias; when used with *guanethidine, MAO inhibitors, methyldopa, parenteral ergot alkaloids, some antihistamines,* and *tricyclic antidepressants,* norepinephrine may cause severe, prolonged hypertension.

ADVERSE REACTIONS
CNS: anxiety, weakness, dizziness, tremor, restlessness, insomnia.
CV: bradycardia, *severe hypertension, arrhythmias.*
Respiratory: respiratory difficulties, *asthmatic episodes.*
Other: *anaphylaxis,* irritation or necrosis with extravasation.

▣ KEY CONSIDERATIONS
Besides the recommendations relevant to all adrenergics, consider the following:
• Geriatric patients are more sensitive to the effects of norepinephrine. Decreased

---

cardiac output may be harmful to geriatric patients with poor cerebral or coronary circulation.
• Correct blood volume depletion before administration. Drug isn't a substitute for blood, plasma, fluid, or electrolyte replacement.
• Select injection site carefully. Administration by I.V. infusion requires an infusion pump or other device to control flow rate. If possible, infuse into antecubital vein of the arm or the femoral vein. Change injection sites for prolonged therapy. Must be diluted before use with D_5W or normal saline solution. (Dilution with normal saline solution alone isn't recommended.) Monitor infusion rate. Withdraw drug gradually; recurrent hypotension may follow abrupt withdrawal.
• Prepare infusion solution by adding 4 mg drug to 1 L D_5W. The resulting solution contains 4 mcg/ml.
• To treat extravasation, infiltrate site promptly with 10 to 15 ml normal saline solution containing 5 to 10 mg of phentolamine, using a fine needle.
• To prevent sloughing should extravasation occur, some health care providers add 5 to 10 mg of phentolamine to each liter of infusion solution.
• Monitor intake and output. Drug reduces renal blood flow, which may cause decreased urine output initially.
• Monitor patient constantly during drug administration. Obtain baseline blood pressure and pulse before therapy, and repeat every 2 minutes until stabilization; repeat every 5 minutes during drug administration.
• In addition to vital signs, monitor patient's mental state, skin temperature of extremities, and skin color (especially earlobes, lips, and nail beds).
• In patients with previously normal blood pressure, adjust flow rate to maintain blood pressure at low normal (usually 80 to 100 mm Hg systolic); in hypertensive patients, maintain systolic no more than 40 mm Hg below preexisting pressure level.
• Protect solution from light. Discard solution that's discolored or contains a precipitate.

Patient education
• Inform patient of need for frequent monitoring of vital signs.
• Tell patient to report adverse reactions.

Overdose & treatment
• Signs and symptoms of overdose include severe hypertension, photophobia, retrosternal or pharyngeal pain, intense sweating, vomiting, cerebral hemorrhage, seizures, and arrhythmias. Monitor vital signs closely.
• Use supportive and symptomatic measures. Use atropine for reflex bradycardia, phentolamine for extravasation, and propranolol for tachyarrhythmias.

norfloxacin (systemic)
Noroxin

Fluoroquinolone, broad-spectrum antibiotic

Available by prescription only
Tablets: 400 mg

INDICATIONS & DOSAGE
Complicated and uncomplicated urinary tract infections caused by various gram-negative and gram-positive bacteria
Adults: For complicated infection, 400 mg P.O. b.i.d. for 10 to 21 days; for uncomplicated infection, 400 mg P.O. b.i.d. for 3 to 10 days. Don't exceed 800 mg/day. Patients with creatinine clearance less than 30 ml/minute should receive 400 mg/day for appropriate duration of therapy.
Uncomplicated gonorrhea
Adults: 800 mg P.O. as a single dose.
Prostatitis
Adults: 400 mg P.O. q 12 hours for 28 days.
◊ *Gastroenteritis*
Adults: 400 mg P.O. b.i.d. for 5 days.
◊ *Treatment of traveler's diarrhea*
Adults: 400 mg P.O. b.i.d. for up to 3 days.

PHARMACODYNAMICS
Antibacterial action: Norfloxacin is generally bactericidal. It inhibits DNA gyrase, blocking DNA synthesis. Spectrum

---

Reactions may be *common,* uncommon, *life-threatening,* or COMMON AND LIFE-THREATENING.

of activity includes most aerobic gram-positive and gram-negative urinary pathogens, including *Pseudomonas aeruginosa.*

PHARMACOKINETICS
Absorption: About 30% to 40% of dose is absorbed from the GI tract (as dose increases, percentage of absorbed drug decreases). Food may reduce absorption.
Distribution: Norfloxacin is distributed into renal tissue, liver, gallbladder, prostatic fluid, testicles, seminal fluid, bile, and sputum. About 10% to 15% binds to plasma proteins.
Metabolism: Unknown.
Excretion: Most systemically absorbed drug is excreted from the kidneys, with about 30% appearing in feces. In patients with normal renal function, plasma half-life is 3 to 4 hours; with severe renal impairment, up to 8 hours.

CONTRAINDICATIONS & PRECAUTIONS
Contraindicated in patients with hypersensitivity to fluoroquinolones. Use cautiously in patients with renal impairment or conditions predisposing them to seizure disorders, such as cerebral arteriosclerosis.

INTERACTIONS
Drug-drug. Use with *antacids* isn't recommended by manufacturer. *Multivitamins* containing *divalent* or *trivalent cations* may interfere with the absorption of norfloxacin. Use with *nitrofurantoin* antagonizes antibacterial activity of norfloxacin. *Probenecid* may increase serum norfloxacin levels. Norfloxacin may prolong PT in patients also receiving *warfarin* therapy. Use with *xanthine derivatives*—such as *aminophylline* and *theophylline*—may increase theophylline levels and the risk for xanthine-related toxic effects.
Drug-food. *Food* interferes with the absorption of norfloxacin.

ADVERSE REACTIONS
CNS: fatigue, somnolence, headache, dizziness, *seizures,* depression, insomnia.
GI: nausea, constipation, flatulence, heartburn, dry mouth, abdominal pain, diarrhea, vomiting, anorexia.

GU: increased serum creatinine and BUN levels, crystalluria.
Hematologic: decreased hematocrit, eosinophilia, neutropenia.
Hepatic: transient elevations of AST, ALT, and alkaline phosphatase levels.
Musculoskeletal: back pain, tendinitis.
Skin: photosensitivity.
Other: hypersensitivity reactions (rash, *anaphylactoid reaction*), fever, hyperhidrosis.

▣ KEY CONSIDERATIONS
• Obtain culture and sensitivity tests before starting therapy; repeat as needed throughout therapy.
• Make sure patient is well hydrated before and during therapy to avoid crystalluria.
• Arrange for baseline and follow-up BUN, creatinine clearance, CBC, and liver function tests.
• Evaluate patient for signs and symptoms of resistant infection or reinfection.

Patient education
• Instruct patient to continue taking norfloxacin as directed, even if he feels better.
• Advise patient to take drug 1 hour before or 2 hours after meals and antacids.
• Warn patient that drug may cause dizziness and impaired ability to perform tasks that require alertness and coordination.
• Instruct patient to avoid excessive exposure to sunlight.

nortriptyline hydrochloride
Aventyl, Pamelor

Tricyclic antidepressant

Available by prescription only
Capsules: 10 mg, 25 mg, 50 mg, 75 mg
Solution: 10 mg/5 ml (4% alcohol)

INDICATIONS & DOSAGE
Depression, ◇ panic disorder
Adults: 25 mg P.O. t.i.d. or q.i.d., gradually increasing to a maximum of 150 mg/day. Alternatively, entire dosage may be given h.s.
Geriatric patients: 30 to 50 mg P.O. daily or in divided doses.

PHARMACODYNAMICS

Antidepressant action: Nortriptyline is thought to inhibit reuptake of norepinephrine and serotonin in CNS nerve terminals (presynaptic neurons), which results in increased levels and enhanced activity of these neurotransmitters in the synaptic cleft. Drug inhibits reuptake of serotonin more actively than norepinephrine; it's less likely than other tricyclic antidepressants to cause orthostatic hypotension.

PHARMACOKINETICS

Absorption: Nortriptyline is absorbed rapidly from the GI tract after oral administration.
Distribution: Drug is distributed widely into the body, including CNS. It's 95% protein-bound. Plasma levels peak within 8 hours after a given dose; steady-state serum levels, within 2 to 4 weeks. Therapeutic serum level ranges from 50 to 150 ng/ml.
Metabolism: Drug is metabolized in the liver; a significant first-pass effect may account for variability of serum levels in different patients taking the same dosage.
Excretion: Drug is mostly excreted in urine; some excreted in feces via the biliary tract.

CONTRAINDICATIONS & PRECAUTIONS

Contraindicated during acute recovery phase of a MI and in patients with hypersensitivity to nortriptyline or MAO inhibitor therapy within past 14 days.

Use cautiously in patients with history of urine retention or seizures, glaucoma, suicidal tendencies, CV disease, or hyperthyroidism and in those receiving thyroid drugs.

INTERACTIONS

Drug-drug. Use with *antiarrhythmics (disopyramide, procainamide,* or *quinidine), pimozide,* or *thyroid drugs* may increase incidence of arrhythmias and conduction defects. *Barbiturates* induce nortriptyline metabolism and decrease therapeutic efficacy; *haloperidol* and *phenothiazines* decrease its metabolism, decreasing therapeutic efficacy; *beta blockers, cimetidine, methylphenidate, oral contraceptives,* and *propoxyphene* may inhibit nortriptyline metabolism, increasing plasma levels and toxicity. Drug may decrease hypotensive effects of *centrally acting antihypertensives,* such as *clonidine, guanabenz, guanadrel, guanethidine, methyldopa,* and *reserpine.* Use with *disulfiram* or *ethchlorvynol* may cause delirium and tachycardia. Use with *sympathomimetics*—including *ephedrine* (found in many nasal sprays), *epinephrine, phenylephrine,* and *phenylpropanolamine*—may increase blood pressure. Use with *warfarin* may increase PT and cause bleeding.

Additive effects are likely after use with the following drugs: *atropine* and other *anticholinergics,* including *antihistamines, antiparkinsonians, meperidine,* and *phenothiazines* (oversedation, paralytic ileus, visual changes, and severe constipation); *CNS depressants,* including *analgesics, anesthetics, barbiturates, narcotics,* and *tranquilizers* (oversedation); and *metrizamide* (increased risk of seizures).
Drug-lifestyle. Use of drug with *alcohol* may cause additive effects. *Smoking* decreases therapeutic efficacy.

ADVERSE REACTIONS

CNS: *drowsiness, dizziness, **seizures,*** tremor, weakness, confusion, headache, nervousness, EEG changes, extrapyramidal reactions, insomnia, nightmares, hallucinations, paresthesia, ataxia, agitation.
CV: *tachycardia,* conduction disturbances, hypertension, hypotension, heart block.
EENT: *blurred vision,* tinnitus, mydriasis.
GI: dry mouth, *constipation,* nausea, vomiting, anorexia, paralytic ileus.
GU: *urine retention.*
Hematologic: bone marrow depression, ***agranulocytosis,*** eosinophilia, ***thrombocytopenia.***
Skin: rash, urticaria, photosensitivity.
Other: *diaphoresis,* hypersensitivity reaction.
After abrupt withdrawal of long-term therapy: nausea, headache, malaise.

Reactions may be *common,* uncommon, *life-threatening*, or COMMON AND LIFE-THREATENING.

▣ KEY CONSIDERATIONS

Besides the recommendations relevant to all tricyclic antidepressants, consider the following:

• Geriatric patients are at greater risk for adverse cardiac effects. Lower dosages may be indicated.

• Nortriptyline is less likely than other tricyclic antidepressants to cause orthostatic hypotension.

• Drug may be administered at bedtime to reduce daytime sedation. Tolerance to sedative effects usually develops over the initial weeks of therapy.

• Withdraw drug gradually over a few weeks; however, it should be discontinued at least 48 hours before surgical procedures.

• Drug is available in liquid form.

• In patients with bipolar disorders, drug may cause symptoms of the manic phase.

Patient education

• Inform patient that full effects of nortriptyline therapy may not be seen for up to 4 weeks after start of therapy.

• Warn patient about sedative effects.

• Recommend taking full daily dose at bedtime to prevent daytime sedation.

• Instruct patient to avoid drinking alcoholic beverages, double dosing after missed dose, and discontinuing drug abruptly, unless instructed.

• Warn patient about possible dizziness. Tell patient to lie down for about 30 minutes after each dose at start of therapy and to avoid sudden postural changes to avoid dizziness. Orthostatic hypotension is usually less severe than with amitriptyline.

• Urge patient to report unusual reactions promptly, such as confusion, movement disorders, fainting, rapid heartbeat, or difficulty urinating.

• Tell patient to store drug away from children.

• Suggest relieving dry mouth with sugarless chewing gum or candy.

• Advise patient to avoid activities that require physical and mental alertness, such as driving a car or operating machinery.

Overdose & treatment

• The first 12 hours after acute ingestion are a stimulatory phase characterized by excessive anticholinergic activity (agitation, irritation, confusion, hallucinations, hyperthermia, parkinsonian signs and symptoms, seizures, urine retention, dry mucous membranes, pupillary dilation, constipation, and ileus). This is followed by CNS depressant effects, including hypothermia, decreased or absent reflexes, sedation, hypotension, cyanosis, and cardiac irregularities, including tachycardia, conduction disturbances, and quinidine-like effects on the ECG.

• Severity of overdose is best indicated by prolonged QRS complex beyond 100 milliseconds, which usually indicates a serum level greater than 1,000 ng/ml. Metabolic acidosis may follow hypotension, hypoventilation, and seizures.

• Treatment is symptomatic and supportive, including maintaining a patent airway, stable body temperature, and fluid and electrolyte balance. Induce vomiting with ipecac syrup if patient is conscious; follow with gastric lavage and activated charcoal to prevent further absorption. Dialysis is usually ineffective.

• Consider using cardiac glycosides or physostigmine if serious CV abnormalities or cardiac failure occurs. Treat seizures with parenteral diazepam or phenytoin; arrhythmias with parenteral phenytoin or lidocaine; and acidosis with sodium bicarbonate. Don't use quinidine, procainamide, or disopyramide to treat arrhythmias because these may further depress myocardial conduction and contractility. Don't give barbiturates; they may enhance CNS and respiratory depressant effects.

---

nystatin
Mycostatin, Nilstat, Nystex

Polyene macrolide, antifungal

Available by prescription only
Tablets: 500,000 U
Suspension: 100,000 U/ml
Vaginal suppositories: 100,000 U
Cream: 100,000 U/g
Ointment: 100,000 U/g
Powder: 100,000 U/g
Lozenges: 200,000 U

INDICATIONS & DOSAGE

GI infections
Adults: 500,000 to 1 million U as oral tablets, t.i.d.

Oral, vaginal, and intestinal infections caused by susceptible organisms
Adults: 500,000 to 1 million U of oral suspension t.i.d. for oral candidiasis. Alternatively, give 200,000 to 400,000 U (lozenges) four to five times daily; allow to dissolve in mouth.

Cutaneous or mucocutaneous candidal infections
Topical use: Apply to affected area b.i.d. or t.i.d. until healing is complete.
Vaginal use: 100,000 U, as vaginal tablets, inserted high into vagina daily or b.i.d. for 14 days.

PHARMACODYNAMICS

Antifungal action: Nystatin is both fungistatic and fungicidal. It binds to sterols in the fungal cell membrane, altering its permeability and allowing leakage of intracellular components. It acts against various yeasts and fungi, including *Candida albicans.*

PHARMACOKINETICS

Absorption: Nystatin isn't absorbed from the GI tract or through intact skin or mucous membranes.
Distribution: None.
Metabolism: None.
Excretion: Oral drug is excreted almost entirely unchanged in feces.

CONTRAINDICATIONS & PRECAUTIONS

Contraindicated in patients with hypersensitivity to nystatin.

ADVERSE REACTIONS

GI: transient nausea, diarrhea (usually with large oral dosage), vomiting (with oral administration or vaginal tablets).
Skin: occasional contact dermatitis from preservatives in some forms (with topical administration or vaginal tablets).

◙ KEY CONSIDERATIONS

• Avoid hand contact with nystatin; hypersensitivity is rare but can occur.
• For treatment of oral candidiasis, patient should have clean mouth and should hold suspension in mouth for several minutes before swallowing.
• May give immunosuppressed patient vaginal tablets (100,000 U) orally to provide prolonged drug contact with oral mucosa; alternatively, use clotrimazole troche.
• For candidiasis of the feet, patient should dust powder on shoes, stockings, and feet for maximal contact and effectiveness.
• Avoid occlusive dressings or ointment on moist covered body areas that favor yeast growth.
• To prevent maceration, use cream on intertriginous areas and powder on moist lesions.
• Clean affected skin gently before topical application; cool, moist compresses applied for 15 minutes between applications help soothe dry skin.
• Douches may be used; use only preparations that don't contain antibacterials, which may alter flora and promote reinfection.
• Protect drug from light, air, and heat.
• Drug is ineffective in systemic fungal infection.

Patient education
• Teach patient signs and symptoms of candidal infection. Inform patient about predisposing factors: drugs (antibiotics, oral contraceptives, and corticosteroids), diabetes, infected sexual partners, and tight-fitting pantyhose and undergarments.
• Teach good oral hygiene. Explain that overuse of mouthwash and poorly fitting dentures, especially in geriatric patients, may alter flora and promote infection.
• Emphasize importance of washing vaginal applicator thoroughly after each use.
• Advise patient to change stockings and undergarments daily; teach good skin care.
• Tell patient to continue nystatin for at least 48 hours after symptoms clear, to prevent reinfection.

Reactions may be *common,* uncommon, *life-threatening,* or COMMON AND LIFE-THREATENING.

O

ofloxacin
Floxin, Ocuflox

Fluoroquinolone, antibiotic

Available by prescription only
Tablets: 200 mg, 300 mg, 400 mg
Injection: 200 mg/50 ml D_5W; 400 mg
in water for injection in 10-ml and 20-ml
single-use vials; 400 mg/100 ml D_5W
Ophthalmic solution: 0.3%

INDICATIONS & DOSAGE
Conjunctivitis caused by known organism
Adults: Instill 1 or 2 gtt in conjunctival
sac q 2 to 4 hours while awake for first 2
days, then q.i.d. for up to 5 additional
days.
Acute bacterial exacerbations of chronic bronchitis and pneumonia caused by susceptible organisms, mild to moderate skin and skin-structure infections, and community-acquired pneumonia
Adults: 400 mg P.O. or I.V. q 12 hours
for 10 days.
Sexually transmitted diseases, such as acute uncomplicated urethral and cervical gonorrhea, nongonococcal urethritis and cervicitis, and mixed infections of urethra and cervix
Adults: for acute uncomplicated gonorrhea, 400 mg P.O. or I.V. once as a single
dose; for cervicitis and urethritis,
300 mg P.O. or I.V. q 12 hours for 7
days.
Urinary tract infections
Adults: for cystitis caused by *Escherichia coli* or *Klebsiella pneumoniae,*
200 mg P.O. or I.V. q 12 hours for 3
days; for cystitis caused by other organisms, 200 mg P.O. or I.V. q 12 hours for
7 days.
Complicated urinary tract infections
Adults: 200 mg P.O. or I.V. q 12 hours
for 10 days.
Prostatitis
Adults: 300 mg P.O. or I.V. q 12 hours
for 6 weeks.
◊***Adjunct in* Brucella *infections***
Adults: 400 mg P.O. daily.

◊***Peritonitis in patients receiving continuous ambulatory peritoneal dialysis***
Adults: 400 mg P.O. loading dose, then
300 mg P.O. daily for 7 to 10 days.
◊***Typhoid fever***
Adults: 200 to 400 mg P.O. q 12 hours
for 7 to 14 days.
◊***Prevention of tuberculosis***
Adults: 300 mg P.O. daily.
◊***Treatment of postoperative sternotomy or soft-tissue wounds caused by* Mycobacterium fortuitum**
Adults: 300 to 600 mg P.O. daily for 3 to
6 months.
◊***Leprosy***
Adults: 400 mg P.O. daily for 8 weeks.
◊***Acute Q fever pneumonia***
Adults: 600 mg P.O. daily for up to 16
days.
◊***Mediterranean spotted fever***
Adults: 200 mg P.O. q 12 hours for 7
days.
✦ ***Dosage adjustment.*** In patients with
renal failure and creatinine clearance of
50 ml/minute or less, adjust dosage.
Give initial dose as recommended; additional doses as follows: If creatinine
clearance is 10 to 50 ml/minute, no
dosage adjustment at 24-hour intervals;
if less than 10 ml/minute, 50% of recommended dose q 24 hours. Maximum
daily dose in patients with hepatic function disorders is 400 mg.

PHARMACODYNAMICS
Antibacterial action: Ofloxacin interferes with DNA gyrase, which is needed
for synthesis of bacterial DNA.

PHARMACOKINETICS
Absorption: Ofloxacin is well absorbed
after oral administration, with maximum
serum levels within 1 to 2 hours. Because the oral bioavailability is about
98%, oral and I.V. dosages are the same.
Distribution: Drug is widely distributed
to body tissues and fluids.
Metabolism: Less than 10% of a single
dose is metabolized.
Excretion: About 70% to 80% is excreted unchanged in urine; less than 5% in
feces.

CONTRAINDICATIONS & PRECAUTIONS

Contraindicated in patients with hypersensitivity to ofloxacin or other fluoroquinolones. Use oral and I.V. forms cautiously in patients with seizure disorders, CNS diseases (such as cerebral arteriosclerosis), hepatic disorders, or renal failure.

INTERACTIONS

Drug-drug. Administration with *antacids* interferes with GI absorption of ofloxacin, resulting in decreased serum levels; separate administration by 2 to 4 hours. Ofloxacin taken with *antidiabetics* may affect blood glucose levels, causing hypoglycemia or hyperglycemia. Therapy with *theophylline* may prolong theophylline half-life, increase serum theophylline levels, and increase the risk for theophylline-related adverse effects; monitor closely and adjust theophylline dosage as needed. Patients receiving *warfarin* may have a prolonged PT or INR.
Drug-lifestyle. *Sun exposure* may cause a photosensitivity reaction; take appropriate precautions.

ADVERSE REACTIONS

CNS: dizziness; headache, fatigue, lethargy, malaise, drowsiness, sleep disorders, nervousness, insomnia, visual disturbances, *seizures* (with oral or I.V. form).
CV: chest pain, phlebitis (with oral or I.V. form).
EENT: *transient ocular burning or discomfort,* stinging, redness, itching, photophobia, lacrimation, eye dryness (with ophthalmic form).
GI: *nausea, pseudomembranous colitis,* anorexia, abdominal pain or discomfort, diarrhea, vomiting, constipation, dry mouth, flatulence, dysgeusia (with oral or I.V. form).
GU: vaginitis, vaginal discharge, genital pruritus (with oral or I.V. form).
Hepatic: elevated liver enzyme levels.
Metabolic: increased blood glucose levels.
Skin: rash, pruritus, photosensitivity (with oral or I.V. form).
Other: trunk pain (with oral or I.V. form), hypersensitivity reactions *(anaphylactoid reaction),* fever.

◙ KEY CONSIDERATIONS

● Periodically assess organ system functions during prolonged therapy.
● Give I.V. ofloxacin by slow infusion only; don't give I.M., S.C., intrathecally, or by intraperitoneal injection. Administer over at least 60 minutes and avoid rapid or bolus injection. Compatible with most common I.V. solutions, including D_5W injection, normal saline injection, dextrose 5% in normal saline injection, dextrose 5% in half-normal saline injection, 5% dextrose in lactated Ringer's solution, and 5% sodium bicarbonate injection.
● Drug isn't recommended for treatment of syphilis.

Patient education

● Advise patient to drink fluids liberally.
● Instruct patient to separate doses of antacids, vitamins, and ofloxacin by 2 hours.
● Advise patient to take on an empty stomach, ½ hour before or 2 hours after meals.
● Tell patient dizziness and light-headedness may occur. Advise caution when driving or operating hazardous machinery until effects of drug are known.
● Warn patient that hypersensitivity reactions may follow first dose. Instruct patient to discontinue drug at first sign of rash or other allergic reaction and notify health care provider immediately.
● Advise patient to avoid prolonged exposure to direct sunlight and to use a sunscreen when outdoors.

olanzapine
Zyprexa

Thienobenzodiazepine derivative, antipsychotic

Available by prescription only
Tablets: 2.5 mg, 5 mg, 7.5 mg, 10 mg

INDICATIONS & DOSAGE
Management of signs and symptoms of psychotic disorders
Adults: initially, 5 to 10 mg P.O. once daily. Adjust dosage in 5-mg daily increments at intervals of not less than 1

Reactions may be *common,* uncommon, *life-threatening,* or COMMON AND LIFE-THREATENING.

week. Most patients respond to 10 mg/day; don't exceed 20 mg/day.

PHARMACODYNAMICS
Antipsychotic action: Mechanism of action is unknown. Acts as an antagonist at dopamine (D_{1-4}) and serotonin (5-$HT_{2A/2C}$) receptors; may also exhibit antagonist binding at adrenergic, cholinergic, and histaminergic receptors.

PHARMACOKINETICS
Absorption: Olanzapine levels peak about 6 hours after oral dose. Food doesn't affect rate or extent of absorption. About 40% of dose is eliminated by first-pass metabolism.
Distribution: Drug is extensively distributed throughout the body, with a volume of distribution of about 1,000 L. Drug is 93% protein-bound, primarily to albumin and alpha$_1$-acid glycoprotein.
Metabolism: Direct glucuronidation and cytochrome P-450–mediated oxidation.
Excretion: About 57% of drug excreted in urine and 30% in feces as metabolites. Only 7% of dose is recovered in the urine unchanged. Elimination half-life ranges from 21 to 54 hours.

CONTRAINDICATIONS & PRECAUTIONS
Contraindicated in patients with known hypersensitivity to olanzapine. Use cautiously in patients with heart disease, cerebrovascular disease, conditions that predispose to hypotension (gradual adjustment of dosage minimizes the risk), history of seizures or conditions that might lower the seizure threshold, and hepatic impairment. Also, use cautiously in geriatric patients, in those with history of paralytic ileus, significant prostatic hyperplasia, or angle-closure glaucoma, or those at risk for aspiration pneumonia.

INTERACTIONS
Drug-drug. *Antihypertensives* and *diazepam* may potentiate hypotensive effects; monitor blood pressure closely. Coadministration with *carbamazepine, omeprazole,* and *rifampin* may cause increased clearance of olanzapine; monitor patient. Use with *dopamine agonists* or *levodopa* may cause antagonized effects of these drugs; monitor patient. *Fluvoxamine* may inhibit olanzapine elimination.
Drug-lifestyle. *Alcohol* may potentiate hypotensive effects.

ADVERSE REACTIONS
CNS: *somnolence, agitation, insomnia, headache, nervousness, hostility, parkinsonism, dizziness,* anxiety, personality disorder, *akathisia,* hypertonia, tremor, amnesia, articulation impairment, euphoria, stuttering, dystonic or dyskinetic events, tardive dyskinesia, neck rigidity, twitching.
CV: orthostatic hypotension, tachycardia, chest pain, hypotension, edema.
EENT: amblyopia, blepharitis, corneal lesion.
GI: constipation, dry mouth, abdominal pain, increased appetite, increased salivation, nausea, vomiting, thirst.
GU: hematuria, metrorrhagia, urinary incontinence, urinary tract infection.
Metabolic: weight gain or loss.
Musculoskeletal: joint pain, extremity pain, back pain.
Respiratory: *rhinitis,* increased cough, pharyngitis, dyspnea.
Skin: vesiculobullous rash.
Other: fever, intentional injury, flulike syndrome, suicide attempt.

▣ KEY CONSIDERATIONS
• Olanzapine may cause asymptomatic increases in ALT, AST, GGT, serum prolactin, and CK levels and eosinophil count.
• Drug may be initiated at lower dose because drug clearance may be decreased. Half-life is 1.5 times greater in geriatric patients.
• Monitor patient for signs of neuroleptic malignant syndrome (hyperpyrexia, muscle rigidity, altered mental status, autonomic instability), a rare but frequently fatal adverse reaction that can occur with the administration of antipsychotics. Drug should be stopped immediately and patient monitored and treated.
• Initiate therapy with 5 mg in patients who are debilitated; predisposed to hypotension; who have an alteration in metabolism because of smoking status, sex, or age; or who are pharmacologically sensitive to drug.

• Efficacy for long-term use (more than 6 weeks) hasn't been established.
• Obtain baseline and periodic liver function tests.

Patient education

• Warn patient to avoid hazardous tasks until adverse CNS effects of olanzapine are known.
• Caution patient against exposure to extreme heat; drug may impair body's ability to reduce core temperature.
• Instruct patient to avoid alcohol.
• Tell patient to rise slowly to avoid orthostatic hypotension.
• Advise patient to use ice chips or sugarless candy or gum to relieve dry mouth.
• Inform patient not to take prescription or OTC drugs without medical approval because of potential drug interactions.

Overdose & treatment

• Signs and symptoms of overdose may include drowsiness and slurred speech.
• No specific antidote to olanzapine exists; treatment should be symptomatic. Monitor patient for hypotension, circulatory collapse, obtundation, seizures, or dystonic reactions. Gastric lavage with activated charcoal and sorbitol may be effective. Dialysis doesn't remove drug from circulation. Avoid epinephrine, dopamine, or other sympathomimetics with beta-agonist activity.

olsalazine sodium
Dipentum

Salicylate, anti-inflammatory

Available by prescription only
Capsules: 250 mg

INDICATIONS & DOSAGE
Maintenance of remission of ulcerative colitis in patients intolerant of sulfasalazine
Adults: 1 g P.O. daily in two divided doses.

PHARMACODYNAMICS
Anti-inflammatory action: Mechanism of action is unknown but appears to be topical rather than systemic. Olsalazine is converted to mesalamine (5-aminosalicylic acid; 5-ASA) in the colon. Presumably, 5-ASA diminishes inflammation by blocking cyclooxygenase and inhibiting prostaglandin production in the colon.

PHARMACOKINETICS
Absorption: After oral administration, about 2.4% of a single dose is absorbed; maximum levels appear in about 2 hours.
Distribution: Once metabolized to 5-ASA, olsalazine is absorbed slowly from the colon, resulting in very high local levels.
Metabolism: About 0.1% is metabolized in the liver; remainder will reach the colon, where it's rapidly converted to 5-ASA by colonic bacteria.
Excretion: Less than 1% is recovered in urine.

CONTRAINDICATIONS & PRECAUTIONS
Contraindicated in patients hypersensitive to salicylates. Use cautiously in patients with renal disease.

INTERACTIONS
Drug increases PT and INR in patients taking *warfarin.*

ADVERSE REACTIONS
CNS: headache, depression, vertigo, dizziness, fatigue.
GI: *diarrhea,* nausea, *abdominal pain,* dyspepsia, bloating, anorexia, stomatitis.
Musculoskeletal: arthralgia.
Skin: rash, itching.

KEY CONSIDERATIONS
• Diarrhea was noted in 17% of patients, but it's difficult to distinguish from underlying condition.
• Monitor CBC with differential and liver function tests periodically.

Patient education
• Advise patient to take olsalazine with food and in evenly divided doses.
• Inform patient to call if diarrhea develops.

Reactions may be *common,* uncommon, *life-threatening,* or COMMON AND LIFE-THREATENING.

omeprazole
Prilosec

Substituted benzimidazole, gastric acid suppressant

Available by prescription only
Capsules (delayed-release): 10 mg, 20 mg

INDICATIONS & DOSAGE
Active duodenal ulcer
Adults: 20 mg P.O. daily for 4 to 8 weeks.
Helicobacter pylori *eradication to reduce the risk of duodenal ulcer recurrence*
Triple therapy (omeprazole/clarithromycin/amoxicillin)
Adults: 20 mg P.O. b.i.d. plus 500 mg clarithromycin P.O. b.i.d. plus 1,000 mg amoxicillin P.O. b.i.d. for 10 days. In patients with an ulcer present at the time of initiation of therapy, an additional 18 days of omeprazole 20 mg once daily is recommended alone for ulcer healing and symptom relief.
Note: Refer to entries on clarithromycin and amoxicillin.
Dual therapy (omeprazole/clarithromycin)
Adults: 40 mg each morning plus 500 mg clarithromycin t.i.d. for 14 days, followed by 14 days of omeprazole 20 mg daily.
Note: Refer to entry on clarithromycin.
Severe erosive esophagitis; symptomatic, poorly responsive gastroesophageal reflux disease (GERD)
Adults: 20 mg P.O. daily for 4 to 8 weeks. Patients with GERD should have failed initial therapy with an H_2 antagonist.
Pathological hypersecretory conditions (such as Zollinger-Ellison syndrome)
Adults: Initial dosage is 60 mg P.O. daily; adjust dosage based on patient response. Administer daily dosages exceeding 80 mg in divided doses. Doses up to 120 mg t.i.d. have been administered. Continue therapy as long as indicated.
Gastric ulcer
Adults: 40 mg P.O. daily for 4 to 8 weeks.

PHARMACODYNAMICS
Antisecretory action: Omeprazole inhibits the activity of the acid (proton) pump, H^+/K^+ adenosine triphosphatase, located at the secretory surface of the gastric parietal cell. This blocks the formation of gastric acid.

PHARMACOKINETICS
Absorption: Omeprazole is acid labile, and the formulation contains enteric-coated granules that permit absorption after drug leaves the stomach. Absorption is rapid; levels peak in less than 3½ hours. Bioavailability is about 40% because of instability in gastric acid and a substantial first-pass effect. Bioavailability increases slightly with repeated dosing, possibly because of the effect of the drug on gastric acidity.
Distribution: Drug is about 95% protein-bound.
Metabolism: Drug is metabolized primarily in the liver.
Excretion: Drug is excreted primarily in the kidneys. Plasma half-life is ¼ to 1 hour, but drug effects may persist for days.

CONTRAINDICATIONS & PRECAUTIONS
Contraindicated in patients hypersensitive to omeprazole or its components.

INTERACTIONS
Drug-drug. Elimination of *drugs metabolized by hepatic oxidation*—including *diazepam, phenytoin,* and *warfarin*—may be impaired by omeprazole; patients taking these drugs or other *drugs metabolized by the hepatic microsomal enzyme system,* including *propranolol* and *theophylline,* should be monitored closely. *Drugs that depend on low gastric pH for absorption*—including *ampicillin esters, iron derivatives, itraconazole,* and *ketoconazole* —may exhibit poor bioavailability in patients taking omeprazole.

ADVERSE REACTIONS
CNS: headache, dizziness, asthenia.
GI: diarrhea, abdominal pain, nausea, vomiting, constipation, flatulence, increased serum gastrin levels in most patients during first 2 weeks of therapy.

Musculoskeletal: back pain.
Respiratory: cough, upper respiratory tract infection.
Skin: rash.

▣ KEY CONSIDERATIONS

• Omeprazole increases its own bioavailability with repeated administration. It's labile in gastric acid; less drug is lost to hydrolysis because it increases gastric pH.
• Dosage adjustments aren't required for patients with impaired renal function; however, they're needed in those with hepatic impairment.
• Capsule shouldn't be crushed.

Patient education

• Explain importance of taking omeprazole exactly as prescribed.
• Tell patient to take before meals and not to crush capsules.

ondansetron hydrochloride
Zofran

Serotonin (5-HT₃) receptor antagonist, antiemetic

Available by prescription only
Tablets: 4 mg, 8 mg
Injection: 2 mg/ml in 20-ml multidose vials, 2-ml single-dose vials
Injection, premixed: 32 mg/50 ml in D_5W single-dose vial

INDICATIONS & DOSAGE
Prevention of nausea and vomiting resulting from initial or repeat courses of emetogenic cancer chemotherapy, including high-dose cisplatin
Adults: Three I.V. doses of 0.15 mg/kg, with first dose infused over 15 minutes beginning 30 minutes before start of chemotherapy, and subsequent doses of 0.15 mg/kg administered 4 and 8 hours after first dose. May also administer as a single dose of 32 mg infused over 15 minutes, 30 minutes before start of chemotherapy.
Adults: 8 mg P.O. b.i.d. starting 30 minutes before start of chemotherapy, with subsequent dose 8 hours after first dose,

then 8 mg q 12 hours for 1 to 2 days after completion of chemotherapy.
Prevention of radiation-induced nausea and vomiting
Adults: 8 mg P.O. t.i.d.
Prevention of postoperative nausea and vomiting
Adults: 16 mg P.O. 1 hour before anesthesia or 4 mg I.V. immediately before anesthesia or shortly postoperatively.

PHARMACODYNAMICS
Antiemetic action: Mechanism of action isn't fully defined; however, ondansetron isn't a dopamine-receptor antagonist. Because serotonin receptors of the 5-HT₃ type are present both peripherally on vagal nerve terminals and centrally in the chemoreceptor trigger zone, it isn't certain if the action of the drug is mediated centrally, peripherally, or both.

PHARMACOKINETICS
Absorption: Absorption is variable with oral administration, with levels peaking within 2 hours and bioavailability of 50% to 60%.
Distribution: Ondansetron is 70% to 76% plasma protein-bound.
Metabolism: Drug is extensively metabolized by hydroxylation on the indole ring, followed by glucuronide or sulfate conjugation.
Excretion: About 5% of dose is recovered in urine as parent compound. Half-life in adults is 3½ to 6 hours.

CONTRAINDICATIONS & PRECAUTIONS
Contraindicated in patients hypersensitive to ondansetron. Use cautiously in patients with hepatic failure.

INTERACTIONS
Drug-drug. Ondansetron is metabolized by cytochrome P-450; thus, *inducers or inhibitors of cytochrome P-450 enzyme* may change clearance and half-life of ondansetron; however, no dosage adjustment is required.

ADVERSE REACTIONS
CNS: *headache, malaise, fatigue, dizziness, sedation.*
CV: chest pain.

Reactions may be *common,* uncommon, *life-threatening,* or **COMMON AND LIFE-THREATENING.**

GI: *diarrhea, constipation,* abdominal pain, xerostomia.
GU: urine retention, gynecologic disorders.
Hepatic: transient elevations in AST and ALT levels.
Musculoskeletal: *pain.*
Skin: rash.
Other: chills, injection-site reaction, fever, hypoxia.

▣ KEY CONSIDERATIONS

• No age-related problems have been reported in geriatric patients.
• Ondansetron is stable at room temperature for 48 hours after dilution with normal saline solution, D_5W, dextrose 5% in normal saline solution, dextrose 5% in half-normal saline solution, or sodium chloride 3%.

oxacillin sodium
Bactocill

Penicillinase-resistant penicillin, antibiotic

Available by prescription only
Capsules: 250 mg, 500 mg
Oral solution: 250 mg/5 ml (after reconstitution)
Injection: 250 mg, 500 mg, 1 g, 2 g, 4 g
I.V. infusion: 1 g, 2 g, 4 g

INDICATIONS & DOSAGE

***Systemic infections caused by* Staphylococcus aureus**
Adults: 2 to 6 g P.O. daily, divided into doses given q 4 to 6 hours; 1 to 12 g I.M. or I.V. daily, divided into doses given q 4 to 6 hours. Doses vary based on severity of infection.
✦ *Dosage adjustment.* In adults with creatinine clearance less than 10 ml/minute, give 1 g I.M. or I.V. q 4 to 6 hours.

PHARMACODYNAMICS

Antibiotic action: Oxacillin is bactericidal; it adheres to bacterial penicillin-binding proteins, thus inhibiting bacterial cell wall synthesis. Drug resists the effects of penicillinases—enzymes that inactivate penicillin—and is thus active

against many strains of penicillinase-producing bacteria. This activity is most important against penicillinase-producing staphylococci; some strains may remain resistant. Drug is also active against a few gram-positive aerobic and anaerobic bacilli but has no significant effect on gram-negative bacilli.

PHARMACOKINETICS

Absorption: Oxacillin is absorbed rapidly but incompletely from the GI tract; it's stable in an acid environment. Serum levels peak ¼ to 2 hours after an oral dose and 30 minutes after an I.M. dose. Food decreases absorption.
Distribution: Drug is distributed widely. CSF penetration is poor but enhanced by meningeal inflammation. It's 89% to 94% protein-bound.
Metabolism: Drug is partially metabolized.
Excretion: Drug and metabolites are excreted primarily in urine through renal tubular secretion and glomerular filtration; a small amount is also excreted in bile. Elimination half-life in adults is ½ to 1 hour, extended to 2 hours in severe renal impairment. Dosage adjustments aren't required in patients with creatinine clearance less than 10 ml/minute.

CONTRAINDICATIONS & PRECAUTIONS

Contraindicated in patients with hypersensitivity to oxacillin or other penicillins. Use cautiously in patients with other drug allergies (especially to cephalosporins).

INTERACTIONS

Drug-drug. Use of oxacillin with *aminoglycosides* produces synergistic bactericidal effects against *S. aureus.* However, the drugs are physically and chemically incompatible and are inactivated when mixed or given together. In vivo inactivation has been reported when aminoglycosides and penicillins are used concomitantly.
  Probenecid blocks renal tubular secretion of penicillins, increasing their serum levels.

ADVERSE REACTIONS

CNS: neuropathy, neuromuscular irritability, *seizures,* lethargy, hallucinations, anxiety, confusion, agitation, depression, dizziness, fatigue.
CV: *thrombophlebitis.*
GI: oral lesions, nausea, vomiting, diarrhea, enterocolitis, pseudomembranous colitis.
GU: interstitial nephritis, nephropathy.
Hematologic: *thrombocytopenia,* eosinophilia, *hemolytic anemia, neutropenia,* anemia, *agranulocytosis.*
Hepatic: elevated liver function test results.
Other: hypersensitivity reactions (fever, chills, rash, urticaria, *anaphylaxis,* overgrowth of nonsusceptible organisms).

▣ KEY CONSIDERATIONS

Besides the recommendations relevant to all penicillins, consider the following:
• Give oral oxacillin with water only; acid in fruit juice or carbonated beverages may inactivate drug.
• Give oral dose on empty stomach; food decreases absorption.
• Except in osteomyelitis, don't give I.M. or I.V. unless patient can't take oral dose.
• Elevations in liver function test results may indicate drug-induced hepatitis or cholestasis.
• Assess renal and hepatic function; watch for elevated AST and ALT levels and report significant changes.
• Drug alters test results for urine and serum proteins; turbidimetric urine and serum proteins are often falsely positive or elevated in tests using sulfosalicylic acid or trichloroacetic acid.
• Half-life may be prolonged in geriatric patients because of impaired renal function.

Patient education

• Explain need to take oral preparations without food and to follow with water only because of acid content of fruit juice and carbonated beverages.
• Tell patient to report allergic reactions or severe diarrhea promptly.
• Emphasize importance of completing the full course of therapy.

oxaprozin
Daypro

NSAID, nonnarcotic analgesic, antipyretic, anti-inflammatory

Available by prescription only
Caplets: 600 mg

INDICATIONS & DOSAGE

Management of acute or chronic osteoarthritis or rheumatoid arthritis
Adults: Initially, 1,200 mg P.O. daily. Individualize to smallest effective dosage to minimize adverse reactions. Smaller patients or those with mild symptoms may require only 600 mg daily. Maximum daily dosage is 1,800 mg or 26 mg/kg, whichever is less, in divided doses.

PHARMACODYNAMICS

Analgesic, antipyretic, and *anti-inflammatory actions:* Exact mechanism of action isn't clearly defined. It inhibits several steps along the arachidonic acid pathway of prostaglandin synthesis. One of the modes of action is presumed to result from the inhibition of cyclooxygenase activity and prostaglandin synthesis at the site of inflammation.

PHARMACOKINETICS

Absorption: Oxaprozin demonstrates high oral bioavailability (95%); plasma levels peak 3 to 5 hours after dosing. Food may reduce the rate, but not extent, of absorption.
Distribution: Drug is about 99.9% bound to albumin in plasma.
Metabolism: Drug is primarily metabolized in the liver through microsomal oxidation (65%) and glucuronic acid conjugation (35%).
Excretion: Glucuronide metabolites are excreted in urine (65%) and feces (35%).

CONTRAINDICATIONS & PRECAUTIONS

Contraindicated in patients with hypersensitivity to oxaprozin or with the syndrome of nasal polyps, angioedema, and bronchospastic reaction to aspirin or other NSAIDs. Use cautiously in patients with renal or hepatic dysfunction, history of peptic ulcer, hypertension, CV disease, or conditions predisposing the patient to fluid retention.

INTERACTIONS

Drug-drug. Use with *aspirin* isn't recommended because oxaprozin displaces salicylates from plasma protein binding, increasing the risk of salicylate toxicity.

Use with *beta blockers* such as *metoprolol* may cause a transient increase in blood pressure after 14 days of therapy. Routine blood pressure monitoring should be considered when starting oxaprozin therapy. *Oral anticoagulants* may increase the risk of bleeding when administered with oxaprozin.

ADVERSE REACTIONS

CNS: depression, sedation, somnolence, confusion, sleep disturbances.
EENT: tinnitus, blurred vision.
GI: *nausea, dyspepsia, diarrhea, constipation,* abdominal pain or distress, anorexia, flatulence, vomiting, ***hemorrhage,*** stomatitis, ulcer.
GU: dysuria, urinary frequency.
Hepatic: elevated liver function test results (with long-term use), ***severe hepatic dysfunction*** (rare).
Skin: *rash,* photosensitivity.

▣ KEY CONSIDERATIONS

• Serious GI toxicity, including peptic ulceration and bleeding, can occur in patients taking NSAIDs despite the absence of GI symptoms. Patients at risk for peptic ulceration and bleeding are those with history of serious GI events, alcoholism, smoking, or other factors associated with peptic ulcer disease.
• Elevations of liver function test results can occur after long-term use. These abnormal findings may persist, worsen, or resolve with continued therapy. Rarely, patients may progress to severe hepatic dysfunction. Periodically monitor liver function tests in patients receiving long-term therapy and closely monitor patients with abnormal test results.
• Anemia may occur in patients receiving oxaprozin. Obtain hemoglobin level or hematocrit in patients with prolonged

therapy at intervals appropriate for their situation.
• Dosages greater than 1,200 mg/day should be used for patients who weigh more than 50 kg (110 lb) and have normal renal and hepatic function, are at low risk for peptic ulceration, and have disease severity that justifies maximal therapy.
• Most patients tolerate once-daily dosing. Divided doses may be tried in patients unable to tolerate single doses.
• Geriatric patients may need a reduced dose because of low body weight or disorders associated with aging.
• Geriatric patients are less likely to tolerate adverse effects of oxaprozin.

Patient education

• Warn patient to call health care provider immediately for signs and symptoms of GI bleeding or visual or auditory adverse reactions.
• Tell patient to take drug with milk or meals if adverse GI reactions occur.
• Because photosensitivity reactions may occur, advise patient to use a sunblock, wear protective clothing, and avoid prolonged exposure to sunlight.

---

oxazepam
Apo-Oxazepam*, Novoxapam*, Oxpam*, Serax, Zapex*

Benzodiazepine, anxiolytic, sedative-hypnotic
Controlled substance schedule IV

Available by prescription only
Tablets: 15 mg
Capsules: 10 mg, 15 mg, 30 mg

INDICATIONS & DOSAGE

Alcohol withdrawal, severe anxiety
Adults: 15 to 30 mg P.O. t.i.d. or q.i.d.
Tension, mild to moderate anxiety
Adults: 10 to 15 mg P.O. t.i.d. or q.i.d.
Geriatric patients: 10 mg P.O. t.i.d.; then increase to 15 mg t.i.d. or q.i.d., p.r.n.

PHARMACODYNAMICS

Anxiolytic and sedative-hypnotic action:
Oxazepam depresses the CNS at the limbic and subcortical levels of the brain. It

reduces anxiety by enhancing the effect of the neurotransmitter gamma-aminobutyric acid on its receptor in the ascending reticular activating system, which increases inhibition and blocks both cortical and limbic arousal.

PHARMACOKINETICS

Absorption: When administered orally, oxazepam is well absorbed through the GI tract. Levels peak 3 hours after dosing; onset of action is 1 to 2 hours.
Distribution: Drug is distributed widely throughout the body. It's 85% to 95% protein-bound.
Metabolism: Drug is metabolized in the liver to inactive metabolites.
Excretion: Metabolites of oxazepam are excreted in urine as glucuronide conjugates. Half-life of drug is 5.7 to 10.9 hours.

CONTRAINDICATIONS & PRECAUTIONS

Contraindicated in patients with psychosis or hypersensitivity to drug. Use cautiously in geriatric or debilitated patients, in those with history of drug abuse, and in those in whom a decrease in blood pressure is associated with cardiac problems.

INTERACTIONS

Drug-drug. *Antacids* may decrease the rate of oxazepam absorption. Oxazepam potentiates the CNS depressant effects of *antidepressants, antihistamines, barbiturates, general anesthetics, MAO inhibitors, narcotics,* and *phenothiazines.* Use with *cimetidine* and possibly *disulfiram* causes diminished hepatic metabolism of oxazepam, which increases its plasma levels. Oxazepam may inhibit the therapeutic effects of *levodopa.*
Drug-lifestyle. Oxazepam potentiates the CNS depressant effects of *alcohol. Heavy smoking* accelerates drug metabolism, thus reducing clinical effectiveness.

ADVERSE REACTIONS

CNS: *drowsiness, lethargy,* dizziness, vertigo, headache, syncope, tremor, slurred speech, changes in EEG patterns (usually low voltage, fast activity may occur during and after oxazepam therapy).
CV: edema.
GI: nausea.
Hematologic: *leukopenia* (rare).
Hepatic: elevated liver function test results, *hepatic dysfunction.*
Skin: rash.
Other: altered libido.

◙ KEY CONSIDERATIONS

Besides the recommendations relevant to all benzodiazepines, consider the following:
● Geriatric patients are more susceptible to the CNS depressant effects of oxazepam. Some may require supervision with ambulation and activities of daily living during initiation of therapy or after an increase in dose.
● Lower doses are usually effective in geriatric patients because of decreased elimination.
● Monitor hepatic and renal function studies to ensure normal function.
● Oxazepam tablets contain tartrazine dye; check patient's history for allergy to this substance.
● Store drug in a cool, dry place away from light.
● Inform patient to reduce dosage gradually (over 8 to 12 weeks) after long-term use.

Patient education

● Advise patient not to change oxazepam regimen without medical approval.
● Instruct patient in safety measures, such as gradual position changes and supervised ambulation, to prevent injury.
● Because sleepiness may not occur for up to 2 hours after taking drug, tell patient to wait before taking an additional dose.
● Advise patient of potential for physical and psychological dependence with long-term use of drug.
● Tell patient not to discontinue drug suddenly after prolonged therapy.

Overdose & treatment

● Signs and symptoms of overdose include somnolence, confusion, coma, hypoactive reflexes, dyspnea, labored breathing, hypotension, bradycardia, slurred speech, and unsteady gait or impaired coordination.

Reactions may be *common*, uncommon, *life-threatening*, or COMMON AND LIFE-THREATENING.

• Support blood pressure and respiration until the drug effects subside; monitor vital signs. Mechanical ventilation via endotracheal tube may be required. Flumazenil, a specific benzodiazepine antagonist, may be useful. Use I.V. fluids and such vasopressors as dopamine and phenylephrine to treat hypotension. If the patient is conscious, induce vomiting; use gastric lavage if ingestion was recent, but only if an endotracheal tube is present to prevent aspiration. Then, administer activated charcoal with a cathartic as a single dose. Dialysis has limited value.

oxybutynin chloride
Ditropan

Synthetic tertiary amine, antispasmodic

Available by prescription only
Tablets: 5 mg
Syrup: 5 mg/5 ml

INDICATIONS & DOSAGE
For the relief of bladder instability associated with voiding in patients with uninhibited and reflex neurogenic bladder
Adults: 5 mg P.O. b.i.d. to t.i.d., to maximum of 5 mg q.i.d.

PHARMACODYNAMICS
Antispasmodic action: Oxybutynin reduces the urge to void, increases bladder capacity, and reduces the frequency of contractions to the detrusor muscle. Drug exerts a direct spasmolytic action and an antimuscarinic action on smooth muscle.

PHARMACOKINETICS
Absorption: Oxybutynin is absorbed rapidly; levels peak in 3 to 6 hours. Action begins in 30 to 60 minutes and persists for 6 to 10 hours.
Distribution: Unknown.
Metabolism: Drug is metabolized in the liver.
Excretion: Drug is excreted principally in urine.

CONTRAINDICATIONS & PRECAUTIONS
Contraindicated in geriatric or debilitated patients with intestinal atony; in patients with hypersensitivity to oxybutynin, myasthenia gravis, GI obstruction, glaucoma, adynamic ileus, megacolon, severe colitis, ulcerative colitis when megacolon is present, or obstructive uropathy; and in hemorrhaging patients with unstable CV status.

Use cautiously in geriatric patients and in those with impaired renal or hepatic function, autonomic neuropathy, or reflux esophagitis.

INTERACTIONS
Drug-drug. Use with other *CNS depressants* may cause additive sedative effects. Use with *digoxin* may increase digoxin levels. Use with *haloperidol* may worsen schizophrenia, decrease serum haloperidol levels, and cause tardive dyskinesia. Increased incidence of anticholinergic adverse effects with *phenothiazine* may occur.

ADVERSE REACTIONS
CNS: dizziness, insomnia, restlessness, hallucinations, asthenia.
CV: *palpitations, tachycardia,* vasodilation.
EENT: mydriasis, cycloplegia, decreased lacrimation, amblyopia.
GI: nausea, vomiting, *constipation, dry mouth,* decreased GI motility.
GU: *urinary hesitancy, urine retention.*
Skin: rash.
Other: decreased diaphoresis, fever.

▣ KEY CONSIDERATIONS
• Geriatric patients may be more sensitive to the antimuscarinic effects. Oxybutynin is contraindicated in geriatric and debilitated patients with intestinal atony.
• Discontinue drug periodically to determine if patient still requires the drug.

Patient education
• Instruct patient regarding oxybutynin and dosage schedule; tell him to take a missed dose as soon as possible and not to double-dose.

• Warn patient about possibility of decreased mental alertness or visual changes.

• Remind patient to use drug cautiously in warm climates to minimize risk of heatstroke that may occur because of decreased sweating.

Overdose & treatment

• Signs and symptoms of overdose include restlessness, excitement, psychotic behavior, flushing, hypotension, circulatory failure, and fever. In severe cases, paralysis, respiratory failure, and coma may occur.

• Treatment requires gastric lavage. Activated charcoal and a cathartic may be administered. Physostigmine may be considered to reverse symptoms of anticholinergic intoxication. Treat hyperpyrexia symptomatically with ice bags or other cold applications and alcohol sponges. Maintain artificial respiration if paralysis of respiratory muscles occurs.

---

oxycodone hydrochloride
OxyContin, Roxicodone, Supeudol*, OxyFast, OxyIR

Opioid, analgesic
Controlled substance schedule II

Available by prescription only
Tablets: 5 mg
Tablets (sustained-release): 10 mg, 20 mg, 40 mg, 80 mg
Oral solution: 5 mg/ml, 20 mg/ml
Suppositories: 10 mg*, 20 mg*

INDICATIONS & DOSAGE
Moderate to severe pain
Adults: 5 mg P.O. q 6 hours; alternatively, 10 to 40 mg P.R., p.r.n., t.i.d. or q.i.d.
Chronic pain
Adults: initially, 10-mg sustained-release tablet q 12 hours; may increase dose q 1 to 2 days. Dosing frequency shouldn't be increased.

PHARMACODYNAMICS
Analgesic action: Oxycodone acts on opiate receptors, providing analgesia for moderate to moderately severe pain. Episodes of acute rather than chronic pain appear to be more responsive to treatment with drug.

PHARMACOKINETICS
Absorption: Onset of analgesic effect after oral administration within 15 to 30 minutes; effect peaks within 1 hour.
Distribution: Drug is distributed rapidly.
Metabolism: Drug is metabolized in the liver.
Excretion: Drug is excreted principally in the kidneys. Duration of analgesia is 6 hours; for sustained-release tablets, 12 hours.

CONTRAINDICATIONS & PRECAUTIONS
Contraindicated in patients with hypersensitivity to oxycodone. Use cautiously in geriatric or debilitated patients and in those with head injury, increased intracranial pressure, seizures, asthma, COPD, prostatic hyperplasia, severe hepatic or renal disease, acute abdominal conditions, urethral stricture, hypothyroidism, Addison's disease, or arrhythmias.

INTERACTIONS
Drug-drug. Use with *anticholinergics* may cause paralytic ileus. Oxycodone products containing *aspirin* may increase the effect of the anticoagulant; monitor clotting times, and use together cautiously. Use with *cimetidine* may increase respiratory and CNS depression, causing confusion, disorientation, apnea, or seizures. Administration with other *CNS depressants*—including *antihistamines, barbiturates, benzodiazepines, general anesthetics, muscle relaxants, narcotic analgesics, phenothiazines, sedative-hypnotics,* and *tricyclic antidepressants*—potentiates the respiratory and CNS depressant, sedative, and hypotensive effects of oxycodone. Drug accumulation and enhanced effects may result from use with other *drugs that are extensively metabolized in the liver*—such as *digitoxin, phenytoin,* and *rifampin.* Severe CV depression may result from use with *general anesthetics.* Patients who become physically dependent on drug may experience acute withdrawal syndrome if given high doses of an *opioid agonist-antagonist* or a *single dose of an antagonist.*

Reactions may be *common,* uncommon, *life-threatening,* or COMMON AND LIFE-THREATENING.

Drug-lifestyle. *Alcohol* potentiates the respiratory and CNS effects of oxycodone.

ADVERSE REACTIONS

CNS: *sedation, somnolence, clouded sensorium, euphoria, dizziness, lightheadedness, seizures.*
CV: *hypotension,* bradycardia.
GI: *nausea, vomiting, constipation,* ileus.
GU: *urine retention.*
Hepatic: increased plasma amylase, lipase, and liver enzyme levels.
Respiratory: *respiratory depression.*
Skin: *diaphoresis,* pruritus, rash.
Other: physical dependence.

▣ KEY CONSIDERATIONS

Besides the recommendations relevant to all opioids, consider the following:
• Lower doses are usually indicated for geriatric patients, who may be more sensitive to the therapeutic and adverse effects of oxycodone.
• Single-drug solution or tablets are ideal for patients who can't take aspirin or acetaminophen.
• Drug has high abuse potential.
• Drug may obscure signs and symptoms of an acute abdominal condition or worsen gallbladder pain.
• Consider prescribing a stool softener for patients on long-term therapy.
• The 80-mg controlled-release tablets are for use in opioid-tolerant patients only.

Patient education
• Instruct patient to take drug before intense pain occurs for full analgesic effect.
• Warn patient about possibility of decreased alertness or visual changes.

Overdose & treatment
• The most common signs and symptoms of a severe overdose are CNS depression, respiratory depression, and miosis (pinpoint pupils). Other acute toxic effects include hypotension, bradycardia, hypothermia, shock, apnea, cardiopulmonary arrest, circulatory collapse, pulmonary edema, and convulsions.
• To treat acute overdose, first establish adequate respiratory exchange via a patent airway and ventilation as needed; administer an opioid antagonist (nalox-

one) to reverse respiratory depression. (Because the duration of action of oxycodone is longer than that of naloxone, repeated naloxone dosing is necessary.) Naloxone shouldn't be given unless patient has significant respiratory or CV depression. Monitor vital signs closely.
• If patient presents within 2 hours of ingestion of an oral overdose, immediately induce vomiting with ipecac syrup or perform gastric lavage. Use caution to avoid risk for aspiration. Administer activated charcoal via NG tube to further remove drug.
• Provide symptomatic and supportive treatment (continued respiratory support, correction of fluid or electrolyte imbalance). Monitor laboratory values, vital signs, and neurologic status closely.
• If acetaminophen-containing product was consumed in overdose, treat as in acetaminophen overdose.

oxymetazoline hydrochloride

Afrin, Allerest 12-Hour Nasal Spray, Chlorphed-LA, Dristan Long Lasting, Duramist Plus, Duration, 4-Way Long Lasting Spray, Neo-Synephrine 12 Hour Nasal Spray, Nostrilla, Nostrilla Long Acting Nasal Decongestant, NTZ Long Acting Decongestant Nasal Spray, OcuClear, Sinarest 12 Hour Nasal Spray, Sinex Long-Acting, Visine L.R.

Sympathomimetic, decongestant, vasoconstrictor

Available without prescription
Nasal drops or spray: 0.05%
Ophthalmic solution: 0.025%

INDICATIONS & DOSAGE

Nasal congestion
Adults: Apply 2 or 3 gtt or sprays of 0.05% solution in each nostril b.i.d.; shouldn't be used for more than 3 to 5 days.

Relief of minor eye redness
Adults: Apply 1 or 2 gtt in the conjunctival sac b.i.d. to q.i.d. (space at least 6 hours apart).

PHARMACODYNAMICS
Decongestant and vasoconstrictive actions: Oxymetazoline produces local vasoconstriction of arterioles through alpha receptors to reduce blood flow and nasal congestion.

PHARMACOKINETICS
Absorption: Following intranasal application, local vasoconstriction occurs within 5 to 10 minutes and persists for 5 to 6 hours, with a gradual decline over the next 6 hours.
Distribution: Unknown.
Metabolism: Unknown.
Excretion: Unknown.

CONTRAINDICATIONS & PRECAUTIONS
Contraindicated in patients with hypersensitivity to oxymetazoline. Ophthalmic form contraindicated in patients with angle-closure glaucoma.

Use cautiously in patients with hyperthyroidism, cardiac disease, or hypertension and in those receiving MAO inhibitors. Use nasal solution cautiously in patients with diabetes mellitus. Ophthalmic form should be used cautiously in those with eye disease, infection, or injury.

INTERACTIONS
Drug-drug. In ophthalmic form, *beta blockers* can increase systemic adverse effects and *local anesthetics* can increase absorption. Oxymetazoline may potentiate the pressor effects of *tricyclic antidepressants* from significant systemic absorption of the decongestant.

ADVERSE REACTIONS
CNS: headache, insomnia, drowsiness, dizziness, possible sedation (with nasal form), light-headedness, nervousness (with ophthalmic form).
CV: palpitations, *CV collapse,* hypertension (with nasal form), tachycardia, *bradycardia,* irregular heartbeat (with ophthalmic form).
EENT: rebound nasal congestion or irritation with excessive or long-term use, dryness of nose and throat, increased nasal discharge, stinging, sneezing (with nasal form), *transient stinging on instillation,* blurred vision, reactive hyperemia, keratitis, lacrimation, increased intraocular pressure (with ophthalmic form).

▣ KEY CONSIDERATIONS
• Use oxymetazoline with caution in geriatric patients with cardiac disease, poorly controlled hypertension, or diabetes mellitus.
• Monitor carefully for adverse reactions in patients with CV disease, diabetes mellitus, or prostatic hyperplasia because systemic absorption can occur.

Patient education
• Emphasize that only one person should use dropper bottle or nasal spray.
• Advise patient not to exceed recommended dosage and to use oxymetazoline only when needed.
• Tell patient to discontinue drug use and call doctor if symptoms persist after 3 days of self-medication.
• Tell patient nasal mucosa may sting, burn, or become dry.
• Warn patient that excessive use may cause bradycardia, hypotension, dizziness, and weakness.
• Show patient how to apply: bend head forward and sniff spray briskly or apply light pressure on lacrimal sac after instillation of eyedrops.

Overdose & treatment
• Signs and symptoms of overdose include somnolence, sedation, sweating, CNS depression with hypertension, bradycardia, decreased cardiac output, rebound hypertension, CV collapse, depressed respirations, coma.
• Because of rapid onset of sedation, don't induce vomiting to treat overdose unless you do so early. Activated charcoal or gastric lavage may be used initially. Monitor vital signs and ECG. Treat seizures with I.V. diazepam.

Reactions may be *common,* uncommon, *life-threatening,* or COMMON AND LIFE-THREATENING.

P

paclitaxel
Taxol

Novel antimicrotubule, antineoplastic

Available by prescription only
Injection: 30 mg/5 ml

INDICATIONS & DOSAGE
Metastatic ovarian cancer after failure of first-line or subsequent chemotherapy
Adults: 135 or 175 mg/m² I.V. over 3 hours q 3 weeks. Subsequent courses shouldn't be repeated until neutrophil count is at least 1,500 cells/mm³ and platelet count is at least 100,000 cells/mm³.
Breast cancer after failure of combination chemotherapy for metastatic disease or relapse within 6 months of adjuvant chemotherapy (prior therapy should have included an anthracycline unless contraindicated)
Adults: 175 mg/m² I.V. over 3 hours q 3 weeks.
Second-line treatment of AIDS-related Kaposi's sarcoma
Adults: 135 mg/m² given I.V. over 3 hours every 3 weeks, or 100 mg/m² over 3 hours every 2 weeks.

PHARMACODYNAMICS
Antineoplastic action: Paclitaxel prevents depolymerization of cellular microtubules, thus inhibiting the normal reorganization of the microtubule network necessary for mitosis and other vital cellular functions.

PHARMACOKINETICS
Absorption: Unknown.
Distribution: Paclitaxel is 89% to 98% bound to serum proteins.
Metabolism: Drug may be metabolized in the liver.
Excretion: Excretion in humans isn't fully understood.

CONTRAINDICATIONS & PRECAUTIONS
Contraindicated in patients with hypersensitivity to paclitaxel or polyoxyethylated castor oil, a vehicle used in drug solution, and in those with baseline neutrophil counts less than 1,500/mm³. Use cautiously in patients who have received radiation therapy.

INTERACTIONS
Drug-drug. Myelosuppression may be greater when *cisplatin* is administered before rather than after paclitaxel. *Cyclosporine, dexamethasone, diazepam, etoposide, ketoconazole, quinidine, teniposide, verapamil,* and *vincristine* may inhibit paclitaxel metabolism; use these drugs cautiously.

ADVERSE REACTIONS
CNS: *peripheral neuropathy.*
CV: *bradycardia, hypotension, phlebitis, abnormal ECG.*
GI: *nausea, vomiting, diarrhea, mucositis.*
Hematologic: NEUTROPENIA, LEUKOPENIA, THROMBOCYTOPENIA, anemia, *bleeding.*
Hepatic: *elevated liver enzyme levels.*
Musculoskeletal: *myalgia, arthralgia.*
Skin: *alopecia.*
Other: *hypersensitivity reactions (**anaphylaxis**), cellulitis at injection site, infections.*

▣ KEY CONSIDERATIONS
• Severe hypersensitivity reactions characterized by dyspnea, hypotension, angioedema, and generalized urticaria have occurred in 2% of patients receiving paclitaxel. To reduce the incidence or severity of these reactions, pretreat patients with corticosteroids (such as dexamethasone), antihistamines (such as diphenhydramine), and H₂-receptor antagonists (such as cimetidine or ranitidine).
• Don't challenge patients who experience severe hypersensitivity reactions to drug.
• In patients who experience severe neutropenia (neutrophil count less than

500 cells/mm³ for 1 week or longer) or severe peripheral neuropathy during drug therapy, reduce dosage by 20% for subsequent courses. Incidence and severity of neurotoxicity and hematologic toxicity increase with dose, especially if greater then 190 mg/m².
• Bone marrow toxicity is the most common and dose-limiting toxicity. Frequent blood count monitoring is necessary during therapy. Packed RBCs or platelet transfusions may be necessary in severe cases. Institute bleeding precautions as appropriate.
• If patient develops significant conduction abnormalities during drug administration, give appropriate therapy and monitor cardiac function continuously during subsequent drug therapy.
• Use caution during preparation and administration of drug. Use gloves. If solution contacts skin, wash skin immediately and thoroughly with soap and water. If drug contacts mucous membranes, flush membranes thoroughly with water. Mark all waste materials with "Chemotherapy Hazard" labels.
• Concentrate must be diluted before infusion. Compatible solutions include normal saline injection, D_5W, dextrose 5% in normal saline injection, and dextrose 5% in lactated Ringer's injection. Dilute to a final concentration of 0.3 to 1.2 mg/ml. Diluted solutions are stable for 27 hours at room temperature.
• Prepare and store infusion solutions in glass containers. Undiluted concentrate shouldn't contact polyvinyl chloride I.V. bags or tubing. Store diluted solution in glass or polypropylene bottles or use polypropylene or polyolefin bags. Administer through polyethylene-lined administration sets, and use an in-line filter with a microporous membrane not exceeding 0.22 microns.
• Continuously monitor patient for 30 minutes after initiating the infusion. Continue close monitoring throughout infusion.

Patient education
• Warn patient that alopecia occurs in almost all patients.
• Teach patient to recognize and immediately report signs and symptoms of peripheral neuropathy, such as tingling, burning, or numbness in the extremities. Although mild symptoms are common, severe symptoms occur infrequently. Dosage may need to be reduced.

Overdose & treatment
• Primary complications of overdose include bone marrow suppression, peripheral neurotoxicity, and mucositis.
• No specific antidote is known.

pamidronate disodium
Aredia

Biphosphonate, pyrophosphate analogue, antihypercalcemic drug

Available by prescription only
Injection: 30 mg/vial, 60 mg/vial, 90 mg/vial

INDICATIONS & DOSAGE
Moderate to severe hypercalcemia associated with malignancy (with or without metastases)
Adults: Dosage depends on severity of hypercalcemia. Serum calcium levels should be corrected for serum albumin. Corrected serum calcium (CCa) is calculated using the following formula:

$$CCa = serum\ Ca + 0.8\ (4 - serum\ albumin)$$
$$(mg/dl)\quad (mg/dl)\qquad\qquad (g/dl)$$

✦ *Dosage adjustment.* Patients with moderate hypercalcemia (CCa levels, 12 to 13.5 mg/dl) may receive 60 to 90 mg by I.V. infusion. The 60-mg dose is given as an initial, single dose I.V. infusion over at least 4 hours. The 90-mg dose must be given as an initial, single-dose I.V. infusion over 24 hours. The recommended dose for severe hypercalcemia (CCa levels greater than 13.5 mg/dl) is 90 mg. This is given as an initial, single-dose I.V. infusion over 24 hours. Repeat doses shouldn't be given sooner than 7 days to allow full response to the initial dose.
Paget's disease
Adults: 30 mg I.V. daily over 4 hours for 3 consecutive days, for total dose of 90 mg.

Reactions may be *common*, uncommon, *life-threatening*, or COMMON AND LIFE-THREATENING.

Osteolytic bone lesions of multiple myeloma
Adults: 90 mg I.V. daily over 4 hours once monthly.

PHARMACODYNAMICS

Antihypercalcemic action: Pamidronate inhibits the resorption of bone. Drug adsorbs to hydroxyapatite crystals in bone and may directly block the dissolution of calcium phosphate. Drug apparently doesn't inhibit bone formation or mineralization.

PHARMACOKINETICS

Absorption: Rapid onset of action; duration of action is up to 6 months in bone.
Distribution: After I.V. administration in animals, 50% to 60% of dose is rapidly absorbed by bone; pamidronate is also taken up by kidneys, liver, spleen, teeth, and tracheal cartilage.
Metabolism: None.
Excretion: Drug is excreted from the kidneys; an average of 51% of dose is excreted in urine within 72 hours of administration.

CONTRAINDICATIONS & PRECAUTIONS

Contraindicated in patients hypersensitive to pamidronate or other biphosphonates such as etidronate. Use with extreme caution in patients with impaired renal function.

INTERACTIONS

Drug-drug. Pamidronate may form a precipitate when mixed with *solutions that contain calcium.*

ADVERSE REACTIONS

CNS: seizures, fatigue, headache, somnolence, *generalized pain.*
CV: atrial fibrillation, syncope, tachycardia, *hypertension.*
GI: *abdominal pain, anorexia, constipation, nausea, vomiting,* GI hemorrhage.
Hematologic: *leukopenia,* **thrombocytopenia,** anemia.
Metabolic: *hypophosphatemia, hypokalemia, hypomagnesemia, hypocalcemia.*
Musculoskeletal: *bone pain.*
Other: *fever, infusion-site reaction.*

🔲 KEY CONSIDERATIONS

• Because pamidronate can cause electrolyte disturbances, careful monitoring of serum electrolyte levels (especially calcium, phosphate, and magnesium) is essential. Short-term administration of calcium may be necessary in patients with severe hypocalcemia. Also, monitor CBC and differential, hematocrit, and creatinine and hemoglobin levels.
• Carefully monitor patients with preexisting anemia, leukopenia, or thrombocytopenia during first 2 weeks after therapy.
• Monitor patient's temperature. In trials, 27% of patients experienced a slightly elevated temperature for 24 to 48 hours after therapy.
• Reconstitute vial with 10 ml sterile water for injection. Once drug is completely dissolved, add to 1,000 ml half-normal or normal saline injection or D₅W. Don't mix with infusion solutions that contain calcium, such as Ringer's injection or lactated Ringer's injection. Administer in a single I.V. solution in a separate line from all other drugs. Inspect for precipitate before administering.
• Injection solution is stable for 24 hours when refrigerated. Give only by I.V. infusion. Animal studies have shown evidence of nephropathy when drug is given as a bolus.
• Consider retreatment if hypercalcemia recurs; allow a minimum of 7 days to elapse before retreatment to allow for full response to the initial dose.

Overdose & treatment

• Symptomatic hypocalcemia could result from overdose.
• Treat with I.V. calcium. In one reported case, a 95-kg (209-lb) woman who received 285 mg daily for 3 days experienced hyperpyrexia (temperature, 103°F [39.4°C]), hypotension, and transient taste perversion. Fever and hypotension were rapidly corrected with corticosteroids.

pancreatin
Dizymes, Donnazyme, Entozyme,
Hi-Vegi-Lip, 4X Pancreatin, 8X
Pancreatin, Pancrezyme 4X

Pancreatic enzyme, digestant

Available without prescription
Dizymes
Tablets (enteric-coated): 250 mg pancreatin; 6,750 U lipase; 41,250 U protease; 43,750 U amylase
Hi-Vegi-Lip
Tablets (enteric-coated): 2,400 mg pancreatin; 4,800 U lipase; 60,000 U protease; 60,000 U amylase
4X Pancreatin, Pancrezyme 4X
Tablets (enteric-coated): 2,400 mg pancreatin; 12,000 U lipase; 60,000 U protease; 60,000 U amylase
8X Pancreatin
Tablets (enteric-coated): 7,200 mg pancreatin; 22,500 U lipase; 180,000 U protease; 180,000 U amylase
Available by prescription only
Donnazyme
Tablets: 500 mg pancreatin; 1,000 U lipase; 12,500 U protease; 12,500 U amylase
Entozyme
Tablets: 300 mg pancreatin; 600 U lipase; 7,500 U protease; 7,500 U amylase

INDICATIONS & DOSAGE
Exocrine pancreatic secretion insufficiency, digestive aid in cystic fibrosis, steatorrhea, and other disorders of fat metabolism secondary to insufficient pancreatic enzyme levels
Adults: 1 to 2 tablets P.O. with meals.

PHARMACODYNAMICS
Digestive action: Proteolytic, amylolytic, and lipolytic enzymes enhance the digestion of proteins, starches, and fats. Pancreatin is sensitive to acids and is more active in neutral or slightly alkaline environments.

PHARMACOKINETICS
Absorption: Pancreatin isn't absorbed; it acts locally in the GI tract.
Distribution: None.
Metabolism: None.

Excretion: Drug is excreted in feces.

CONTRAINDICATIONS & PRECAUTIONS
Contraindicated in patients with hypersensitivity to pancreatin or pork protein or enzymes, acute pancreatitis, and acute exacerbations of chronic pancreatitis.

INTERACTIONS
Drug-drug. Pancreatin activity may be reduced by *calcium-* or *magnesium-containing antacids*; however, *antacids* or *H_2 blockers* (such as *cimetidine*) may reduce the inactivation of the enzymes by gastric acid. Pancreatin decreases absorption of *iron-containing products*.

ADVERSE REACTIONS
GI: nausea, diarrhea (with high doses), perianal irritation.
Skin: rash.
Other: allergic reactions, increased uric acid levels.

▣ KEY CONSIDERATIONS
• For maximum effect, administer dose just before or during a meal.
• Tablets may not be crushed or chewed; follow with a glass of water to ensure complete swallowing.
• Diet should balance fat, protein, and starch intake properly to avoid indigestion. Dosage varies according to degree of maldigestion and malabsorption, amount of fat in diet, and enzyme activity of individual preparations.
• Adequate replacement decreases number of bowel movements and improves stool consistency.
• Use only after confirmed diagnosis of exocrine pancreatic insufficiency. Not effective in GI disorders unrelated to pancreatic enzyme deficiency.
• Enteric coating may reduce availability of enzyme in upper portion of jejunum.
• Retention in the mouth may cause mucosal irritation. Pancreatin should be swallowed promptly.

Patient education
• Explain use of pancreatin and advise storage away from heat and light.
• Make sure patient or family understands special dietary instructions for the particular disease.

Reactions may be *common*, uncommon, **life-threatening**, or COMMON AND LIFE-THREATENING.

• Instruct patient not to change brands without medical approval.

pancrelipase

Cotazym, Cotazym-S, Creon 10, Creon 20, Ilozyme, Ku-Zyme HP, Pancrease, Pancrease MT 4, Pancrease MT 10, Pancrease MT 16, Pancrease MT 20, Pancrelipase, Protilase, Ultrase MT 12, Ultrase MT 20, Ultrase MT 24, Viokase, Zymase

Pancreatic enzyme, digestant

Available by prescription only
Cotazym
Capsules: 8,000 U lipase; 30,000 U protease; 30,000 U amylase
Cotazym-S
Capsules (enteric-coated spheres): 5,000 U lipase; 20,000 U protease; 20,000 U amylase
Creon 5
Enteric-coated minimicrospheres: 5,000 U lipase, 16,600 U amylase, 18,750 U protease
Creon 10
Capsules (delayed-release): 10,000 U lipase; 37,500 U protease; 33,200 U amylase
Creon 20
Capsules (delayed-release): 20,000 U lipase; 75,000 U protease; 66,400 U amylase
Ilozyme
Tablets: 11,000 U lipase; 30,000 U protease; 30,000 U amylase
Ku-Zyme HP
Capsules: 8,000 U lipase; 30,000 U protease; 30,000 U amylase
Pancrease
Capsules (enteric-coated minispheres): 4,000 U lipase; 25,000 U protease; 20,000 U amylase
Pancrease MT 4
Capsules (enteric-coated minitablets): 4,000 U lipase; 12,000 U protease; 12,000 U amylase
Pancrease MT 10
Capsules (enteric-coated microtablets): 10,000 U lipase; 30,000 U protease; 30,000 U amylase

Pancrease MT 16
Capsules (enteric-coated minitablets): 16,000 U lipase; 48,000 U protease; 48,000 U amylase
Pancrease MT 20
Capsules (enteric-coated minitablets): 20,000 U lipase; 44,000 U protease; 56,000 U amylase
Pancrelipase and Protilase
Capsules: 4,000 U lipase; 25,000 U protease; 20,000 U amylase
Ultrase MT 12
Capsules (enteric-coated minitablets): 12,000 U lipase; 39,000 U protease; 39,000 U amylase
Ultrase MT 20
Capsules: 20,000 U lipase; 65,000 U protease; 65,000 U amylase
Ultrase MT 24
Capsules: 24,000 U lipase; 78,000 U protease; 78,000 U amylase
Viokase
Tablets: 8,000 U lipase; 30,000 U protease; 30,000 U amylase
Powder: 16,800 U lipase; 70,000 U protease; 70,000 U amylase
Zymase
Capsules: 12,000 U lipase; 24,000 U protease; 24,000 U amylase

INDICATIONS & DOSAGE
Exocrine pancreatic secretion insufficiency, cystic fibrosis in adults, steatorrhea and other disorders of fat metabolism secondary to insufficient pancreatic enzymes
Adults: 8,000 to 24,000 USP U of lipase activity with meals and snacks. Dosage must be adjusted to patient's response.

PHARMACODYNAMICS
Digestive action: Proteolytic, amylolytic, and lipolytic enzymes enhance the digestion of proteins, starches, and fats. Pancrelipase is sensitive to acids and is more active in neutral or slightly alkaline environments.

PHARMACOKINETICS
Absorption: Pancrelipase isn't absorbed and acts locally in the GI tract.
Distribution: None.
Metabolism: None.
Excretion: Drug is excreted in feces.

---

*Canada only   ◊ Unlabeled clinical use

CONTRAINDICATIONS & PRECAUTIONS

Contraindicated in patients with severe hypersensitivity to pork, acute pancreatitis, or acute exacerbations of chronic pancreatic diseases.

INTERACTIONS

Drug-drug. Pancrelipase activity may be reduced by *calcium-* or *magnesium-containing antacids*; however, *antacids* or *H_2 blockers* (such as *cimetidine*) may reduce inactivation of the enzymes by gastric acid. Pancrelipase decreases absorption of *iron-containing products.*

ADVERSE REACTIONS

GI: *nausea,* cramping, diarrhea (high doses).

Other: allergic reaction; increased serum uric acid levels, particularly with large doses.

◙ KEY CONSIDERATIONS

• For maximal effect, administer dose just before or during a meal. Patient should drink a glass of water or juice to ensure he completely swallows drug.

• Preparations may not be crushed or chewed.

• Use only after confirmed diagnosis of exocrine pancreatic insufficiency. Pancrelipase is ineffective in GI disorders unrelated to enzyme deficiency.

• Dosage varies with degree of maldigestion and malabsorption, amount of fat in diet, and enzyme activity of individual preparations.

• Adequate replacement decreases number of bowel movements and improves stool consistency.

• Enteric coating on some products may reduce availability of enzyme in upper portion of jejunum.

Patient education

• Teach patient or family proper use of pancrelipase and advise storage away from heat and light.

• Make sure patient or family understands special dietary instructions for the particular disease.

• Tell patient not to change brands without medical approval.

Overdose & treatment

• Signs and symptoms of overdose include hyperuricosuria, hyperuricemia, diarrhea, and transient GI upset.

• Treatment of overdose includes supportive care.

---

paroxetine hydrochloride
Paxil

Selective serotonin reuptake inhibitor (SSRI), antidepressant

---

Available by prescription only
Tablets: 10 mg, 20 mg, 30 mg, 40 mg
Oral suspension: 10 mg/5 ml

INDICATIONS & DOSAGE

Depression

Adults: initially, 20 mg P.O. daily, preferably in the morning. Increase dosage by 10 mg/day at 1-week intervals to maximum of 50 mg daily, if necessary.

Geriatric patients: 10 mg P.O. daily, preferably in the morning. Increase dosage by 10 mg/day at 1-week intervals, as necessary, to maximum of 40 mg daily.

✦ *Dosage adjustment.* For debilitated patients or patients with severe hepatic or renal disease, 10 mg P.O. daily, preferably in the morning. Increase dosage by 10 mg/day at 1-week intervals, as necessary, to maximum of 40 mg daily.

Obsessive-compulsive disorder

Adults: initially, 20 mg P.O. daily, preferably in the morning. Increase by 10 mg/day at 1-week intervals to target dose of 40 mg/day. Maximum dose is 60 mg/day.

Panic disorder

Adults: initially, 10 mg P.O. daily, preferably in the morning. Increase by 10 mg/day at 1-week intervals, to target dose of 40 mg/day. Maximum dose is 60 mg/day.

PHARMACODYNAMICS

Antidepressant action: Action is presumed to be linked to potentiation of serotonergic activity in the CNS, resulting from inhibition of neuronal reuptake of serotonin.

Reactions may be *common,* uncommon, *life-threatening,* or COMMON AND LIFE-THREATENING.

PHARMACOKINETICS

Absorption: Paroxetine is completely absorbed after oral dosing.

Distribution: Drug distributes throughout the body, including the CNS, with only 1% remaining in the plasma; 93% to 95% is bound to plasma protein.

Metabolism: About 36% of drug is metabolized in the liver. The principal metabolites are polar and conjugated products of oxidation and methylation, which are readily cleared.

Excretion: About 64% is excreted in urine (2% as parent compound and 62% as metabolite).

CONTRAINDICATIONS & PRECAUTIONS

Contraindicated in patients taking MAO inhibitors; drug shouldn't be given to patients within 14 days of discontinuing an MAO inhibitor. Use cautiously in patients with history of seizures or mania; in those with severe, concurrent systemic illness; or in those at risk for volume depletion. Also contraindicated in patients with hypersensitivity to SSRIs.

INTERACTIONS

Drug-drug. *Cimetidine* decreases hepatic metabolism of paroxetine, leading to risk of toxicity; dosage adjustments may be necessary. Paroxetine may decrease *digoxin* levels; monitor patient closely. Use with a *MAO inhibitor* may increase the risk for serious, sometimes fatal, adverse reactions and should be avoided. *Phenobarbital* induces paroxetine metabolism, thereby reducing plasma levels of drug. Paroxetine may alter the pharmacokinetics of *phenytoin,* requiring dosage adjustment. Paroxetine may increase *procyclidine* levels; monitor the patient for excessive anticholinergic effects. Use with *tryptophan* may increase the incidence of adverse reactions, such as diaphoresis, headache, nausea, and dizziness; avoid use. Paroxetine may increase risk of bleeding when used concomitantly with *warfarin;* monitor INR.

ADVERSE REACTIONS

CNS: *asthenia, somnolence, dizziness, insomnia, tremor, nervousness,* anxiety, paresthesia, confusion, *headache,* agita-

tion, decreased concentration, abnormal dreams.

CV: *chest pain,* palpitations, vasodilation, postural hypotension.

EENT: lump or tightness in throat, dysgeusia, visual disturbances, blurred vision.

GI: *dry mouth, nausea, constipation, diarrhea,* flatulence, vomiting, dyspepsia, increased or decreased appetite, abdominal pain.

GU: ejaculatory disturbances, male genital disorders (including anorgasmia, erectile difficulties, delayed ejaculation or orgasm, impotence, and sexual dysfunction), urinary frequency, other urinary disorders, female genital disorders (including anorgasmia, difficulty with orgasm).

Hematologic: altered platelet function.

Musculoskeletal: myopathy, myalgia, myasthenia.

Skin: rash, pruritus, sweating.

Other: *diaphoresis,* decreased libido, yawning.

▣ KEY CONSIDERATIONS

• Use cautiously and in lower dosages in geriatric patients because of possible decreased renal function and baseline hearing impairment in this age-group.

• At least 14 days should elapse between discontinuation of an MAO inhibitor and initiation of drug therapy. Similarly, at least 14 days should elapse between discontinuation of paroxetine and initiation of a MAO inhibitor.

• Hyponatremia may occur with drug use, especially in geriatric patients, those who are taking diuretics, and those who are otherwise volume depleted. Monitor serum sodium levels.

• If signs of psychosis occur or increase, reduce dosage. Monitor patients for suicidal tendencies and allow them only a minimum supply of drug.

Patient education

• Caution patient not to operate hazardous machinery, including automobiles, until reasonably certain that paroxetine therapy doesn't affect ability to engage in such activity.

• Tell patient that he may notice improvement in 1 to 4 weeks but to contin-

---

ue with the prescribed regimen to obtain continued benefits.

• Instruct patient to call before taking other drugs, including OTC preparations, while receiving drug.

• Tell patient to abstain from alcohol while taking drug.

Overdose & treatment

• Signs and symptoms of overdose may include dizziness, sweating, nausea, vomiting, drowsiness, sinus tachycardia, and dilated pupils.

• Treatment should consist of general measures used to manage overdose with any antidepressant. Induced vomiting, gastric lavage, or both should be performed. In most cases, 20 to 30 g activated charcoal may then be administered every 4 to 6 hours during the first 24 to 48 hours after ingestion. Supportive care, frequent monitoring of vital signs, and careful observation are indicated. ECG and cardiac function monitoring are warranted with evidence of an abnormality.

• Take special caution with a patient who receives or recently received paroxetine if the patient ingests an excessive quantity of a tricyclic antidepressant. In such cases, accumulation of the parent tricyclic and its active metabolite may increase the possibility of clinically significant sequelae and extend the time needed for close medical observation.

penicillamine
Cuprimine, Depen

Chelating drug, heavy metal antagonist, antirheumatic

Available by prescription only
Capsules: 125 mg, 250 mg
Tablets: 250 mg

INDICATIONS & DOSAGE
Wilson's disease
Adults: 250 mg P.O. q.i.d. 0.5 to 1 hour before meals and at least 2 hours after evening meal. Adjust dosage to achieve urine copper excretion of 0.5 to 1 mg daily. A dose exceeding 2 g is seldom necessary.

Cystinuria
Adults: 250 mg P.O. daily in four divided doses, then gradually increase dosage. Usual dosage, 2 g daily (range, 1 to 4 g daily). Adjust dosage to achieve urine cystine excretion of less than 100 mg daily when renal calculi are present, or 100 to 200 mg daily when no calculi are present.
Rheumatoid arthritis, ◊ Felty's syndrome
Adults: initially, 125 to 250 mg P.O. daily, with increases of 125 to 250 mg daily at 1- to 3-month intervals if necessary. Maximum dosage is 1.5 g daily. Onset of effect may not be seen for 1 to 3 months.
◊ Adjunctive treatment of heavy metal poisoning
Adults: 500 to 1,500 mg P.O. daily for 1 to 2 months.
◊ Primary biliary cirrhosis
Adults: initially, 250 mg P.O. daily, with increases of 250 mg q 2 weeks. Maximum dosage, 1 g daily in divided doses.

PHARMACODYNAMICS
Antirheumatic action: Mechanism of action in rheumatoid arthritis is unknown; penicillamine depresses circulating immunoglobulin M rheumatoid factor (but not total circulating immunoglobulin levels) and depresses T-cell, but not B-cell, activity. It also depolymerizes some macroglobulins (for example, rheumatoid factor).

Chelating action: Penicillamine forms stable, soluble complexes with copper, iron, mercury, lead, and other heavy metals excreted in urine; it's particularly useful in chelating copper in patients with Wilson's disease. Drug also combines with cystine to form a complex more soluble than cystine alone, thereby reducing free cystine below the level of urinary calculi formation.

PHARMACOKINETICS
Absorption: Penicillamine is well absorbed after oral administration; serum levels peak at 3 hours.
Distribution: Unknown.
Metabolism: Drug is metabolized in liver to inactive compounds.
Excretion: Only small amounts of drug are excreted unchanged; after 24 hours,

about 50% of drug is excreted in urine and about 50% in feces.

CONTRAINDICATIONS & PRECAUTIONS

Contraindicated in patients with known hypersensitivity to penicillamine, history of drug-related aplastic anemia or agranulocytosis or significant renal or hepatic insufficiency, and in patients receiving gold salts, immunosuppressants, antimalarials, or phenylbutazone because of the increased risk of serious hematologic effects.

Use cautiously in patients allergic to penicillin (cross-reaction is rare); in those who receive a second course of therapy and who may have become sensitized and are more likely to have allergic reactions; and in patients who develop proteinuria not associated with Goodpasture's syndrome.

INTERACTIONS

Drug-drug. Antacids and *iron salts* decrease absorption of penicillamine. *Antimalarials, cytotoxic drugs, gold therapy, oxyphenbutazone,* and *phenylbutazone* shouldn't be given concurrently; these are associated with serious hematologic and renal effects. *Digoxin* levels may be decreased when given concurrently.

ADVERSE REACTIONS

EENT: alteration in sense of taste (salty and sweet), metallic taste, oral ulcerations, glossitis, cheilosis, tinnitus, optic neuritis.
GI: anorexia, nausea, vomiting, dyspepsia, diarrhea, dysgeusia, *hypogeusia.*
GU: *proteinuria.*
Hematologic: eosinophilia, leukopenia, *thrombocytopenia, aplastic anemia, agranulocytosis,* thrombotic thrombocytopenia, purpura, hemolytic anemia or iron deficiency anemia, lupus-like syndrome.
Hepatic: cholestatic jaundice, *pancreatitis,* hepatic dysfunction.
Musculoskeletal: arthralgia.
Skin: *pruritus; erythematous rash;* intensely pruritic rash with scaly, macular lesions on trunk; pemphigoid reactions; urticaria; *exfoliative dermatitis;* increased skin friability; purpuric or vesicular ecchymoses; wrinkling; alopecia.

Other: lymphadenopathy, pneumonitis, Goodpasture's syndrome, drug fever, thyroiditis, myasthenia gravis (with prolonged use).

▣ KEY CONSIDERATIONS

● Lower doses may be indicated in geriatric patients. Monitor renal and hepatic function closely. Penicillamine toxicity may be twice as common in geriatric patients.
● Perform urinalysis and CBC including differential every 2 weeks for 4 to 6 months, then monthly; kidney and liver functions studies also should be performed, usually every 6 months. Report fever or allergic reactions—such as rash, joint pain, and easy bruising—immediately. Check routinely for proteinuria, and handle patient carefully to avoid skin damage.
● About one-third of patients receiving penicillamine experience an allergic reaction. Monitor patient for signs and symptoms of allergic reaction.
● Patients with Wilson's disease or cystinuria may require daily pyridoxine (vitamin B_6) supplementation.
● Prescribe drug to be taken 1 hour before or 2 hours after meals or other drugs to facilitate absorption.
● For initial treatment of Wilson's disease, 10 to 40 mg of sulfurated potash should be administered with each meal during penicillamine therapy for 6 months to 1 year, then discontinued.
● Drug therapy may cause positive test results for antinuclear antibody with or without systemic lupus-like syndrome.
● Discontinue drug if patient has signs of hypersensitivity or drug fever, usually in conjunction with other allergic signs and symptoms (if Wilson's disease, may rechallenge), or if the following occur: rash developing 6 months or more after start of therapy; pemphigoid reaction; hematuria or proteinuria with hemoptysis or pulmonary infiltrates; gross or persistent microscopic hematuria or proteinuria greater than 2 g/day in patients with rheumatoid arthritis; platelet count less than 100,000/mm³ or leukocyte count less than 3,500/mm³; or if either shows three consecutive decreases (even within normal range).

Patient education

• Provide health education for patients with Wilson's disease, rheumatoid arthritis, or cystinuria; explain disease process and rationale for therapy and explain that results may not be evident for 3 months.
• Encourage patient compliance with therapy and follow-up visits.
• Stress importance of immediately reporting fever, chills, sore throat, bruising, bleeding, or allergic reaction.
• Tell patient to take penicillamine on an empty stomach 30 minutes to 1 hour before meals or 2 hours after ingesting food, antacids, mineral supplements, vitamins, or other drugs. Tell patient to drink large amounts of water, especially at night.
• Advise patient receiving drug for rheumatoid arthritis that disease may be exacerbated during therapy. This usually can be controlled with NSAIDs.
• Advise patient taking drug for Wilson's disease to maintain a low-copper (less than 2 mg daily) diet by excluding foods with high copper content, such as chocolate, nuts, liver, and broccoli. Also, sulfurated potash may be administered with meals to minimize copper absorption.

penicillin G benzathine
Bicillin L-A, Megacillin Suspension*, Permapen

penicillin G benzathine and procaine
Bicillin CR, Bicillin CR 900/300

penicillin G potassium
Pfizerpen

penicillin G procaine
Ayercillin*, Pfizerpen-AS, Wycillin

penicillin G sodium

Natural penicillin, antibiotic

Available by prescription only
penicillin G benzathine
Suspension: 250,000 U/5 ml*, 500,000 U/ml*
Injection: 300,000 U/ml, 600,000 U/ml, 1.2 million U/2 ml, 2.4 million U/4 ml

penicillin G benzathine and procaine
Bicillin CR
Injection: 300,000 U/ml
Tubex: 600,000 U/dose, 1,200,000 U/dose, 2,400,000 U/dose
Bicillin CR 900/300
Tubex injection: 1,200,000 U/dose
penicillin G potassium
Powder for injection: 1 million U, 5 million U, 10 million U, 20 million U
Injection (premixed, frozen): 1 million U/50 ml, 2 million U/50 ml, 3 million U/50 ml
penicillin G procaine
Injection: 300,000 U/ml, 500,000 U/ml, 600,000 U/ml
penicillin G sodium
Powder for injection: 1 million U*, 5 million U, 10 million U*

INDICATIONS & DOSAGE
Group A streptococcal upper respiratory tract infections, ◊ diphtheria, ◊ yaws, pinta, and bejel
penicillin G benzathine
Adults: 1.2 million U I.M. in a single injection.
Prophylaxis of poststreptococcal rheumatic fever
penicillin G benzathine
Adults: 1.2 million U I.M. once monthly.
Syphilis of less than 1-year duration
penicillin G benzathine
Adults: 2.4 million U I.M. in a single dose.
Syphilis of more than 1-year duration
penicillin G benzathine
Adults: 2.4 million U I.M. weekly for 3 successive weeks.
Moderate to severe systemic infections
penicillin G potassium, sodium
Adults: 12 to 24 million U I.M. or I.V. daily, given in divided doses q 4 hours.
Moderate to severe systemic infections, pneumococcal pneumonia
penicillin G procaine
Adults: 600,000 to 1.2 million U I.M. daily as a single dose.
Uncomplicated gonorrhea
penicillin G procaine
Adults: 1 g probenecid P.O., then 30 minutes later, 4.8 million U penicillin G procaine I.M., divided into two injection sites.

Reactions may be *common*, uncommon, *life-threatening*, or COMMON AND LIFE-THREATENING.

✦ *Dosage adjustment.* For patients with renal failure, refer to the following table.

Creatinine clearance (ml/min)	Dosage (after full loading dose)
10-50	50% of usual dose q 4 to 5 hr; or give usual dose q 8 to 12 hr
< 10	50% of usual dose q 8 to 12 hr; or give usual dose q 12 to 18 hr

PHARMACODYNAMICS

Antibiotic action: Penicillin G is bactericidal; it adheres to penicillin-binding proteins, thus inhibiting bacterial cell wall synthesis. Spectrum of activity includes most nonpenicillinase-producing strains of gram-positive and gram-negative aerobic cocci, spirochetes, and some gram-positive aerobic and anaerobic bacilli.

PHARMACOKINETICS

Penicillin G is available as four salts, each having the same bactericidal action, but designed to offer greater oral stability (potassium salt) or to prolong duration of action by slowing absorption after I.M. injection (benzathine and procaine salts).
Absorption: Potassium and sodium salts of penicillin G are absorbed rapidly after I.M. injection; serum levels peak within 15 to 30 minutes. Absorption of other salts is slower. Serum penicillin G procaine levels peak at 1 to 4 hours, with drug detectable in serum for 1 to 2 days; serum penicillin G benzathine levels peak at 13 to 24 hours, with serum levels detectable for 1 to 4 weeks.
Distribution: Drug is distributed widely into synovial, pleural, pericardial, and ascitic fluids and bile and into liver, skin, lungs, kidneys, muscle, intestines, tonsils, maxillary sinuses, saliva, and erythrocytes. CSF penetration is poor but is enhanced in patients with inflamed meninges. Drug is 45% to 68% protein-bound.
Metabolism: Between 16% and 30% of an I.M. dose is metabolized to inactive compounds.
Excretion: Drug is excreted primarily in urine through tubular secretion; 20% to 60% of dose is recovered in 6 hours. Elimination half-life in adults is about ½

to 1 hour. Severe renal impairment prolongs half-life; drug is removed through hemodialysis and is only minimally removed through peritoneal dialysis.

CONTRAINDICATIONS & PRECAUTIONS

Contraindicated in patients with hypersensitivity to penicillin G or other penicillins. Use cautiously in patients with drug allergies (especially to cephalosporins or imipenem). Penicillin G potassium is contraindicated in patients with renal failure.

INTERACTIONS

Drug-drug. Use with *aminoglycosides* produces synergistic therapeutic effects, chiefly against enterococci; this combination is most effective in enterococcal bacterial endocarditis; however, drugs are physically and chemically incompatible and are inactivated when mixed or given together. In vivo inactivation has been reported when aminoglycosides and penicillins are used together.

Use of penicillin G with *clavulanate* appears to enhance the effect of penicillin G against certain beta-lactamase–producing bacteria. Penicillins may increase risk for bleeding with use of *heparin* or *oral anticoagulants.* Large doses of drug may interfere with renal tubular secretion of *methotrexate*, thus delaying elimination and elevating serum methotrexate levels. Use of drug with some *NSAIDs* prolongs penicillin half-life by competition for urine excretion or displacement of penicillin from protein-binding sites; similarly, use with *sulfinpyrazone*, which inhibits tubular secretion of penicillin G, also prolongs its half-life. Penicillins may decrease effectiveness of *oral contraceptives.* Use of parenteral penicillin G potassium with *potassium sparing diuretics* may cause hyperkalemia. *Probenecid* blocks tubular secretion of penicillin, increasing its serum levels.

ADVERSE REACTIONS

CNS: neuropathy, *seizures* (with high doses), lethargy, hallucinations, anxiety, confusion, agitation, depression, dizziness, fatigue, pain at injection site.

CV: thrombophlebitis (with penicillin G potassium only).

GI: nausea, vomiting, enterocolitis, pseudomembranous colitis.

GU: interstitial nephritis, nephropathy.

Hematologic: eosinophilia, hemolytic anemia, *thrombocytopenia,* leukopenia, anemia, *agranulocytosis.*

Other: hypersensitivity reactions (maculopapular and *exfoliative dermatitis,* chills, fever, edema, *anaphylaxis*), sterile abscess at injection site, overgrowth of nonsusceptible organisms (with penicillin G potassium and procaine), possible severe potassium poisoning with high doses (hyperreflexia, *seizures, coma*).

▣ KEY CONSIDERATIONS

Besides the recommendations relevant to all penicillins, consider the following:
• Half-life is prolonged in geriatric patients because of impaired renal function. Monitor closely for adverse effects.
• Monitor closely for possible hypernatremia with sodium salt or hyperkalemia with potassium salt.
• Patients with poor renal function are predisposed to high blood levels, which may cause seizures. Monitor renal function.
• Have emergency equipment on hand to manage possible anaphylaxis.
• Because penicillins are dialyzable, patients undergoing hemodialysis may need dosage adjustments.
• Administer by deep I.M. injection in outer upper quadrant of buttock.
• Penicillin G can be administered as a continuous infusion for meningitis.
• Drug alters test results for urine and serum protein levels; it interferes with turbidimetric methods using sulfosalicylic acid, trichloracetic acid, acetic acid, and nitric acid. Drug doesn't interfere with tests using bromophenol blue (Albustix, Albutest, Multistix).
• Drug alters urine glucose testing using cupric sulfate (Benedict's reagent); use Diastix, Chemstrip uG, or glucose enzymatic test strip instead. Drug may cause falsely elevated results of urine specific gravity tests in patients with low urine output and dehydration and falsely elevated Norymberski and Zimmermann test results for 17-ketogenic steroids; it causes false-positive CSF protein test results (Folin-Ciocalteau method) and may cause positive Coombs' test results.
• Drug may falsely decrease serum aminoglycoside levels. Adding beta-lactamase to the sample inactivates the penicillin, rendering the assay more accurate. Alternatively, the sample can be spun down and frozen immediately after collection.

Overdose & treatment

• Signs and symptoms of overdose include neuromuscular irritability or seizures.
• No specific recommendations are available. Treatment is supportive. After recent ingestion (within 4 hours), induce vomiting or perform gastric lavage. Follow with activated charcoal to decrease absorption. Hemodialysis removes penicillin G.

penicillin V

penicillin V potassium
Beepen VK, Betapen-VK, Ledercillin VK, Nadopen-V*, Pen Vee K, PVF K*, Robicillin VK, V-Cillin K, Veetids

Natural penicillin, antibiotic

Available by prescription only
penicillin V
Tablets: 125 mg, 250 mg, 500 mg
Solution: 125 mg/5 ml, 250 mg/5 ml (after reconstitution)
penicillin V potassium
Tablets: 500 mg
Tablets (film-coated): 250 mg, 500 mg
Solution: 125 mg/5 ml, 250 mg/5 ml (after reconstitution)

INDICATIONS & DOSAGE
Mild to moderate susceptible infections
Adults: 125 to 500 mg (200,000 to 800,000 U) P.O. q 6 hours for 10 days.
Endocarditis prophylaxis for dental surgery
Adults: 2 g P.O. 30 to 60 minutes before procedure, then 1 g 6 hours later.

Necrotizing ulcerative gingivitis
Adults: 250 to 500 mg P.O. q 6 to 8 hours.
◊ *Lyme disease*
Adults: 250 to 500 mg P.O. q.i.d. for 10 to 20 days.
◊ *Prophylaxis for pneumococcal infection*
Adults: 250 mg P.O. b.i.d.

PHARMACODYNAMICS
Antibiotic action: Penicillin V is bactericidal; it adheres to penicillin-binding proteins, thus inhibiting bacterial cell wall synthesis. Spectrum of activity includes most nonpenicillinase-producing strains of gram-positive and gram-negative aerobic cocci, spirochetes, and some gram-positive aerobic and anaerobic bacilli.

PHARMACOKINETICS
Absorption: Penicillin V has greater acid stability and is absorbed more completely than penicillin G after oral administration. Some 60% to 75% of oral dose is absorbed. Serum levels peak at 60 minutes in fasting subjects; food doesn't significantly affect absorption.
Distribution: Drug is distributed widely into synovial, pleural, pericardial, and ascitic fluids and bile and into liver, skin, lungs, kidneys, muscle, intestines, tonsils, maxillary sinuses, saliva, and erythrocytes. CSF penetration is poor but is enhanced in patients with inflamed meninges. It's 75% to 89% protein-bound.
Metabolism: Between 35% and 70% of a dose is metabolized to inactive compounds.
Excretion: Drug is excreted primarily in urine by tubular secretion; 26% to 65% of dose is recovered in 6 hours. Elimination half-life in adults is ½ hour. Severe renal impairment prolongs half-life.

CONTRAINDICATIONS & PRECAUTIONS
Contraindicated in patients with hypersensitivity to penicillin V or other penicillins. Use cautiously in patients with drug allergies (especially to cephalosporins or imipenem).

INTERACTIONS
Drug-drug. Use with *aminoglycosides* produces synergistic therapeutic effects, chiefly against enterococci; however, drugs are physically and chemically incompatible and are inactivated when given together. In vivo inactivation has been reported when aminoglycosides and penicillins are used concomitantly.
Penicillin V may decrease the efficacy of *estrogen-containing oral contraceptives;* breakthrough bleeding may occur. Use with *heparin* or *some anticoagulants* can increase the risk of bleeding. *Probenecid* blocks tubular secretion of penicillin, resulting in higher serum drug levels. Use with *sulfinpyrazone,* which inhibits tubular secretion of penicillin V, prolongs its half-life.

ADVERSE REACTIONS
CNS: neuropathy.
GI: *epigastric distress,* vomiting, diarrhea, *nausea,* black hairy tongue.
GU: nephropathy.
Hematologic: eosinophilia, hemolytic anemia, leukopenia, ***thrombocytopenia.***
Other: hypersensitivity reactions (rash, urticaria, fever, laryngeal edema, ***anaphylaxis***), overgrowth of nonsusceptible organisms.

▣ KEY CONSIDERATIONS
Besides the recommendations relevant to all penicillins, consider the following:
● Half-life may be prolonged in geriatric patients because of impaired renal function. Monitor closely for adverse effects.
● Give oral dose 1 hour before or 2 hours after meals for maximum absorption.
● After reconstitution, oral solution is stable for 14 days if refrigerated.
● Penicillin V alters test results for urine and serum protein levels; it interferes with turbidimetric methods using sulfosalicylic acid, trichloracetic acid, acetic acid, and nitric acid. Drug doesn't interfere with tests using bromophenol blue (Albustix, Albutest, MultiStix). Drug may falsely decrease serum aminoglycoside levels.

Overdose & treatment
● Signs and symptoms of overdose include neuromuscular sensitivity and seizures.
● No specific recommendations are available. Treatment is supportive. After recent ingestion (within 4 hours), induce vomiting or perform gastric lavage; follow with activated charcoal to reduce absorption.

---

pentazocine hydrochloride
Talacen (with Acetaminophen), Talwin Compound (with Aspirin), Talwin*, Talwin-Nx (with naloxone hydrochloride)

pentazocine lactate
Talwin

Narcotic agonist-antagonist, opioid partial agonist, analgesic adjunct to anesthesia
Controlled substance schedule IV

Available by prescription only
Tablets: 50 mg
Injection: 30 mg/ml
Combinations:
Talacen: 25 mg of pentazocine hydrochloride and 650 mg of acetaminophen
Talwin Compound: 12.5 mg of pentazocine hydrochloride and 325 mg of aspirin
Talwin-Nx: 50 mg of pentazocine hydrochloride and 0.5 mg base of naloxone hydrochloride

INDICATIONS & DOSAGE
Moderate to severe pain
Adults: 50 to 100 mg P.O. q 3 to 4 hours, p.r.n., or around the clock. Maximum oral dosage, 600 mg daily. Or 30 mg I.M., I.V., or S.C. q 3 to 4 hours, p.r.n., or around the clock. Maximum parenteral dosage, 360 mg daily. Doses greater than 30 mg I.V. or 60 mg I.M. or S.C. aren't recommended.

PHARMACODYNAMICS
Analgesic action: Exact mechanism of action is unknown. It's believed to be a competitive antagonist at some receptors and an agonist at others, thus relieving moderate pain.
    Pentazocine can produce respiratory depression, sedation, miosis, and antitussive effects. It also may cause psychotomimetic and dysphoric effects. In patients with coronary artery disease, it elevates mean aortic pressure, left ventricular end-diastolic pressure, and mean pulmonary artery pressure. In patients with an acute MI, I.V. pentazocine increases systemic and pulmonary arterial pressures and systemic vascular resistance.

PHARMACOKINETICS
Absorption: Pentazocine is well absorbed after oral or parenteral administration. However, orally administered drug undergoes first-pass-metabolism in the liver; less than 20% of a dose reaches the systemic circulation unchanged. Bioavailability is increased in patients with hepatic dysfunction; patients with cirrhosis absorb 60% to 70% of drug. Onset of analgesia is 15 to 30 minutes; effect peaks at 15 to 60 minutes.
Distribution: Drug appears to be widely distributed in the body.
Metabolism: Drug is metabolized in the liver, mainly by oxidation and secondarily by glucuronidation. Metabolism may be prolonged in patients with impaired hepatic function.
Excretion: Duration of effect is 3 hours. Urine excretion varies considerably among patients. A small amount of drug is excreted in feces after oral or parenteral administration.

CONTRAINDICATIONS & PRECAUTIONS
Contraindicated in patients with hypersensitivity to pentazocine or its components. Use cautiously in patients with impaired renal or hepatic function, an acute MI, head injury, increased intracranial pressure, or respiratory depression.

INTERACTIONS
Drug-drug. If administered within a few hours of *barbiturates* such as *thiopental*, pentazocine may produce additive CNS and respiratory depressant effects and possibly apnea. *Cimetidine* may increase

---

Reactions may be *common*, uncommon, *life-threatening*, or COMMON AND LIFE-THREATENING.

pentazocine toxicity, causing disorientation, respiratory depression, apnea, and seizures; because data are limited, this combination isn't contraindicated, but be prepared to administer naloxone if patient has a toxic reaction. Reduced doses of pentazocine usually are necessary when drug is used with other *CNS depressants*—including *antihistamines, barbiturates, benzodiazepines, muscle relaxants, narcotic analgesics, phenothiazines, sedative-hypnotics,* and *tricyclic antidepressants*—because such use potentiates the respiratory and CNS depressant, sedative, and hypotensive effects of the drug. Drug accumulation and enhanced effects may result from use with other *drugs that are extensively metabolized in the liver*—such as *digitoxin, phenytoin,* and *rifampin.* Use with *general anesthetics* may cause severe CV depression. Patients who become physically dependent on drug may experience acute withdrawal syndrome if given high doses of a *narcotic agonist-antagonist* or a single dose of an antagonist; use with caution, and monitor closely.

Drug-lifestyle. *Alcohol* may potentiate the respiratory and CNS effects of drug.

ADVERSE REACTIONS

CNS: *sedation,* visual disturbances, hallucinations, drowsiness, *dizziness, lightheadedness,* confusion, *euphoria,* headache, syncope, psychotomimetic effects.

CV: circulatory depression, *shock,* hypertension, hypotension.

EENT: dry mouth, blurred vision, nystagmus.

GI: *nausea, vomiting,* taste alteration, constipation.

GU: urine retention.

Hematologic: leukocyte depression, transient eosinophilia.

Respiratory: *respiratory depression,* dyspnea, apnea.

Skin: induration, nodules, sloughing, and sclerosis of injection site; diaphoresis; pruritus; facial edema; sweating.

Other: hypersensitivity reactions *(anaphylaxis),* physical and psychological dependence.

KEY CONSIDERATIONS

Besides the recommendations relevant to all opioid (narcotic) agonist-antagonists, consider the following:

• Lower doses are usually indicated for geriatric patients, who may be more sensitive to the therapeutic and adverse effects of pentazocine.

• Tablets aren't well absorbed.

• Don't mix in same syringe with soluble barbiturates.

• Drug may obscure the signs and symptoms of acute abdominal condition or worsen gallbladder pain.

• Drug may cause orthostatic hypotension in ambulatory patients. Have patient sit down to relieve symptoms.

• Drug possesses narcotic antagonist properties. May precipitate abstinence syndrome in narcotic-dependent patients.

• Talwin-Nx contains the narcotic antagonist naloxone, which prevents illicit I.V. use.

• Use S.C. route only when necessary; severe tissue damage is possible at injection site.

Patient education

• Tell patient to report rash, confusion, disorientation, or other serious adverse effects.

• Warn patient that Talwin-Nx is for oral use only. Severe reactions may result if tablets are crushed, dissolved, and injected.

• Tell patient to avoid use of alcohol and other CNS depressants.

Overdose & treatment

• The signs and symptoms of pentazocine hydrochloride overdose haven't been defined because of a lack of experience with overdose.

• If overdose occurs, supportive measures (for example, oxygen, I.V. fluids, vasopressors) should be used as necessary. Mechanical ventilation should be considered. Parenteral naloxone is an effective antagonist for respiratory depression caused by pentazocine.

pentobarbital sodium
Nembutal

*Barbiturate, anticonvulsant,
sedative-hypnotic*
*Controlled substance schedule II
(suppositories, schedule III)*

Available by prescription only
Elixir: 18.2 mg/5 ml
Capsules: 50 mg, 100 mg
Injection: 50 mg/ml, 2-ml disposable syringes; 2-ml, 20-ml, and 50-ml vials
Suppositories: 30 mg, 60 mg, 120 mg,
200 mg

INDICATIONS & DOSAGE
Sedation
Adults: 20 to 40 mg P.O., b.i.d. to q.i.d.
Insomnia
Adults: 100 mg P.O. h.s. or 150 to
200 mg deep I.M.; 120 to 200 mg P.R.
Preanesthetic drug
Adults: 150 to 200 mg I.M. or P.O. in
two divided doses.
Anticonvulsant
Adults: Initially, 100 mg I.V.; after 1
minute, additional doses may be given.
Maximum dose is 500 mg.

PHARMACODYNAMICS
Anticonvulsant action: Pentobarbital suppresses the spread of seizure activity produced by epileptogenic foci in the cortex,
thalamus, and limbic systems by enhancing the effect of gamma-aminobutyric
acid (GABA). Both presynaptic and
postsynaptic excitability are decreased,
and the seizure threshold is raised.
Sedative-hypnotic action: Exact cellular
site and mechanism of action are unknown. Drug acts throughout the CNS
as a nonselective depressant with a fast
onset and short duration of action. The
reticular activating system, which controls CNS arousal, is particularly sensitive to this drug. Drug decreases both
presynaptic and postsynaptic membrane
excitability by facilitating the action of
GABA.

PHARMACOKINETICS
Absorption: Pentobarbital is absorbed
rapidly after oral or rectal administration; onset of action is 10 to 15 minutes.
Serum levels peak 30 to 60 minutes after
oral administration. After I.M. injection,
onset of action is within 10 to 25 minutes. After I.V. administration, onset of
action occurs immediately. Serum levels
needed for sedation and hypnosis are 1
to 5 µg/ml and 5 to 15 µg/ml, respectively. After oral or rectal administration, duration of hypnosis is 1 to 4 hours.
Distribution: Drug is distributed widely
throughout the body; 35% to 45% is protein-bound. Drug accumulates in fat
with long-term use.
Metabolism: Drug is metabolized in the
liver by penultimate oxidation.
Excretion: About 99% of drug is eliminated as glucuronide conjugates and other metabolites in the urine. Terminal
half-life is from 35 to 50 hours. Duration
of action is 3 to 4 hours.

CONTRAINDICATIONS & PRECAUTIONS
Contraindicated in patients with hypersensitivity to barbiturates, porphyria, or
with severe respiratory disease when
dyspnea or obstruction is evident. Use
cautiously in geriatric or debilitated patients and in those with acute or chronic
pain, mental depression, suicidal tendencies, history of drug abuse, or impaired
hepatic function.

INTERACTIONS
Drug-drug. Pentobarbital may potentiate or add to CNS and respiratory depressant effects of other *antidepressants,
antihistamines, opioids, sedative-hypnotics,* and *tranquilizers.* Drug also
enhances hepatic metabolism of some
drugs, including *corticosteroids, digitoxin* (not digoxin), *doxycycline, oral contraceptives* and *other estrogens,* and
theophylline and *other xanthines. Disulfiram, MAO inhibitors,* and *valproic acid*
decrease the metabolism of pentobarbital and can increase its toxicity. Pentobarbital impairs the effectiveness of
griseofulvin by decreasing absorption
from the GI tract. Pentobarbital enhances the enzymatic degradation of
other oral anticoagulants and *warfarin;*
patients may require increased doses of
the anticoagulants. *Rifampin* may de-

Reactions may be *common,* uncommon, **life-threatening,** or **COMMON AND LIFE-THREATENING.**

crease pentobarbital levels by increasing hepatic metabolism.

Drug-lifestyle. *Alcohol* may potentiate the respiratory and CNS depressant effects of drug.

ADVERSE REACTIONS

CNS: *drowsiness, confusion, disorientation, lethargy, hangover,* paradoxical excitement in geriatric patients, somnolence, syncope, hallucinations. EEG patterns show a change in low-voltage, fast activity; changes persist for a time after discontinuation of therapy.

CV: bradycardia, hypotension.

GI: nausea, vomiting.

Hematologic: exacerbation of porphyria.

Respiratory: *respiratory depression.*

Skin: rash, urticaria, *Stevens-Johnson syndrome.*

Other: *angioedema,* physical and psychological dependence.

▣ KEY CONSIDERATIONS

Besides the recommendations relevant to all barbiturates, consider the following:

• Geriatric patients usually require lower doses because of increased susceptibility to CNS depressant effects of pentobarbital. Use with caution.

• Reserve I.V. injection for emergency treatment. Be prepared for emergency resuscitative measures.

• To prevent hypotension and respiratory depression, avoid I.V. administration at a rate exceeding 50 mg/minute.

• High-dose therapy for elevated intracranial pressure may require mechanically assisted ventilation.

• Administer I.M. dose deep into large muscle mass. Don't administer more than 5 ml into one site.

• Discard solution that's discolored or contains precipitate.

• Administration of full loading doses over short periods of time to treat status epilepticus requires ventilatory support in adults.

• To ensure accuracy of dosage, don't divide suppository.

• Drug has no analgesic effect and may cause restlessness or delirium in patients with pain.

• Nembutal tablets contain tartrazine dye, which may cause allergic reactions in susceptible persons.

• To prevent rebound of rapid-eye-movement sleep after prolonged therapy, discontinue gradually over 5 to 6 days.

• Drug may cause a false-positive phentolamine test result. The physiological effects of the drug may impair the absorption of cyanocobalamin ^{57}Co; it may decrease serum bilirubin levels in patients with epilepsy and those with congenital nonhemolytic unconjugated hyperbilirubinemia.

Patient education

• Tell patient not to take pentobarbital continuously for longer than 2 weeks.

• Emphasize the dangers of combining drug with alcohol. An excessive depressant effect is possible even if drug is taken the evening before ingestion of alcohol.

Overdose & treatment

• Signs and symptoms of overdose include unsteady gait, slurred speech, sustained nystagmus, somnolence, confusion, respiratory depression, pulmonary edema, areflexia, and coma. Typical shock syndrome with tachycardia and hypotension may occur. Jaundice, hypothermia followed by fever, and oliguria also may occur. Serum levels greater than 10 µg/ml may produce profound coma; concentrations greater than 30 µg/ml may be fatal.

• To treat, maintain and support ventilation and pulmonary function and support cardiac function and circulation with vasopressors and I.V. fluids, as needed. If patient is conscious, gag reflex is intact, and ingestion is recent, induce vomiting with ipecac syrup. If vomiting is contraindicated, perform gastric lavage while a cuffed endotracheal tube is in place to prevent aspiration. Follow with administration of activated charcoal or sodium chloride cathartic. Measure intake and output, vital signs, and laboratory parameters. Maintain body temperature.

• Alkalinization of urine may help remove drug from the body. Hemodialysis may be useful in severe overdose.

pentoxifylline
Trental

Xanthine derivative, intermittent claudication therapy

Available by prescription only
Tablets (extended-release): 400 mg

INDICATIONS & DOSAGE
Intermittent claudication from chronic occlusive vascular disease
Adults: 400 mg P.O. t.i.d. with meals. Continue treatment for at least 8 weeks.

PHARMACODYNAMICS
Hemorrheleogic action: Pentoxifylline improves capillary blood flow by increasing erythrocyte flexibility and reducing blood viscosity.

PHARMACOKINETICS
Absorption: Pentoxifylline is absorbed almost completely from the GI tract but undergoes first-pass hepatic metabolism. Food slows absorption. Levels peak in 2 to 4 hours, but therapeutic effect requires 2 to 4 weeks of continued therapy.
Distribution: Unknown; drug is bound to erythrocyte membrane.
Metabolism: Erythrocytes and the liver metabolize the drug extensively.
Excretion: Metabolites are excreted principally in urine; less than 4% of drug is excreted in feces. Half-life of unchanged drug is approximately ½ to ¾ hour; half-life of metabolites is 1 to 1½ hours.

CONTRAINDICATIONS & PRECAUTIONS
Contraindicated in patients who are intolerant to pentoxifylline or methylxanthines, such as caffeine, theophylline, and theobromine, and in patients with recent cerebral or retinal hemorrhage. Use cautiously in geriatric patients.

INTERACTIONS
Drug-drug. Use with *antihypertensives* may increase hypotensive response; some patients taking pentoxifylline have had small decreases in blood pressure. Although a causal relationship hasn't been proved, bleeding and prolonged PT have been reported in patients treated with drug; patients taking *drugs that inhibit platelet aggregation* or *oral anticoagulants* (such as *warfarin*) with pentoxifylline may have bleeding abnormalities.

ADVERSE REACTIONS
CNS: headache, dizziness.
CV: angina, chest pain.
GI: dyspepsia, nausea, vomiting, flatus, bloating.

◙ KEY CONSIDERATIONS
• Geriatric patients may have increased bioavailability and decreased excretion of pentoxifylline and thus are at higher risk for toxicity; adverse reactions may be more common in geriatric patients.
• Monitor blood pressure regularly, especially in patients taking antihypertensives; also monitor INR, especially in patients taking anticoagulants such as warfarin.
• If patient experiences GI and CNS adverse reactions, decrease dosage to twice daily. If they persist, discontinue drug.
• Drug is useful in patients who aren't good candidates for surgery.
• Don't crush or break timed-release tablets; make sure patient swallows them whole.
• Theophylline levels may increase when pentoxifylline is used concomitantly. Monitor patient closely.

Patient education
• Explain need for continuing therapy for at least 8 weeks; warn patient not to discontinue pentoxifylline during this period without medical approval.
• Advise taking drug with meals to minimize GI distress.
• Tell patient to report GI and CNS adverse reactions; they may require dosage reduction.

Overdose & treatment
• Signs and symptoms of overdose include flushing, hypotension, seizures, somnolence, loss of consciousness, fever, and agitation.
• No known antidote exists. Perform gastric lavage and administer activated charcoal; treat symptoms and support respiration and blood pressure.

Reactions may be *common,* uncommon, *life-threatening,* or COMMON AND LIFE-THREATENING.

pergolide mesylate
Permax

Dopaminergic agonist, antiparkinsonian

Available by prescription only
Tablets: 0.05 mg, 0.25 mg, 1 mg

INDICATIONS & DOSAGE
Adjunct to levodopa-carbidopa in the management of Parkinson's disease
Adults: Initially, 0.05 mg P.O. daily for first 2 days. Gradually increase dosage by 0.1 to 0.15 mg q 3rd day over next 12 days of therapy. Subsequent dosage can be increased by 0.25 mg q 3rd day until optimum response occurs. Mean therapeutic daily dose is 3 mg.

Drug is usually administered in divided doses t.i.d. Gradual reductions in levodopa-carbidopa dosage may be made during dosage adjustment.

PHARMACODYNAMICS
Antiparkinsonian action: Pergolide stimulates dopamine receptors at both D_1 and D_2 sites. It acts by directly stimulating postsynaptic receptors in the nigrostriatal system.

PHARMACOKINETICS
Absorption: Pergolide is well absorbed after oral administration.
Distribution: About 90% of drug binds to plasma proteins.
Metabolism: Drug is metabolized to at least 10 different compounds, some of which retain pharmacologic activity.
Excretion: Drug is excreted primarily from the kidneys.

CONTRAINDICATIONS & PRECAUTIONS
Contraindicated in patients hypersensitive to pergolide or to ergot alkaloids. Use cautiously in patients prone to arrhythmias.

INTERACTIONS
Drug-drug. Use of *dopamine antagonists*—including *butyrophenones, metoclopramide, phenothiazines,* and *thioxanthenes*—may antagonize the effects of pergolide. Pergolide is extensively protein-bound; use caution if it's administered with other *drugs known to affect protein binding.*

ADVERSE REACTIONS
CNS: headache, asthenia, *dyskinesia, dizziness, hallucinations, dystonia, confusion, somnolence,* insomnia, anxiety, depression, tremor, abnormal dreams, personality disorder, psychosis, abnormal gait, akathisia, extrapyramidal syndrome, incoordination, akinesia, hypertonia, neuralgia, speech disorder, twitching, paresthesia.
CV: *orthostatic hypotension,* vasodilation, chest pain, palpitations, hypotension, syncope, hypertension, *arrhythmias, MI.*
EENT: *rhinitis,* epistaxis, abnormal vision, diplopia, eye disorder.
GI: dry mouth, taste perversion, abdominal pain, *nausea, constipation,* diarrhea, dyspepsia, anorexia, vomiting.
GU: urinary frequency, urinary tract infection, hematuria.
Metabolic: weight gain.
Musculoskeletal: arthralgia, bursitis, myalgia, neck and back pain.
Respiratory: dyspnea.
Skin: rash, diaphoresis.
Other: flulike syndrome; chills; infection; facial, peripheral, or generalized edema; anemia.
Note: The preceding adverse reactions, although not always attributable to pergolide, occurred in more than 1% of the study population.

▣ KEY CONSIDERATIONS
• Use cautiously in patients with underlying psychiatric disturbances, especially hallucinations, confusion, and delirium.
• Adverse effects such as dizziness and nausea may subside with time.
• Give with food.

Patient education
• Inform patient of potential for adverse effects. Warn patient to avoid activities that could expose him to injury secondary to orthostatic hypotension and syncope.
• Caution patient to rise slowly to avoid orthostatic hypotension, particularly at the beginning of therapy.

Overdose & treatment
• Signs and symptoms of overdose include hypotension, vomiting, hallucinations, involuntary movements, palpitations, and arrhythmias.
• Provide supportive treatment. Monitor cardiac function and protect the patient's airway. Antiarrhythmics and sympathomimetics may be necessary to support CV function. Adverse CNS effects may be treated with dopaminergic antagonists (such as phenothiazines). If indicated, perform gastric lavage or induce vomiting and administer activated charcoal.

permethrin
Elimite, Nix

Synthetic pyrethroid, scabicide, pediculicide

Available by prescription only
Elimite
Cream: 5%
Available without prescription
Nix
Liquid: 60 ml (1%)

INDICATIONS & DOSAGE
Pediculosis
Adults: Apply sufficient volume to saturate the hair and scalp. Allow to remain on the hair for 10 minutes before rinsing.
Scabies
Adults: Thoroughly massage into skin from head to soles of feet. Remove cream by washing after 8 to 14 hours. One application is curative.

PHARMACODYNAMICS
Scabicide action: Permethrin acts on the parasites' nerve cell membranes to disrupt the sodium channel current and paralyze them.

PHARMACOKINETICS
Absorption: Not entirely investigated but probably less than 2% of the amount applied is absorbed.
Distribution: Systemic distribution is unknown.
Metabolism: Permethrin is rapidly metabolized by ester hydrolysis to inactive metabolites.

Excretion: Metabolites are excreted in urine. Residual persistence on the hair is detectable for up to 10 days.

CONTRAINDICATIONS & PRECAUTIONS
Contraindicated in patients hypersensitive to pyrethrins or chrysanthemums.

INTERACTIONS
None reported.

ADVERSE REACTIONS
Skin: pruritus, *burning, stinging,* edema, tingling, numbness or scalp discomfort, mild erythema, scalp rash.

🔲 KEY CONSIDERATIONS
• A single treatment is usually effective. Although combing of nits isn't required for effectiveness, drug package supplies a fine-tooth comb.
• A second application may be necessary if lice are observed 7 days after the initial application.

Patient education
• Tell patient or caregiver to wash hair with shampoo, rinse it thoroughly, and then towel dry.
• Tell patient or caregiver to apply sufficient volume to saturate the hair and scalp.
• Instruct patient to report itching, redness, or swelling of the scalp.
• Advise patient that permethrin is for external use only and to avoid contact with mucous membranes.

Overdose & treatment
• With accidental ingestion, perform gastric lavage and use general supportive measures.

perphenazine
Apo-Perphenazine*, Etrafon, Triavil, Trilafon

Phenothiazine (piperazine derivative), antipsychotic, antiemetic

Available by prescription only
Tablets: 2 mg, 4 mg, 8 mg, 16 mg
Oral concentrate: 16 mg/5 ml
Injection: 5 mg/ml

Reactions may be *common*, uncommon, *life-threatening*, or COMMON AND LIFE-THREATENING.

INDICATIONS & DOSAGE
Psychosis
Adults: Initially, 8 to 16 mg P.O. b.i.d., t.i.d., or q.i.d., increasing to 64 mg daily. Alternatively, administer 5 to 10 mg I.M.; change to P.O. as soon as possible.

Mental disturbances, acute alcoholism, nausea, vomiting, hiccups
Adults: 5 to 10 mg I.M., p.r.n. Maximum dosage is 15 mg daily in ambulatory patients; 30 mg daily in hospitalized patients; or 8 to 16 mg P.O. daily in divided doses.

Perphenazine may be given slowly by I.V. drip at a rate of 1 mg/2 minutes with continuous blood pressure monitoring (rarely used). A maximum of 5 mg I.V. diluted to 0.5 mg/ml with normal saline solution may be given for severe hiccups or vomiting.

PHARMACODYNAMICS
Antipsychotic and antiemetic actions: Perphenazine is thought to exert its antipsychotic effects via postsynaptic blockade of CNS dopamine receptors, thus inhibiting dopamine-mediated effects; antiemetic effects are attributed to dopamine receptor blockade in the medullary chemoreceptor trigger zone. Drug has many other central and peripheral effects: It produces both alpha and ganglionic blockade and counteracts histamine- and serotonin-mediated activity. Its most serious adverse reactions are extrapyramidal.

PHARMACOKINETICS
Absorption: Rate and extent of absorption vary with administration route: Oral tablet absorption is erratic and variable, with onset of action from ½ to 1 hour; oral concentrate absorption is much more predictable. I.M. drug is absorbed rapidly.
Distribution: Perphenazine is distributed widely into the body. Drug is 91% to 99% protein-bound. After oral tablet administration, effect peaks at 2 to 4 hours; steady-state serum levels are within 4 to 7 days.
Metabolism: Drug is metabolized extensively in the liver, but no active metabolites are formed.

Excretion: Drug is mostly excreted in urine from the kidneys, with some in feces from the biliary tract.

CONTRAINDICATIONS & PRECAUTIONS
Contraindicated in patients with hypersensitivity to perphenazine; in patients experiencing coma; in those with CNS depression, blood dyscrasia, bone marrow depression, liver damage, or subcortical damage; and in those receiving large doses of CNS depressants.

Use cautiously in geriatric or debilitated patients; in those with alcohol withdrawal, psychic depression, suicidal tendencies, adverse reaction to other phenothiazines, impaired renal function, respiratory disorders; and in patients receiving other CNS depressants or anticholinergics.

Contraindicated in patients with suspected subcortical brain damage, with or without hypothalamic damage, because hyperthermic reaction may occur.

INTERACTIONS
Drug-drug. Pharmacokinetic alterations and subsequent decreased therapeutic response to perphenazine may follow use with *aluminum-* and *magnesium-containing antacids, antidiarrheals* (decreased absorption), and *phenobarbital* (enhanced renal excretion). Use of perphenazine with *appetite suppressants* or *sympathomimetics*—including *ephedrine* (found in many nasal sprays), *epinephrine, phenylephrine,* and *phenylpropanolamine*—may decrease their stimulatory and pressor effects. *Beta blockers* may inhibit perphenazine metabolism, increasing plasma levels and toxicity. Perphenazine may antagonize therapeutic effect of *bromocriptine* on prolactin secretion; it may also decrease vasoconstrictive effects of *high-dose dopamine* and may decrease effectiveness and increase toxicity of *levodopa* (by dopamine blockade). Perphenazine may inhibit blood pressure response to *centrally acting antihypertensives,* such as *clonidine, guanabenz, guanadrel, guanethidine, methyldopa,* and *reserpine.* Phenothiazines can cause *epinephrine* reversal and a hypotensive response when epinephrine is used for its pressor

effects. Use with *lithium* may result in severe neurologic toxicity with an encephalitis-like syndrome and a decreased therapeutic response to perphenazine. Perphenazine may inhibit the metabolism and increase toxicity of *phenytoin.* Use with *propylthiouracil* increases risk for agranulocytosis.

Additive effects are likely after use with the following drugs: *antiarrhythmics, disopyramide, procainamide,* and *quinidine* (increased incidence of arrhythmias and conduction defects); *atropine* or *other anticholinergics,* including *antidepressants, antihistamines, antiparkinsonians, MAO inhibitors, meperidine,* and *phenothiazines* (oversedation, paralytic ileus, visual changes, and severe constipation); *CNS depressants,* including *analgesics, anesthetics (epidural, general,* or *spinal), barbiturates, narcotics,* or *tranquilizers*—or *parenteral magnesium sulfate* (oversedation, respiratory depression, and hypotension); *metrizamide* (increased risk for seizures); and *nitrates* (hypotension).
Drug-lifestyle. Additive effects are likely after use of drug with *alcohol. Caffeine* and *heavy smoking* may cause a decrease in therapeutic response because of increased drug metabolism.

ADVERSE REACTIONS

CNS: *extrapyramidal reactions, tardive dyskinesia,* sedation, pseudoparkinsonism, EEG changes, dizziness, adverse behavioral effects, **seizures,** drowsiness.
CV: *orthostatic hypotension,* tachycardia, ECG changes, **cardiac arrest.**
EENT: ocular changes, *blurred vision,* nasal congestion.
GI: *dry mouth, constipation,* nausea, vomiting, diarrhea, ileus, elevated liver enzyme levels.
GU: *urine retention,* dark urine, gynecomastia, inhibited ejaculation.
Hematologic: leukopenia, **agranulocytosis,** eosinophilia, **hemolytic anemia, thrombocytopenia.**
Hepatic: jaundice, abnormal liver function test results.
Metabolic: hyperglycemia, hypoglycemia.

Skin: *mild photosensitivity,* allergic reactions, pain at I.M. injection site, sterile abscess.
Other: weight gain, SIADH, **neuroleptic malignant syndrome.**
After abrupt withdrawal of long-term therapy: gastritis, nausea, vomiting, dizziness, tremors, feeling of warmth or cold, diaphoresis, tachycardia, headache, insomnia.

▣ KEY CONSIDERATIONS
Besides the recommendations relevant to all phenothiazines, consider the following:
• Use lower doses in geriatric patients. Dosage must be adjusted based on effects; 30% to 50% of the usual dose may be effective. Geriatric patients are at greater risk for adverse effects, especially tardive dyskinesia and other extrapyramidal effects.
• Oral formulations may cause stomach upset; administer with food or fluid.
• Dilute the concentrate in 2 to 4 oz (60 to 120 ml) liquid (water, carbonated drinks, fruit juice, tomato juice, milk, or puddings). Dilute every 5 ml concentrate with 60 ml suitable fluid.
• Liquid formulation may cause rash on contact with skin.
• I.M. injection may cause skin necrosis; avoid extravasation.
• Administer I.M. injection deep into outer upper quadrant of buttocks. Massaging the injection site may prevent formation of abscesses.
• Don't administer perphenazine for injection if it's excessively discolored or contains precipitate.
• Monitor blood pressure before and after parenteral administration.
• Shake oral concentrate before administration.
• Drug causes false-positive test results for urine porphyrins, urobilinogen, amylase, and 5-hydroxyindoleacetic acid because of darkening of urine by metabolites.
• Drug elevates test results for protein-bound iodine.

Reactions may be common, uncommon, *life-threatening*, or COMMON AND LIFE-THREATENING.

Patient education
• Explain the risks for dystonic reactions and tardive dyskinesia, and tell patient to report abnormal body movements.
• Instruct patient to avoid sun exposure, to wear sunscreen when going outdoors to prevent photosensitivity reactions, and to avoid using sun lamps and tanning beds, which may cause burning of the skin or skin discoloration.
• Tell patient to avoid spilling the liquid; contact with skin may cause rash and irritation.
• Warn patient not to take extremely hot or cold baths and to avoid exposure to temperature extremes, sun lamps, or tanning beds; perphenazine may cause thermoregulatory changes.
• Advise patient to take drug exactly as prescribed and not to double-dose for missed doses.
• Inform patient that interactions with many other drugs are possible. Advise patient to seek medical approval before self-medicating.
• Instruct patient not to stop taking drug suddenly; adverse reactions may be alleviated with a dosage reduction. Patient should promptly report difficulty urinating, sore throat, dizziness, or fainting.
• Tell patient to avoid hazardous activities that require alertness until effect of drug is established. Reassure patient that sedative effects of drug should become tolerable in several weeks.
• Tell patient not to drink alcohol or take other drugs that may cause excessive sedation.
• Explain which fluids are appropriate for diluting the concentrate (not apple juice or caffeine-containing drinks); explain dropper technique of measuring dose.
• Recommend sugarless hard candy or chewing gum, ice chips, or artificial saliva to relieve dry mouth.
• Tell patient not to crush or chew sustained-release form.

Overdose & treatment
• CNS depression is characterized by deep sleep (in which the patient can't be aroused) and possible coma, hypotension or hypertension, extrapyramidal symptoms, dystonia, abnormal involuntary muscle movements, agitation, seizures, arrhythmias, ECG changes, hypothermia or hyperthermia, and autonomic nervous system dysfunction.
• Treatment is symptomatic and supportive, including maintaining vital signs, airway, stable body temperature, and fluid and electrolyte balance.
• Don't induce vomiting if consciousness is impaired. Perphenazine inhibits cough reflex; aspiration may occur. Perform gastric lavage, then administer activated charcoal and sodium chloride cathartics; dialysis is usually ineffective. Regulate body temperature as needed. Treat hypotension with I.V. fluids: Don't give epinephrine. Treat seizures with parenteral diazepam or barbiturates, arrhythmias with 1 mg/kg of parenteral phenytoin with rate titrated to blood pressure, and extrapyramidal reactions with 1 to 2 mg of benztropine or 10 to 50 mg of parenteral diphenhydramine.

phenazopyridine hydrochloride
Azo-Standard, Baridium, Geridium, Phenazo*, Phenazodine, Prodium, Pyridiate, Pyridium, Urodine, Urogesic

Azo dye, urinary analgesic

Available without prescription
Tablets: 95 mg
Available by prescription only
Tablets: 100 mg, 200 mg

INDICATIONS & DOSAGE
Pain with urinary tract irritation or infection
Adults: 200 mg P.O. t.i.d. after meals.

PHARMACODYNAMICS
Analgesic action: Phenazopyridine has a local anesthetic effect on urinary tract mucosa via an unknown mechanism.

PHARMACOKINETICS
Absorption: Unknown.
Distribution: Traces of phenazopyridine are thought to enter CSF.
Metabolism: Drug is metabolized in the liver.

Excretion: Drug is excreted by the kidneys; 65% unchanged in urine. Average time of total excretion is 20.4 hours.

CONTRAINDICATIONS & PRECAUTIONS

Contraindicated in patients with hypersensitivity to phenazopyridine, glomerulonephritis, severe hepatitis, uremia, or renal insufficiency.

INTERACTIONS

None significant.

ADVERSE REACTIONS

CNS: headache.
GI: nausea, GI disturbances.
Hematologic: hemolytic anemia.
Skin: rash, pruritus.
Other: *anaphylactoid reactions,* methemoglobinemia.

▣ KEY CONSIDERATIONS

• Use with caution in geriatric patients because of possible decreased renal function.
• Administer with food or fluids to reduce GI upset.
• Evaluate response to drug therapy; assess urinary function, such as output and complaints of burning, pain, and frequency.
• Monitor vital signs, especially temperature.
• Encourage patient to increase fluid intake (if not contraindicated). Monitor intake and output.
• Use drug only as an analgesic.
• May be used with an antibiotic to treat urinary tract infections.
• Discontinue phenazopyridine in 2 days with concurrent antibiotic use.
• Drug may alter results of Diastix, Chemstrip uG, glucose enzymatic test strip, Acetest, and Ketostix. Clinitest should be used to obtain accurate urine glucose test results.
• Drug may also interfere with Ehrlich's test for urine urobilinogen; phenolsulfonphthalein excretion tests of kidney function; sulfobromophthalein excretion tests of liver function; and urine tests for protein, steroids, or bilirubin.

Patient education

• Instruct patient in measures to prevent urinary tract infection.
• Advise patient of possible adverse reactions; caution that phenazopyridine colors urine red or orange and may stain clothing.
• Tell patient that stains on clothing may be removed with a 0.25% solution of sodium dithionite or hydrosulfite.
• Advise patient to take missed dose as soon as possible and to not double-dose.
• Instruct patient to report symptoms that worsen or don't resolve.

Overdose & treatment

• Signs and symptoms of overdose include methemoglobinemia (most obvious as cyanosis) and renal and hepatic impairment and failure.
• To treat overdose, immediately induce vomiting with ipecac syrup or perform gastric lavage. To reverse methemoglobinemia, administer 1 to 2 mg/kg of methylene blue I.V. or 100 to 200 mg of ascorbic acid P.O. Provide symptomatic and supportive measures (respiratory support and correction of fluid and electrolyte imbalances). Monitor laboratory parameters and vital signs closely. Contact local or regional poison information center for specific instructions.

phenelzine sulfate
Nardil

MAO inhibitor, antidepressant

Available by prescription only
Tablets: 15 mg

INDICATIONS & DOSAGE
Severe depression
Adults: 15 mg P.O. t.i.d. Increase rapidly to 60 mg/day; maximum daily dose is 90 mg. Onset of maximum therapeutic effect is 2 to 6 weeks. Some health care providers reduce dosage after response occurs; maintenance dosage may be as low as 15 mg daily or every other day.

PHARMACODYNAMICS
Antidepressant action: Depression is thought to result from low CNS levels of

neurotransmitters, including norepinephrine and serotonin. Phenelzine inhibits MAO, an enzyme that normally inactivates amine-containing substances, thus increasing the level and activity of these drugs.

PHARMACOKINETICS
Absorption: Phenelzine is absorbed rapidly and completely from the GI tract.
Distribution: Unknown.
Metabolism: Drug is metabolized in the liver.
Excretion: Drug is excreted primarily in urine within 24 hours; some drug is excreted in feces from the biliary tract. Half-life is relatively short, but enzyme inhibition is prolonged and unrelated to half-life.

CONTRAINDICATIONS & PRECAUTIONS
Contraindicated in patients with hypersensitivity to phenelzine, heart failure, pheochromocytoma, hypertension, liver disease, and CV disease. Also contraindicated during therapy with other MAO inhibitors (such as isocarboxazid and tranylcypromine) or within 10 days of such therapy or within 10 days of elective surgery requiring general anesthesia, cocaine use, or local anesthesia containing sympathomimetic vasoconstrictors. Contraindicated within 2 weeks of using a selective serotonin reuptake inhibitor. Contraindicated by some manufacturers in patients older than age 60 because of possibility of existing cerebrosclerosis with damaged vessels.

Use cautiously in patients at risk for diabetes, suicide, or seizures and in those receiving thiazide diuretics or spinal anesthetics.

INTERACTIONS
Drug-drug. Phenelzine enhances pressor effects of *amphetamines, ephedrine, phenylephrine, phenylpropanolamine*, and related drugs and may result in serious CV toxicity; most *hay fever, OTC cold*, and *weight-reduction products* contain these drugs. Use with *general* or *spinal anesthetics*, which are normally metabolized by MAO, may cause severe hypotension and excessive CNS depression; phenelzine decreases effectiveness

of *local anesthetics* (such as *lidocaine* and *procaine),* resulting in poor nerve block, and should be discontinued for at least 1 week before use of these drugs. Use cautiously and in reduced dosage with *barbiturates* and *dextromethorphan, narcotics, other sedatives*, and *tricyclic antidepressants*. Use with *disulfiram* may cause tachycardia, flushing, or palpitations. Use with *serotonergic drugs*—including *fluoxetine, fluvoxamine, paroxetine,* and *sertraline*—can result in serious adverse effects; at least a 2-week waiting period between drug use is recommended.
Drug-food. Use with foods high in *caffeine, tryptophan,* or *tyramine* may precipitate hypertensive crisis; avoid use.
Drug-lifestyle. *Alcohol* should be avoided when taking phenelzine and for 2 weeks after it's discontinued.

ADVERSE REACTIONS
CNS: *dizziness,* vertigo, headache, hyperreflexia, tremor, muscle twitching, *insomnia,* drowsiness, weakness, fatigue.
CV: postural hypotension, edema.
GI: dry mouth, *anorexia,* nausea, constipation, elevated liver function test results.
Metabolic: weight gain.
Other: diaphoresis, sexual disturbances.

▣ KEY CONSIDERATIONS
• Phenelzine isn't recommended for patients older than age 60 because of the potential for increased adverse effects. Monitor patient closely.
• Exercise precautions for use of MAO inhibitors, given alone or with other drugs, for 14 days after stopping drug.
• Consider the inherent risk for suicide until significant improvement of depressive state occurs. High-risk patients should have close supervision during initial drug therapy. To reduce risk of suicidal overdose, prescribe the smallest quantity of tablets consistent with good management.
• At start of therapy, patient should lie down for 1 hour after taking phenelzine; to prevent dizziness from orthostatic blood pressure changes, sudden changes to standing position should be avoided.

• Unlike that with other MAO inhibitors, combination therapy with phenelzine and tricyclic antidepressants is generally well tolerated.

Patient education
• Warn patient not to take alcohol, other CNS depressants, or self-prescribed drugs (such as cold, hay fever, or diet preparations) without medical approval.
• Explain that many foods and beverages (such as wine, beer, cheeses, and preserved fruits, meats, and vegetables) may interact with drug. Patient can obtain a list of foods to avoid from the dietary department or pharmacy at most hospitals.
• Tell patient to avoid hazardous activities that require alertness until the full effect of phenelzine on the CNS is known. Suggest taking drug at bedtime to minimize daytime sedation.
• Instruct patient to take drug exactly as prescribed and not to double-dose if a dose is missed.
• Tell patient not to discontinue drug abruptly and to report problems; dosage reduction can relieve most adverse reactions.

Overdose & treatment
• Signs and symptoms of overdose include exacerbations of adverse reactions or exaggerated responses to normal pharmacologic activity; such symptoms become apparent slowly (within 24 to 48 hours) and may persist for up to 2 weeks. Agitation, flushing, tachycardia, hypotension, hypertension, palpitations, increased motor activity, twitching, increased deep tendon reflexes, seizures, hyperpyrexia, cardiorespiratory arrest, and coma may occur. Doses of 375 mg to 1.5 g have been ingested with fatal and nonfatal results.
• Treat symptomatically and supportively: Give 5 to 10 mg of phentolamine I.V. push for hypertensive crisis; I.V. diazepam for seizures, agitation, or tremors; beta blockers for tachycardia; and cooling blankets for fever. Monitor vital signs and fluid and electrolyte balance. Sympathomimetics (such as norepinephrine or phenylephrine) are contraindicated in hypotension caused by MAO inhibitors.

phenobarbital
Solfoton

phenobarbital sodium
Luminal

Barbiturate, anticonvulsant, sedative-hypnotic
Controlled substance schedule IV

Available by prescription only
Tablets: 15 mg, 16 mg, 30 mg, 60 mg, 100 mg
Capsules: 16 mg
Elixir: 15 mg/ ml, 20 mg/5 ml
Injection: 30 mg/ml, 60 mg/ml, 65 mg/ml, 130 mg/ml
Powder for injection: 120 mg/ampule

INDICATIONS & DOSAGE
All forms of epilepsy except absence seizures
Adults: 60 to 100 mg P.O. daily, divided t.i.d. or given as single dose h.s. Alternatively, give 200 to 300 mg I.M. or I.V. and repeat q 6 hours, p.r.n.
Status epilepticus
Adults: 10 to 20 mg/kg I.V. over 10 to 15 minutes. Repeat if necessary.
Sedation
Adults: 30 to 120 mg P.O., I.M., or I.V. daily in two or three divided doses.
Insomnia
Adults: 100 to 200 mg P.O. or 100 to 320 mg I.M.
Preoperative sedation
Adults: 100 to 200 mg I.M. 60 to 90 minutes before surgery.

PHARMACODYNAMICS
Anticonvulsant action: By enhancing the effect of gamma-aminobutyric acid (GABA), phenobarbital suppresses the spread of seizure activity that the epileptogenic foci in the cortex, thalamus, and limbic systems produce. Both presynaptic and postsynaptic excitability are decreased; also, drug raises the seizure threshold.
Sedative-hypnotic action: Drug acts throughout the CNS as a nonselective depressant with a slow onset and long duration of action. The reticular activating system, which controls CNS arousal,

is particularly sensitive to this drug. Drug decreases both presynaptic and postsynaptic membrane excitability by facilitating the action of GABA. The exact cellular site and mechanism of action are unknown.

PHARMACOKINETICS

Absorption: Phenobarbital is well absorbed after oral and rectal administration, with 70% to 90% reaching the bloodstream. Absorption after I.M. administration is 100%. After oral administration, serum levels peak in 1 to 2 hours, and CNS levels peak in 20 to 60 minutes. Onset of action is 1 hour or longer after oral dosing; after I.V. administration, about 5 minutes. A serum level of 10 µg/ml is needed to produce sedation; 40 µg/ml usually produces sleep. Levels of 20 to 40 µg/ml are considered therapeutic for anticonvulsant therapy. *Distribution:* Drug is distributed widely throughout the body; 25% to 30% is protein-bound.
Metabolism: Drug is metabolized by the hepatic microsomal enzyme system.
Excretion: About 25% to 50% of dose is eliminated unchanged in urine; remainder is excreted as metabolites of glucuronic acid. Half-life is 5 to 7 days.

CONTRAINDICATIONS & PRECAUTIONS

Contraindicated in patients with barbiturate hypersensitivity, history of manifest or latent porphyria, hepatic dysfunction, respiratory disease with dyspnea or obstruction, and nephritis.

Use cautiously in geriatric or debilitated patients and in those with acute or chronic pain, depression, suicidal tendencies, history of drug abuse, blood pressure alterations, CV disease, shock, or uremia. S.C. administration is contraindicated.

INTERACTIONS

Drug-drug. Phenobarbital may add to or potentiate CNS and respiratory depressant effects of other *antidepressants, antihistamines, narcotics, phenothiazines, sedative-hypnotics,* and *tranquilizers.* Drug also enhances hepatic metabolism of some drugs— including *corticosteroids, digitoxin* (not digoxin), *doxycycline, oral contraceptives* and *other estrogens,* and *other xanthines* and *theophylline. Disulfiram, MAO inhibitors,* and *valproic acid* decrease the metabolism of phenobarbital and can increase its toxicity. Phenobarbital impairs the effectiveness of *griseofulvin* by decreasing absorption from the GI tract. Drug enhances the enzymatic degradation of *other oral anticoagulants* and *warfarin;* patients may require increased doses of the anticoagulant. *Rifampin* may decrease phenobarbital levels by increasing hepatic metabolism.
Drug-lifestyle. Drug potentiates the CNS and respiratory effects of *alcohol.*

ADVERSE REACTIONS

CNS: *drowsiness, lethargy, hangover,* paradoxical excitement, somnolence, pain at injection site. EEG patterns show a change in low-voltage, fast activity; changes persist for a time after discontinuation of therapy.
CV: bradycardia, hypotension, thrombophlebitis.
GI: nausea, vomiting.
Hematologic: exacerbation of porphyria.
Respiratory: *respiratory depression, apnea.*
Skin: rash, *erythema multiforme, Stevens-Johnson syndrome,* urticaria; swelling, necrosis, nerve injury at injection site.
Other: *angioedema,* physical and psychological dependence.

▣ KEY CONSIDERATIONS

Besides the recommendations relevant to all barbiturates, consider the following:
• Geriatric patients are more sensitive to the effects of phenobarbital—such as confusion, disorientation, and excitability—and usually require lower doses.
• Drug may cause a false-positive phentolamine test result. The physiological effects of drug may impair the absorption of cyanocobalamin ^{57}Co.
• Oral solution may be mixed with water or juice to improve taste.
• Don't crush or break extended-release form because this will impair drug action.

• Reconstitute powder for injection with 2.5 to 5 ml sterile water for injection. Roll vial in hands; don't shake.
• To prevent extravasation, use a larger vein for I.V. administration.
• To prevent hypotension and respiratory depression, avoid I.V. administration at a rate exceeding 60 mg/minute. It may take up to 30 minutes after I.V. administration to achieve maximum effect.
• Administer parenteral dose within 30 minutes of reconstitution because drug hydrolyzes in solution and on exposure to air.
• Keep emergency resuscitation equipment on hand when administering drug I.V.
• Administer I.M. dose deep into a large muscle mass to prevent tissue injury.
• Don't use injectable solution if it contains a precipitate.
• Administration of full loading doses over short periods of time to treat status epilepticus will require ventilatory support in adults.
• Unless a loading dose is used, full therapeutic effects aren't seen for 2 to 3 weeks.

Patient education
• Advise patient of potential for physical and psychological dependence with prolonged use.
• Warn patient to avoid alcohol and other CNS depressants while taking phenobarbital. An excessive depressant effect is possible even if drug is taken the evening before ingestion of alcohol.
• Caution patient not to stop taking drug suddenly because this could cause a withdrawal reaction.
• Advise patient to avoid driving and other hazardous activities that require alertness until the adverse CNS effects of drug are known.

Overdose & treatment
• Signs and symptoms of overdose include unsteady gait, slurred speech, sustained nystagmus, somnolence, confusion, respiratory depression, pulmonary edema, areflexia, and coma. Typical shock syndrome with tachycardia and hypotension, along with jaundice, oliguria, and chills followed by fever, may occur.

• Treatment includes maintenance and support of ventilation and pulmonary function and support of cardiac function and circulation with vasopressors and I.V. fluids, as needed. If patient is conscious, gag reflex is intact, and ingestion was recent, induce vomiting with ipecac syrup. If vomiting is contraindicated, perform gastric lavage while a cuffed endotracheal tube is in place to prevent aspiration. Then administer activated charcoal or sodium chloride cathartic. Measure intake and output, vital signs, and laboratory parameters. Maintain body temperature.
• Alkalinization of urine may help remove phenobarbital from the body; hemodialysis may be useful in severe overdose. Oral activated charcoal may enhance drug elimination regardless of its route of administration.
• Hemodialysis or hemoperfusion may be used in severe barbiturate intoxication or if the patient is anuric or in shock.

phenylephrine hydrochloride
Nasal products
Alconefrin 12, Alconefrin 25, Neo-Synephrine, Rhinall Nostril, Sinex

Parenteral
Neo-Synephrine

Ophthalmic
Ak-Dilate, Ak-Nefrin, Mydfrin, Neo-Synephrine, Prefrin Liquifilm, Relief, Phenoptic

Adrenergic, vasoconstrictor

Available by prescription only
Injection: 10 mg/ml parenteral
Ophthalmic solution: 2.5%, 10%
Available without prescription
Nasal solution: 0.125%, 0.16%, 0.25%, 0.5%, 1%
Nasal spray: 0.25%, 0.5%, 1%
Ophthalmic solution: 0.12%

INDICATIONS & DOSAGE
Hypotensive emergencies during spinal anesthesia
Adults: initially, 0.1 to 0.2 mg I.V.; subsequent doses should be 0.1 mg.

Prevention of hypotension during spinal or inhalation anesthesia
Adults: 2 to 3 mg S.C. or I.M. 3 to 4 minutes before anesthesia.

Mild to moderate hypotension
Adults: 1 to 10 mg S.C. or I.M. (initial dose shouldn't exceed 5 mg). Additional doses may be given in 1 to 2 hours if needed. Or, 0.1 to 0.5 mg slow I.V. injection (initial dose shouldn't exceed 0.5 mg). Additional doses may be given q 10 to 15 minutes.

Paroxysmal supraventricular tachycardia
Adults: Initially, 0.5 mg rapid I.V.; subsequent doses may be increased in increments of 0.1 to 0.2 mg. Maximum dose shouldn't exceed 1 mg.

Prolongation of spinal anesthesia
Adults: 2 to 5 mg added to anesthetic solution.

Adjunct in the treatment of severe hypotension or shock
Adults: 0.1 to 0.18 mcg/minute I.V. infusion. After blood pressure stabilizes, maintain at 0.04 to 0.06 mcg/minute, adjusted to patient response.

Vasoconstrictor for regional anesthesia
Adults: 1 mg phenylephrine added to 20 ml local anesthetic.

Mydriasis (without cycloplegia)
Adults: Instill 1 or 2 gtt 2.5% or 10% solution in eye before procedure. May be repeated in 10 to 60 minutes if needed.

Posterior synechia (adhesion of iris)
Adults: Instill 1 gtt 10% solution in eye three or more times daily with atropine sulfate.

Diagnosis of Horner's or Raeder's syndrome
Adults: Instill a 1% or 10% solution in both eyes.

Initial treatment of postoperative malignant glaucoma
Adults: Instill 1 gtt 10% solution with 1 gtt 1% to 4% atropine sulfate solution three or more times daily.

Nasal, ◇ sinus, or eustachian tube congestion
Adults: Apply 2 or 3 gtt or 1 or 2 sprays of 0.25% to 1% solution in each nostril; or a small quantity of 0.5% nasal jelly applied into each nostril. Apply jelly or spray to nasal mucosa.

Conjunctival congestion
Adults: 1 or 2 gtt 0.08% to 0.25% solution applied to conjunctiva q 3 to 4 hours, p.r.n.

PHARMACODYNAMICS

Vasopressor action: Phenylephrine directly stimulates alpha-adrenergic receptors, which constrict resistance and capacitance blood vessels, resulting in increased total peripheral resistance; increases systolic and diastolic blood pressure; decreases blood flow to vital organs, skin, and skeletal muscle; and constricts renal blood vessels, which reduces renal blood flow. Its main therapeutic effect is vasoconstriction.

It may also act indirectly by releasing norepinephrine from its storage sites. Drug doesn't stimulate beta receptors except in large doses (activates beta$_1$ receptors). Drug tolerance may follow repeated injections.

Other alpha-adrenergic effects include action on the dilator muscle of the pupil (producing contraction) and local decongestant action in the arterioles of the conjunctiva (producing constriction).

Drug acts directly on alpha-adrenergic receptors in the arterioles of conjunctiva nasal mucosa, producing constriction. Its vasoconstrictive action on skin, mucous membranes, and viscera slows the vascular absorption rate of local anesthetics, which prolongs their action, localizes anesthesia, and decreases the risk of toxicity.

PHARMACOKINETICS

Absorption: Pressor effects occur almost immediately after I.V. injection and persist 15 to 20 minutes; after I.M. injection, onset is within 10 to 15 minutes, lasting ½ to 2 hours; after S.C. injection, within 10 to 15 minutes, with effects lasting 50 to 60 minutes. Nasal or conjunctival decongestant effects last 30 minutes to 4 hours. Effects peak for mydriasis at 15 to 60 minutes for the 2.5% solution; 10 to 90 minutes for the 10% solution. Mydriasis recovery time is 3 hours for the 2.5% solution; 3 to 7 hours for the 10% solution.
Distribution: Unknown.

Metabolism: MAOs in the liver and intestine metabolize phenylephrine.
Excretion: Unknown.

CONTRAINDICATIONS & PRECAUTIONS
All forms are contraindicated in patients with hypersensitivity to phenylephrine. Injected form is also contraindicated in those with severe hypertension or ventricular tachycardia. Ophthalmic form is also contraindicated in patients with angle-closure glaucoma and in those who wear soft contact lenses.

Use all forms cautiously in geriatric patients and in those with hyperthyroidism or cardiac disease. Use nasal and ophthalmic forms cautiously in patients with type 1 diabetes mellitus, hypertension, or advanced arteriosclerotic changes. Use injectable form cautiously in patients with severe atherosclerosis, bradycardia, partial heart block, myocardial disease, or allergy to sulfites.

INTERACTIONS
Drug-drug. Decreased pressor response (hypotension) may result when phenylephrine is used with *alpha-adrenergic blockers, antihypertensives, diuretics used as antihypertensives, guanadrel* or *guanethidine, nitrates,* or *rauwolfia alkaloids.* Phenylephrine may increase risk for arrhythmias, including tachycardia, when used with *cardiac glycosides, epinephrine* or *other sympathomimetics, general anesthetics* (such as *cyclopropane* and *halothane), guanadrel* or *guanethidine, levodopa, MAO inhibitors,* or *tricyclic antidepressants.* The mydriatic response to drug is increased when used with *cycloplegic antimuscarinics* such as *atropine* and is decreased when used with *levodopa.* Pressor effects are potentiated used with *doxapram, ergot alkaloids, MAO inhibitors, mazindol, methyldopa,* or *oxytocic drugs.* Use with *nitrates,* may reduce antianginal effects. Use with *thyroid hormones* may increase effects of either drug.

ADVERSE REACTIONS
CNS: *headache;* excitability (with injected form); brow ache (with ophthalmic form); tremor, dizziness, nervousness (with nasal form).

CV: bradycardia, *arrhythmias,* hypertension (with injected form); *hypertension* (with 10% solution), tachycardia, palpitations, *PVCs, MI* (with ophthalmic form); *palpitations, tachycardia, PVCs,* hypertension, pallor (with nasal form).
EENT: transient eye burning or stinging on instillation, blurred vision, increased intraocular pressure, keratitis, lacrimation, reactive hyperemia of eye, allergic conjunctivitis, rebound miosis (with ophthalmic form); transient burning or stinging, dryness of nasal mucosa, rebound nasal congestion with continued use (with nasal form).
GI: nausea (with nasal form).
Skin: pallor, dermatitis (with ophthalmic form).
Other: tachyphylaxis (may occur with continued use); *anaphylaxis, asthmatic episodes,* decreased organ perfusion (with prolonged use); tissue sloughing with extravasation (with injected form); trembling, diaphoresis (with ophthalmic form).

▣ KEY CONSIDERATIONS
Besides the recommendations relevant to all adrenergics, consider the following:
• Effects may be exaggerated in geriatric patients. In patients older than age 50, phenylephrine (ophthalmic solution) appears to alter the response of the dilator muscle of the pupil so that rebound miosis may occur the day after drug is administered.
• Give I.V. through large veins and monitor flow rate. To treat extravasation ischemia, infiltrate site promptly and liberally with 10 to 15 ml sodium chloride solution containing 5 to 10 mg phentolamine through fine needle. Topical nitroglycerin has also been used.
• During I.V. administration, pulse, blood pressure, and central venous pressure should be monitored every 2 to 5 minutes. Control flow rate and dosage to prevent excessive increases. I.V. overdoses can induce ventricular arrhythmias.
• Hypovolemic states should be corrected before administration; drug shouldn't be used in place of fluid, blood, plasma, and electrolyte replacement.

Reactions may be *common,* uncommon, *life-threatening,* or COMMON AND LIFE-THREATENING.

• Drug is chemically incompatible with butacaine, sulfate, alkalies, ferric salts, and oxidizing drugs and metals.
• Drug may reduce intraocular pressure in healthy eyes or in open-angle glaucoma. Drug also may cause false-normal tonometry readings

Ophthalmic
• Apply digital pressure to lacrimal sac during and for 1 to 2 minutes after instillation to prevent systemic absorption.
• Prolonged exposure to air or strong light may cause oxidation and discoloration. Don't use if solution is brown or contains precipitate.
• To prevent contamination, don't touch applicator tip to a surface. Instruct patient in proper technique.

Nasal
• Prolonged or long-term use may result in rebound congestion and chronic swelling of nasal mucosa.
• To reduce risk for rebound congestion, use weakest effective dose.
• After use, rinse tip of spray bottle or dropper with hot water and dry with clean tissue. Wipe tip of nasal jelly container with clean, damp tissues.

Patient education
• Tell patient to store away from heat, light, and humidity (not in bathroom medicine cabinet) and out of children's reach.
• Warn patient to use only as directed. If using OTC product, patient should follow directions on label and not use more often or in larger doses than prescribed or recommended.
• Caution patient not to exceed recommended dosage, regardless of formulation; patient shouldn't double, decrease, or omit doses or change dosage intervals unless so instructed.
• Tell patient to call if phenylephrine provides no relief within 2 days after using ophthalmic solution or 3 days after using the nasal solution.
• Explain that systemic absorption from nasal and conjunctival membranes can occur. Patient should report systemic reactions, such as dizziness and chest pain, and discontinue drug.

Ophthalmic
• Instruct patient not to use if solution is brown or contains a precipitate.
• Tell patient to wash hands before applying and to use finger to apply pressure to lacrimal sac during and for 1 to 2 minutes after instillation to decrease systemic absorption.
• Warn patient to avoid touching tip to a surface to prevent contamination.
• Inform patient that after applying drops, pupils will become unusually large. Patient should use sunglasses to protect eyes from sunlight and other bright lights and call if effects persist 12 hours or more.

Nasal
• After use, tell patient to rinse tip of spray bottle or dropper with hot water and dry with clean tissue or wipe tip of nasal jelly container with clean, damp tissues.
• Instruct patient to blow nose gently (with both nostrils open) to clear nasal passages well before using drug.
• Teach patient correct instillation. For drops, tilt head back while sitting or standing up, or lie on bed and hang head over side; stay in position a few minutes to permit drug to spread through nose. For spray, with head upright, squeeze bottle quickly and firmly to produce 1 or 2 sprays into each nostril; wait 3 to 5 minutes, blow nose and repeat dose.
• Tell patient that increased fluid intake helps keep secretions liquid.
• Warn patient to avoid using OTC drugs with drug to prevent possible hazardous interactions.

Overdose & treatment
• Signs and symptoms of overdose include exaggeration of common adverse reactions, palpitations, paresthesia, vomiting, arrhythmias, and hypertension.
• To treat, discontinue phenylephrine and provide symptomatic and supportive measures. Monitor vital signs closely. Use atropine sulfate to block reflex bradycardia; phentolamine to treat excessive hypertension; and propranolol to treat cardiac arrhythmias, or levodopa to reduce an excessive mydriatic effect of an ophthalmic preparation as necessary.

---

phenytoin, phenytoin sodium, phenytoin sodium (extended)
Dilantin, Dilantin Infatab, Dilantin 125, Dilantin Kapseals

phenytoin sodium (prompt)

Hydantoin derivative, anticonvulsant

Available by prescription only
phenytoin
Tablets (chewable): 50 mg
Oral suspension: 30 mg/5 ml*, 125 mg/5 ml
phenytoin sodium
Injection: 50 mg/ml
phenytoin sodium (extended)
Capsules: 30 mg, 100 mg
phenytoin sodium (prompt)
Capsules: 30 mg, 100 mg

INDICATIONS & DOSAGE
Generalized tonic-clonic seizures, status epilepticus, nonepileptic seizures (post–head trauma, Reye's syndrome)
Adults: Loading dose is 10 to 15 mg/kg I.V. slowly, not to exceed 50 mg/minute; oral loading dosage consists of 1 g divided into three doses (400 mg, 300 mg, 300 mg) given at 2-hour intervals. Maintenance dosage once controlled is 300 mg P.O. daily (extended only); initially use a dose divided t.i.d. (extended or prompt).
Neuritic pain (migraine, trigeminal neuralgia, and Bell's palsy)
Adults: 200 to 600 mg P.O. daily in divided doses.
Skeletal muscle relaxant
Adults: 200 to 600 mg P.O. daily, p.r.n.
◊ ***Ventricular arrhythmias unresponsive to lidocaine or procainamide, and arrhythmias induced by cardiac glycosides***
Adults: 50 to 100 mg q 10 to 15 minutes, p.r.n., not to exceed 15 mg/kg. Infusion rate should never exceed 50 mg/minute (slow I.V. push).
Alternate method: 100 mg I.V. q 15 minutes until adverse effects develop, arrhythmias are controlled, or 1 g has been given. Also, may administer entire load-ing dose of 1 g I.V. slowly at 25 mg/minute. Can be diluted in normal saline solution. I.M. dosage isn't recommended because of pain and erratic absorption.
Prophylactic control of seizures during neurosurgery
Adults: 100 to 200 mg I.V. at intervals of about 4 hours during perioperative and postoperative periods.

PHARMACODYNAMICS
Anticonvulsant action: Like other hydantoin derivatives, phenytoin stabilizes neuronal membranes and limits seizure activity by either increasing efflux or decreasing influx of sodium ions across cell membranes in the motor cortex during generation of nerve impulses. Drug exerts its antiarrhythmic effects by normalizing sodium influx to Purkinje's fibers in patients with cardiac glycoside–induced arrhythmias. It's indicated for generalized tonic-clonic and partial seizures.
Other actions: Drug inhibits excessive collagenase activity in patients with epidermolysis bullosa.

PHARMACOKINETICS
Absorption: Phenytoin is absorbed slowly from the small intestine; absorption is formulation dependent and bioavailability may differ among products. With extended-release capsules, serum levels peak at 4 to 12 hours; with prompt-release products, $1\frac{1}{4}$ to 3 hours. I.M. doses are absorbed erratically; about 50% to 75 in 24 hours.
Distribution: Drug is distributed widely throughout the body. In most patients, therapeutic plasma levels are 10 to 20 µg/ml; however, in some patients, they're 5 to 10 µg/ml. Lateral nystagmus may occur at levels greater than 20 µg/ml; ataxia usually occurs at levels greater than 30 µg/ml; significantly decreased mental capacity occurs at 40 µg/ml. Drug is about 90% protein-bound, less so in uremic patients.
Metabolism: Drug is metabolized in the liver to inactive metabolites.
Excretion: Drug is excreted in urine and exhibits dose-dependent (zero-order) elimination kinetics; above a certain

dosage level, small increases in dosage disproportionately increase serum levels.

CONTRAINDICATIONS & PRECAUTIONS
Contraindicated in patients with hydantoin hypersensitivity, sinus bradycardia, SA block, second- or third-degree AV block, or Stokes-Adams syndrome.

Use cautiously in geriatric or debilitated patients; in those with hepatic dysfunction, hypotension, myocardial insufficiency, diabetes, or respiratory depression; and in those receiving hydantoin derivatives.

INTERACTIONS
Drug-drug. Phenytoin interacts with many drugs. Diminished therapeutic effects and toxic reactions commonly are the result of recent changes in drug therapy. The therapeutic effects of the drug may be increased when drug is used with *allopurinol, amiodarone, chloramphenicol, chlorpheniramine, cimetidine, diazepam, disulfiram, ethanol (acute), ibuprofen, imipramine, isoniazid, miconazole, phenacemide, phenylbutazone, salicylates, succinimides, trimethoprim,* or *valproic acid.* The therapeutic effects of the drug may be decreased when drug is used with *antacids, antineoplastics, barbiturates, calcium, calcium gluconate, carbamazepine, charcoal, diazoxide, ethanol (chronic), folic acid, loxapine, nitrofurantoin, pyridoxine, rifampin, sucralfate,* or *theophylline.* Other drugs that lower seizure threshold (such as *antipsychotics*) may attenuate the therapeutic effects of phenytoin.

By stimulating hepatic metabolism, phenytoin may decrease the effects of *amiodarone, carbamazepine, corticosteroids, cyclosporine, dicumarol, digitoxin, disopyramide, dopamine, doxycycline, estrogens, furosemide, haloperidol, levodopa, mebendazole, meperidine, methadone, metyrapone, oral contraceptives, phenothiazines, quinidine,* and *sulfonylureas.*

ADVERSE REACTIONS
CNS: *ataxia, slurred speech,* dizziness, insomnia, nervousness, twitching, headache, *mental confusion, decreased coordination.*

CV: periarteritis nodosa, hypotension.
EENT: *nystagmus, diplopia,* blurred vision, *gingival hyperplasia.*
GI: *nausea, vomiting,* constipation.
Hematologic: ***thrombocytopenia, leukopenia, agranulocytosis, pancytopenia,*** macrocythemia, megaloblastic anemia.
Hepatic: *toxic hepatitis.*
Skin: scarlatiniform or morbilliform rash; bullous, *exfoliative* or purpuric dermatitis; ***Stevens-Johnson syndrome;*** lupus erythematosus; *hirsutism;* ***toxic epidermal necrolysis;*** photosensitivity; pain, necrosis, and inflammation at injection site; discoloration of skin (purple-glove syndrome) if given by I.V. push in back of hand.
Other: lymphadenopathy, hyperglycemia, osteomalacia, hypertrichosis.

▣ KEY CONSIDERATIONS
Besides the recommendations relevant to all hydantoin derivatives, consider the following:
• Geriatric patients metabolize and excrete phenytoin slowly; they may require lower doses.
• Monitoring serum levels is essential because of dose-dependent excretion.
• Drug commonly is abbreviated as DPH (diphenylhydantoin), an older drug name.
• Only extended-release capsules are approved for once-daily dosing; all other forms are given in divided doses every 8 to 12 hours.
• Oral or NG feeding may interfere with absorption of oral suspension; separate doses as much as possible from feedings, but by no less than 1 hour. During continuous tube feeding, tube should be flushed before and after dose.
• If suspension is used, shake well.
• Avoid I.M. administration; it's painful and drug absorption is erratic.
• Mix I.V. doses in normal saline solution and use within ½ hour; mixtures with D_5W will precipitate. Don't refrigerate solution; don't mix with other drugs.
• Manufacturer recommends using in line filter during administration.

- When giving I.V., continuously monitor ECG, blood pressure, and respiratory status.
- Abrupt withdrawal may precipitate status epilepticus.
- If using I.V. bolus, use slow (50 mg/minute) I.V. push or constant infusion; too-rapid I.V. injection may cause hypotension and circulatory collapse. Don't use I.V. push in veins on back of hand; larger veins are needed to prevent discoloration associated with purple-glove syndrome.
- Drug may increase blood glucose levels by inhibiting pancreatic insulin release; it may decrease serum levels of protein-bound iodine and may interfere with the 1-mg dexamethasone suppression test.

Patient education
- Tell patient to use same brand of phenytoin consistently. Changing brands may change therapeutic effect.
- Instruct patient to take drug with food or milk to minimize GI distress.
- Warn patient not to discontinue drug unless with medical supervision, to avoid hazardous activities that require alertness until CNS effect is determined, and to avoid alcoholic beverages, which can decrease effectiveness of drug and increase adverse reactions.
- Encourage patient to wear a medical identification bracelet or necklace.
- Stress good oral hygiene to minimize overgrowth and sensitivity of gums.

Overdose & treatment
- Early signs and symptoms of overdose include drowsiness, nausea, vomiting, nystagmus, ataxia, dysarthria, tremor, and slurred speech. Hypotension, arrhythmias, respiratory depression, and coma may follow. Death is caused by respiratory and circulatory depression. Estimated lethal dose in adults is 2 to 5 g.
- To treat overdose, induce vomiting or perform gastric lavage and follow with supportive treatment. Carefully monitor vital signs and fluid and electrolyte balance. Forced diuresis is of little or no value. Hemodialysis or peritoneal dialysis may be helpful.

physostigmine salicylate
Antilirium

physostigmine sulfate
Eserine, Isopto Eserine

Anticholinesterase, antimuscarinic antidote, antiglaucoma drug

Available by prescription only
Injection: 1 mg/ml
Ophthalmic ointment: 0.25%
Ophthalmic solution: 0.25%, 0.5%

INDICATIONS & DOSAGE
Tricyclic antidepressant and anticholinergic poisoning
Adults: 0.5 to 2 mg I.M. or I.V. given slowly (not to exceed 1 mg/minute I.V.). Dosage individualized and repeated, p.r.n., q 10 minutes.
Postanesthesia care
Adults: 0.5 to 1 mg I.M. or I.V. given slowly (not to exceed 1 mg/minute I.V.). Dosage individualized and repeated, p.r.n., q 10 to 30 minutes.
Open-angle glaucoma
Adults: Instill 2 gtt into eye(s) up to q.i.d., or apply ointment to lower fornix up to t.i.d.

PHARMACODYNAMICS
Antimuscarinic and antiglaucoma actions: Physostigmine competitively blocks cholinesterase from hydrolyzing acetylcholine, causing acetylcholine to accumulate at cholinergic synapses. This accumulation antagonizes the muscarinic effects of overdose with antidepressants and anticholinergics. With ophthalmic use, miosis and ciliary muscle contraction increase aqueous humor outflow and decrease intraocular pressure.

PHARMACOKINETICS
Absorption: Physostigmine is well absorbed from the GI tract, mucous membranes, and subcutaneous tissues when given I.M. or I.V.; effects peak within 5 minutes. After ophthalmic use, drug may be absorbed orally after passage through the nasolacrimal duct.
Distribution: Drug is distributed widely and crosses the blood-brain barrier.

Metabolism: Cholinesterase hydrolyzes drug relatively quickly. Duration of effect is 1 to 2 hours after I.V. administration, 12 to 48 hours after ophthalmic use.
Excretion: Only a small amount of drug is excreted in urine. Following topical application, miosis occurs within 10 to 30 minutes and persists 12 to 48 hours.

CONTRAINDICATIONS & PRECAUTIONS

Injected form contraindicated in patients with mechanical obstruction of the intestine or urogenital tract, asthma, gangrene, diabetes, CV disease, or vagotonia and in those receiving choline esters or depolarizing neuromuscular blockers.

Ophthalmic form is contraindicated in patients with intolerance to drug, active uveitis, or corneal injury.

INTERACTIONS

Drug-drug. Use with *succinylcholine* may prolong respiratory depression by inhibiting plasma esterases from hydrolyzing succinylcholine. Use with *systemic cholinergics* may cause additive toxicity.

ADVERSE REACTIONS

CNS: weakness, headache (with ophthalmic form), *seizures, restlessness, excitability* (with injected form).
CV: slow or irregular heartbeat (with ophthalmic form), bradycardia, hypotension (with injected form).
EENT: blurred vision, eye pain, burning, redness, stinging, eye irritation, twitching of eyelids, watering of eyes (with ophthalmic form); miosis (with injected form).
GI: nausea, vomiting, diarrhea; epigastric pain, *excessive salivation* (with injected form).
GU: loss of bladder control (with ophthalmic form), urinary urgency (with injected form).
Respiratory: *bronchospasm,* bronchial constriction, shortness of breath, dyspnea (with injected form).
Other: diaphoresis.

▣ KEY CONSIDERATIONS

Besides the recommendations relevant to all anticholinesterases, consider the following:
• Use caution when administering to geriatric patients because they may be more sensitive to the effects of physostigmine.

• Observe solution for discoloration. Don't use if darkened.
• Atropine injection should always be available as an antagonist and antidote for most of the effects of physostigmine.
• The commercially available formulation of physostigmine salicylate injection contains sodium bisulfite, a sulfite that can cause allergic-type reactions, including anaphylaxis and life-threatening or less severe asthma episodes in certain susceptible individuals.
Ophthalmic
• If using the solution, have patient lie down or tilt head back to facilitate administration of eyedrops. Gently pinch patient's nasal bridge for 1 to 2 minutes after administering each dose of eyedrops to minimize systemic absorption. Wait at least 5 minutes before administering other eyedrops.
• If using the ointment, have patient close eyelids and roll eyes after application.

Patient education

• Teach patient how to administer ophthalmic ointment or solution.
• Instruct patient not to close eyes tightly or blink unnecessarily after instilling the ophthalmic solution.
• Warn patient that he may experience blurred vision and difficulty seeing after initial doses.
• Instruct patient to report abdominal cramps, diarrhea, or excessive salivation.
• Remind patient to wait 5 minutes (if using eyedrops) or 10 minutes (if using ointment) before using another eye preparation.

Overdose & treatment

• Signs and symptoms of overdose include headache, nausea, vomiting, diarrhea, blurred vision, miosis, myopia, excessive tearing, bronchospasm, increased bronchial secretions, hypotension, incoordination, excessive sweating, muscle weakness, bradycardia, excessive salivation, restlessness or agitation, and confusion.
• Support respiration; bronchial suctioning may be necessary. Physostigmine should be discontinued immediately. Atropine may be given to block muscarinic

◊ Unlabeled clinical use

effects. Avoid atropine overdose because it may cause bronchial plug formation.

pilocarpine hydrochloride
Adsorbocarpine, Akarpine, Isopto Carpine, Minims Pilocarpine*, Miocarpine*, Ocusert Pilo, Pilocar, Pilopine HS

pilocarpine nitrate
P.V. Carpine Liquifilm

Cholinergic agonist, miotic

Available by prescription only
pilocarpine hydrochloride
Solution: 0.25%, 0.5%, 1%, 2%, 3%, 4%, 5%, 6%, 8%, 10%
Gel: 4%
Releasing-system insert: 20 mcg/hour, 40 mcg/hour
pilocarpine nitrate
Solution: 1%, 2%, 4%

INDICATIONS & DOSAGE
Chronic open-angle glaucoma; before or instead of emergency surgery in acute angle-closure glaucoma
Adults: Instill 1 or 2 gtt 1% to 4% solution in the lower conjunctival sac q 4 to 12 hours (dosage should be based on periodic tonometric readings) or apply ½″ (1.3 cm) ribbon of 4% gel (Pilopine HS) h.s.

Alternatively, apply one Ocusert Pilo System (20 or 40 mcg/hour) q 7 days.
Emergency treatment of acute narrow-angle glaucoma
Adults: 1 gtt 2% solution q 5 minutes for three to six doses, followed by 1 gtt q 1 to 3 hours until pressure is controlled.
To counteract mydriatic effects of sympathomimetics
Adults: 1 gtt 1% solution in affected eye.

PHARMACODYNAMICS
Miotic action: Pilocarpine stimulates cholinergic receptors of the sphincter muscles of the iris, resulting in miosis. It also produces ciliary muscle contraction, resulting in accommodation with deepening of the anterior chamber and vasodilation of conjunctival vessels of the outflow tract.

PHARMACOKINETICS
Absorption: Pilocarpine drops act within 10 to 30 minutes; effect peaks at 2 to 4 hours. With the Ocusert Pilo System, 0.3 to 7 mg pilocarpine is released during the initial 6-hour period; during the remainder of the 1-week insertion period, the release rate is within ± 20% of the rated value. Effect occurs in 1½ to 2 hours and is maintained for the 1-week life of the insertion.
Distribution: Unknown.
Metabolism: Unknown.
Excretion: Duration of effect of pilocarpine drops is 4 to 6 hours.

CONTRAINDICATIONS & PRECAUTIONS
Contraindicated in patients with hypersensitivity to pilocarpine or when cholinergic effects such as constriction are undesirable (for example, acute iritis, some forms of secondary glaucoma, pupillary block glaucoma, acute inflammatory disease of the anterior chamber).

Use cautiously in patients with acute cardiac failure, bronchial asthma, peptic ulcer, hyperthyroidism, GI spasm, urinary obstruction, and Parkinson's disease.

INTERACTIONS
Drug-drug. *Demecarium, echothiophate,* and *isoflurophate* decrease the pharmacologic effects of pilocarpine. Pilocarpine can enhance the intraocular pressure–lowering effects of *epinephrine derivatives* and *timolol.*

ADVERSE REACTIONS
CV: hypertension, tachycardia.
EENT: periorbital or supraorbital headache, *myopia,* ciliary spasm, *blurred vision,* conjunctival irritation, transient stinging and burning, keratitis, lens opacity, retinal detachment, lacrimation, changes in visual field, *brow pain.*
GI: nausea, vomiting, diarrhea, salivation.
Respiratory: ***bronchoconstriction, pulmonary edema.***
Other: hypersensitivity reactions, diaphoresis.

Reactions may be *common,* uncommon, *life-threatening,* or COMMON AND LIFE-THREATENING.

▣ KEY CONSIDERATIONS
• Pilocarpine may be used alone or with mannitol, urea, glycerol, or acetazolamide. It also may be used to counteract effects of mydriatic and cycloplegic drugs after surgery or ophthalmoscopic examination and may be used alternately with atropine to break adhesions.

Patient education
• Warn patient that vision will be temporarily blurred, that miotic pupil may make surroundings appear dim and reduce peripheral field of vision, and that transient brow ache and myopia are common at first. Ensure patient that adverse effects subside 10 to 14 days after therapy begins.
• Instruct patient to check for the pilocarpine ocular system at bedtime and on arising.
• Tell patient that if systems in both eyes are lost, they should be replaced as soon as possible. If one system is lost, it may either be replaced with a fresh system or the system remaining in the other eye may be removed and both replaced with fresh systems so that both systems will subsequently be replaced on the same schedule.
• Instruct patient that if the Ocusert System falls out of the eye during sleep, he should wash hands, then rinse Ocusert in cool tap water and reposition it in the eye. Don't use the insert if it's deformed.
• Inform patient that systems should be replaced every 7 days.
• Provide patient with a copy of the manufacturer's instructions for the pilocarpine ocular system.
• Tell patient to use caution when driving at night or performing other activities in poor light because miotic pupil diminishes side vision and illumination.
• Stress importance of complying with prescribed medical regimen.
• Reassure patient that adverse effects will subside.
• Teach patient the correct way to instill drops and to apply light finger pressure on lacrimal sac for 1 minute after administration to minimize systemic absorption.

• Instruct patient to apply gel at bedtime because it'll cause blurred vision.

Overdose & treatment
• Signs and symptoms of overdose include flushing, vomiting, bradycardia, bronchospasm, increased bronchial secretion, sweating, tearing, involuntary urination, hypotension, and tremors.
• Vomiting is usually spontaneous with accidental ingestion; if not, induce vomiting and follow with activated charcoal or a cathartic. Treat dermal exposure by washing the areas twice with water. Use epinephrine to treat the CV responses. Atropine sulfate is the antidote of choice. Flush the eye with water or sodium chloride to treat a local overdose. Doses up to 20 mg are generally considered nontoxic.

pilocarpine hydrochloride
Salagen

Cholinergic agonist, antixerostomia drug

Available by prescription only
Tablets: 5 mg

INDICATIONS & DOSAGE
Treatment of symptoms of xerostomia from salivary gland hypofunction caused by radiotherapy for cancer of the head and neck
Adults: 5 mg P.O. t.i.d. Dosage may be increased to 10 mg P.O. t.i.d., p.r.n.

PHARMACODYNAMICS
Antixerostomia action: Oral pilocarpine increases secretion of the salivary glands, eliminating dryness.

PHARMACOKINETICS
Absorption: Pilocarpine is absorbed in the GI tract. A high-fat meal may decrease rate of absorption.
Distribution: Unknown.
Metabolism: Inactivation of drug is believed to occur at neuronal synapses and probably in plasma.

Excretion: Drug and its minimally active or inactive degradation products are excreted in urine.

CONTRAINDICATIONS & PRECAUTIONS

Contraindicated in patients with uncontrolled asthma or known hypersensitivity to pilocarpine and in patients in whom miosis is undesirable, such as those with acute iritis or angle-closure glaucoma.

Use cautiously in patients with CV disease, controlled asthma, chronic bronchitis, COPD, cholelithiasis, biliary tract disease, nephrolithiasis, and cognitive or psychiatric disturbances.

INTERACTIONS

Drug-drug. *Beta blockers* may increase the risk of conduction disturbances; use together cautiously. *Drugs with anticholinergic effects* may antagonize the anticholinergic effects of oral pilocarpine; use together cautiously. *Drugs with parasympathomimetic effects* may result in additive pharmacologic effects; monitor patient closely.

ADVERSE REACTIONS

CNS: *dizziness, headache,* tremor, *asthenia.*
CV: hypertension, tachycardia, *flushing,* edema.
GI: *nausea,* dyspepsia, taste perversion, diarrhea, abdominal pain, vomiting, dysphagia.
GU: *urinary frequency.*
EENT: *rhinitis,* lacrimation, amblyopia, pharyngitis, voice alteration, conjunctivitis, epistaxis, sinusitis, abnormal vision.
Musculoskeletal: myalgia.
Skin: rash, pruritus.
Other: *sweating, chills.*

▣ KEY CONSIDERATIONS

• Patient should undergo careful examination of the fundus before therapy is initiated because retinal detachment has been reported with pilocarpine use in patients with preexisting retinal disease.

Patient education

• Warn patient that pilocarpine may cause visual disturbances, especially at night, that could impair his ability to drive safely.

• Tell patient to drink plenty of fluids to prevent dehydration if drug causes excessive sweating. If adequate fluid intake can't be maintained, tell patient to notify doctor.

Overdose & treatment

• Taking 100 mg oral pilocarpine is potentially fatal.
• Signs and symptoms of toxicity, characterized by exaggerated parasympathomimetic effects of the drug, include headache, visual disturbance, lacrimation, sweating, respiratory distress, GI spasm, nausea, vomiting, diarrhea, AV block, tachycardia, bradycardia, hypotension, hypertension, shock, mental confusion, cardiac arrhythmia, and tremors.
• Treatment is with atropine titration (0.5 mg to 1 mg S.C. or I.V.) and supportive measures to maintain respiration and circulation. Epinephrine (0.3 mg to 1 mg S.C. or I.M.) may also be useful during severe CV depression or bronchoconstriction. It's unknown if drug is dialyzable.

---

pimozide
Orap

Diphenylbutylpiperidine, antipsychotic

Available by prescription only
Tablets: 2 mg

INDICATIONS & DOSAGE

Suppression of severe motor and phonic tics in patients with Tourette syndrome
Adults: Initially, 1 to 2 mg/day in divided doses. Then, increase dosage, p.r.n., every other day.
Maintenance dose: 7 to 16 mg/day.
Maximum dosage is 20 mg/day.

PHARMACODYNAMICS

Antipsychotic action: Mechanism of action in treating Tourette syndrome is unknown; it's thought to act by postsynaptic and/or presynaptic blockade of CNS dopamine receptors, thus inhibiting dopamine-mediated effects. Pimozide also has anticholinergic, antiemetic, and

---

Reactions may be *common,* uncommon, *life-threatening*, or COMMON AND LIFE-THREATENING.

anxiolytic effects and produces alpha blockade.

PHARMACOKINETICS

Absorption: Pimozide is absorbed slowly and incompletely from the GI tract; bioavailability is about 50%. Plasma levels may peak from 4 to 12 hours (usually in 6 to 8 hours).

Distribution: Drug is distributed widely into the body.

Metabolism: Drug is metabolized by the liver; a significant first-pass effect exists.

Excretion: About 40% of a given dose is excreted in urine as parent drug and metabolites in 3 to 4 days; about 15% is excreted in feces by the biliary tract within 3 to 6 days.

CONTRAINDICATIONS & PRECAUTIONS

Contraindicated in patients with hypersensitivity to pimozide, congenital long QT-interval syndrome or history of arrhythmias, or severe toxic CNS depression; in patients experiencing coma; in patients being treated for simple tics or tics other than those associated with Tourette syndrome; and in patients taking a drug causing motor and phonic tics.

Use cautiously in patients with impaired renal or hepatic function, glaucoma, prostatic hyperplasia, seizure disorders, or EEG abnormalities.

INTERACTIONS

Drug-drug. Use with *amphetamines, methylphenidate,* or *pemoline* may induce Tourette-like tic and may exacerbate existing tics. Use with *anticonvulsants*—including *carbamazepine, phenobarbital,* and *phenytoin*—may induce seizures, even in patients previously stabilized on anticonvulsants; an anticonvulsant dosage increase may be required. Use of pimozide with *antidepressants, disopyramide, other antipsychotics, phenothiazines, procainamide,* or *quinidine* or *other antiarrhythmics* may further depress cardiac conduction and prolong QT interval, resulting in serious arrhythmias. Use with *CNS depressants*—including *analgesics, anesthetics (epidural, general, or spinal), anxiolytics, barbiturates, narcotics, parenteral magnesium sulfate,* and *tranquilizers*—may cause oversedation and respiratory depression because of additive CNS depressant effects.

Drug-lifestyle. Use with *alcohol* may enhance respiratory and CNS effects.

ADVERSE REACTIONS

CNS: *parkinsonian-like symptoms,* drowsiness, headache, insomnia, other extrapyramidal signs and symptoms (dystonia, akathisia, hyperreflexia, opisthotonos, oculogyric crisis), *tardive dyskinesia, sedation, adverse behavioral effects.*

CV: *ECG changes (prolonged QT interval, flattening or inversion of T wave),* hypotension, hypertension, tachycardia.

EENT: visual disturbances.

GI: *dry mouth, constipation.*

GU: impotence, urinary frequency.

Musculoskeletal: muscle rigidity.

Skin: rash, diaphoresis.

Other: *neuroleptic malignant syndrome.*

▣ KEY CONSIDERATIONS

• Geriatric patients are more likely to develop cardiac toxicity and tardive dyskinesia, even at normal doses.

• Geriatric patients may be at greater risk for adverse CV effects.

• Obtain baseline ECG before therapy begins and then periodically to monitor CV effects.

• Maintain patient's serum potassium level within normal range; decreased potassium levels increase the risk of arrhythmias. Monitor potassium level in patients with diarrhea and those who are taking diuretics.

• Assess patient periodically for abnormal body movement.

• Extrapyramidal reactions develop in 10% to 15% of patients at normal doses. They're especially likely to occur during early days of therapy.

• If excessive restlessness and agitation occur, therapy with a beta blocker such as propranolol or metoprolol may be helpful.

Patient education

• Inform patient of risks, signs, and symptoms of dystonic reactions and tardive dyskinesia.

• Advise patient to take pimozide exactly as prescribed, not to double-dose for missed doses, not to share drug with others, and not to stop taking it suddenly.
• Explain that the therapeutic effect of the drug may not be apparent for several weeks.
• Urge patient to report unusual effects promptly.
• Tell patient not to take drug with alcohol, sleeping aids, or other drugs that may cause drowsiness without medical approval.
• Recommend use of sugarless hard candy or chewing gum, ice chips, or artificial saliva to relieve dry mouth.
• To prevent dizziness at start of therapy, tell patient to lie down for 30 minutes after taking each dose and avoid sudden changes in posture, especially when rising to upright position.
• To minimize daytime sedation, suggest taking entire daily dose at h.s.
• Warn patient to avoid hazardous activities that require alertness until the effects of the drug are known.

Overdose & treatment
• Signs and symptoms of overdose include severe extrapyramidal reactions, hypotension, respiratory depression, coma, and ECG abnormalities, including prolongation of QT interval, inversion or flattening of T waves, and new appearance of U waves.
• Use gastric lavage to remove unabsorbed drug. Maintain blood pressure with I.V. fluids, plasma expanders, or norepinephrine. Don't use epinephrine.
• Don't induce vomiting because of the potential for aspiration.
• Treat extrapyramidal symptoms with parenteral diphenhydramine. Monitor for adverse effects for at least 4 days because of prolonged half-life of drug.

pindolol
Visken

Beta blocker, antihypertensive

Available by prescription only
Tablets: 5 mg, 10 mg

INDICATIONS & DOSAGE
Hypertension
Adults: initially, 5 mg P.O. b.i.d. increased by 10 mg/day q 3 to 4 weeks up to maximum of 60 mg/day. Usual dosage is 10 to 30 mg daily, given in two or three divided doses. In some patients, once-daily dosing may be possible.
◇ **Angina**
Adults: 15 to 40 mg daily P.O. in three or four divided doses.

PHARMACODYNAMICS
Antihypertensive action: Exact mechanism is unknown. Pindolol doesn't consistently affect cardiac output or renin release, and its other mechanisms, such as decreased peripheral resistance, probably contribute to its hypotensive effect. Because drug has some intrinsic sympathomimetic activity—that is, beta-agonist sympathomimetic activity—it may be useful in patients who develop bradycardia with other beta-blockers. It's a nonselective beta blocker that inhibits both $beta_1$ and $beta_2$ receptors.

PHARMACOKINETICS
Absorption: After oral administration, pindolol is absorbed rapidly from the GI tract; plasma levels peak in 1 to 2 hours. Effect on heart rate usually occurs in 3 hours. Food doesn't reduce bioavailability but may increase the rate of GI absorption.
Distribution: Drug is distributed widely throughout the body; 40% to 60% protein-bound.
Metabolism: About 60% to 65% of a given dose is metabolized by the liver.
Excretion: In adults with normal renal function, 35% to 50% of a given dose is excreted unchanged in urine; half-life is about 3 to 4 hours. Antihypertensive effect usually persists for 24 hours.

CONTRAINDICATIONS & PRECAUTIONS
Contraindicated in patients with hypersensitivity to pindolol, bronchial asthma, severe bradycardia, heart block greater than first degree, cardiogenic shock, or overt cardiac failure.
    Use cautiously in patients with heart failure, nonallergic bronchospastic dis-

---

Reactions may be *common*, uncommon, *life-threatening*, or COMMON AND LIFE-THREATENING.

ease, diabetes, hyperthyroidism, and impaired renal or hepatic function.

INTERACTIONS
Drug-drug. Pindolol may potentiate the antihypertensive effects of *other antihypertensives.*

ADVERSE REACTIONS
CNS: *insomnia, fatigue, dizziness, nervousness,* vivid dreams, weakness, paresthesia.
CV: *edema,* bradycardia, *heart failure,* chest pain.
GI: *nausea,* abdominal discomfort.
Musculoskeletal: *muscle pain, joint pain.*
Respiratory: *increased airway resistance,* dyspnea.
Skin: rash, pruritus.

▣ KEY CONSIDERATIONS
Besides the recommendations relevant to all beta blockers, consider the following:
• Geriatric patients may require lower maintenance doses because of increased bioavailability or delayed metabolism; they also may experience enhanced adverse effects. Half-life of pindolol may be increased in geriatric patients.
• Maximum therapeutic response may not be seen for 2 weeks or more.

Overdose & treatment
• Signs and symptoms of overdose include severe hypotension, bradycardia, heart failure, and bronchospasm.
• After acute ingestion, induce vomiting or perform gastric lavage and give activated charcoal to reduce absorption. Subsequent treatment is usually symptomatic and supportive.

piperacillin sodium
Pipracil

Extended-spectrum penicillin, acylaminopenicillin, antibiotic

Available by prescription only
Injection: 2 g, 3 g, 4 g
Infusion: 2 g, 3 g, 4 g

INDICATIONS & DOSAGE
Infections caused by susceptible organisms
Adults: Serious infection: 12 to 18 g/day I.V. in divided doses q 4 to 6 hours; uncomplicated urinary tract infection (UTI) and community-acquired pneumonia: 6 to 8 g/day I.V. in divided doses q 6 to 12 hours; complicated UTI: 8 to 16 g/day I.V. in divided doses q 6 to 8 hours; and uncomplicated gonorrhea: 2 g I.M. as single dose. Maximum daily dose is 24 g.
Prophylaxis of surgical infections
Adults: Intra-abdominal surgery: 2 g I.V. before surgery, 2 g during surgery, and 2 g q 6 hours after surgery for no more than 24 hours; vaginal hysterectomy: 2 g I.V. before surgery, 2 g 6 hours after first dose, then 2 g 12 hours after second dose; abdominal hysterectomy: 2 g I.V. before surgery, 2 g in postanesthesia care unit, and 2 g after 6 hours.
✦ *Dosage adjustment.* For adult patients with renal failure, refer to this table.

Creatinine clearance (ml/min)	Dosage for uncomplicated UTI	Dosage for complicated UTI	Dosage for serious systemic infection
20-40	*	3 g q 8 hr	4 g q 8 hr
< 20	3 g q 12 hr	3 g q 12 hr	4 g q 12 hr

* No dosage adjustment necessary

PHARMACODYNAMICS
Antibiotic action: Piperacillin is bactericidal; it adheres to bacterial penicillin-binding proteins, thus inhibiting bacterial cell wall synthesis.

Extended-spectrum penicillins are more resistant to inactivation by certain beta-lactamases, especially those produced by gram-negative organisms, but are still susceptible to inactivation by certain others. Because bacterial resistance can develop rapidly, piperacillin shouldn't be used alone to treat an infection.

Drug's spectrum of activity includes many gram-negative aerobic and anaerobic bacilli, many gram-positive and gram-negative aerobic cocci, and some gram-positive aerobic and anaerobic bacilli. Drug may be effective against some strains of carbenicillin-resistant and ticarcillin-resistant gram-negative bacilli. Drug is more active against *Pseudomonas aeruginosa* than other extended-spectrum penicillins.

PHARMACOKINETICS
Absorption: Plasma levels peak 30 to 50 minutes after an I.M. dose.
Distribution: Piperacillin is distributed widely after parenteral administration. It penetrates minimally into noninflamed meninges and slightly into bone and sputum. Drug is 16% to 22% protein-bound.
Metabolism: Drug isn't significantly metabolized.
Excretion: Drug is excreted primarily (42% to 90%) in urine through renal tubular secretion and glomerular filtration; it's also excreted in bile. Elimination half-life in adults is ½ to 1½ hours; in extensive renal impairment, half-life is extended to 2 to 6 hours; in combined hepatorenal dysfunction, half-life may extend from 11 to 32 hours. Drug is removed by hemodialysis but not by peritoneal dialysis.

CONTRAINDICATIONS & PRECAUTIONS
Contraindicated in patients with hypersensitivity to piperacillin or other penicillins. Use cautiously in patients with other drug allergies (especially to cephalosporins), bleeding tendencies, uremia, or hypokalemia.

INTERACTIONS
Drug-drug. Use with *aminoglycosides* results in synergistic bactericidal effects against *P. aeruginosa; Escherichia coli; Klebsiella, Citrobacter, Enterobacter* and *Serratia* species; and *Proteus mirabilis;* however, drugs are physically and chemically incompatible and are inactivated when mixed or given together. In vivo inactivation has been reported when aminoglycosides and extended-spectrum penicillins are used concomitantly.
   Use with *clavulanic acid, sulbactam,* or *tazobactam* also produces a synergistic bactericidal effect against certain beta-lactamase–producing bacteria. Large doses of piperacillin may interfere with renal tubular secretion of *methotrexate,* thus delaying elimination and elevating serum methotrexate levels. *Probenecid* blocks tubular secretion of piperacillin, increasing serum drug levels.

ADVERSE REACTIONS
CNS: *seizures,* headache, dizziness, fatigue, pain at injection site.
CV: phlebitis.
GI: nausea, diarrhea, vomiting, pseudomembranous colitis.
GU: interstitial nephritis.
Hematologic: *bleeding (with high doses),* neutropenia, eosinophilia, leukopenia, *thrombocytopenia.*
Metabolic: *hypokalemia.*
Musculoskeletal: prolonged muscle relaxation.
Other: hypersensitivity reactions (edema, fever, chills, rash, pruritus, urticaria, *anaphylaxis*), overgrowth of nonsusceptible organisms, vein irritation.

▣ KEY CONSIDERATIONS
Besides the recommendations relevant to all penicillins, consider the following:
• Half-life may be prolonged in geriatric patients because of impaired renal function. Monitor patient closely for adverse effects.
• Piperacillin is almost always used with another antibiotic such as an aminoglycoside in life-threatening situations.
• Drug may be more suitable than carbenicillin or ticarcillin for patients on salt-free diets; piperacillin contains only 1.85 mEq/g sodium.
• Drug may be administered by direct I.V. injection, given slowly over at least 5 minutes; chest discomfort occurs if injection is given too rapidly.
• Patients with cystic fibrosis are most susceptible to fever or rash from piperacillin.
• Monitor serum electrolyte levels, especially potassium.
• Monitor neurologic status. High serum drug levels may cause seizures.
• Use reduced dosage in patients with creatinine clearance less than 40 ml/minute.
• Drug may cause positive Coombs' test result.

Reactions may be *common,* uncommon, *life-threatening,* or COMMON AND LIFE-THREATENING.

• Monitor CBC and differential and platelet counts. Drug may cause thrombocytopenia. Observe patient carefully for signs of occult bleeding.
• Because drug is dialyzable, patients undergoing hemodialysis may need dosage adjustments.

Overdose & treatment
• Signs and symptoms of overdose include neuromuscular hypersensitivity or seizures resulting from CNS irritation from high drug levels.
• A 4- to 6-hour hemodialysis removes 10% to 50% of piperacillin.

piperacillin sodium and tazobactam sodium
Zosyn

Extended-spectrum penicillin, beta-lactamase inhibitor, antibiotic

Available by prescription only
Powder for injection (equivalent to piperacillin/tazobactam in a ratio of 8:1): 2.25 g, 3.375 g, 4.5 g

INDICATIONS & DOSAGE
Treatment of moderate to severe infections caused by piperacillin-resistant, piperacillin/tazobactam-susceptible, beta-lactamase–producing strains of microorganisms in the following conditions: appendicitis (complicated by rupture or abscess) and peritonitis caused by Escherichia coli, Bacteroides fragilis, Bacteroides ovatus, Bacteroides thetaiotaomicron, Bacteroides vulgatus; *skin and skin-structure infections caused by* Staphylococcus aureus; *pelvic inflammatory disease caused by* E. coli; *moderately severe community-acquired pneumonia caused by* Haemophilus influenzae
Adults: 3.375 g (3.0 g piperacillin/0.375 g tazobactam) q 6 hours as a 30-minute I.V. infusion.
♦ *Dosage adjustment.* For patients with renal dysfunction, refer to the table.

Creatinine clearance (ml/min)	Recommended dosage
> 40	12 g/1.5 g/day in divided doses of 3.375 g q 6 hr
20-40	8 g/1 g/day in divided doses of 2.25 g q 6 hr
< 20	6 g/0.75 g/day in divided doses of 2.25 g q 8 hr

Note: Discontinue therapy if hypersensitivity reactions or signs or symptoms of bleeding occur.

PHARMACODYNAMICS
Antibiotic action: Piperacillin is an extended-spectrum penicillin that inhibits cell wall synthesis during microorganism multiplication. By inactivating beta-lactamases, which destroy penicillins, tazobactam increases the effectiveness of piperacillin.

PHARMACOKINETICS
Absorption: Unknown.
Distribution: Both piperacillin and tazobactam are about 30% bound to plasma proteins.
Metabolism: Piperacillin is metabolized to a minor microbiologically active desethyl metabolite. Tazobactam is metabolized to a single metabolite that lacks pharmacologic and antibacterial activities.
Excretion: Both drugs are eliminated from the kidneys through glomerular filtration and tubular secretion. Piperacillin is excreted rapidly as unchanged drug (68% of dose) and tazobactam is excreted as unchanged drug (80%) in urine. Piperacillin, tazobactam, and desethyl piperacillin also are secreted into bile.

CONTRAINDICATIONS & PRECAUTIONS
Contraindicated in patients with hypersensitivity to piperacillin, tazobactam, or other penicillins. Use cautiously in patients with drug allergies (especially to cephalosporins), bleeding tendencies, uremia, or hypokalemia.

INTERACTIONS
Drug-drug. Mixing piperacillin/tazobactam with an *aminoglycoside* can substan-

---

tially inactivate the aminoglycoside; don't mix in the same I.V. container. Coagulation parameters should be tested more frequently and monitored regularly during simultaneous administration of high doses of *heparin, oral anticoagulants,* or other *drugs that may affect the blood coagulation system or the thrombocyte function.* Administration with *probenecid* increases blood piperacillin/tazobactam levels. When used with *vecuronium,* piperacillin may prolong the neuromuscular blockade of vecuronium; piperacillin/tazobactam could produce the same phenomenon if given with vecuronium, so monitor patient closely.

ADVERSE REACTIONS

CNS: *headache, insomnia,* pain, agitation, dizziness, anxiety.
CV: hypertension, tachycardia, chest pain, phlebitis at I.V. site, edema.
EENT: rhinitis.
GI: *diarrhea, nausea, constipation,* vomiting, dyspepsia, stool changes, abdominal pain.
GU: interstitial nephritis.
Hematologic: leukopenia, anemia, eosinophilia, ***thrombocytopenia.***
Respiratory: dyspnea.
Skin: rash (including maculopapular, bullous, urticarial, and eczematoid), pruritus.
Other: fever, candidiasis, inflammation at I.V. site, ***anaphylaxis.***

▣ KEY CONSIDERATIONS

• Obtain specimen for culture and sensitivity tests before giving first dose. Therapy may begin pending results.
• Pseudomembranous colitis has been reported with nearly all antibacterials, including piperacillin/tazobactam, and may range in severity from mild to life-threatening. Therefore, consider this diagnosis in patients presenting with diarrhea after drug administration.
• Bacterial and fungal superinfection may occur and warrants appropriate measures.
• Use piperacillin/tazobactam in combination with an aminoglycoside to treat infections caused by *Pseudomonas aeruginosa.*
• Piperacillin/tazobactam contains 2.35 mEq (54 mg) sodium/g piperacillin in the combination product. This should be considered when treating patients requiring restricted sodium intake.
• Perform periodic electrolyte determinations in patients with low potassium reserves; hypokalemia can occur when patient with potentially low potassium reserves receives cytotoxic therapy or diuretics.
• As with other semisynthetic penicillins, piperacillin has been associated with increased incidence of fever and rash in patients with cystic fibrosis.
• Reconstitute piperacillin/tazobactam with 5 ml diluent/1 g piperacillin. Appropriate diluents include sterile or bacteriostatic water for injection, normal saline injection, bacteriostatic normal saline injection, D_5W, dextrose 5% in normal saline injection, or dextran 6% in normal saline injection. Don't use lactated Ringer's injection. Shake until dissolved. Further dilution can be made to a final desired volume.
• Infuse over at least 30 minutes. Discontinue primary infusion during administration if possible. Don't mix with other drugs.
• Use single-dose vials immediately after reconstitution. Discard unused drug after 24 hours if kept at room temperature; 48 hours if refrigerated. Once diluted, drug is stable in I.V. bags for 24 hours at room temperature or 1 week if refrigerated.
• Change I.V. site every 48 hours.
• As with other penicillins, piperacillin/tazobactam may result in a false-positive reaction for urine glucose using a copper-reduction method such as Clinitest. Glucose tests based on enzymatic glucose oxidase reactions (such as Diastix or glucose enzymatic test strip) are recommended.

---

piroxicam
Apo-Piroxicam*, Feldene, Novo-Pirocam*

NSAID, nonnarcotic analgesic, antipyretic, anti-inflammatory

Available by prescription only
Capsules: 10 mg, 20 mg

INDICATIONS & DOSAGE

Osteoarthritis and rheumatoid arthritis
Adults: 20 mg P.O. once daily. If desired, dose may be divided.

PHARMACODYNAMICS
Analgesic, antipyretic, and anti-inflammatory actions: Exact mechanisms of action are unknown, but piroxicam is thought to inhibit prostaglandin synthesis.

PHARMACOKINETICS
Absorption: Piroxicam is absorbed rapidly from the GI tract. Effect peaks 3 to 5 hours after dosing. Food delays absorption.
Distribution: Drug is highly protein-bound.
Metabolism: Drug is metabolized in the liver.
Excretion: Drug is excreted in urine. Its long half-life (about 50 hours) allows for once-daily dosing.

CONTRAINDICATIONS & PRECAUTIONS
Contraindicated in patients with hypersensitivity to piroxicam or with bronchospasm or angioedema precipitated by aspirin or NSAIDs.

Use cautiously in geriatric patients and in patients with GI disorders; history of renal, peptic ulcer, or cardiac disease; hypertension; or conditions predisposing to fluid retention.

INTERACTIONS
Drug-drug. Use with *acetaminophen, gold compounds,* or other *anti-inflammatories* may increase nephrotoxicity. Use of piroxicam with *anticoagulants* or *thrombolytics*—including *coumarin derivatives, heparin*, and other *highly protein-bound drugs*—may potentiate anticoagulant effects. Piroxicam may decrease the effectiveness of *antihypertensives* and *diuretics;* furthermore, use with diuretics may increase risk for nephrotoxicity. Use with *anti-inflammatories, corticotropin, salicylates,* or *steroids* may cause increased GI adverse effects, including ulceration and hemorrhage. *Aspirin* may decrease the bioavailability of piroxicam. Toxicity may occur with *coumarin derivatives,*

nifedipine, phenytoin, or *verapamil.* Bleeding problems may occur if used with other *drugs that inhibit platelet aggregation,* such as *aspirin, cefamandole, cefoperazone, dextran, dipyridamole, mezlocillin,* other *anti-inflammatories piperacillin, plicamycin, salicylates, sulfinpyrazone, ticarcillin,* or *valproic acid.* Piroxicam may displace *highly protein-bound drugs* from binding sites. Piroxicam may decrease the renal clearance of *lithium* and *methotrexate.* Because of the influence of prostaglandins on glucose metabolism, use with *insulin* or *oral antidiabetics* may potentiate hypoglycemic effects.
Drug-lifestyle. Use with *alcohol* may cause increased adverse GI effects.

ADVERSE REACTIONS
CNS: headache, drowsiness, dizziness, somnolence, vertigo.
CV: peripheral edema.
EENT: auditory disturbances.
GI: *epigastric distress, nausea, occult blood loss,* **peptic ulceration, severe GI bleeding,** diarrhea, constipation, abdominal pain, dyspepsia, flatulence, anorexia, stomatitis.
GU: *nephrotoxicity;* elevated BUN, creatinine, and uric acid levels.
Hematologic: prolonged bleeding time, increased PT, decreased hemoglobin level, anemia, leukopenia, **aplastic anemia, agranulocytosis,** eosinophilia, **thrombocytopenia.**
Hepatic: elevated liver enzyme levels.
Metabolic: increased potassium and serum glucose levels.
Skin: pruritus, rash, urticaria, *photosensitivity.*

▣ KEY CONSIDERATIONS
Besides the recommendations relevant to all NSAIDs, consider the following:
• Patients older than age 60 are more sensitive to the adverse effects of piroxicam. Use with caution.
• Through its effect on renal prostaglandins, drug may cause fluid retention and edema. This may be significant in geriatric patients and those with heart failure.
• Drug is usually administered as a single dose.

• Adverse skin reactions are more common with piroxicam than with other NSAIDs; photosensitivity reactions are the most common.
• Effectiveness of drug usually isn't seen for at least 2 weeks after therapy begins. Evaluate response to drug as evidenced by reduced symptoms.

Patient education
• Advise patient to seek medical approval before taking OTC drugs.
• Caution patient to avoid hazardous activities requiring alertness until CNS effects are known. Instruct patient in safety measures to prevent injury.
• Instruct patient in signs and symptoms of adverse effects. Tell patient to report them immediately.
• Encourage patient to comply with recommended medical follow-up.
• Tell patient to avoid aspirin and alcoholic beverages during therapy.

Overdose & treatment
• Signs and symptoms of overdose include vomiting, irritability, acidosis, and dehydration. May progress to GI bleeding, hyponatremia, hypocalcemia, mental confusion, and generalized seizures. Subsequently, hematologic, hepatic, and renal toxicity may develop.
• To treat overdose, immediately induce vomiting with ipecac syrup or perform gastric lavage. Administer activated charcoal via NG tube. Provide symptomatic and supportive measures (respiratory support and correction of fluid and electrolyte imbalances). Monitor laboratory parameters and vital signs closely.

pneumococcal vaccine, polyvalent
Pneumovax 23, Pnu-Imune 23

Bacterial vaccine

Available by prescription only
Injection: 25 mcg each of 23 polysaccharide isolates of *Streptococcus pneumoniae* per 0.5-ml dose, in 1-ml and 5-ml vials and disposable syringes.

INDICATIONS & DOSAGE
Pneumococcal immunization
Adults: 0.5 ml I.M. or S.C. as a one-time dose.

PHARMACODYNAMICS
Pneumonia prophylaxis: Pneumococcal vaccine promotes active immunity against the 23 most prevalent pneumococcal types.

PHARMACOKINETICS
Absorption: Protective antibodies are produced within 3 weeks after injection. Duration of vaccine-induced immunity is at least 5 years in adults.
Distribution: Unknown.
Metabolism: Unknown.
Excretion: Unknown.

CONTRAINDICATIONS & PRECAUTIONS
Contraindicated in patients hypersensitive to pneumococcal vaccine or its components (phenol). Also contraindicated in patients with Hodgkin's disease who have received extensive chemotherapy or nodal irradiation.

INTERACTIONS
Drug-drug. Use of pneumococcal vaccine with *corticosteroids* or other *immunosuppressants* may impair the immune response to vaccine; vaccination should be avoided.

ADVERSE REACTIONS
CNS: headache.
GI: nausea, vomiting.
Musculoskeletal: arthralgia, myalgia.
Other: adenitis, *anaphylaxis,* rash, serum sickness, *slight fever, soreness at injection site,* severe local reaction associated with revaccination within 3 years.

▣ KEY CONSIDERATIONS
• Candidates for pneumococcal vaccine include geriatric patients.
• Obtain a thorough history of allergies and reactions to immunizations.
• Persons with asplenia who received the 14-valent vaccine should be revaccinated with the 23-valent vaccine.
• Epinephrine solution 1:1,000 should be available to treat allergic reactions.

Reactions may be *common*, uncommon, *life-threatening*, or COMMON AND LIFE-THREATENING.

• Use the deltoid or midlateral thigh. Don't inject I.V. Avoid I.D. administration because this may cause severe local reactions.
• Vaccine also is recommended for patients awaiting organ transplants, those receiving radiation therapy or cancer chemotherapy, patients in nursing homes, and patients who are bedridden.
• If different sites and separate syringes are used, vaccine may be administered simultaneously with influenza; diphtheria, tetanus, pertussis; poliovirus; or *Haemophilus* b polysaccharide vaccines.
• Store vaccine at 36°F to 46°F (2°C to 8°C). Reconstitution or dilution is unnecessary.

Patient education
• Tell patient to expect redness, soreness, swelling, and pain at the injection site after vaccination. Patient may also develop fever, joint or muscle aches and pains, rash, itching, general weakness, or difficulty breathing.
• Encourage patient to report distressing adverse reactions promptly.
• Advise patient to use acetaminophen to relieve adverse reactions promptly.

polyethylene glycol-electrolyte solution (PEG-ES)
Colovage, Colyte, GoLYTELY, NuLYTELY, OCL

Polyethylene glycol 3350 nonabsorbable solution, laxative and bowel evacuant

Available by prescription only
Powder for oral solution: polyethylene glycol (PEG) 3350 (6 g), anhydrous sodium sulfate (568 mg), sodium chloride (146 mg), potassium chloride (74.5 mg/100 ml) (Colovage); PEG 3350 (120 g), sodium sulfate (3.36 g), sodium chloride (2.92 g), potassium chloride (1.49 g/2 L) (Colyte); PEG 3350 (236 g), sodium sulfate (22.74 g), sodium bicarbonate (6.74 g), sodium chloride (5.86 g), potassium chloride (2.97 g/4.8 L) (GoLYTELY); PEG 3350

(420 g), sodium bicarbonate (5.72 g), sodium chloride (11.2 g), potassium chloride (1.48 g/4 L) (NuLYTELY); PEG 3350 (6 g), sodium sulfate decahydrate (1.29 g), sodium chloride (146 mg), potassium chloride (75 mg), polysorbate-80 (30 mg/100 ml) (OCL)

INDICATIONS & DOSAGE
Bowel preparation before GI examination
Adults: 240 ml P.O. q 10 minutes until 4 L are consumed or the rectal effluent is clear. Typically, administer 4 hours before examination, allowing 3 hours for drinking and 1 hour for bowel evacuation.
Note: If a patient experiences severe bloating, distention, or abdominal pain, slow or temporarily discontinue administration until symptoms abate.

PHARMACODYNAMICS
Laxative and bowel evacuant action: PEG-ES acts as an osmotic drug. With sodium sulfate as the major sodium source, active sodium absorption is markedly reduced. Diarrhea results, which rapidly cleans the bowel, usually within 4 hours.

PHARMACOKINETICS
Absorption: PEG-ES is a nonabsorbable solution. Onset of action occurs within 30 to 60 minutes.
Distribution: Drug isn't absorbed.
Metabolism: Drug isn't metabolized.
Excretion: PEG-ES is excreted in the GI tract.

CONTRAINDICATIONS & PRECAUTIONS
Contraindicated in patients with GI obstruction or perforation, gastric retention, toxic colitis, ileus, or megacolon.

INTERACTIONS
Drug-drug. *Oral drugs given within 1 hour before start of therapy* may be flushed from the GI tract and not absorbed.

ADVERSE REACTIONS
EENT: rhinorrhea.
GI: anal irritation, *nausea, bloating, cramps, vomiting, abdominal fullness.*

Skin: urticaria, dermatitis.
Other: *anaphylaxis.*

▣ KEY CONSIDERATIONS
• Patient preparation for barium enema may be less satisfactory with this solution because it may interfere with the barium coating of the colonic mucosa using the double-contrast technique.
• PEG-ES may be given through an NG tube (at 20 to 30 ml/minute or 1.2 to 1.8 L/hour) to patients unwilling or unable to drink the preparation. The first bowel movement should occur within 1 hour.
• Tap water may be used to reconstitute the solution. Shake container vigorously several times to ensure that the powder is completely dissolved. After reconstitution to 4 L with water, the solution contains PEG 3350, 17.6 mmol/L; sodium, 125 mmol/L; sulfate, 40 mmol/L (Colyte 80 mmol/L); chloride, 35 mmol/L; bicarbonate, 20 mmol/L; and potassium, 10 mmol/L (1 mmol/L = 1 mEq/L).
• Store reconstituted solution in refrigerator (chilling before administration improves palatability); use within 48 hours.
• Don't add flavorings or additional ingredients to solution before use.
• No major shifts in fluid or electrolyte balance have been reported.

Patient education
• Instruct patient to fast 3 to 4 hours before ingesting the solution.
• Inform him that no foods except clear liquids are permitted after administration of solution until the examination is completed.

polysaccharide-iron complex
Hytinic, Niferex, Niferex-150, Nu-Iron, Nu-Iron 150

Oral iron supplement, hematinic

Available without prescription
Tablets (film-coated): 50 mg
Capsules: 150 mg
Solution: 100 mg/5 ml

INDICATIONS & DOSAGE
Treatment of uncomplicated iron-deficiency anemia
Adults: 150 to 300 mg P.O. daily as capsules or tablets or 1 to 2 tsp of elixir P.O. daily.

PHARMACODYNAMICS
Hematinic action: Polysaccharide-iron complex provides elemental iron, an essential component in the formation of hemoglobin.

PHARMACOKINETICS
Absorption: Although iron is absorbed from entire length of GI tract, the duodenum and proximal jejunum are the primary absorption sites. Up to 10% of iron is absorbed by healthy individuals; patients with iron-deficiency anemia may absorb up to 60%. Enteric-coated and some extended-release formulas have decreased absorption because they're designed to release iron past points in GI tract of highest absorption. Food may decrease absorption by 33% to 50%.
Distribution: Iron is transported through GI mucosal cells directly into the blood, where it's immediately bound to a carrier protein, transferrin, and transported to the bone marrow for incorporation into hemoglobin. Iron is highly protein-bound.
Metabolism: Iron is liberated by the destruction of hemoglobin, but is conserved and reused by the body.
Excretion: Healthy individuals lose only a small amount of iron each day. Men and postmenopausal women lose about 1 mg/day. Loss usually occurs in nails, hair, feces, and urine; trace amounts are lost in bile and sweat.

CONTRAINDICATIONS & PRECAUTIONS
Contraindicated in patients with hypersensitivity to a component of polysaccharide-iron complex and in those with hemochromatosis and hemosiderosis.

INTERACTIONS
Drug-drug. *Antacids, cholestyramine resin, cimetidine, tetracycline,* and *vitamin E* decrease iron absorption; separate doses by 2 to 4 hours. *Chloramphenicol* causes a delayed response to iron thera-

py; monitor patient carefully. Iron decreases absorption of *fluoroquinolones, levodopa, methyldopa,* and *penicillamine,* possibly resulting in decreased serum levels or efficacy. *Vitamin C* may increase iron absorption.

ADVERSE REACTIONS

Although nausea, constipation, black stools, and epigastric pain are common adverse reactions to iron therapy, few, if any, occur with polysaccharide-iron complex. Iron-containing liquids may temporarily stain teeth.

▣ KEY CONSIDERATIONS

• Because iron-induced constipation is common in geriatric patients, stress proper diet to minimize this adverse effect. Geriatric patients may need higher doses of iron because reduced gastric secretions and achlorhydria may reduce capacity for iron absorption.

• Administer iron with juice (preferably orange juice) or water, but not with milk or antacids.

• Polysaccharide-iron complex is nontoxic, and there are relatively few, if any, of the GI adverse effects associated with other iron preparations.

• Monitor hemoglobin level and hematocrit and reticulocyte counts during therapy.

• Be aware that oral iron may turn stools black. This unabsorbed iron is harmless; however, it could mask melena.

• Drug may interfere with test for occult blood in stool; guaiac and orthotoluidine tests may yield false-positive results. Benzidine test is usually unaffected. Iron overload may decrease uptake of technetium-99m and thus interfere with skeletal imaging.

Patient education

• Inform patients that as few as three or four tablets can cause serious iron poisoning in children.

• If patient misses a dose, tell him to take it as soon as he remembers, but not to double-dose.

• Advise patient to avoid certain foods that may impair oral iron absorption, including yogurt, cheese, eggs, milk, whole grain breads and cereals, tea, and coffee.

• Teach patient dietary measures to prevent constipation.

Overdose & treatment

• The lethal dose of iron is between 200 and 250 mg/kg; fatalities have occurred with lower doses. Symptoms may follow ingestion of 20 to 60 mg/kg. Signs and symptoms of acute overdose may occur as follows: Between ½ and 8 hours after ingestion, patient may experience lethargy, nausea and vomiting, green then tarry stools, weak and rapid pulse, hypotension, dehydration, acidosis, and coma. If death doesn't immediately ensue, symptoms may clear for about 24 hours. At 12 to 48 hours, symptoms may return, accompanied by diffuse vascular congestion, pulmonary edema, shock, seizures, anuria, and hyperthermia. Death may follow.

• Treatment requires immediate support of airway, respiration, and circulation. Induce vomiting with ipecac in conscious patients with intact gag reflex; for unconscious patients, perform gastric lavage. Follow emesis with lavage, using 1% sodium bicarbonate solution to convert iron to less irritating, poorly absorbed form. (Phosphate solutions have been used, but carry the risk of other adverse effects.) Perform radiographic evaluation of abdomen to determine continued presence of excess iron; if serum iron levels exceed 350 mg/dl, deferoxamine may be used for systemic chelation.

• Survivors are likely to sustain organ damage, including pyloric or antral stenosis, hepatic cirrhosis, CNS damage, and intestinal obstruction.

---

*Canada only   ◊ Unlabeled clinical use

potassium salts, oral

potassium acetate

potassium bicarbonate
K⁺ Care ET, K-Electrolyte, K-Ide, Klor-Con/EF, K-Lyte, K-Vescent

potassium chloride
Apo-K*, Cena-K, Gen-K, K-8, K-10*, Kalium Durules*, Kaochlor S-F, Kaon-Cl, Kaon-Cl-10, Kato, Kay Ciel, K⁺ Care, KCL*, K-Dur, K-Ide, K-Lease, K-Long*, K-Lor, Klor-Con, Klorvess, Klotrix, K-Lyte/Cl Powder, K-Med 900*, K-Norm, K-Sol, K-Tab, Micro-K Extencaps, Micro-K 10 Extencaps, Potasalan, Rum-K, Slow-K, Ten-K

potassium gluconate

Potassium supplement, therapeutic drug for electrolyte balance

Available by prescription only
potassium acetate
Vials: 2 mEq/ml and 4 mEq/ml in 20-ml vials
potassium bicarbonate
Tablets (effervescent): 6.5 mEq, 20 mEq, 25 mEq, 50 mEq
potassium chloride
Tablets (sustained-release): 6.7 mEq, 8 mEq, 10 mEq, 20 mEq
Powder: 15 mEq/package, 20 mEq/package, and 25 mEq/package
potassium gluconate
Liquid: 15 mEq/15 ml, 20 mEq/15 ml

INDICATIONS & DOSAGE
Hypokalemia
Adults: 40- to 100-mEq tablets divided into two to four doses daily. Use I.V. potassium chloride when oral replacement is unfeasible or when hypokalemia is life-threatening. Dosage up to 20 mEq/hour in concentrations of 60 mEq/L or less. Further dose based on serum potassium levels. Don't exceed total daily dose of 150 mEq.

Further doses are based on serum potassium levels and blood pH. I.V. potassium replacement should be performed only with ECG monitoring and frequent serum potassium levels.
Prevention of hypokalemia
Adults: initially, 20 mEq of potassium supplement P.O. daily, in divided doses. Adjust dosage, p.r.n., based on serum potassium levels.
Potassium replacement
Adults: Potassium chloride should be diluted in a suitable I.V. solution (not more than 40 mEq/L) and administered at rate not exceeding 20 mEq/hour. Don't exceed total dosage of 400 mEq/day. I.V. potassium replacement should be performed only with ECG monitoring and frequent serum potassium levels.

PHARMACODYNAMICS
Potassium replacement action: Potassium, the main cation in body tissue, is necessary for physiological processes, such as maintaining intracellular tonicity, maintaining a balance with sodium across cell membranes, transmitting nerve impulses, maintaining cellular metabolism, contracting cardiac and skeletal muscle, maintaining acid-base balance, and maintaining normal renal function.

PHARMACOKINETICS
Absorption: Potassium is well absorbed from the GI tract. It should be taken with meals and sipped slowly over a 5- to 10-minute period to decrease irritation. Potassium bicarbonate doesn't correct hypochloremic alkalosis.
Distribution: The normal serum potassium levels range from 3.8 to 5 mEq/L. Up to 60 mEq/L of potassium may be found in gastric secretions and diarrhea.
Metabolism: Insignificant.
Excretion: Potassium is excreted largely from the kidneys. A small amount may be excreted from the skin and intestinal tract, but intestinal potassium usually is reabsorbed. A healthy patient on a potassium-free diet excretes 40 to 50 mEq of potassium daily.

CONTRAINDICATIONS & PRECAUTIONS
Contraindicated in patients with severe renal impairment with oliguria, anuria, or azotemia; in those with untreated Ad-

---

dison's disease; and in those with acute dehydration, heat cramps, hyperkalemia, hyperkalemic form of familial periodic paralysis, and conditions associated with extensive tissue breakdown.

Use cautiously in patients with cardiac or renal disease.

INTERACTIONS

Drug-drug. Use of potassium with *ACE inhibitors (captopril), potassium sparing diuretics,* or *salt substitutes containing potassium salts* can cause severe hyperkalemia. When used with potassium, *anticholinergics* that slow GI motility may increase the chance of GI irritation and ulceration. Potassium isn't recommended in patients with severe or complete heart block who are receiving *digoxin* because of potential for arrhythmias. Administration with *potassium-containing products* may cause hyperkalemia within 1 to 2 days.

ADVERSE REACTIONS

CNS: paresthesia of the extremities, listlessness, mental confusion, weakness or heaviness of legs, flaccid paralysis, pain at infusion site.
CV: hypotension, *arrhythmias, cardiac arrest,* heart block, ECG changes.
GI: nausea, vomiting, abdominal pain, diarrhea.
Respiratory: *respiratory paralysis.*
Skin: redness at infusion site.
Other: fever, hyperkalemia.

◎ KEY CONSIDERATIONS

• In patients receiving cardiac glycosides, removing potassium too rapidly may result in digitalis toxicity.
• Monitor serum potassium, BUN, and serum creatinine levels; pH; and intake and output.
• Don't give potassium during immediate postoperative period until urine flow is established.
• Give parenteral potassium by slow infusion only, never by I.V. push or I.M. Dilute I.V. potassium preparations with large volume of parenteral solutions.
• Give oral potassium supplements with extreme caution because its many forms deliver varying amounts of potassium.

Patient may tolerate one product better than another.
• Potassium gluconate doesn't correct hypokalemic hypochloremic alkalosis.
• Enteric-coated tablets aren't recommended because of the potential for GI bleeding and small-bowel ulcerations.
• Tablets in wax matrix sometimes lodge in esophagus and cause ulceration in cardiac patients who have esophageal compression from an enlarged left atrium. In such patients and in those with esophageal or GI stasis or obstruction, use liquid form.
• Often used orally with diuretics that cause potassium excretion. Potassium chloride is the most useful because diuretics waste chloride ions. Hypokalemic alkalosis is treated best with potassium chloride.
• Monitor ECG, pH, and serum potassium and other electrolyte levels during therapy.
• Don't crush sustained-released potassium products.

Patient education

• Tell patient potassium is available only with a prescription because the wrong amount may cause severe reactions.
• Suggest diluting liquid potassium product in at least 4 to 8 oz (120 to 240 ml) water, taking it after meals, and sipping it slowly to minimize GI irritation.
• Tell patient to dissolve powder, soluble tablets, or granules completely in at least 4 oz (120 ml) water or juice, and to allow fizzing to finish before drinking.
• Instruct patient not to crush or chew sustained-release capsules; contents of capsule can be opened and sprinkled onto applesauce or other soft food.
• If the patient experiences confusion; irregular heartbeat; numbness of feet, fingers or lips; shortness of breath; anxiety, excessive tiredness, or weakness of legs; unexplained diarrhea; nausea and vomiting; stomach pain; or bloody or black stools, tell him to stop taking the drug immediately and report the reactions to his health care provider. Such reactions are rare.
• Tell patient that expelling a whole tablet in the stool (sustained-release

tablet) is normal. The body eliminates the shell after absorbing the potassium.
• Warn patient to avoid salt substitutes except when prescribed.

Overdose & treatment
• Signs and symptoms of overdose include increased serum potassium level and characteristic ECG changes, including tall peaked T waves, depression of ST segment, disappearance of P wave, prolonged QT interval, and widening and slurring of QRS complex. Late signs and symptoms include weakness, paralysis of voluntary muscles, respiratory distress, and dysphagia. These may precede severe or fatal cardiac toxicity. Hyperkalemia produces symptoms paradoxically similar to those of hypokalemia.
• Treatment of overdose includes discontinuation of the potassium supplement and, if necessary, lavage of the GI tract. In patients with a potassium level greater then 6.5 mEq/L, supportive therapy may include continuous ECG monitoring and infusion of 40 to 160 mEq sodium bicarbonate I.V. over a 5-minute interval (repeated in 10 to 15 minutes if ECG abnormalities persist) or infusion of 300 to 500 ml of $D_{10}W$ to $D_{25}W$ over 1 hour (insulin [5 to 10 U/20 g dextrose] should be added to the infusion or, ideally, administered as a separate injection).
• Patients with absent P waves or broad QRS complexes who aren't receiving cardiotonic glycosides should immediately be given 0.5 to 1 g calcium gluconate or another calcium salt I.V. over a 2-minute period (with continuous ECG monitoring) to antagonize the cardiotoxic effect of the potassium. May be repeated in 1 to 2 minutes if ECG abnormalities persist.
• To remove potassium from the body, use sodium polystyrene sulfonate resin, hemodialysis, or peritoneal dialysis. Administer potassium-free I.V. fluids when hyperkalemia is associated with water loss.

pramipexole dihydrochloride
Mirapex

Nonergot dopamine agonist, antiparkinsonian

Available by prescription only
Tablets: 0.125 mg, 0.25 mg, 0.5 mg, 1 mg, 1.5 mg

INDICATIONS & DOSAGE
Treatment of idiopathic Parkinson's disease
Adults: initially, 0.375 mg P.O. daily given in three divided doses; don't increase more than q 5 to 7 days. Increase dose by 0.75 mg in divided doses weekly until maximum dosage of 1.5 mg t.i.d. is reached after 7 weeks of therapy. Maintenance dosing ranges from 1.5 to 4.5 mg daily administered in three divided doses.
♦ **Dosage adjustment.** In patients with impaired renal function and creatinine clearance of 35 to 59 ml/minute, initial dosage is 0.125 mg P.O. b.i.d., and maintenance maximum dosage is 1.5 mg b.i.d. For patients with creatinine clearance of 15 to 34 ml/minute, initial dose is 0.125 mg P.O. daily and maintenance maximum dose is 1.5 mg daily.

PHARMACODYNAMICS
Antiparkinsonian action: Pramipexole is thought to stimulate dopamine receptors in striatum; in animal studies, drug influences striatal neuronal firing rates via activation of dopamine receptors in the striatum and the substantia nigra, the site of neurons that send projections to the striatum.

PHARMACOKINETICS
Absorption: Pramipexole is rapidly absorbed; levels peak in about 2 hours. Absolute bioavailability of drug is more than 90%, suggesting that it's well absorbed and undergoes little presystemic metabolism. Food doesn't affect extent of absorption, but maximum plasma level peaks about 1 hour later than usual when drug is taken with meals.
Distribution: Drug is extensively distributed, with a volume of distribution of

---

Reactions may be *common*, uncommon, **life-threatening**, or COMMON AND LIFE-THREATENING.

about 500 L. About 15% is bound to plasma proteins. Drug also distributes into RBCs. Terminal half-life is 8 to 12 hours; steady-state is reached within 2 days of dosing. In a study in which drug was administered to patients 60 years and older, systemic exposure was twice that of patients 18 to 30 years of age. *Metabolism:* Drug is thought to be metabolized through cytochrome P-450–mediated oxygenation in the liver. A small amount of metabolism also occurs in the lungs.

Excretion: About 90% of dose is excreted unchanged in urine. Nonrenal routes may contribute to a small extent to elimination, although no metabolites have been identified in plasma or urine. Drug is secreted from the renal tubules, probably through the organic transport system.

CONTRAINDICATIONS & PRECAUTIONS

Contraindicated in patients with hypersensitivity to pramipexole or its components. Use cautiously in patients who have renal impairment, such as those with Parkinson's disease, because dosing may need to be adjusted.

INTERACTIONS

Drug-drug. *Cimetidine* causes an increase in bioavailability and half-life of pramipexole. *Dopamine antagonists*—such as *butyrophenones, metoclopramide, phenothiazines,* and *thiothixenes*—may diminish the effectiveness of pramipexole. *Drugs eliminated via renal secretion*—including *cimetidine, diltiazem, quinidine, quinine, ranitidine, triamterene,* and *verapamil*—decrease oral clearance of pramipexole by about 20%. Administration with *levodopa* causes an increase in maximum plasma levodopa levels.

ADVERSE REACTIONS

CNS: malaise, *dizziness,* somnolence, *insomnia,* hallucinations, *confusion,* amnesia, hypesthesia, dystonia, akathisia, thought abnormalities, myoclonus, *asthenia, dyskinesia, extrapyramidal syndrome, dream abnormalities,* gait abnormalities, hypertonia, paranoid reaction, delusions, sleep disorders.

CV: chest pain, general edema, peripheral edema, *orthostatic hypotension.*
EENT: accommodation abnormalities, diplopia, rhinitis, vision abnormalities.
GI: dry mouth, anorexia, *constipation,* dysphagia, nausea.
GU: impotence, urinary frequency, urinary tract infection, urinary incontinence.
Musculoskeletal: arthritis, twitching, bursitis, myasthenia.
Respiratory: dyspnea, pneumonia.
Skin: skin disorders.
Other: fever, unassessable reaction, decreased libido, *accidental injury.*

▣ KEY CONSIDERATIONS

• Pramipexole clearance decreases with age because half-life and clearance are about 40% longer and about 30% lower, respectively, in patients age 65 or older. Monitor patient closely for adverse effects.
• If drug needs to be discontinued, it should be done over a 1-week period.
• Drug may cause orthostatic hypotension, especially during dose escalation; monitor patient carefully.
• Neuroleptic malignant syndrome (elevated temperature, muscular rigidity, altered consciousness, and autonomic instability) without obvious cause has occurred with rapid dose reduction or withdrawal of or changes in antiparkinsonian therapy.
• Adjust dosage gradually. Increase dosage to achieve maximum therapeutic effect balanced against the main adverse effects of dyskinesia, hallucinations, somnolence, and dry mouth.

Patient education

• Tell patient to take pramipexole only as prescribed and not to discontinue it abruptly.
• Instruct patient not to rise rapidly after sitting or lying down because of risk for orthostatic hypotension.
• Caution patient not to drive a car or operate complex machinery until response to drug is known.
• Tell patient to use caution before taking drug with other CNS depressants.
• Advise patient to take drug with food if nausea develops.

pravastatin sodium
Pravachol

3-hydroxy-3-methylglutaryl coen-zyme A (HMG-CoA) reductase in-hibitor, antilipemic

Available by prescription only
Tablets: 10 mg, 20 mg, 40 mg

INDICATIONS & DOSAGE
Reduction of low-density lipoprotein and total cholesterol levels in patients with primary hypercholesterolemia (types IIa and IIb), primary prevention of coronary events
Adults: initially, 10 to 20 mg daily h.s. Adjust dosage q 4 weeks based on patient tolerance and response; maximum daily dosage is 40 mg.
Geriatric patients: Most geriatric patients respond to a daily dosage of 20 mg or less.

PHARMACODYNAMICS
Antilipemic action: Pravastatin inhibits the enzyme HMG-CoA reductase. This hepatic enzyme is an early (and rate-limiting) step in the synthetic pathway of cholesterol.

PHARMACOKINETICS
Absorption: Pravastatin is rapidly absorbed; plasma levels peak in 1 to 1½ hours. Average oral absorption is 34%, with absolute bioavailability of 17%. Although food reduces bioavailability, drug effects are the same if drug is taken with or 1 hour before meals.
Distribution: Plasma levels are proportional to dose, but don't necessarily correlate perfectly with lipid-lowering effects. About 50% is bound to plasma proteins. Drug experiences extensive first-pass extraction, possibly because of an active transport system into hepatocytes.
Metabolism: Drug is metabolized by the liver; at least six metabolites have been identified. Some are active.
Excretion: Drug is excreted from the liver and kidneys.

CONTRAINDICATIONS & PRECAUTIONS
Contraindicated in patients with hypersensitivity to pravastatin and in those with active liver disease or conditions that cause unexplained, persistent elevations of serum transaminase levels.

Use cautiously in patients who consume large quantities of alcohol or have history of liver disease.

INTERACTIONS
Drug-drug. Use with *cholestyramine* or *colestipol* may decrease plasma pravastatin levels; administer pravastatin 1 hour before or 4 hours after these drugs. *Drugs that decrease levels or activity of endogenous steroids*—including *cimetidine, ketoconazole,* and *spironolactone*—may increase risk for endocrine dysfunction, but no intervention appears necessary; take complete drug history in patients who develop endocrine dysfunction. Use with *erythromycin, fibric acid derivatives* (such as *clofibrate* and *gemfibrozil*), *immunosuppressants* (such as *cyclosporine*), or *high doses of niacin* (1 g or more *nicotinic acid* daily) may increase risk for rhabdomyolysis; monitor patient closely if use can't be avoided. Avoid use with *gemfibrozil* because it decreases protein binding and urine clearance of pravastatin. *Hepatotoxic drugs* may increase risk for hepatotoxicity.
Drug-lifestyle. Chronic *alcohol* abuse may increase risk for hepatotoxicity. Exposure to *sunlight* may cause photosensitivity reaction.

ADVERSE REACTIONS
CNS: headache, dizziness, fatigue.
CV: chest pain.
EENT: rhinitis, myositis, myopathy.
GI: vomiting, diarrhea, heartburn, abdominal pain, constipation, flatulence, nausea.
GU: renal failure secondary to myoglobinuria.
Hepatic: increased AST, ALT, CK, alkaline phosphatase, and bilirubin levels.
Musculoskeletal: *localized muscle pain,* myalgia, ***rhabdomyolysis.***
Respiratory: cough, influenza, common cold.

Reactions may be *common*, uncommon, *life-threatening*, or COMMON AND LIFE-THREATENING.

Skin: rash, photosensitivity.
Other: flulike syndrome, *abnormal thyroid function tests.*

🔲 KEY CONSIDERATIONS

• Maximum effectiveness is usually evident with daily doses of 20 mg or less.
• Discontinue pravastatin temporarily in patient with an acute condition that suggests a developing myopathy or in patient with risk factors that may predispose him to renal failure secondary to rhabdomyolysis (including severe acute infection; severe endocrine, metabolic, or electrolyte disorders; hypotension; major surgery; or uncontrolled seizures).
• Watch for signs of myositis. Rarely, myopathy and markedly elevated CK levels, possibly leading to rhabdomyolysis and renal failure secondary to myoglobinuria, have been reported.
• Initiate drug therapy only after diet and other nonpharmacologic therapies have proved ineffective. Patients should continue a cholesterol-lowering diet during therapy.
• Give drug in the evening, preferably at bedtime. Drug may be given without regard to meals.
• Dosage adjustments should be made about every 4 weeks. May reduce dosage if cholesterol levels fall below target range.

Patient education

• Teach patient appropriate dietary management (restricting total fat and cholesterol intake), weight control, and exercise. Explain importance of these interventions in controlling serum lipid levels.
• Because pravastatin may affect liver function, advise patient to restrict alcohol intake.
• Tell patient to call if he experiences adverse reactions, particularly muscle aches and pains.
• Inform patient to take drug at bedtime.

prazosin hydrochloride
Minipress

Alpha-adrenergic blocker, antihypertensive

Available by prescription only
Capsules: 1 mg, 2 mg, 5 mg

INDICATIONS & DOSAGE
Hypertension
Adults: initially, 1 mg P.O. b.i.d. or t.i.d., gradually increased to maximum of 20 mg daily. Usual maintenance dosage is 6 to 15 mg daily in divided doses. If other antihypertensives or diuretics are added to prazosin therapy, reduce dosage of prazosin to 1 or 2 mg t.i.d. and then gradually increase as necessary.
◇ **BPH**
Adults: initially, 2 mg P.O. b.i.d. Dosage may range from 1 to 9 mg/day.

PHARMACODYNAMICS
Antihypertensive action: Prazosin selectively and competitively inhibits alpha-adrenergic receptors, causing arterial and venous dilation, reducing peripheral vascular resistance and blood pressure.
Hypertrophic action: Drug's alpha blockade in nonvascular smooth muscle causes relaxation, notably in prostatic tissue, thereby reducing urinary symptoms in men with BPH.

PHARMACOKINETICS
Absorption: Absorption from the GI tract is variable. Antihypertensive effect begins in about 2 hours, peaks in 2 to 4 hours; full effect may not occur for 4 to 6 weeks.
Distribution: Prazosin is distributed throughout the body and is highly protein-bound (about 97%).
Metabolism: Drug is metabolized extensively in the liver.
Excretion: More than 90% of a given dose is excreted in feces by bile; remainder is excreted in urine. Plasma half-life is 2 to 4 hours. Antihypertensive effect lasts less than 24 hours.

CONTRAINDICATIONS & PRECAUTIONS
No known contraindications. Use cautiously in patients receiving antihypertensives and in those with chronic renal failure.

INTERACTIONS
Drug-drug. The hypotensive effects of prazosin may be increased when administered with *diuretics* or other *antihypertensives*. Because prazosin is highly bound to plasma proteins, it may interact with other *highly protein-bound drugs*.

ADVERSE REACTIONS
CNS: *dizziness,* headache, drowsiness, nervousness, paresthesia, weakness, *first-dose syncope,* depression.
CV: orthostatic hypotension, *palpitations*.
EENT: blurred vision, tinnitus, conjunctivitis, nasal congestion, epistaxis.
GI: vomiting, diarrhea, abdominal cramps, constipation, *nausea*.
GU: priapism, impotence, urinary frequency, incontinence.
Musculoskeletal: arthralgia, myalgia.
Respiratory: dyspnea.
Other: pruritus, edema, fever.

▣ KEY CONSIDERATIONS
Besides the recommendations relevant to all alpha-adrenergic blockers, consider the following:
• Geriatric patients may be more sensitive to hypotensive effects and may require lower doses because of altered prazosin metabolism.
• First-dose syncope—dizziness, lightheadedness, and syncope—may occur within ½ to 1 hour after initial dose. It may be severe, with loss of consciousness, if initial dose exceeds 2 mg. Effect is transient and may be diminished by giving drug at bedtime, by limiting the initial dose to 1 mg, by subsequently increasing the dosage gradually, and by introducing other antihypertensives into the patient's regimen cautiously. Effect is more common during febrile illness and more severe if patient has hyponatremia. Always increase dosage gradually and have patient sit or lie down if he experiences dizziness.

• The drug affects diastolic blood pressure more than systolic pressure.
• Drug has been used to treat vasospasm associated with Raynaud's syndrome. It also has been used with diuretics and cardiac glycosides to treat severe heart failure, to manage the signs and symptoms of pheochromocytoma preoperatively, and to treat ergotamine-induced peripheral ischemia.
• Drug alters results of screening tests for pheochromocytoma and causes increases in levels of the urine metabolite of norepinephrine and vanillylmandelic acid; it may cause positive antinuclear antibody titer.

Patient education
• Teach patient about his disease and therapy, and explain that he must take prazosin exactly as prescribed, even when feeling well. Advise him never to discontinue drug suddenly because severe rebound hypertension may occur, and instruct him to promptly report malaise or unusual adverse effects.
• Tell patient to avoid hazardous activities that require mental alertness until tolerance develops to sedation, drowsiness, and other CNS effects, to avoid sudden position changes to minimize orthostatic hypotension, and to use ice chips, candy, or gum to relieve dry mouth.
• Warn patient to seek medical approval before taking OTC cold preparations.

Overdose & treatment
• Signs and symptoms of overdose are hypotension and drowsiness.
• After acute ingestion, induce vomiting or perform gastric lavage, and give activated charcoal to reduce absorption. Further treatment is usually symptomatic and supportive. Drug isn't dialyzable.

Reactions may be *common,* uncommon, *life-threatening*, or COMMON AND LIFE-THREATENING.

prednisolone (systemic)
Delta-Cortef, Prelone

prednisolone acetate
Key-Pred-25, Predalone-50,
Predate, Predcor-50

prednisolone acetate and prednisolone sodium phosphate
Predicort-RP

prednisolone sodium phosphate
Hydeltrasol, Key-Pred SP,
Pediapred, Predate S

prednisolone tebutate
Hydeltra-T.B.A., Nor-Pred T.B.A.,
Predate TBA, Predcor-TBA

Glucocorticoid, mineralocorticoid, anti-inflammatory, immunosuppressant

---

Available by prescription only
prednisolone
Tablets: 5 mg
Syrup: 15 mg/5 ml
prednisolone acetate
Injection: 25 mg/ml, 50 mg/ml,
100 mg/ml suspension
prednisolone acetate and prednisolone sodium phosphate
Injection: 80 mg acetate and 20 mg sodium phosphate/ml suspension
prednisolone sodium phosphate
Oral liquid: 6.7 mg (5 mg base)/5 ml
Injection: 20 mg/ml solution
prednisolone tebutate
Injection: 20 mg/ml suspension

INDICATIONS & DOSAGE
Severe inflammation, modification of body's immune response to disease
Adults: 2.5 to 15 mg P.O. b.i.d., t.i.d., or q.i.d.
prednisolone acetate
Adults: 2 to 30 mg I.M. q 12 hours.
prednisolone acetate and prednisolone sodium phosphate suspension
Adults: 0.25 to 1 ml into joints weekly, p.r.n.

prednisolone sodium phosphate
Adults: 2 to 30 mg I.M. or I.V. q 12 hours, or into joints, lesions and soft tissue, p.r.n.
prednisolone tebutate
Adults: 4 to 40 mg into joints and lesions, p.r.n.

PHARMACODYNAMICS
Anti-inflammatory and immunosuppressant actions: Prednisolone stimulates the synthesis of enzymes needed to decrease the inflammatory response. It suppresses the immune system by reducing activity and volume of the lymphatic system, thus producing lymphocytopenia (primarily of T lymphocytes), decreasing immunoglobulin and complement levels, decreasing passage of immune complexes through basement membranes, and possibly by depressing reactivity of tissue to antigen-antibody interactions.

The mineralocorticoids regulate electrolyte homeostasis by acting at the renal distal tubules to enhance the reabsorption of sodium ions (and thus water) from the tubular fluid into the plasma and enhance the excretion of both potassium and hydrogen ions.

Drug is an adrenocorticoid with both glucocorticoid and mineralocorticoid properties. It's a weak mineralocorticoid with only half the potency of hydrocortisone but it's a more potent glucocorticoid, with four times the potency of equal weight of hydrocortisone. It's used primarily as an anti-inflammatory and immunosuppressant. It isn't used for mineralocorticoid replacement therapy because of the availability of more specific and potent drugs.

Drug may be administered orally. Prednisolone sodium phosphate is highly soluble, has a rapid onset and short duration of action, and may be given I.M. or I.V. Prednisolone acetate and tebutate are suspensions that may be administered by intra-articular, intrasynovial, intrabursal, intralesional, or soft-tissue injection. They have a slow onset but long duration of action.

Prednisolone acetate and prednisolone sodium phosphate is a combination product of the rapid-acting phosphate salt and the slightly soluble, slowly released acetate salt. This product provides rapid anti-inflammatory effects with a sustained duration of action. It's a suspension and shouldn't be given I.V. It's particularly useful as an anti-inflammatory in intra-articular, I.D., and intralesional injections.

PHARMACOKINETICS

Absorption: Prednisolone is absorbed readily after oral administration. After oral and I.V. administration, effects peak in about 1 to 2 hours. Acetate and tebutate suspensions for injection have a variable absorption rate over 24 to 48 hours, depending on whether they are injected into an intra-articular space or a muscle, and on the blood supply to that muscle. Systemic absorption occurs slowly after intra-articular injection.

Distribution: Drug is removed rapidly from the blood and distributed to muscle, liver, skin, intestines, and kidneys. It's extensively bound to plasma proteins (transcortin and albumin). Only the unbound portion is active.

Metabolism: Drug is metabolized in the liver to inactive glucuronide and sulfate metabolites.

Excretion: The inactive metabolites and small amounts of unmetabolized drug are excreted in urine. Insignificant quantities of drug are excreted in feces. Biologic half-life is 18 to 36 hours.

CONTRAINDICATIONS & PRECAUTIONS

Contraindicated in patients with hypersensitivity to prednisolone or its ingredients and systemic fungal infections.

Use cautiously in patients with a recent MI, GI ulcer, renal disease, hypertension, osteoporosis, diabetes mellitus, hypothyroidism, cirrhosis, diverticulitis, nonspecific ulcerative colitis, recent intestinal anastomoses, thromboembolic disorders, seizures, myasthenia gravis, heart failure, tuberculosis, ocular herpes simplex, emotional instability, or psychotic tendencies.

INTERACTIONS

Drug-drug. *Antacids, cholestyramine,* and *colestipol* adsorb the corticosteroid, thus decreasing the amount of drug absorbed as well as the effect of the drug.

Barbiturates, phenytoin, and *rifampin* may cause decreased corticosteroid effects because of increased hepatic metabolism. Use with *estrogens* may reduce the metabolism of prednisolone by increasing transcortin levels; the half-life of the corticosteroid is then prolonged because of increased protein binding. Glucocorticoids cause hyperglycemia, requiring dosage adjustment of *insulin* or *oral antidiabetics* in patients with diabetes and may enhance hypokalemia associated with *amphotericin B* or *diuretic* therapy; the hypokalemia may increase the risk of toxicity in patients receiving *cardiac glycosides*. Glucocorticoids increase the metabolism of *isoniazid* and *salicylates*. Prednisolone may decrease the effects of *oral anticoagulants* by unknown mechanisms (rare). Administration with *ulcerogenic drugs* such as *NSAIDs* may increase risk of GI ulceration.

ADVERSE REACTIONS

Most adverse reactions to corticosteroids are dose- or duration-dependent.

CNS: *euphoria, insomnia,* psychotic behavior, pseudotumor cerebri, vertigo, headache, paresthesia, *seizures.*

CV: *heart failure, thromboembolism,* hypertension, edema, *arrhythmias,* thrombophlebitis.

EENT: cataracts, glaucoma.

GI: *peptic ulceration,* GI irritation, increased appetite, pancreatitis, nausea, vomiting.

Metabolic: cushingoid state (moonface, buffalo hump, central obesity), hypokalemia, hyperglycemia, carbohydrate intolerance.

Musculoskeletal: muscle weakness, osteoporosis.

Skin: delayed wound healing, acne, various skin eruptions, hirsutism.

Other: susceptibility to infections; *acute adrenal insufficiency may occur with increased stress (infection, surgery, or trauma) or abrupt withdrawal after long-term therapy.*

After abrupt withdrawal: rebound inflammation, fatigue, weakness, arthralgia, fever, dizziness, lethargy, depression, fainting, orthostatic hypotension, dyspnea, anorexia, hypoglycemia. *After*

Reactions may be *common,* uncommon, *life-threatening,* or **COMMON AND LIFE-THREATENING.**

prolonged use, sudden withdrawal may be fatal.

▣ KEY CONSIDERATIONS

Besides the recommendations relevant to all systemic adrenocorticoids, consider the following:

• Geriatric patients may be more susceptible to osteoporosis with long-term use.

• Drug suppresses reactions to skin tests; causes false-negative results in the nitroblue tetrazolium test for systemic bacterial infections; decreases ^{131}I uptake and protein-bound iodine levels in thyroid function tests; may increase glucose and cholesterol levels; may decrease serum potassium, calcium, T_4, and T_3 levels; and may increase urine glucose and calcium levels.

• Always adjust to lowest effective dose.

• Give oral dose with food when possible to reduce GI irritation. Patient may require drug to prevent GI irritation.

• Give I.M. injection deeply into gluteal muscle. To prevent muscle atrophy, rotate injection sites. Avoid S.C. injection because atrophy and sterile abscesses may occur.

• Monitor patient's weight, blood pressure, and serum electrolyte levels.

• Watch for depression or psychotic episodes, especially in high-dose therapy.

• Drug may mask or exacerbate infections, including latent amebiasis.

Patient teaching

• Tell patient not to discontinue prednisolone abruptly or without consent.

• Instruct patient to take oral form of drug with food or milk.

• Teach patient the signs and symptoms of early adrenal insufficiency: fatigue, muscular weakness, joint pain, fever, anorexia, nausea, dyspnea, dizziness, and fainting.

• Instruct patient to carry a card identifying his need for supplemental systemic glucocorticoids during stress. This card should indicate the prescriber's name, drug, and dose taken.

• Instruct patient to avoid exposure to infections.

• Tell patient to avoid immunizations while taking drug.

prednisolone acetate (ophthalmic)
AK-Tate, Econopred Ophthalmic, Ocu-Pred-A, Predair A, Pred Forte, Pred Mild Ophthalmic

prednisolone sodium phosphate
AK-Pred, Inflamase Forte, Inflamase Mild Ophthalmic, I-Pred, Ocu-Pred, Predair

Corticosteroid, ophthalmic anti-inflammatory

Available by prescription only
prednisolone acetate
Suspension: 0.12%, 0.125%, 0.25%, 1%
prednisolone sodium phosphate
Solution: 0.125%, 0.5%, 1%

INDICATIONS & DOSAGE
Inflammation of palpebral and bulbar conjunctiva, cornea, and anterior segment of globe; corneal injury; graft rejection
Adults: Instill 1 or 2 gtt in eye. In severe conditions, may be used hourly, tapering to discontinuation as inflammation subsides. In mild conditions, may be used four to six times daily.

PHARMACODYNAMICS
Anti-inflammatory action: Corticosteroids stimulate the synthesis of enzymes needed to decrease the inflammatory response. Prednisolone, a synthetic corticosteroid, has about four times the anti-inflammatory potency of an equal weight of hydrocortisone. Prednisolone acetate is poorly soluble and has a slower onset but longer duration of action when applied in a liquid suspension. The sodium phosphate salt is highly soluble and has a rapid onset but short duration of action.

PHARMACOKINETICS
Absorption: After ophthalmic administration, prednisolone is absorbed through the aqueous humor. Systemic absorption rarely occurs.
Distribution: After ophthalmic application, drug is distributed throughout the

local tissue layers. Drug that is absorbed into circulation is rapidly removed from the blood and distributed into muscle, liver, skin, intestines, and kidneys.
Metabolism: After ophthalmic administration, corticosteroids are primarily metabolized locally. The small amount that is absorbed into systemic circulation is metabolized primarily in the liver to inactive compounds.
Excretion: Inactive metabolites are excreted by the kidneys, primarily as glucuronides and sulfates, but also as unconjugated products. Small amounts of the metabolites are excreted in feces.

CONTRAINDICATIONS & PRECAUTIONS
Contraindicated in patients with acute, untreated, purulent ocular infections; acute superficial herpes simplex (dendritic keratitis); vaccinia, varicella, or other viral or fungal eye diseases; or ocular tuberculosis. Use cautiously in patients with corneal abrasions that may be contaminated (especially with herpes).

ADVERSE REACTIONS
EENT: increased intraocular pressure; thinning of cornea, interference with corneal wound healing, increased susceptibility to viral or fungal corneal infection, corneal ulceration. With excessive or long-term use: discharge, discomfort, foreign body sensation, glaucoma exacerbation, cataracts, visual acuity and visual field defects, optic nerve damage.
Other: systemic effects and adrenal suppression with excessive or long-term use.

▣ KEY CONSIDERATIONS
• Shake suspension and check dosage before administering. Store in tightly covered container.

Patient education
• Teach patient how to instill drops. Advise him to wash hands before and after applying, and warn him not to touch tip of dropper to eye or surrounding area.
• Advise patient to apply light finger pressure on lacrimal sac for 1 minute after instillation.

• Tell patient on long-term therapy to have frequent tonometric examinations.
• Warn patient not to use leftover medication for a new eye inflammation because serious problems may occur.
• Tell patient not to share drug, washcloths, or towels with family members and to notify prescriber if anyone develops same signs or symptoms.
• Stress importance of compliance with recommended therapy.

---

prednisone
Apo-Prednisone*, Deltasone, Meticorten, Orasone, Prednicen-M, Sterapred, Winpred*

Adrenocorticoid, anti-inflammatory, immunosuppressant

Available by prescription only
Tablets: 1 mg, 2.5 mg, 5 mg, 10 mg, 20 mg, 25 mg, 50 mg
Oral solution: 5 mg/ml; 5 mg/5 ml
Syrup: 5 mg/5 ml

INDICATIONS & DOSAGE
Severe inflammation, modification of body's immune response to disease
Adults: 5 to 60 mg P.O. daily in single dose or divided doses. (Maximum daily dose is 250 mg.) Maintenance dose given once daily or every other day. Dosage must be individualized.
Acute exacerbations of multiple sclerosis
Adults: 200 mg P.O. daily for 1 week, then 80 mg every other day for 1 month.
◊ ***Adjunct to anti-infective therapy in the treatment of moderate to severe*** Pneumocystis carinii *pneumonia*
Adults with AIDS: 40 mg P.O. b.i.d. for 5 days; then 40 mg. P.O. once daily for 5 days; then 20 mg P.O. once daily for 11 days (or until completion of the concurrent anti-infective regimen).

PHARMACODYNAMICS
Anti-inflammatory action: Prednisone is an intermediate-acting glucocorticoid, with greater glucocorticoid activity than cortisone and hydrocortisone, but less anti-inflammatory activity than betamethasone, dexamethasone, or para-

---

methasone. Prednisone is about four to five times more potent as an anti-inflammatory than hydrocortisone, but it has only half the mineralocorticoid activity of an equal weight of hydrocortisone. Prednisone is the oral glucocorticoid of choice for anti-inflammatory or immunosuppressant effects.

Immunosuppressant action: Prednisone stimulates the synthesis of enzymes needed to decrease the inflammatory response. It suppresses the immune system by reducing activity and volume of the lymphatic system, thus producing lymphocytopenia (primarily of T lymphocytes), decreasing immunoglobulin and complement levels, decreasing passage of immune complexes through basement membranes, and possibly by depressing reactivity of tissue to antigen-antibody interactions.

For those patients who can't swallow tablets, a liquid form is available. The oral concentrate (5 mg/ml) may be diluted in juice or another flavored diluent or mixed in semisolid food (such as applesauce) before administration.

PHARMACOKINETICS

Absorption: Prednisone is absorbed readily after oral administration; effects peak in 1 to 2 hours.
Distribution: Drug is distributed rapidly to muscle, liver, skin, intestines, and kidneys. Drug is extensively bound to plasma proteins (transcortin and albumin); only the unbound portion is active.
Metabolism: Drug is metabolized in the liver to the active metabolite prednisolone, which in turn is then metabolized to inactive glucuronide and sulfate metabolites.
Excretion: The inactive metabolites and a small amount of unmetabolized drug are excreted from the kidneys. Insignificant quantities of drug are also excreted in feces. Biological half-life is 18 to 36 hours.

CONTRAINDICATIONS & PRECAUTIONS

Contraindicated in patients with hypersensitivity to prednisone or systemic fungal infections.

Use cautiously in patients with GI ulcer, renal disease, hypertension, osteo-porosis, diabetes mellitus, hypothyroidism, cirrhosis, diverticulitis, nonspecific ulcerative colitis, recent intestinal anastomoses, thromboembolic disorders, seizures, myasthenia gravis, heart failure, tuberculosis, ocular herpes simplex, emotional instability, and psychotic tendencies.

INTERACTIONS

Drug-drug. *Antacids, cholestyramine,* and *colestipol* decrease the effect of prednisone by adsorbing the corticosteroid, decreasing the amount absorbed. *Barbiturates, phenytoin,* and *rifampin* may cause decreased effects because of increased hepatic metabolism. Use with *estrogens* may reduce the metabolism of prednisone by increasing transcortin levels; the half-life of prednisone is then prolonged because of increased protein binding. Drug causes hyperglycemia, requiring dosage adjustment of *insulin* or *oral antidiabetics* in patients with diabetes and may enhance hypokalemia associated with *amphotericin B* or *diuretic* therapy; the hypokalemia may increase the risk for toxicity in patients receiving *cardiac glycosides.* Drug increases the metabolism of *isoniazid* and *salicylates.* Use of prednisone rarely may decrease the effects of *oral anticoagulants* by unknown mechanisms. Use with *ulcerogenic drugs* such as *NSAIDs* may increase the risk for GI ulceration.

ADVERSE REACTIONS

Most adverse reactions to corticosteroids are dose dependent or duration dependent.
CNS: *euphoria, insomnia,* psychotic behavior, pseudotumor cerebri, vertigo, headache, paresthesia, *seizures.*
CV: hypertension, edema, *arrhythmias,* thrombophlebitis, *thromboembolism, heart failure.*
EENT: cataracts, glaucoma.
GI: *peptic ulceration,* GI irritation, increased appetite, pancreatitis, nausea, vomiting.
Metabolic: cushingoid state (moonface, buffalo hump, central obesity), hypokalemia, hyperglycemia, and carbohydrate intolerance.

Musculoskeletal: muscle weakness, osteoporosis.

Skin: delayed wound healing, acne, various skin eruptions, hirsutism.

Other: susceptibility to infections; *acute adrenal insufficiency may occur with increased stress (infection, surgery, or trauma) or abrupt withdrawal after long-term therapy.*

After abrupt withdrawal: rebound inflammation, fatigue, weakness, arthralgia, fever, dizziness, lethargy, depression, fainting, orthostatic hypotension, dyspnea, anorexia, hypoglycemia. *After prolonged use, sudden withdrawal may be fatal.*

▣ KEY CONSIDERATIONS

Beside the recommendations relevant to all systemic adrenocorticoids, consider the following:

• Geriatric patients may be more susceptible to osteoporosis with long-term use.

• Prednisone suppresses reactions to skin tests; causes false-negative results in the nitroblue tetrazolium test for systemic bacterial infections; decreases ^{131}I uptake and protein-bound iodine levels in thyroid function tests; may increase glucose and cholesterol levels; may decrease serum potassium, calcium, T_3, and T_4 levels; and may increase urine glucose and calcium levels.

• Always adjust to the lowest effective dose.

• For better results and less toxicity, give a once-daily dose in the morning.

• Monitor patient's blood pressure, sleep patterns, and serum potassium levels.

• Watch for depression or psychotic episodes, especially in high-dose therapy.

• Drug may mask or exacerbate infections, including latent amebiasis.

Patient teaching

• Tell patient not to discontinue prednisone abruptly or without consent.

• Instruct patient to take drug with food or milk.

• Teach patient the signs and symptoms of early adrenal insufficiency: fatigue, muscular weakness, joint pain, fever, anorexia, nausea, dyspnea, dizziness, and fainting.

• Instruct patient to carry a card identifying his need for supplemental systemic glucocorticoids during stress. This card should indicate the prescriber's name, drug, and dose taken.

• Tell patient to report slow healing.

• Advise patient receiving long-term therapy to have periodic ophthalmic examinations.

---

primidone
Myidone, Mysoline, Sertan

Barbiturate analogue, anticonvulsant

Available by prescription only
Tablets: 50 mg, 250 mg
Suspension: 250 mg/5 ml

INDICATIONS & DOSAGE

Generalized tonic-clonic seizures, focal seizures, complex-partial (psychomotor) seizures

Adults: 100 to 125 mg P.O. h.s. on days 1 to 3; 100 to 125 mg P.O. b.i.d. on days 4 to 6; 100 to 125 mg P.O. t.i.d. on days 7 to 9; and maintenance dose of 250 mg P.O. t.i.d. on day 10. May require up to 2 g/day.

Benign familial tremor (essential tremor)

Adults: 750 mg P.O. daily.

PHARMACODYNAMICS

Anticonvulsant action: Primidone acts as a nonspecific CNS depressant used alone or with other anticonvulsants to control refractory tonic-clonic seizures and to treat psychomotor or focal seizures. Mechanism of action is unknown; some activity may be from phenobarbital, an active metabolite.

PHARMACOKINETICS

Absorption: Primidone is absorbed readily from the GI tract; serum levels peak at about 3 hours. Phenobarbital appears in plasma after several days of continuous therapy; most laboratory assays detect both phenobarbital and primidone. Therapeutic levels are 5 to 12 µg/ml for primidone and 10 to 30 µg/ml for phenobarbital.

Reactions may be *common*, uncommon, *life-threatening*, or COMMON AND LIFE-THREATENING.

Distribution: Drug is distributed widely throughout the body.
Metabolism: Drug is metabolized slowly by the liver to phenylethylmalonamide (PEMA) and phenobarbital; PEMA is the major metabolite.
Excretion: Drug is excreted in urine.

CONTRAINDICATIONS & PRECAUTIONS
Contraindicated in patients with phenobarbital hypersensitivity or porphyria.

INTERACTIONS
Drug-drug. Coadministration with *acetazolamide* or *succinimides* may decrease primidone levels. *Carbamazepine* and *phenytoin* may decrease effects of primidone and increase its conversion to phenobarbital; monitor serum levels to prevent toxicity. *CNS depressants,* including *narcotic analgesics,* cause excessive depression in patients taking primidone.
Drug-lifestyle. *Alcohol* causes excessive depression in patients taking primidone.

ADVERSE REACTIONS
CNS: *drowsiness, ataxia,* emotional disturbances, vertigo, hyperirritability, fatigue, paranoia.
EENT: *diplopia,* nystagmus.
GI: anorexia, nausea, vomiting.
GU: impotence, polyuria.
Hematologic: megaloblastic anemia, *thrombocytopenia.*
Hepatic: *abnormal liver function test results.*
Skin: morbilliform rash.

▣ KEY CONSIDERATIONS
Besides the recommendations relevant to all barbiturates, consider the following:
• Reduce dose in geriatric patients; many have decreased renal function.
• Perform CBC and liver function tests every 6 months.
• Abrupt withdrawal of primidone may cause status epilepticus; dosage should be reduced gradually.
• Barbiturates impair ability to perform tasks requiring mental alertness, such as driving a car.

Patient education
• Explain rationale for therapy and the potential risks and benefits.
• Teach patient signs and symptoms of adverse reactions.
• Tell patient to avoid alcohol and other sedatives to prevent added CNS depression.
• Instruct patient not to discontinue primidone or to alter dosage without medical approval.
• Advise patient to avoid hazardous tasks that require mental alertness until degree of sedative effect is determined. Tell the patient that dizziness and incoordination are common at first but will disappear.
• Recommend that patient wear a medical identification bracelet or necklace identifying him as having a seizure disorder and listing drug.
• Tell patient to shake oral suspension well before use.

Overdose & treatment
• Signs and symptoms of overdose resemble those of barbiturate intoxication, including CNS and respiratory depression, areflexia, oliguria, tachycardia, hypotension, hypothermia, and coma. Shock may occur.
• Treat overdose supportively. In conscious patient with intact gag reflex, induce vomiting with ipecac; follow in 30 minutes with repeated doses of activated charcoal. Use lavage if vomiting isn't feasible. Alkalinization of urine and forced diuresis may hasten excretion. Hemodialysis may be necessary. Monitor vital signs and fluid and electrolyte balance.

probenecid
Benemid, Probalan

Sulfonamide-derivative, uricosuric

Available by prescription only
Tablets: 500 mg

INDICATIONS & DOSAGE
Adjunct to penicillin therapy
Adults: 500 mg P.O. q.i.d.

Single-dose penicillin treatment of gonorrhea

Adults: 1 g P.O. given together with penicillin treatment, or 1 g P.O. 30 minutes before I.M. dose of penicillin.

Hyperuricemia associated with gout

Adults: 250 mg P.O. b.i.d. for first week, then 500 mg b.i.d., to maximum of 2 to 3 g daily.

◇ To diagnose parkinsonian syndrome or mental depression

Adults: 500 mg P.O. q 12 hours for five doses.

PHARMACODYNAMICS

Uricosuric action: Probenecid competitively inhibits the active reabsorption of uric acid at the proximal convoluted tubule, thereby increasing urine excretion of uric acid.

Adjunctive action in antibiotic therapy: Drug competitively inhibits secretion of weak organic acids, including penicillins, cephalosporins, and other beta-lactam antibiotics, thereby increasing serum levels of these drugs.

PHARMACOKINETICS

Absorption: Probenecid is completely absorbed after oral administration; serum levels peak at 2 to 4 hours.

Distribution: Distributes throughout the body; drug is about 75% protein-bound. CSF levels are about 2% of serum levels.

Metabolism: Drug is metabolized in the liver to active metabolites, with some uricosuric effect.

Excretion: Drug and metabolites are excreted in urine; probenecid (but not metabolites) is actively reabsorbed.

CONTRAINDICATIONS & PRECAUTIONS

Contraindicated in patients with hypersensitivity to probenecid, uric acid kidney stones, or blood dyscrasias; or in acute gout attack. Use cautiously in patients with impaired renal function or peptic ulcer.

INTERACTIONS

Drug-drug. Use increases serum levels (thus increasing risk of toxicity) of *aminosalicylic acid, dapsone, methotrexate,* and *nitrofurantoin.* Use significantly increases or prolongs effects of *cephalosporins,* other *beta-lactam antibiotics, penicillins,* and *sulfonamides,* and possibly *ketamine* and *thiopental.* Use enhances hypoglycemic effects of *chlorpropamide* and other *oral sulfonylureas.* The uricosuric action of drug is antagonized by *diuretics* and *pyrazinamide;* increased doses of probenecid may be required. *Salicylates* inhibit the uricosuric effect of probenecid only in doses that achieve levels of 50 μg/ml or more; occasional use of low-dose *aspirin* doesn't interfere. Probenecid inhibits urine excretion of *weak organic acids;* it impairs naturietic effects of *bumetanide, ethacrynic acid,* and *furosemide;* and it also decreases excretion of *indomethacin* and *naproxen,* permitting use of lower doses. Administration with *zidovudine* may increase bioavailability of zidovudine, resulting in cutaneous eruptions accompanied by systemic symptoms, including malaise, myalgia, and fever.

Drug-lifestyle. *Alcohol* decreases the uricosuric action of probenecid.

ADVERSE REACTIONS

CNS: *headache,* dizziness.

CV: flushing.

GI: anorexia, nausea, vomiting, sore gums.

GU: urinary frequency, renal colic, nephrotic syndrome.

Hematologic: *hemolytic anemia, aplastic anemia,* anemia.

Hepatic: *hepatic necrosis.*

Skin: dermatitis, pruritus.

Other: fever, exacerbation of gout, hypersensitivity reactions (including *anaphylaxis*).

▣ KEY CONSIDERATIONS

• Lower doses are indicated in geriatric patients because of increased potential for adverse effects.

• When used for hyperuricemia associated with gout, probenecid has no analgesic or anti-inflammatory actions and no effect on acute attacks; start therapy after attack subsides. Because drug may increase the frequency of acute attacks during the first 6 to 12 months of therapy, prophylactic doses of colchicine or

---

Reactions may be *common*, uncommon, *life-threatening*, or COMMON AND LIFE-THREATENING.

NSAIDs should be administered during the first 3 to 6 months of therapy.
• Monitor BUN and serum creatinine levels closely; drug is ineffective in severe renal insufficiency.
• Monitor uric acid levels and adjust dose to the lowest dose that maintains normal uric acid levels.
• Give with food, milk, or prescribed antacids to lessen GI upset.
• Maintain adequate hydration with high fluid intake to prevent formation of uric acid renal calculi. Also maintain alkalinization of urine.
• Drug has been used to help diagnose parkinsonian syndrome and mental depression.
• Drug causes false-positive test results for urine glucose with tests using cupric sulfate reagent (Benedict's reagent, Clinitest, and Fehling's test); perform tests with glucose oxidase reagent (Diastix, Chemstrip uG, or glucose enzymatic test strip) instead.

Patient education
• Instruct patient not to discontinue probenecid without medical approval.
• Warn patient not to use drug for pain or inflammation and not to increase dose during gouty attack.
• Tell patient to drink 8 to 10 glasses of fluid daily and to take drug with food to minimize GI upset.
• Warn patient to avoid aspirin and other salicylates, which may antagonize uricosuric effect of the drug.
• Caution patients with diabetes to use glucose enzymatic test strip, Diastix, or Chemstrip uG for urine glucose testing.

Overdose & treatment
• Signs and symptoms of overdose include nausea, copious vomiting, stupor, coma, and tonic-clonic seizures.
• Treat supportively, using mechanical ventilation if needed; induce vomiting or perform gastric lavage, as appropriate. Control seizures with I.V. phenobarbital and phenytoin.

procainamide hydrochloride
Procanbid, Promine, Pronestyl, Pronestyl-SR

Procaine derivative, ventricular antiarrhythmic, supraventricular antiarrhythmic

Available by prescription only
Tablets: 250 mg, 375 mg, 500 mg
Tablets (extended-release): 500 mg, 1 g
Tablets (sustained-release): 250 mg, 500 mg, 750 mg
Capsules: 250 mg, 375 mg, 500 mg
Injection: 100 mg/ml, 500 mg/ml

INDICATIONS & DOSAGE
Symptomatic PVCs; life-threatening ventricular tachycardia; ◊ atrial fibrillation and flutter unresponsive to quinidine; ◊ paroxysmal atrial tachycardia
Adults: 50 to 100 mg q 5 minutes by slow I.V. push, no faster than 25 to 50 mg/minute, until arrhythmias disappear, adverse effects develop, or 500 mg has been given. When arrhythmias disappear, give continuous infusion of 1 to 6 mg/minute. Usual effective loading dose is 500 to 600 mg. If arrhythmias recur, repeat bolus as above and increase infusion rate. For I.M. administration, give 50 mg/kg divided q 3 to 6 hours; during surgery, 100 to 500 mg I.M. For oral therapy, initiate dosage at 50 mg/kg P.O. in divided doses q 3 hours until therapeutic levels are reached. Once patient is stable, may substitute sustained-release form q 6 hours or extended-release form at dose of 50 mg/kg in two divided doses q 12 hours.
◊ Loading dose to prevent atrial fibrillation or paroxysmal atrial tachycardia
Adults: 1 to 1.25 g P.O. If arrhythmias persist after 1 hour, give additional 750 mg. If no change occurs, give 500 mg to 1 g q 2 hours until arrhythmias disappear or adverse effects occur.
Loading dose to prevent ventricular tachycardia
Adults: 1 g P.O. Maintenance dosage is 50 mg/kg/day given at 3-hour intervals; average is 250 to 500 mg q 4 hours but may require 1 to 1.5 g q 4 to 6 hours.

◊ *Treatment of malignant hyperthermia*
Adults: 200 to 900 mg I.V. followed by an infusion.

PHARMACODYNAMICS

Antiarrhythmic action: A class IA antiarrhythmic, procainamide depresses phase 0 of the action potential. It's considered a myocardial depressant because it decreases myocardial excitability and conduction velocity and may depress myocardial contractility. It also possesses anticholinergic activity, which may modify its direct myocardial effects. In therapeutic doses, it reduces conduction velocity in the atria, ventricles, and His-Purkinje system. Its effectiveness in controlling atrial tachyarrhythmias stems from its ability to prolong the effective refractory period and increase the action potential duration in the atria, ventricles, and His-Purkinje system. Because prolongation of the effective refractory period exceeds action potential duration, tissue remains refractory even after returning to resting membrane potential (membrane-stabilizing effect).

Drug shortens the effective refractory period of the AV node. Its anticholinergic action also may increase AV node conductivity. Suppression of automaticity in the His-Purkinje system and ectopic pacemakers accounts for drug's effectiveness in treating PVCs. At therapeutic doses, procainamide prolongs the PR and QT intervals. (This effect may be used as an index of drug effectiveness and toxicity.) The QRS complex usually isn't prolonged beyond normal range; the QT interval isn't prolonged to the extent achieved with quinidine.

Drug exerts a peripheral vasodilative effect; with I.V. administration, it may cause hypotension, which limits the administration rate and amount of drug deliverable.

PHARMACOKINETICS

Absorption: Rate and extent of absorption from intestines vary; usually 75% to 95% of an orally administered dose. With administration of tablets and capsules, plasma levels peak in about 1 hour. Extended-release tablets are formulated to provide a sustained and relatively constant rate of release and absorption throughout the small intestine. After drug release, extended wax matrix isn't absorbed and may appear in feces after 15 minutes to 1 hour. With I.M. injection, onset of action is 10 to 30 minutes; levels peak in about 1 hour.
Distribution: Drug is distributed widely in most body tissues, including CSF, liver, spleen, kidneys, lungs, muscles, brain, and heart. Only about 15% binds to plasma proteins. Usual therapeutic range for serum levels is 4 to 8 µg/ml. Some experts suggest a range of 10 to 30 µg/ml for the sum of procainamide and N-acetyl procainamide serum levels is therapeutic.
Metabolism: Drug is acetylated in the liver to form N-acetyl procainamide. Acetylation rate is determined genetically and affects N-acetyl procainamide formation. (N-acetyl procainamide also exerts antiarrhythmic activity.)
Excretion: Drug and N-acetyl procainamide metabolite are excreted in urine. The half-life of the drug is about 2½ to 4¾ hours; the half-life of N-acetyl procainamide is about 6 hours. In patients with heart failure or renal dysfunction, half-life increases; in such patients, dosage reduction is required to avoid toxicity.

CONTRAINDICATIONS & PRECAUTIONS

Contraindicated in patients with hypersensitivity to procaine and related drugs; in those with complete, second- or third-degree heart block in the absence of an artificial pacemaker; and in patients with myasthenia gravis or systemic lupus erythematosus. Also contraindicated in patients with atypical ventricular tachycardia (torsades de pointes) because drug may aggravate this condition.

Use cautiously in patients with ventricular tachycardia during coronary occlusion, heart failure or other conduction disturbances (bundle-branch heart block, sinus bradycardia, cardiac glycoside intoxication), impaired renal or hepatic function, preexisting blood dyscrasia, or bone marrow suppression.

INTERACTIONS

Drug-drug. Use with other *antiarrhythmics* may result in additive or antagonistic cardiac effects and with possible additive toxic effects. Use with *antihypertensives* may cause additive hypotensive effects (most common with I.V. procainamide). Use with *anticholinergics*—including *atropine, diphenhydramine,* and *tricyclic antidepressants*—may cause additive anticholinergic effects. Use with *cimetidine* may result in impaired renal clearance of procainamide and N-acetyl procainamide, with elevated serum drug levels. Use with *cholinergics*—such as *neostigmine* and *pyridostigmine,* which are used to treat myasthenia gravis—may negate the effects of these drugs, requiring increased dosage. Use of procainamide with *neuromuscular blockers*—such as *decamethonium bromide, gallium triethiodide, metocurine iodide, pancuronium bromide, succinylcholine chloride,* and *tubocurarine chloride*—may potentiate the effects of the neuromuscular blockers.

ADVERSE REACTIONS

CNS: hallucinations, confusion, *seizures,* depression, dizziness.
CV: *hypotension, ventricular asystole, bradycardia,* AV block, *ventricular fibrillation* (after parenteral use).
GI: nausea, vomiting, anorexia, diarrhea, bitter taste.
Hematologic: *thrombocytopenia, neutropenia* (especially with sustained-release forms), *agranulocytosis, hemolytic anemia.*
Hepatic: increased bilirubin, LD, alkaline phosphatase, ALT, and AST levels.
Skin: *maculopapular rash, urticaria, pruritus, flushing, angioneurotic edema.*
Other: *fever, lupus-like syndrome* (especially after prolonged administration).

▣ KEY CONSIDERATIONS

• Geriatric patients may require reduced dosage. Because metabolism varies from patient to patient, monitor serum levels.
• Procainamide will invalidate bentiromide test results; discontinue at least 3 days before bentiromide test. Drug may alter edrophonium test results.

• In treating atrial fibrillation and flutter, ventricular rate may accelerate from vagolytic effects on the AV node; to prevent this effect, a cardiac glycoside may be administered before drug therapy begins.
• Monitor patient receiving infusions at all times.
• Infusion pump or microdrip system and timer should be used to monitor infusion precisely.
• Monitor blood pressure and ECG continuously during I.V. administration. Watch for prolonged QT interval and widened QRS complex (50% or greater widening), heart block, or increased arrhythmias. When these ECG signs appear, drug should be discontinued and the patient monitored closely.
• Monitor serum levels of drug: Therapeutic level is 3 to 10 µg/ml (most patients are controlled at 4 to 8 µg/ml); patient may exhibit toxicity at levels greater than 16 µg/ml). Monitor N-acetyl procainamide levels as well; some health care providers believe that procainamide and N-acetyl procainamide levels should be 10 to 30 µg/ml.
• Baseline and periodic determinations of antinuclear antibody titers, lupus erythematosus cell preparations, and CBC may be indicated because drug therapy (usually long-term) has been associated with syndrome resembling systemic lupus erythematosus.
• For initial oral therapy, use conventional capsules and tablets; use extended-release tablets only for maintenance therapy.
• I.V. drug form is more likely to cause adverse cardiac effects, possibly resulting in severe hypotension.
• In prolonged use of oral form, perform ECGs occasionally to determine continued need for drug.
• Drug may cause positive antinuclear antibody titers, positive direct antiglobulin (Coombs') tests.

Overdose & treatment

• Signs and symptoms of overdose include severe hypotension, widening QRS complex, junctional tachycardia, intraventricular conduction delay, ven-

tricular fibrillation, oliguria, confusion and lethargy, and nausea and vomiting.
• Treatment involves general supportive measures (including respiratory and CV support) with hemodynamic and ECG monitoring. After recent ingestion of oral form, gastric lavage, induced vomiting, and activated charcoal may be used to decrease absorption. Phenylephrine or norepinephrine may be used to treat hypotension after ensuring adequate hydration. Hemodialysis may be effective in removing drug and N-acetyl procainamide. A 1/6 M solution of sodium lactate may reduce the cardiotoxic effect of the drug.

prochlorperazine
Compazine, Stemetil*

prochlorperazine edisylate
Compazine

prochlorperazine maleate
Compazine, Compazine Spansule, Stemetil*

Phenothiazine (piperazine derivative), antipsychotic, antiemetic, anxiolytic

Available by prescription only
prochlorperazine edisylate
Spansules (sustained-release): 10 mg, 15 mg, 30 mg
Syrup: 1 mg/ml
Injection: 5 mg/ml
Suppositories: 2.5 mg, 5 mg, 25 mg
prochlorperazine maleate
Tablets: 5 mg, 10 mg, 25 mg

INDICATIONS & DOSAGE
Preoperative nausea control
Adults: 5 to 10 mg I.M. 1 to 2 hours before induction of anesthesia, repeat once in 30 minutes if necessary; or 5 to 10 mg I.V. 15 to 30 minutes before induction of anesthesia, repeat once if necessary; or 20 mg/L D₅W and normal saline solution by I.V. infusion, added to infusion 15 to 30 minutes before induction. Maximum parenteral dosage is 40 mg daily.

Severe nausea, vomiting
Adults: 5 to 10 mg P.O. t.i.d. or q.i.d.; or 15 mg of sustained-release form P.O. on arising; or 10 mg of sustained-release form P.O. q 12 hours; or 25 mg P.R. b.i.d.; or 5 to 10 mg I.M. injected deeply into outer upper quadrant of gluteal region. Repeat q 3 to 4 hours, p.r.n. May be given I.V. Maximum parenteral dosage, 40 mg daily.
Adults: 5 mg P.O. t.i.d. or q.i.d.
Psychotic disorders
Adults: 5 to 10 mg P.O. or 10 to 20 mg I.M. t.i.d. or q.i.d.; up to 150 mg daily P.O. for hospitalized patients.

PHARMACODYNAMICS
Antipsychotic action: Prochlorperazine is thought to exert its effects via postsynaptic blockade of CNS dopamine receptors, thus inhibiting dopamine-mediated effects.
Antiemetic action: Antiemetic effects are attributed to dopamine receptor blockade in the medullary chemoreceptor trigger zone.

Drug has many other central and peripheral effects. It produces alpha and ganglionic blockade and counteracts histamine- and serotonin-mediated activity. Its most prevalent adverse reactions are extrapyramidal. It's used primarily as an antiemetic; it's ineffective against motion sickness.

PHARMACOKINETICS
Absorption: Rate and extent of absorption vary with administration route: oral tablet absorption is erratic and variable, with onset of action from ½ to 1 hour; oral concentrate absorption is more predictable. I.M. prochlorperazine is absorbed rapidly.
Distribution: Drug is distributed widely into the body; 91% to 99% protein-bound. Effect peaks at 2 to 4 hours; steady-state serum levels, within 4 to 7 days.
Metabolism: Drug is metabolized extensively by the liver, but no active metabolites are formed; duration of action is about 3 to 4 hours and 10 to 12 hours for the extended-release form.

Excretion: Drug is mostly excreted in urine by the kidneys; some is excreted in feces from the biliary tract.

CONTRAINDICATIONS & PRECAUTIONS
Contraindicated in patients hypersensitive to phenothiazines; in those with CNS depression, including coma; and when using spinal or epidural anesthetic, adrenergic blockers, or ethanol.

Use cautiously in patients with impaired CV function, glaucoma, seizure disorders; and in those who have been exposed to extreme heat.

INTERACTIONS
Drug-drug. Pharmacokinetic alterations and subsequent decreased therapeutic response to prochlorperazine may follow use with *aluminum-* or *magnesium-containing antacids* or *antidiarrheals* (decreased absorption) or *phenobarbital* (enhanced renal excretion). Use with *appetite suppressants* or *sympathomimetics*—including *ephedrine* (found in many nasal sprays), *epinephrine, phenylephrine,* and *phenylpropanolamine*—may decrease their stimulatory and pressor effects and may cause epinephrine reversal (hypotensive response to epinephrine). *Beta blockers* may inhibit prochlorperazine metabolism, increasing plasma levels and toxicity. Drug may antagonize therapeutic effect of *bromocriptine* on prolactin secretion; it also may decrease the vasoconstrictive effects of *high-dose dopamine* and may decrease effectiveness and increase toxicity of *levodopa* (by dopamine blockade). Drug may inhibit blood pressure response to *centrally acting antihypertensives,* such as *clonidine, guanabenz, guanadrel, guanethidine, methyldopa,* and *reserpine.* Use with *lithium* may result in severe neurological toxicity with an encephalitis-like syndrome and in decreased therapeutic response to prochlorperazine. Prochlorperazine may inhibit metabolism and increase toxicity of *phenytoin.* Use with *propylthiouracil* increases risk of agranulocytosis.

Additive effects are likely after use of prochlorperazine with *antiarrhythmics, disopyramide, procainamide,* and *quinidine* (increased incidence of arrhythmias

and conduction defects); *CNS depressants,* including *anesthetics (epidural, general, or spinal), barbiturates, narcotics,* and *tranquilizers*—or *parenteral magnesium sulfate* (oversedation, respiratory depression, and hypotension); *atropine* and other *anticholinergics,* including *antidepressants, antihistamines, antiparkinsonians, MAO inhibitors, meperidine,* and *phenothiazines* (oversedation, paralytic ileus, visual changes, and severe constipation); *metrizamide* (increased risk of seizures); or *nitrates* (hypotension).

Drug-lifestyle. *Alcohol* causes additive CNS depressant effects. Pharmacokinetic alterations and subsequent decreased therapeutic response to drug may follow use with *caffeine* or *heavy smoking* (increased metabolism).

ADVERSE REACTIONS
CNS: *extrapyramidal reactions,* sedation, pseudoparkinsonism, EEG changes, dizziness.
CV: *orthostatic hypotension,* tachycardia, quinidine-like ECG changes.
EENT: *ocular changes, blurred vision.*
GI: *dry mouth, constipation,* ileus, increased appetite.
GU: *urine retention,* gynecomastia, dark urine, inhibited ejaculation.
Hematologic: *transient leukopenia,* **agranulocytosis, thrombocytopenia, hemolytic anemia.**
Hepatic: *cholestatic jaundice, elevated liver enzyme levels.*
Metabolic: hyperglycemia, hypoglycemia, weight gain.
Skin: mild photosensitivity, allergic reactions, exfoliative dermatitis.
Other: elevated protein-bound iodine test results.

▣ KEY CONSIDERATIONS
Besides the recommendations relevant to all phenothiazines, consider the following:
• Geriatric patients tend to require lower doses, individualized to the patient. These patients are at greater risk for adverse reactions, especially tardive dyskinesia, other extrapyramidal effects, and hypotension.

- Liquid and injectable formulations may cause a rash after contact with skin.
- Prochlorperazine may cause a pink to brown discoloration of urine.
- Drug is associated with a high incidence of extrapyramidal effects and, in institutionalized psychiatric patients, photosensitivity reactions; patient should avoid exposure to sunlight and heat lamps.
- Oral formulations may cause stomach upset. Administer with food or fluid.
- Dilute the concentrate in 2 to 4 oz (60 to 120 ml) water. The suppository form should be stored in a cool place.
- Give I.V. dose slowly (5 mg/minute). I.M. injection may cause skin necrosis; take care to prevent extravasation. Don't mix with other medications in the syringe. Don't administer S.C.
- Administer I.M. injection deep into the outer upper quadrant of the buttock. Massaging the area after administration may prevent formation of abscesses.
- Solution for injection may be slightly discolored. Don't use if excessively discolored or if a precipitate is evident. Contact pharmacist.
- Monitor patient's blood pressure before and after parenteral administration.
- Drug is ineffective in treating motion sickness.
- Chewing gum, hard candy, or ice may help relieve dry mouth.
- Protect the liquid formulation from light.
- Prochlorperazine causes false-positive test results for urine porphyrins, urobilinogen, 5-hydroxyindoleacetic acid, and amylase because metabolites darken the urine.

Patient education
- Explain risks for dystonic reactions and tardive dyskinesia. Tell patient to report abnormal body movements promptly.
- Tell patient to avoid sun exposure and to wear sunscreen when going outdoors to prevent photosensitivity reactions. (Note that heat lamps and tanning beds also may burn or discolor the skin.)
- Tell patient to avoid spilling the liquid form. Contact with skin may cause rash and irritation.

- Warn patient to avoid extremely hot or cold baths and exposure to temperature extremes, sunlamps, or tanning beds; prochlorperazine may cause thermoregulatory changes.
- Advise patient to take drug exactly as prescribed, not to double-dose after missing dose, and not to share drug with others.
- Warn patient to avoid alcohol and not take other drugs that may cause excessive sedation.
- Tell patient to dilute the concentrate in water; explain the dropper technique of measuring dose; teach correct use of suppository.
- Tell patient that hard candy, chewing gum, or ice chips can alleviate dry mouth.
- Urge patient to store drug safely away from children.
- Inform patient that drug interacts with many other drugs. Warn him to seek medical approval before taking self-medicating.
- Warn patient not to stop taking drug suddenly and to promptly report difficulty urinating, sore throat, dizziness, or fainting. Reassure patient that most reactions can be relieved by reducing dose.
- Caution patient to avoid hazardous activities that require alertness until the effect of the drug is established. Reassure patient that sedative effects subside and become tolerable in several weeks.

Overdose & treatment
- CNS depression is characterized by deep sleep (in which the patient can't be aroused) and possible coma, hypotension or hypertension, extrapyramidal symptoms, dystonia, abnormal involuntary muscle movements, agitation, seizures, arrhythmias, ECG changes, hypothermia or hyperthermia, and autonomic nervous system dysfunction.
- Treatment is symptomatic and supportive and includes maintaining vital signs, airway, stable body temperature, and fluid and electrolyte balance.
- Don't induce vomiting: Prochlorperazine inhibits cough reflex, and aspiration may occur. Perform gastric lavage, then administer activated charcoal and sodium chloride cathartics; dialysis

---

Reactions may be *common*, uncommon, *life-threatening*, or COMMON AND LIFE-THREATENING.

doesn't help. Regulate body temperature as needed. Treat hypotension with I.V. fluids: Don't give epinephrine. Treat seizures with parenteral diazepam or barbiturates, arrhythmias with 1 mg/kg of parenteral phenytoin (with rate titrated to blood pressure), and extrapyramidal reactions with 2 mg/kg/minute of benztropine or parenteral diphenhydramine.

promethazine hydrochloride
Anergan 25, Anergan 50, Histantil*, Pentazine, Phencen-50, Phenergan, Phenergan Fortis, Phenergan Plain, Phenoject-50, Promet, Prorex-25, Prorex-50, Prothazine, Prothazine Plain, V-Gan-25, V-Gan-50

Phenothiazine derivative, antiemetic, antivertigo drug, antihistamine (H_1-receptor antagonist), preoperative or postoperative sedative, adjunct to analgesics

Available by prescription only
Tablets: 12.5 mg, 25 mg, 50 mg
Syrup: 6.25 mg/5 ml, 10 mg/5 ml, 25 mg/5 ml
Suppositories: 12.5 mg, 25 mg, 50 mg
Injection: 25 mg/ml, 50 mg/ml

INDICATIONS & DOSAGE
Motion sickness
Adults: 25 mg P.O. b.i.d.
Nausea
Adults: 12.5 to 25 mg P.O., I.M., or P.R. q 4 to 6 hours, p.r.n.
Rhinitis, allergy symptoms
Adults: 12.5 to 25 mg P.O. before meals and h.s., or 25 mg P.O. h.s.
Sedation
Adults: 25 to 50 mg P.O. or I.M. h.s. or p.r.n.
Routine preoperative or postoperative sedation or as an adjunct to analgesics
Adults: 25 to 50 mg I.M., I.V., or P.O.

PHARMACODYNAMICS
Antiemetic and antivertigo actions: The central antimuscarinic actions of antihistamines probably are responsible for their antivertigo and antiemetic effects; promethazine also is believed to inhibit the medullary chemoreceptor trigger zone.
Antihistamine action: Drug competes with histamine for the H_1-receptor, thereby suppressing allergic rhinitis and urticaria; drug doesn't prevent histamine release.
Sedative action: CNS depressant mechanism of drug is unknown; phenothiazines probably cause sedation by reducing stimuli to the brain-stem reticular system.

PHARMACOKINETICS
Absorption: Promethazine is well absorbed from the GI tract. Onset begins 20 minutes after P.O., P.R., or I.M. administration and within 3 to 5 minutes after I.V. administration. Effects usually last 4 to 6 hours but may persist for 12 hours.
Distribution: Drug is distributed widely throughout the body.
Metabolism: Drug is metabolized in the liver.
Excretion: Metabolites are excreted in urine and feces.

CONTRAINDICATIONS & PRECAUTIONS
Contraindicated in patients with hypersensitivity to promethazine; in those with intestinal obstruction, prostatic hyperplasia, bladder neck obstruction, seizure disorders, coma, CNS depression, and stenosing peptic ulcerations.
    Use cautiously in patients with asthma or cardiac, pulmonary, or hepatic disease.

INTERACTIONS
Drug-drug. Additive CNS depression may occur when promethazine is given with *CNS depressants,* such as *anxiolytics, barbiturates, sleeping aids,* and *tranquilizers* or *other antihistamines.* Don't give promethazine with *epinephrine* because it may result in partial adrenergic blockade, producing further hypotension, or with *MAO inhibitors,* which interfere with the detoxification of antihistamines and phenothiazines and thus prolong and intensify their sedative and anticholinergic effects. Promethazine may block the antiparkinsonian action of *levodopa.*

Drug-lifestyle. *Alcohol* causes additive CNS depressant effects.

ADVERSE REACTIONS

CNS: *sedation,* confusion, sleepiness, dizziness, disorientation, extrapyramidal symptoms, *drowsiness.*
CV: hypotension, hypertension.
EENT: blurred vision.
GI: nausea, vomiting, *dry mouth.*
GU: urine retention.
Hematologic: leukopenia, *agranulocytosis, thrombocytopenia.*
Skin: photosensitivity, rash.

▣ KEY CONSIDERATIONS

Besides the recommendations relevant to all phenothiazines, consider the following:
● Geriatric patients are usually more sensitive to adverse effects of antihistamines and are especially likely to experience a greater degree of dizziness, sedation, hyperexcitability, dry mouth, and urine retention than younger patients. Symptoms usually respond to a decrease in dosage.
● Pronounced sedative effects may limit use in some ambulatory patients.
● The 50-mg/ml concentration is for I.M. use only; inject deep into large muscle mass. Don't administer drug S.C.; this may cause chemical irritation and necrosis. Drug may be administered I.V. in concentrations not to exceed 25 mg/ml and at a rate not to exceed 25 mg/minute; when using I.V. drip, wrap in aluminum foil to protect drug from light.
● Promethazine and meperidine (Demerol) may be mixed in the same syringe.
● Discontinue drug 4 days before diagnostic skin tests to avoid preventing, reducing, or masking test response.

Patient education

● Warn patient about possible photosensitivity and ways to avoid it.
● When treating motion sickness, tell patient to take first dose 30 to 60 minutes before travel; on succeeding days, he should take dose on arising and with evening meal.
● Advise patient to limit alcohol use during drug therapy.

Overdose & treatment

● Signs and symptoms of overdose may include those of CNS depression—including sedation, reduced mental alertness, apnea, and CV collapse—or CNS stimulation—including insomnia, hallucinations, tremors, or seizures. Atropine-like signs and symptoms—such as dry mouth, flushed skin, fixed and dilated pupils, and GI symptoms—are common.
● Perform gastric lavage; don't induce vomiting. Treat hypotension with vasopressors, and control seizures with diazepam or phenytoin; correct acidosis and electrolyte imbalance. Urinary acidification promotes excretion of drug. Don't give stimulants.

propafenone hydrochloride
Rythmol

Sodium channel antagonist, antiarrhythmic

Available by prescription only
Tablets: 150 mg, 225 mg, 300 mg

INDICATIONS & DOSAGE
Suppression of documented life-threatening ventricular arrhythmias
Adults: Initially, 150 mg P.O. q 8 hours. Dosage may be increased to 225 mg q 8 hours after 3 or 4 days; if necessary, increase dosage to 300 mg q 8 hours. Maximum daily dosage, 900 mg.
✦ *Dosage adjustment.* For patients with hepatic failure, reduce usual dosage by 20% to 30%.

PHARMACODYNAMICS
Antiarrhythmic action: Propafenone reduces the inward sodium current in myocardial cells and Purkinje fibers; it also has weak beta blocking effects. It slows the upstroke velocity of the action potential (phase 0 depolarization) and slows conduction in the AV node, His-Purkinje system, and intraventricular conduction system and prolongs the refractory period in the AV node.

PHARMACOKINETICS
Absorption: Propafenone is well absorbed from the GI tract; food doesn't

affect absorption. Because of a significant first-pass effect, bioavailability is limited; however, it increases with dosage. Absolute bioavailability is 3.4% with the 150-mg tablet and 10.6% with the 300-mg tablet.

Distribution: Plasma levels peak about 3.5 hours after administration.

Metabolism: Drug is metabolized in the liver, with a significant first-pass effect. Two active metabolites have been identified: 5-hydroxypropafenone and N-depropylpropafenone. Some patients (10% of all patients and all patients receiving quinidine) metabolize drug more slowly. Little (if any) 5-hydroxypropafenone is present in the plasma.

Excretion: Elimination half-life is 2 to 10 hours in patients with normal metabolism (about 90% of patients); it can be as long as 10 to 32 hours in patients with slow metabolism.

CONTRAINDICATIONS & PRECAUTIONS

Contraindicated in patients with hypersensitivity to propafenone and in those with severe or uncontrolled heart failure; cardiogenic shock; SA, AV, or intraventricular disorders of impulse conduction in the absence of a pacemaker; bradycardia; marked hypotension; bronchospastic disorders; and electrolyte imbalance.

Use cautiously in patients with renal or hepatic failure or heart failure, and in those receiving other cardiac depressant drugs.

INTERACTIONS

Drug-drug. Propafenone may increase plasma levels of some *beta blockers,* including *metoprolol* and *propranolol,* and of *warfarin,* resulting in increased INR; monitor appropriately. *Cimetidine* may increase plasma propafenone levels, so monitor patient closely. Drug causes a dose-related increase in plasma *digoxin* levels, ranging from 35% at 450 mg/day to 85% at 900 mg/day; monitor plasma digoxin levels closely and adjust dosage of digoxin as necessary. Use of *local anesthetics* may increase the risk for CNS toxicity. Use of *quinidine* competitively inhibits one of the metabolic pathways for propafenone, thereby increasing its half-life, and isn't recommended.

ADVERSE REACTIONS

CNS: anxiety, ataxia, *dizziness,* drowsiness, fatigue, headache, insomnia, syncope, tremor.

CV: atrial fibrillation, bradycardia, bundle-branch block, angina, chest pain, edema, first-degree AV block, hypotension, increased QRS duration, intraventricular conduction delay, palpitations, ***heart failure, proarrhythmic events (ventricular tachycardia, PVCs, ventricular fibrillation).***

EENT: blurred vision.

GI: abdominal pain or cramps, constipation, diarrhea, dyspepsia, anorexia, flatulence, *nausea, vomiting,* dry mouth, unusual taste.

Musculoskeletal: joint pain.

Respiratory: dyspnea.

Skin: rash.

Other: diaphoresis.

▣ KEY CONSIDERATIONS

• In geriatric patients and patients with substantial heart disease, increase dosage more gradually during the initial phase of treatment.

• Propafenone pharmacokinetics are complex; a threefold increase in daily dosage (from 300 to 900 mg/day) may produce a tenfold increase in plasma levels. Dosage must be individualized.

Patient education

• Instruct patient to report signs and symptoms of infection, such as sore throat, chills, or fever.

Overdose & treatment

• Signs and symptoms usually develop within 3 hours of ingestion. They include hypotension, somnolence, bradycardia, conduction disturbances, ventricular arrhythmias, and seizures.

• Provide supportive treatment and assist respirations as necessary. Rhythm and blood pressure may be controlled with dopamine and isoproterenol; seizures may respond to I.V. diazepam.

propantheline bromide
Pro-Banthine, Propanthel*

Anticholinergic, antimuscarinic, GI antispasmodic

Available by prescription only
Tablets: 7.5 mg, 15 mg

INDICATIONS & DOSAGE
Adjunctive treatment of peptic ulcer, irritable bowel syndrome, and other GI disorders; to reduce duodenal motility during diagnostic radiologic procedures
Adults: 15 mg P.O. t.i.d. before meals and 30 mg h.s.; up to 60 mg q.i.d.
Geriatric patients: 7.5 mg P.O. t.i.d. before meals.

PHARMACODYNAMICS
Anticholinergic action: Propantheline competitively blocks the actions of acetylcholine at cholinergic neuroeffector sites, decreasing GI motility and inhibiting gastric acid secretion.

PHARMACOKINETICS
Absorption: Only 10% to 25% of propantheline is absorbed (absorption varies among patients).
Distribution: Drug doesn't cross the blood-brain barrier; little else is known about its distribution.
Metabolism: Drug appears to undergo considerable metabolism in the upper small intestine and liver.
Excretion: Absorbed drug is excreted in urine as metabolites and unchanged drug.

CONTRAINDICATIONS & PRECAUTIONS
Contraindicated in patients with angle-closure glaucoma, obstructive uropathy, obstructive disease of the GI tract, severe ulcerative colitis, myasthenia gravis, hypersensitivity to anticholinergics, paralytic ileus, intestinal atony, unstable CV status in acute hemorrhage, or toxic megacolon.

Use cautiously in patients with impaired renal or hepatic function, autonomic neuropathy, hyperthyroidism, coronary artery disease, arrhythmias, heart failure, hypertension, hiatal hernia associated with gastric reflux, or ulcerative colitis and in those living in a hot or humid environment.

INTERACTIONS
Drug-drug. Administration of *antacids* decreases oral absorption of anticholinergics; administer propantheline at least 1 hour before antacids. *Anticholinergics* decrease GI absorption of many drugs, such as *ketoconazole* and *levodopa;* conversely, use with *digoxin* may yield higher serum digoxin levels. Propantheline may increase *atenolol* absorption, thereby enhancing the effects of atenolol. Administration of *drugs with anticholinergic effects* may cause additive toxicity. Use cautiously with *oral potassium supplements* (especially *wax-matrix formulations*) because they may increase the risk of potassium-induced GI ulcerations.

ADVERSE REACTIONS
CNS: headache, insomnia, drowsiness, dizziness, *confusion or excitement in geriatric patients,* nervousness, weakness.
CV: *palpitations,* tachycardia.
EENT: *blurred vision,* mydriasis, increased intraocular pressure, cycloplegia, drying of salivary secretions.
GI: *dry mouth,* constipation, loss of taste, nausea, vomiting, paralytic ileus, bloated feeling.
GU: *urinary hesitancy, urine retention,* impotence.
Skin: urticaria, decreased sweating or possible anhidrosis, other dermal manifestations.
Other: allergic reactions *(anaphylaxis).*

🔲 KEY CONSIDERATIONS
Besides the recommendations relevant to all anticholinergics, consider the following:
• Administer propantheline cautiously to geriatric patients. Lower doses are recommended because of increased risk for adverse effects in this population.
• Drug may be used with H_2 receptor to treat Zollinger-Ellison syndrome as an unlabeled use.
• Adjust dosage until therapeutic effect is obtained or adverse effects become intolerable.

Reactions may be *common,* uncommon, *life-threatening,* or COMMON AND LIFE-THREATENING.

Patient education
• Instruct patient to swallow tablets whole rather than chewing or crushing them.

Overdose & treatment
• Signs and symptoms of overdose include curare-like symptoms and such peripheral effects as headache; dilated, nonreactive pupils; blurred vision; flushed, hot, dry skin; dryness of mucous membranes; dysphagia; decreased or absent bowel sounds; urine retention; hyperthermia; tachycardia; hypertension; and increased respirations.
• Treatment is primarily symptomatic and supportive, as needed. If the patient is alert, induce vomiting (or perform gastric lavage) and follow with a sodium chloride cathartic and activated charcoal to prevent further drug absorption. In severe cases, physostigmine may be administered to block the antimuscarinic effects of the drug. Give fluids, as needed, to treat shock. If urine retention develops, catheterization may be necessary.

propoxyphene hydrochloride
Darvon, Dolene

propoxyphene napsylate
Darvon-N

Opioid, analgesic
Controlled substance schedule IV

Available by prescription only
propoxyphene hydrochloride
Tablets: 65 mg
Capsules: 65 mg
propoxyphene napsylate
Tablets: 50 mg, 100 mg
Capsules: 50 mg, 100 mg
Suspension: 50 mg/5 ml

INDICATIONS & DOSAGE
Mild to moderate pain
Adults: 65 mg (hydrochloride) P.O. q 4 hours, p.r.n., or 100 mg (napsylate) P.O. q 4 hours, p.r.n.

PHARMACODYNAMICS
Analgesic action: Propoxyphene exerts its analgesic effect via opiate agonist activity and alters the patient's response to painful stimuli, particularly mild to moderate pain.

PHARMACOKINETICS
Absorption: After oral administration, propoxyphene is absorbed primarily in the upper small intestine. Equimolar doses of the hydrochloride and napsylate salts provide similar plasma levels. Onset of analgesia occurs in 20 to 60 minutes, and analgesic effects peak at 2 to 2½ hours.
Distribution: Drug enters the CSF.
Metabolism: Drug is degraded mainly in the liver; about one-quarter of a dose is metabolized to norpropoxyphene, an active metabolite.
Excretion: Drug is excreted in the urine. Duration of effect is 4 to 6 hours.

CONTRAINDICATIONS & PRECAUTIONS
Contraindicated in patients with hypersensitivity to propoxyphene. Use cautiously in patients with impaired renal or hepatic function, emotional instability, or history of drug or alcohol abuse.

INTERACTIONS
Drug-drug. Patients who become physically dependent on drug may experience acute withdrawal syndrome when given a single dose of an *antagonist;* use with caution and monitor closely.

Propoxyphene may inhibit the metabolism of *antidepressants,* such as *doxepin,* necessitating a lower dose of antidepressant. Use with *carbamazepine* increases the effects of carbamazepine; monitor serum carbamazepine levels. Use with *cimetidine* may enhance respiratory and CNS depression, resulting in confusion, disorientation, apnea, or seizures. Reduced doses of propoxyphene are usually needed when given with other *CNS depressants*—such as *antidepressants, antihistamines, barbiturates, benzodiazepines, general anesthetics, muscle relaxants, opioid analgesics, phenothiazines,* and *sedative-hypnotics*—to avoid potentiation of adverse effects (respiratory depression, sedation, hypotension). Use propoxyphene with caution with *drugs that are highly metabolized in the liver*—including *digitoxin, phenytoin,* and *rifampin*—because accumulation of either drug may occur; withdrawal symptoms may result if used together. Severe CV depression may result from use with *general anesthetics.*

Drug-lifestyle. *Alcohol* may intensify respiratory and CNS depressant effects.

ADVERSE REACTIONS

CNS: *dizziness, sedation,* headache, euphoria, light-headedness, weakness, hallucinations.

GI: *nausea, vomiting,* constipation, abdominal pain.

GU: false decrease in test for urine steroid excretion.

Hepatic: abnormal liver function test results.

Respiratory: *respiratory depression.*

Other: psychological and physical dependence.

▣ KEY CONSIDERATIONS

Besides the recommendations relevant to all opioids, consider the following:

• Lower doses are usually indicated for geriatric patients because they may be more sensitive to the therapeutic and adverse effects of propoxyphene.

• Drug may obscure the signs and symptoms of an acute abdominal condition or worsen gallbladder pain.

• Don't prescribe drug for maintenance purposes in narcotic addiction.

• Drug can be considered a mild narcotic analgesic, but pain relief is equivalent to aspirin.

Patient education

• Warn patient not to exceed recommended dosage.

• Tell patient to avoid use of alcohol because it will cause additive CNS depressant effects.

• Warn patient of additive depressant effect that can occur if propoxyphene is prescribed for medical conditions requiring use of sedatives, tranquilizers, muscle relaxants, antidepressants, or other CNS-depressants.

• Tell patient to take drug with food if GI upset occurs.

Overdose & treatment

• The most common signs and symptoms of overdose are CNS depression, respiratory depression, and miosis (pinpoint pupils). Others include hypotension, bradycardia, hypothermia, shock, apnea, cardiopulmonary arrest, circulatory collapse, pulmonary edema, and seizures.

• Propoxyphene is known to cause ECG changes (prolonged QRS complex) and nephrogenic diabetes insipidus with acute toxic doses. Death from acute overdose is most likely to occur within the 1st hour. Signs and symptoms of overdose with propoxyphene combination products include salicylism from aspirin and acetaminophen toxicity.

• To treat acute overdose, first establish adequate respiratory exchange via a patent airway and ventilation as needed; administer a narcotic antagonist (naloxone) to reverse respiratory depression. (Because the duration of action of drug is longer than naloxone, repeated dosing is necessary.) Don't give naloxone unless the patient has significant respiratory or CV depression. Monitor vital signs closely.

• If patient presents within 2 hours of ingestion of an oral overdose, immediately induce vomiting with ipecac syrup or perform gastric lavage. Use caution to avoid risk of aspiration. Administer activated charcoal via NG tube to further remove drug.

• Provide symptomatic and supportive treatment (continued respiratory support, correction of fluid or electrolyte imbalance). Anticonvulsants may be needed; monitor laboratory parameters, vital signs, and neurologic status closely. Dialysis may be helpful in the treatment of overdose with propoxyphene combination products containing aspirin or acetaminophen.

propranolol hydrochloride
Inderal, Inderal LA

Beta blocker, antihypertensive, antianginal, antiarrhythmic, adjunctive therapy for migraine, adjunctive therapy of MI

Available by prescription only
Tablets: 10 mg, 20 mg, 40 mg, 60 mg, 80 mg, 90 mg
Capsules (extended-release): 60 mg, 80 mg, 120 mg, 160 mg
Injection: 1 mg/ml
Solution: 4 mg/ml, 8 mg/ml, 20 mg/5 ml, 40 mg/5 ml, 80 mg/ml (concentrated)

INDICATIONS & DOSAGE
Hypertension
Adults: Initially, 80 mg P.O. daily in two to four divided doses or sustained-release form once daily. Increase at 3- to 7-day intervals to maximum daily dosage of 640 mg. Usual maintenance dosage is 160 to 480 mg daily.
Management of angina pectoris
Adults: 10 to 20 mg t.i.d. or q.i.d., or one 80-mg sustained-release capsule daily. Dosage may be increased at 7- to 10-day intervals. Average optimum dosage is 160 to 240 mg daily.
Supraventricular, ventricular, and atrial arrhythmias; tachyarrhythmias caused by excessive catecholamine action during anesthesia, hyperthyroidism, and pheochromocytoma
Adults: 1 to 3 mg I.V. diluted in 50 ml D_5W or normal saline solution infused slowly, not to exceed 1 mg/minute. After 3 mg have been infused, another dose may be given in 2 minutes; subsequent doses no sooner than q 4 hours. Usual maintenance dosage is 10 to 30 mg P.O. t.i.d. or q.i.d.
Prevention of frequent, severe, uncontrollable, or disabling migraine or vascular headache
Adults: initially, 80 mg daily in divided doses or one sustained-release capsule once daily. Usual maintenance dosage is 160 to 240 mg daily, divided t.i.d. or q.i.d.

To reduce mortality after an MI
Adults: 180 to 240 mg P.O. daily in divided doses. Usually administered in three or four doses daily, beginning 5 to 21 days after infarct.
Hypertrophic subaortic stenosis
Adults: 10 to 20 mg P.O. t.i.d. or q.i.d. before meals and h.s.
Preoperative pheochromocytoma
Adults: 60 mg P.O. daily.
◇ *Adjunctive treatment for anxiety*
Adults: 10 to 80 mg P.O. 1 hour before anxiety-provoking activity.
◇ *Treatment of essential, familial, or senile movement tremors*
Adults: 40 mg P.O. b.i.d., as tolerated and needed.

PHARMACODYNAMICS
Antihypertensive action: Exact mechanism of action is unknown; drug may reduce blood pressure by blocking adrenergic receptors (thus decreasing cardiac output), by decreasing sympathetic outflow from the CNS, and by suppressing renin release.
Antianginal action: Drug decreases myocardial oxygen consumption by blocking catecholamine access to beta receptors, thus relieving angina.
Antiarrhythmic action: Drug decreases heart rate and prevents exercise-induced increases in heart rate. It also decreases myocardial contractility, cardiac output, and SA and AV nodal conduction velocity.
Migraine prophylactic action: Effect is thought to result from inhibition of vasodilation.
MI prophylactic action: Exact mechanism by which drug decreases mortality after an MI is unknown.

PHARMACOKINETICS
Absorption: Propranolol is absorbed almost completely from the GI tract. Absorption is enhanced when given with food. Plasma levels peak 60 to 90 minutes after administration of regular-release tablets. After I.V. administration, levels peak in about 1 minute, with virtually immediate onset of action.
Distribution: Drug is distributed widely throughout the body; more than 90% protein-bound.

Metabolism: Hepatic metabolism is almost total; oral form undergoes extensive first-pass metabolism.

Excretion: About 96% to 99% of a given dose is excreted in urine as metabolites; remainder is excreted in feces as unchanged drug and metabolites. Biological half-life is about 4 hours.

CONTRAINDICATIONS & PRECAUTIONS

Contraindicated in patients with bronchial asthma, sinus bradycardia and heart block greater than first-degree, cardiogenic shock, and heart failure (unless failure is secondary to a tachyarrhythmia that can be treated with propranolol).

Use cautiously in geriatric patients; in those with impaired renal or hepatic function, nonallergic bronchospastic disease, diabetes mellitus, or thyrotoxicosis; and in those receiving other antihypertensives.

INTERACTIONS

Drug-drug. *Aluminum hydroxide ant-acid* decreases GI absorption; *ethanol* slows the rate of absorption. Use with *antidiabetics* or *insulin* can alter dosage requirements in patients with previously stable diabetes. Propranolol may potentiate antihypertensive effects of other *antihypertensives,* especially *catecholamine-depleting drugs* such as *reserpine. Atropine,* other *drugs with anticholinergic effects,* and *tricyclic antidepressants* may antagonize propranolol-induced bradycardia; *NSAIDs* may antagonize its hypotensive effects. Use with *calcium channel blockers,* especially *I.V. verapamil,* may depress myocardial contractility or AV conduction (on rare occasions, the I.V. use of a beta blocker and verapamil has resulted in serious adverse reactions, especially in patients with severe cardiomyopathy, heart failure, or recent MI). *Cimetidine* may decrease clearance of propranolol by inhibiting hepatic metabolism and thus also enhancing its beta-blocking effects. *Phenytoin* and *rifampin* accelerate clearance of propranolol. Propranolol may antagonize beta stimulating effects of *sympathomimetics* such as *isoproterenol* and of *MAO inhibitors;* use with *epinephrine*

causes severe vasoconstriction. High doses of propranolol may potentiate neuromuscular blocking effect of *tubocurarine* and related compounds.

ADVERSE REACTIONS

CNS: *fatigue, lethargy,* vivid dreams, hallucinations, mental depression, lightheadedness, insomnia.

CV: *bradycardia, hypotension,* **heart failure,** intermittent claudication, intensification of AV block.

GI: nausea, vomiting, diarrhea, abdominal cramping.

GU: elevated BUN levels in patients with severe heart disease.

Hepatic: elevated serum transaminase, alkaline phosphatase, and LD levels.

Respiratory: *bronchospasm.*

Skin: rash.

Other: fever, *agranulocytosis.*

🔲 KEY CONSIDERATIONS

Besides the recommendations relevant to all beta blockers, consider the following:
● Geriatric patients may require lower maintenance doses of propranolol because of increased bioavailability or delayed metabolism; they also may experience enhanced adverse effects.
● Drug also has been used to treat aggression and rage, stage fright, recurrent GI bleeding in cirrhotic patients, and menopausal symptoms.
● Never administer drug as an adjunct in treatment of pheochromocytoma unless patient has been pretreated with alpha-adrenergic blockers.
● Drug may mask signs of hypoglycemia.

Patient education

● Warn patient not to abruptly stop taking propranolol.
● Instruct patient on proper use, dosage, and potential adverse effects of drug.
● Tell patient to call before taking OTC drugs that may interact with propranolol, such as nasal decongestants or cold preparations.

Overdose & treatment

● Signs and symptoms of overdose include severe hypotension, bradycardia, heart failure, and bronchospasm.

Reactions may be *common,* uncommon, **life-threatening,** or COMMON AND LIFE-THREATENING.

• After acute ingestion, induce vomiting or perform gastric lavage; follow with activated charcoal to reduce absorption, and administer symptomatic and supportive care. Treat bradycardia with atropine (0.25 to 1 mg); if no response, administer isoproterenol cautiously. Treat cardiac failure with cardiac glycosides and diuretics and hypotension with glucagon and/or vasopressors: epinephrine is preferred. Treat bronchospasm with isoproterenol and aminophylline.

---

propylthiouracil (PTU)
Propyl-Thyracil*

Thyroid hormone antagonist, antihyperthyroid drug

Available by prescription only
Tablets: 50 mg

INDICATIONS & DOSAGE
Hyperthyroidism
Adults: 300 to 450 mg P.O. daily in divided doses. Continue until patient is euthyroid; then start maintenance dosage of 100 mg daily to t.i.d.

PHARMACODYNAMICS
Antithyroid action: Used to treat hyperthyroidism, PTU inhibits synthesis of thyroid hormone by interfering with the incorporation of iodine into thyroglobulin; it also inhibits the formation of iodothyronine. Besides blocking hormone synthesis, it also inhibits the peripheral deiodination of T_4 to T_3 (liothyronine). Effects become evident only when the preformed hormone is depleted and circulating hormone levels decline.

As preparation for thyroidectomy, PTU inhibits synthesis of the thyroid hormone and causes a euthyroid state, reducing surgical problems during thyroidectomy; as a result, the mortality for a single-stage thyroidectomy is low. Iodide reduces the vascularity of the gland and makes it less friable.

Used in treating thyrotoxic crisis, PTU inhibits peripheral deiodination of T_4 to T_3. It's preferred over methimazole in thyroid storm because of its peripheral action.

PHARMACOKINETICS
Absorption: PTU is absorbed rapidly and readily (about 80%) from the GI tract. Levels peak at 1 to 1½ hours.
Distribution: Drug appears to be concentrated in the thyroid gland. It's 75% to 80% protein-bound.
Metabolism: Drug is metabolized rapidly in the liver.
Excretion: About 35% of a dose is excreted in urine. Half-life is 1 to 2 hours in patients with normal renal function and 8½ hours in anuric patients.

CONTRAINDICATIONS & PRECAUTIONS
Contraindicated in patients with hypersensitivity to PTU.

INTERACTIONS
Drug-drug. Use of PTU with *adrenocorticoids* or *corticotropin* may require a dosage adjustment of the steroid when thyroid status changes. Use with *bone marrow depressants* increases the risk of agranulocytosis; use with *hepatotoxic drugs* increases the risk of hepatotoxicity; use with *iodinated glycerol, lithium,* or *potassium iodide* may potentiate hypothyroid effects.

The anti–vitamin K activity of PTU may potentiate the effects of *oral anticoagulants.*

ADVERSE REACTIONS
CNS: headache, drowsiness, vertigo, paresthesia, neuritis, neuropathies, CNS stimulation, depression.
CV: vasculitis.
EENT: visual disturbances.
GI: diarrhea, *nausea, vomiting (may be dose-related),* epigastric distress, salivary gland enlargement, loss of taste.
GU: nephritis.
Hematologic: *agranulocytosis, thrombocytopenia, aplastic anemia,* leukopenia.
Hepatic: jaundice, *hepatotoxicity.*
Musculoskeletal: arthralgia, myalgia.
Skin: rash, urticaria, skin discoloration, pruritus, erythema nodosum, exfoliative dermatitis, lupus-like syndrome.

Other: fever, lymphadenopathy; dose-related hypothyroidism (mental depression; hypoprothrombinemia, bleeding, cold intolerance, hard, nonpitting edema).

◰ **KEY CONSIDERATIONS**
• Best response occurs when PTU is administered around the clock and given at the same time each day with respect to meals.
• A beta blocker, usually propranolol, commonly is given to manage the peripheral signs of hyperthyroidism, which are primarily cardiac related (tachycardia).
• Observe for signs and symptoms of hypothyroidism (mental depression; cold intolerance; hard, nonpitting edema; hair loss).
• Discontinue drug if patient develops severe rash or enlarged cervical lymph nodes.
• PTU therapy alters selenomethionine levels and INR; it also alters AST, ALT, and LD levels as well as liothyronine uptake.

Patient education
• Warn patient to avoid using self-prescribed antitussives; many contain iodine.
• Suggest taking PTU with meals to reduce GI adverse effects.
• Instruct patient to store drug in a light-resistant container. Warn patient not to store drug in the bathroom; heat and humidity may cause drug to deteriorate.
• Tell patient to promptly report fever, sore throat, malaise, unusual bleeding, yellowing of eyes, nausea, or vomiting.
• Advise patient to have medical review of thyroid status before undergoing surgery (including dental surgery).
• Teach patient how to recognize the signs of hyperthyroidism and hypothyroidism and what to do if they occur.

Overdose & treatment
• Signs and symptoms of overdose include nausea, vomiting, epigastric distress, fever, headache, arthralgia, pruritus, edema, and pancytopenia.

• For agranulocytosis, pancytopenia, hepatitis, fever, or exfoliative dermatitis, withdraw the drug. For depression of bone marrow, treatment may require antibiotics and transfusions of fresh whole blood. For hepatitis, treatment includes rest, adequate diet, and symptomatic support, including analgesics, gastric lavage, I.V. fluids, and mild sedation.

protamine sulfate

Antidote, heparin antagonist

Available by prescription only
Injection: 10 mg/ml in 5-ml ampule, 25-ml ampule, 5-ml vial, 10-ml vial, 25-ml vial

INDICATIONS & DOSAGE
Heparin overdose
Adults: Dosage based on venous blood coagulation studies, usually 1 mg for each 90 U heparin derived from lung tissue or 1 mg for each 115 U heparin derived from intestinal mucosa. Give by slow I.V. injection over 1 to 3 minutes. Maximum dosage is 50 mg in a 10-minute period.

PHARMACODYNAMICS
Heparin antagonism: Protamine has weak anticoagulant activity; however, when given in the presence of heparin, it forms a salt that neutralizes the anticoagulant effects of both drugs.

PHARMACOKINETICS
Absorption: Heparin-neutralizing effect of protamine occurs within 30 to 60 seconds.
Distribution: Unknown.
Metabolism: Fate of the heparin-protamine complex is unknown; however, it appears to be partially degraded, with release of some heparin.
Excretion: The terminal elimination half-life is 2 hours.

CONTRAINDICATIONS & PRECAUTIONS
Contraindicated in patients with hypersensitivity to protamine. Use cautiously after cardiac surgery.

Reactions may be *common*, uncommon, *life-threatening*, or COMMON AND LIFE-THREATENING.

ADVERSE REACTIONS

CNS: lassitude.
CV: transitory flushing, feeling of warmth, decreased blood pressure, bradycardia, *circulatory collapse.*
GI: nausea, vomiting.
Hematologic: shortens heparin-prolonged PTT.
Respiratory: dyspnea, *pulmonary edema, acute pulmonary hypertension.*
Other: *anaphylaxis, anaphylactoid reactions.*

▣ KEY CONSIDERATIONS

- Check for possible fish allergy.
- Don't mix protamine with other drugs.
- Reconstitute powder by adding 5 ml sterile water to 50-mg vial (25 ml to 250-mg vial); discard unused solution.
- Slow I.V. administration (over 1 to 3 minutes) decreases adverse effects; have antishock equipment available.
- Monitor patient continually and check vital signs frequently; blood pressure may decrease suddenly.
- Dosage is based on blood coagulation studies as well as on route of administration of heparin and time elapsed since heparin was administered.

Patient education

- Advise patient that he may experience transitory flushing or feel warm after I.V. administration.

Overdose & treatment

- Overdose may cause bleeding secondary to interaction with platelets and proteins, including fibrinogen.
- Replace blood loss with blood transfusions or fresh frozen plasma. If hypotension occurs, consider treating with fluids, epinephrine, dobutamine, or dopamine.

pseudoephedrine hydrochloride

pseudoephedrine sulfate

Cenafed, Decofed, Efidac/24, Myfedrine, Novafed, PediaCare Infants' Decongestant Drops, Pseudogest, Sinufed Timecelles, Sudafed

Adrenergic, decongestant

Available without prescription
Oral solution: 7.5 mg/0.8 ml, 15 mg/5 ml, 30 mg/5 ml
Tablets: 30 mg, 60 mg
Tablets (extended-release): 120 mg, 240 mg
Capsules: 60 mg
Capsules (extended-release): 120 mg

INDICATIONS & DOSAGE

Nasal and eustachian tube decongestant
Adults: 60 mg P.O. q 4 to 6 hours. Maximum dosage is 240 mg daily, or 120 mg P.O. extended-release tablet q 12 hours.

PHARMACODYNAMICS

Decongestant action: Pseudoephedrine directly stimulates alpha-adrenergic receptors of respiratory mucosa to produce vasoconstriction; shrinkage of swollen nasal mucous membranes; reduction of tissue hyperemia, edema, and nasal congestion; an increase in airway (nasal) patency and drainage of sinus excretions; and opening of obstructed eustachian ostia. Relaxation of bronchial smooth muscle may result from direct stimulation of beta receptors. Mild CNS stimulation may also occur.

PHARMACOKINETICS

Absorption: Nasal decongestion occurs within 30 minutes and persists 4 to 6 hours after oral dose of 60-mg tablet or oral solution. Effects persist 8 hours after 60-mg dose and up to 12 hours after 120-mg dose of extended-release form.
Distribution: Pseudoephedrine is widely distributed throughout the body.

Metabolism: N-demethylation in the liver completely metabolizes the drug to inactive compounds.
Excretion: About 55% to 75% of a dose is excreted unchanged in urine; remainder is excreted as unchanged drug and metabolites.

CONTRAINDICATIONS & PRECAUTIONS
Contraindicated in patients with severe hypertension or severe coronary artery disease and in those receiving MAO inhibitors.

Use cautiously in geriatric patients and in those with hypertension, cardiac disease, diabetes, glaucoma, hyperthyroidism, or prostatic hyperplasia.

INTERACTIONS
Drug-drug. *Beta blockers* may increase pressor effects of pseudoephedrine. *MAO inhibitors* potentiate pressor effects of pseudoephedrine. Use with other *sympathomimetics* may produce additive effects and toxicity; with *methyldopa* and *reserpine,* may reduce their antihypertensive effects. *Tricyclic antidepressants* may antagonize effects of pseudoephedrine.

ADVERSE REACTIONS
CNS: *anxiety,* transient stimulation, tremor, dizziness, headache, insomnia, *nervousness.*
CV: *arrhythmias, palpitations,* tachycardia.
GI: anorexia, nausea, vomiting, dry mouth.
GU: difficulty urinating.
Respiratory: respiratory difficulties.
Skin: pallor.

▣ KEY CONSIDERATIONS
Besides the recommendations relevant to all adrenergics, consider the following:
● Geriatric patients may be sensitive to effects of pseudoephedrine; lower dose may be needed. Overdosage may cause hallucinations, CNS depression, seizures, and death in patients older than age 60. Use extended-release preparations with caution in geriatric patients.
● To minimize insomnia, administer last daily dose several hours before bedtime.

● If symptoms persist longer than 5 days or fever is present, reevaluate therapy.
● Observe patient for complaints of headache or dizziness; monitor blood pressure.

Patient education
● If patient finds swallowing the drug difficult, suggest opening capsules and mixing contents with applesauce, jelly, honey, or syrup. Mixture must be swallowed without chewing.
● Tell patient that dry mouth may occur and suggest using ice chips, sugarless gum, or hard candy for relief.
● Instruct patient to take missed dose if remembered within 1 hour. If beyond 1 hour, patient should skip and resume regular schedule; he shouldn't double-dose.
● Tell patient to store pseudoephedrine away from heat and light (not in bathroom medicine cabinet) and safely out of reach of children.
● Caution patient that many OTC preparations may contain sympathomimetics, which can cause additive, hazardous reactions.
● Advise patient to take last dose at least 2 to 3 hours before bedtime to avoid insomnia.

Overdose & treatment
● Signs and symptoms of overdose include exaggeration of common adverse reactions, particularly seizures, arrhythmias, and nausea and vomiting.
● Treatment may include induced vomiting or gastric lavage within 4 hours of ingestion. Activated charcoal is effective only if administered within 1 hour, unless extended-release form was used. If renal function is adequate, forced diuresis increases elimination. Don't force diuresis in severe overdose. Monitor vital signs, cardiac state, and electrolyte levels. I.V. propranolol may control cardiac toxicity; I.V. diazepam may be helpful to manage delirium or seizures; dilute potassium chloride solutions (I.V.) may be given for hypokalemia.

psyllium

Cillium, Fiberall, Hydrocil Instant,
Konsyl, Konsyl-D, Metamucil,
Naturacil, Reguloid, Serutan, Siblin,
Syllact, V-Lax

Adsorbent, bulk laxative

Available without prescription
Powder: 3.3 g/tsp, 3.4 g/tsp, 3.5 g/tsp,
4.94 g/tsp
Powder (effervescent): 3.4 g/packet,
3.7 g/packet
Granules: 2.5 g/tsp, 4.03 g/tsp
Chewable pieces: 1.7 g/piece
Wafers: 1.7 g/wafer, 3.4 g/wafer

INDICATIONS & DOSAGE
Constipation, bowel management, irritable bowel syndrome
Adults: 1 to 2 rounded tsp P.O. in full
glass of liquid daily, b.i.d. or t.i.d., followed by second glass of liquid; or 1
packet P.O. dissolved in water daily; or 2
wafers b.i.d. or t.i.d.

PHARMACODYNAMICS
Laxative action: Psyllium adsorbs water
in the gut; it also serves as a source of
indigestible fiber, increasing stool bulk
and moisture, thus stimulating peristaltic
activity and bowel evacuation.

PHARMACOKINETICS
Absorption: None; onset of action varies
from 12 hours to 3 days.
Distribution: Psyllium is distributed locally in the gut.
Metabolism: None.
Excretion: Drug is excreted in feces.

CONTRAINDICATIONS & PRECAUTIONS
Contraindicated in patients with hypersensitivity to psyllium, abdominal pain,
nausea, vomiting, or other symptoms of
appendicitis and in those with intestinal
obstruction or ulceration, disabling adhesions, or difficulty swallowing.

INTERACTIONS
Drug-drug. Psyllium may adsorb oral
drugs, such as *anticoagulants, cardiac
glycosides,* and *salicylates.*

ADVERSE REACTIONS
GI: nausea, vomiting, diarrhea (with excessive use); esophageal, gastric, small-intestinal, and rectal obstruction when
psyllium is taken in dry form; abdominal
cramps, especially in severe constipation.

▣ KEY CONSIDERATIONS
• Before administering psyllium, add at
least 8 oz (240 ml) water or juice and stir
for a few seconds (improves taste). Have
patient drink mixture immediately to
prevent it from congealing; then have
him drink another glass of fluid.
• Separate administration of psyllium
and oral anticoagulants, cardiac glycosides, and salicylates by at least 2 hours.
• Drug may reduce appetite if administered before meals.
• Psyllium and other bulk laxatives most
closely mimic natural bowel function
and don't cause laxative dependence;
they're especially useful for patients
with diverticular disease, for debilitated
patients, for irritable bowel syndrome,
and for patients who use laxatives regularly.
• Give patients with diabetes a sugar-and sodium-free psyllium product.

Patient education
• Warn patient not to swallow psyllium
in dry form; he should mix it with at
least 8 oz (240 ml) of fluid, stir briefly,
drink immediately (to prevent mixture
from congealing), and follow it with another 8 oz of fluid.
• Explain that drug may reduce appetite
if taken before meals; recommend taking
drug 2 hours after meals and other oral
drugs.
• Advise patients with diabetes and
those with restricted sodium or sugar intake to avoid psyllium products containing salt or sugar. Advise patients who
must restrict phenylalanine intake to
avoid psyllium products containing aspartame.

pyrazinamide
PMS-Pyrazinamide*, Tebrazid*

Synthetic pyrazine analogue of nicotinamide, antituberculotic

Available by prescription only
Tablets: 500 mg

INDICATIONS & DOSAGE
Adjunctive treatment of tuberculosis (when primary and secondary antituberculotics can't be used or have failed)
Adults: 15 to 30 mg/kg P.O. daily, in one or more doses. Maximum dosage is 3 g daily. Alternatively, a twice-weekly dose of 50 to 70 mg/kg (based on lean body weight) has been developed to promote patient compliance. Lower dosage is recommended in decreased renal function.

PHARMACODYNAMICS
Antibiotic action: Mechanism of action is unknown; pyrazinamide may be bactericidal or bacteriostatic, depending on organism susceptibility and drug level at infection site. Drug is active only against *Mycobacterium tuberculosis.* Drug is considered adjunctive in tuberculosis therapy and is given with other drugs to prevent or delay development of resistance to pyrazinamide by *M. tuberculosis.*

PHARMACOKINETICS
Absorption: Pyrazinamide is well absorbed after oral administration; serum levels peak 2 hours after an oral dose.
Distribution: Distributed widely into body tissues and fluids, including lungs, liver, and CSF; drug is 50% protein-bound.
Metabolism: Drug is hydrolyzed in the liver; some hydrolysis occurs in stomach.
Excretion: Drug is excreted almost completely in urine through glomerular filtration. Elimination half-life in adults is 9 to 10 hours. Half-life is prolonged in renal and hepatic impairment.

CONTRAINDICATIONS & PRECAUTIONS
Contraindicated in patients with hypersensitivity to pyrazinamide, severe hepatic disease, or acute gout. Use cautiously in patients with diabetes mellitus, renal failure, or gout.

ADVERSE REACTIONS
CNS: malaise.
GI: anorexia, nausea, vomiting.
GU: dysuria, may interfere with urine ketone determinations, increased urate levels, hyperuricemia, interstitial nephritis.
Hematologic: sideroblastic anemia, *thrombocytopenia.*
Hepatic: increased liver enzyme levels.
Musculoskeletal: gout, *arthralgia, myalgia.*
Skin: rash, urticaria, pruritus, photosensitivity.
Other: fever, porphyria, *hepatitis.*

▣ KEY CONSIDERATIONS
• Because geriatric patients commonly have diminished renal function, which decreases pyrazinamide excretion, drug should be used with caution
• Monitor liver function, especially enzyme and bilirubin levels, and renal function, especially serum uric acid levels, before therapy and thereafter at 2- to 4-week intervals; observe patient for signs of liver damage or decreased renal function.
• In patients with diabetes mellitus, drug therapy may hinder stabilization of serum glucose levels.
• In many cases, drug elevates serum uric acid levels. Although usually asymptomatic, a uricosuric drug such as probenecid or allopurinol may be necessary.
• Patients with concomitant infection HIV may require a longer course of treatment.

Patient education
• Explain the disease and the rationale for long-term therapy.
• Teach signs and symptoms of hypersensitivity and other adverse reactions and emphasize need to report them; urge patient to report unusual reactions, especially signs of gout.
• Be sure patient understands how and when to take drugs; urge patient to complete entire prescribed regimen, to com-

ply with instructions for around-the-clock dosage, and to keep follow-up appointments.

Overdose & treatment
• Hepatotoxicity is dose related and may occur with overdose.
• No specific recommendations are available. Treatment is supportive. After recent ingestion (4 hours or less), induce vomiting or perform gastric lavage. Follow with activated charcoal to decrease absorption.

pyridoxine hydrochloride (vitamin B₆)
Beesix, Nestrex

Water-soluble vitamin, nutritional supplement

Available by prescription only
Injection: 10-ml vial (100 mg/ml), 30-ml vial (100 mg/ml), 10-ml vial (100 mg/ml, with 1.5% benzyl alcohol), 30-ml vial (100 mg/ml, with 1.5% benzyl alcohol), 10-ml vial (100 mg/ml, with 0.5% chlorobutanol), 1-ml vial (100 mg/ml)
Available without prescription
Tablets: 10 mg, 25 mg, 50 mg, 100 mg, 200 mg, 250 mg, 500 mg
Tablets (timed-release): 500 mg

INDICATIONS & DOSAGE
Dietary vitamin B₆ deficiency
Adults: 2.5 to 10 mg P.O., I.M., or I.V. daily for 3 weeks, then 2 to 5 mg daily as a supplement to a proper diet.
Seizures related to vitamin B₆ deficiency or dependency
Adults: 100 mg I.M. or I.V. in single dose.
Vitamin B₆–responsive anemias or dependency syndrome (inborn errors of metabolism)
Adults: 100 to 200 mg daily for 3 weeks then 2.5 to 100 mg daily until symptoms subside; then 50 mg daily for life.
◊ *Hyperoxaluria type I*
Adults: 25 to 300 mg P.O., I.M., or I.V. daily.

Seizures secondary to isoniazid overdose
Adults: A dose of pyridoxine equal to the amount of isoniazid ingested is usually given; generally, 1 to 4 g I.V. initially and then 1 g I.M. every 30 minutes until the entire dose has been given.

PHARMACODYNAMICS
Metabolic action: Natural vitamin B₆ contained in plant and animal foodstuffs is converted to physiologically active forms of vitamin B₆, pyridoxal phosphate, and pyridoxamine phosphate. Exogenous forms of the vitamin are metabolized in humans. Vitamin B₆ acts as a coenzyme in protein, carbohydrate, and fat metabolism and participates in the decarboxylation of amino acids in protein metabolism. Vitamin B₆ also helps convert tryptophan to niacin or serotonin and it helps with the deamination, transamination, and transulfuration of amino acids. Vitamin B₆ is responsible for the breakdown of glycogen to glucose-1-phosphate in carbohydrate metabolism. The total adult body store consists of 16 to 27 mg pyridoxine. The need for the drug increases with the amount of protein in the diet.

PHARMACOKINETICS
Absorption: After oral administration, pyridoxine and its substituents are absorbed readily from the GI tract. GI absorption may be diminished in patients who have malabsorption syndromes or who have had gastric resection. Normal serum levels of drug are 30 to 80 ng/ml.
Distribution: Drug is stored mainly in the liver. The total body store is 16 to 27 mg. Pyridoxal and pyridoxal phosphate are the most common forms found in the blood and are highly protein-bound.
Metabolism: Drug is degraded to 4-pyridoxic acid in the liver.
Excretion: In erythrocytes, pyridoxine is converted to pyridoxal phosphate, and pyridoxamine is converted to pyridoxamine phosphate. The phosphorylated form of pyridoxine is transaminated to pyridoxal and pyridoxamine, which is phosphorylated rapidly. The conversion of pyridoxine phosphate to pyridoxal

phosphate requires riboflavin. Biological half-life is 15 to 20 days.

CONTRAINDICATIONS & PRECAUTIONS
Contraindicated in patients hypersensitive to pyridoxine.

INTERACTIONS
Drug-drug. *Cycloserine, hydralazine, isoniazid, oral contraceptives,* and *penicillamine* may increase pyridoxine requirements. Pyridoxine reverses the therapeutic effects of *levodopa* by accelerating peripheral metabolism. Use of drug with *phenobarbital* or *phenytoin* may cause a 50% decrease in serum levels of these *anticonvulsants.*

ADVERSE REACTIONS
CNS: paresthesia, unsteady gait, numbness, somnolence.

▣ KEY CONSIDERATIONS
• Prepare a dietary history. A single vitamin deficiency is unusual; lack of one vitamin commonly indicates a deficiency of others.
• Monitor protein intake; excessive protein intake increases pyridoxine requirements.
• A dosage of 25 mg/kg/day is well tolerated. Adults consuming 200 mg/day for 33 days and on a normal dietary intake develop vitamin B_6 dependency.
• Don't mix with sodium bicarbonate in the same syringe.
• Patients receiving levodopa shouldn't take more than 5 mg/day of pyridoxine.
• Store in a tight, light-resistant container.
• Don't use injection solution if it contains precipitate. Slight darkening is acceptable.
• Drug therapy alters determinations for urobilinogen in the spot test using Ehrlich's reagent, resulting in a false-positive reaction.

Patient education
• Teach patient about dietary sources of vitamin B_6, such as yeast, wheat germ, liver, whole grain cereals, bananas, and legumes.

Overdose & treatment
• Signs and symptoms of overdose include ataxia and severe sensory neuropathy after long-term use of high daily doses of pyridoxine (2 to 6 g).
• These neurologic deficits usually resolve after drug is discontinued.

Q

quetiapine fumarate
Seroquel

*Dibenzothiazepine derivative,
antipsychotic*

Available by prescription only
Tablets: 25 mg, 100 mg, 200 mg

INDICATIONS & DOSAGE
Management of psychotic disorders
Adults: Initially, 25 mg P.O. b.i.d.; increase in increments of 25 to 50 mg
b.i.d. or t.i.d. on days 2 and 3 as tolerated to a target dose range of 300 to
400 mg daily by day 4, divided into two or three doses. Further dosage adjustments, if indicated, should generally occur at intervals of not less than 2 days.
Dosages can be increased or decreased by 25 to 50 mg b.i.d. Antipsychotic efficacy is generally in dosage range of 150 to 750 mg/day. Safety of dosages more than 800 mg/day hasn't been evaluated.
✦ **Dosage adjustment.** In geriatric or debilitated patients or those with hepatic impairment or a predisposition to hypotensive reactions, consider lower doses, longer intervals between doses, and careful monitoring during initial dosing period. No specific dosing recommendations are given.

PHARMACODYNAMICS
Antipsychotic action: Exact mechanism of action is unknown. Quetiapine is a dibenzothiazepine derivative that is thought to act through antagonism of dopamine type 2 (D_2) and serotonin type 2 (5-HT_2) receptors. Antagonism at serotonin 5-HT_{1A}, D_1, and H_1 and alpha$_1$- and alpha$_2$-adrenergic receptors may explain other effects.

PHARMACOKINETICS
Absorption: Quetiapine is rapidly absorbed after oral administration. Plasma levels peak in about 1½ hours. Food affects absorption, with maximum level increasing 25% and bioavailability increasing 15%.

Distribution: Apparent volume of distribution is 10 ± 4 L/kg. Drug is 83% plasma protein-bound, with steady-state levels within 2 days.
Metabolism: Drug is extensively metabolized by the liver through sulfoxidation and oxidation. Cytochrome P-450 3A4 is the major isoenzyme involved.
Excretion: Less than 1% of dose is excreted as unchanged drug; about 73% is recovered in urine and 20% in feces. Mean terminal half-life is about 6 hours.

CONTRAINDICATIONS & PRECAUTIONS
Contraindicated in patients hypersensitive to quetiapine or its ingredients.

Use cautiously in patients with known CV or cerebrovascular disease or conditions that would predispose patient to hypotension, history of seizures or with conditions that potentially lower the seizure threshold, and in those at risk for aspiration pneumonia because of associated esophageal dysmotility and aspiration. Also use cautiously in patients with conditions that may elevate core body temperature.

INTERACTIONS
Drug-drug. Use with *antihypertensives* may potentiate the hypotensive effect of both drugs. Use cautiously with other *centrally acting drugs.* Multiple daily doses of *cimetidine* result in a 20% decrease in mean oral clearance of quetiapine. Use with caution when administering with a potent *cytochrome P-450 3A inhibitor (erythromycin, fluconazole, itraconazole, ketoconazole).* Drug may antagonize the effect of *dopamine agonists* and *levodopa.* Mean oral clearance of *lorazepam* is reduced by 20% when administered together. *Phenytoin* increases the mean oral clearance of quetiapine fivefold. *Thioridazine* increases oral clearance of quetiapine by 65%.
Drug-lifestyle. Use with *alcohol* may potentiate cognitive and motor effects; avoid use during drug therapy.

ADVERSE REACTIONS

CNS: *dizziness, headache, somnolence,* asthenia, hypertonia, dysarthria.
CV: postural hypotension, tachycardia, palpitations, peripheral edema.
EENT: pharyngitis, rhinitis, ear pain.
GI: dry mouth, dyspepsia, abdominal pain, constipation, anorexia.
Hematologic: *leukopenia.*
Metabolic: *weight gain.*
Musculoskeletal: back pain.
Respiratory: increased cough, dyspnea.
Skin: rash, diaphoresis.
Other: fever, flulike syndrome.

▣ KEY CONSIDERATIONS

• No difference appears in tolerability in patients ages 65 or older. Factors that may decrease pharmacokinetic clearance, increase pharmacodynamic response to quetiapine, or cause poor tolerance or orthostasis indicate use of a lower starting dose, slower titration, and careful monitoring during the initial dosing period.

• Examine the lens before therapy begins or shortly thereafter and at 6-month intervals during long-term treatment for possible cataract formation.

• Total and free T_4 levels may decrease but this decrease is usually insignificant. Although rare, some patients experience increased thyroid-stimulating hormone levels and require thyroid hormone replacement.

• Drug may increase cholesterol and triglyceride levels.

• Asymptomatic, transient, and reversible increases in serum transaminase levels (primarily ALT) have been reported. These elevations usually occur within the first 3 weeks of therapy and promptly return to pretreatment levels with continued use.

• Neuroleptic malignant syndrome, a potentially fatal syndrome, has been reported with use of antipsychotics. Signs and symptoms include hyperpyrexia, muscle rigidity, altered mental status, and evidence of autonomic instability. Carefully monitor at-risk patients.

• Use smallest effective dose for shortest duration to minimize the risk of tardive dyskinesia.

• Closely monitor schizophrenic patients during drug therapy because of the inherent risk of a suicide attempt.

Patient education

• Advise patient of risk of orthostatic hypotension, especially during the initial 3- to 5-day period of dose titration and during dosage increase or treatment reinitiation.

• Tell patient to avoid becoming overheated or dehydrated.

• Warn patient to avoid activities that require mental alertness during initial dose titration or dosage increase, such as driving a car or operating hazardous machinery, until CNS effects of quetiapine are known.

• Advise patient to avoid alcohol while taking drug.

• Remind patient to have an initial eye examination at the beginning of drug therapy and every 6 months during treatment to monitor for cataract formation.

• Tell patient to call doctor before taking other prescription or OTC drugs.

Overdose & treatment

• Signs and symptoms of overdose include an exaggeration of the pharmacologic effects of the drug—such as drowsiness, sedation, tachycardia, and hypotension. Hypokalemia and first-degree heart block may also occur.

• For acute overdose, treatment includes establishing and maintaining an airway to ensure adequate oxygenation and ventilation. Consider gastric lavage and administration of activated charcoal or a laxative. Begin CV monitoring, including ECG monitoring, immediately. Avoid use of disopyramide, procainamide, quinidine, and bretylium if antiarrhythmic therapy is indicated. Administer I.V. fluids or sympathomimetics (not epinephrine or dopamine) to treat hypotension and circulatory collapse. For severe extrapyramidal symptoms, administer anticholinergics.

Reactions may be *common*, uncommon, *life-threatening*, or COMMON AND LIFE-THREATENING.

quinapril hydrochloride
Accupril

ACE inhibitor, antihypertensive

Available by prescription only
Tablets: 5 mg, 10 mg, 20 mg, 40 mg

INDICATIONS & DOSAGE
Hypertension
Adults: Initially, 10 mg P.O. daily. Adjust dosage based on response at intervals of about 2 weeks. Most patients are controlled at 20, 40, or 80 mg daily, as a single dose or in two divided doses.
Hypertension in patients receiving diuretics, management of heart failure
Adults: Initially, 5 mg P.O. b.i.d. when added to diuretic and cardiac glycoside therapy. Adjust dosage weekly based on response. Usual dosage is 20 to 40 mg daily in two equally divided doses.
✦ *Dosage adjustment.* In adults with renal impairment, initial dose is 10 mg P.O. daily if creatinine clearance exceeds 60 ml/minute, 5 mg if it's 30 to 60 ml/minute, and 2.5 mg if it's 10 to 30 ml/minute. No dose recommendations are available for creatinine clearance less than 10 ml/minute.

PHARMACODYNAMICS
Antihypertensive action: Quinapril and its active metabolite, quinaprilat, inhibit ACE, preventing conversion of angiotensin I to angiotensin II, a potent vasoconstrictor. Reduced formation of angiotensin II decreases peripheral arterial resistance, aldosterone secretion, sodium and water retention, and blood pressure. Drug also has antihypertensive activity in patients with low-renin hypertension.

PHARMACOKINETICS
Absorption: At least 60% of quinapril is absorbed; plasma levels peak within 1 hour. Rate and extent of absorption are decreased 25% to 30% when drug is administered during a high-fat meal.
Distribution: About 97% of drug and active metabolite are bound to plasma proteins.
Metabolism: About 38% of oral dose is deesterified in the liver to quinaprilat, the active metabolite.
Excretion: Drug is primarily excreted in urine; terminal elimination half-life is about 25 hours.

CONTRAINDICATIONS & PRECAUTIONS
Contraindicated in patients with hypersensitivity to ACE inhibitors or history of angioedema related to treatment with an ACE inhibitor. Use cautiously in patients with impaired renal function.

INTERACTIONS
Drug-drug. *Diuretics* and *other antihypertensives* increase risk of excessive hypotension; discontinue diuretic or reduce dose of quinapril as needed. Increased serum *lithium* levels and lithium toxicity have been reported when used with ACE inhibitors. *Potassium sparing diuretics* and *potassium supplements* may increase the risk of hyperkalemia; avoid using together. Each tablet of quinapril contains magnesium carbonate and magnesium stearate; administration with *tetracycline* significantly impairs absorption of tetracycline.
Drug-food. *High-fat meals* may impair absorption. *Sodium substitutes* may contain potassium and cause hyperkalemia.
Drug-lifestyle. *Sun exposure* can increase the risk of photosensitivity reactions.

ADVERSE REACTIONS
CNS: somnolence, vertigo, nervousness, headache, dizziness, fatigue, depression.
CV: palpitations, tachycardia, angina, hypertensive crisis, orthostatic hypotension, chest pain, *rhythm disturbances.*
GI: dry mouth, abdominal pain, constipation, vomiting, nausea, **hemorrhage.**
Hematologic: *thrombocytopenia, agranulocytosis.*
Hepatic: elevated liver enzyme levels.
Metabolic: hyperkalemia.
Respiratory: *dry, persistent, tickling, nonproductive cough.*
Skin: pruritus, *exfoliative dermatitis, photosensitivity,* diaphoresis.
Other: *angioedema.*

▣ KEY CONSIDERATIONS

• Geriatric patients have shown higher peak plasma levels and slower elimination of quinapril; these changes are related to decreased renal function that occurs in many geriatric patients.

• Blood pressure measurements should be made when drug levels peak (2 to 6 hours after dosing) and trough (just before a dose) to verify adequate blood pressure control.

• Because administration with diuretics may increase the risk of excessive hypotension, diuretic therapy should be discontinued 2 to 3 days before start of quinapril, if possible. If quinapril alone doesn't adequately control blood pressure, a diuretic may be carefully added to the regimen.

• Like other ACE inhibitors, drug may cause a dry, persistent, tickling cough that's reversible when therapy is discontinued.

• Assess renal and hepatic function before and periodically throughout therapy. Also, monitor CBC and serum potassium levels.

Patient education

• Tell patient quinapril should be taken on an empty stomach because meals, particularly high-fat meals, can impair absorption.

• Tell patient to immediately report signs or symptoms of angioedema, such as swelling of face, eyes, lips, tongue, or difficulty breathing. If these occur, patient should stop taking the drug and seek immediate medical attention.

• Warn patient that light-headedness may occur, especially during first few days of therapy. Tell him to arise slowly to minimize this effect and to report persistent or severe symptoms. If syncope occurs, patient should stop taking drug and call immediately.

• Inadequate fluid intake, vomiting, diarrhea, and excessive perspiration can lead to light-headedness and syncope. Patient should avoid dehydration and overheating in hot weather and during periods of exercise.

• Tell patient not to use sodium substitutes because they contain potassium and can cause hyperkalemia.

• Tell patient to report immediately signs or symptoms of infection (sore throat, fever) or easy bruising or bleeding. Other ACE inhibitors have been associated with development of agranulocytosis and neutropenia.

Overdose & treatment

• Peritoneal dialysis or hemodialysis wouldn't be beneficial; no data are available to support use of certain physiological maneuvers such as urine acidification. Treat symptomatically. Infusions of normal saline solution have been suggested to treat hypotension.

---

quinidine gluconate
Quinaglute Dura-Tabs, Quinalan

quinidine polygalacturonate
Cardioquin

quinidine sulfate
Apo-Quinidine,* Quinidex Extentabs, Quinora

Cinchona alkaloid, ventricular antiarrhythmic, supraventricular antiarrhythmic, atrial antitachyarrhythmic

---

Available by prescription only
Tablets: 325 mg* (gluconate); 275 mg (polygalacturonate); 200 mg, 300 mg (sulfate); 300 mg (extended-release, sulfate); 324 mg (extended-release, gluconate)
Injection: 80 mg/ml (gluconate); 200 mg/ml (sulfate); 190 mg/ml (sulfate)*

INDICATIONS & DOSAGE
Atrial flutter or fibrillation
Adults: 200 mg (sulfate or equivalent base) P.O. q 2 to 3 hours for five to eight doses, with subsequent daily increases until sinus rhythm is restored or toxic effects develop. Administer quinidine only after giving digoxin to avoid increasing AV conduction. Maximum dose is 3 to 4 g/day.

Maintenance dosage is 200 to 400 mg P.O. t.i.d. or q.i.d. or 600 mg P.O. q 8 to 12 hours daily (extended-release).

Paroxysmal supraventricular tachycardia
Adults: 400 to 600 mg (sulfate) P.O. q 2 to 3 hours until toxic effects develop or arrhythmia subsides.
Premature atrial contractions, PVCs, paroxysmal AV junctional rhythm or atrial or ventricular tachycardia, maintenance of cardioversion
Adults: Give test dose of 50 to 200 mg P.O. sulfate (or 200 mg gluconate I.M.), then monitor vital signs before beginning therapy with 200 to 400 mg P.O. sulfate or equivalent base q 4 to 6 hours; or initially 600 mg gluconate I.M., then up to 400 mg q 2 hours p.r.n.; or 800 mg I.V. gluconate diluted in 40 ml D_5W infused at 16 mg (1 ml)/minute. Alternatively, give 300 to 600 mg sulfate (extended-release), or 324 to 648 mg gluconate (extended-release) q 8 to 12 hours.
◇ *Malaria (when quinine dihydrochloride is unavailable)*
Adults: Administer quinidine gluconate by continuous I.V. infusion. Initial loading dose of 10 mg/kg diluted in 250 ml normal saline injection infused over 1 to 2 hours, followed by a continuous maintenance infusion of 0.02 mg/kg/minute (20 mcg/kg/minute) for 72 hours or until parasitemia is reduced to less than 1% or oral therapy can be started; or 10 mg/kg quinidine sulfate P.O. q 8 hours for 5 to 7 days. Contact the Malaria Branch of the Centers for Disease Control and Prevention (CDC) for protocol instructions for recommendations.

PHARMACODYNAMICS

Antiarrhythmic action: A class IA antiarrhythmic, quinidine depresses phase 0 of the action potential. It's considered a myocardial depressant because it decreases myocardial excitability and conduction velocity and may depress myocardial contractility. It also exerts anticholinergic activity, which may modify its direct myocardial effects. In therapeutic doses, quinidine reduces conduction velocity in the atria, ventricles, and His-Purkinje system. It helps control atrial tachyarrhythmias by prolonging the effective refractory period (ERP) and increasing the action potential duration in the atria, ventricles, and His-Purkinje system. Because ERP prolongation exceeds action potential duration, tissue remains refractory even after returning to resting membrane potential (membrane-stabilizing effect). Quinidine shortens the ERP of the AV node. Because the anticholinergic action of the drug may increase AV node conductivity, a cardiac glycoside should be administered for atrial tachyarrhythmias before quinidine therapy begins to prevent ventricular tachyarrhythmias. Quinidine also suppresses automaticity in the His-Purkinje system and ectopic pacemakers, making it useful in treating PVCs. At therapeutic doses, quinidine prolongs the QRS complex and QT interval; these ECG effects may be used as an index of drug effectiveness and toxicity.

PHARMACOKINETICS

Absorption: Although all quinidine salts are well absorbed from the GI tract, individual serum drug levels vary greatly. Onset of action of quinidine sulfate is from 1 to 3 hours. For extended-release forms, onset of action may be slightly slower, but duration of effect is longer because drug delivery system allows longer-than-usual dosing intervals. Plasma levels peak in 3 to 4 hours for quinidine gluconate and 6 hours for quinidine polygalacturonate.
Distribution: Drug is well distributed in all tissues except brain. It concentrates in the heart, liver, kidneys, and skeletal muscle. Distribution volume decreases in patients with heart failure, possibly requiring reduction in maintenance dosage. About 80% of drug is bound to plasma proteins; the unbound (active) fraction may increase in patients with hypoalbuminemia from various causes, including hepatic insufficiency. Usual therapeutic serum levels depend on assay method and ranges as follows: For specific assay (enzyme multiplied immunoassay technique, high-performance liquid chromatography, fluorescence polarization), 2 to 5 µg/ml; for nonspecific assay (fluorometric), 4 to 8 µg/ml.
Metabolism: About 60% to 80% of drug is metabolized in the liver to two

metabolites that may have some pharmacologic activity.

Excretion: About 10% to 30% of administered dose is excreted in urine within 24 hours as unchanged drug. Urine acidification increases drug excretion; alkalinization decreases excretion. Most of administered dose is eliminated in urine as metabolites; elimination half-life is from 5 to 12 hours (usual half-life, about 6½ hours). Duration of effect ranges from 6 to 8 hours.

CONTRAINDICATIONS & PRECAUTIONS

Contraindicated in patients with hypersensitivity to quinidine or related cinchona derivatives, intraventricular conduction defects, cardiac glycoside toxicity when AV conduction is grossly impaired, abnormal rhythms resulting from escape mechanisms, and history of drug-induced torsades de pointes or QT syndrome.

Use cautiously in patients with impaired renal or hepatic function, asthma, muscle weakness, or infection accompanied by a fever because hypersensitivity reactions may be masked.

INTERACTIONS

Drug-drug. Use with some *antacids, sodium bicarbonate,* and *thiazide diuretics* may decrease quinidine elimination when urine pH increases, requiring close monitoring of therapy. Use with *anticholinergics* may lead to additive anticholinergic effects. The anticholinergic effects of quinidine may negate the effects of such *anticholinesterases* as *neostigmine* and *pyridostigmine* when these drugs are used to treat myasthenia gravis. Use with *anticonvulsants* (such as *phenobarbital* and *phenytoin*) increases the rate of quinidine metabolism, leading to decreased quinidine levels. Use with *antihypertensives* may cause additive hypotensive effects (mainly when administered I.V.). When used together, *cholinergics* may fail to terminate paroxysmal supraventricular tachycardia because quinidine antagonizes the vagal excitation effect of cholinergics on the atria and AV node. Use with *coumarin* may potentiate the anticoagulant effect of coumarin, possibly leading to hypoprothrombinemic hemorrhage. Use with *digitoxin* or *digoxin* may cause increased (possibly toxic) serum digoxin levels; some experts recommend a 50% reduction in digoxin dosage when quinidine therapy is initiated, with subsequent monitoring of serum levels. Use with *neuromuscular blockers* (such as *metocurine iodide, pancuronium bromide, succinylcholine chloride,* and *tubocurarine chloride*) may potentiate anticholinergic effects; use of quinidine should be avoided immediately after use of these drugs, and if quinidine must be used, respiratory support may be needed. Use with *nifedipine* may result in decreased quinidine levels. Use with *other antiarrhythmics* (such as *amiodarone, lidocaine, phenytoin, procainamide,* and *propranolol*) may cause additive or antagonistic cardiac effects and additive toxic effects. For example, use with *other antiarrhythmics that increase the QT interval* may further prolong the QT interval and lead to torsades de pointes tachycardia. Use with *phenothiazines* or *reserpine* may cause additive cardiac depressant effects. Use with *rifampin* may increase quinidine metabolism and decrease serum quinidine levels, possibly necessitating dosage adjustment when rifampin therapy is initiated or discontinued. Use with *verapamil* may result in significant hypotension in some patients with hypertrophic cardiomyopathy.

ADVERSE REACTIONS

CNS: *vertigo, headache,* confusion, *light-headedness,* ataxia, depression, dementia.

CV: *PVCs,* **ventricular tachycardia, torsades de pointes,** hypotension, **complete AV block,** tachycardia, ECG changes *(particularly widening of QRS complex, widened QT and PR intervals).*

EENT: *tinnitus,* excessive salivation, blurred vision, diplopia, photophobia.

GI: *diarrhea, nausea, vomiting,* anorexia, abdominal pain.

Hematologic: **hemolytic anemia, thrombocytopenia, agranulocytosis.**

Hepatic: **hepatotoxicity.**

Respiratory: acute asthma attack, **respiratory arrest.**

Reactions may be *common,* uncommon, **life-threatening,** or COMMON AND LIFE-THREATENING.

Skin: rash, petechial hemorrhage of buccal mucosa, pruritus, urticaria, lupus erythematosus, photosensitivity.
Other: *angioedema, fever, cinchonism.*

▣ KEY CONSIDERATIONS

• Dosage reduction may be necessary in geriatric patients. Because of highly variable metabolism, monitor serum levels.
• When quinidine is used to treat atrial tachyarrhythmias, the anticholinergic effects of the drug on the AV node may accelerate the ventricular rate.
• Because conversion of chronic atrial fibrillation may be associated with embolism, anticoagulant should be administered for several weeks before quinidine therapy begins.
• Check apical pulse rate, blood pressure, and ECG tracing before starting therapy.
• I.V. route should be used for acute arrhythmias only; it's generally avoided because of the potential of severe hypotension.
• Don't use discolored (brownish) quinidine solution.
• For maintenance, give only by oral or I.M. route. Dosage requirements vary. Some patients may require drug q 4 hours, others q 6 hours. Titrate dose based on response and blood levels.
• When changing administration route, alter dosage to compensate for variations in quinidine base content.
• Decrease dosage in patients with heart failure and hepatic disease.
• Monitor ECG, especially when administering large doses of drug. Quinidine-induced cardiotoxicity is evidenced by conduction defects (50% widening of the QRS complex), ventricular tachycardia or flutter, frequent PVCs, and complete AV block. When these ECG signs appear, discontinue drug and monitor patient closely.
• Monitor liver function test results during first 4 to 8 weeks of therapy.
• Drug may increase toxicity of cardiac glycoside derivatives. Use cautiously in patients receiving cardiac glycosides. Monitor digoxin levels and expect to reduce dosage of cardiac glycoside derivatives (many health care providers recom-

mend reducing digoxin dosage by 50% when quinidine therapy is initiated).
• GI adverse effects, especially diarrhea, are signs of toxicity. Check blood quinidine levels; suspect toxicity when greater than 8 μg/ml. GI symptoms may be decreased by giving drug with meals.
• Lidocaine may be effective in treating quinidine-induced arrhythmias because it increases AV conduction.
• Quinidine may cause hemolysis in patients with G6PD deficiency.
• Hemodialysis removes a small amount of quinidine; peritoneal dialysis doesn't remove any.
• Amount of quinidine in the various salt forms varies as follows:
Gluconate: 62% quinidine (324 mg gluconate, 202 mg sulfate).
Polygalacturonate: 60% quinidine (275 mg polygalacturonate, 166 mg sulfate).
Sulfate: 83% quinidine. The sulfate form is considered the standard dosage preparation.
• Quinidine gluconate is reported to be as or more active in vitro against *Plasmodium falciparum* than quinine dihydrochloride. Because the latter drug is only available through the CDC, quinidine gluconate may be useful in the treatment of severe malaria when delay of therapy may be life-threatening. Follow up treatment with either tetracycline or sulfadoxine and pyrimethamine.

Patient education

• Instruct patient to report rash, fever, unusual bleeding, bruising, ringing in ears, or visual disturbance.

Overdose & treatment

• The most serious signs and symptoms of overdose include severe hypotension, ventricular arrhythmias (including torsades de pointes), and seizures. QRS complexes and QT and PR intervals may be prolonged, and ataxia, anuria, respiratory distress, irritability, and hallucinations may develop.
• If ingestion was recent, perform gastric lavage, induce vomiting, or administer activated charcoal to decrease absorption. Urine acidification may be used to help increase quinidine elimination.

Treatment involves general supportive measures (including CV and respiratory support) with hemodynamic and ECG monitoring. Metaraminol or norepinephrine may be used to reverse hypotension (after ensuring adequate hydration). CNS depressants should be avoided because CNS depression may occur, possibly with seizures. Cardiac pacing may be necessary. Isoproterenol or ventricular pacing possibly may be used to treat torsades de pointes tachycardia. I.V. infusion of 1/6 M sodium lactate solution reduces the cardiotoxic effect of quinidine. Hemodialysis, although rarely warranted, also may be effective.

quinine sulfate

Cinchona alkaloid, antimalarial

Available by prescription only
Tablets: 260 mg, 325 mg
Capsules: 260 mg

INDICATIONS & DOSAGE
Malaria (chloroquine-resistant)
Adults: 650 mg P.O. q 8 hours for 10 days, with 25 mg pyrimethamine q 12 hours for 3 days and 500 mg sulfadiazine q.i.d. for 5 days.
Babesia microti *infections*
Adults: 650 mg P.O. q 6 to 8 hours for 7 days.
◇ *Nocturnal recumbency leg muscle cramps*
Adults: 200 to 300 mg P.O. h.s. Discontinue if leg cramps don't occur after several days to determine if continued therapy is necessary.

PHARMACODYNAMICS
Antimalarial action: Quinine intercalates into DNA, disrupting replication and transcription of the parasite; drug also depresses its oxygen uptake and carbohydrate metabolism. It's active against the asexual erythrocytic forms of *Plasmodium falciparum, P. malariae,* and *P. ovale* and is used for chloroquine-resistant malaria.
Skeletal muscle relaxant action: Quinine increases the refractory period, decreases excitability of the motor end plate, and affects calcium distribution within muscle fibers.

PHARMACOKINETICS
Absorption: Quinine is almost completely absorbed; serum levels peak at 1 to 3 hours.
Distribution: Drug is distributed widely into the liver, lungs, kidneys, and spleen; CSF levels reach 2% to 5% of serum levels. Drug is about 70% bound to plasma proteins.
Metabolism: Drug is metabolized in the liver.
Excretion: Less than 5% of a single dose is excreted unchanged in urine; small amounts of metabolites appear in feces, gastric juice, bile, and saliva. Half-life is 7 to 21 hours in healthy patients or convalescents, longer in patients with malaria. Urine acidification hastens elimination.

CONTRAINDICATIONS & PRECAUTIONS
Contraindicated in patients with known hypersensitivity to quinine, G6PD deficiency, optic neuritis, tinnitus, or history of blackwater fever or thrombocytopenic purpura associated with previous quinine ingestion.

Use cautiously in patients with arrhythmias and in those taking sodium bicarbonate.

INTERACTIONS
Drug-drug. Use with *acetazolamide* or *sodium bicarbonate* may increase level of quinine by decreasing urine excretion. Use with *aluminum-containing antacids* may delay or decrease absorption of quinine. Quinine may increase plasma levels of *digitoxin* and *digoxin*. Use with *mefloquine* may cause additive adverse cardiac effects. Drug may potentiate the effects of *neuromuscular blockers*. Drug may potentiate the action of *warfarin* by depressing synthesis of vitamin K–dependent clotting factors.

ADVERSE REACTIONS
CNS: severe headache, apprehension, excitement, confusion, delirium, vertigo, syncope, hypothermia, *seizures.*
CV: hypotension, *CV collapse,* conduction disturbances, flushing.

Reactions may be *common,* uncommon, *life-threatening,* or COMMON AND LIFE-THREATENING.

EENT: altered color perception, photophobia, blurred vision, night blindness, amblyopia, scotoma, diplopia, mydriasis, optic atrophy, tinnitus, impaired hearing.
GI: epigastric distress, diarrhea, nausea, vomiting.
GU: renal tubular damage, anuria.
Hematologic: *hemolytic anemia, thrombocytopenia, agranulocytosis,* hypoprothrombinemia, thrombosis at infusion site.
Metabolic: hypoglycemia.
Respiratory: asthma, dyspnea.
Skin: rash, pruritus.
Other: fever, facial edema.

▣ KEY CONSIDERATIONS

• Use with caution in geriatric patients with conduction disturbances.
• Administer quinine after meals to minimize gastric distress; don't crush tablets because drug irritates gastric mucosa.
• Discontinue drug if signs of hypersensitivity or toxicity occur.
• Serum levels of 10 µg/ml or more may confirm toxicity as the cause of tinnitus or hearing loss.
• Drug is no longer used for acute malarial attack by *P. vivax* or for suppression of malaria from resistant organisms.
• Drug may falsely elevate urine catecholamine levels and may interfere with 17-hydroxycorticosteroid and 17-ketogenic steroid tests.

Patient education

• Teach patient about adverse reactions and the need to report them immediately—especially tinnitus and hearing impairment.
• Tell patient to avoid use with aluminum-containing antacids because these may alter drug absorption.
• Instruct patient to keep drug out of reach of children.

Overdose & treatment

• Signs and symptoms of overdose include tinnitus, vertigo, headache, fever, rash, CV effects, GI distress (including vomiting), blindness, apprehension, confusion, and seizures.
• Treatment includes gastric lavage followed by supportive measures, which may include fluid and electrolyte replacement, artificial respiration, and stabilization of blood pressure and renal function. Anaphylactic reactions may require epinephrine, corticosteroids, or antihistamines. Urine acidification may increase elimination of quinine but will also augment renal obstruction. Hemodialysis or hemoperfusion may be helpful. Vasodilator therapy or stellate blockage may relieve visual disturbances.

rabies immune globulin, human (RIG)
Hyperab, Imogam Rabies Immune Globulin

Immune serum, rabies prophylaxis

Available by prescription only
Injection: 150 IU/ml in 2-ml and 10-ml vials

INDICATIONS & DOSAGE
Rabies exposure
Adults: 20 IU/kg at time of first dose of rabies vaccine. Use half of dose to infiltrate wound area. Give remainder I.M. (gluteal area preferred). Don't give rabies vaccine and RIG in same syringe or at same site.

PHARMACODYNAMICS
Postexposure rabies prophylaxis: RIG provides passive immunity to rabies.

PHARMACOKINETICS
Absorption: After slow I.M. absorption, rabies antibody appears in serum within 24 hours and peaks within 2 to 13 days.
Distribution: Unknown.
Metabolism: Unknown.
Excretion: Serum half-life for rabies antibody titer is about 24 days.

CONTRAINDICATIONS & PRECAUTIONS
Don't give repeated doses once vaccine treatment has been started.

Use cautiously in patients with immunoglobulin A deficiency or history of systemic allergic reactions after administration of human immunoglobulin preparations and in those with known hypersensitivity to thimerosal.

INTERACTIONS
Drug-drug. Antirabies serum may partially suppress the antibody response to rabies vaccine; use only the recommended dose of *antirabies vaccine*. Use with *corticosteroids* and *immunosuppressants* may interfere with the immune response to RIG; when possible, avoid using these drugs during the postexposure immunization period. RIG may interfere with the immune response to *live virus vaccine*, such as *measles, mumps,* and *rubella*; don't administer live virus vaccines within 3 months after administration of RIG.

ADVERSE REACTIONS
CNS: pain.
GU: *nephrotic syndrome.*
Skin: *rash,* redness, induration at injection site.
Other: slight fever, *anaphylaxis, angioedema.*

▣ KEY CONSIDERATIONS
• Obtain a thorough history of the animal bite, allergies, and reactions to immunizations.
• Epinephrine solution 1:1,000 should be available to treat allergic reactions.
• Repeated doses of RIG shouldn't be given after rabies vaccine is started.
• Don't administer more than 5 ml I.M. at one injection site; divide I.M. doses exceeding 5 ml and administer them at different sites.
• Don't confuse drug with rabies vaccine, which is a suspension of attenuated or killed microorganisms used to confer active immunity. These two drugs are commonly given together prophylactically after exposure to known or suspected rabid animals.
• Ask patient when he received his last tetanus immunization; a booster may be indicated.
• Patients previously immunized with a tissue culture–derived rabies vaccine and those who have confirmed adequate rabies antibody titers should receive only the vaccine.
• Drug hasn't been associated with an increased frequency of AIDS. The immune globulin is devoid of HIV. Immune globulin recipients don't develop antibodies to HIV.
• Store between 36° F to 46° F (2° C to 8° C). Don't freeze.

Patient education
• Explain that about 1 week is needed to develop immunity to rabies after vaccine is administered; therefore, patients receive RIG to provide antibodies in their blood for immediate protection against rabies.
• Inform patient that reactions to antirabies serum may occur up to 12 days after administration; patient should report skin changes, difficulty breathing, or headache.
• Tell patient that local pain, swelling, and tenderness at injection site may occur; recommend acetaminophen to alleviate these minor effects.

rabies vaccine, adsorbed

Viral vaccine

Available by prescription only
Injection: 1-ml single-dose vial

INDICATIONS & DOSAGE
Preexposure prophylaxis rabies immunization for persons in high-risk groups
Adults: 1 ml I.M. at 0, 7, and 21 or 28 days for a total of three injections. Patients at increased risk for rabies should be checked every 6 months and given a booster vaccination—1 ml I.M. p.r.n.— to maintain adequate serum titer.
Postexposure rabies prophylaxis
Adults not previously vaccinated against rabies: 20 IU/kg human rabies immune globulin (HRIG) I.M. and five 1-ml injections of rabies vaccine, adsorbed, given I.M. one each on days 0, 3, 7, 14, and 28.
Adults previously vaccinated against rabies: Two 1-ml injections of rabies vaccine, adsorbed, given I.M. one each on days 0 and 3. Don't give HRIG.

PHARMACODYNAMICS
Vaccine action: Rabies vaccine promotes active immunity to rabies.

PHARMACOKINETICS
Absorption: Antibodies can be detected consistently in serum about 2 weeks after last injection in series. People at high risk should be retested for rabies antibody titer every 6 months.
Distribution: Unknown.
Metabolism: Unknown.
Excretion: Unknown.

CONTRAINDICATIONS & PRECAUTIONS
Contraindicated in patients with a history of life-threatening allergic reactions to previous injections of vaccine or its components, including thimerosal.

Use cautiously in patients with history of non–life-threatening allergic reactions to previous injections of vaccine or hypersensitivity to monkey proteins.

INTERACTIONS
Drug-drug. *Antimalarials, corticosteroids,* and *immunosuppressants* decrease response to rabies vaccine; don't use together.

ADVERSE REACTIONS
CNS: *headache, dizziness, fatigue,* transient pain (at injection site).
GI: *nausea, abdominal pain.*
Musculoskeletal: *myalgia,* aching of injected muscle.
Skin: erythema, pruritus (at injection site).
Other: *anaphylaxis, slight fever,* serum sickness–like reactions, swelling and mild inflammatory reaction (at injection site).

🔲 KEY CONSIDERATIONS
• Keep epinephrine 1:1,000 readily available.
• Administer I.M. into deltoid region in adults; vaccine shouldn't be administered I.D. Don't inject vaccine close to a peripheral nerve or in adipose and subcutaneous tissue.
• Vaccine is normally a light pink because of presence of phenol red in the suspension.
• Preexposure immunization should be delayed in patient with acute intercurrent illness.
• If patient experiences a serious adverse reaction to the vaccine, report it promptly to the manufacturer: Michigan Department of Public Health, (517) 335-8050 during working hours or (517) 335-9030 at other times.

Patient education
- Tell patient that pain, swelling, and itching at injection site; headache; stomach upset; or fever may occur.
- Recommend acetaminophen to alleviate headache, fever, and muscle aches.

---

rabies vaccine, human diploid cell (HDCV)
Imovax Rabies I.D. Vaccine (inactivated whole virus), Imovax Rabies Vaccine

Vaccine, viral vaccine

Available by prescription only
I.M. injection: 2.5 IU rabies antigen/ml, in single-dose vial with diluent
I.D. injection: 0.25 IU rabies antigen/dose

INDICATIONS & DOSAGE
Preexposure prophylaxis immunization for persons in high-risk groups
Adults: Three 0.1-ml injections I.D. or three 1-ml injections I.M. Give first dose day 0 (1st day vaccination), second dose day 7, and third dose either day 21 or 28.
Booster: Patients exposed to rabies virus at their workplace should have antibody titers checked q 6 months. Those persons with continued risk of exposure should have antibody titers checked q 2 years. When titers are inadequate, administer a booster dose.
Primary postexposure dosage
Adults: Five 1-ml doses I.M. on each of days 3, 7, 14, and 28 (in conjunction with rabies immune globulin day 0). A sixth dose may be given on day 90. For patients who previously received the full HDCV vaccination regimen or who have demonstrated rabies antibody, give two 1-ml doses I.M. Give first dose day 0 and second dose 3 days later. Rabies immune globulin shouldn't be given.

PHARMACODYNAMICS
Rabies prophylaxis action: Vaccine promotes active immunity to rabies.

PHARMACOKINETICS
Absorption: After I.D. injection, rabies antibodies appear in serum within 7 to 10 days and peak at 30 to 60 days. Vaccine-induced immunity persists for about 1 year.
Distribution: Unknown.
Metabolism: Unknown.
Excretion: Unknown.

CONTRAINDICATIONS & PRECAUTIONS
No contraindications reported for persons after exposure. An acute febrile illness contraindicates use of vaccine for persons previously exposed. Use cautiously in patients with history of hypersensitivity.

INTERACTIONS
Drug-drug. Use of rabies vaccine with *corticosteroids* or *immunosuppressants* may interfere with the development of active immunity to rabies vaccine; avoid its use in this situation when possible.

ADVERSE REACTIONS
CNS: *headache,* dizziness, *pain (at injection site), fatigue.*
GI: *nausea,* abdominal pain, diarrhea.
Musculoskeletal: muscle aches.
Skin: *erythema, pruritus* (at injection site).
Other: *anaphylaxis,* fever, serum sickness, *swelling (at injection site).*

▣ KEY CONSIDERATIONS
- I.D. form is for preexposure use only.
- Obtain a thorough history of allergies, especially to antibiotics, and reactions to immunizations.
- Epinephrine solution 1:1,000 should be available to treat allergic reactions.
- I.M. injections should be administered in the deltoid or outer upper quadrant of the gluteus muscle in adults.
- Reconstitute with diluent provided. Gently shake vial until vaccine is completely dissolved.
- Store vaccine at 36° F to 46° F (2° C to 8° C). Don't freeze.

Patient education
- Tell patient that headache, stomach upset, and fever and pain, swelling, and itching at injection site may occur after vaccination.
- Recommend acetaminophen to alleviate headache, fever, and muscle aches.

Reactions may be *common,* uncommon, *life-threatening,* or COMMON AND LIFE-THREATENING.

raloxifene hydrochloride
Evista

Selective estrogen receptor modulator, antiosteoporotic drug

Available by prescription only
Tablets: 60 mg

INDICATIONS & DOSAGE
Prevention of osteoporosis in post-menopausal women
Adults: One 60-mg tablet P.O. once daily.

PHARMACODYNAMICS
Antiosteoporotic action: Raloxifene decreases bone turnover and reduces bone resorption. These effects are evident in reduced serum and urine levels of bone turnover markers and increased bone mineral density. Biological actions are mediated through binding to estrogen receptors, resulting in differential expression of multiple estrogen-regulated genes in different tissues.

PHARMACOKINETICS
Absorption: Raloxifene is rapidly absorbed. Peak levels depend on systemic interconversion and enterohepatic cycling of drug and its metabolites. After oral administration, about 60% of raloxifene is absorbed. Due to extensive presystemic glucuronide conjugation, absolute bioavailability is 2%.
Distribution: Apparent volume of distribution is 2,348 L/kg and doesn't depend on dose. Drug is highly bound to plasma proteins, both albumin and alpha-1 acid glycoprotein, but doesn't appear to interact with the binding of warfarin, phenytoin, or tamoxifen to plasma proteins.
Metabolism: Drug undergoes extensive first-pass metabolism to glucuronide conjugates.
Excretion: Drug is primarily excreted in feces, with less than 6% of dose eliminated as glucuronide conjugates in urine. Less than 0.2% of dose is excreted unchanged in urine.

CONTRAINDICATIONS & PRECAUTIONS
Contraindicated in patients hypersensitive to raloxifene or its components. Also contraindicated in women with history of or current venous thromboembolic events, including pulmonary embolism, retinal vein thrombosis, and deep vein thrombosis. Use of drug with hormone replacement therapy or systemic estrogen hasn't been evaluated and therefore isn't recommended.

Use with caution in patients with severe hepatic impairment.

INTERACTIONS
Drug-drug. *Ampicillin* may decrease absorption of raloxifene by up to 14%. Although raloxifene is highly protein-bound, it doesn't appear to affect the pharmacokinetics of digoxin, phenytoin, tamoxifen, or warfarin. *Cholestyramine* significantly reduces raloxifene absorption; don't use together. Use caution when administering raloxifene with *other highly protein-bound drugs (clofibrate, diazepam, diazoxide, ibuprofen, indomethacin, naproxen)*. Administration with *warfarin* causes a decrease in PT; monitor PT and INR.

ADVERSE REACTIONS
CNS: depression, insomnia, migraine.
CV: *hot flashes,* chest pain.
EENT: *sinusitis,* pharyngitis, laryngitis.
GI: nausea, dyspepsia, vomiting, flatulance, GI disorder, gastroenteritis, abdominal pain.
GU: vaginitis, urinary tract infection, cystitis, leukorrhea, endometrial disorder, vaginal bleeding, breast pain.
Hematologic: decreased platelet count.
Metabolic: weight gain; hypocalcemia; decreased inorganic phosphate, total protein, and albumin levels.
Musculoskeletal: *arthralgia,* myalgia, arthritis, leg cramps.
Respiratory: cough, pneumonia.
Skin: rash, sweating.
Other: *infection, flulike syndrome,* fever, peripheral edema.

▣ KEY CONSIDERATIONS
• The greatest risk of thromboembolic events (deep-vein thrombosis, pulmonary embolism, retinal vein thrombo-

sis) occurs during first 4 months of treatment.
• Discontinue raloxifene at least 72 hours before prolonged immobilization.
• Endometrial proliferation hasn't been associated with drug use. Evaluate unexplained uterine bleeding.
• No association between breast enlargement, breast pain, or increased risk of breast cancer has been shown. Evaluate breast abnormalities that occur during treatment.
• Safety and efficacy haven't been evaluated in men.
• Effect on bone mineral density beyond 2 years of drug treatment is unknown.
• Drug therapy causes increased apolipoprotein A1 levels and reduced serum total cholesterol, low-density lipoprotein cholesterol, fibrinogen, apolipoprotein B, and lipoprotein (a) levels. No effect on high-density lipoprotein or triglyceride levels has been shown.
• Drug modestly increases hormone-binding globulin levels.

Patient education
• Tell patient to avoid long periods of restricted movement (such as during travel) because the risk of venous thromboembolic events (such as deep-vein thrombosis and pulmonary embolism) increases.
• Inform patient that hot flashes or flushing may occur and won't disappear with raloxifene use.
• Tell patient to take supplemental calcium and vitamin D if dietary intake is inadequate.
• Encourage patient to perform weight-bearing exercises.
• Advise patient to stop alcohol consumption and smoking.
• Tell patient that drug may be taken without regard for food.
• Drug may be taken with antacids.

ramipril
Altace

ACE inhibitor, antihypertensive

Available by prescription only
Capsules: 1.25 mg, 2.5 mg, 5 mg, 10 mg

INDICATIONS & DOSAGE
Treatment of hypertension either alone or with thiazide diuretics
Adults: Initially, 2.5 mg P.O. daily in patients not receiving diuretic therapy. Adjust dose based on blood pressure response. Usual maintenance dosage is 2.5 to 20 mg daily as a single dose or in two equal doses.

In patients receiving diuretic therapy, symptomatic hypotension may occur. To minimize this, discontinue diuretic, if possible, 2 to 3 days before starting ramipril. When this isn't possible, initial dose of ramipril should be 1.25 mg.
✦ *Dosage adjustment.* In renally impaired patients with creatinine clearance less than 40 ml/minute (serum creatinine level greater than 2.5 mg/dl), recommended initial dosage is 1.25 mg daily, adjusted upward to maximum dose of 5 mg based on blood pressure response.
Heart failure post-MI
Adults: Initially, 2.5 mg P.O. b.i.d. Titrate to target dose of 5 mg P.O. b.i.d.

PHARMACODYNAMICS
Antihypertensive action: Ramipril and its active metabolite, ramiprilat, inhibit ACE, preventing conversion of angiotensin I to angiotensin II, a potent vasoconstrictor. Reduced formation of angiotensin II decreases peripheral arterial resistance and, in turn, decreases aldosterone secretion, sodium and water retention, and blood pressure. Ramipril also has antihypertensive activity in patients with low-renin hypertension.

PHARMACOKINETICS
Absorption: Between 50% and 60% of ramipril is absorbed after oral administration; levels peak within 1 hour. Plasma ramiprilat levels peak in 2 to 4 hours.
Distribution: Drug is 73% is serum protein-bound; ramiprilat, 56%.
Metabolism: Drug is almost completely metabolized to ramiprilat, which has six times more ACE inhibitory effects than parent drug.
Excretion: About 60% is excreted in urine; 40%, in feces. Less than 2% of dose is excreted in urine as unchanged drug.

Reactions may be *common*, uncommon, *life-threatening*, or COMMON AND LIFE-THREATENING.

CONTRAINDICATIONS & PRECAUTIONS

Contraindicated in patients with hypersensitivity to ACE inhibitors or history of angioedema related to treatment with an ACE inhibitor. Use cautiously in patients with impaired renal function.

INTERACTIONS

Drug-drug. Excessive hypotension may result with use of *diuretics;* discontinue diuretic or reduce dosage of ramipril as needed. Drug may increase serum *lithium* levels and lithium toxicity. Use with *potassium sparing diuretics* or *potassium supplements* may result in hyperkalemia.

Drug-food. *Sodium substitutes containing potassium* may contribute to hyperkalemia.

Drug-lifestyle. *Sun exposure* may increase the risk of photosensitivity reactions.

ADVERSE REACTIONS

CNS: asthenia, dizziness, fatigue, headache, malaise, light-headedness, anxiety, amnesia, *seizures,* depression, insomnia, nervousness, neuralgia, neuropathy, paresthesia, somnolence, tremor, vertigo.

CV: orthostatic hypotension, syncope, angina, *arrhythmias, MI,* chest pain, palpitations, edema.

EENT: epistaxis, tinnitus.

GI: nausea, vomiting, abdominal pain, anorexia, constipation, diarrhea, dyspepsia, dry mouth, gastroenteritis.

GU: impotence, transient increases in BUN and creatinine levels.

Hematologic: *hemolytic anemia, pancytopenia, neutropenia, thrombocytopenia.*

Hepatic: elevated liver enzyme, serum bilirubin, and uric acid levels; *hepatitis.*

Metabolic: hyperglycemia, hyperkalemia, weight gain.

Musculoskeletal: arthralgia, arthritis, myalgia.

Respiratory: *dry, persistent, tickling, nonproductive cough;* dyspnea.

Skin: hypersensitivity reactions, rash, dermatitis, pruritus, photosensitivity, diaphoresis.

Other: *angioedema.*

▣ KEY CONSIDERATIONS

● Diuretic therapy should be discontinued 2 to 3 days before starting ramipril therapy, if possible, to decrease potential for excessive hypotensive response.

● Like other ACE inhibitors, drug may cause a dry, persistent, tickling, nonproductive cough that's reversible when drug is stopped.

● Assess renal and hepatic function before and periodically throughout therapy.

● Monitor serum potassium levels.

Patient education

● Tell patient to report signs or symptoms of angioedema immediately: swelling of face, eyes, lips, or tongue or difficulty breathing. Tell patient to stop taking ramipril and seek medical attention.

● Warn patient that light-headedness can occur, especially during first few days of therapy. Tell him to change positions slowly to reduce hypotensive effect and to report these symptoms. If syncope occurs, instruct patient to stop drug and call immediately.

● Warn patient that inadequate fluid intake, vomiting, diarrhea, or excessive perspiration can lead to light-headedness and syncope. Advise caution in excessive heat and during exercise.

● Tell patient to avoid using sodium substitutes containing potassium unless instructed.

● Tell patient to immediately report signs or symptoms of infection, such as sore throat or fever.

ranitidine

Zantac, Zantac 75, Zantac
EFFERdose, Zantac GELdose

H₂-receptor antagonist, antiulcerative

Available by prescription only
Tablets: 150 mg, 300 mg
Tablets (effervescent): 150 mg
Capsules: 150 mg, 300 mg
Granules (effervescent): 150 mg
Injection: 25 mg/ml
Injection (premixed): 50 mg/50 ml, 50 mg/100 ml

Syrup: 15 mg/ml
Available without prescription
Tablets: 75 mg

INDICATIONS & DOSAGE

Duodenal and gastric ulcer (short-term treatment); pathological hypersecretory conditions such as Zollinger-Ellison syndrome
Adults: 150 mg P.O. b.i.d. or 300 mg h.s.
Dosages up to 6 g/day may be given to patients with Zollinger-Ellison syndrome. May give drug parenterally, 50 mg I.V. or I.M. q 6 to 8 hours.
Maintenance therapy in duodenal ulcer
Adults: 150 mg P.O. h.s.
Prophylaxis of gastric ulcer
Adults: Continuous I.V. infusion of 150 mg/250 ml compatible solution delivered at a rate of 6.25 mg/hour using an infusion pump.
Gastroesophageal reflux disease
Adults: 150 mg P.O. b.i.d.
Erosive esophagitis
Adults: 150 mg or 10 ml (2 tsp equivalent to 150 mg ranitidine) P.O. q.i.d.
Self-medication for relief of occasional heartburn, acid indigestion, and sour stomach
Adults: 75 mg once daily or b.i.d.; maximum daily dose, 150 mg.

PHARMACODYNAMICS

Antiulcerative action: Ranitidine competitively inhibits histamine's action at H_2-receptors in gastric parietal cells. This reduces basal and nocturnal gastric acid secretion as well as that caused by histamine, food, amino acids, insulin, and pentagastrin.

PHARMACOKINETICS

Absorption: 50% to 60% of oral dose is absorbed; food doesn't significantly affect absorption. After I.M. injection, ranitidine is absorbed rapidly from parenteral sites.
Distribution: Drug is distributed to many body tissues and appears in CSF; 10% to 19% is protein-bound.
Metabolism: Drug is metabolized in the liver.
Excretion: Drug is excreted in urine and feces; half-life is 2 to 3 hours.

CONTRAINDICATIONS & PRECAUTIONS

Contraindicated in patients hypersensitive to ranitidine or in those with history of acute porphyria.
Use cautiously in patients with impaired renal or hepatic function.

INTERACTIONS

Drug-drug. *Antacids* decrease ranitidine absorption; separate drugs by at least 1 hour. Use with *diazepam* decreases absorption of diazepam. Use with *glipizide* may increase hypoglycemic effect; dosage adjustment of glipizide may be necessary. Drug may decrease renal clearance of *procainamide* and may interfere with clearance of *warfarin*.

ADVERSE REACTIONS

CNS: malaise, vertigo.
EENT: blurred vision.
GU: increased serum creatinine levels.
Hematologic: *reversible leukopenia, pancytopenia, granulocytopenia, thrombocytopenia.*
Hepatic: elevated liver enzyme levels, jaundice.
Skin: pruritus (at injection site).
Other: burning (at injection site), *anaphylaxis,* angioneurotic edema.

▣ KEY CONSIDERATIONS

● Geriatric patients may experience more adverse reactions because of reduced renal clearance. Debilitated patients may experience reversible confusion, agitation, depression, and hallucinations.
● When administering I.V. push, dilute to total volume of 20 ml and inject over 5 minutes. Dilution is unnecessary when administering I.M. Drug may also be administered by intermittent I.V. infusion. Dilute 50 mg ranitidine in 100 ml D_5W and infuse over 15 to 20 minutes.
● Dosage adjustment may be required in patients with impaired renal function.
● Dialysis removes drug; administer drug after treatment.
● Drug may cause false-positive results in urine protein tests using Multistix.

Patient education

● Instruct patient to take ranitidine as directed, even after pain subsides, to ensure proper healing.

Reactions may be *common*, uncommon, *life-threatening*, or COMMON AND LIFE-THREATENING.

- Advise patient taking a single daily dose to take it at bedtime.
- Instruct patient not to take OTC preparations continuously for longer than 2 weeks without medical supervision.
- Tell patient to swallow the oral drug whole with water.

ranitidine bismuth citrate
Tritec

H₂-receptor antagonist, antimicrobial, antiulcerative

Available by prescription only
Tablets: 400 mg

INDICATIONS & DOSAGE
Treatment with clarithromycin for active duodenal ulcer caused by Helicobacter pylori *infection*
Adults: 400 mg P.O. b.i.d for 28 days in conjunction with clarithromycin, 500 mg P.O. t.i.d. for first 14 days.

PHARMACODYNAMICS
Antiulcerative action: Ranitidine reduces gastric acid secretion by competitively inhibiting histamine at the H₂-receptor of the gastric parietal cells. Bismuth is a topical drug that disrupts the integrity of bacterial cell walls, prevents adhesion of *H. pylori* to gastric epithelium, decreases the development of resistance, and inhibits urease, phospholipase, and proteolytic activities of *H. pylori*.

PHARMACOKINETICS
Absorption: Ranitidine bismuth citrate dissociates to ranitidine and bismuth after ingestion. Mean plasma ranitidine levels peak within ½ to 5 hours. Oral bioavailability of bismuth is variable; mean plasma level peaks 15 to 60 minutes after 400-mg dose.
Distribution: Volume of distribution of ranitidine is 1.7 L/kg. Ranitidine and bismuth are 15% and 98% protein-bound, respectively.
Metabolism: Drug is metabolized in the liver. It's unknown if bismuth undergoes biotransformation.
Excretion: Ranitidine is primarily eliminated from the kidneys; elimination half-

life is about 3 hours. Although bismuth is excreted primarily in feces, a small amount is excreted in bile and urine; terminal elimination half-life is 11 to 28 days.

CONTRAINDICATIONS & PRECAUTIONS
Contraindicated in patients with known hypersensitivity to ranitidine bismuth citrate or its components.

INTERACTIONS
Drug-drug. Drug shouldn't be used with *clarithromycin* in patients with history of acute porphyria; this combination isn't recommended in patients with creatinine clearance less than 25 ml/minute. Use with *diazepam* may decrease diazepam absorption; stagger administration times. Ranitidine may increase hypoglycemic effects of *glipizide*. Administration with *high-dose antacids* (170 mEq) may decrease plasma levels of ranitidine and bismuth. Ranitidine may increase plasma levels of *procainamide*. Use with *warfarin* may increase the hypoprothrombinemic effects of warfarin.

ADVERSE REACTIONS
CNS: headache.
GI: constipation, diarrhea.

▣ KEY CONSIDERATIONS
- Serum ranitidine bismuth citrate levels may be increased in geriatric patients.
- Drug shouldn't be prescribed alone for treatment of active duodenal ulcers.
- If drug therapy in combination with clarithromycin isn't successful, patient is considered to have clarithromycin-resistant *H. pylori* and shouldn't be retreated with another regimen containing clarithromycin.
- Dialysis removes ranitidine; administer drug after treatment.
- Drug may cause false-positive results in urine protein tests using Multistix; test with sulfosalicylic acid if necessary.

Patient education
- Inform patient that ranitidine bismuth citrate may be administered without regard to food.
- Instruct patient to take drug as directed, even after pain subsides.

• Tell patient it's important to take clarithromycin with drug for specified length of time.

• Inform patient that temporary and harmless darkening of the tongue or stool may occur with drug use.

---

repaglinide
Prandin

Meglitinide, antidiabetic

Available by prescription only
Tablets: 0.5 mg, 1 mg, 2 mg

INDICATIONS & DOSAGE
Adjunct to diet and exercise in reducing blood glucose levels in patients with type 2 diabetes mellitus that isn't controlled by diet and exercise alone
Adults: For patients not previously treated with an antidiabetic or for patients with hemoglobin A_{1c} (HbA_{1c}) levels less than 8%, starting dose is 0.5 mg P.O. with each meal given 15 minutes before meal; however, time may vary from immediately before to as long as 30 minutes before meal. For patients previously treated with glucose-reducing drugs with HbA_{1c} levels of 8% or more, initial dosage is 1 to 2 mg P.O. with each meal. Recommended dosage range is 0.5 to 4 mg with meals b.i.d., t.i.d., or q.i.d. Maximum daily dose is 16 mg.

Dosage should be determined by blood glucose response. Dosage may be doubled up to 4 mg with each meal until satisfactory blood glucose response is achieved. At least 1 week should elapse between dosage adjustments to assess response to each dose.

Metformin may be added if repaglinide monotherapy is inadequate.

PHARMACODYNAMICS
Antidiabetic action: Repaglinide stimulates the release of insulin from pancreatic beta cells. Drug closes adenosine triphosphate–dependent potassium channels in the beta cell membrane, which causes depolarization of the beta cell and opening of the calcium channels. The increased calcium influx induces insulin

secretion; the overall effect is to reduce the blood glucose level.

PHARMACOKINETICS
Absorption: Repaglinide is rapidly and completely absorbed with oral administration; plasma levels peak within 1 hour.
Distribution: Mean volume of distribution after I.V. administration is 31 L; protein-binding to albumin exceeds 98%.
Metabolism: Drug is completely metabolized by oxidative biotransformation and conjugation with glucuronic acid. The cytochrome P-450 (CYP) isoenzyme system (specifically, CYP 3A4) is also involved in N-dealkylation of drug. Because all metabolites are inactive, they don't help lower the blood glucose level.
Excretion: About 90% of dose appears in feces as metabolites; about 8% of dose is recovered in urine as metabolites, and less than 0.1% as parent drug. Half-life is about 1 hour.

CONTRAINDICATIONS & PRECAUTIONS
Contraindicated in patients with hypersensitivity to repaglinide or its inactive ingredients and in those with type 1 diabetes mellitus or ketoacidosis.

Use cautiously in patients with hepatic insufficiency in whom reduced metabolism could cause elevated blood drug levels and hypoglycemia.

INTERACTIONS
Drug-drug. *Beta blockers, chloramphenicol, coumarins, MAO inhibitors, NSAIDs* and *other highly protein-bound drugs, probenecid, salicylates,* and *sulfonamides* may potentiate the hypoglycemic action of repaglinide. *Calcium channel blockers, corticosteroids, estrogens, isoniazid, nicotinic acid, oral phenothiazines, phenytoin, sympathomimetics, thiazides* and *other diuretics,* and *thyroid products* may produce hyperglycemia, resulting in a loss of glycemic control. Repaglinide metabolism may be inhibited by *erythromycin, ketoconazole, miconazole,* and similar *inhibitors of CYP 3A4. Inducers of CYP3A4*—such as *barbiturates, carbamazepine, rifampin,*

---

and *troglitazone*—may increase the metabolism of repaglinide.

ADVERSE REACTIONS
CNS: *headache.*
CV: chest pain, angina.
EENT: tooth disorder, rhinitis.
GI: nausea, diarrhea, constipation, vomiting, dyspepsia.
GU: urinary tract infection.
Metabolic: HYPOGLYCEMIA.
Musculoskeletal: arthralgia, back pain.
Respiratory: bronchitis, sinusitis, *upper respiratory tract infection.*

⊡ KEY CONSIDERATIONS
• Studies show no increase in the frequency or severity of hypoglycemia in geriatric patients.
• Administration of other oral antidiabetics has been associated with increased CV mortality compared with diet treatment alone. Although not specifically evaluated for repaglinide, this warning may also apply.
• Loss of glycemic control can occur during stress, such as fever, trauma, infection, or surgery. If this occurs, discontinue drug and administer insulin.
• Hypoglycemia may be difficult to recognize in geriatric patients and in those taking beta blockers.
• Use caution when increasing drug dosage in patients with impaired renal function or renal failure requiring dialysis.
• To determine minimum effective dose, monitor patient's blood glucose levels periodically.

Patient education
• Instruct patient on importance of diet and exercise.
• Discuss symptoms of hypoglycemia with patient and family.
• Monitor long-term efficacy by measuring HbA_{1c} levels every 3 months.
• Tell patient to take drug before meals, usually 15 minutes before start of meal; however, time can vary from immediately before a meal to up to 30 minutes before a meal.
• Tell patient that if a meal is skipped or an extra meal added, he should skip the dose or add an extra dose of drug for that meal.

Overdose & treatment
• Overdose causes few adverse effects other than those associated with the intended effect of reducing the patient's blood glucose level.
• Treat hypoglycemia without loss of consciousness or neurologic findings aggressively with oral glucose and dosage or meal pattern adjustments. Monitor patient closely for minimum of 24 to 48 hours because hypoglycemia may reoccur after apparent recovery. Treat severe hypoglycemia with coma, seizure, or other neurologic impairment immediately with I.V. dextrose 50% solution followed by a continuous infusion of glucose 10% solution. Carefully monitor blood glucose levels.

reteplase, recombinant
Retavase

Tissue-plasminogen activator, thrombolytic enzyme

Available by prescription only
Injection: 10.8 U (18.8 mg)/vial (supplied in kit with components for reconstitution and administration of two single-use vials)

INDICATIONS & DOSAGE
Management of acute MI
Adults: Double-bolus injection of 10 + 10 U. Give each bolus I.V. over 2 minutes. If such complications as serious bleeding or anaphylactoid reactions don't occur after first bolus, give second bolus 30 minutes after start of first bolus. Initiate treatment soon after onset of symptoms of acute MI. There's no experience with repeated courses of reteplase.

PHARMACODYNAMICS
Thrombolytic action: Reteplase catalyzes the cleavage of plasminogen to generate plasmin, which leads to fibrinolysis.

PHARMACOKINETICS
Absorption: Reteplase is given I.V.
Distribution: Drug is cleared from plasma at a rate of 250 to 450 ml/minute.
Metabolism: Drug is metabolized primarily by the liver and kidney.
Excretion: Plasma half-life is 13 to 16 minutes.

CONTRAINDICATIONS & PRECAUTIONS
Contraindicated in patients with active internal bleeding, known bleeding diathesis, history of CVA, recent intracranial or intraspinal surgery or trauma, severe uncontrolled hypertension, intracranial neoplasm, arteriovenous malformation, or aneurysm.

Use cautiously in patients with recent (within 10 days) major surgery, organ biopsy, or trauma; previous puncture of noncompressible vessels; cerebrovascular disease; recent GI or GU bleeding; hypertension (systolic pressure 180 mm Hg or more or diastolic pressure 110 mm Hg or more); likelihood of left-sided heart thrombus; subacute bacterial endocarditis; acute pericarditis; hemostatic defects; diabetic hemorrhagic retinopathy; or septic thrombophlebitis. Use cautiously in patients with other conditions in which bleeding would be difficult to manage and in those ages 75 or older.

INTERACTIONS
Drug-drug. *Heparin, oral anticoagulants, platelet inhibitors (abciximab, aspirin,* and *dipyridamole),* and *vitamin K antagonists* may increase risk of bleeding; use together cautiously.

ADVERSE REACTIONS
CNS: *intracranial hemorrhage.*
CV: *arrhythmias, cholesterol embolization.*
GI: *hemorrhage.*
GU: hematuria.
Hematologic: anemia, *bleeding tendency.*
Other: *bleeding* (at puncture site), *hemorrhage.*

◙ KEY CONSIDERATIONS
● Use cautiously in geriatric patients; risk of intracranial hemorrhage increases with age.
● Carefully monitor ECG during treatment. Coronary thrombolysis may result in arrhythmias associated with reperfusion; be prepared to treat bradycardia or ventricular irritability.
● Monitor for bleeding. Avoid I.M. injections, invasive procedures, and nonessential handling of patient. Bleeding is the most common adverse reaction and may occur internally or at external puncture sites. If local measures don't control serious bleeding, discontinue anticoagulation therapy. Withhold second bolus of reteplase.
● Drug is administered I.V. as a double-bolus injection. If bleeding or anaphylactoid reactions occur after first bolus; second bolus may be withheld.
● Reconstitute drug according to manufacturer's instructions, using items provided in the kit.
● Don't administer with other I.V. drugs through same I.V. line. Heparin and reteplase are incompatible in solution.
● Potency is expressed in terms of units specific for reteplase and not similar to other thrombolytics.
● Avoid use of noncompressible pressure sites during therapy. If an arterial puncture is needed, use an upper extremity. Apply pressure for at least 30 minutes, then apply pressure dressing. Check site frequently.
● Drug may alter coagulation study results; it remains active in vitro and can lead to degradation of fibrinogen in sample. Take precautions to prevent fibrinolytic artifacts.

Patient education
● Explain to patient and family about use and administration of reteplase.
● Tell patient to report adverse reactions, such as signs and symptoms of bleeding or allergic reaction, immediately.
● Advise patient about proper dental care to avoid excessive gum trauma.

Reactions may be *common,* uncommon, *life-threatening,* OR COMMON AND LIFE-THREATENING.

riboflavin (vitamin B₂)

Water-soluble vitamin, vitamin B complex vitamin

Available without prescription
Tablets: 10 mg, 25 mg, 50 mg, 100 mg, 250 mg

INDICATIONS & DOSAGE

Riboflavin deficiency or adjunct to thiamine treatment for polyneuritis or cheilosis secondary to pellagra
Adults: 5 to 30 mg P.O. daily, depending on severity.
Microcytic anemia associated with splenomegaly and glutathione reductase deficiency
Adults: 10 mg P.O. daily for 10 days.
Dietary supplementation
Adults: 1 to 4 mg P.O. daily. For maintenance, increase nutritional intake and supplement with vitamin B complex.

PHARMACODYNAMICS

Metabolic action: Riboflavin, a coenzyme, functions in the forms of flavin adenine dinucleotide (FAD) and flavin mononucleotide (FMN) and has a vital metabolic role in numerous tissue respiration systems. FAD and FMN act as hydrogen-carrier molecules for several flavoproteins involved in intermediary metabolism. Riboflavin is directly involved in maintaining erythrocyte integrity.
Vitamin replacement action: Administration of riboflavin reverses riboflavin deficiency. Signs and symptoms—cheilosis, angular stomatitis, glossitis, keratitis, scrotal skin changes, ocular changes, and seborrheic dermatitis—generally become evident after 3 to 8 months of inadequate riboflavin intake. In severe deficiency, normochromic normocytic anemia and neuropathy may occur. Riboflavin deficiency rarely occurs alone and is commonly associated with deficiency of other B vitamins and protein.

PHARMACOKINETICS

Absorption: Although riboflavin is absorbed readily from the GI tract, extent of absorption is limited. Absorption occurs at a specialized segment of the mucosa and is limited by duration of drug's contact with this area. Before absorption, riboflavin-5-phosphate is rapidly dephosphorylated in the GI lumen. GI absorption increases when drug is administered with food and decreases when hepatitis, cirrhosis, biliary obstruction, or probenecid administration is present.
Distribution: FAD and FMN are distributed widely to body tissues. Free riboflavin is present in the retina. Riboflavin is stored in limited amounts in the liver, spleen, kidneys, and heart, mainly in the form of FAD. FAD and FMN are about 60% protein-bound in blood.
Metabolism: Drug is metabolized to FMN in erythrocytes, GI mucosal cells, and the liver; FMN is converted to FAD in the liver.
Excretion: After a single oral dose, biological half-life is about 66 to 84 minutes in healthy individuals. About 9% of drug is excreted unchanged in urine after normal ingestion. Excretion involves renal tubular secretion and glomerular filtration. Amount renally excreted unchanged is directly proportional to dose. Drug removal by hemodialysis is slower than by natural renal excretion.

CONTRAINDICATIONS & PRECAUTIONS

No known contraindications.

INTERACTIONS

Drug-drug. Use with *propantheline bromide* delays absorption rate of riboflavin but increases total amount absorbed.
Drug-lifestyle. *Alcohol* impairs intestinal absorption of riboflavin.

ADVERSE REACTIONS

GU: bright yellow urine.

▣ KEY CONSIDERATIONS

• RDA of riboflavin is 1.2 to 1.7 mg/day in adults.
• Give oral preparation of riboflavin with food to increase absorption.
• Obtain dietary history because other vitamin deficiencies may coexist.
• Drug therapy alters urinalysis based on spectrophotometry or color reactions.

---

*Canada only   ◊ Unlabeled clinical use

Large doses of drug result in bright yellow urine. Riboflavin produces fluorescent substances in urine and plasma, which can falsely elevate fluorometric determinations of catecholamine and urobilinogen levels.

Patient education
• Inform patient that riboflavin may discolor urine, making it more yellow.
• Teach patient good dietary sources of riboflavin, such as whole grain cereals and green vegetables. Liver, kidney, heart, eggs, and dairy products are dietary sources but may not be appropriate, based on patient's serum cholesterol and triglyceride levels.
• Tell patient to store riboflavin in a tight, light-resistant container.

---

rifabutin
Mycobutin

Semisynthetic ansamycin, antibiotic

Available by prescription only
Capsules: 150 mg

INDICATIONS & DOSAGE
Prevention of disseminated **Mycobacterium avium** *complex disease in patients with advanced HIV infection*
Adults: 300 mg P.O. daily as a single dose or divided b.i.d. with food.

PHARMACODYNAMICS
Antibiotic action: Rifabutin inhibits DNA-dependent RNA polymerase in susceptible strains of *Escherichia coli* and *Bacillus subtilis,* but not in mammalian cells. It's unknown whether drug inhibits this enzyme in *M. avium* or *Mycobacterium intracellulare,* which cause *M. avium* complex disease.

PHARMACOKINETICS
Absorption: Rifabutin is readily absorbed from the GI tract. Plasma levels peak 2 to 4 hours after oral dose.
Distribution: Because of its high lipophilicity, drug shows a high propensity for distribution and intracellular tissue uptake. About 85% is bound to plasma proteins.

Metabolism: Drug is metabolized in the liver to five identified metabolites. The 25-0-desacetyl metabolite has an activity equal to parent drug and contributes up to 10% of total antimicrobial activity.
Excretion: Less than 10% is excreted in urine as unchanged drug. About 53% of oral dose is excreted in urine, primarily as metabolites; about 30%, in feces.

CONTRAINDICATIONS & PRECAUTIONS
Contraindicated in patients with hypersensitivity to rifabutin or other rifamycin derivatives (such as rifampin) and in patients with active tuberculosis because single-drug therapy with rifabutin increases the risk of inducing bacterial resistance to both rifabutin and rifampin.

Use cautiously in patients with preexisting neutropenia and thrombocytopenia.

INTERACTIONS
Drug-drug. Rifabutin may decrease serum *zidovudine* levels, but rifabutin doesn't affect zidovudine's inhibition of HIV. Because rifabutin has liver enzyme-inducing properties, it may reduce serum levels of other drugs as well. Although dosage adjustments may be necessary, further study is needed.

ADVERSE REACTIONS
CNS: headache, insomnia.
GI: dyspepsia, eructation, flatulence, diarrhea, nausea, vomiting, abdominal pain, altered taste.
GU: *brown-orange urine.*
Hematologic: NEUTROPENIA, LEUKOPENIA, ***thrombocytopenia,*** eosinophilia.
Musculoskeletal: myalgia.
Skin: *rash.*
Other: fever.

▣ KEY CONSIDERATIONS
• Evaluate patient who develops symptoms consistent with active tuberculosis during rifabutin prophylaxis immediately so that active disease may be treated with an effective combination regimen of antituberculotics. Single-drug rifabutin therapy in patients with active tuberculosis likely leads to resistance to rifabutin and rifampin.

Reactions may be *common,* uncommon, *life-threatening,* or COMMON AND LIFE-THREATENING.

- Because drug may cause neutropenia and more rarely thrombocytopenia, consider obtaining hematologic studies periodically in patients receiving drug prophylaxis.
- High-fat meals slow rate but not extent of drug absorption.

Patient education
- Tell patient with difficulty swallowing to mix drug with soft foods such as applesauce.
- Advise patient with nausea, vomiting, or other GI upset to take drug with food in two divided doses.
- Warn patient that drug may discolor urine and other body fluids to brown-orange and may permanently discolor clothes and soft contact lenses.

rifampin
Rifadin, Rimactane

Semisynthetic rifamycin B derivative (macrocyclic antibiotic), antituberculotic

Available by prescription only
Capsules: 150 mg, 300 mg
Injection: 600 mg/vial

INDICATIONS & DOSAGE
Primary treatment in pulmonary tuberculosis
Adults: 600 mg P.O. or I.V. daily as single dose (give P.O. dose 1 hour before or 2 hours after meals).
Administration with other effective antituberculotics is recommended. Treatment usually lasts 6 to 9 months.
Asymptomatic meningococcal carriers
Adults: 600 mg P.O. b.i.d. for 2 days.
Prophylaxis of **Haemophilus influenzae type B**
Adults: 20 mg/kg (up to 600 mg) once daily for 4 consecutive days.
◇ *Leprosy*
Adults: 600 mg P.O. once monthly, usually with other drugs.
✦ *Dosage adjustment.* Reduce dosage in patients with hepatic dysfunction.

PHARMACODYNAMICS
Antibiotic and antituberculotic actions:
Rifampin impairs RNA synthesis by inhibiting DNA-dependent RNA polymerase. Drug may be bacteriostatic or bactericidal, depending on organism susceptibility and drug level at infection site. It acts against *Mycobacterium tuberculosis, M. bovis, M. marinum, M. kansasii,* some strains of *M. fortuitum, M. avium,* and *M. avium-intracellulare,* and many gram-positive and some gram-negative bacteria. Resistance to drug by *M. tuberculosis* can develop rapidly; drug is usually given with other antituberculotics to prevent or delay resistance.

PHARMACOKINETICS
Absorption: Rifampin is absorbed completely from the GI tract after oral administration; serum levels peak 1 to 4 hours after ingestion. Food delays absorption.
Distribution: Drug is distributed widely into body tissues and fluids, including CSF; ascitic, pleural, and seminal fluids; tears; and saliva, and into liver, prostate, lungs, and bone. Drug is 84% to 91% protein-bound.
Metabolism: Drug is metabolized extensively in the liver by deacetylation. It undergoes enterohepatic circulation.
Excretion: Drug and metabolite are excreted primarily in bile; drug, but not metabolite, is reabsorbed. From 6% to 30% of drug and metabolite appear unchanged in urine in 24 hours; about 60% excreted in feces. Plasma half-life in adults is 1½ to 5 hours; serum levels increase in obstructive jaundice. Dosage adjustment isn't necessary for patients with renal failure. Neither hemodialysis nor peritoneal dialysis remove drug.

CONTRAINDICATIONS & PRECAUTIONS
Contraindicated in patients with hypersensitivity to rifampin.
Use cautiously in patients with hepatic disease.

INTERACTIONS
Drug-drug. Rifampin-induced hepatic microsomal enzymes inactivate the following drugs: *anticoagulants, barbitu-*

rates, beta blockers, chloramphenicol, clofibrate, corticosteroids, cyclosporine, cardiac glycoside derivatives, dapsone, disopyramide, estrogens, methadone, oral sulfonylureas, phenytoin, quinidine, tocainide, and *verapamil;* decreased serum levels of those drugs require dosage adjustments. Rifampin-induced enzyme activity may accelerate metabolic conversion of *isoniazid* to hepatotoxic metabolites, increasing hazard of isoniazid hepatotoxicity. Use with *para-aminosalicylate* may decrease oral absorption of rifampin, reducing serum levels; administer drugs 8 to 12 hours apart.

Drug-food. *Food* may interfere with drug absorption; give 1 hour before or 2 hours after a meal.

Drug-lifestyle. Daily use of *alcohol* while using rifampin may increase risk of hepatotoxicity.

ADVERSE REACTIONS

CNS: headache, fatigue, drowsiness, behavioral changes, dizziness, ataxia, mental confusion, generalized numbness.
EENT: visual disturbances, exudative conjunctivitis.
GI: epigastric distress, anorexia, nausea, vomiting, abdominal pain, diarrhea, flatulence, sore mouth and tongue, pseudomembranous colitis, *pancreatitis.*
GU: hemoglobinuria, hematuria, *acute renal failure.*
Hematologic: eosinophilia, *thrombocytopenia, transient leukopenia, hemolytic anemia.*
Hepatic: *hepatotoxicity, transient abnormalities in liver function test results.*
Metabolic: hyperuricemia.
Respiratory: shortness of breath, wheezing.
Skin: pruritus, urticaria, rash.
Other: osteomalacia, flulike syndrome, discoloration of body fluids, *shock,* porphyria exacerbation.

▣ KEY CONSIDERATIONS

• Usual dose in geriatric and debilitated patients is 10 mg/kg once daily.
• Give rifampin 1 hour before or 2 hours after meals for maximum absorption; capsule contents may be mixed with food or fluid to enhance swallowing.

• Obtain specimens for culture and sensitivity testing before giving first dose but don't delay therapy; repeat periodically to detect drug resistance.
• To minimize toxicity, observe patient for adverse reactions and monitor hematologic, renal, and liver function study results and serum electrolyte levels. Watch for signs and symptoms of hepatic impairment, including anorexia, fatigue, malaise, jaundice, dark urine, and liver tenderness.
• Increased liver enzyme activity inactivates certain drugs (especially warfarin, corticosteroids, and oral antidiabetics), requiring dosage adjustments.
• Reconstituted solution is stable for 24 hours at room temperature. Infusion solutions of 100 to 500 ml should be used within 4 hours.
• Drug alters standard serum folate and vitamin B_{12} assay results.
• Drug may cause temporary retention of sulfobromophthalein in the liver excretion test; it may also interfere with contrast material in gallbladder studies and urinalysis based on spectrophotometry.

Patient education

• Explain the disease and the rationale for long-term therapy.
• Teach signs and symptoms of hypersensitivity and other adverse reactions, and emphasize need to call if these occur; urge patient to report *any* unusual reactions.
• Tell patient to take rifampin on an empty stomach, at least 1 hour before or 2 hours after a meal. If GI irritation occurs, patient may need to take drug with food.
• Urge patient to comply with prescribed regimen, not to miss doses, and not to discontinue drug without medical approval. Explain importance of follow-up appointments.
• Encourage patient to report promptly any flulike signs or symptoms, weakness, sore throat, loss of appetite, unusual bruising, rash, itching, tea-colored urine, clay-colored stools, or yellow discoloration of eyes or skin.
• Explain that drug turns all body fluids red-orange; advise patient of possible

---

Reactions may be *common,* uncommon, *life-threatening,* or COMMON AND LIFE-THREATENING.

permanent stains on clothes and soft contact lenses.

Overdose & treatment
• Signs and symptoms of overdose include lethargy, nausea, and vomiting; hepatotoxicity from massive overdose includes hepatomegaly, jaundice, elevated liver function test results and bilirubin levels, and loss of consciousness. Redorange discoloration of skin, urine, sweat, saliva, tears, and feces may occur.
• Perform gastric lavage, and then administer activated charcoal; if necessary, force diuresis. Perform bile drainage if hepatic dysfunction persists beyond 24 to 48 hours.

---

riluzole
Rilutek

Benzothiazole, neuroprotector

Available by prescription only
Tablets: 50 mg

INDICATIONS & DOSAGE
Amyotrophic lateral sclerosis (ALS)
Adults: 50 mg P.O. q 12 hours on an empty stomach.

PHARMACODYNAMICS
Neuroprotector action: It's unknown how riluzole improves signs and symptoms of ALS.

PHARMACOKINETICS
Absorption: Riluzole is well absorbed from GI tract (about 90%), with average absolute oral bioavailability of about 60%. A high-fat meal decreases absorption.
Distribution: Drug is 96% protein-bound.
Metabolism: Drug is extensively metabolized in the liver to six major and several minor metabolites, not all identified.
Excretion: Drug is excreted primarily in urine and a small amount in feces. Half-life is 12 hours with repeated doses.

CONTRAINDICATIONS & PRECAUTIONS
Contraindicated in patients with history of severe hypersensitivity reactions to riluzole or components in tablets.

Use cautiously in patients with hepatic or renal dysfunction and in geriatric patients. Also use cautiously in female and Japanese patients, who may have a lower metabolic capacity to eliminate drug compared with male and white patients, respectively.

INTERACTIONS
Drug-drug. Use cautiously with potentially *hepatotoxic drugs*—such as *allopurinol, methyldopa,* or *sulfasalazine.*

ADVERSE REACTIONS
CNS: headache, aggravation reaction, hypertonia, depression, dizziness, insomnia, somnolence, malaise, vertigo, *asthenia,* circumoral paresthesia.
CV: hypertension, tachycardia, palpitation, phlebitis, orthostatic hypotension.
EENT: rhinitis, dry mouth, sinusitis.
GI: abdominal pain, *nausea,* vomiting, dyspepsia, anorexia, diarrhea, flatulence, stomatitis, tooth disorder, oral candidiasis.
GU: urinary tract infection, dysuria.
Metabolic: weight loss.
Musculoskeletal: back pain, arthralgia.
Respiratory: *decreased lung function,* increased cough.
Skin: pruritus, eczema, alopecia, exfoliative dermatitis.
Other: peripheral edema.

◙ KEY CONSIDERATIONS
• Age-related decreased renal and hepatic function may reduce riluzole clearance; administer drug cautiously in geriatric patients.
• Baseline elevations in liver function test results (especially elevated bilirubin level) should preclude use of drug; perform liver function studies periodically during therapy. In many patients, drug may cause elevated serum aminotransferase levels; discontinue drug if levels exceed 10 times upper limit of normal range or if jaundice develops.
• Give drug at least 1 hour before or 2 hours after a meal to avoid a food-related decrease in bioavailability.

Patient education

• Tell patient or caregiver that riluzole must be taken regularly and at the same time each day. If a dose is missed, tell patient to take the next tablet as originally scheduled.

• Instruct patient to report febrile illness so that his WBC count can be checked.

• Warn patient to avoid hazardous activities until CNS effects of drug are known.

• Advise patient to avoid excessive alcohol intake while taking drug.

• Tell patient to store drug at room temperature and protect from bright light.

• Stress importance of keeping drug out of reach of children.

rimantadine hydrochloride
Flumadine

Adamantine, antiviral

Available by prescription only
Tablets: 100 mg
Syrup: 50 mg/5 ml

INDICATIONS & DOSAGE

Prophylaxis against influenza A virus
Adults: 100 mg P.O. b.i.d.
Geriatric patients in long-term care facilities: 100 mg P.O. daily is recommended.

✦ *Dosage adjustment.* For patients with severe hepatic dysfunction or renal failure (creatinine clearance 10 ml/minute or less), 100 mg P.O. daily is recommended.

Treatment of illness caused by various strains of influenza A virus
Adults: 100 mg P.O. b.i.d. for 7 days from initial onset of symptoms.
Geriatric patients in long-term care facilities: 100 mg P.O. daily is recommended.

✦ *Dosage adjustment.* For patients with severe hepatic dysfunction or renal failure (creatinine clearance 10 ml/minute or less), 100 mg P.O. daily is recommended.

PHARMACODYNAMICS

Antiviral action: Rimantadine's mechanism of action isn't fully understood. It appears to exert its inhibitory effect early in the viral replicative cycle, possibly inhibiting the uncoating of the virus. Genetic studies suggest a virus protein specified by the virion M^2 gene has an important role in the susceptibility of influenza A virus to inhibition by drug.

PHARMACOKINETICS

Absorption: Tablet and syrup formulations are equally absorbed after oral administration. Levels peak about 6 hours in an otherwise healthy adult.
Distribution: Rimantadine is about 40% plasma protein-bound.
Metabolism: Drug is extensively metabolized in the liver.
Excretion: Less than 25% of drug is excreted unchanged in urine; elimination half-life is about 25.4 to 32 hours. Hemodialysis doesn't eliminate drug.

CONTRAINDICATIONS & PRECAUTIONS

Contraindicated in patients with hypersensitivity to rimantadine or amantadine. Use cautiously in patients with impaired renal or hepatic function or seizure disorders (especially epilepsy).

INTERACTIONS

Drug-drug. Administration with *acetaminophen* reduces peak level and area under the curve for rimantadine by 11%, and administration with *aspirin* reduces values by 10%; monitor effectiveness of rimantadine. *Cimetidine* may decrease total rimantadine clearance by about 16%; monitor patient for adverse effects associated with rimantadine use.

ADVERSE REACTIONS

CNS: insomnia, headache, dizziness, nervousness, fatigue, asthenia.
GI: nausea, vomiting, anorexia, dry mouth, abdominal pain.

▣ KEY CONSIDERATIONS

• Adverse reactions associated with rimantadine are more common in geriatric patients than in patients in other age-groups; monitor these patients closely.

• For illnesses associated with various strains of influenza A, treatment should begin as soon as possible (preferably within 48 hours after onset of signs and

---

symptoms) to reduce duration of fever and systematic symptoms.

• Because of risk for drug metabolite accumulation during multiple dosing, monitor patient with renal insufficiency for adverse reactions and adjust dosage as necessary.

• An increased incidence of seizures has been observed in some patients with history of seizures who weren't taking anticonvulsants during drug therapy; if seizures develop, discontinue drug.

• Influenza A–resistant strains can emerge during therapy. Patients taking drug may still be able to spread the disease.

Patient education

• Tell patient to take rimantadine several hours before bedtime to prevent insomnia.

• Inform patient that taking drug doesn't prevent the spread of disease and he should limit contact with others until fully recovered.

• Warn patient that drug may cause adverse CNS effects; he shouldn't drive or perform activities that require mental alertness until these effects are known.

• Tell patient with history of epilepsy to stop taking drug and call if seizure activity occurs.

Overdose & treatment

• Overdose of a related drug, amantadine, has been reported; signs and symptoms include agitation, hallucinations, cardiac arrhythmia, and death.

• Administration of I.V. physostigmine (1 to 2 mg in adults, repeated as needed but not exceeding 2 mg/hour) has been reported anecdotally to benefit patients with CNS effects from overdose of amantadine.

risperidone
Risperdal

Benzisoxazole derivative, antipsychotic drug

Available by prescription only
Tablets: 1 mg, 2 mg, 3 mg, 4 mg

INDICATIONS & DOSAGE
Psychosis

Adults: Initially, 1 mg P.O. b.i.d. Increase in increments of 1 mg b.i.d. days 2 and 3 of treatment to a target dose of 3 mg b.i.d. Wait at least 1 week before adjusting dosage further. Dosages more than 6 mg/day aren't more effective than lower doses and are associated with more extrapyramidal effects.

✦ *Dosage adjustment.* Geriatric, debilitated, or hypotensive patients or those with severe renal or hepatic impairment should initially receive 0.5 mg P.O. b.i.d. Increase dosage in increments of 0.5 mg b.i.d. days 2 and 3 of treatment to a target dosage of 1.5 mg P.O. b.i.d. Wait at least 1 week before further increasing dosage.

PHARMACODYNAMICS
Antipsychotic action: Risperidone's exact mechanism of action is unknown. Activity may be mediated through a combination of dopamine type 2 (D_2) and serotonin type 2 (5-HT_2) antagonism. Antagonism at receptors other than D_2 and 5-HT_2 may explain other effects of drug.

PHARMACOKINETICS
Absorption: Risperidone is well absorbed after oral administration. Absolute oral bioavailability is 70%. Food doesn't affect rate or extent of absorption.

Distribution: Plasma protein-binding is about 90% for drug and 77% for its major active metabolite, 9-hydroxyrisperidone.

Metabolism: Drug is metabolized in the liver to 9-hydroxyrisperidone, the predominant circulating species, which appears about equally effective with risperidone in receptor-binding activity. (About 6% to 8% of whites and a low percentage of Asians show little or no receptor-binding activity and are poor metabolizers.)

Excretion: Metabolite is excreted from the kidney. Clearance of drug and its metabolite is reduced in renally impaired patients.

CONTRAINDICATIONS & PRECAUTIONS
Contraindicated in patients hypersensitive to risperidone.

Use cautiously in patients with prolonged QT interval, CV disease, cerebrovascular disease, dehydration, hypovolemia, history of seizures, or exposure to extreme heat or conditions that could affect metabolism or hemodynamic responses.

INTERACTIONS
Drug-drug. Because risperidone may induce hypotension, it may enhance the effects of certain *antihypertensives. Carbamazepine* may increase the clearance of risperidone, thereby decreasing the effectiveness of risperidone; monitor patient closely. *Clozapine* may decrease the clearance of risperidone, increasing the risk of toxicity; monitor patient closely. Risperidone may antagonize the effects of *dopamine agonists* and *levodopa.* Administration with *ethanol* and *other CNS depressants* may cause additive CNS depression; administer together with caution.

Drug-lifestyle. Use with *alcohol* causes additive CNS depression.

ADVERSE REACTIONS
CNS: *somnolence, extrapyramidal symptoms, headache, insomnia, agitation, anxiety,* tardive dyskinesia, aggressiveness.
CV: tachycardia, chest pain, orthostatic hypotension, prolonged QT interval.
EENT: *rhinitis,* sinusitis, pharyngitis, abnormal vision.
GI: *constipation, nausea, vomiting, dyspepsia.*
Metabolic: increased serum prolactin levels.
Musculoskeletal: arthralgia, back pain.
Respiratory: cough, upper respiratory tract infection.
Skin: rash, dry skin, photosensitivity.
Other: fever, *neuroleptic malignant syndrome.*

▣ KEY CONSIDERATIONS
• A lower starting dose is recommended for geriatric patients because of decreased pharmacokinetic clearance; a greater incidence of hepatic, renal, or cardiac dysfunction; and a greater tendency to orthostatic hypotension.
• Risperidone and 9-hydroxyrisperidone appear to lengthen the QT interval in some patients, although no average increase in treated patients—even in those taking 12 to 16 mg/day (well above recommended dose)—exists. Other drugs that prolong the QT interval may cause torsades de pointes, a life-threatening arrhythmia. Bradycardia, electrolyte imbalance, use with other drugs that prolong the QT interval, or congenital prolongation of the QT interval can increase the risk of occurrence of this arrhythmia.
• Drug has an antiemetic effect in animals that may occur in humans, masking signs and symptoms of overdose or of such conditions as intestinal obstruction, Reye's syndrome, and brain tumor.
• Tardive dyskinesia may occur after prolonged drug therapy. It may not appear until months or years later and may disappear spontaneously or persist for life, despite discontinuation of drug.
• Neuroleptic malignant syndrome is rare, but fatal in many cases. It isn't necessarily related to length of drug use or type of neuroleptic. Monitor patient closely for symptoms, including hyperpyrexia, muscle rigidity, altered mental status, irregular pulse, alteration in blood pressure, and diaphoresis.
• When restarting drug therapy for patients who have been off drug, follow initial 3-day dose initiation schedule.
• When switching patient from other antipsychotic drugs to risperidone, immediately discontinue other antipsychotic drug on initiation of risperidone therapy when appropriate.

Patient education
• Advise patient to rise slowly from a recumbent or seated position to minimize light-headedness.
• Warn patient not to operate hazardous machinery or drive a car until the effects of risperidone are known.
• Tell patient to call before taking new drugs, including OTC drugs, because of potential for interactions.
• Advise patient to avoid alcohol use during drug therapy.

Reactions may be *common,* uncommon, *life-threatening,* or COMMON AND LIFE-THREATENING.

Overdose & treatment

• Signs and symptoms of overdose result from an exaggeration of the known pharmacologic effects of risperidone, including drowsiness and sedation, tachycardia and hypotension, and extrapyramidal symptoms. Hyponatremia, hypokalemia, prolonged QT interval, widened QRS complex, and seizures also have been reported.

• No specific antidote to overdose exists; institute appropriate supportive measures. Consider performing gastric lavage (after intubation, if patient is unconscious) and administering activated charcoal with a laxative. CV monitoring is essential to detect possible arrhythmias. If antiarrhythmic therapy is administered, disopyramide, procainamide, and quinidine may cause QT-prolonging effects that might be additive to those of risperidone. Similarly, the bretylium's alpha-blocking properties might be additive to those of risperidone, resulting in problematic hypotension.

---

rizatriptan benzoate
Maxalt, Maxalt-MLT

Selective 5-hydroxtryptamine $_{1B/1D}$ (5-HT $_{1B/1D}$) receptor agonist, antimigraine drug

Tablets: 5 mg, 10 mg
Tablets (orally disintegrating): 5 mg, 10 mg

INDICATIONS & DOSAGE

Treatment of acute migraine headaches with or without aura
Adults: Initially, 5 or 10 mg P.O. If first dose is ineffective, another dose can be given at least 2 hours after first dose. Maximum dose is 30 mg within a 24-hour period. For patients receiving propranolol, 5 mg P.O. up to maximum of three doses (15 mg) in 24 hours.

PHARMACODYNAMICS

Antimigraine action: Rizatriptan is believed to act as an agonist at serotonin receptors on the extracerebral intracranial blood vessels, which results in vasoconstriction of the affected vessels, inhi-

bition of neuropeptide release, and reduction of pain transmission in the trigeminal pathways.

PHARMOCOKINETICS

Absorption: Rizatriptan is completely absorbed. Mean absolute bioavailability is about 45%; plasma levels peak in 1 to 1½ hours.
Distribution: A large volume of drug distributes, but only 14% binds to plasma proteins.
Metabolism: Drug is metabolized by oxidative deaminiation to an inactive metabolite.
Excretion: About 82% is recovered in urine and 12% in feces; elimination half-life is 2 to 3 hours.

CONTRAINDICATIONS & PRECAUTIONS

Contraindicated in patients with ischemic heart disease (angina pectoris, history of MI, or documented silent ischemia) or in those with symptoms or findings consistent with ischemic heart disease, coronary artery vasospasm (Prinzmetal's variant angina), or other significant underlying CV disease. Also contraindicated in patients with uncontrolled hypertension or within 24 hours of treatment with another 5-HT$_1$ agonist or an ergotamine-containing or ergot-type drug such as dihydroergotamine or methysergide. Don't use within 2 weeks of discontinuation of MAO inhibitor. Also contraindicated in patients hypersensitive to rizatriptan or its inactive ingredients.

Use cautiously in patients with hepatic or renal impairment. Use cautiously in those with risk factors for coronary artery disease—such as hypertension, hypercholesterolemia, smoking, obesity, diabetes, strong family history of coronary artery disease, women with surgical or physiological menopause, or men older than age 40—unless a cardiac evaluation provides evidence that patient is free from heart disease.

INTERACTIONS

Drug-drug. *Ergot-containing* or *ergot-type drugs (dihydroergotamine, methysergide)* and *other 5-HT$_1$ agonists* cause prolonged vasospastic reactions; don't use within 24 hours of rizatriptan. *MAO inhibitors (moclobemide* and *nonselective MAO inhibitors [types A and B; isocarboxazid, pargyline, phenelzine, tranylcypromine])* cause increased plasma levels of rizatriptan; don't use together and allow at least 14 days to elapse between discontinuation of MAO inhibitor and taking rizatriptan. *Propranolol* causes increased rizatriptan levels; reduce rizatriptan dose to 5 mg. *Selective serotonin reuptake inhibitors (fluoxetine, fluvoxamine, paroxetine, sertraline)* may cause weakness, hyperreflexia, and incoordination; monitor patient.

ADVERSE REACTIONS

CNS: dizziness, headache, somnolence, paresthesia, asthenia, fatigue, hypesthesia, decreased mental acuity, euphoria, pain, tremor.
CV: chest pain, pressure, or heaviness; flushing; palpitations.
EENT: neck, throat, and jaw pain, pressure, or heaviness.
GI: dry mouth, nausea, diarrhea, vomiting.
Respiratory: dyspnea.
Other: warm or cold sensations, hot flashes.

▣ KEY CONSIDERATIONS

• Rizatriptan is as safe and effective for use in geriatric patients as in younger patients.
• For patients with risk factors for coronary artery disease who have a satisfactory cardiac evaluation, monitor closely after first dose.
• Assess CV status in patients who develop risk factors for coronary artery disease during treatment.
• Drug should be used only after a definite diagnosis of migraine is established.
• Don't use for prophylactic therapy of migraines or in patients with hemiplegic or basilar migraine or cluster headaches.
• The safety of treating on average more than four headaches in a 30-day period hasn't been established.
• The orally disintegrating tablets contain phenylalanine.

Patient education

• Inform patient that rizatriptan doesn't prevent migraine headache from occurring.
• For Maxalt-MLT, tell patient to remove blister pack from pouch, then remove drug from blister pack immediately before use. Tablet shouldn't be popped out of blister pack, but pack should be carefully peeled away with dry hands, and tablet placed on tongue and allowed to dissolve. Tablet is then swallowed with the saliva. No water is necessary or recommended. Tell patient that orally dissolving tablet doesn't provide more rapid headache relief.
• Advise patient that if headache returns after initial dose, a second dose may be taken with medical approval at least 2 hours after the first dose. Don't take more than 30 mg in a 24-hour period.
• Inform patient that drug may cause somnolence and dizziness and warn him to avoid hazardous activities until effects are known.
• Tell patient that food may delay drug's onset of action.

---

ropinirole hydrochloride
Requip

Nonergoline dopamine agonist, antiparkinsonian

Available by prescription only
Tablets: 0.25 mg, 0.5 mg, 1 mg, 2 mg, 5 mg

INDICATIONS & DOSAGE
Treatment of idiopathic Parkinson's disease
Adults: Initially, 0.25 mg P.O. t.i.d. Based on patient response, dosage should be titrated at weekly intervals: 0.5 mg t.i.d. after week 1, 0.75 mg t.i.d. after week 2, and 1 mg t.i.d. after week 3. After week 4, dosage may be increased by 1.5 mg/day on a weekly basis up to 9 mg/day and then increased weekly by up to 3 mg/day to maximum dose of 24 mg/day.

PHARMACODYNAMICS

Antiparkinsonian action: Exact mechanism of action is unknown. Ropinirole is a nonergoline dopamine agonist thought to stimulate postsynaptic dopamine D_2 receptors within the caudate-putamen in the brain.

PHARMACOKINETICS

Absorption: Ropinirole is rapidly absorbed; levels peak in about 1 to 2 hours. Absolute bioavailability is 55%.
Distribution: Drug is widely distributed throughout the body, with an apparent volume of distribution of 7.5 L/kg; up to 40% is plasma protein-bound.
Metabolism: Drug is extensively metabolized by cytochrome P-450 1A2 (CYP 1A2) isoenzyme to inactive metabolites.
Excretion: Less than 10% of administered dose is excreted unchanged in urine; elimination half-life is 6 hours.

CONTRAINDICATIONS & PRECAUTIONS

Contraindicated in patients with known hypersensitivity to ropinirole or its components.

Use cautiously in patients with severe renal or hepatic impairment.

INTERACTIONS

Drug-drug. Administration with *ciprofloxacin* causes increased ropinirole levels. *CNS depressants (antidepressants, antipsychotic drugs, benzodiazepines)* increase CNS effects; use cautiously. Administration with *dopamine antagonists (butyrophenones, metoclopramide, phenothiazines, thioxanthenes)* may decrease the effectiveness of ropinirole. *Estrogens* reduce the clearance of ropinirole; adjust ropinirole dose if estrogens are started or stopped during ropinirole treatment. *Inhibitors or substrates of CYP 1A2 (ciprofloxacin, fluvoxamine, mexiletine, norfloxacin)* alter clearance; dosage adjustment of ropinirole may be required.
Drug-lifestyle. Use with *alcohol* increases CNS effects. *Smoking* may increase clearance of ropinirole; monitor closely.

ADVERSE REACTIONS

Early Parkinson's disease (without levodopa)—
CNS: asthenia, hallucinations, *dizziness, aggravated Parkinson's disease, somnolence, fatigue,* headache, confusion, hyperkinesia, hypesthesia, vertigo, pain, amnesia, impaired concentration, malaise.
CV: orthostatic hypotension, orthostatic symptoms, hypertension, *syncope,* edema, flushing, chest pain, extrasystoles, **atrial fibrillation,** palpitation, tachycardia.
EENT: pharyngitis, abnormal vision, eye abnormality, xerophthalmia, rhinitis, sinusitis.
GI: *nausea, vomiting, dyspepsia,* flatulence, abdominal pain, anorexia, dry mouth, abdominal pain.
GU: urinary tract infection, impotence.
Respiratory: bronchitis, dyspnea.
Skin: increased sweating.
Other: *viral infection,* yawning, peripheral ischemia.
Advanced Parkinson's disease (with levodopa)—
CNS: *dizziness,* pain, aggravated parkinsonism, *somnolence, headache,* insomnia, *hallucinations,* abnormal dreaming, confusion, tremor, *dyskinesia,* anxiety, nervousness, amnesia, hypokinesia, paresthesia, paresis.
CV: hypotension, syncope.
EENT: diplopia.
GI: *nausea,* abdominal pain, vomiting, dry mouth, constipation, diarrhea, dysphagia, flatulence, increased saliva.
GU: urinary tract infection, pyuria, urinary incontinence.
Hematologic: anemia.
Metabolic: weight loss.
Musculoskeletal: arthralgia, arthritis.
Respiratory: upper respiratory tract infection, dyspnea.
Skin: increased sweating.
Other: *falls,* viral infection, increased drug level.

▣ KEY CONSIDERATIONS

• Geriatric patients are at a greater risk for CNS disturbances and orthostatic hypotension.
• Dosage adjustment isn't needed for patients with mild to moderate renal im-

---

pairment; adjust ropinirole dose with caution in patients with severe renal or hepatic impairment.

• Drug may cause increased alkaline phosphatase and BUN levels.

• Although not reported with ropinirole, a symptom complex resembling neuroleptic malignant syndrome (elevated temperature, muscular rigidity, altered consciousness, and autonomic instability) has been reported with rapid dose reduction or withdrawal of antiparkinsonians. If this occurs, stop drug gradually over 7 days and reduce frequency of administration to twice daily for 4 days, then once daily over the remaining 3 days.

• Symptomatic hypotension caused by impairment of systemic regulation of blood pressure by dopamine agonist may occur; monitor patient for orthostatic hypotension, especially when increasing drug dosage.

• Syncope, with or without bradycardia, has been reported; monitor patient carefully, especially after 4 weeks of initiation of therapy and with dosage increases.

• Other adverse events reported with dopaminergic therapy may occur with drug; these include withdrawal-emergent hyperpyrexia, confusion, and complications from fibrosis.

• Drug can potentiate the dopaminergic adverse effects of levodopa and may cause or exacerbate existing dyskinesia. If this occurs, the dosage of levodopa may need to be decreased.

Patient education
• Inform patient to take ropinirole with food to reduce nausea.

• Advise patient that hallucinations may occur; geriatric patients are at greater risk than younger patients with Parkinson's disease.

• Instruct patient to rise slowly after sitting or lying down because of risk of orthostatic hypotension, which may occur during initial therapy or after a dosage increase.

• Advise patient to use caution when driving or operating machinery until CNS effects of drug are known.

• Advise patient to avoid alcohol and other CNS depressants.

Overdose & treatment
• Signs and symptoms of overdose include mild or facial dyskinesia, agitation, increased dyskinesia, grogginess, sedation, orthostatic hypotension, chest pain, confusion, vomiting, and nausea.

• Treatment involves general supportive measures and removal of unabsorbed ropinirole.

Reactions may be *common*, uncommon, *life-threatening*, or COMMON AND LIFE-THREATENING.

salmeterol xinafoate
Serevent

Selective beta₂ agonist, bronchodilator

Available by prescription only
Inhalation aerosol: 25 mcg/activation in 6.5-g canister (60 activations), 25 mcg/activation in 13-g canister (120 activations)

INDICATIONS & DOSAGE
Long-term maintenance treatment of asthma; prevention of bronchospasm in patients with nocturnal asthma or reversible obstructive airway disease who require regular treatment with short-acting beta agonists
Adults: Two inhalations b.i.d. in the morning and evening.
Prevention of exercise-induced bronchospasm
Adults: Two inhalations at least 30 to 60 minutes before exercise.

Note: Paradoxical bronchospasms (which can be life-threatening) have been reported after use of salmeterol. If they occur, drug should be discontinued immediately and alternative therapy instituted.
◇ *COPD or emphysema*
Adults: Single oral inhalation of 42 to 63 mcg.

PHARMACODYNAMICS
Bronchodilator action: Salmeterol selectively stimulates beta₂ receptors, resulting in bronchodilation. Drug also blocks the release of histamine from mast cells lining the respiratory tract, which produces vasodilation and increases ciliary motility.

PHARMACOKINETICS
Absorption: Because of the low therapeutic dose, systemic levels of salmeterol are low or undetectable after inhalation of recommended dose.
Distribution: Drug is highly bound to human plasma proteins (94% to 99%).

Metabolism: Drug is extensively metabolized by hydroxylation.
Excretion: Drug is excreted primarily in feces.

CONTRAINDICATIONS & PRECAUTIONS
Contraindicated in patients with hypersensitivity to salmeterol or its formulation.

Use cautiously in patients with coronary insufficiency, arrhythmias, hypertension, other CV disorders, thyrotoxicosis, or seizure disorders and in those unusually responsive to sympathomimetics.

INTERACTIONS
Drug-drug. Administration with *beta agonists, other methylxanthines,* or *theophylline* may result in possible adverse cardiac effects with excessive use of salmeterol; monitor patient closely. Use with *MAO inhibitors* or *tricyclic antidepressants* carries a risk of severe adverse CV effects; avoid use of salmeterol within 14 days of MAO therapy.

ADVERSE REACTIONS
CNS: *headache,* sinus headache, tremor, nervousness, giddiness.
CV: tachycardia, palpitations, ***ventricular arrhythmias.***
EENT: *nasopharyngitis,* nasal cavity or sinus disorder.
GI: nausea, vomiting, diarrhea, heartburn.
Musculoskeletal: joint and back pain, myalgia.
Respiratory: cough, *upper respiratory tract infection,* lower respiratory tract infection, ***bronchospasm.***
Other: ***hypersensitivity reactions*** (rash, urticaria).

🔲 KEY CONSIDERATIONS
• As with other beta₂ agonists, use salmeterol with extreme caution in geriatric patients with CV disease that could be adversely affected by this class of drugs.
• Don't use drug in patients with asthma that can be managed by occasional use

of a short-acting, inhaled beta₂ agonist such as albuterol.

• Drug inhalation shouldn't be used more than twice daily (morning and evening) at the recommended dose. Provide patient with a short-acting inhaled beta₂ agonist for treatment of symptoms that occur despite regular twice-daily use of salmeterol.

• Patients taking a short-acting inhaled beta₂ agonist daily should be advised to use it only as needed if they develop asthma symptoms while taking salmeterol.

• Drug isn't a substitute for oral or inhaled corticosteroids.

• Patients receiving drug twice daily shouldn't use additional doses to prevent exercise-induced bronchospasm.

Patient education

• Instruct patient on the proper use of the salmeterol inhalation device; tell him to review the illustrated instructions in the package insert.

• Remind patient to shake the container well before using.

• Remind patient to take drug at about 12-hour intervals for optimum effect and to take it even when he's feeling better.

• Inform patient that drug isn't meant to relieve acute symptoms. Acute symptoms should be treated with an inhaled, short-acting bronchodilator prescribed for symptomatic relief.

• Tell patient to call if the short-acting agonist no longer provides sufficient relief or if more than four inhalations are being used daily; this may be a sign that asthma symptoms are worsening.

• Instruct patient already receiving short-acting beta₂ agonist to discontinue the regular daily dosing regimen for the drug and to use the short-acting drug only if he experiences asthma symptoms while taking salmeterol.

• Tell patient taking an inhaled corticosteroid to continue to use it regularly. Warn patient not to take other drugs without medical approval.

• If drug is being used to prevent exercise-induced bronchospasm, tell patient to take it 30 to 60 minutes before exercise.

Overdose & treatment

• Signs and symptoms of overdose include exaggerated pharmacologic adverse effects of beta-adrenoceptor agonists: tachycardia, arrhythmias, tremor, headache, and muscle cramps. Overdose can lead to significant prolongation of the QT interval, which can produce ventricular arrhythmias. Abuse of salmeterol may cause cardiac arrest and death. Other signs of overdose include hypokalemia and hyperglycemia.

• Therapy with salmeterol and all beta stimulant drugs should be stopped, supportive therapy should be provided, and judicious use of a beta blocker should be considered, bearing in mind the possibility that such drugs can produce bronchospasm. Cardiac monitoring is recommended in cases of overdose. Dialysis isn't appropriate treatment.

saquinavir
Fortovase

saquinavir mesylate
Invirase

HIV-1 and HIV-2 proteinase inhibitor, antiviral

Available by prescription only
saquinavir
Capsules (soft gelatin): 200 mg
saquinavir mesylate
Capsules (hard gelatin): 200 mg

INDICATIONS & DOSAGE

Adjunct treatment of advanced HIV infection in selected patients
Adults: 600 mg (Invirase, three 200-mg capsules) P.O. t.i.d. taken within 2 hours after a full meal and in combination with a nucleoside analogue such as zalcitabine at a dosage of 0.75 mg P.O. t.i.d. or 200 mg zidovudine P.O. t.i.d. Or, 1,200 mg (Fortovase, six 200-mg capsules) t.i.d. within 2 hours after a full meal in combination with a nucleoside analogue.

✦ *Dosage adjustment.* For toxicities that occur with saquinavir or saquinavir mesylate, interrupt drug therapy. In combination therapy with nucleoside analogues, dosage adjustments of the nucleoside analogue should be based on the known toxicity profile of specific drug.

PHARMACODYNAMICS

Antiviral action: Saquinavir inhibits the activity of HIV protease and prevents the cleavage of HIV polyproteins, which are essential for the maturation of HIV.

PHARMACOKINETICS

Absorption: Saquinavir is poorly absorbed from the GI tract. Higher saquinavir levels are achieved with Fortovase than with Invirase. (Fortovase has a relative bioavailability of 331% of Invirase.)
Distribution: Drug is about 98% bound to plasma proteins.
Metabolism: Drug is rapidly metabolized.
Excretion: Drug is excreted mainly in feces.

CONTRAINDICATIONS & PRECAUTIONS

Contraindicated in patients with hypersensitivity to saquinavir or components contained in the capsule.

INTERACTIONS

Drug-drug. Use with *cisapride* may cause serious CV events; don't use together. *Rifabutin* and *rifampin* reduce the steady-state level of saquinavir; use together cautiously.
Drug-food. *Food* increases bioavailability of drug; give within 2 hours after a meal.

ADVERSE REACTIONS

CNS: paresthesia, headache, asthenia.
EENT: pharyngitis, rhinitis, epistaxis.
GI: diarrhea, ulcerated buccal mucosa, abdominal pain, nausea, increased liver function test results.
Musculoskeletal: arthralgia; arthritis; leg cramps; muscle cramps; spasms; stiffness; weakness; back, leg, facial, or jaw pain.
Respiratory: bronchitis, dyspnea, hemoptysis, upper respiratory tract disorder, cough.
Skin: rash.

☐ KEY CONSIDERATIONS

• Evaluate CBC, platelet count, and electrolyte, uric acid, liver enzyme, and bilirubin levels before therapy starts and then at appropriate intervals during therapy.
• If a serious or severe toxicity occurs during treatment, discontinue saquinavir until the cause is identified or toxicity resolves. Dosage doesn't need to be modified when drug is resumed.
• Invirase will be phased out and Fortovase will replace it. Be aware of the dosing differences.

Patient education

• Inform patient that saquinavir should be taken within 2 hours after a full meal.
• Tell patient to report adverse reactions.
• Inform patient that drug is usually administered with other AIDS-related antivirals.
• Tell patient to use Fortovase within 3 months when stored at room temperature or refer to expiration date on the label if capsules are refrigerated.

scopolamine hydrobromide
Isopto Hyoscine, Transderm Scop

Anticholinergic, antimuscarinic, cycloplegic mydriatic

Available by prescription only
Injection: 0.3 mg/ml and 1 mg/ml in 1-ml vials and ampules; 0.4 mg/ml and 0.86 mg/ml in 0.5-ml ampules
Ophthalmic solution: 0.25%
Topical: Transdermal system

INDICATIONS & DOSAGE

Antimuscarinic; adjunct to anesthesia; prevention of nausea and vomiting
Adults: 0.3 to 0.6 mg I.M., S.C., or I.V. (after dilution with sterile water for injection) as a single dose.
Prevention of motion sickness
Adults: Apply 1 patch behind the ear 4 hours before anticipated exposure to motion. Delivers 1 mg/72 hours. Remove patch when the antiemetic effect is no longer desired or in 72 hours (replace current system if antiemetic effects are still desired).

Cycloplegic refraction
Adults: 1 or 2 gtt 0.25% solution in eye 1 hour before refraction.
Iritis, uveitis
Adults: 1 or 2 gtt 0.25% solution daily or up to t.i.d.

PHARMACODYNAMICS

Antimuscarinic action: Scopolamine inhibits the action of acetylcholine on autonomic effectors, resulting in decreased secretions and GI motility; it also blocks vagal inhibition of the SA node.
Mydriatic action: Drug competitively blocks acetylcholine at cholinergic neuroeffector sites, antagonizing the effects of acetylcholine on the sphincter muscle and ciliary body, thus producing mydriasis and cycloplegia; these effects are used to produce cycloplegic refraction and pupil dilation to treat preoperative and postoperative iridocyclitis.

PHARMACOKINETICS

Absorption: Scopolamine is rapidly absorbed when administered I.M. or S.C.; effects occur 15 to 30 minutes after I.M. or S.C. administration. Drug may be systemically absorbed from drug passage through the nasolacrimal duct and is well absorbed percutaneously. Ophthalmic mydriatic effect peaks at 20 to 30 minutes after administration; cycloplegic effects peak 30 to 60 minutes after administration.
Distribution: Drug is distributed widely throughout body tissues; probably crosses blood-brain barrier.
Metabolism: Drug is probably metabolized completely in the liver; however, its exact metabolic fate is unknown. Mydriatic and cycloplegic effects persist for 3 to 7 days.
Excretion: Drug is probably excreted in urine as metabolites.

CONTRAINDICATIONS & PRECAUTIONS

Systemic form is contraindicated in patients with angle-closure glaucoma, obstructive uropathy, obstructive disease of the GI tract, asthma, chronic pulmonary disease, myasthenia gravis, paralytic ileus, intestinal atony, unstable CV status in acute hemorrhage, or toxic megacolon. Ophthalmic form is contraindicated in patients with shallow anterior chamber and angle-closure glaucoma or hypersensitivity to scopolamine.

Use systemic form cautiously in patients with autonomic neuropathy, hyperthyroidism, coronary artery disease, arrhythmias, heart failure, hypertension, hiatal hernia associated with reflux esophagitis, hepatic or renal disease, or ulcerative colitis; or in patients in a hot or humid environment. Use ophthalmic form cautiously in geriatric patients and in those with cardiac disease.

INTERACTIONS

Drug-drug. Use with *CNS depressants (sedative-hypnotics, tranquilizers)* may increase CNS depression. Administration with *drugs with anticholinergic effects* may cause additive toxicity. Decreased GI absorption of many drugs has been reported after the use of anticholinergics (for example, *ketoconazole, levodopa*). Use cautiously with *oral potassium supplements (especially wax-matrix formulations)* because the incidence of potassium-induced GI ulcerations may be increased. *Slowly dissolving digoxin tablets* may yield higher serum digoxin levels when administered with anticholinergics.
Drug-lifestyle. Use with *alcohol* may increase CNS depression.

ADVERSE REACTIONS

CNS: disorientation, restlessness, irritability, dizziness, drowsiness, headache, confusion, hallucinations, delirium.
CV: tachycardia; flushing (with systemic form); palpitations, ***paradoxical bradycardia (with systemic form).***
EENT: blurred vision, photophobia, increased intraocular pressure; dilated pupils, difficulty swallowing (with systemic form); ocular congestion (with prolonged use); conjunctivitis, eye dryness, transient stinging and burning, edema (with ophthalmic form).
GI: dry mouth; *constipation, nausea, vomiting, epigastric distress* (with systemic form).
GU: urinary hesitancy, urine retention (with systemic form).

Reactions may be *common*, uncommon, *life-threatening*, or COMMON AND LIFE-THREATENING.

Respiratory: bronchial plugging, *depressed respirations* (with systemic form).

Skin: rash (with systemic form), dryness or contact dermatitis (with ophthalmic form).

Other: fever (with systemic form).

▣ KEY CONSIDERATIONS

Besides the recommendations relevant to all anticholinergics, consider the following:

• Geriatric patients may experience transient excitement or disorientation.

• Use caution when administering scopolamine to geriatric patients; lower doses are indicated.

• Adverse reactions may be caused by pending atropine-like toxicity and are dose related. Individual tolerance varies.

• Many adverse reactions (such as dry mouth, constipation) are an expected extension of drug's pharmacologic activity.

• Therapeutic doses may produce amnesia, drowsiness, and euphoria (desired effects for use as an adjunct to anesthesia). As necessary, reorient patient.

Ophthalmic

• Apply pressure to the lacrimal sac for 1 minute after instillation to reduce the risk of systemic drug absorption.

• Have patient lie down, tilt head back, or look at ceiling to aid instillation.

Patient education
Ophthalmic

• Instruct patient to apply pressure to bridge of nose for about 1 minute after instillation.

• Advise patient not to close eyes tightly or blink for about 1 minute after instillation.

Topical

• Instruct patient to wash hands after applying patch.

• Tell patient to apply only one patch at a time.

Overdose & treatment

• Signs and symptoms of overdose include excitability, seizures, CNS stimulation followed by depression, and such psychotic symptoms as disorientation, confusion, hallucinations, delusions, anxiety, agitation, and restlessness. Peripheral effects include dilated, nonreactive pupils; blurred vision; flushed, hot, dry skin; dryness of mucous membranes; dysphagia; decreased or absent bowel sounds; urine retention; hyperthermia; tachycardia; hypertension; and increased respiration.

• Treatment is primarily symptomatic and supportive, as needed. Maintain patent airway. If patient is awake and alert, induce vomiting (or perform gastric lavage) and follow with a sodium chloride cathartic and activated charcoal to prevent further drug absorption. In severe life-threatening cases, physostigmine may be administered to block the antimuscarinic effects of scopolamine. Give fluids as needed to treat shock, diazepam to control psychotic symptoms, and pilocarpine (instilled into the eyes) to relieve mydriasis. If urine retention develops, catheterization may be necessary.

---

secobarbital sodium
Novosecobarb,* Seconal

Barbiturate, sedative-hypnotic, anticonvulsant
Controlled substance schedule II

Available by prescription only
Capsules: 50 mg, 100 mg
Injection: 50 mg/ml in 2-ml disposable syringe

INDICATIONS & DOSAGE
Preoperative sedation
Adults: 200 to 300 mg P.O. 1 to 2 hours before surgery or 1 mg/kg I.M. 15 minutes before procedure.
Insomnia
Adults: 100 mg P.O., 100 to 200 mg I.M., or 50 to 250 mg I.V.
Status epilepticus
Adults: 250 to 350 mg I.M. or I.V.
  Note: No more than 250 mg (5 ml) should be injected at one site.

PHARMACODYNAMICS
Sedative-hypnotic action: Secobarbital acts throughout the CNS as a nonselective depressant with a rapid onset and short duration of action. The reticular ac-

tivating system, which controls CNS arousal, is particularly sensitive to this drug. Drug decreases both presynaptic and postsynaptic membrane excitability by facilitating the action of gamma-aminobutyric acid. The exact cellular site and mechanisms of action are unknown.

PHARMACOKINETICS

Absorption: After oral administration, 90% of secobarbital is absorbed rapidly. After rectal administration, drug is nearly 100% absorbed. Serum levels peak after oral or rectal administration between 2 and 4 hours. Onset of action is rapid; within 15 minutes when administered orally. Effects peak 15 to 30 minutes after oral and rectal administration, 7 to 10 minutes after I.M. administration, and 1 to 3 minutes after I.V. administration. Levels of 1 to 5 μg/ml are needed to produce sedation; 5 to 15 μg/ml are needed for hypnosis. Hypnosis lasts for 1 to 4 hours after oral doses of 100 to 150 mg.
Distribution: Drug is distributed rapidly throughout body tissues and fluids; 30% to 45% is protein-bound.
Metabolism: Drug is oxidized in the liver to inactive metabolites. Duration of action is 3 to 4 hours.
Excretion: Drug has elimination half-life of about 30 hours; 95% of dose is eliminated as glucuronide conjugates and other metabolites in urine.

CONTRAINDICATIONS & PRECAUTIONS

Contraindicated in patients with respiratory disease with evidence of dyspnea or obstruction or those with hypersensitivity to barbiturates or porphyria.

Use cautiously in patients with acute or chronic pain, depression, suicidal tendencies, history of drug abuse, or impaired hepatic or renal function.

INTERACTIONS

Drug-drug. Secobarbital may add to or potentiate CNS and respiratory depressant effects of *antidepressants, antihistamines, narcotics,* other *sedative-hypnotics,* and *tranquilizers.* Drug also enhances hepatic metabolism of some drugs, including *corticosteroids, digitoxin* (not digoxin), *doxycycline, estrogens, theophylline,* and other *xanthines. Disulfiram, MAO inhibitors,* and *valproic acid* decrease the metabolism of secobarbital and can increase its toxicity. Secobarbital impairs the effectiveness of *griseofulvin* by decreasing absorption from the GI tract. *Rifampin* may decrease secobarbital levels by increasing metabolism. Secobarbital enhances the enzymatic degradation of other *oral anticoagulants* and *warfarin;* patients may require increased doses of anticoagulant.
Drug-lifestyle. *Alcohol* use may add to or potentiate CNS and respiratory depressant effects.

ADVERSE REACTIONS

CNS: *drowsiness, lethargy, hangover,* change in EEG patterns, paradoxical excitement in geriatric patients, somnolence.
CV: hypotension (with I.V. use).
GI: nausea, vomiting.
Hematologic: exacerbation of porphyria.
Respiratory: *respiratory depression.*
Skin: rash, urticaria, **Stevens-Johnson syndrome,** tissue reactions, injection-site pain.
Other: *angioedema,* physical and psychological dependence.

▣ KEY CONSIDERATIONS

Besides the recommendations relevant to all barbiturates, consider the following:
• Geriatric patients are more susceptible to the effects of secobarbital and usually require a lower dosage; further, these patients may experience confusion, disorientation, and excitability.
• Administer I.V. only in emergencies or when other routes are unavailable.
• Dilute secobarbital injection with sterile water for injection, normal saline injection, or Ringer's injection solution. Total I.V. dose shouldn't exceed 500 mg. Don't use if solution is discolored or if a precipitate forms.
• To prevent hypotension and respiratory depression, avoid I.V. administration at rate greater than 50 mg/15 seconds. Have emergency resuscitative equipment on hand.
• To prevent tissue injury, administer I.M. dose deep into large muscle mass.

Reactions may be *common,* uncommon, **life-threatening**, or COMMON AND LIFE-THREATENING.

- To prevent possible toxicity, monitor hepatic and renal studies frequently.
- Drug may cause a false-positive phentolamine test result.
- The physiological effects of the drug may impair the absorption of cyanocobalamin C57.
- Drug may decrease serum bilirubin levels in epileptic patients and in those with congenital nonhemolytic unconjugated hyperbilirubinemia.

Patient education
- Emphasize danger of combining drug with alcohol. An excessive depressive effect is possible even if drug is taken the evening before ingestion of alcohol.

Overdose & treatment
- Signs and symptoms of overdose include unsteady gait, slurred speech, sustained nystagmus, somnolence, confusion, respiratory depression, pulmonary edema, areflexia, and coma. Typical shock syndrome with tachycardia and hypotension, jaundice, hypothermia followed by fever, and oliguria may occur.
- Maintain and support ventilation and pulmonary function as necessary; support cardiac function and circulation with vasopressors and I.V. fluids as needed. If patient is conscious and gag reflex is intact, induce vomiting (if ingestion was recent) by administering ipecac syrup. If vomiting is contraindicated, perform gastric lavage while a cuffed endotracheal tube is in place to prevent aspiration. Then administer activated charcoal or a sodium chloride cathartic. Measure intake and output, vital signs, and laboratory parameters; maintain body temperature. Patient should be rolled from side to side every 30 minutes to avoid pulmonary congestion. Alkalinization of urine may be helpful in removing drug from body; hemodialysis may be useful in severe overdose.

selegiline hydrochloride (L-deprenyl hydrochloride)
Eldepryl

MAO inhibitor, antiparkinsonian

Available by prescription only
Capsules: 5 mg

INDICATIONS & DOSAGE
Adjunctive treatment to carbidopa-levodopa in the management of Parkinson's disease
Adults: 10 mg P.O. daily, taken as 5 mg at breakfast and 5 mg at lunch. After 2 to 3 days of therapy, begin gradual decrease of carbidopa-levodopa dosage.

PHARMACODYNAMICS
Antiparkinsonian action: Probably acts by selectively inhibiting MAO type B (found mostly in the brain). At doses higher than recommended, it's a nonselective inhibitor of MAO, including MAO type A found in the GI tract. It may also directly increase dopaminergic activity by decreasing the reuptake of dopamine into nerve cells. It has pharmacologically active metabolites (amphetamine and methamphetamine) that may contribute to this effect.

PHARMACOKINETICS
Absorption: Selegiline is rapidly absorbed; about 73% of dose is absorbed.
Distribution: After a single dose, plasma levels are less than detectable levels (less than 10 ng/ml).
Metabolism: Three metabolites have been detected in serum and urine: N-desmethyldeprenyl, amphetamine, and methamphetamine.
Excretion: About 45% of drug appears as metabolite in urine after 48 hours.

CONTRAINDICATIONS & PRECAUTIONS
Contraindicated in patients with hypersensitivity to selegiline and in those receiving meperidine and other opioids.

INTERACTIONS
Drug-drug. Use with *adrenergics* may increase the pressor response, particularly in patients who have taken an over-

dose of selegiline. Contraindicated for use with *meperidine* because fatal interactions have been reported.

Drug-lifestyle. Use with *alcohol* causes excessive depressant effects.

ADVERSE REACTIONS

CNS: malaise, *dizziness,* increased tremor, chorea, loss of balance, restlessness, increased bradykinesia, facial grimacing, stiff neck, dyskinesia, involuntary movements, twitching, increased apraxia, behavioral changes, fatigue, headache, confusion, vivid dreams, anxiety, insomnia, lethargy, hallucinations.
CV: orthostatic hypotension, hypertension, hypotension, *arrhythmias,* palpitations, new or increased anginal pain, tachycardia, peripheral edema, syncope.
EENT: blepharospasm.
GI: dry mouth, *nausea,* vomiting, constipation, weight loss, abdominal pain, anorexia or poor appetite, dysphagia, diarrhea, heartburn.
GU: slow urination, transient nocturia, prostatic hyperplasia, urinary hesitancy, urinary frequency, urine retention, sexual dysfunction.
Skin: rash, hair loss, diaphoresis.

⬚ KEY CONSIDERATIONS

• In some cases, levodopa causes more adverse reactions (including dyskinesias), and dosage of carbidopa-levodopa needs to be reduced; most patients require a 10% to 30% reduction.

Patient education

• Advise patient not to take more than 10 mg daily. No evidence exists that higher dosage improves efficacy, and it may increase adverse reactions.
• Warn patient to move about cautiously at the start of therapy because dizziness may occur, which can cause falls.
• Because selegiline is a MAO inhibitor, tell patient that the drug may interact with tyramine-containing foods. Tell patient to immediately report signs or symptoms of hypertension, including severe headache. This interaction isn't reported to occur at the recommended dosage; at 10 mg daily, drug inhibits only MAO type B. Thus, dietary restrictions appear unnecessary, provided pa-

tient doesn't exceed the recommended dose.
• Emphasize danger of combining drug with alcohol. An excessive depressant effect is possible even if drug is taken the evening before ingestion of alcohol.
• Advise patient to take second dose with lunch to prevent nighttime insomnia.

Overdose & treatment

• Limited experience with overdose suggests symptoms may include hypotension and psychomotor agitation. Because selegiline becomes a nonselective MAO inhibitor in high doses, consider the possibility of MAO inhibitor poisoning; signs and symptoms include drowsiness, dizziness, hyperactivity, agitation, seizures, coma, hypertension, hypotension, cardiac conduction disturbances, and CV collapse. These signs and symptoms may not develop immediately after ingestion (delays of 12 hours or more are possible).
• Provide supportive treatment and closely monitor the patient for worsening of signs and symptoms. Inducing vomiting or performing gastric lavage may be helpful in the early stages of treatment. Avoid phenothiazine derivatives and CNS stimulants; adrenergics may provoke an exaggerated response. Diazepam may be useful in treating seizures.

senna
Black-Draught, Fletcher's Castoria, Gentlax S, Nytilax, Senexon, Senokot, Senolax, X-Prep

Anthraquinone derivative, stimulant laxative

Available without prescription
Tablets: 187 mg, 217 mg, 374 mg, 600 mg
Granules: 326 mg/tsp, 1.65 g/¼ tsp
Liquid: 33.3 mg/ml
Suppositories: 652 mg
Syrup: 218 mg/5 ml

Reactions may be *common,* uncommon, *life-threatening,* or COMMON AND LIFE-THREATENING.

INDICATIONS & DOSAGE
Acute constipation, preparation for bowel examination
Black-Draught
Adults: 2 tablets or ¼ to ½ level tsp granules mixed with water.
Other preparations
Adults: Usual dose is 2 tablets, 1 tsp of granules dissolved in water, 1 suppository, or 10 to 15 ml syrup h.s. Maximum dosage varies with preparation used.

PHARMACODYNAMICS
Laxative action: Senna has a local irritant effect on the colon, which promotes peristalsis and bowel evacuation. It also enhances intestinal fluid accumulation, increasing the stool's moisture content.

PHARMACOKINETICS
Absorption: Senna is absorbed minimally. With oral administration, laxative effect occurs in 6 to 10 hours; with suppository administration, laxative effect occurs in 30 minutes to 2 hours.
Distribution: Drug may be distributed in bile, saliva, and colonic mucosa.
Metabolism: Absorbed portion is metabolized in the liver.
Excretion: Unabsorbed drug is excreted mainly in feces; absorbed drug is excreted in urine and feces.

CONTRAINDICATIONS & PRECAUTIONS
Contraindicated in patients with ulcerative bowel lesions; nausea, vomiting, abdominal pain, or other symptoms of appendicitis or acute surgical abdomen; fecal impaction; or intestinal obstruction or perforation.

INTERACTIONS
None reported.

ADVERSE REACTIONS
GI: *nausea,* vomiting, diarrhea, loss of normal bowel function (with excessive use), *abdominal cramps* (especially in severe constipation), malabsorption of nutrients, cathartic colon (syndrome resembling ulcerative colitis radiologically) with chronic misuse, possible constipation after catharsis, yellow or yellow-green cast to feces, darkened pigmentation of rectal mucosa with long-term use (usually reversible within 4 to 12 months after stopping drug), laxative dependence (with excessive use).
GU: red-pink discoloration in alkaline urine, yellow-brown discoloration in acidic urine.
Metabolic: protein-losing enteropathy, electrolyte imbalance (such as hypokalemia).

▣ KEY CONSIDERATIONS
• Many geriatric patients overuse laxatives and are prone to laxative dependency.
• Protect senna from excessive heat or light.
• In the phenolsulfonphthalein excretion test, drug may turn urine pink, red, violet, or brown.

Patient education
• Warn patient that senna may turn urine pink, red, violet, or brown, depending on urine pH.
• Instruct patient that he shouldn't use laxatives for more than a week because excessive use may cause dependence or electrolyte imbalance.
• Tell patient that bowel movement may have a yellow or yellow-green cast.

sertraline hydrochloride
Zoloft

Serotonin uptake inhibitor, antidepressant

Available by prescription only
Tablets: 50 mg, 100 mg

INDICATIONS & DOSAGE
Depression, obsessive-compulsive disorder
Adults: 50 mg P.O. daily. Adjust dosage as needed and tolerated; clinical trials involved dosages of 50 to 200 mg daily. Dosage adjustments should be made at intervals of no less than 1 week.
✦ *Dosage adjustment.* Reduced dosage should be used in patients with hepatic impairment. Particular care should be used in patients with renal failure.

PHARMACODYNAMICS

Antidepressant action: Sertraline probably acts by blocking the reuptake of serotonin (5-hydroxy-tryptamine; 5-HT) into presynaptic neurons in the CNS, prolonging the action of 5-HT.

PHARMACOKINETICS

Absorption: Sertraline is well absorbed after oral administration; absorption rate and extent are enhanced when taken with food. Serum levels peak between 4.5 and 8.4 hours after dose.

Distribution: In vitro studies indicate drug is highly protein-bound (more than 98%).

Metabolism: Metabolism is probably hepatic; drug undergoes significant first-pass metabolism. N-desmethylsertraline is substantially less active than the parent compound.

Excretion: Drug is excreted mostly as metabolites in urine and feces; mean elimination half-life is 26 hours. Steady-state levels are reached within 1 week of daily dosing in young, healthy patients.

CONTRAINDICATIONS & PRECAUTIONS

Contraindicated in patients receiving MAO inhibitors.

Use cautiously in patients at risk for suicide and in those with seizure disorders, major affective disorder, or diseases or conditions that affect metabolism or hemodynamic responses.

INTERACTIONS

Drug-drug. In one study, *cimetidine* increased sertraline bioavailability, peak plasma level, and half-life; significance is unknown. Sertraline decreases clearance of *diazepam* and *tolbutamide;* although significance is unknown, monitor patient for increased drug effects. Use with *MAO inhibitors* may cause serious mental status changes, hyperthermia, autonomic instability, rapid fluctuations of vital signs, delirium, coma, and death; don't administer within 14 days after discontinuing a MAO inhibitor and wait 14 days after discontinuing sertraline before starting a MAO inhibitor. *Other highly protein-bound drugs* and *warfarin* and may cause interactions, increasing plasma levels of sertraline or the other highly bound drug. Small (8%) increases in PT have occurred with use of warfarin; monitor PT and INR closely.

Drug-lifestyle. *Alcohol* use may increase CNS effects; don't use together.

ADVERSE REACTIONS

CNS: *headache, tremor, dizziness, insomnia, somnolence,* paresthesia, hypoesthesia, *fatigue,* nervousness, anxiety, agitation, hypertonia, twitching, confusion.

CV: palpitations, chest pain, hot flashes.

GI: *dry mouth, nausea, diarrhea, loose stools, dyspepsia,* vomiting, constipation, thirst, flatulence, anorexia, abdominal pain, increased appetite.

GU: *male sexual dysfunction,* polyuria, nocturia, dysuria.

Hepatic: elevated liver enzyme levels.

Musculoskeletal: myalgia.

Skin: rash, pruritus, *diaphoresis.*

▣ KEY CONSIDERATIONS

• Plasma clearance of sertraline is slower in geriatric patients; studies indicate it may take 2 to 3 weeks of daily dosing before steady-state levels are reached. Monitor closely for dose-related adverse effects.

• Patients who respond during the first 8 weeks of therapy will probably continue to respond to drug, although there are limited studies of drug use in depressed patients for periods longer than 16 weeks. For prolonged therapy, periodically monitor drug effectiveness. It's unknown if periodic dosage adjustments are necessary to maintain effectiveness.

• Drug may activate mania or hypomania in patients with cyclic disorders.

Patient education

• Tell patient to take sertraline once daily, either in the morning or evening, with or without food.

• Advise patient to avoid use of alcohol while taking drug and to call before taking OTC drugs.

• Although problems haven't been reported to date, advise patient to use caution when performing hazardous tasks that require alertness, such as driving and operating heavy machinery. Drugs

---

that influence the CNS may impair judgment.

Overdose & treatment
• Experience with overdose is limited.
• Treatment is supportive. Establish airway and maintain adequate ventilation. Because recent studies question the value of forced vomiting and gastric lavage, consider using activated charcoal in sorbitol to bind drug in the GI tract.

sildenafil citrate
Viagra

Selective inhibitor of cyclic guanosine monophosphate (cGMP)– specific phosphodiesterase type 5, therapy for erectile dysfunction

Available by prescription only
Tablets: 25 mg, 50 mg, 100 mg

INDICATIONS & DOSAGE
Treatment of erectile dysfunction
Adults: 50 mg P.O. as a single dose p.r.n. 1 hour before sexual activity, or may take drug 30 minutes to 4 hours before sexual activity. Based on effectiveness and tolerance by patient, may increase to maximum single dose of 100 mg or decrease dose to 25 mg. A maximum recommended dosing frequency is once daily.
Geriatric patients: Consider a starting dose of 25 mg.
✦ *Dosage adjustment.* In patients with hepatic impairment or severe renal impairment and in those taking potent cytochrome P-450 3A4 (CYP 3A4) inhibitors, consider a starting dose of 25 mg.

PHARMACODYNAMICS
Erectile action: Sildenafil has no direct relaxant effect on isolated human corpus cavernosum, but enhances the effect of nitric oxide by inhibiting phosphodiesterase type 5 (PDE5), which is responsible for degradation of cGMP in the corpus cavernosum. When sexual stimulation causes local release of nitric oxide, inhibition of PDE5 by drug causes increased levels of cGMP in the corpus cavernosum, resulting in smooth-muscle relaxation and inflow of blood to the corpus cavernosum.

PHARMACOKINETICS
Absorption: Sildenafil is rapidly absorbed after oral administration. Plasma levels peak in ½ to 2 hours (median, 1 hour); a high-fat meal delays the rate of absorption by about 1 hour and reduces peak levels by one-third. Absolute bioavailability is about 40%.
Distribution: Drug is widely distributed to body tissues, with a mean steady-state volume of distribution of 105 L. Both drug and its major active metabolite are 96% bound to plasma proteins; protein-binding is independent of drug levels.
Metabolism: The primary pathway for drug elimination is metabolism by the CYP 3A4 and CYP 2C9 hepatic microsomal isoenzymes. N-desmethylation converts drug into the major circulating metabolite, which accounts for about 20% of pharmacologic effects of the drug.
Excretion: About 80% of oral dose is metabolized and excreted in feces; about 13% is excreted in urine.

CONTRAINDICATIONS & PRECAUTIONS
Contraindicated in patients also using organic nitrates and in those with known hypersensitivity to sildenafil or its components.

Use cautiously in patients with an MI, stroke, or life-threatening arrhythmias within the last 6 months; in patients with history of heart failure, coronary artery disease, or uncontrolled high or low blood pressure; in those with anatomic deformation of the penis; and in those predisposed to priapism (sickle cell anemia, multiple myeloma, leukemia), retinitis pigmentosa, bleeding disorders, or active peptic ulcers.

INTERACTIONS
Drug-drug. *Inhibitors of CYP 3A4 (cimetidine, erythromycin, itraconazole, ketoconazole)* may reduce the clearance of sildenafil. Sildenafil enhances the hypotensive effects of *nitrates. Rifampin* may reduce sildenafil plasma levels.

ADVERSE REACTIONS

CNS: *headache*, dizziness.
CV: *flushing*.
EENT: nasal congestion, abnormal vision (photophobia, color blindness).
GI: dyspepsia, diarrhea.
GU: urinary tract infection.
Skin: rash.

▣ KEY CONSIDERATIONS

• Sildenafil clearance may be reduced in healthy patients ages 65 or older, which results in plasma levels about 40% greater than those in younger patients.
• Because sexual activity poses some cardiac risk, evaluate patient's CV status before initiating therapy.

Patient education

• Advise patient that a high-fat meal will delay sildenafil absorption by 60 minutes.
• Tell patient drug doesn't protect against sexually transmitted diseases and that he should use protective measures to prevent infection.
• Instruct patient not to take drug with nitrates.
• Tell patient to notify health care provider of visual changes.
• Urge patient to seek medical attention if erection persists for more than 4 hours.
• Advise patient that drug has no effect in the absence of sexual stimulation.

silver sulfadiazine

Silvadene, SSD AF, SSD Cream, Thermazene

Synthetic anti-infective, topical antibacterial

Available by prescription only
Cream: 1%

INDICATIONS & DOSAGE

Adjunct in the prevention and treatment of wound infection for second- and third-degree burns
Adults: Apply ¹⁄₁₆" (16-mm) thickness of ointment to cleaned and debrided burn wound once or twice daily. Reapply if accidentally removed.

PHARMACODYNAMICS

Antibacterial action: Silver sulfadiazine acts on bacterial cell membrane and bacterial cell wall. Drug has a broad spectrum of activity, including against gram-negative and gram-positive organisms.

PHARMACOKINETICS

Absorption: Limited with topical use.
Distribution: None.
Metabolism: None.
Excretion: Silver sulfadiazine is excreted in urine.

CONTRAINDICATIONS & PRECAUTIONS

Contraindicated in patients with hypersensitivity to silver sulfadiazine.
    Use cautiously in patients with sulfonamide sensitivity.

INTERACTIONS

Drug-drug. *Collagenase*, *papain*, and *sutilains* may be inactivated if used with silver sulfadiazine.

ADVERSE REACTIONS

CNS: pain.
Hematologic: *neutropenia, reversible leukopenia.*
Skin: burning, rash, pruritus, skin necrosis, *erythema multiforme,* skin discoloration.

▣ KEY CONSIDERATIONS

• If silver sulfadiazine is used on several areas of the body, systemic absorption may result in decreased neutrophil count, indicating reversible leukopenia.
• Avoid drug contact with eyes and mucous membranes.
• Apply drug with a sterile gloved hand; the burned area should be covered with cream at all times.
• Daily bathing aids in debridement of burn wounds.
• Continue treatment until site is healed or ready for skin grafting.
• Monitor for signs of fungal superinfection.
• Delayed eschar separation may result when drug is used.
• Monitor CBC, drug levels, and urine for crystalluria and calculi formation.

Reactions may be *common*, uncommon, *life-threatening*, or COMMON AND LIFE-THREATENING.

Patient education
• Teach patient about wound care.
• Advise patient that silver sulfadiazine doesn't stain the skin.
• Teach patient proper application.
• Warn patient of potential photosensitivity.

simethicone
Gas-X, Mylicon, Phazyme

Antiflatulent

Available without prescription
Tablets (delayed-release; enteric-coated core): 60 mg, 95 mg
Tablets (chewable): 40 mg, 80 mg, 125 mg
Capsules: 125 mg
Drops: 40 mg/0.6 ml

INDICATIONS & DOSAGE
Flatulence, functional gastric bloating
Adults: 40 to 125 mg P.O. after each meal and h.s.

PHARMACODYNAMICS
Antiflatulent action: Simethicone acts as a defoaming drug by decreasing the surface tension of gas bubbles, thereby preventing the formation of mucus-coated gas bubbles.

PHARMACOKINETICS
Absorption: None.
Distribution: None.
Metabolism: None.
Excretion: Simethicone is excreted in feces.

CONTRAINDICATIONS & PRECAUTIONS
Contraindicated in patients hypersensitive to simethicone.

INTERACTIONS
Drug-drug. Simethicone may decrease the effectiveness of *alginic acid.*

ADVERSE REACTIONS
GI: belching, rectal flatus.

▣ KEY CONSIDERATIONS
• Simethicone is found in many combination antacid products.

Patient education
• Tell patient to chew tablets thoroughly or to shake suspension well before using.

simvastatin
Zocor

3-hydroxy-3-methylglutaryl-coenzyme A (HMG-CoA) reductase inhibitor, antilipemic

Available by prescription only
Tablets: 5 mg, 10 mg, 20 mg, 40 mg

INDICATIONS & DOSAGE
Reduction of low-density lipoprotein (LDL) and total cholesterol levels in patients with primary hypercholesterolemia (types IIa and IIb)
Adults: Initially, 5 to 10 mg daily in the evening. Adjust dosage q 4 weeks based on patient tolerance and response; maximum daily dose for adults is 40 mg; for geriatric patients, 20 mg.
✦ *Dosage adjustment.* For patients receiving immunosuppressants, start with 5 mg/day; maximum daily dose is 10 mg. For patients with mild to moderate renal insufficiency, give usual daily dose; in those with severe renal impairment, start therapy with 5 mg P.O. daily and closely monitor patient.

PHARMACODYNAMICS
Antilipemic action: Simvastatin inhibits HMG-CoA reductase. This hepatic enzyme is an early (and rate-limiting) step in the synthetic pathway of cholesterol.

PHARMACOKINETICS
Absorption: Simvastatin is readily absorbed; however, extensive hepatic extraction limits plasma availability of active inhibitors to 5% of dose or less. Individual absorption varies considerably.
Distribution: Parent drug and active metabolites are more than 95% bound to plasma proteins.
Metabolism: Hydrolysis occurs in plasma; at least three major metabolites have been identified.
Excretion: Drug is primarily excreted in bile.

CONTRAINDICATIONS & PRECAUTIONS

Contraindicated in patients with hypersensitivity to simvastatin and in those with active hepatic disease or conditions that cause unexplained persistent elevations of serum transaminase levels.

Use cautiously in patients with history of liver disease or in those who consume excessive amounts of alcohol.

INTERACTIONS

Drug-drug. Limit daily dose of simvastatin to 10 mg if patient must take *cyclosporine*. Simvastatin may slightly elevate *digoxin* levels; closely monitor plasma digoxin levels at the start of simvastatin therapy. Drugs that decrease the level or activity of *endogenous steroids* (such as *cimetidine, ketoconazole, spironolactone*) may increase the risk of developing endocrine dysfunction; no intervention appears necessary, but obtain complete drug history in patients who develop endocrine dysfunction. Use with *erythromycin, fibric acid derivatives* (such as *clofibrate, gemfibrozil*), *immunosuppressants* (such as *cyclosporine*), or high doses of *niacin (nicotinic acid;* 1 g or more daily) may increase risk of rhabdomyolysis; monitor patient closely if use can't be avoided. Patients taking *hepatotoxic drugs* may be at increased risk of hepatotoxicity. Simvastatin may slightly enhance the anticoagulant effect of *warfarin;* monitor PT and INR at the start of therapy and during dosage adjustment.

Drug-lifestyle. Patients who abuse *alcohol* may be at increased risk for hepatotoxicity.

ADVERSE REACTIONS

CNS: headache, asthenia.
GI: abdominal pain, constipation, diarrhea, dyspepsia, flatulence, nausea, vomiting.
Hepatic: elevated liver enzyme levels.
Respiratory: upper respiratory tract infection.

🔲 KEY CONSIDERATIONS

● Most geriatric patients respond to daily dose of 20 mg or less.
● Dosage adjustments should be made about q 4 weeks. If cholesterol levels de-crease to less than the target range, dosage may be reduced.
● Perform liver function tests frequently at the start of therapy and periodically thereafter.
● Initiate simvastatin only after diet and other nonpharmacologic therapies have proved ineffective. Patient should continue a cholesterol-reducing diet during therapy.
● As an expected pharmacologic effect, drug reduces total plasma cholesterol, very low-density lipoprotein, and LDL levels and may variably increase high-density lipoprotein (HDL) levels. The ratios of total cholesterol to HDL, total cholesterol to LDL, and LDL to HDL are reduced. Modest decreases in triglyceride levels may also occur.
● Toxic effects of drug may be evident by marked, persistent elevations of serum transaminase levels. During clinical trials, about 5% of patients had asymptomatic, marked elevations in the noncardiac fraction of CK.

Patient education

● Tell patient that simvastatin should be taken in the evening and may be taken without regard to meals.
● Because of the possible impact of drug on liver function, advise patient to restrict alcohol intake.
● Tell patient to report adverse reactions, particularly muscle aches and pains.
● Explain importance of controlling serum lipid levels for CV health. Teach appropriate dietary management (restricting total fat and cholesterol intake), weight control, and exercise.

sodium bicarbonate
Bell/ans, Neut, Soda Mint

Systemic and urinary alkalizer, systemic hydrogen ion buffer, oral antacid

Available by prescription only
Injection: 4% (2.4 mEq/5 ml), 4.2% (5 mEq/10 ml), 5% (297.5 mEq/500 ml), 7.5% (8.92 mEq/10 ml and 44.6 mEq/ 50 ml), 8.4% (10 mEq/10 ml and 50 mEq/50 ml)

Reactions may be *common,* uncommon, ***life-threatening,*** or **COMMON AND LIFE-THREATENING.**

Available without prescription
Tablets: 325 mg, 500 mg, 520 mg,
650 mg

INDICATIONS & DOSAGE
Cardiac arrest
Adults: Although no longer routinely
recommended, 1 mEq/kg I.V. of 7.5% or
8.4% solution, followed by 0.5 mEq/kg
I.V. q 10 minutes, depending on arterial
blood gas (ABG) levels. Further dosages
based on results of ABG analysis. If
ABG results are unavailable, use 0.5
mEq/kg I.V. q 10 minutes until spontaneous circulation returns.
Metabolic acidosis
Adults: Dose depends on blood carbon
dioxide content, pH, and patient's condition. Generally, administer 90 to 180
mEq/L I.V. during 1st hour, then adjust
p.r.n.
Urinary alkalization
Adults: 325 mg to 2 g P.O. up to q.i.d.
Don't exceed 8 g in patients older than
age 60.
Antacid
Adults: 300 mg to 2 g P.O. one to four
times daily.

PHARMACODYNAMICS
Alkalizing buffering action: Sodium bicarbonate is an alkalizing drug that dissociates to provide bicarbonate ion. Bicarbonate in excess of that needed to
buffer hydrogen ions causes systemic alkalization and, when excreted, urinary
alkalization.
Oral antacid action: Taken orally, drug
neutralizes stomach acid by the above
mechanism.

PHARMACOKINETICS
Absorption: Sodium bicarbonate is well
absorbed after oral administration as
sodium ion and bicarbonate.
Distribution: Bicarbonate occurs naturally and is confined to the systemic circulation.
Metabolism: None.
Excretion: Bicarbonate is filtered and reabsorbed in the kidney; less than 1% of
filtered bicarbonate is excreted.

CONTRAINDICATIONS & PRECAUTIONS
Contraindicated in patients with metabolic or respiratory alkalosis; in those
losing chlorides by vomiting or continuous GI suction; in those receiving diuretics known to produce hypochloremic alkalosis; and in patients with hypocalcemia in whom alkalosis may produce
tetany, hypertension, seizures, or heart
failure. Orally administered sodium bicarbonate is contraindicated in patients
with acute ingestion of strong mineral
acids.
  Use with extreme caution in patients
with heart failure, renal insufficiency, or
other edematous or sodium-retaining
conditions.

INTERACTIONS
Drug-drug. If urinary alkalization occurs, sodium bicarbonate increases half-
life of *amphetamines, ephedrine, pseudoephedrine,* and *quinidine* and increases urine excretion of *chlorpropamide,
lithium, salicylates,* and *tetracyclines.*
Use with *corticosteroids* may increase
sodium retention.

ADVERSE REACTIONS
CNS: pain at injection site.
GI: gastric distention, belching, flatulence.
Metabolic: altered serum electrolyte
levels, increased serum lactate levels,
metabolic alkalosis, hypernatremia, hyperosmolarity (with overdose).
Other: irritation at injection site.

▣ KEY CONSIDERATIONS
• Geriatric patients with heart failure or
other fluid-retaining conditions are at
greater risk for increased fluid retention;
use sodium bicarbonate with caution.
• Monitor vital signs regularly; when
drug is used as urinary alkalizer, monitor
urine pH.
• Avoid extravasation of I.V. solutions.
Addition of calcium salts may cause precipitate; bicarbonate may inactivate catecholamines in solution (epinephrine,
phenylephrine, and dopamine).
• Discourage use as oral antacid because
of hazardous excessive systemic absorption.

• If the patient has taken the drug for a long time, assess him for milk-alkali syndrome.

• Drug may be used as an adjunct to treat hyperkalemia (with dextrose and insulin).

Patient education

• Advise patient to avoid continual or long-term use as oral antacid; recommend nonabsorbable antacids.

• Tell patient taking oral dosage form to take sodium bicarbonate 1 hour before or 2 hours after enteric-coated drugs, because sodium bicarbonate may cause enteric-coated products to dissolve in the stomach.

Overdose & treatment

• Signs and symptoms of overdose include depressed consciousness and obtundation from hypernatremia, tetany from hypocalcemia, arrhythmias from hypokalemia, and seizures from alkalosis.

• Correct fluid, electrolyte, and pH abnormalities. Monitor vital signs and fluid and electrolytes closely.

sodium chloride (NaCl)

Electrolyte, sodium and chloride replacement

Available by prescription only
Injection: Half-normal saline in 25 ml, 50 ml, 150 ml, 250 ml, 500 ml, 1,000 ml; normal saline in 2 ml, 3 ml, 5 ml, 10 ml, 20 ml, 25 ml, 30 ml, 50 ml, 100 ml, 150 ml, 250 ml, 500 ml, 1,000 ml; 3% NaCl in 500 ml; 5% NaCl in 500 ml
Available without prescription
Tablets: 650 mg, 1 g
Tablets (slow-release): 600 mg

INDICATIONS & DOSAGE

Water and electrolyte replacement in hyponatremia from electrolyte loss or severe NaCl depletion
Adults: Treatment is highly individualized based on frequent laboratory values and patient's condition. See manufacturer's recommendations for P.O. dosing.

PHARMACODYNAMICS

Electrolyte replacement: NaCl solution replaces deficiencies of sodium and chloride ions in blood plasma.

PHARMACOKINETICS

Absorption: Oral and parenteral NaCl are absorbed readily.
Distribution: Drug is distributed widely.
Metabolism: None significant.
Excretion: Drug is eliminated primarily in urine, but also in sweat, tears, and saliva.

CONTRAINDICATIONS & PRECAUTIONS

Contraindicated in patients with conditions in which NaCl administration is detrimental. NaCl 3% and 5% injections are contraindicated in patients with increased, normal, or only slightly decreased serum electrolyte levels.

Use cautiously in patients with heart failure, renal dysfunction, circulatory insufficiency, or hypoproteinemia and in geriatric or postoperative patients.

INTERACTIONS

None reported.

ADVERSE REACTIONS

CV: thrombophlebitis, aggravation of heart failure, edema (if given too rapidly or in excess).
Metabolic: hypernatremia and aggravation of existing metabolic acidosis (with excessive infusion), serious electrolyte disturbances, loss of potassium.
Respiratory: *pulmonary edema* (if given too rapidly or in excess).
Skin: tissue necrosis at injection site.
Other: local tenderness, abscess.

🔲 KEY CONSIDERATIONS

• Use concentrated solutions (3% and 5%) only for correcting severe sodium deficits (sodium level less than 120 mEq/ml). Infuse solutions very slowly and with caution to avoid pulmonary edema; observe patient constantly.

• Concentrated solutions (3.5 and 4 mEq/ml) are available for addition to parenteral nutrition solutions.

• Monitor changes in fluid balance, serum electrolyte disturbances, and acid-base imbalances.

Reactions may be *common,* uncommon, *life-threatening,* or COMMON AND LIFE-THREATENING.

• Monitor for hypokalemia with administration of potassium-free solutions.
• Normal saline solution may be used in managing extreme dilution of hyponatremia and hypochloremia resulting from administration of sodium-free fluids during fluid and electrolyte therapy and in managing extreme dilution of extracellular fluid after excessive water intake (for example, after multiple enemas).

Overdose & treatment
• NaCl overdose causes serious electrolyte disturbances. Oral ingestion of large quantities irritates the GI mucosa and may cause nausea and vomiting, diarrhea, and abdominal cramps.
• Treatment of oral overdose consists of emptying the stomach, giving magnesium sulfate as cathartic, and providing supportive therapy. Provide airway and ventilation if necessary. Excessive I.V. administration requires discontinuation of NaCl infusion.

sodium lactate

Systemic alkalizer

Available by prescription only
Injection: 1/6 M solution
Injection for preparations of I.V. admixtures: 5 mEq/ml

INDICATIONS & DOSAGE
To alkalize urine
Adults: 30 ml of 1/6 M solution/kg of body weight given in divided doses over 24 hours.
Mild to moderate metabolic acidosis
Adults: Dosage is highly individualized and depends on the severity of acidosis; patient's age, weight, and clinical condition; and laboratory determinants. Use the following formula to determine dosage for administration by I.V. infusion.

$$\text{Dose in ml of 1/6 M solution} = (60 - \text{plasma } CO_2) \times (0.8 \times \text{body weight in lb})$$

PHARMACODYNAMICS
Alkalizing action: Sodium lactate is metabolized in the liver, producing bicar-

bonate, the primary extracellular alkalotic buffer for the body's acid-base system, and glycogen. The simultaneous removal of lactate and hydrogen ion during metabolism also produces alkalization.

PHARMACOKINETICS
Absorption: Not applicable.
Distribution: Lactate ion occurs naturally throughout the body.
Metabolism: Lactate is metabolized in the liver to glycogen.
Excretion: None.

CONTRAINDICATIONS & PRECAUTIONS
Contraindicated in patients with hypernatremia, lactic acidosis, or conditions in which sodium administration is detrimental.
   Use extreme caution in patients with metabolic or respiratory alkalosis, severe renal or hepatic disease, shock, hypoxia, or beriberi.

INTERACTIONS
None reported.

ADVERSE REACTIONS
Metabolic: *metabolic alkalosis,* hypernatremia, hyperosmolarity (with overdose).
Other: fever, infection or thrombophlebitis at injection site.

▣ KEY CONSIDERATIONS
• Use cautiously in geriatric patients with heart failure and other fluid- and sodium-retaining states.
• To prevent alkalosis, assess electrolyte, fluid, and acid-base status throughout infusion.
• Monitor injection site for infiltration, extravasation, or both.
• Sodium lactate shouldn't be used to treat severe metabolic acidosis because the production of bicarbonate from lactate may take 1 to 2 hours.
• I.V. infusion rate shouldn't exceed 300 ml/hour.
• Drug is physically incompatible with sodium bicarbonate solutions.

Overdose & treatment
• Signs and symptoms of overdose include tetany from hypocalcemia,

seizures from alkalosis, and arrhythmias from hypokalemia.
• Correct fluid, electrolyte, and pH abnormalities. Monitor vital signs and fluid status closely.

sodium phosphates (sodium phosphate and sodium biphosphate)
Fleet Phospho-Soda

Acid salt, sodium chloride laxative

Available without prescription
Solution: 18 g sodium phosphate and 48 g sodium biphosphate/100 ml

INDICATIONS & DOSAGE
Constipation
Adults: 20 to 30 ml solution mixed with 4 oz (120 ml) cold water.
Purgative action
Adults: 45 ml solution mixed with 4 oz cold water.

PHARMACODYNAMICS
Laxative action: Sodium phosphate and sodium biphosphate exert an osmotic effect in the small intestine by drawing water into the intestinal lumen, producing distention that promotes peristalsis and bowel evacuation.

PHARMACOKINETICS
Absorption: About 1% to 20% of oral dose of sodium phosphates is absorbed; action begins in 3 to 6 hours.
Distribution: Unknown.
Metabolism: Unknown.
Excretion: Unknown; probably in feces and urine.

CONTRAINDICATIONS & PRECAUTIONS
Contraindicated in patients with abdominal pain, nausea, vomiting, or other symptoms of appendicitis or acute surgical abdomen; intestinal obstruction or perforation; edema; heart failure; megacolon; or impaired renal function and in patients on sodium-restricted diets.
    Use cautiously in patients with large hemorrhoids or anal excoriations.

INTERACTIONS
Drug-drug. Administration with *antacids* may inactivate both.

ADVERSE REACTIONS
GI: *abdominal cramping.*
Metabolic: fluid and electrolyte disturbances (hypernatremia, hyperphosphatemia) with daily use.
Other: laxative dependence with long-term or excessive use.

▣ KEY CONSIDERATIONS
• Dilute sodium phosphates with water before giving orally (add 30 ml drug to 120 ml water). After the patient takes the drug have him drink a full glass of water.
• Monitor serum electrolyte levels; when drug is given as sodium chloride laxative, up to 10% of sodium content may be absorbed.
• Drug isn't routinely used to treat constipation but is commonly used to evacuate the bowel.

Patient education
• Instruct patient how to mix sodium phosphates and on dosage schedule.
• Warn patient that frequent or prolonged use of drug may lead to laxative dependence.

sodium polystyrene sulfonate
Kayexalate, SPS

Cation-exchange resin, potassium-removing resin

Available by prescription only
Oral powder: 1.25 g/5-ml suspension
Powder for oral or rectal administration: 453.6 g in 1-lb jar
Rectal administration: 1.25 g/5-ml, 15 g/60-ml suspension

INDICATIONS & DOSAGE
Hyperkalemia
Adults: 15 g P.O. daily to q.i.d. in water or sorbitol. Alternatively, give 30 to 50 g q.i.d. or q 6 hours as retention enema.

PHARMACODYNAMICS

Potassium-removing action: Sodium polystyrene sulfonate is a cation-exchange resin that releases sodium in exchange for other cations in the GI tract. High levels of potassium ion are found in the large intestine and therefore are exchanged and eliminated.

PHARMACOKINETICS

Absorption: Sodium polystyrene sulfonate isn't absorbed; onset of action varies from hours to days.
Distribution: None.
Metabolism: None.
Excretion: Drug is excreted unchanged in feces.

CONTRAINDICATIONS & PRECAUTIONS

Contraindicated in patients with hypokalemia or hypersensitivity to sodium polystyrene sulfonate.

Use cautiously in patients with marked edema or severe heart failure or hypertension.

INTERACTIONS

Drug-drug. When used concomitantly, *calcium-* and *magnesium-containing antacids* are bound by the resin, possibly causing metabolic alkalosis in patients with renal impairment. Toxic effects of *cardiac glycosides* are exaggerated by hypokalemia, even when serum digoxin levels are in the normal range.

ADVERSE REACTIONS

GI: *constipation,* fecal impaction, anorexia, gastric irritation, nausea, vomiting, *diarrhea* (with sorbitol emulsions).
Metabolic: *hypokalemia,* hypocalcemia, sodium retention.

▣ KEY CONSIDERATIONS

• Fecal impaction is more likely in geriatric patients.
• For oral administration, mix resin only with water or sorbitol; never mix with orange juice (high potassium content).
• To increase palatability, chill the oral suspension; don't heat because that inactivates the resin.
• P.R. route is recommended when the patient is vomiting or has P.O. restrictions or upper GI tract problems.

• To prevent fecal impaction, administer the resin P.R.; a cleansing enema should precede P.R. administration.
• For P.R. administration, mix polystyrene resin only with water and sorbitol for rectal use. Don't use other vehicles (mineral oil) for P.R. administration to prevent impactions. Ion exchange requires aqueous medium. Sorbitol content prevents impaction. Prepare rectal dose at room temperature. Stir emulsion gently during administration.
• Monitor serum potassium level at least once daily. Watch for other signs of hypokalemia.
• Monitor for symptoms of other electrolyte deficiencies (magnesium, calcium) because drug is nonselective. Monitor serum calcium level in patients receiving sodium polystyrene therapy for more than 3 days; supplementary calcium may be needed.
• Constipation is more likely to occur when drug is given with phosphate binders (such as aluminum hydroxide). Monitor patient's bowel habits.
• If hyperkalemia is severe, more drastic modalities should be added; for example, dextrose 50% with regular insulin I.V. push. Don't depend solely on polystyrene resin to reduce serum potassium levels in severe hyperkalemia.

Patient education

• Instruct patient in the importance of following a prescribed low-potassium diet.
• Explain necessity of retaining enema to patient; retention for 6 to 10 hours is ideal, but 30 to 60 minutes is acceptable.

Overdose & treatment

• Signs and symptoms of overdose include those of hypokalemia (irritability, confusion, arrhythmias, ECG changes, severe muscle weakness, and sometimes paralysis) and digitalis toxicity in patients receiving digoxin.
• Sodium polystyrene sulfonate may be discontinued or the dose reduced when serum potassium level decreases to the 4- to 5-mEq/L range.

sotalol
Betapace

Beta blocker, antiarrhythmic

Available by prescription only
Tablets: 80 mg, 120 mg, 160 mg,
240 mg

INDICATIONS & DOSAGE
Documented, life-threatening ventricular arrhythmias
Adults: Initially, 80 mg P.O. b.i.d. Increase dosage q 2 to 3 days as needed and tolerated. Most patients respond to daily dose of 160 to 320 mg. A few patients with refractory arrhythmias have received as much as 640 mg daily.
✦ ***Dosage adjustment.*** For adults with renal failure and creatinine clearance greater than 60 ml/minute, no adjustment in dosage interval is necessary. If creatinine clearance is 30 to 60 ml/minute, give q 24 hours; 10 to 30 ml/minute, q 36 to 48 hours; and if less than 10 ml/minute, individualize dosage.

PHARMACODYNAMICS
Antiarrhythmic action: Sotalol is a nonselective beta blocker that depresses sinus heart rate, slows AV node conduction, increases AV nodal refractoriness, prolongs the refractory period of atrial and ventricular muscle and AV accessory pathways in anterograde and retrograde directions, decreases cardiac output, and reduces systolic and diastolic blood pressure.

PHARMACOKINETICS
Absorption: Sotalol is well absorbed after oral administration, with a bioavailability of 90% to 100%. After oral administration, plasma levels peak in 2½ to 4 hours and plasma levels reach steady state in 2 to 3 days (after 5 or 6 doses when administered b.i.d.).
Distribution: Drug doesn't bind to plasma proteins and crosses the blood-brain barrier poorly.
Metabolism: Drug isn't metabolized.
Excretion: Drug is excreted primarily in urine unchanged.

CONTRAINDICATIONS & PRECAUTIONS
Contraindicated in patients with hypersensitivity to sotalol, severe sinus node dysfunction, sinus bradycardia, second- or third-degree AV block in the absence of an artificial pacemaker, congenital or acquired long QT interval syndrome, cardiogenic shock, uncontrolled heart failure or bronchial asthma.
Use cautiously in patients with impaired renal function or diabetes mellitus.

INTERACTIONS
Drug-drug. *Antiarrhythmics* cause additive effects when administered with sotalol; don't use together. *Calcium channel antagonists* enhance myocardial depression and shouldn't be given with sotalol. *Catecholamine-depleting drugs,* such as *guanethidine* and *reserpine,* enhance the hypotensive effects of sotalol; monitor patient closely. Sotalol may enhance the rebound hypertensive effect seen after withdrawal of *clonidine*; discontinue sotalol several days before withdrawing *clonidine.* Sotalol may require dosage adjustments with *insulin* or *oral antidiabetics* because it may increase blood glucose levels and mask symptoms of hypoglycemia.

ADVERSE REACTIONS
CNS: *asthenia, light-headedness, headache, dizziness, weakness, fatigue,* sleep problems.
CV: *bradycardia, palpitations, chest pain,* **arrhythmias, heart failure, AV block, proarrhythmic events (ventricular tachycardia, PVCs, ventricular fibrillation),** edema, ECG abnormalities, hypotension.
GI: *nausea, vomiting,* diarrhea, dyspepsia.
Hepatic: elevated liver enzyme levels.
Metabolic: hyperglycemia.
Respiratory: *dyspnea,* **bronchospasm.**

▣ KEY CONSIDERATIONS
• Make dosage adjustments slowly, allowing 2 to 3 days between dosage increments for adequate monitoring of QT intervals and for sotalol plasma levels to reach steady state.

Reactions may be *common,* uncommon, *life-threatening,* or COMMON AND LIFE-THREATENING.

• Because proarrhythmic events such as sustained ventricular tachycardia or ventricular fibrillation may occur at start of therapy and during dosage adjustments, patient should be hospitalized. Facilities and personnel should be available for cardiac rhythm monitoring and ECG interpretation.

• Although patients receiving I.V. lidocaine have begun sotalol therapy without ill effect, other antiarrhythmics should be withdrawn before sotalol therapy begins. Sotalol therapy typically is delayed until two or three half-lives of the withdrawn drug have elapsed. After withdrawal of amiodarone, sotalol shouldn't be administered until the QT interval normalizes.

• Monitor serum electrolyte levels regularly, especially if patient is receiving diuretics. Electrolyte imbalances, such as hypokalemia or hypomagnesemia, may further prolong the QT interval and increase risk of serious arrhythmias, such as torsades de pointes.

Patient education

• Explain importance of taking sotalol as prescribed, even when patient is feeling well.

• Caution patient not to discontinue drug suddenly.

Overdose & treatment

• The most common signs and symptoms of overdose are bradycardia, heart failure, hypotension, bronchospasm, and hypoglycemia.

• Sotalol should be discontinued and the patient observed closely. Because of the lack of protein-binding, hemodialysis is useful in reducing plasma levels. Patient should be carefully observed until QT intervals are normalized. Atropine, another anticholinergic, a beta agonist, or transvenous cardiac pacing may also be used to treat bradycardia. Use transvenous cardiac pacing to treat second- or third-degree heart block; epinephrine to treat hypotension (depending on associated factors); aminophylline or an aerosol beta$_2$-receptor stimulant to treat bronchospasm; and direct current cardioversion, transvenous cardiac pacing,

epinephrine, or magnesium sulfate to treat torsades de pointes.

---

sparfloxacin
Zagam

Fluorinated quinolone, broad-spectrum antibacterial

Available by prescription only
Tablets: 200 mg

INDICATIONS & DOSAGE

Acute bacterial exacerbation of chronic bronchitis caused by **Staphylococcus aureus, Streptococcus pneumoniae, Chlamydia pneumoniae, Enterobacter cloacae, Klebsiella pneumoniae, Moraxella catarrhalis, Haemophilus influenzae,** *or* **H. parainfluenzae**
Adults: 400 mg P.O. 1st day as loading dose, then 200 mg daily for 10 days of therapy (total of 11 tablets).

Community-acquired pneumonia caused **by S. pneumoniae, M. catarrhalis, H. influenzae, H. parainfluenzae, C. pneumoniae,** *or* **Mycoplasma pneumoniae**
Adults: 400 mg P.O. 1st day as a loading dose, then 200 mg daily for total of 10 days of therapy (total of 11 tablets).

✦ *Dosage adjustment.* In patients with renal impairment, if creatinine clearance is less than 50 ml/minute, give loading dose of 400 mg P.O.; then 200 mg P.O. q 48 hours for total of 9 days of therapy (total of 6 tablets).

PHARMACODYNAMICS

Antibacterial action: Sparfloxacin inhibits bacterial DNA gyrase and prevents DNA replication, transcription, repair, and deactivation in susceptible bacteria.

PHARMACOKINETICS

Absorption: Sparfloxacin is well absorbed after oral administration; absolute bioavailability of 92%. Plasma levels peak 3 to 6 hours after dosing.
Distribution: Drug's volume of distribution is about 3.9 L/kg, indicating distribution well into the tissues. Level in respiratory tissues at 2 to 6 hours after dos-

---

ing is about three to six times greater than plasma.

Metabolism: Drug is metabolized by the liver, primarily by phase II glucuronidation. Its metabolism doesn't interfere with or use the cytochrome P-450 system.

Excretion: Drug is excreted in urine (50%) and feces (50%). Terminal elimination half-life varies between 16 and 30 hours; mean, 20 hours.

CONTRAINDICATIONS & PRECAUTIONS

Contraindicated in patients with history of hypersensitivity or photosensitivity reactions to drugs and those who can't stay out of the sun. Don't use in patients with cardiac conditions that predispose to them arrhythmias.

Use with caution in patients with known or suspected CNS disorders, such as seizures, toxic psychoses, or tremors.

INTERACTIONS

Drug-drug. *Antacids containing aluminum* or *magnesium, iron salts, sucralfate,* or *zinc* may interfere with GI absorption of sparfloxacin; administer at least 4 hours apart. *Drugs that prolong the QTc interval and may cause torsades de pointes* (including *amiodarone, bepridil,* class Ia antiarrhythmics *[procainamide, quinidine],* class III drugs *[sotalol],* and *disopyramide)* are contraindicated in these patients. Other *QTc-prolonging drugs* include *cisapride, erythromycin, pentamidine,* some *antipsychotic drugs* (including *phenothiazines*), and *tricyclic antidepressants.*
Drug-lifestyle. *Sun exposure* may exacerbate photosensitivity reactions.

ADVERSE REACTIONS

CNS: asthenia, dizziness, headache, insomnia, *seizures,* somnolence.
CV: *QT interval prolongation*, vasodilation.
GI: abdominal pain, diarrhea, dyspepsia, flatulence, nausea, pseudomembranous colitis, vomiting, dry mouth, taste perversion.
GU: vaginal candidiasis.
Hematologic: increased WBC count.
Hepatic: elevated liver enzyme levels.
Musculoskeletal: tendon rupture.

Skin: photosensitivity, pruritus, rash.
Other: *hypersensitivity reactions.*

▣ KEY CONSIDERATIONS

• Because moderate to severe phototoxic reactions have occurred, avoid exposure to sun, bright natural light, or ultraviolet light during therapy and for 5 days after therapy is completed.
• Drug may produce false-negative culture results for *Mycobacterium tuberculosis.*

Patient education

• Inform patient that sparfloxacin may be taken with food, milk, or products that contain caffeine.
• Tell patient to take drug as prescribed, even if symptoms disappear.
• Advise patient to take drug with plenty of fluids and to avoid antacids, sucralfate, and products containing iron or zinc for at least 4 hours after each dose.
• Warn patient to avoid hazardous tasks until adverse CNS effects of drug are known.
• Advise patient to avoid direct, indirect, and artificial ultraviolet light, even with sunscreen, during treatment and for 5 days after treatment. Patient should stop drug and call if signs or symptoms of phototoxicity (skin burning, redness, swelling, blisters, rash, itching) occur.
• Tell patient to discontinue drug and report pain or inflammation; tendon rupture can occur. Tell patient to rest and refrain from exercise until a diagnosis is made.
• Instruct patient to drink fluids liberally.

---

spironolactone
Aldactone

Potassium sparing diuretic, antihypertensive, diagnosis of primary hyperaldosteronism, treatment of diuretic-induced hypokalemia

Available by prescription only
Tablets: 25 mg, 50 mg, 100 mg

INDICATIONS & DOSAGE
Edema
Adults: 25 to 200 mg P.O. daily in divided doses.
Hypertension
Adults: 50 to 100 mg P.O. daily in divided doses.
Diuretic-induced hypokalemia
Adults: 25 to 100 mg P.O. daily when oral potassium supplements are considered inappropriate.
Detection of primary hyperaldosteronism
Adults: 400 mg P.O. daily for 4 days (short test) or for 3 to 4 weeks (long test). If hypokalemia and hypertension are corrected, a presumptive diagnosis of primary hyperaldosteronism is made.
◊ Hirsutism
Adults: 50 to 200 mg P.O. daily.

PHARMACODYNAMICS
Diuretic and potassium sparing actions: Spironolactone competitively inhibits aldosterone effects on the distal renal tubules, increasing sodium and water excretion and decreasing potassium excretion. Drug is used to treat edema associated with excessive aldosterone secretion, such as that associated with hepatic cirrhosis, nephrotic syndrome, and heart failure. It's also used to treat diuretic-induced hypokalemia.
Antihypertensive action: Mechanism of action is unknown; drug may block the effect of aldosterone on arteriolar smooth muscle.
Diagnosis of primary hyperaldosteronism: Drug inhibits the effects of aldosterone, so correction of hypokalemia and hypertension is presumptive evidence of primary hyperaldosteronism.

PHARMACOKINETICS
Absorption: About 90% of spironolactone is absorbed after oral administration. Onset of action is gradual; maximum effect occurs on the 3rd day of therapy.
Distribution: Drug and its major metabolite, canrenone, are more than 90% plasma protein-bound.
Metabolism: Drug is rapidly and extensively metabolized to canrenone.

Excretion: Canrenone and other metabolites are excreted primarily in urine, and small amount is excreted in feces through the biliary tract; half-life of canrenone is 13 to 24 hours. Half-life of parent compound is 1 to 2 hours.

CONTRAINDICATIONS & PRECAUTIONS
Contraindicated in patients with anuria, acute or progressive renal insufficiency, or hyperkalemia.
  Use cautiously in patients with impaired renal function, hepatic disease, or fluid and electrolyte imbalances.

INTERACTIONS
Drug-drug. Spironolactone increases the risk of hyperkalemia when administered with *ACE inhibitors, other potassium sparing diuretics, potassium-containing drugs (parenteral penicillin G),* and *potassium supplements.* Aspirin may slightly decrease response to spironolactone. *NSAIDs* such as *ibuprofen* or *indomethacin* may impair renal function and thus affect potassium excretion. Spironolactone may potentiate the hypotensive effects of *other antihypertensives;* this may be used to therapeutic advantage.
Drug-food. Use with *sodium substitutes* increases the risk of hyperkalemia.

ADVERSE REACTIONS
CNS: headache, drowsiness, lethargy, confusion, ataxia.
GI: diarrhea, gastric bleeding, ulceration, cramping, gastritis, vomiting.
GU: transient elevation in BUN level, inability to maintain erection, breast soreness in women, gynecomastia.
Hematologic: *agranulocytosis.*
Metabolic: *hyperkalemia,* dehydration, hyponatremia, metabolic acidosis.
Skin: urticaria, maculopapular eruptions.
Other: hirsutism, drug fever.

▣ KEY CONSIDERATIONS
Besides the recommendations relevant to all potassium sparing diuretics, consider the following:
• Geriatric patients are more susceptible to diuretic effects and may require a lower dosage to prevent excessive diuresis.

• Give spironolactone with meals to enhance absorption.

• Diuretic effect may be delayed 2 to 3 days if drug is used alone; maximum antihypertensive effect may be delayed 2 to 3 weeks.

• Protect drug from light.

• Adverse reactions are related to dosage levels and duration of therapy and usually disappear with withdrawal of drug; however, gynecomastia may persist.

• Drug is antiandrogenic and has been used to treat hirsutism in dosages of 200 mg/day.

• Avoid unnecessary use of drug; it's been shown to induce tumors in laboratory animals.

• Drug therapy alters plasma and urine 17-hydroxycorticosteroid levels on fluorometry and may falsely elevate serum digoxin level on radioimmunoassay.

Patient education

• Explain that maximal diuresis may not occur until the third day of therapy and that diuresis may continue for 2 to 3 days after spironolactone is withdrawn.

• Instruct patient to report mental confusion or lethargy immediately.

• Explain that adverse reactions usually disappear after drug is discontinued; gynecomastia may persist.

• Caution patient to avoid such hazardous activities as driving until response to drug is known.

Overdose & treatment

• Signs and symptoms of overdose are consistent with dehydration and electrolyte disturbance.

• Treatment is supportive and symptomatic. In acute ingestion, induce vomiting or perform gastric lavage. In severe hyperkalemia (more than 6.5 mEq/L), reduce serum potassium levels with I.V. sodium bicarbonate or glucose with insulin. A cation-exchange resin, sodium polystyrene sulfonate, given orally or as a retention enema, may also reduce serum potassium levels.

stavudine (d4T)
Zerit

Synthetic thymidine nucleoside analogue, antiviral

Available by prescription only
Capsules: 15 mg, 20 mg, 30 mg, 40 mg

INDICATIONS & DOSAGE
Treatment of HIV infection in patients who received prior prolonged zidovudine therapy
Adults: For patients weighing 60 kg (132 lb) or more, 40 mg P.O. q 12 hours; for patients weighing less than 60 kg, 30 mg P.O. q 12 hours.

✦ *Dosage adjustment.* For patients with renal impairment, refer to table.

Creatinine clearance (ml/min)	Dosage for patients weighing ≥ 60 kg	Dosage for patients weighing < 60 kg
> 50	40 mg q 12 hr	30 mg q 12 hr
26-50	20 mg q 12 hr	15 mg q 12 hr
10-25	20 mg q 24 hr	15 mg q 24 hr

PHARMACODYNAMICS
Antiviral action: Stavudine is phosphorylated by cellular kinases to stavudine triphosphate, which exerts antiviral activity. Stavudine triphosphate inhibits HIV replication by two known mechanisms. It inhibits HIV reverse transcriptase by competing with the natural substrate deoxythymidine triphosphate, and it inhibits viral DNA synthesis by causing DNA chain termination because stavudine lacks the 3"-hydroxyl group necessary for DNA elongation. Stavudine triphosphate also inhibits cellular DNA polymerase beta and gamma and markedly reduces mitochondrial DNA synthesis.

PHARMACOKINETICS
Absorption: Stavudine is rapidly absorbed, with a mean absolute bioavailability of 86.4%. Plasma levels peak in 1 hour or less.
Distribution: Mean volume of distribution is 58 L, suggesting distribution into extravascular space. Drug is distributed

equally between RBCs and plasma; it binds poorly to plasma proteins.
Metabolism: Unknown.
Excretion: Renal elimination accounts for about 40% of overall clearance, regardless of administration route; active tubular secretion in addition to glomerular filtration occurs.

CONTRAINDICATIONS & PRECAUTIONS
Contraindicated in patients with hypersensitivity to stavudine. Use cautiously in patients with impaired renal function or history of peripheral neuropathy.

INTERACTIONS
None significant.

ADVERSE REACTIONS
CNS: *peripheral neuropathy, asthenia, headache, malaise, insomnia, anxiety, depression, nervousness,* dizziness.
CV: chest pain.
EENT: conjunctivitis.
GI: *abdominal pain, diarrhea, nausea, vomiting, anorexia,* dyspepsia, constipation.
Hematologic: *neutropenia, thrombocytopenia,* anemia.
Hepatic: elevated liver enzyme levels, *hepatotoxicity.*
Metabolic: weight loss.
Musculoskeletal: *myalgia, back pain, arthralgia.*
Respiratory: *dyspnea.*
Skin: *rash, diaphoresis, pruritus,* maculopapular rash.
Other: *chills, fever.*

▣ KEY CONSIDERATIONS
● Monitor patient for peripheral neuropathy, usually characterized by numbness, tingling, or pain in the feet or hands. If symptoms develop, interrupt drug therapy. Symptoms may resolve if therapy is withdrawn promptly. Symptoms may worsen temporarily after drug is discontinued. If symptoms resolve completely, resume treatment using the following dosage schedule: patients weighing 60 kg or more, 20 mg b.i.d.; patients weighing less than 60 kg, 15 mg b.i.d. Manage significant elevations of hepatic transaminase levels in same way.

Patient education
● Inform patient that stavudine isn't a cure for HIV infection and patient may continue to acquire illnesses associated with AIDS or AIDS-related complex, including opportunistic infections.
● Inform patient that drug doesn't reduce risk of transmitting HIV to others through sexual contact or blood contamination.
● Instruct patient to report signs of peripheral neuropathy—such as tingling, burning, pain, or numbness in the hands or feet—because dosage adjustments may be necessary. Counsel patient that this toxicity occurs with greater frequency in those with a history of peripheral neuropathy. Advise patient not to use other drugs, including OTC preparations, without calling first; some drugs can exacerbate peripheral neuropathy.
● Explain that long-term effects of drug are unknown.

streptokinase
Kabikinase, Streptase

Plasminogen activator, thrombolytic enzyme

Available by prescription only
Injection: 250,000 IU, 600,000 IU, 750,000 IU, 1,500,000 IU in vials for reconstitution

INDICATIONS & DOSAGE
Lysis of coronary artery thrombi after an acute MI
Adults: 1,500,000 IU by I.V. infusion over 60 minutes; intracoronary loading dose of 20,000 IU via coronary catheter, followed by a maintenance dose of 2,000 IU/minute for 60 minutes as infusion.
Arteriovenous cannula occlusion
Adults: 250,000 IU in 2 ml I.V. solution by I.V. infusion pump into each occluded limb of the cannula over 25 to 35 minutes. Clamp off cannula for 2 hours, then aspirate contents of cannula, flush with sodium chloride solution, and reconnect.

Venous thrombosis, pulmonary embolism, and arterial thrombosis and embolism
Adults: Loading dose of 250,000 IU I.V. infusion over 30 minutes. Sustaining dose of 100,000 IU/hour I.V. infusion for 72 hours for deep vein thrombosis and 100,000 IU/hour over 24 hours by I.V. infusion pump for pulmonary embolism.

PHARMACODYNAMICS
Thrombolytic action: Streptokinase promotes thrombolysis by activating plasminogen in two steps. First, plasminogen and streptokinase form a complex, exposing plasminogen-activating site, and second, cleavage of peptide bond converts plasminogen to plasmin.

To treat an acute MI, streptokinase prevents primary or secondary thrombus formation in microcirculation surrounding the necrotic area.

PHARMACOKINETICS
Absorption: Plasminogen activation begins promptly after infusion or instillation of streptokinase; adequate activation of fibrinolytic system occurs in 3 to 4 hours.
Distribution: Unknown.
Metabolism: Insignificant.
Excretion: Antibodies and the reticuloendothelial system remove drug from circulation. Half-life is biphasic; initially it's 18 minutes (from antibody action), then extends up to 83 minutes. Anticoagulant effect may persist for 12 to 24 hours after infusion is discontinued.

CONTRAINDICATIONS & PRECAUTIONS
Contraindicated in patients with ulcers, active internal bleeding, recent CVA, recent trauma with possible internal injuries, visceral or intracranial malignant neoplasms, ulcerative colitis, diverticulitis, severe hypertension, acute or chronic hepatic or renal insufficiency, uncontrolled hypocoagulation, chronic pulmonary disease with cavitation, subacute bacterial endocarditis or rheumatic valvular disease, or recent cerebral embolism, thrombosis, or hemorrhage. Also contraindicated within 10 days after intra-arterial diagnostic procedure or any surgery, including liver or kidney biopsy,

lumbar puncture, thoracentesis, paracentesis, or extensive or multiple cutdowns. I.M. injections and other invasive procedures are contraindicated during streptokinase therapy.

Use cautiously in patients with arterial embolism that originates from the left side of the heart.

INTERACTIONS
Drug-drug. *Aminocaproic acid* inhibits streptokinase-induced activation of plasminogen. Use with *anticoagulants* may cause hemorrhage; it may also be necessary to reverse effects of oral anticoagulants before beginning therapy. Use with *aspirin, indomethacin, other drugs affecting platelet activity* or *phenylbutazone* increases risk of bleeding.

ADVERSE REACTIONS
CNS: polyradiculoneuropathy, headache.
CV: *reperfusion arrhythmias,* hypotension, vasculitis, flushing.
EENT: periorbital edema.
GI: nausea.
Hematologic: *bleeding;* increased thrombin time, activated partial thromboplastin time, and PT; moderately decreased hematocrit.
Musculoskeletal: pain.
Respiratory: minor breathing difficulty, *bronchospasm.*
Skin: urticaria, pruritus.
Other: phlebitis at injection site, hypersensitivity reactions *(anaphylaxis), delayed hypersensitivity reactions* (interstitial nephritis, serum sickness-like reactions), *angioedema, fever.*

▣ KEY CONSIDERATIONS
Besides the recommendations relevant to all thrombolytic enzymes, consider the following:
• Patients ages 75 or older are at greater risk for cerebral hemorrhage because they're likely to have preexisting cerebrovascular disease.
• Reconstitute vial with 5 ml normal saline injection and further dilute to 45 ml; roll gently to mix. Don't shake. Use immediately; refrigerate remainder, and discard after 8 hours. Store powder at room temperature.

Reactions may be *common*, uncommon, *life-threatening*, or COMMON AND LIFE-THREATENING.

• Rate of I.V. infusion depends on thrombin time and streptokinase resistance; higher loading dose may be necessary in patients with recent streptococcal infection or recent treatment with streptokinase to compensate for antibody drug neutralization.

• Don't discontinue therapy for minor allergic reactions that can be treated with antihistamines or corticosteroids; about one-third of patients experience a slight temperature elevation and some have chills. Symptomatic treatment with acetaminophen (but not aspirin or other salicylates) is indicated if temperature reaches 104° F (40° C). Patients may be pretreated with corticosteroids, repeating doses during therapy, to minimize pyrogenic or allergic reactions.

• If minor bleeding can be controlled with local pressure, don't decrease dose so that more plasminogen is available for conversion to plasmin.

• Antibodies to drug can persist for 3 to 6 months or longer after the initial dose; if further thrombolytic therapy is needed, consider urokinase.

sucralfate
Carafate

Pepsin inhibitor, antiulcerative

Available by prescription only
Tablets: 1 g
Suspension: 1 g/10 ml

INDICATIONS & DOSAGE
Short-term (up to 8 weeks) treatment of duodenal ulcer, ◊ aspirin-induced gastric erosion
Adults: 1 g P.O. q.i.d. 1 hour before meals and h.s.
Maintenance therapy of duodenal ulcer
Adults: 1 g P.O. b.i.d.

PHARMACODYNAMICS
Antiulcerative action: Sucralfate has a unique mechanism of action. It adheres to proteins at the ulcer site, forming a protective coating against gastric acid, pepsin, and bile salts. It also inhibits pepsin, exhibits a cytoprotective effect, and forms a viscous, adhesive barrier on the surface of the intact intestinal mucosa and stomach.

PHARMACOKINETICS
Absorption: Only 3% to 5% of dose is absorbed. Sucralfate activity isn't related to amount absorbed.
Distribution: Drug acts locally at the ulcer site; absorbed drug is distributed to many body tissues, including liver and kidneys.
Metabolism: None.
Excretion: About 90% of dose is excreted in feces; absorbed drug is excreted unchanged in urine. Duration of effect is 6 hours.

CONTRAINDICATIONS & PRECAUTIONS
No known contraindications. Use cautiously in patients with chronic renal failure.

INTERACTIONS
Drug-drug. *Antacids* may decrease binding of sucralfate to gastroduodenal mucosa, impairing effectiveness; separate dosing of sucralfate and antacids by 30 minutes. Sucralfate decreases absorption of *cimetidine, digoxin, fat-soluble vitamins A, D, E, and K, phenytoin, quinidine, quinolones, ranitidine, tetracycline,* and *theophylline.*

ADVERSE REACTIONS
CNS: dizziness, sleepiness, headache, vertigo.
GI: *constipation,* nausea, gastric discomfort, diarrhea, bezoar formation, vomiting, flatulence, dry mouth, indigestion.
Musculoskeletal: back pain.
Skin: rash, pruritus.

▣ KEY CONSIDERATIONS
• Sucralfate may inhibit absorption of other drugs; schedule other drugs 2 hours before or after sucralfate.
• Drug is poorly water soluble. For administration via an NG tube, have pharmacist prepare water-sorbitol suspension of sucralfate. Alternatively, place tablet in 60-ml syringe, add 20 ml water, and let stand with tip up for about 5 minutes, occasionally shaking gently. The resultant suspension may be administered

from the syringe. After administration, tube should be flushed several times to ensure that the patient receives the entire dose.
• Patients who have difficulty swallowing tablet may place it in 15 to 30 ml water at room temperature, allow it to disintegrate, and ingest the resulting suspension. This is particularly useful for patients with esophagitis and painful swallowing.
• Monitor patient for constipation.
• Therapy exceeding 8 weeks isn't recommended.
• Some experts believe that 2 g given b.i.d. is as effective as the standard regimen.
• Drug treats ulcers as effectively as H_2-receptor antagonists.

Patient education
• Remind patient to take sucralfate on an empty stomach and at least 1 hour before meals.
• Advise patient to continue taking drug as directed even after pain begins to subside to ensure adequate healing.
• Tell patient he may take an antacid 30 minutes before or 2 hours after sucralfate.
• Warn patient not to take drug for more than 8 weeks.

sulfamethoxazole
Gantanol

Sulfonamide, antibiotic

Available by prescription only
Tablets: 500 mg
Suspension: 500 mg/5 ml

INDICATIONS & DOSAGE
Urinary tract and systemic infections
Adults: Initially, 2 g P.O.; then 1 g P.O. b.i.d., up to t.i.d. for severe infections.
Lymphogranuloma venereum (genital, inguinal, or anorectal infection)
Adults: 1 g P.O. b.i.d. for 21 days.

PHARMACODYNAMICS
Antibacterial action: Sulfamethoxazole is bacteriostatic. It inhibits formation of tetrahydrofolic acid from PABA, thus preventing bacterial cell synthesis of folic acid.
   Spectrum of action includes some gram-positive bacteria, *Chlamydia trachomatis,* many Enterobacteriaceae, and some strains of *Toxoplasma* and *Plasmodium.*

PHARMACOKINETICS
Absorption: Sulfamethoxazole is absorbed from the GI tract after oral administration; serum levels peak in 3 to 4 hours.
Distribution: Drug is distributed widely into most body tissues and fluids, including CSF, synovial, pleural, prostatic, peritoneal, and seminal fluids. It's 50% to 70% protein-bound.
Metabolism: Drug is partially metabolized in the liver.
Excretion: Both unchanged drug and metabolites are excreted primarily in urine through glomerular filtration and, to a lesser extent, renal tubular secretion. Urinary solubility of unchanged drug increases as urine pH increases. Elimination half-life in patients with normal renal function is 7 to 12 hours.

CONTRAINDICATIONS & PRECAUTIONS
Contraindicated in patients with porphyria or hypersensitivity to sulfonamides.
   Use cautiously in patients with renal or hepatic impairment, bronchial asthma, severe allergies, G6PD deficiency, or blood dyscrasia.

INTERACTIONS
Drug-drug. Sulfamethoxazole may inhibit hepatic metabolism of *oral anticoagulants,* displacing them from binding sites and enhancing anticoagulant effects. Use with *oral antidiabetics (sulfonylureas)* enhances their hypoglycemic effects, probably by displacing sulfonylureas from protein-binding sites; with *PABA,* antagonizes sulfonamide effects; and with either *pyrimethamine* or *trimethoprim (folic acid antagonists* with different mechanisms of action), results in synergistic antibacterial effects and delays or prevents bacterial resistance.

Drug-lifestyle. Prolonged or unprotected *exposure to the sun* may cause photosensitivity reactions.

ADVERSE REACTIONS

CNS: headache, mental depression, *seizures,* hallucinations, aseptic meningitis, tinnitus, apathy.
GI: *nausea, vomiting, diarrhea,* abdominal pain, anorexia, stomatitis, *pancreatitis,* pseudomembranous colitis.
GU: *toxic nephrosis with oliguria and anuria,* crystalluria, hematuria, interstitial nephritis.
Hematologic: *agranulocytosis, hemolytic anemia, aplastic anemia,* megaloblastic anemia, *thrombocytopenia, leukopenia.*
Hepatic: elevated liver function test results, *jaundice.*
Skin: *erythema multiforme (Stevens-Johnson syndrome),* generalized skin eruption, *epidermal necrolysis, exfoliative dermatitis,* photosensitivity, urticaria, pruritus.
Other: hypersensitivity reactions *(serum sickness, drug fever, anaphylaxis*).

▣ KEY CONSIDERATIONS

• Recommendations for administration, preparation and storage, and patient care and teaching during therapy with sulfamethoxazole are those common to all sulfonamides.
• Sulfamethoxazole alters results of urine glucose tests using cupric sulfate (Benedict's reagent or Clinitest).

Overdose & treatment

• Signs and symptoms of overdose include dizziness, drowsiness, headache, unconsciousness, anorexia, abdominal pain, nausea, and vomiting. More severe complications, including hemolytic anemia, agranulocytosis, dermatitis, acidosis, sensitivity reactions, and jaundice, may be fatal.
• Perform gastric lavage if ingestion occurred within the preceding 4 hours. Then, correct acidosis, force fluids, and administer I.V. fluids if urine output is low and renal function is normal. Treatment of renal failure and transfusion of appropriate blood products (in severe hematologic toxicity) may be required.

sulfasalazine
Azulfidine, Azulfidine EN-tabs

Sulfonamide, antibiotic

Available by prescription only
Tablets (with or without enteric coating): 500 mg
Suspension: 250 mg/5 ml

INDICATIONS & DOSAGE
Mild to moderate ulcerative colitis, adjunctive therapy in severe ulcerative colitis
Adults: Initially, 3 to 4 g P.O. daily in evenly divided doses. Maintenance dosage is 2 g P.O. daily in divided doses q 6 hours. May need to start with 1 to 2 g initially, with a gradual increase in dose to minimize adverse reactions.

PHARMACODYNAMICS
Antibacterial action: Exact mechanism of action of sulfasalazine in ulcerative colitis is unknown; it may be a prodrug metabolized by intestinal flora in the colon. One metabolite (5-aminosalicylic acid, or mesalamine) is responsible for the anti-inflammatory effect; the other metabolite (sulfapyridine) may be responsible for antibacterial action and some adverse effects.

PHARMACOKINETICS
Absorption: Sulfasalazine is poorly absorbed from the GI tract after oral administration; 70% to 90% is transported to the colon, where intestinal flora metabolize drug to its active ingredients, sulfapyridine (antibacterial) and 5-aminosalicylic acid (anti-inflammatory), which exert their effects locally. Sulfapyridine is absorbed from the colon, but only a small portion of 5-aminosalicylic acid is absorbed.
Distribution: Human data on drug distribution are lacking; animal studies have identified drug and metabolites in sera, liver, and intestinal walls.
Metabolism: Drug is cleaved by intestinal flora in the colon.
Excretion: Systemically absorbed drug is excreted chiefly in urine. Plasma half-life is about 6 to 8 hours.

CONTRAINDICATIONS & PRECAUTIONS

Contraindicated in patients with known hypersensitivity to salicylates or sulfonamides or to other drugs containing sulfur (such as thiazides, furosemide, or oral sulfonylureas) and in those with porphyria or severe renal or hepatic dysfunction. Sulfasalazine is also contraindicated in patients with intestinal or urinary tract obstructions because of the risk of local GI irritation and crystalluria.

Use cautiously in patients with mild to moderate renal or hepatic dysfunction, severe allergies, asthma, blood dyscrasia, or G6PD deficiency.

INTERACTIONS

Drug-drug. Use with *antacids* may cause enteric-coated tablets (designed to dissolve in the intestines) to dissolve prematurely, thus increasing systemic absorption and risk of toxicity. Use with *antibiotics that alter intestinal flora* may interfere with conversion of sulfasalazine to sulfapyridine and 5-aminosalicylic acid, decreasing its effectiveness. Sulfasalazine may reduce GI absorption of *digoxin* and *folic acid.* Sulfasalazine may inhibit hepatic metabolism of *oral anticoagulants*, displacing them from binding sites and enhancing anticoagulant effects. Use with *oral antidiabetics (sulfonylureas)* enhances hypoglycemic effects, probably by displacing sulfonylureas from protein-binding sites. Use with *urine-acidifying drugs (ammonium chloride, ascorbic acid)* decreases urine pH and sulfonamide solubility, thus increasing risk of crystalluria.
Drug-lifestyle. *Sun exposure* may cause photosensitivity reactions.

ADVERSE REACTIONS

CNS: headache, mental depression, *seizures,* hallucinations, tinnitus.
GI: *nausea, vomiting, diarrhea, abdominal pain, anorexia,* stomatitis.
GU: *toxic nephrosis* with oliguria and anuria, crystalluria, hematuria, oligospermia, infertility.
Hematologic: *agranulocytosis, aplastic anemia,* megaloblastic anemia, *thrombocytopenia, leukopenia,* hemolytic anemia.

Hepatic: jaundice, elevated liver function test results.
Skin: *erythema multiforme (Stevens-Johnson syndrome),* generalized skin eruption, *epidermal necrolysis, exfoliative dermatitis,* photosensitivity, urticaria, pruritus.
Other: *hypersensitivity reactions,* serum sickness, drug fever, *anaphylaxis,* bacterial and fungal superinfection.

▣ KEY CONSIDERATIONS

Besides the recommendations relevant to all sulfonamides, consider the following:
● Most adverse effects involve the GI tract; minimize reactions and facilitate absorption by spacing doses evenly and administering sulfasalazine after food.
● Drug turns urine orange-yellow; may also turn skin orange-yellow.
● Don't administer antacids with enteric-coated drug; they may alter drug absorption.
● Discontinue drug in patients with signs of toxicity or hypersensitivity; hematologic abnormalities accompanied by sore throat, pallor, fever, jaundice, purpura, or weakness; crystalluria accompanied by renal colic, hematuria, oliguria, proteinuria, urinary obstruction, urolithiasis, increased BUN levels, or anuria; severe diarrhea indicating pseudomembranous colitis; or severe persistent nausea, vomiting, or diarrhea.
● Drug alters results of urine glucose tests using cupric sulfate (Benedict's reagent or Clinitest).

Patient education

● Tell patient that sulfasalazine normally turns urine orange-yellow; skin may also turn orange-yellow, and drug may permanently stain soft contact lenses yellow.
● Advise patient not to take antacids with drug.
● Advise patient to take drug after meals to reduce GI distress and facilitate passage into intestines.
● Tell patient to avoid prolonged exposure to sunlight and to wear protective clothing and sunscreen because photosensitivity may occur.

Reactions may be *common*, uncommon, *life-threatening*, or COMMON AND LIFE-THREATENING.

Overdose & treatment
• Signs and symptoms of overdose include dizziness, drowsiness, headache, unconsciousness, anorexia, abdominal pain, nausea, and vomiting. More severe complications—including hemolytic anemia, agranulocytosis, dermatitis, acidosis, sensitivity reactions, and jaundice—may be fatal.
• Perform gastric lavage if ingestion occurred within the preceding 4 hours. Then, correct acidosis, force fluids, and alkalize urine to enhance solubility and excretion. Treatment of renal failure and transfusion of appropriate blood products (in severe hematologic toxicity) may be required.

sulfinpyrazone
Anturane

Uricosuric, renal tubular-blocker, platelet aggregation inhibitor

Available by prescription only
Tablets: 100 mg
Capsules: 200 mg

INDICATIONS & DOSAGE
Chronic and intermittent gouty arthritis, or hyperuricemia associated with gout
Adults: Initially, 200 to 400 mg P.O. daily in two divided doses, gradually increasing to maintenance dosage in 1 week. Maintenance dosage is 400 mg P.O. daily in two divided doses; may increase to 800 mg daily or decrease to 200 mg daily.
◊ ***Prophylaxis of thromboembolic disorders—including angina, an MI, and transient (cerebral) ischemic attacks—and in patients with prosthetic heart valves***
Adults: 600 to 800 mg daily in divided doses to decrease platelet aggregation.

PHARMACODYNAMICS
Uricosuric action: Sulfinpyrazone competitively inhibits renal tubule reabsorption of uric acid. Drug inhibits adenosine diphosphate and 5-HT, resulting in decreased platelet adhesiveness and increased platelet survival time.

PHARMACOKINETICS
Absorption: Sulfinpyrazone is absorbed completely after oral administration; plasma levels peak in 2 hours. Effects usually last 4 to 6 hours but may persist up to 10 hours.
Distribution: Drug is 98% to 99% protein-bound.
Metabolism: Drug is metabolized rapidly in the liver.
Excretion: Drug and its metabolites are eliminated in urine; about 50% is excreted unchanged.

CONTRAINDICATIONS & PRECAUTIONS
Contraindicated in patients with hypersensitivity to pyrazolone derivatives (including oxyphenbutazone and phenylbutazone), blood dyscrasia, active peptic ulcer, or symptoms of GI inflammation or ulceration.

Use cautiously in patients with healed peptic ulcer.

INTERACTIONS
Drug-drug. *Cholestyramine* decreases absorption of sulfinpyrazone; sulfinpyrazone should be taken 1 hour before or 4 to 6 hours after cholestyramine. *Diazoxide, diuretics,* and *pyrazinamide* may increase serum uric acid and thus increase sulfinpyrazone dosage requirements. Reduced excretion of *nitrofurantoin* decreases the efficacy of sulfinpyrazone in urinary tract infections and increases systemic toxicity; decreased excretion of *sulfonylureas* may cause hypoglycemia. Sulfinpyrazone decreases renal tubular secretion of *nitrofurantoin, other beta-lactam antibiotics, penicillin,* and *sulfonylureas.* Sulfinpyrazone may potentiate effects of *oral antidiabetics* such as *sulfonylureas. Probenecid* inhibits renal excretion of sulfinpyrazone. *Salicylates* block the uricosuric effects of sulfinpyrazone only in high doses; small occasional doses usually don't interact significantly. Sulfinpyrazone decreases the metabolism of *warfarin,* enhancing its hypoprothrombinemic effect and the risk of bleeding; increased bleeding in these patients also may result from the antiplatelet effect of sulfinpyrazone.

Drug-lifestyle. *Alcohol* may increase serum uric acid levels and thus increase sulfinpyrazone dosage requirements.

ADVERSE REACTIONS

GI: *nausea, dyspepsia,* epigastric pain, reactivation of peptic ulcerations.
Hematologic: *blood dyscrasia* (such as anemia, *leukopenia, agranulocytosis, thrombocytopenia, aplastic anemia*).
Respiratory: *bronchoconstriction* in patients with aspirin-induced asthma.
Skin: rash.

▣ KEY CONSIDERATIONS

• Geriatric patients are more likely to have glomerular filtration rates less than 50 ml/minute; sulfinpyrazone may be ineffective.
• Drug doesn't accumulate and tolerance doesn't develop; it's suitable for long-term use.
• Drug has no analgesic or anti-inflammatory effects.
• Drug may be ineffective and should be avoided when creatinine clearance is less than 50 ml/minute.
• Monitor renal function and CBC routinely.
• Monitor serum uric acid levels and adjust dosage accordingly.
• Give with food, milk, or prescribed antacids to lessen GI upset.
• Sulfinpyrazone is used investigationally to increase platelet survival time, treat thromboembolic phenomena, and prevent MI recurrence.
• Maintain adequate hydration with high fluid intake to prevent formation of uric acid kidney stones.
• Drug decreases urine excretion of aminohippuric acid and phenolsulfonphthalein and may alter renal function test results.

Patient education

• Explain that gouty attacks may increase during first 6 to 12 months of therapy; patient shouldn't discontinue sulfinpyrazone without medical approval.
• Encourage patient to comply with dosage regimen and to keep scheduled follow-up visits.

• Tell patient to drink 8 to 10 glasses of fluid each day and to take drug with food to minimize GI upset; warn patient to avoid alcoholic beverages, which decrease the therapeutic effect of sulfinpyrazone.

sulfisoxazole
Gantrisin

sulfisoxazole diolamine
Gantrisin (Ophthalmic Solution)

Sulfonamide, antibiotic

Available by prescription only
Tablets: 500 mg
Liquid: 500 mg/5 ml
Ophthalmic solution: 4%

INDICATIONS & DOSAGE

Urinary tract and systemic infections
Adults: Initially, 2 to 4 g P.O., then 4 to 8 g P.O. daily in divided doses q 4 to 6 hours.
Maximum dose shouldn't exceed 6 g/24 hours.
Lymphogranuloma venereum (genital, inguinal, or anorectal infection)
Adults: 500 mg to 1 g q.i.d. for 3 weeks.
Conjunctivitis, corneal ulcer, superficial ocular infections; adjunct in systemic treatment of trachoma
Adults: Instill 1 or 2 gtt in the lower conjunctival sac of affected eye daily q 1 to 4 hours.

PHARMACODYNAMICS

Antibacterial action: Sulfisoxazole is bacteriostatic. It inhibits formation of tetrahydrofolic acid from PABA, thus preventing bacterial cell synthesis of folic acid. It acts synergistically with folic acid antagonists such as trimethoprim, which block folic acid synthesis at a later stage, thus delaying or preventing bacterial resistance.

Drug is active against some gram-positive bacteria, *Chlamydia trachomatis,* many Enterobacteriaceae, and some strains of *Toxoplasma* and *Plasmodium.*

Reactions may be *common,* uncommon, *life-threatening,* or COMMON AND LIFE-THREATENING.

PHARMACOKINETICS

Absorption: Sulfisoxazole is absorbed readily from the GI tract after oral administration; serum levels peak in 2 to 4 hours.

Distribution: Drug is distributed into extracellular compartments; CSF penetration is 8% to 57% of blood levels in uninflamed meninges. Drug is 85% protein-bound.

Metabolism: Drug is metabolized partially in the liver.

Excretion: Both unchanged drug and metabolites are excreted primarily in urine through glomerular filtration and, to a lesser extent, renal tubular secretion. Urinary solubility of unchanged drug increases as urine pH increases. Plasma half-life in patients with normal renal function is about 4½ to 8 hours.

CONTRAINDICATIONS & PRECAUTIONS

Contraindicated in patients with hypersensitivity to sulfonamines.

Use oral form cautiously in patients with impaired renal or hepatic function, severe allergies, bronchial asthma, or G6PD deficiency. Use ophthalmic form cautiously in patients with severely dry eyes.

INTERACTIONS

Drug-drug. Sulfisoxazole may inhibit hepatic metabolism of *oral anticoagulants*, displacing them from binding sites and exaggerating anticoagulant effects. Use with *oral antidiabetics (sulfonylureas)* enhances hypoglycemic effects, probably by displacing sulfonylureas from protein-binding sites; with *PABA*, antagonizes effects of sulfonamides; with either *pyrimethamine* or *trimethoprim (folic acid antagonists* with different mechanisms of action), results in synergistic antibacterial effects and delays or prevents bacterial resistance. Use with *urine-acidifying drugs (ammonium chloride, ascorbic acid)* decreases urine pH and sulfonamide solubility, thus increasing risk of crystalluria.

Drug-lifestyle. *Sun exposure* may cause photosensitivity reactions.

ADVERSE REACTIONS

CNS: headache; mental depression, hallucinations, *seizures* (with oral administration).

CV: tachycardia, palpitations, syncope, cyanosis (with oral administration).

EENT: *ocular irritation, itching, chemosis, periorbital edema* (with ophthalmic form).

GI: *nausea, vomiting, diarrhea,* abdominal pain, anorexia, stomatitis, pseudomembranous colitis (with oral administration).

GU: *toxic nephrosis with oliguria and anuria, acute renal failure,* crystalluria, hematuria (with oral administration).

Hematologic: *agranulocytosis, aplastic anemia, thrombocytopenia, hemolytic anemia,* megaloblastic anemia, *leukopenia* (with oral administration).

Hepatic: elevated liver function test results, jaundice (with oral administration), *hepatitis*.

Skin: *erythema multiforme, epidermal necrolysis, exfoliative dermatitis, Stevens-Johnson syndrome, generalized skin eruption,* photosensitivity, urticaria, pruritus (with oral administration).

Other: hypersensitivity reactions (*serum sickness, drug fever, anaphylaxis*), overgrowth of nonsusceptible organisms (with ophthalmic form).

▣ KEY CONSIDERATIONS

Besides the recommendations relevant to all sulfonamides, consider the following:
- Sulfisoxazole-pyrimethamine is used to treat toxoplasmosis.
- Sulfisoxazole alters results of urine glucose tests using cupric sulfate (Benedict's reagent or Clinitest).

Patient education
- Tell patient to drink 8 oz (240 ml) water with each oral dose and to take sulfisoxazole on an empty stomach.
- Tell patient to complete prescribed drug therapy.
- Teach patient how to use ophthalmic preparations; warn patient not to touch tip of dropper or tube to any surface.
- Warn patient that ophthalmic solution may cause blurred vision immediately after application. Tell patient to gently

close eyes and keep closed for 1 to 2 minutes.

• Tell patient to avoid prolonged exposure to sunlight because photosensitivity may occur and to wear protective clothing and sunscreen.

Overdose & treatment
• Signs and symptoms of overdose include dizziness, drowsiness, headache, unconsciousness, anorexia, abdominal pain, nausea, and vomiting. More severe complications, including hemolytic anemia, agranulocytosis, dermatitis, acidosis, sensitivity reactions, and jaundice, may be fatal.
• Perform gastric lavage if ingestion occurred within the preceding 4 hours. Then, correct acidosis, force fluids, and alkalize urine to enhance solubility and excretion. Treatment of renal failure and transfusion of appropriate blood products (in severe hematologic toxicity) may be required.

sulindac
Clinoril

NSAID, nonnarcotic analgesic, antipyretic

Available by prescription only
Tablets: 150 mg, 200 mg

INDICATIONS & DOSAGE
Osteoarthritis, rheumatoid arthritis, ankylosing spondylitis
Adults: 150 mg P.O. b.i.d. initially; may increase to 200 mg P.O. b.i.d.
Acute subacromial bursitis or supraspinatus tendinitis, acute gouty arthritis
Adults: 200 mg P.O. b.i.d. for 7 to 14 days. Dose may be reduced as symptoms subside.

PHARMACODYNAMICS
Analgesic, antipyretic, and anti-inflammatory actions: Mechanisms of action are unknown but are thought to inhibit prostaglandin synthesis.

PHARMACOKINETICS
Absorption: Sulindac is rapidly and completely absorbed from the GI tract.
Distribution: Drug is highly protein-bound.
Metabolism: Drug is inactive and is metabolized in the liver to the active sulfide metabolite.
Excretion: Drug is excreted in urine; half-life of parent drug is about 8 hours, half-life of active metabolite is about 16 hours.

CONTRAINDICATIONS & PRECAUTIONS
Contraindicated in patients with hypersensitivity to sulindac or in whom acute asthma attacks, urticaria, or rhinitis are precipitated by use of aspirin or NSAIDs.

Use cautiously in patients with history of ulcer or GI bleeding, renal dysfunction, compromised cardiac function, hypertension, or conditions predisposing to fluid retention.

INTERACTIONS
Drug-drug. *Antacids* delay and decrease the absorption of sulindac. Sulindac may potentiate the platelet-inhibiting effect of *anticoagulants* and *thrombolytics*. *Aspirin* and *diflunisal* decrease plasma levels of the active sulfide metabolite. *Dimethyl sulfoxide* may interact with sulindac, causing decreased plasma levels of the active sulfide metabolite; peripheral neuropathies have also been reported with this combination. Use with other *GI irritants (antibiotics, NSAIDs, steroids)* may potentiate the adverse GI effects of sulindac; use together with caution. Use with *highly protein-bound drugs (phenytoin, sulfonylureas, warfarin)* may cause displacement of either drug and adverse effects; monitor therapy closely for both drugs. NSAIDs decrease renal clearance of *lithium carbonate*, thus increasing lithium serum levels and risk of adverse effects. *Probenecid* increases plasma levels of sulindac and its inactive sulfane metabolite; sulindac may decrease the uricosuric effect of probenecid.
Drug-food. *Food* may delay and decrease the absorption of sulindac.

Reactions may be *common*, uncommon, **life-threatening**, or COMMON AND LIFE-THREATENING.

ADVERSE REACTIONS

CNS: dizziness, headache, nervousness, psychosis.

CV: edema, hypertension, *heart failure,* palpitations.

EENT: tinnitus, transient visual disturbances.

GI: *epigastric distress, peptic ulceration, GI bleeding, pancreatitis,* occult blood loss, nausea, constipation, dyspepsia, flatulence, anorexia, vomiting, diarrhea.

GU: interstitial nephritis, increased BUN and serum creatinine levels, *nephrotic syndrome, renal failure.*

Hematologic: prolonged bleeding time, *aplastic anemia, thrombocytopenia, agranulocytosis, neutropenia,* hemolytic anemia.

Hepatic: elevated liver enzyme levels.

Metabolic: hyperkalemia.

Skin: *rash,* pruritus.

Other: drug fever, *anaphylaxis, hypersensitivity syndrome, angioedema.*

▣ KEY CONSIDERATIONS

● Patients older than age 60 are more sensitive to the adverse effects of sulindac; use cautiously.

● Because of its effect on renal prostaglandins, drug may cause fluid retention and edema; this may be significant in geriatric patients and those with heart failure.

● Drug may be the safest NSAID for patients with mild renal impairment and may be less likely to cause further renal toxicity.

● Assess cardiopulmonary status frequently. Monitor vital signs, especially heart rate and blood pressure, to detect abnormalities.

● Assess fluid balance status. Monitor intake and output and daily weight. Observe for presence and amount of edema.

● Impose safety measures to prevent injury, such as using side rails and supervised ambulation.

● Symptomatic improvement may take 7 days or longer. Evaluate patient's response as evidenced by a reduction in symptoms.

Patient education

● Caution patient to avoid use of OTC drugs unless medically approved.

● Teach patient how to recognize signs and symptoms of possible adverse reactions; instruct patient to report such adverse reactions.

● Instruct patient to check weight two or three times weekly and to report weight gain of 1.5 kg (3 lb) or more within 1 week.

● Because drug causes sodium retention, advise patient to report edema and to have blood pressure checked routinely.

● Instruct patient in safety measures; advise him to avoid hazardous activities that require alertness until CNS effects of drug are known.

Overdose & treatment

● Signs and symptoms of overdose include dizziness, drowsiness, mental confusion, disorientation, lethargy, paresthesia, numbness, vomiting, gastric irritation, nausea, abdominal pain, headache, stupor, coma, and hypotension.

● To treat overdose, immediately induce vomiting with ipecac syrup or perform gastric lavage. Administer activated charcoal via an NG tube. Provide symptomatic and supportive measures (respiratory support and correction of fluid and electrolyte imbalances). Dialysis is thought to be of minimal value because drug is highly protein-bound. Monitor laboratory parameters and vital signs closely.

sumatriptan succinate
Imitrex

Selective 5-hydroxytryptamine (5HT$_1$)-receptor agonist, antimigraine drug

Available by prescription only
Tablets: 25 mg, 50 mg
Injection: 12 mg/ml (0.5 ml in 1-ml prefilled syringe), 6-mg single-dose (0.5 ml in 2 ml) vial, and self-dose system kit
Nasal spray: 5 mg and 20 mg unit dose nasal spray device

INDICATIONS & DOSAGE

Acute migraine attacks (with or without aura)

Adults: 6 mg S.C. Maximum recommended dosage is two 6-mg injections in 24 hours, separated by at least 1 hour, or 25 to 100 mg P.O. initially. If response isn't achieved in 2 hours, may give second dose of 25 to 100 mg. Additional doses may be used in at least 2-hour intervals. Maximum daily dose is 300 mg.

For nasal spray, administer single dose of 5 mg, 10 mg, or 20 mg once in one nostril; may repeat once after 2 hours under guidance of health care provider for maximum daily dose of 40 mg. (A 10-mg dose may be given by administering a single 5-mg dose in each nostril.)

PHARMACODYNAMICS

Antimigraine action: Sumatriptan selectively binds to a 5-HT$_1$ receptor subtype found in the basilar artery and vasculature of dura mater, where it presumably exerts its antimigraine effect. In these tissues, sumatriptan activates the receptor to cause vasoconstriction, an action in humans correlating with the relief of migraine.

PHARMACOKINETICS

Absorption: Bioavailability by S.C. injection is 97% of that obtained by I.V. injection. Level after S.C. injection of sumatriptan peaks in about 12 minutes.
Distribution: Drug has a low protein-binding capacity (about 14% to 21%).
Metabolism: About 80% of drug is metabolized in the liver, primarily to an inactive indoleacetic acid metabolite.
Excretion: Drug is excreted primarily in urine, partly (20%) as unchanged drug and partly as the indoleacetic acid metabolite; elimination half-life is about 2 hours.

CONTRAINDICATIONS & PRECAUTIONS

Contraindicated in patients with hypersensitivity to sumatriptan; in those with uncontrolled hypertension, ischemic heart disease (such as angina pectoris, Prinzmetal's angina, history of MI, or documented silent ischemia), or hemiplegic or basilar migraine; within 14 days of MAO therapy; and in patients taking ergotamine.

Use cautiously in patients who may be at risk for coronary artery disease (CAD) (such as postmenopausal women or men older than age 40) or those with risk factors such as hypertension, hypercholesterolemia, obesity, diabetes, smoking, or family history.

INTERACTIONS

Drug-drug. *Ergot* and *ergot derivatives* prolong vasospastic effects when given with sumatriptan; these drugs shouldn't be used within 24 hours of sumatriptan therapy.

ADVERSE REACTIONS

CNS: *dizziness, vertigo,* drowsiness, headache, anxiety, malaise, fatigue, anxious feeling, tight feeling in head, cold sensation.
CV: *atrial fibrillation, ventricular fibrillation, ventricular tachycardia,* flushing, pressure or tightness in chest, *MI, ECG changes such as ischemic ST segment elevation.*
EENT: discomfort of throat, nasal cavity or sinus, mouth, jaw, or tongue; altered vision.
GI: abdominal discomfort, dysphagia.
Musculoskeletal: myalgia, muscle cramps, neck pain.
Skin: diaphoresis.
Other: *tingling, warm or hot sensation, burning sensation, injection site reaction.*

▣ KEY CONSIDERATIONS

• Don't use sumatriptan to manage hemiplegic or basilar migraine. Safety and effectiveness also haven't been established for cluster headache, which occurs in an older, predominantly male population.
• Don't give drug I.V. because coronary vasospasm may occur.
• Nasal spray is generally well tolerated; however, adverse reactions seen with the other forms of the drug can still occur.
• Drug injection may cause serious or life-threatening arrhythmias—such as atrial and ventricular fibrillation, ventricular tachycardia, an MI, or marked ischemic ST elevations—or chest and

arm discomfort, which may indicate angina pectoris. Because such coronary events can occur, consider administering first dose in an outpatient setting to patients in whom unrecognized CAD is comparatively likely (such as postmenopausal women; men older than age 40; and patients with risk factors for CAD, such as hypertension, hypercholesterolemia, obesity, diabetes, smoking, and strong family history of CAD).

• Patient response to nasal spray may be varied. The choice of dose should be made individually, weighing the possible benefit of the 20-mg dose with the potential of a greater risk of adverse events.

Patient education

• Tell patient that sumatriptan may be given at any time during a migraine attack, but preferably as soon as symptoms begin. A second injection may be given if symptoms recur. Tell patient not to use more than two injections in 24 hours and to allow at least 1 hour between doses. Pain or redness at the injection site may occur but usually lasts less than 1 hour.

• Explain that drug is intended to relieve migraine, not to prevent or reduce the number of attacks.

• Tell patient not to use a second dose if he doesn't respond to the initial dose, unless he contacts the health care provider first.

• Explain that drug is available in a spring-loaded injector system that facilitates self-administration. Review detailed information with patient. Be sure he understands how to load the injector, administer the injection, and dispose of the used syringes.

• Tell patient who feels persistent or severe chest pain to call immediately. Tell patient who experiences pain or tightness in the throat, wheezing, heart throbbing, rash, lumps, hives, or swollen eyelids, face, or lips to stop using the drug and call at once.

Overdose & treatment

• Signs and symptoms include seizures, tremor, inactivity, erythema of the extremities, reduced respiratory rate, cyanosis, ataxia, mydriasis, injection site reactions, and paralysis.

• Continue monitoring patient while signs and symptoms persist and for at least 10 hours thereafter. Effect of hemodialysis or peritoneal dialysis on serum levels of sumatriptan is unknown.

---

tacrine hydrochloride
Cognex

Centrally acting reversible cholinesterase inhibitor, psychotherapeutic drug

Available by prescription only
Capsules: 10 mg, 20 mg, 30 mg, 40 mg

INDICATIONS & DOSAGE
Mild to moderate dementia of the Alzheimer's type
Adults: Initially, 10 mg P.O. q.i.d. Maintain dose for at least 4 weeks; monitor transaminase levels every other week, beginning the fourth week of therapy. If patient tolerates treatment and transaminase levels remain normal, increase to 20 mg P.O. q.i.d. After 4 weeks, adjust dosage to 30 mg P.O. q.i.d. If still tolerated, increase to 40 mg P.O. q.i.d. after another 4 weeks.

✦ *Dosage adjustment.* In patients with ALT levels two to three times the upper limit of normal, monitor ALT level weekly. If ALT level is three to five times the upper limit of normal, reduce daily dose by 40 mg and monitor ALT level weekly. When ALT level returns to normal, continue to adjust dosage and monitor level every other week. If ALT level is more than five times the upper limit of normal, stop treatment and monitor ALT level and for signs and symptoms of hepatitis. Rechallenge when ALT level is normal and monitor weekly.

PHARMACODYNAMICS
Psychotherapeutic action: Tacrine presumably slows degradation of acetylcholine released by still intact cholinergic neurons, thereby elevating acetylcholine levels in the cerebral cortex. If this theory is correct, drug effects may lessen as the disease progresses and fewer cholinergic neurons remain functionally intact. No evidence suggests drug alters the course of the underlying dementia.

PHARMACOKINETICS
Absorption: Tacrine is rapidly absorbed after oral administration; plasma levels peak within 1 to 2 hours. Absolute bioavailability of drug is about 17%. Food reduces bioavailability by 30% to 40%; there's no food effect if drug is administered at least 1 hour before meals.
Distribution: Drug is about 55% bound to plasma proteins.
Metabolism: Drug undergoes first-pass metabolism, which is dose-dependent. It's extensively metabolized by the cytochrome P-450 system to multiple metabolites, not all identified.
Excretion: Elimination half-life is 2 to 4 hours.

CONTRAINDICATIONS & PRECAUTIONS
Contraindicated in patients hypersensitive to tacrine or acridine derivatives. Also contraindicated in patients with drug-related jaundice confirmed by an elevated total bilirubin level of more than 3 mg/dl and in patients with hypersensitivity reactions associated with elevated ALT levels.

Use cautiously in patients with sick sinus syndrome, bradycardia, history of hepatic disease, renal disease, Parkinson's disease, asthma, prostatic hyperplasia, or other urine outflow impairment and in those at risk for peptic ulcer.

INTERACTIONS
Drug-drug. Because of its mechanism of action, tacrine has the potential to interfere with the activity of *anticholinergics*. A synergistic effect is expected when tacrine is given with *cholinergic agonists* such as *bethanechol, cholinesterase inhibitors,* or *succinylcholine.* Use with *cimetidine* increases the plasma tacrine level. Drug interactions may occur when administered with *drugs that undergo extensive metabolism by cytochrome P-450.* Use with *NSAIDs* may contribute to GI irritation and gastric bleeding. Administration with *theophylline* increases theophylline elimination half-life and average plasma levels; monitoring of plasma theophylline levels

and appropriate reduction of theophylline dose are recommended.

ADVERSE REACTIONS

CNS: agitation, ataxia, insomnia, abnormal thinking, somnolence, depression, anxiety, *headache, dizziness,* fatigue, confusion, seizures.
CV: bradycardia, hypertension, palpitations, chest pain.
GI: *nausea, vomiting, diarrhea,* dyspepsia, loose stools, changes in stool color, anorexia, abdominal pain, flatulence, constipation.
Hepatic: *elevated transaminase levels (especially ALT).*
Metabolic: weight loss.**Musculoskeletal:** myalgia.
Respiratory: rhinitis, upper respiratory tract infection, cough.
Skin: rash, jaundice, facial flushing, diaphoresis.

▣ KEY CONSIDERATIONS

• Tacrine, a cholinesterase inhibitor, is likely to exaggerate succinylcholine-type muscle relaxation during anesthesia.
• Because of its cholinomimetic action, drug may have vagotonic effects on heart rate (such as bradycardia), which may be particularly important to patients with sick sinus syndrome.
• Monitor serum ALT levels every other week from at least the fourth to the 16th week after initiation of therapy, after which monitoring may be decreased to every 3 months if ALT level is two times the upper limit of normal or less. With each dosage adjustment, resume monitoring every other week. Elevated transaminase levels are more common in women. No other predictors for the risk of hepatocellular injury exist.
• Dosage may be adjusted at a slower rate if patient is intolerant to the recommended schedule; however, don't adjust the dosage quicker than recommended.
• If drug is discontinued for 4 weeks or more, restart full dosage adjustment and monitoring schedule.
• Cognitive function can worsen if drug is abruptly discontinued or dosage is reduced by 80 mg/day or more.

Patient education

• Tell patient and caregiver that tacrine should be taken between meals when possible. If GI upset occurs, drug may be taken with meals but may reduce plasma levels.
• Inform patient and family that drug doesn't alter the underlying degenerative disease but can alleviate symptoms; for therapy to be effective, drug must be administered regularly.
• Remind patient and caregiver that dosage adjustment is an integral part of the safe use of drug but that abruptly discontinuing or reducing daily dose by 80 mg/day or more may precipitate behavioral disturbances and a decline in cognitive function.
• Advise patient and caregiver to report significant adverse effects or change in status immediately.

Overdose & treatment

• Overdose with cholinesterase inhibitors can cause a cholinergic crisis characterized by severe nausea, vomiting, salivation, sweating, bradycardia, hypotension, and seizures. Increasing muscle weakness may occur and can result in death if respiratory muscles are involved.
• Use general supportive measures. Tertiary anticholinergics such as atropine may be used as an antidote for tacrine overdose. I.V. atropine sulfate titrated to effect is recommended (initial dose of 1 to 2 mg I.V., with subsequent doses based on response). It's unknown whether dialysis eliminates tacrine or its metabolites.

tamoxifen citrate
Nolvadex, Nolvadex-D,* Tamofen*

Nonsteroidal antiestrogen, antineoplastic

Available by prescription only
Tablets: 10 mg, 20 mg
Tablets (enteric-coated): 20 mg*

INDICATIONS & DOSAGE

Dosage and indications vary. Check current literature for recommended protocol.

Advanced breast cancer (men and postmenopausal women)
Adults: 10 to 20 mg P.O. b.i.d.

Adjunct treatment for breast cancer
Adults: 10 mg P.O. b.i.d. to t.i.d. for no more than 2 years.

Prevention of breast cancer in high-risk women
Adults: 20 mg P.O. daily for 5 years.

◇ ***Mastalgia***
Adults: 10 mg P.O. daily for 4 months.

PHARMACODYNAMICS

Antineoplastic action: Exact mechanism of action is unclear. Tamoxifen may block estrogen receptors within tumor cells that require estrogen to thrive. The estrogen receptor–tamoxifen complex may be translocated into the nucleus of the tumor cell, where it inhibits DNA synthesis.

PHARMACOKINETICS

Absorption: Tamoxifen appears to be well absorbed across the GI tract after oral administration. Serum levels reach steady state after 3 to 4 weeks.
Distribution: Distribution of drug and its metabolites into body tissues and fluids isn't fully established.
Metabolism: Drug is metabolized extensively in the liver to several metabolites.
Excretion: Drug is excreted primarily in feces, mostly as metabolites; distribution phase half-life is 7 to 14 hours. Secondary plasma levels peak 4 days after dose, probably because of enterohepatic circulation. Half-life of the terminal elimination phase is more than 7 days.

CONTRAINDICATIONS & PRECAUTIONS

Contraindicated in patients hypersensitive to tamoxifen. Also contraindicated in women who require coumarin-type anticoagulants or have a history of deep vein thrombosis or pulmonary embolism.

Use cautiously in patients with leukopenia or thrombocytopenia.

INTERACTIONS

Drug-drug. *Bromocriptine* may elevate serum tamoxifen and N-desmethyltamoxifen levels. Use with *coumadin* may significantly increase in anticoagulation effect. Administration with *cytotoxic drugs* increases the risk of thromboembolic events. Use with *estrogens* may interfere with the therapeutic effect of tamoxifen.

ADVERSE REACTIONS

GI: *nausea, vomiting, diarrhea.*
GU: *vaginal discharge* and bleeding, *increased BUN level.*
Hematologic: transient decrease in WBC or platelet counts, *leukopenia, thrombocytopenia.*
Hepatic: elevated liver enzyme levels.
Metabolic: increased serum calcium, triglyceride, cholesterol, and T_4 levels; *fluid retention; weight gain or loss.*
Musculoskeletal: temporary bone pain, brief exacerbation of pain from osseous metastases.
Skin: *skin changes.*
Other: temporary tumor pain, *hot flashes.*

▣ KEY CONSIDERATIONS

• Initial adverse reaction (increased bone pain) may be associated with a good tumor response shortly after starting tamoxifen therapy.
• Analgesics are indicated to relieve pain.
• Adverse reactions are usually minor and well tolerated; reducing the drug dosage should help minimize them.
• Clotting factor abnormalities may occur with prolonged drug therapy at usual dosages.
• Monitor WBC and platelet counts and periodic liver function test results.
• Monitor serum calcium levels; hypercalcemia may occur during initial therapy in patients with bone metastases.
• Drug acts as an antiestrogen; best results occur in patients with positive estrogen receptors.
• Drug is also used to treat breast cancer in men and advanced ovarian cancer in women.
• Some postmenopausal women have shown variations on karyopyknotic in-

---

Reactions may be common, uncommon, *life-threatening*, or COMMON AND LIFE-THREATENING.

dex in vaginal smears and various degrees of estrogen effect on Papanicolaou smears.

Patient education
• Emphasize importance of continuing tamoxifen therapy despite nausea and vomiting.
• Tell patient to promptly report vomiting if it occurs shortly after he takes a dose.
• Reassure patient that acute exacerbation of bone pain during drug therapy usually indicates drug will produce good response.
• Stress importance of swallowing enteric-coated tablets without crushing or breaking them.

tamsulosin hydrochloride
Flomax

Alpha₁ₐ-antagonist, anti-BPH drug

Available by prescription only
Capsules: 0.4 mg

INDICATIONS & DOSAGE
BPH
Adults: 0.4 mg P.O. once daily, administered 30 minutes after same meal each day. For those who fail to respond after 2 to 4 weeks, increase dosage to 0.8 mg P.O. once daily. If either dosing regimen is interrupted for several days, restart therapy with the 0.4-mg once-daily dose.

PHARMACODYNAMICS
Anti-BPH action: Drug selectively blocks alpha₁-receptors in the prostate, leading to relaxation of smooth muscles in the bladder neck and prostate, improved urine flow, and reduced BPH symptoms.

PHARMACOKINETICS
Absorption: Essentially complete after oral administration under fasting conditions. Steady state is achieved by day 5 of once-daily dosing. Levels peak 4 to 5 hours under fasting conditions and 6 to 7 hours when administered with food.
Distribution: Studies suggest distribution into extracellular fluids and most tissues, including kidney, prostate, gallbladder, heart, aorta, and brown fat, with minimal distribution into brain, spinal cord, and testes. Tamsulosin is extensively bound to plasma proteins but isn't thought to affect other highly protein-bound drugs.
Metabolism: Drug is metabolized by cytochrome P-450 in the liver, with less than 10% excreted unchanged; however, pharmacokinetic profile of metabolites hasn't been established. Drug's metabolites undergo extensive conjugation to glucuronide or sulfate before renal excretion.
Excretion: Drug is excreted primarily in urine (76%); about 21% excreted in feces. Elimination half-life is 5 to 7 hours, with apparent half-life from 9 to 15 hours secondary to rate-controlled absorption pharmacokinetics.

CONTRAINDICATIONS & PRECAUTIONS
Contraindicated in patients with hypersensitivity to tamsulosin or its components.

INTERACTIONS
Drug-drug. *Alpha blockers* are presumed to interact with tamsulosin; don't use together. *Cimetidine* decreases clearance of tamsulosin; use together with caution, particularly if tamsulosin dose is more than 0.4 mg. Use drug cautiously with *cytochrome P-450–metabolized drugs*. Studies with *warfarin* are inconclusive; use together with caution.

ADVERSE REACTIONS
CNS: *dizziness, headache,* insomnia, asthenia, somnolence.
CV: chest pain, syncope.
EENT: amblyopia, pharyngitis, *rhinitis,* sinusitis.
GI: diarrhea, nausea, tooth disorder.
GU: abnormal ejaculation.
Musculoskeletal: back pain.
Respiratory: increased cough.
Other: decreased libido, *infection.*

▣ KEY CONSIDERATIONS
• Geriatric patients may be more prone to syncopal episodes.
• Monitor patient for decreased blood pressure.

• Symptoms of BPH and prostate cancer are similar; rule out cancer before starting therapy with tamsulosin.

• If treatment is interrupted for several days or more, restart therapy at 1 capsule daily.

Patient education

• Instruct patient not to crush, chew, or open capsules.

• Tell patient to get up slowly from chair or bed during initiation of therapy.

• Instruct patient not to drive or perform hazardous tasks during initiation if therapy and for 12 hours after the initial dose or changes in dose until response can be monitored.

• Tell patient to take tamsulosin about 30 minutes after same meal each day.

• Caution patient to avoid situations where injury could occur as a result of syncope.

temazepam
Restoril

Benzodiazepine, sedative-hypnotic
Controlled substance schedule IV

Available by prescription only
Capsules: 7.5 mg, 15 mg, 30 mg

INDICATIONS & DOSAGE
Insomnia
Adults: 7.5 to 30 mg P.O. 30 minutes before bedtime.
Geriatric patients: 7.5 mg P.O. h.s. until individual response is determined.

PHARMACODYNAMICS
Sedative-hypnotic action: Temazepam depresses the CNS at the limbic and subcortical levels of the brain. It produces a sedative-hypnotic effect by potentiating the effect of the neurotransmitter gamma-aminobutyric acid on its receptor in the ascending reticular activating system, which increases inhibition and blocks both cortical and limbic arousal.

PHARMACOKINETICS
Absorption: When administered orally, temazepam is well absorbed through the GI tract. Levels peak in 1.2 to 1.6 hours (mean, 1.5 hours). Onset of action occurs at 30 to 60 minutes.
Distribution: Drug is widely distributed throughout the body and is 96% protein-bound.
Metabolism: Drug is metabolized in the liver primarily to inactive metabolites.
Excretion: Metabolites are excreted in urine as glucuronide conjugates. Half-life of drug is between 4 and 20 hours.

CONTRAINDICATIONS & PRECAUTIONS
Contraindicated in patients with hypersensitivity to temazepam or other benzodiazepines.
Use cautiously in patients with impaired renal or hepatic function, chronic pulmonary insufficiency, severe or latent mental depression, suicidal tendencies, or history of drug abuse.

INTERACTIONS
Drug-drug. Temazepam potentiates the CNS depressant effects of *antidepressants, antihistamines, barbiturates, general anesthetics, MAO inhibitors, narcotics,* and *phenothiazines.* Temazepam may decrease plasma *haloperidol* levels. Benzodiazepines block the therapeutic effects of *levodopa.*
Drug-lifestyle. Temazepam potentiates the CNS depressant effects of *alcohol. Heavy smoking* accelerates temazepam metabolism, reducing effectiveness.

ADVERSE REACTIONS
CNS: *drowsiness, dizziness, lethargy,* disturbed coordination, daytime sedation, confusion, nightmares, vertigo, euphoria, weakness, headache, fatigue, nervousness, anxiety, depression, minor changes in EEG patterns.
EENT: blurred vision.
GI: diarrhea, nausea, dry mouth.
Hepatic: elevated liver function test results.
Other: physical and psychological dependence.

▣ KEY CONSIDERATIONS
Besides the recommendations relevant to all benzodiazepines, consider the following:
• Lower doses are usually effective in

Reactions may be *common*, uncommon, *life-threatening*, or COMMON AND LIFE-THREATENING.

geriatric patients because of decreased elimination.

• Geriatric patients are more susceptible to the CNS depressant effects of temazepam. Use with caution.

• Geriatric patients who receive the drug require supervision with ambulation and activities of daily living during initiation of therapy or after a dosage increase.

• Evaluate patient for cause of insomnia, which is commonly a symptom of an underlying disorder such as depression.

• Drug is useful for patients who have difficulty falling asleep or who awaken frequently in the night.

• Prolonged use is discouraged; however, drug has proven effective for up to 4 weeks of continuous use.

• Remove all potential safety hazards such as cigarettes from patient's reach.

• To prevent possible injury, impose safety measures, such as call bell within reach and side rails raised.

• Monitor hepatic function studies to prevent toxicity; lower doses are indicated in patients with hepatic dysfunction.

• After long-term use, avoid abrupt withdrawal and follow a gradual tapering dosing schedule.

• Store drug in a cool, dry place away from light.

Patient education

• Instruct patient to seek medical approval before making changes in temazepam regimen.

• As necessary, teach patient safety measures to prevent injury, such as gradual position changes and supervised ambulation.

• Inform patient of the risk of physical and psychological dependence with long-term use.

• Emphasize potential for excessive CNS depression if drug is taken with alcohol.

• Tell patient that rebound insomnia may occur after stopping drug.

Overdose & treatment

• Signs and symptoms of overdose include somnolence, confusion, hypoactive or absent reflexes, dyspnea, labored breathing, hypotension, bradycardia, slurred speech, unsteady gait or impaired coordination, and coma.

• Support blood pressure and respirations until temazepam effects subside; monitor vital signs. Mechanical ventilatory assistance by endotracheal tube may be required to maintain a patent airway and support adequate oxygenation. Flumazenil, a specific benzodiazepine antagonist, may be useful. Use I.V. fluids and vasopressors such as dopamine and phenylephrine to treat hypotension as needed. If patient is conscious, induce vomiting, or perform gastric lavage if ingestion was recent, but only if an endotracheal tube is present to prevent aspiration. Then, administer activated charcoal with a cathartic as a single dose. Don't use barbiturates if excitation occurs. Dialysis is of limited value.

---

terazosin hydrochloride
Hytrin

Selective alpha$_1$ blocker, antihypertensive

Available by prescription only
Capsules: 1 mg, 2 mg, 5 mg, 10 mg

INDICATIONS & DOSAGE
Mild to moderate hypertension
Adults: Initially, 1 mg P.O. h.s. Adjust dose and schedule according to patient response. Recommended range is 1 to 5 mg daily or divided b.i.d.

If therapy is discontinued for several days or longer, reinstitute using the initial dosing regimen of 1 mg P.O. h.s. Slowly increase dose until desired blood pressure is attained. Doses more than 20 mg don't appear to further affect blood pressure.
BPH
Adults: Initially, 1 mg P.O. h.s. Dosage may be adjusted upward based on patient response. Increase to 2 mg, 5 mg, and then 10 mg. A daily dose of 10 mg may be required.

PHARMACODYNAMICS
Antihypertensive action: Terazosin reduces blood pressure by selectively inhibiting alpha$_1$ receptors in vascular

smooth muscle, thus reducing peripheral vascular resistance. Because of its selectivity for alpha$_1$ receptors, heart rate increases minimally. Serum cholesterol, low-density lipoprotein, and very low-density lipoprotein cholesterol levels decrease significantly during therapy; however, the relevance of these changes is unknown, as is the mechanism by which they occur.

Drug doesn't significantly alter potassium or glucose levels; it has been used successfully with diuretics, beta blockers, and other antihypertensives.
Hypertrophic action: Alpha blockade in nonvascular smooth muscle causes relaxation, notably in prostatic tissue, thereby reducing urinary symptoms in men with BPH.

PHARMACOKINETICS
Absorption: Terazosin is rapidly absorbed after oral administration; plasma levels peak in 1 to 2 hours. About 90% of oral dose is bioavailable; food doesn't appear to alter bioavailability.
Distribution: Drug is 90% to 94% plasma protein-bound.
Metabolism: Drug is metabolized in the liver; pharmacokinetics don't appear to be affected by hypertension, heart failure, or age.
Excretion: About 40% is excreted in urine, 60% in feces, mostly as metabolites; up to 30% may be excreted unchanged. Elimination half-life is about 12 hours.

CONTRAINDICATIONS & PRECAUTIONS
Contraindicated in patients with hypersensitivity to terazosin.

INTERACTIONS
Drug-drug. When adding *another antihypertensive* or a *diuretic,* dosage reduction and adjustment may be necessary. Use caution when administering terazosin with *other antihypertensives.*

ADVERSE REACTIONS
CNS: *asthenia, dizziness, headache,* nervousness, paresthesia, somnolence.
CV: *palpitations, peripheral edema,* postural hypotension, tachycardia, syncope.

EENT: *nasal congestion,* sinusitis, blurred vision.
GI: *nausea.*
GU: impotence.
Hematologic: decreased hematocrit, WBC count, and hemoglobin level.
Metabolic: decreased total protein and albumin levels.
Musculoskeletal: back pain, muscle pain.
Respiratory: dyspnea.

▣ KEY CONSIDERATIONS
Besides the recommendations relevant to all alpha-adrenergic blockers, consider the following:
• Postural adverse effects may be exaggerated in geriatric patients.
• Terazosin can cause marked hypotension, especially orthostatic hypotension, and syncope with the first dose or during the first few days of therapy. A similar response occurs if therapy is interrupted for more than a few doses.

Patient education
• Instruct patient to take first dose at bedtime.
• Warn patient to avoid hazardous tasks that require alertness for 12 hours after first dose, when dose is first increased, or when restarting dose after interruption of therapy.
• Caution patient to rise carefully and slowly from sitting and supine positions and to report dizziness, lightheadedness, or palpitations; dosage adjustment may be necessary.

Overdose & treatment
• Signs and symptoms of overdose are exaggerated adverse reactions, particularly hypotension and shock.
• Treatment is symptomatic and supportive. Dialysis may not be helpful because terazosin is highly protein-bound.

Reactions may be *common*, uncommon, *life-threatening*, or COMMON AND LIFE-THREATENING.

terbinafine hydrochloride
Lamisil

Synthetic allylamine derivative, antifungal

Available by prescription only
Cream: 1% in 15-g and 30-g containers
Tablets: 250 mg

INDICATIONS & DOSAGE

***Interdigital tinea pedis (athlete's foot), tinea cruris (jock itch), or tinea corporis (ringworm) caused by* Epidermophyton floccosum, Trichophyton mentagrophytes, *or* Trichophyton rubrum**
Adults: For interdigital tinea pedis, apply to cover the affected and immediately surrounding areas b.i.d. until signs and symptoms are significantly improved (for most patients, this occurs by the 7th day of therapy); for tinea cruris or tinea corporis, apply to cover the affected and immediately surrounding areas once or twice daily until signs and symptoms are significantly improved (for most patients, this occurs by the 7th day of therapy). Treatment shouldn't exceed 4 weeks.
Note: If irritation or sensitivity develops, discontinue treatment and institute appropriate therapy.
Onychomycosis of fingernails or toenails caused by dermatophytes (tinea unguium)
Adults: For treatment of fingernails, give 250 mg/day P.O. for 6 weeks; for toenails, give 250 mg/day P.O. for 12 weeks.

PHARMACODYNAMICS

Antifungal action: Terbinafine inhibits squalene epoxidase, a key enzyme in sterol biosynthesis in fungi. This action results in a deficiency in ergosterol and a corresponding accumulation of squalene within the fungal cell and causes fungal cell death.

PHARMACOKINETICS
Topical
Absorption: Systemic absorption of terbinafine is highly variable.
Distribution: Unknown.

Metabolism: Unknown.
Excretion: About 75% of cutaneously absorbed drug is eliminated in urine, predominantly as metabolites.
Oral
Absorption: More than 70% of drug is absorbed; food enhances absorption. Peak plasma level is 1 mcg/ml within 2 hours of first dose.
Distribution: Drug is distributed to serum and skin. Plasma half-life is about 36 hours; half-life in tissue is 200 to 400 hours. More than 99% of drug binds to plasma proteins.
Metabolism: First-pass metabolism is about 40%.
Excretion: About 70% of dose is eliminated in urine; clearance is decreased by 50% in patients with hepatic cirrhosis and impaired renal function.

CONTRAINDICATIONS & PRECAUTIONS
Contraindicated in patients hypersensitive to terbinafine. Oral form is also contraindicated in patients with preexisting hepatic disease or impaired renal function (creatinine clearance of 50 ml/minute or less).

INTERACTIONS
None reported for topical form.
Drug-drug. Administration with *cyclosporine* increases cyclosporine clearance by 15%. For oral form, administration with *I.V. caffeine* decreases clearance of caffeine by 19%. *Rifampin* increases clearance of terbinafine by 100%, whereas *cimetidine* decreases terbinafine clearance by 33%.

ADVERSE REACTIONS
CNS: *headache.*
EENT: taste disturbances, visual disturbances.
GI: diarrhea, dyspepsia, abdominal pain, nausea, flatulence.
Hematologic: decreased absolute lymphocyte count.
Hepatic: abnormal liver enzyme levels.
Skin: ***Stevens-Johnson syndrome,*** irritation, burning, pruritus, dryness.

▣ KEY CONSIDERATIONS

- Topical form of terbinafine is for topical use only; it isn't for oral, ophthalmic, or intravaginal use.
- Diagnosis should be confirmed either by direct microscopic examination of scrapings from infected tissue mounted in a solution of potassium hydroxide or by culture.

For topical form

- Minimum duration of therapy is 1 week; maximum, 4 weeks.
- Many patients treated only 1 to 2 weeks continue to improve for 2 to 4 weeks after completing drug therapy; patients shouldn't be considered therapeutic failures until they've been observed for 2 to 4 weeks off therapy. If successful outcome isn't achieved during the posttreatment observation period, review the diagnosis.
- Monitor patient for irritation or sensitivity to drug; if present, discontinue therapy and institute appropriate treatment measures.

For oral form

- Perform liver function tests for patients receiving oral treatment for more than 6 weeks.

Patient education

- Advise patient to use drug as directed and to avoid contact with eyes, nose, mouth, or other mucous membranes.
- Stress importance of using drug for recommended treatment time.
- Tell patient to call if the area of application shows signs or symptoms of increased irritation or possible sensitization (redness, itching, burning, blistering, swelling, or oozing).
- Instruct patient not to use occlusive dressings unless directed.

terbutaline sulfate
Brethaire, Brethine, Bricanyl

Adrenergic (beta₂ agonist), bronchodilator, tocolytic

Available by prescription only
Tablets: 2.5 mg, 5 mg
Aerosol inhaler: 200 mcg/metered spray
Injection: 1 mg/ml parenteral

INDICATIONS & DOSAGE
Relief of bronchospasm in patients with reversible obstructive airway disease
Adults: Administer 5 mg P.O. t.i.d. at 6-hour intervals. Reduce dosage to 2.5 mg P.O. t.i.d. if patient experiences adverse reactions. Maximum daily dose is 15 mg. Alternatively, 0.25 mg S.C. may be repeated in 15 to 30 minutes; maximum, 0.5 mg q 4 hours. Alternatively, two inhalations may be given q 4 to 6 hours with 1 minute between inhalations.

PHARMACODYNAMICS
Bronchodilator action: Terbutaline acts directly on beta₂ receptors to relax bronchial smooth muscle, relieving bronchospasm and reducing airway resistance. Cardiac and CNS stimulation may occur with high doses.

PHARMACOKINETICS
Absorption: About 33% to 50% of oral dose is absorbed through the GI tract. Onset of action occurs within 30 minutes, peaks within 2 to 3 hours, and persists for 4 to 8 hours. After S.C. injection, onset occurs within 15 minutes, peaks within 30 to 60 minutes, and persists for 1½ to 4 hours. After oral inhalation, onset of action occurs within 5 to 30 minutes, peaks within 1 to 2 hours, and persists for 3 to 4 hours.
Distribution: Terbutaline is widely distributed throughout the body.
Metabolism: Drug is partially metabolized in liver to inactive compounds.
Excretion: After parenteral administration, 60% is excreted unchanged in urine, 3% in feces through bile, and the remainder in urine as metabolites. After oral administration, most of drug is excreted as metabolites.

CONTRAINDICATIONS & PRECAUTIONS
Contraindicated in patients with hypersensitivity to terbutaline or sympathomimetic amines.

Use cautiously in patients with CV disorders, hyperthyroidism, diabetes, or seizure disorders.

INTERACTIONS

Drug-drug. *Beta blockers* may antagonize bronchodilator effects of terbutaline. Use of *MAO inhibitors* within 14 days of terbutaline or use of *tricyclic antidepressants* may potentiate effects of terbutaline on the vascular system. When used with *other sympathomimetics,* terbutaline may potentiate adverse CV effects of the other drugs; however, as an aerosol bronchodilator (adrenergic stimulator type), use may relieve acute bronchospasm in patients on long-term oral terbutaline therapy.

ADVERSE REACTIONS

CNS: *nervousness, tremor, drowsiness, dizziness, headache,* weakness.
CV: *palpitations,* tachycardia, **_arrhythmias,_** flushing.
EENT: dry and irritated nose and throat (with inhaled form).
GI: *vomiting, nausea,* heartburn.
Metabolic: hypokalemia (with high doses).
Respiratory: _paradoxical bronchospasm with prolonged usage,_ dyspnea.
Skin: diaphoresis.

▣ KEY CONSIDERATIONS

Besides the recommendations relevant to all adrenergics, consider the following:
• Geriatric patients are more sensitive to the effects of terbutaline; a lower dose may be required.
• Store injection solution away from light; don't use if discolored.
• Double-check dosage: 2.5 mg P.O. or 0.25 mg S.C. A decimal error can be fatal.
• Give S.C. injection in lateral deltoid area.
• CV effects are more likely with S.C. route and when patient has arrhythmias. Check pulse rate and blood pressure before each dose and monitor for changes from baseline.
• Most adverse reactions are transient; however, tachycardia may persist for a relatively long time.
• Patient may use tablets and aerosol together. Carefully monitor patient for toxic reaction.

• Aerosol drug produces minimal cardiac stimulation and tremors.
• Drug may reduce the sensitivity of spirometry for diagnosis of bronchospasm.

Patient education

• Instruct patient taking oral terbutaline on how to take pulse rate and to report if pulse varies significantly from baseline.
• Instruct patient not to administer drug with adrenocorticoid aerosol; separate administration time by 15 minutes.
• Demonstrate and give patient instructions on proper use of inhaler: Shake canister thoroughly to activate; place mouthpiece well into mouth, aimed at back of throat. Close lips and teeth around mouthpiece. Exhale through nose as completely as possible, then inhale through mouth slowly and deeply while actuating the nebulizer to release dose. Hold breath 10 seconds (count "1-100, 2-100, 3-100," up to "10-100"); remove mouthpiece, and then exhale slowly.
• Warn patient not to puncture aerosol drug container. Contents are under pressure. Instruct the patient not to store the container near heat or open flame or to expose it to temperatures exceeding 120° F (49° C), which may burst the container. Tell patient to store containers out of children's reach and to avoid discarding containers into a fire or incinerator.
• Advise patient to take a missed dose within 1 hour. After 1 hour, patient should skip the dose and resume regular schedule. Patient shouldn't double-dose.
• Instruct patient to use drug only as directed. If drug produces no relief or if condition worsens, he should call his health care provider promptly.
• Warn patient not to use OTC drugs without medical approval. Many cold and allergy remedies contain a sympathomimetic, which may be harmful when used with terbutaline.
• Advise patient to report decreased effectiveness. Excessive or prolonged use of aerosol form can lead to tolerance.

Overdose & treatment

• Signs and symptoms of overdose include exaggeration of common adverse reactions, particularly arrhythmias, seizures, nausea, and vomiting.

• Treatment requires supportive measures. If patient is conscious and ingestion was recent, induce vomiting and then perform gastric lavage. If patient is comatose, after endotracheal tube is in place with cuff inflated, perform gastric lavage; then administer activated charcoal to reduce drug absorption. Maintain adequate airway, provide cardiac and respiratory support, and monitor vital signs closely.

terconazole
Terazol 3, Terazol 7

Triazole derivative, antifungal

Available by prescription only
Vaginal cream: 0.4% in 45-g tube, 0.8% in 20-g tube with applicator
Vaginal suppositories: 80 mg

INDICATIONS & DOSAGE
Local treatment of vulvovaginal candidiasis
Adults: 0.4%: 1 full applicator (5 g) intravaginally once daily h.s. for 7 consecutive days; 0.8%: 1 full applicator (5 g) intravaginally once daily h.s. for 3 consecutive days. Alternatively, insert one suppository vaginally h.s. for 3 consecutive days.

PHARMACODYNAMICS
Antifungal action: Exact mechanism of action is unknown. Terconazole may disrupt fungal cell membrane permeability.

PHARMACOKINETICS
Absorption: Minimal; absorption may range from 5% to 16%.
Distribution: Drug effect is mainly local.
Metabolism: Drug is metabolized mainly by oxidative *N*- and *O*-dealkylation, dioxolane ring cleavage, and conjugation pathways.
Excretion: After oral administration, 32% to 56% of dose is excreted in urine and 47% to 52% is excreted in feces within 24 hours.

CONTRAINDICATIONS & PRECAUTIONS
Contraindicated in patients with known sensitivity to terconazole or inactive ingredients in drug.

INTERACTIONS
None reported.

ADVERSE REACTIONS
CNS: *headache.*
GU: pain of female genitalia, vulvovaginal burning.
Musculoskeletal: body aches.
Skin: irritation, *pruritus,* photosensitivity.
Other: fever, chills.

▣ KEY CONSIDERATIONS
• Terconazole is only effective against vulvovaginitis caused by *Candida* species; cultures or potassium hydroxide smears should confirm diagnosis.
• Reinfection may be responsible for a persistent infection; evaluate patient for possible sources.
• Intractable candidiasis may be a sign of diabetes mellitus; check blood and urine glucose levels to rule out undiagnosed diabetes mellitus.

Patient education
• Instruct patient to insert cream high into the vagina.
• Tell patient to complete full course of therapy and to use terconazole continuously.
• Inform patient to report if drug causes burning or irritation.
• Advise patient to refrain from sexual intercourse or suggest partner use a condom to avoid reinfection.
• Advise patient to use a sanitary napkin to prevent staining of clothing.

Reactions may be *common*, uncommon, *life-threatening*, or COMMON AND LIFE-THREATENING.

testosterone
Histerone 100, Malogen in Oil,*
Tesamone, Testandro, Testaqua

testosterone cypionate
depAndro 100, depAndro 200,
Depotest 100, Depotest 200, Depo-
Testosterone, Duratest-100,
Duratest-200, T-Cypionate, Testred
Cypionate 200, Virilon IM

testosterone enanthate
Andro L.A. 200, Andropository 200,
Delatestryl, Durathate-200, Everone
200, Testrin-P.A.

testosterone propionate
Malogen in Oil,* Testex

*Androgen, androgen replacement,
antineoplastic*
Controlled substance schedule III

Available by prescription only
testosterone
Injection (aqueous suspension):
25 mg/ml, 50 mg/ml, 100 mg/ml
testosterone cypionate (in oil)
Injection: 100 mg/ml, 200 mg/ml
testosterone enanthate (in oil)
Injection: 100 mg/ml, 200 mg/ml
testosterone propionate (in oil)
Injection: 50 mg/ml, 100 mg/ml

INDICATIONS & DOSAGE
Male hypogonadism
**testosterone or testosterone propi-
onate**
Adults: 10 to 25 mg I.M. two or three
times weekly.
testosterone cypionate or enanthate
Adults: 50 to 400 mg I.M. q 2 to 4
weeks.
Inoperable breast cancer
testosterone propionate
Adults: 50 to 100 mg I.M. three times
weekly.
testosterone cypionate or enanthate
Adults: 200 to 400 mg I.M. q 2 to 4
weeks.
testosterone
Adults: 100 mg I.M. three times weekly.

PHARMACODYNAMICS
Androgenic action: Testosterone is the
endogenous androgen that stimulates receptors in androgen-responsive organs
and tissues to promote growth and development of male sexual organs and
secondary sexual characteristics.
Antineoplastic action: Drug exerts inhibitory, antiestrogenic effects on
hormone-responsive breast tumors and
metastases.

PHARMACOKINETICS
Absorption: Testosterone and its esters
must be administered parenterally because they're inactivated rapidly by the
liver when given orally. Onset of action
of cypionate and enanthate esters of
testosterone is somewhat slower than
that of testosterone.
Distribution: Drug is normally 98% to
99% plasma protein-bound, primarily to
the testosterone-estradiol binding globulin.
Metabolism: Drug is metabolized to several 17-ketosteroids by two main pathways in the liver. A large portion of these
metabolites then form glucuronide and
sulfate conjugates. Plasma half-life of
drug ranges from 10 to 100 minutes. The
cypionate and enanthate esters of testosterone have longer durations of action
than drug.
Excretion: Very little unchanged drug
appears in urine or feces. About 90% of
metabolized drug is excreted in urine in
the form of sulfate and glucuronide conjugates.

CONTRAINDICATIONS & PRECAUTIONS
Contraindicated in men with breast or
prostate cancer and in patients with hypercalcemia or cardiac, hepatic, or renal
decompensation.
Use cautiously in geriatric patients.

INTERACTIONS
Drug-drug. In patients with diabetes,
decreased blood glucose levels may require adjustment of *insulin* or *oral antidiabetic* dosage. Administration with
oxyphenbutazone may increase serum
oxyphenbutazone levels. Testosterone
may potentiate the effects of *warfarin-*

type anticoagulants, prolonging PT and INR.

ADVERSE REACTIONS

CNS: headache, anxiety, depression, paresthesia, sleep apnea syndrome.
CV: edema.
GI: nausea.
GU: hypoestrogenic effects in women (flushing; diaphoresis; vaginitis, including itching, drying, and burning; vaginal bleeding), excessive hormonal effects in men (testicular atrophy, oligospermia, decreased ejaculatory volume, impotence, gynecomastia, epididymitis).
Hematologic: polycythemia, suppression of clotting factors.
Hepatic: reversible jaundice, *cholestatic hepatitis*, abnormal liver enzyme levels.
Metabolic: increased serum creatinine, sodium, potassium, calcium, phosphate, and cholesterol levels.
Skin: pain and induration at injection site, local edema, *hypersensitivity reactions.*
Other: androgenic effects in women (*acne, edema, oily skin, weight gain, hirsutism, hoarseness,* clitoral enlargement, deepening voice, decreased or increased libido).

◫ KEY CONSIDERATIONS

Besides the recommendations relevant to all androgens, consider the following:
• Observe geriatric men for prostatic hyperplasia; development of symptomatic prostatic hyperplasia or prostate cancer mandates discontinuation of drug.
• When used to treat male hypogonadism, initiate therapy with full therapeutic doses and taper according to patient tolerance and response. Administering long-acting esters (enanthate or cypionate) at intervals greater than q 2 to 3 weeks may cause hormone levels to fall below those found in normal adults.
• Carefully observe female patients for signs of excessive virilization. If possible, discontinue therapy at first sign of virilization because some adverse effects (deepening of voice, clitoral enlargement) are irreversible.
• To avoid serious hypercalcemia, patients with metastatic breast cancer

should have their serum calcium level checked regularly.
• Inject I.M. deeply, preferably into a large muscle mass such as the outer upper quadrant of the gluteal muscle.
• Testosterone enanthate has been used for postmenopausal osteoporosis and to stimulate erythropoiesis.
• Solutions of long-acting esters (enanthate and cypionate) may become cloudy if a wet needle is used to draw up the solution, with no effect on potency.
• Warm (to room temperature) and shake vial to help dissolve crystals that formed after storage.
• Testosterone may cause abnormal results of glucose tolerance tests.
• Thyroid function test results (protein-bound iodine, ^{131}I uptake, thyroid-binding capacity) and serum 17-ketosteroid levels may decrease.

Patient education

• Explain to women that virilization may occur. Tell patient to report androgenic effects immediately; stopping drug prevents further androgenic changes but probably won't reverse those already present.
• Inform men to report too frequent or persistent penile erections.
• Advise patient to report persistent GI distress, diarrhea, or the onset of jaundice.

---

testosterone transdermal system
Androderm, Testoderm

Androgen, androgen replacement
Controlled substance schedule III

Available by prescription only
Transdermal system: 2.5 mg/day (Androderm), 4 mg/day (Testoderm), 6 mg/day (Testoderm)

INDICATIONS & DOSAGE
Primary or hypogonadotropic hypogonadism
Testoderm
Adult men: Apply one 6-mg/day patch to scrotal area daily for 22 to 24 hours. If

---

scrotal area is too small for 6-mg/day patch, start therapy with 4-mg/day patch.

Androderm

Adult men: Two systems applied nightly for 24 hours, providing a total dose of 5 mg/day. Apply on dry area of skin on back, abdomen, upper arms, or thighs. Don't apply to scrotum.

PHARMACODYNAMICS

Androgenic action: Testosterone transdermal system releases testosterone, the endogenous androgen that stimulates receptors in androgen-responsive organs and tissues to promote growth and development of male sex organs and secondary sex characteristics.

PHARMACOKINETICS

Absorption: After placement of testosterone transdermal system on scrotal skin, serum level peaks in 2 to 4 hours and returns toward baseline within about 2 hours after system removal. After application to nonscrotal skin, drug is absorbed during the 24-hour dosing period. Daily application of two Androderm systems at bedtime results in a serum drug level profile that mimics the normal circadian variation in healthy young men.

Distribution: Circulating drug is chiefly bound in the serum to sex hormone–|binding globulin and albumin.

Metabolism: Drug is metabolized to various 17-ketosteroids through two different pathways; the major active metabolites are estradiol and dihydrotestosterone.

Excretion: Little unchanged drug appears in urine or feces.

CONTRAINDICATIONS & PRECAUTIONS

Contraindicated in patients hypersensitive to testosterone, in women, and in men with known or suspected breast or prostate cancer.

Use cautiously in patients with preexisting renal, cardiac, or hepatic disease and in geriatric men.

INTERACTIONS

Drug-drug. In patients with diabetes, testosterone transdermal system may decrease blood glucose levels and therefore requirements for *antidiabetics* such as *insulin.* C-17 substituted derivatives of testosterone have reportedly decreased the anticoagulant requirements of patients receiving *oral anticoagulants;* these patients require close monitoring, especially when drug system is started or stopped. Administration with *oxyphenbutazone* may result in elevated serum oxyphenbutazone levels.

ADVERSE REACTIONS

CNS: *CVA.*

GU: *gynecomastia,* prostatitis, urinary tract infection, breast tenderness.

Skin: acne, *pruritus.*

Other: discomfort, irritation.

▣ KEY CONSIDERATIONS

● Geriatric patients treated with androgens may be at increased risk for developing prostatic hyperplasia and prostate cancer; use testosterone transdermal system cautiously in these patients.

● Testoderm form of drug system doesn't produce adequate serum testosterone if applied to nonscrotal skin.

● Edema with or without heart failure may be a serious complication in patients with preexisting cardiac, renal, or hepatic disease; in addition to discontinuation of drug system, diuretic therapy may be required.

● Gynecomastia commonly develops and occasionally persists in patients receiving treatment for hypogonadism.

● Topical adverse reactions decrease with duration of use.

● Check hemoglobin levels and hematocrit periodically (to detect polycythemia) in patients on long-term androgen therapy.

● Check liver function, prostatic acid phosphatase, prostatic specific antigen, cholesterol, and high-density lipoprotein values periodically.

● After 3 to 4 weeks of daily system use in patients receiving Testoderm, draw blood 2 to 4 hours after system application for determination of serum total drug level. For patients receiving Androderm, monitor serum drug level the morning after regular evening application. Because of variability in analytic values among diagnostic laboratories, this laboratory work and later analyses

for assessing drug effect should be performed at the same laboratory.
• If patient hasn't achieved desired results within 8 weeks, consider another form of drug replacement therapy.
• Store testosterone transdermal system at room temperature.
• Androgens such as testosterone may decrease levels of thyroxin-binding globulin, resulting in decreased total T_4 serum levels and increased resin uptake of T_3 and T_4.

Patient education

• Show patient how to use testosterone transdermal system. For Testoderm, tell him to place system on clean, dry scrotal skin. Scrotal hair should be dry-shaved for optimal skin contact. Chemical depilatories shouldn't be used. For Androderm, tell patient to apply patches to clean, dry designated areas. Avoid bony prominences such as shoulder and hip areas.
• Tell patient to wear the Testoderm transdermal system 22 to 24 hours daily. Tell patient to wear Androderm 24 hours daily and to rotate the site, allowing 7 days between applications to the same site.
• Instruct patient to report if he experiences nausea, vomiting, skin color changes, ankle edema, or too-frequent or persistent penile erections.
• Inform patient that men who use topical testosterone preparations may cause virilization in female partners. Advise him to report if his female partner experiences changes in body hair distribution or a significant increase in acne.

---

tetanus immune globulin, human (TIG)
Hyper-Tet

Immune serum, tetanus prophylaxis

Available by prescription only
Injection: 250 U/ml in 1-ml vial or syringe

INDICATIONS & DOSAGE
Tetanus prophylactic dose
Adults: 250 U I.M.

Tetanus treatment
Adults: Single doses of 3,000 to 6,000 U I.M. have been used. Optimal dosage schedules aren't established. Don't give at same site as toxoid.

PHARMACODYNAMICS
Antitetanus action: TIG provides passive immunity to tetanus. Antibodies remain at effective levels for 3 weeks or longer. TIG protects the patient for the incubation period of most tetanus cases.

PHARMACOKINETICS
Absorption: TIG is absorbed slowly.
Distribution: Unknown.
Metabolism: Unknown.
Excretion: Serum half-life of drug is about 28 days.

CONTRAINDICATIONS & PRECAUTIONS
Contraindicated in patients with thrombocytopenia or coagulation disorder that contraindicates I.M. injection unless potential benefits outweigh risks. Contraindicated for use in patients with hypersensitivity to thimerosal or TIG. Not recommended for patients with immunoglobulin A deficiency. Don't give I.V.

INTERACTIONS
None reported.

ADVERSE REACTIONS
GU: nephrotic syndrome.
Other: slight fever; hypersensitivity reactions; ***anaphylaxis; angioedema;*** erythema, stiffness, and pain at injection site.

▣ KEY CONSIDERATIONS
• Obtain a thorough history of injury, tetanus immunizations, last tetanus toxoid injection, allergies, and reactions to immunizations.
• Have epinephrine solution 1:1,000 available to treat allergic reactions.
• For wound management, use TIG for prophylaxis in patients with dirty wounds if patient had fewer than three previous tetanus toxoid injections or if the immunization history is unknown or uncertain.

- Thoroughly clean and remove all foreign matter and necrotic tissue from wound.
- Give tetanus antitoxin when TIG isn't available.
- Don't confuse drug with tetanus toxoid, which should be given at the same time but at different sites to produce active immunization.
- Administer I.M. in the deltoid muscle for adults. Don't inject I.V.
- TIG hasn't been associated with an increase in AIDS cases. The immune globulin is devoid of HIV. Immune globulin recipients don't develop antibodies to HIV.
- Store TIG between 36° and 46° F (2° and 8° C). Don't freeze.

Patient education
- Tell patient that available data indicate TIG administration doesn't cause AIDS or hepatitis.
- Inform patient that some local pain, swelling, and tenderness may occur at the injection site; recommend acetaminophen to alleviate these minor effects.
- Encourage patient to report headache, skin changes, or difficulty breathing.

tetanus toxoid, adsorbed
tetanus toxoid, fluid

Toxoid, tetanus prophylaxis

Available by prescription only
Adsorbed toxoid
Injection: 5 to 10 Lf U of inactivated tetanus/0.5-ml dose, in 0.5-ml syringes and 5-ml vials
Fluid toxoid
Injection: 4 to 5 Lf U of inactivated tetanus/0.5-ml dose, in 0.5-ml syringes and 7.5-ml vials

INDICATIONS & DOSAGE
Primary immunization (adsorbed formulation)
Adults: 0.5 ml I.M. 4 to 8 weeks apart for two doses, then a third dose 6 to 12 months after the second dose.

Primary immunization (fluid formulation)
Adults: 0.5 ml I.M. or S.C. 4 to 8 weeks apart for three doses, then a fourth dose 6 to 12 months after the third dose. Booster dosage, 0.5 ml I.M. or S.C. q 10 years.

PHARMACODYNAMICS
Tetanus prophylaxis action: Tetanus toxoid promotes active immunity by inducing production of tetanus antitoxin.

PHARMACOKINETICS
Absorption: Tetanus toxoid is slowly absorbed; fluid formulation provides quicker booster effect.
Distribution: Unknown.
Metabolism: Unknown.
Excretion: Unknown. Active immunity usually persists for 10 years. Adsorbed tetanus toxoid usually produces more persistent antitoxin titers than fluid tetanus toxoid.

CONTRAINDICATIONS & PRECAUTIONS
Contraindicated in patients with immunosuppression and in those with immunoglobulin abnormalities or severe hypersensitivity or neurologic reactions to the toxoid or its ingredients, such as thimerosal. Also contraindicated in patients with thrombocytopenia or coagulation disorder that would contraindicate I.M. injection unless the potential benefits outweigh the risks. Vaccination should be deferred in patients with acute illness and during polio outbreaks, except in emergencies.

INTERACTIONS
Drug-drug. Use with *chloramphenicol, corticosteroids,* or *immunosuppressants* theoretically may impair the immune response to tetanus toxoid; avoid elective immunization under these circumstances.

ADVERSE REACTIONS
CNS: malaise.
CV: flushing, tachycardia, hypotension.
Musculoskeletal: aches and pains.
Skin: urticaria, pruritus, erythema, induration, nodule (at injection site).
Other: slight fever, chills, *anaphylaxis.*

▣ KEY CONSIDERATIONS

• Geriatric patients develop lower-than-normal antitoxin levels after tetanus immunization than younger patients. Skin test responsiveness may be delayed or reduced in geriatric patients.

• Obtain a thorough history of allergies and reactions to immunizations.

• Have epinephrine 1:1,000 solution available to treat allergic reactions.

• Determine tetanus immunization status and date of last tetanus immunization.

• The deltoid or midlateral thigh is the preferred I.M. injection site.

• Preferably, tetanus immunization should be completed and maintained using multiple antigen preparations appropriate for patient's age.

• Adsorbed toxoids induce higher antitoxin titers and hence more persistent antitoxin levels; thus, adsorbed tetanus toxoid is strongly recommended over fluid tetanus toxoid for primary and booster immunizations.

• Shake vial vigorously to ensure a uniform suspension before withdrawing the dose.

• Don't confuse drug with tetanus immune globulin.

• These toxoids are used to prevent, not treat, tetanus infections.

• Store at 36° to 46° F (2° to 8° C). Don't freeze.

Patient education

• Tell patient to expect discomfort at injection site, with a nodule that may develop and persist for several weeks after immunization. If fever, general malaise, or body aches and pains develop, advise patient to treat with acetaminophen.

• Instruct patient not to use hot or cold compresses at injection site because this may increase the severity of the local reaction.

• Encourage patient to report distressing adverse reactions.

• Tell patient that immunization requires a series of injections; stress the importance of keeping scheduled appointments for subsequent doses.

tetracycline hydrochloride

Achromycin, Ala-Tet, Novotetra,*
Panmycin, Robitet, Sumycin, Teline,
Tetralan,* Topicycline

Tetracycline, antibiotic

Available by prescription only
Capsules: 100 mg, 250 mg, 500 mg
Tablets: 250 mg, 500 mg
Suspension: 125 mg/5 ml
Topical solution: 2.2 mg/ml
Available without prescription
Topical ointment: 3%*

INDICATIONS & DOSAGE

Infections caused by sensitive organisms
Adults: 1 to 2 g P.O. divided into two to four doses.

Uncomplicated urethral, endocervical, or rectal infection caused by **Chlamydia trachomatis**
Adults: 500 mg P.O. q.i.d. for at least 7 days.

Brucellosis
Adults: 500 mg P.O. q 6 hours for 3 weeks with streptomycin, 1 g I.M. q 12 hours week 1 and daily week 2.

Gonorrhea in patients sensitive to penicillin
Adults: Initially, 1.5 g P.O., then 500 mg q 6 hours for 4 days.

Syphilis in patients sensitive to penicillin
Adults: 500 mg P.O. q.i.d. for 14 days.

◊ *Lyme disease*
Adults: 250 to 500 mg P.O. q.i.d. for 10 to 30 days.

◊ *Acute transmitted epididymitis;*
◊ *pelvic inflammatory disease;*
◊ **Helicobacter pylori** *(all these indications use tetracycline as adjunctive therapy)*
Adults: 500 mg P.O. q.i.d. for 10 to 14 days.

Infection prophylaxis in minor skin abrasions and treatment of superficial infections caused by susceptible organisms
Adults: Apply topical ointment to infected area one to five times daily.

PHARMACODYNAMICS

Antibacterial action: Tetracycline is bacteriostatic; it binds reversibly to ribosomal subunits, thus inhibiting bacterial protein synthesis. Its spectrum of action includes many gram-negative and gram-positive organisms, *Mycoplasma, Rickettsia, Chlamydia,* and spirochetes.

It's useful against brucellosis, glanders, mycoplasma pneumonia infections (some health care providers prefer erythromycin), leptospirosis, early stages of Lyme disease, rickettsial infections (such as Rocky Mountain spotted fever, Q fever, and typhus fever), and chlamydial infections. It's an alternative to penicillin for *Neisseria gonorrhoeae,* but because of a high level of resistance in the United States, other drugs should be considered.

PHARMACOKINETICS

Absorption: Tetracycline is 75% to 80% absorbed after oral administration; serum levels peak at 2 to 4 hours. Food or milk products significantly reduce oral absorption.
Distribution: Drug is widely distributed into body tissues and fluids, including synovial, pleural, prostatic, and seminal fluids, bronchial secretions, saliva, and aqueous humor; CSF penetration is poor. Drug is 20% to 67% protein-bound.
Metabolism: Drug isn't metabolized.
Excretion: Drug is excreted primarily unchanged in urine through glomerular filtration; plasma half-life is 6 to 12 hours in adults with normal renal function. Hemodialysis and peritoneal dialysis remove only minimal amounts of the drug.

CONTRAINDICATIONS & PRECAUTIONS

Contraindicated in patients with hypersensitivity to tetracyclines.

Use cautiously in patients with impaired renal or hepatic function.

INTERACTIONS

Drug-drug. Tetracycline absorption may be decreased by *antacids containing aluminum, calcium,* or *magnesium; laxatives containing magnesium* because of chelation; *oral iron;* and *sodium bicarbonate. Cimetidine* may decrease the GI absorption of tetracycline. Use of tetracycline necessitates reduced dosages of *digoxin* because of increased bioavailability and of *oral anticoagulants* because of enhanced effects. Use of tetracycline increases the risk of nephrotoxicity from *methoxyflurane.* Tetracycline may antagonize bactericidal effects of *penicillin,* inhibiting cell growth from bacteriostatic action; administer penicillin 2 to 3 hours before tetracycline.
Drug-food. Use with *dairy products* or *food* may decrease absorption.
Drug-lifestyle. Prolonged or unprotected *exposure to the sun* may cause sensitivity reactions.

ADVERSE REACTIONS

Unless otherwise noted, the following adverse reactions result from the oral form of drug:
CNS: dizziness, headache, ***intracranial hypertension (pseudotumor cerebri).***
CV: pericarditis.
EENT: sore throat, glossitis, dysphagia.
GI: anorexia, *epigastric distress, nausea,* vomiting, *diarrhea,* esophagitis, oral candidiasis, stomatitis, enterocolitis, inflammatory lesions in anogenital region.
GU: *increased BUN levels.*
Hematologic: *neutropenia,* eosinophilia.
Hepatic: elevated liver enzyme levels.
Skin: *candidal superinfection, maculopapular and erythematous rashes, urticaria, photosensitivity, increased pigmentation,* temporary stinging or burning on application, slight yellowing of treated skin (especially in patients with light complexion), severe dermatitis (with topical administration).
Other: *hypersensitivity reactions.*

▣ KEY CONSIDERATIONS

Besides the recommendations relevant to all tetracyclines, consider the following:
● Discontinue topical use if condition persists or worsens.

- To control the flow of ointment, increase or decrease pressure of applicator against skin.
- Avoid contact with eyes, nose, and mouth.
- Solution should be used within 2 months.
- Tetracycline causes false-negative results in urine tests using glucose oxidase reagent (Diastix, Chemstrip uG, or glucose enzymatic test strip) and falsely elevates fluorometric tests for urine catecholamine levels.

Patient education

- Warn patient to avoid sharing washcloths and towels with family members when using topical form.
- Instruct patient to take tetracycline 1 hour before or 2 hours after eating food or drinking milk.
- Tell patient not to share drug with others.
- Inform patient using topical form that normal use of cosmetics may be continued.
- Explain that floating plug in bottle of topical tetracycline is an inert and harmless result of proper reconstitution of the preparation and shouldn't be removed.
- Tell patient that stinging may occur with topical use but resolves quickly; drug may stain clothing.
- Warn patient to avoid prolonged exposure to sunlight.
- Tell patient to report persistent nausea or vomiting or yellowing of skin or eyes.

---

theophylline

Accurbron, Aerolate, Aquaphyllin, Asmalix, Bronkodyl, Constant-T, Elixophyllin, Lanophyllin, Quibron-T, Respbid, Slo-Bid Gyrocaps, Slo-Phyllin, Sustaire, Theobid Duracaps, Theochron, Theoclear-80, Theo-Dur, Theolair, Theo-Sav, Theo-24, Theospan-SR, Theostat-80, Theovent, Theo-X, T-Phyl, Uniphyl

Xanthine derivative, bronchodilator

Available by prescription only
Capsules: 100 mg, 200 mg

Capsules (extended-release): 50 mg, 60 mg, 65 mg, 75 mg, 100 mg, 125 mg, 130 mg, 200 mg, 250 mg, 260 mg, 300 mg
Tablets: 100 mg, 125 mg, 200 mg, 250 mg, 300 mg
Tablets (extended-release): 100 mg, 200 mg, 250 mg, 300 mg, 400 mg, 450 mg, 500 mg
Elixir: 50 mg/5 ml, 80 mg/15 ml
Syrup: 50 mg/5 ml, 80 mg/15 ml, 150 mg/15 ml
Dextrose 5% injection: 200 mg in 50 ml or 100 ml; 400 mg in 100 ml, 250 ml, 500 ml, or 1,000 ml; 800 mg in 500 ml or 1,000 ml

INDICATIONS & DOSAGE

Symptomatic relief of bronchospasm in patients not receiving theophylline who require rapid relief of acute symptoms
Loading dose: 6 mg/kg anhydrous theophylline, then:
Adult nonsmokers: 3 mg/kg q 6 hours for two doses, then 3 mg/kg q 8 hours.
Older adults with cor pulmonale: 2 mg/kg q 6 hours for two doses, then 2 mg/kg q 8 hours.
Adults with heart failure: 2 mg/kg q 8 hours for two doses, then 1 to 2 mg/kg q 12 hours.
Parenteral theophylline for patients not receiving theophylline
Loading dose: 4.7 mg/kg (equivalent to 6 mg/kg anhydrous aminophylline) I.V. slowly, then maintenance infusion.
Adult nonsmokers: 0.55 mg/kg/hour (equivalent to 0.7 mg/kg/hour anhydrous aminophylline) for 12 hours, then 0.39 mg/kg/hour (equivalent to 0.5 mg/kg/hour anhydrous aminophylline).
Older adults with cor pulmonale: 0.47 mg/kg/hour (equivalent to 0.6 mg/kg/hour anhydrous aminophylline) for 12 hours, then 0.24 mg/kg/hour (equivalent to 0.3 mg/kg/hour anhydrous aminophylline).
Adults with heart failure or liver disease: 0.39 mg/kg/hour (equivalent to 0.5 mg/kg/hour anhydrous aminophylline) for 12 hours, then 0.08 to 0.16 mg/kg/hour (equivalent to 0.1 to 0.2 mg/kg/hour anhydrous aminophylline).

Reactions may be *common*, uncommon, *life-threatening*, or COMMON AND LIFE-THREATENING.

Switch to oral theophylline as soon as patient shows adequate improvement.

Symptomatic relief of bronchospasm in patients receiving theophylline

Adults: Each 0.5 mg/kg I.V. or P.O. (loading dose) increases plasma levels by 1 μg/ml. Ideally, dose is based on current theophylline level and lean body weight. In emergency situations, may use a 2.5-mg/kg P.O. dose of rapidly absorbed form if no obvious signs of theophylline toxicity are present.

Prophylaxis of bronchial asthma, bronchospasm of chronic bronchitis, and emphysema

Adults: Using rapidly absorbed dosage forms, initial dosage is 16 mg/kg or 400 mg P.O. daily (whichever is less) divided q 6 to 8 hours; dosage may be increased in approximate increments of 25% at 2- to 3-day intervals. Using extended-release dosage forms, initial dose is 12 mg/kg or 400 mg P.O. daily (whichever is less) divided q 8 to 12 hours; dosage may be increased, if tolerated, by 2 to 3 mg/kg daily at 3-day intervals. Regardless of dosage form used, dosage may be increased, if tolerated, up to the following maximum daily doses without measurements of serum theophylline level.

Adults: 13 mg/kg P.O. or 900 mg P.O. daily in divided doses.

Note: Dosage individualization is required. Use peak plasma and trough levels to estimate dose. Therapeutic range is 10 to 20 mcg/ml. All doses are based on theophylline anhydrous and lean body weight.

◇ *Promotion of diuresis;* ◇ *treatment of Cheyne-Stokes respirations;* ◇ *paroxysmal nocturnal dyspnea*

Adults: 200 to 400 mg I.V. bolus (single dose).

PHARMACODYNAMICS

Bronchodilator action: Theophylline may act by inhibiting phosphodiesterase, elevating cellular cAMP levels, or antagonizing adenosine receptors in the bronchi, resulting in relaxation of the smooth muscle.

Drug also increases sensitivity of the medullary respiratory center to carbon dioxide to reduce apneic episodes. It prevents muscle fatigue, especially that of the diaphragm. It also causes diuresis and cardiac and CNS stimulation.

PHARMACOKINETICS

Absorption: Theophylline is well absorbed. Rate and onset of action depend on dosage form; food may further alter rate of absorption, especially of some extended-release preparations.

Distribution: Drug is distributed throughout the extracellular fluids; equilibrium between fluid and tissues occurs within an hour of I.V. loading dose. Therapeutic plasma levels are 10 to 20 μg/ml, but many patients respond to lower levels.

Metabolism: Drug is metabolized in the liver to inactive compounds. Half-life is 7 to 9 hours in adults and 4 to 5 hours in smokers.

Excretion: About 10% of dose is excreted in urine unchanged; the other metabolites include 1-methyluric acid, 3-methylxanthine, and 1,3 dimethyluric acid.

CONTRAINDICATIONS & PRECAUTIONS

Contraindicated in patients with hypersensitivity to xanthine compounds (caffeine, theobromine) and in those with active peptic ulcer and seizure disorders.

Use cautiously in geriatric patients and in those with COPD, cardiac failure, cor pulmonale, renal or hepatic disease, peptic ulcer, hyperthyroidism, diabetes mellitus, glaucoma, severe hypoxemia, hypertension, compromised cardiac or circulatory function, angina, an acute MI, or sulfite sensitivity.

INTERACTIONS

Drug-drug. *Allopurinol (high dose), calcium channel blockers, cimetidine, corticosteroids, erythromycin, interferon, mexiletine, propranolol, quinolones,* and *troleandomycin* may cause increased serum theophylline levels by decreasing the hepatic clearance. *Barbiturates* and *phenytoin* enhance hepatic metabolism of theophylline, decreasing plasma levels. *Beta blockers* exert an antagonistic pharmacologic effect. *Carbamazepine, isoniazid,* and *loop diuretics* may increase or decrease theophylline levels.

Charcoal and *ketoconazole* may decrease theophylline levels. Theophylline increases the excretion of *lithium*. *Rifampin* may decrease serum theophylline levels by increasing hepatic clearance of theophylline.

Drug-food. Avoid excessive use of *caffeine-containing beverages* and *xanthine-containing foods.*

ADVERSE REACTIONS

CNS: *restlessness, dizziness, insomnia,* headache, irritability, *seizures,* muscle twitching.
CV: *palpitations, sinus tachycardia,* extrasystoles, flushing, marked hypotension, *arrhythmias.*
GI: *nausea, vomiting,* diarrhea, epigastric pain.
Metabolic: increased plasma free fatty acid and urine catecholamine levels.
Respiratory: tachypnea, *respiratory arrest.*

▣ KEY CONSIDERATIONS

• Theophylline may increase the risk of vertigo in geriatric patients.
• Don't crush extended-release tablets; some capsules are formulated to be opened and sprinkled on food.
• Monitor vital signs and observe for signs and symptoms of toxic reaction.
• Obtain serum theophylline levels in patients receiving long-term therapy. Ideal levels are between 10 and 20 µg/ml, although some patients may respond adequately with lower serum levels. Check every 6 months. If levels are less than 10 µg/ml, increase dose by about 25% each day. If levels are 20 to 25 µg/ml, decrease dose by about 10% each day. If levels are 25 to 30 µg/ml, skip next dose and decrease by 25% each day. If levels are more than 30 µg/ml, skip next two doses and decrease by 50% each day. Check serum theophylline level again.
• Depending on assay used, furosemide, phenylbutazone, probenecid, theobromine, caffeine, tea, chocolate, cola beverages, and acetaminophen may falsely elevate theophylline levels.

Patient education

• Instruct patient regarding theophylline and dosage schedule; if dose is missed, he should take it as soon as possible, but he shouldn't double-dose.
• Advise patient to take drug at regular intervals as instructed, around the clock.
• Inform patient of adverse effects and possible signs of toxic reaction.
• Tell patient to avoid excessive use of xanthine-containing foods and caffeine-containing beverages.
• Warn geriatric patient of dizziness, a common reaction at start of therapy.
• Tell patient to take drug with food if GI upset occurs with liquid preparations or nonsustained release forms.
• Instruct patient to continue to use the same brand of theophylline.

Overdose & treatment

• Signs and symptoms of overdose include nausea, vomiting, insomnia, irritability, tachycardia, extrasystoles, tachypnea, or tonic-clonic seizures. The onset of toxicity may be sudden and severe, with arrhythmias and seizures as the first signs.
• Induce vomiting except in convulsing patients, then use activated charcoal and cathartics. Treat arrhythmias with lidocaine and seizures with I.V. diazepam; support respiratory and CV systems.

thiamine hydrochloride (vitamin B$_1$)
Biamine, Thiamilate

Water-soluble vitamin, nutritional supplement

Available by prescription only
Injection: 1-ml ampules (100 mg/ml), 1-ml vials (100 mg/ml), 2-ml vials (100 mg/ml), 10-ml vials (100 mg/ml), 30-ml vials (100 mg/ml), 30-ml vials (200 mg/ml), 30-ml vials (100 mg/ml, with 0.5% chlorobutanol)
Available without prescription
Tablets: 25 mg, 50 mg, 100 mg, 250 mg, 500 mg
Tablets (enteric-coated): 20 mg

INDICATIONS & DOSAGE
Beriberi
Adults: 10 to 20 mg I.M., depending on severity (can receive up to 100 mg I.M.

or I.V. for severe cases), t.i.d. for 2 weeks, followed by dietary correction and multivitamin supplement containing 5 to 30 mg thiamine daily in single or three divided doses for 1 month.

Anemia secondary to thiamine deficiency; polyneuritis secondary to alcoholism, or pellagra
Adults: P.O. dosage is based on RDA for age-group.

Wernicke's encephalopathy
Adults: Initially, 100 mg I.V., followed by 50 to 100 mg I.M. or I.V. daily.

Wet beriberi with myocardial failure
Adults: 10 to 30 mg I.V. for emergency treatment.

PHARMACODYNAMICS

Metabolic action: Exogenous thiamine is required for carbohydrate metabolism. Drug combines with adenosine triphosphate to form thiamine pyrophosphate, a coenzyme in carbohydrate metabolism and transketolation reactions. This coenzyme is also necessary in the hexose monophosphate shunt during pentose use. One sign of thiamine deficiency is increased pyruvic acid levels. The body's need for thiamine is greater when the carbohydrate content of the diet is high. Within 3 weeks of total absence of dietary thiamine, significant vitamin depletion can occur. Thiamine deficiency can cause beriberi.

PHARMACOKINETICS

Absorption: Thiamine is absorbed readily after oral administration of small doses; after oral administration of a large dose, the total amount absorbed is limited to 4 to 8 mg. In alcoholics and in patients with cirrhosis or malabsorption, GI absorption of drug is decreased. When given with meals, drug's GI rate of absorption decreases, but total absorption remains the same. After I.M. administration, drug is absorbed rapidly and completely.
Distribution: Drug is distributed widely into body tissues. When intake exceeds minimal requirements, tissue stores become saturated.
Metabolism: Drug is metabolized in the liver.

Excretion: Excess drug is excreted in urine. After administration of doses exceeding 10 mg, both unchanged drug and metabolites are excreted in urine after tissue stores become saturated.

CONTRAINDICATIONS & PRECAUTIONS

Contraindicated in patients hypersensitive to thiamine products.

INTERACTIONS

Drug-drug. Don't use with *alkaline solutions (bicarbonates, carbonates, citrates);* thiamine is unstable in *alkaline* or *neutral solutions.* Use with *neuromuscular blockers* may enhance the effects of neuromuscular blockers. Solutions containing *sulfites* are incompatible with thiamine.

ADVERSE REACTIONS

CNS: weakness, restlessness.
CV: *angioedema, CV collapse,* cyanosis.
EENT: tightness of throat (allergic reaction).
GI: nausea, hemorrhage.
Respiratory: pulmonary edema.
Skin: feeling of warmth, pruritus, urticaria, diaphoresis.
Other: tenderness and induration after I.M. administration.

▣ KEY CONSIDERATIONS

• The RDA of thiamine is as follows: men ages 51 and older, 1.2 mg daily; women ages 51 and older, 1 mg daily.
• Give I.D. skin test before I.V. drug administration if sensitivity is suspected because anaphylaxis can occur; keep epinephrine available when administering large parenteral doses.
• I.M. injection may be painful. Rotate injection sites and apply cold compresses to ease discomfort.
• Accurate dietary history is important during vitamin replacement therapy. Help patient develop a practical plan for adequate nutrition.
• Total absence of dietary thiamine can produce a deficiency state in about 3 weeks.
• Subclinical deficiency of thiamine or other B vitamins is common in patients

who are poor, have chronic alcoholism, or follow fad diets.

• Store drug in light-resistant, nonmetallic container.

• Drug therapy may produce false-positive results in the phosphotungstate method for determining uric acid and in the urine spot tests with Ehrlich's reagent for urobilinogen.

• Large doses of drug interfere with the Schack and Waxler spectrophotometric method of determining serum theophylline levels.

Patient education

• Inform patient about dietary sources of thiamine, such as yeast, pork, beef, liver, whole grains, peas, and beans.

thioridazine
Mellaril-S

thioridazine hydrochloride
Apo-Thioridazine,* Mellaril, Novo-Ridazine,* PMS Thioridazine*

Phenothiazine (piperidine derivative), antipsychotic drug

Available by prescription only
Tablets: 10 mg, 15 mg, 25 mg, 50 mg, 100 mg, 150 mg, 200 mg
Oral concentrate: 30 mg/ml, 100 mg/ml (3% to 4.2% alcohol)
Suspension: 25 mg/5 ml, 100 mg/5 ml

INDICATIONS & DOSAGE
Psychosis
Adults: Initially, 50 to 100 mg P.O. t.i.d., with gradual increments up to 800 mg daily in divided doses, if needed. Dosage varies.
Dysthymic disorder (neurotic depression), dementia
Adults: Initially, 25 mg P.O. t.i.d. Maintenance dosage is 20 to 200 mg daily.

PHARMACODYNAMICS
Antipsychotic action: Thioridazine is thought to act by postsynaptic blockade of CNS dopamine receptors, inhibiting dopamine-mediated effects.

Drug has many other central and peripheral effects. It produces both alpha and ganglionic blockade and counteracts histamine- and serotonin-mediated activity. Its most prevalent adverse reactions are antimuscarinic and sedative; it causes fewer extrapyramidal effects than other antipsychotic drugs.

PHARMACOKINETICS
Absorption: Rate and extent of absorption vary with administration route. Oral tablet absorption is erratic and variable, with onset from ½ to 1 hour. Oral concentrates and suspensions are much more predictable.
Distribution: Thioridazine is distributed widely into the body; effects peak at 2 to 4 hours, serum level reaches steady state within 4 to 7 days. Drug is 91% to 99% protein-bound.
Metabolism: Drug is metabolized extensively in the liver and forms the active metabolite mesoridazine; duration of action is 4 to 6 hours.
Excretion: Drug is mostly excreted as metabolites in urine; some excreted in feces through biliary tract.

CONTRAINDICATIONS & PRECAUTIONS
Contraindicated in patients with hypersensitivity to thioridazine or in those experiencing coma, CNS depression, or severe hypertensive or hypotensive heart disease.

Use cautiously in geriatric or debilitated patients and in those with hepatic or CV disease, respiratory or seizure disorders, hypocalcemia, severe reactions to insulin or electroconvulsive therapy, and exposure to extreme cold or heat or to organophosphate insecticides.

INTERACTIONS
Drug-drug. Pharmacokinetic alterations and subsequent decreased therapeutic response to thioridazine may follow use with *aluminum-* and *magnesium-containing antacids* and *antidiarrheals* (decreased absorption) and *phenobarbital* (enhanced renal excretion). Additive effects are likely after use of thioridazine with *antiarrhythmics,* including *disopyramide* and *procainamide* (increased incidence of arrhythmias and conduction defects), and *quinidine; atropine* and other *anticholinergics,* including *antide-*

Reactions may be *common,* uncommon, **life-threatening**, or COMMON AND LIFE-THREATENING.

pressants, antihistamines, antiparkinso-nians (oversedation, paralytic ileus, visu-al changes, severe constipation), *MAO inhibitors, meperidine,* and *pheno-thiazines; CNS depressants,* including *analgesics, anesthetics (epidural, gener-al,* or *spinal), barbiturates, narcotics,* and *tranquilizers;* and *parenteral magne-sium sulfate* (oversedation, respiratory depression, and hypotension); *metriza-mide* (increased risk for seizures); and *nitrates* (hypotension).

Use of thioridazine with *appetite sup-pressants* and with *sympathomimetics,* including *ephedrine* (found in many nasal sprays), *epinephrine, phenyl-ephrine,* and *phenylpropanolamine,* may decrease their stimulatory and pressor effects; thioridazine may cause *epineph-rine reversal. Beta blockers* may inhibit thioridazine metabolism, increasing plasma levels and toxic effects.

Thioridazine may antagonize thera-peutic effect of *bromocriptine* on pro-lactin secretion; it also may decrease the vasoconstrictive effects of *high-dose dopamine* and may decrease effective-ness and increase toxicity of *levodopa* (by dopamine blockade). Thioridazine may inhibit blood pressure response to *centrally acting antihypertensives,* such as *clonidine, guanabenz, guanadrel, guanethidine, methyldopa,* and *reserpine.* Use with *lithium* may result in severe neurologic toxicity with an encephalitis-like syndrome and in de-creased therapeutic response to thiori-dazine. Thioridazine may inhibit metab-olism and increase toxic effects of *phenytoin.* Use with *propylthiouracil* in-creases risk of agranulocytosis.

Drug-food. Use with *caffeine* may in-crease metabolism of drug.

Drug-lifestyle. *Alcohol* use may cause additive effects after use of thioridazine. Prolonged or unprotected exposure to the *sun* may cause photosensitivity reac-tions. Use with *heavy smoking* may in-crease metabolism of drug.

ADVERSE REACTIONS

CNS: extrapyramidal reactions, *tardive dyskinesia, sedation,* EEG changes, dizziness.

CV: *orthostatic hypotension,* tachycar-dia, ECG changes.

EENT: *ocular changes, blurred vision,* retinitis pigmentosa.

GI: increased appetite, *dry mouth, con-stipation.*

GU: *urine retention,* dark urine, gyneco-mastia, inhibited ejaculation.

Hematologic: transient leukopenia, agranulocytosis, hyperprolactinemia.

Hepatic: cholestatic jaundice, elevated liver enzyme levels.

Metabolic: weight gain.

Skin: *mild photosensitivity,* allergic re-actions.

Other: elevated protein-bound iodine levels.

After abrupt withdrawal of long-term therapy: gastritis, nausea, vomiting, dizziness, tremor, feeling of warmth or cold, diaphoresis, tachycardia, headache, insomnia.

▣ KEY CONSIDERATIONS

Besides the recommendations relevant to all phenothiazines, consider the follow-ing:

● Geriatric patients tend to require lower dosages adjusted to individual response. Such patients also are more likely to de-velop adverse reactions, especially tar-dive dyskinesia and other extrapyramidal effects.

● Dosages exceeding 300 mg/day are usually reserved for adults with severe psychosis; don't exceed 800 mg/day be-cause of ophthalmic toxicity.

● Liquid formulations may cause a rash if skin contact occurs.

● Thioridazine can discolor urine pink to brown.

● Drug commonly causes sedation, anti-cholinergic effects, orthostatic hypoten-sion, photosensitivity reactions, and de-layed or absent ejaculation. It has the lowest potential for extrapyramidal reac-tions of all phenothiazines.

● Oral formulations may cause stomach upset; administer with food or fluid.

● Check patient regularly for abnormal body movements (at least every 6 months).

● Concentrate must be diluted in 60 to 120 ml (2 to 4 oz) of liquid—preferably

water, carbonated drinks, fruit juice, tomato juice, or milk—or pudding.
• All liquid formulations must be protected from light.
• Drug causes false-positive test results for urine porphyrins, urobilinogen, amylase, and 5-hydroxyindoleacetic acid levels because of darkening of urine by metabolites.

Patient education
• Explain risks of dystonic reactions and tardive dyskinesia, and tell patient to report abnormal body movements.
• Tell patient to avoid sun exposure and to wear sunscreen when going outdoors to prevent photosensitivity reactions. (Heat lamps and tanning beds also may burn or discolor the skin.)
• Warn patient not to spill liquid thioridazine on the skin; rash and irritation may result.
• Warn patient to avoid extremely hot or cold baths or exposure to temperature extremes, sunlamps, or tanning beds; drug may cause thermoregulatory changes.
• Advise patient to take drug exactly as prescribed and not to double-dose for missed doses.
• Explain that many drug interactions are possible; patient should seek medical approval before taking any nonprescribed drug.
• Tell patient not to stop taking drug suddenly; dosage reduction will alleviate most adverse reactions. However, patient should call promptly if he experiences difficulty urinating, sore throat, dizziness or fainting, or visual changes.
• Warn patient to avoid hazardous activities that require alertness until the effect of drug is established; reassure patient that excessive sedation usually subsides after several weeks.
• Tell patient not to drink alcohol or take other drugs that may cause excessive sedation.
• Advise patient to maintain adequate hydration.
• Explain which fluids are appropriate for diluting the concentrate and the dropper technique of measuring dose.

• Suggest sugarless gum or candy, ice chips, or artificial saliva to relieve dry mouth.
• Tell patient to store drug safely away from children.

Overdose & treatment
• CNS depression is characterized by deep sleep (in which the patient can't be aroused) and possible coma, hypotension or hypertension, extrapyramidal symptoms, abnormal involuntary muscle movements, agitation, seizures, arrhythmias, ECG changes, hypothermia or hyperthermia, and autonomic nervous system dysfunction.
• Treatment is symptomatic and supportive and includes maintaining vital signs, airway, stable body temperature, and fluid and electrolyte balance. Don't induce vomiting. Thioridazine inhibits cough reflex and aspiration may occur. Perform gastric lavage, then administer activated charcoal and sodium chloride cathartics; dialysis doesn't help. Regulate body temperature as needed. Treat hypotension with I.V. fluids. Don't give epinephrine. Treat seizures with parenteral diazepam or barbiturates; arrhythmias with 1 mg/kg of parenteral phenytoin, with the rate titrated to blood pressure; and extrapyramidal reactions with 1 to 2 mg of benztropine or 10 to 50 mg of parenteral diphenhydramine.

thiothixene

thiothixene hydrochloride
Navane

Thioxanthene, antipsychotic drug

Available by prescription only
Capsules: 1 mg, 2 mg, 5 mg, 10 mg, 20 mg
Oral concentrate: 5 mg/ml (7% alcohol)
Injection: 2 mg/ml, 5 mg/ml

INDICATIONS & DOSAGE
Acute agitation
Adults: 4 mg I.M. b.i.d. to q.i.d.; maximum dosage is 30 mg I.M. daily.

Reactions may be *common,* uncommon, ***life-threatening***, or COMMON AND LIFE-THREATENING.

Change to P.O. form as soon as possible; I.M. dosage form causes irritation.

Mild to moderate psychosis
Adults: Initially, 2 mg P.O. t.i.d.; may increase gradually to 15 mg daily.

Severe psychosis
Adults: Initially, 5 mg P.O. b.i.d.; may increase gradually to 20 to 30 mg daily. Maximum recommended daily dose is 60 mg.

PHARMACODYNAMICS

Antipsychotic action: Thiothixene is thought to act by postsynaptic blockade of CNS dopamine receptors, thereby inhibiting dopamine-mediated effects.

Drug has many other central and peripheral effects; it also acts as an alpha blocker. Its most prominent adverse reactions are extrapyramidal.

PHARMACOKINETICS

Absorption: Thiothixene is rapidly absorbed; I.M. onset of action is 10 to 30 minutes.
Distribution: Drug is widely distributed into the body. Effects peak at 1 to 6 hours after I.M. administration; drug is 91% to 99% protein-bound.
Metabolism: Drug is metabolized in the liver.
Excretion: Mostly excreted as parent drug in feces from the biliary tract.

CONTRAINDICATIONS & PRECAUTIONS

Contraindicated in patients with hypersensitivity to thiothixene and in those experiencing circulatory collapse, coma, CNS depression, or blood dyscrasia.

Use cautiously in geriatric or debilitated patients; in those with history of seizure disorders, CV disease, heat exposure, glaucoma, or prostatic hyperplasia; and in those in a state of alcohol withdrawal.

INTERACTIONS

Drug-drug. Pharmacokinetic alterations and subsequent decreased therapeutic response to thiothixene may follow use with *aluminum-* and *magnesium-containing antacids* and *antidiarrheals* (decreased absorption) and *phenobarbital* (enhanced renal excretion). Additive effects are likely when used with *antiar-*

rhythmics, including *disopyramide, quinidine,* and *procainamide* (increased incidence of cardiac arrhythmias and conduction defects); *atropine* and *other anticholinergics,* including *antidepressants, antihistamines, MAO inhibitors, meperidine,* and *phenothiazines; antiparkinsonians* (oversedation, paralytic ileus, visual changes, severe constipation); *CNS depressants,* including *analgesics, anesthetics (epidural, general,* or *spinal), barbiturates, narcotics, tranquilizers; metrizamide* (increased risk of seizures); *nitrates* (hypotension); and *parenteral magnesium sulfate* (oversedation, respiratory depression, hypotension). Use with *appetite suppressants* and *sympathomimetics*—including *ephedrine* (found in nasal sprays), *epinephrine, phenylephrine,* and *phenylpropanolamine*—may decrease their stimulatory and pressor effects.

Thiothixene may cause *epinephrine* reversal; patients taking thiothixene may experience a decrease in blood pressure when epinephrine is used as a pressor drug. *Beta blockers* may inhibit thiothixene metabolism, increasing plasma levels and toxicity. Thiothixene may antagonize therapeutic effect of *bromocriptine* on prolactin secretion; it may also decrease the vasoconstrictive effects of *high-dose dopamine* and may decrease effectiveness and increase toxicity of *levodopa* (by dopamine blockade). Thiothixene may inhibit blood pressure response to *centrally acting antihypertensives,* such as *clonidine, guanabenz, guanadrel, guanethidine, methyldopa,* and *reserpine.*

Use with *lithium* may result in severe neurologic toxicity with an encephalitis-like syndrome and in decreased therapeutic response to thiothixene. Use with *propylthiouracil* increases risk of agranulocytosis. Thiothixene may inhibit metabolism and potentiate the effects of *phenytoin.*

Drug-food. Pharmacokinetic alterations and subsequent decreased therapeutic response to thiothixene may follow use with *caffeine.*

Drug-lifestyle. *Alcohol* may cause additive effects. *Heavy smoking* may cause pharmacokinetic alterations and subsequent decreased therapeutic response to thiothixene because of increased metabolism.

ADVERSE REACTIONS

CNS: *extrapyramidal reactions,* drowsiness, restlessness, agitation, insomnia, *tardive dyskinesia,* sedation, pseudoparkinsonism, EEG changes, dizziness.
CV: *hypotension,* tachycardia, ECG changes.
EENT: ocular changes, *blurred vision,* nasal congestion.
GI: *dry mouth, constipation.*
GU: *urine retention,* gynecomastia, inhibited ejaculation.
Hematologic: *transient leukopenia,* leukocytosis, *agranulocytosis.*
Hepatic: jaundice, elevated liver enzyme levels.
Metabolic: weight gain.
Skin: *mild photosensitivity,* allergic reactions, pain at I.M. injection site, sterile abscess.
Other: elevated protein-bound iodine level, *neuroleptic malignant syndrome.*
After abrupt withdrawal of long-term therapy: gastritis, nausea, vomiting, dizziness, tremor, feeling of warmth or cold, diaphoresis, tachycardia, headache, insomnia.

▣ KEY CONSIDERATIONS

• Geriatric patients tend to require lower dosages adjusted to individual response. Adverse reactions, especially tardive dyskinesia and other extrapyramidal effects, are more likely to develop in such patients.
• Liquid and injectable formulations may cause a rash if skin contact occurs.
• Thiothixene commonly causes extrapyramidal reactions.
• Because stomach upset may occur, administer oral form with food or fluid.
• Check patient regularly for abnormal body movements (at least every 6 months).
• Dilute the concentrate in 2 to 4 oz (60 to 120 ml) of liquid—preferably water, carbonated drinks, fruit juice, tomato juice, or milk—or pudding.

• Photosensitivity reactions may occur; patient should avoid exposure to sunlight or heat lamps.
• Administer I.M. injection deep into outer upper quadrant of the buttock. Massaging the area after administration may prevent abscesses from forming. I.M. injection may cause skin necrosis; avoid extravasation or give drug I.V.
• Solution for injection may be slightly discolored; don't use if excessively discolored or if a precipitate is evident. Contact pharmacist.
• Monitor blood pressure before and after parenteral administration.
• Shake concentrate before administration.
• Patient may use sugarless gum, hard candy, or ice to help relieve dry mouth.
• Drug is stable after reconstitution for 48 hours at room temperature.
• Protect liquid formulation from light.
• Drug causes false-positive test results for urine porphyrins, urobilinogen, amylase, and 5-hydroxyindoleacetic acid levels because of darkening of urine by metabolites.

Patient education
• Explain risks of dystonic reactions and tardive dyskinesia, and tell patient to report abnormal body movements.
• Tell patient to avoid sun exposure and to wear sunscreen when going outdoors to prevent photosensitivity reactions. (Heat lamps and tanning beds also may burn or discolor the skin.)
• Instruct patient not to spill liquid thiothixene on skin; contact with skin may cause rash and irritation.
• Warn patient to avoid extremely hot or cold baths or exposure to temperature extremes, sunlamps, or tanning beds; drug may cause thermoregulatory changes.
• Tell patient to take drug exactly as prescribed, not to double-dose for missed doses, and not to share drug with others.
• Explain that many drug interactions are possible; patient should seek medical approval before taking any nonprescribed drug.
• Tell patient not to stop taking drug suddenly; dosage adjustment alleviates most adverse reactions. However, patient

should call if he experiences difficulty urinating, sore throat, dizziness, or fainting.

• Warn patient against hazardous activities that require alertness until effect of drug is established; reassure patient that sedation usually subsides after several weeks.

• Tell patient not to drink alcohol or take other drugs that may cause excessive sedation.

• Explain which fluids are appropriate for diluting the concentrate and the dropper technique of measuring dose.

• Recommend sugarless hard candy, chewing gum, or ice to alleviate dry mouth.

• Tell patient to shake concentrate before administration.

• Instruct patient to store drug away from children.

Overdose & treatment

• CNS depression is characterized by deep sleep (in which the patient can't be aroused) and possible coma, hypotension or hypertension, extrapyramidal symptoms, abnormal involuntary muscle movements, agitation, seizures, arrhythmias, ECG changes, hypothermia or hyperthermia, and autonomic nervous system dysfunction.

• Treatment is symptomatic and supportive and includes maintaining vital signs, airway, stable body temperature, and fluid and electrolyte balance. *Don't induce vomiting.* Thiothixene inhibits cough reflex and aspiration may occur. Perform gastric lavage, then administer activated charcoal and sodium chloride cathartics; dialysis doesn't help. Regulate body temperature as needed. Treat hypotension with I.V. fluids: *Don't give epinephrine.* Seizures may be treated with parenteral diazepam or barbiturates; arrhythmias with 1 mg/kg of parenteral phenytoin, with rate titrated to blood pressure; and extrapyramidal reactions with 1 to 2 mg of benztropine or 10 to 50 mg of parenteral diphenhydramine.

thyroid, desiccated
Armour Thyroid, S-P-T, Thyrar, Thyroid Strong, Thyroid USP

Thyroid hormone

Available by prescription only
Tablets: 15 mg, 30 mg, 60 mg, 90 mg, 120 mg, 180 mg, 240 mg, 300 mg (Armour Thyroid)
Tablets (bovine): 30 mg, 60 mg, 120 mg (Thyrar)
Tablets (enteric-coated): 60 mg, 120 mg
Thyroid Strong tablets (contain 0.3% iodine): 32.5 mg, 65 mg, 130 mg, 200 mg
Capsules (pork): 60 mg, 120 mg, 180 mg, 300 mg (S-P-T, suspended in soybean oil)

INDICATIONS & DOSAGE
Adult hypothyroidism
Adults: Initially, 30 mg P.O. daily, increased by 15 mg q 14 to 30 days, depending on disease severity until desired response is achieved. Usual maintenance dosage is 60 to 180 mg P.O. daily as single dose.

PHARMACODYNAMICS
Thyrotropic action: Thyroid affects protein and carbohydrate metabolism, promotes gluconeogenesis, increases the use and mobilization of glycogen, stimulates protein synthesis, and regulates cell growth and differentiation. The major effect of drug is that it increases the metabolic rate of tissue.

PHARMACOKINETICS
Absorption: Thyroid is absorbed from the GI tract.
Distribution: Unknown. Drug is highly protein-bound.
Metabolism: Unknown.
Excretion: Unknown.

CONTRAINDICATIONS & PRECAUTIONS
Contraindicated in patients with hypersensitivity to thyroid, an acute MI uncomplicated by hypothyroidism, untreated thyrotoxicosis, or uncorrected adrenal insufficiency.

Use cautiously in geriatric patients and in those with angina pectoris, hypertension, other CV disorders, renal insufficiency, or ischemia.

INTERACTIONS
Drug-drug. Use with *adrenocorticoids* or *corticotropin* causes changes in thyroid status, and changes in thyroid dosages may require adrenocorticoid or corticotropin dosage changes as well. Use with *anticoagulants* may alter anticoagulant effect; an increased thyroid dosage may necessitate a lower anticoagulant dose. *Cholestyramine* and *colestipol* may decrease absorption. *Estrogens,* which increase serum T_4-binding globulin levels, increase thyroid requirements. *I.V. phenytoin* may release free thyroid from thyroglobulin. Use with *insulin* or *oral antidiabetics* may affect dosage requirements of these drugs. Use with *somatrem* may accelerate epiphyseal maturation. Use with *sympathomimetics* or *tricyclic antidepressants* may increase the effects of these drugs or of thyroid, possibly leading to coronary insufficiency or cardiac arrhythmias.

ADVERSE REACTIONS
CNS: *nervousness, insomnia,* tremor, headache.
CV: *tachycardia, arrhythmias, cardiac decompensation and collapse,* angina pectoris.
GI: diarrhea, vomiting.
Metabolic: weight loss.
Skin: *allergic skin reactions,* diaphoresis.
Other: heat intolerance.

▣ KEY CONSIDERATIONS
Besides the recommendations relevant to all thyroid hormones, consider the following:
● Geriatric patients are more sensitive to thyroid effects; in patients older than age 60, initial dosage should be 25% less than usual recommended dosage.
● Levothyroxine is considered drug of choice for thyroid hormone supplementation.
● Commercial preparations may have variable hormonal content and produce fluctuating liothyronine and levothyroxine levels. Because of this variability,

use of thyroid has decreased considerably.
● Thyroid Strong is 50% stronger than Thyroid USP. Each grain is equivalent to 1½ grains Thyroid USP.
● Monitor patient's pulse rate and blood pressure. Drug commonly causes adverse CV effects.
● Enteric-coated tablets give unreliable absorption.
● Digoxin levels should be monitored closely as patient becomes euthyroid.

Patient education
● Encourage patient to take daily dose at the same time each day, preferably in the morning to avoid insomnia.
● Advise patient to call if he experiences headache, diarrhea, nervousness, excessive sweating, heat intolerance, chest pain, increased pulse rate, or palpitations.
● Tell patient not to store drug in warm, humid areas such as the bathroom to prevent deterioration.
● Warn patient not to switch brands or dose.

Overdose & treatment
● Signs and symptoms of overdose include those of hyperthyroidism, including weight loss, increased appetite, palpitations, nervousness, diarrhea, abdominal cramps, sweating, tachycardia, increased pulse and blood pressure, angina, cardiac arrhythmias, tremor, headache, insomnia, heat intolerance, and fever.
● Treatment of acute overdose requires reduction of GI absorption and efforts to counteract central and peripheral effects, primarily sympathetic activity. Perform gastric lavage or induce vomiting (then administer activated charcoal, if less than 4 hours after ingestion). If the patient is comatose or having seizures, inflate cuff on endotracheal tube to prevent aspiration. Treatment may include oxygen and artificial ventilation to support respiration. It also should include appropriate measures to treat heart failure and control fever, hypoglycemia, and fluid loss. Propranolol may be used to combat many of the effects of increased sympathetic activity. Thyroid therapy should be

withdrawn gradually over 2 to 6 days, then resumed at a lower dose.

---

tiagabine hydrochloride
Gabitril

Gamma aminobutyric acid (GABA) enhancer, anticonvulsant

Available by prescription only
Tablets: 4 mg, 12 mg, 16 mg, 20 mg

INDICATIONS & DOSAGE
Adjunctive therapy in the treatment of partial seizures
Adults: Initially, 4 mg P.O. once daily. May increase total daily dose by 4 to 8 mg at weekly intervals until patient responds to drug or up to maximum of 56 mg/day. Give total daily dose in divided doses b.i.d. to q.i.d.
✦ *Dosage adjustment.* In patients with impaired liver function, initial and maintenance doses may be reduced, and dosing intervals may be increased.

PHARMACODYNAMICS
Anticonvulsant action: Exact mechanism is unknown. Tiagabine is thought to enhance the activity of GABA, the major inhibitory neurotransmitter in the CNS. It binds to recognition sites associated with the GABA uptake carrier and may thus permit more GABA to be available for binding to receptors on postsynaptic cells.

PHARMACOKINETICS
Absorption: Tiagabine is rapidly and nearly completely absorbed (more than 95%). Plasma levels peak 45 minutes after oral dose in the fasting state; absolute bioavailability is about 90%.
Distribution: About 96% binds to human plasma proteins, mainly to serum albumin and alpha-1 acid glycoprotein.
Metabolism: Drug is likely metabolized by the cytochrome P-450 3A isoenzymes.
Excretion: About 2% is excreted unchanged, with 25% and 63% of dose excreted into urine and feces, respectively. The average elimination half-life is 7 to 9 hours.

CONTRAINDICATIONS & PRECAUTIONS
Contraindicated in patients with hypersensitivity to tiagabine or its ingredients.

INTERACTIONS
Drug-drug. *Carbamazepine, phenobarbital,* and *phenytoin* increase tiagabine clearance. Tiagabine enhances the effects of *CNS depressants.* Tiagabine slightly decreases *valproate* levels.
Drug-lifestyle. Tiagabine enhances the CNS depressant effects of *alcohol.*

ADVERSE REACTIONS
CNS: *dizziness, asthenia, somnolence, nervousness,* tremor, difficulty with attention, insomnia, ataxia, confusion, speech disorder, difficulty with memory, paresthesia, depression, emotional lability, abnormal gait, hostility, language problems, agitation.
CV: vasodilation.
EENT: amblyopia, nystagmus, pharyngitis.
GI: abdominal pain, *nausea,* diarrhea, vomiting, increased appetite, mouth ulceration.
GU: urinary tract infection.
Musculoskeletal: myalgia, myasthenia.
Respiratory: increased cough.
Skin: rash, pruritus.
Other: flulike syndrome.

▣ KEY CONSIDERATIONS
• Because few patients older than age 65 were exposed to tiagabine during its evaluation, safety and effectiveness in these patients is unknown; observe closely.
• Never withdraw drug suddenly because seizure frequency may increase; withdraw gradually unless safety concerns require a more rapid withdrawal.
• A therapeutic range for plasma drug levels hasn't been established.
• Because of the potential for pharmacokinetic interactions between tiagabine and drugs that induce or inhibit hepatic metabolizing enzymes, obtain plasma tiagabine levels before and after changes are made in the therapeutic regimen.
• Status epilepticus and sudden unexpected death in epilepsy have occurred in patients receiving drug. Patients who aren't also receiving at least one

enzyme-inducing antiepileptic at the time of tiagabine initiation may require lower doses or slower dosage adjustment.

Patient education

● Advise patient to take tiagabine only as prescribed.
● Tell patient to take drug with food.
● Warn patient that drug may cause dizziness, somnolence, and other signs and symptoms of CNS depression; advise patient to avoid driving and other potentially hazardous activities that require mental alertness until drug's CNS effects are known.

Overdose & treatment

● The most common signs and symptoms reported after overdose include somnolence, impaired consciousness, impaired speech, agitation, confusion, speech difficulty, hostility, depression, weakness, and myoclonus.
● No specific antidote for tiagabine exists. If indicated, induce vomiting or perform gastric lavage. Observe usual precautions to maintain the airway, and provide general supportive care.

ticarcillin disodium
Ticar

Extended-spectrum penicillin, alpha-carboxypenicillin, antibiotic

Available by prescription only
Injection: 1 g, 3 g, 6 g
I.V. infusion: 3 g

INDICATIONS & DOSAGE
Serious infections caused by susceptible organisms
Adults: 200 to 300 mg/kg I.V. daily, divided into doses given q 4 or 6 hours.
Urinary tract infection
Adults: For patients with complicated infection, give 150 to 200 mg/kg I.V. daily, divided into doses q 4 to 6 hours; for treating uncomplicated infections, give 1 g I.V. or I.M. q 6 hours.
✦ *Dosage adjustment.* In patients with renal failure, initial loading dose is 3 g I.V., then refer to the table on this page. Patients on hemodialysis should receive

2 g I.V. q 12 hr with 3 g I.V. after each treatment; patients on peritoneal dialysis should receive 3 g I.V. q 12 hr.

Creatinine (clearance ml/min)	Dosage in adults
> 60	3 g I.V. q 4 hr
30-60	2 g I.V. q 4 hr
10-30	2 g I.V. q 8 hr
< 10	2 g I.V. q 12 hr or 1 g I.M. q 6 hr
< 10 with hepatic failure	2 g I.V. q 24 hr or 1 g I.M. q 12 hr

PHARMACODYNAMICS
Antibiotic action: Ticarcillin is bactericidal; it adheres to bacterial penicillin-binding proteins, inhibiting bacterial cell wall synthesis. Extended-spectrum penicillins are more resistant to inactivation by certain beta-lactamases, especially those produced by gram-negative organisms, but are still susceptible to inactivation by certain others.

Spectrum of activity includes many gram-negative aerobic and anaerobic bacilli, many gram-positive and gram-negative aerobic cocci, and some gram-positive aerobic and anaerobic bacilli. Drug may be effective against some strains of carbenicillin-resistant gram-negative bacilli.

In many cases, drug is more active (by weight) against *Pseudomonas aeruginosa* than carbenicillin. Drug is primarily used with an aminoglycoside to treat *P. aeruginosa* infections.

When ticarcillin is used alone, resistance develops rapidly. It's almost always used with other antibiotics (such as aminoglycosides).

PHARMACOKINETICS
Absorption: Plasma levels peak 30 to 75 minutes after I.M. dose; about 86% of dose is absorbed.
Distribution: Ticarcillin is distributed widely; it penetrates minimally into CSF with noninflamed meninges. Drug is 45% to 65% protein-bound.
Metabolism: About 13% of dose is metabolized through hydrolysis to inactive compounds.
Excretion: Drug is excreted primarily (80% to 93%) in urine through renal

---

Reactions may be *common*, uncommon, *life-threatening*, or COMMON AND LIFE-THREATENING.

tubular secretion and glomerular filtration; also excreted in bile. Elimination half-life in adults is about 1 hour; in severe renal impairment, half-life extends to about 3 hours. Peritoneal dialysis removes drug; hemodialysis doesn't.

CONTRAINDICATIONS & PRECAUTIONS
Contraindicated in patients with hypersensitivity to ticarcillin or other penicillins. Use cautiously in patients with other drug allergies, especially allergies to cephalosporins; impaired renal function; hemorrhagic conditions; hypokalemia; and sodium restrictions.

INTERACTIONS
Drug-drug. Use with *aminoglycoside antibiotics* results in synergistic bactericidal effects against *P. aeruginosa, Escherichia coli, Klebsiella, Citrobacter, Enterobacter, Serratia,* and *Proteus mirabilis;* however, drugs are physically and chemically incompatible and are inactivated when mixed or given together. Use of ticarcillin (and other extended-spectrum penicillins) with *clavulanic acid* also produces a synergistic bactericidal effect against certain beta-lactamase–producing bacteria. Large doses of penicillins may interfere with renal tubular secretion of *methotrexate,* thus delaying elimination and elevating serum methotrexate levels. *Probenecid* blocks renal tubular secretion of ticarcillin, increasing serum ticarcillin levels.

ADVERSE REACTIONS
CNS: *seizures,* neuromuscular excitability, pain at injection site.
GI: nausea, diarrhea, vomiting, pseudomembranous colitis.
Hematologic: *leukopenia, neutropenia,* eosinophilia, *thrombocytopenia, hemolytic anemia.*
Hepatic: transient elevations in liver function test results.
Metabolic: hypokalemia, hypernatremia.
Other: hypersensitivity reactions (rash, pruritus, urticaria, chills, fever, edema, *anaphylaxis*), overgrowth of nonsusceptible organisms, vein irritation, phlebitis.

KEY CONSIDERATIONS
Besides the recommendations relevant to all penicillins, consider the following:
• Half-life may be prolonged in geriatric patients because of impaired renal function.
• Ticarcillin is almost always used with another antibiotic such as an aminoglycoside in life-threatening situations.
• Drug contains 5.2 mEq sodium/g; use with caution in patients who require sodium restriction.
• To prevent hypokalemia and hypernatremia, monitor serum electrolyte levels.
• Monitor neurologic status; high levels may cause seizures.
• Check CBC, differential, PT, INR, and PTT. Drug may cause thrombocytopenia; watch for signs of bleeding.
• Because drug is dialyzable, patients undergoing hemodialysis may need dosage adjustments.
• Drug alters test results for urine or serum protein levels; it interferes with turbidimetric methods that use sulfosalicylic acid, trichloroacetic acid, acetic acid, or nitric acid. Ticarcillin doesn't interfere with tests using bromophenol blue (Albustix, Albutest, Multistix).
• Drug may falsely decrease serum aminoglycoside levels and cause a positive Coombs' test.

Overdose & treatment
• Signs and symptoms of overdose include neuromuscular hypersensitivity or seizures resulting from CNS irritation by high drug levels.
• Hemodialysis removes drug.

ticarcillin disodium/ clavulanate potassium
Timentin
Extended-spectrum penicillin, beta-lactamase inhibitor, antibiotic

Available by prescription only
Injection: 3 g ticarcillin and 100 mg clavulanic acid

INDICATIONS & DOSAGE
Infections of the lower respiratory tract, urinary tract, bones and joints,

and skin and soft-tissue, and septi-cemia when caused by susceptible organisms

Adults: 3.1 g (contains 3 g ticarcillin and 0.1 g clavulanate potassium) diluted in 50 to 100 ml D_5W, normal saline, or lactated Ringer's injection and administered by I.V. infusion over 30 minutes q 4 to 6 hours.

✦ *Dosage adjustment.* In patients with renal failure, loading dose is 3.1 g (3 g ticarcillin with 100 mg clavulanate). Patients on hemodialysis should receive 2 g I.V. q 12 hr, then 3.1 g after treatment; patients on peritoneal dialysis should receive 3.1 g I.V. q 12 hr.

Creatinine clearance (ml/min)	Dosage in adults
> 60	3 g I.V. q 4 hr
30-60	2 g I.V. q 4 hr
10-30	2 g I.V. q 8 hr
< 10	2 g I.V. q 12 hr
< 10 with hepatic failure	2 g I.V. q 24 hr

PHARMACODYNAMICS

Antibiotic action: Ticarcillin is bactericidal; it adheres to bacterial penicillin-binding proteins, inhibiting bacterial cell wall synthesis. Extended-spectrum penicillins are more resistant to inactivation by certain beta-lactamases, especially those produced by gram-negative organisms, but are still susceptible to inactivation by certain others.

Clavulanic acid has only weak antibacterial activity and doesn't affect the action of ticarcillin. However, clavulanic acid has a beta-lactam ring and is structurally similar to penicillin and cephalosporins; it binds irreversibly with certain beta-lactamases, preventing inactivation of ticarcillin and broadening its bactericidal spectrum.

Spectrum of activity of ticarcillin includes many gram-negative aerobic and anaerobic bacilli, many gram-positive and gram-negative aerobic cocci, and some gram-positive aerobic and anaerobic bacilli. The combination of ticarcillin and clavulanate potassium is also effective against many beta-lactamase–producing strains, including *Staphylococcus aureus, Haemophilus influenzae, Neisseria*

gonorrhoeae, Escherichia coli, Klebsiella, Providencia, and *Bacteroides fragilis,* but not *Pseudomonas aeruginosa.*

PHARMACOKINETICS

Absorption: Ticarcillin/clavulanate is only administered I.V.; plasma levels peak immediately after infusion is complete.

Distribution: Ticarcillin is distributed widely. It penetrates minimally into CSF with noninflamed meninges. Clavulanic acid penetrates into pleural fluid, lungs, and peritoneal fluid. Ticarcillin achieves high levels in urine. Protein-binding is 45% to 65% for ticarcillin and 22% to 30% for clavulanic acid.

Metabolism: About 13% of ticarcillin dose is metabolized through hydrolysis to inactive compounds; clavulanic acid is thought to undergo extensive metabolism, but its fate is unknown.

Excretion: Ticarcillin is excreted primarily (83% to 90%) in urine through renal tubular secretion and glomerular filtration; it's also excreted in bile. Metabolites of clavulanate are excreted in urine through glomerular filtration. Elimination half-life of ticarcillin in adults is about 1 hour and that of clavulanate is about 1 hour; in severe renal impairment, half-life of ticarcillin is extended to about 8 hours and that of clavulanate to about 3 hours. Both drugs are removed through hemodialysis but only slightly through peritoneal dialysis.

CONTRAINDICATIONS & PRECAUTIONS

Contraindicated in patients with hypersensitivity to ticarcillin/calvulanate or other penicillins. Use cautiously in patients with other drug allergies, especially allergies to cephalosporins; impaired renal function; hemorrhagic conditions; hypokalemia; or sodium restrictions.

INTERACTIONS

Drug-drug. Use with *aminoglycoside antibiotics* results in synergistic bactericidal effects against *P. aeruginosa, E. coli, Klebsiella, Citrobacter, Enterobacter, Serratia,* and *Proteus mirabilis;* however, drugs are physically and chemically incompatible and are inactivated when mixed or given together. In vivo inacti-

---

Reactions may be *common,* uncommon, *life-threatening,* or COMMON AND LIFE-THREATENING.

vation has been reported when *aminoglycosides* and extended-spectrum penicillins are used together. Large doses of penicillin may interfere with renal tubular secretion of *methotrexate,* thus delaying elimination and elevating serum methotrexate levels. *Probenecid* blocks tubular secretion of ticarcillin, elevating its serum level; it has no effect on clavulanate.

ADVERSE REACTIONS

CNS: *seizures,* neuromuscular excitability, headache, giddiness, pain at injection site.
GI: nausea, diarrhea, stomatitis, vomiting, epigastric pain, flatulence, pseudomembranous colitis, taste and smell disturbances.
Hematologic: *leukopenia, neutropenia,* eosinophilia, *thrombocytopenia, hemolytic anemia,* anemia.
Hepatic: transient elevations in liver function test results.
Metabolic: hypokalemia, hypernatremia.
Other: hypersensitivity reactions (rash, pruritus, urticaria, chills, fever, edema, *anaphylaxis*), overgrowth of nonsusceptible organisms, vein irritation, phlebitis.

KEY CONSIDERATIONS

Besides the recommendations relevant to all penicillins, consider the following:
• Half-life may be prolonged in geriatric patients because of impaired renal function.
• Ticarcillin/clavulanate is almost always used with another antibiotic such as an aminoglycoside in life-threatening situations.
• Administer aminogylcosides 1 hour before or after drug.
• Ticarcillin contains 5.2 mEq sodium/g; use with caution in patients with sodium restriction.
• Monitor serum electrolyte levels; observe for signs of hypernatremia and hypokalemia.
• Monitor neurologic status; high blood levels may cause seizures.
• Because drug is dialyzable, patients undergoing hemodialysis may need dosage adjustments.

• Drug alters test results for urine or serum protein levels; it interferes with turbidimetric methods that use sulfosalicylic acid, trichloroacetic acid, acetic acid, or nitric acid. Drug doesn't interfere with tests using bromophenol blue (Albustix, Albutest, Multistix). It may also falsely decrease serum aminoglycoside level.
• Drug may cause positive Coombs' test.

ticlopidine hydrochloride
Ticlid

Platelet aggregation inhibitor, antithrombotic

Available by prescription only
Tablets (film-coated): 250 mg

INDICATIONS & DOSAGE

Reduction of risk of thrombotic stroke in patients with history of stroke, in those who have experienced stroke precursors, or in those who are intolerant to aspirin therapy
Adults: 250 mg P.O. b.i.d. with meals.

PHARMACODYNAMICS

Antithrombotic action: Ticlopidine blocks adenosine diphosphate–induced platelet-fibrinogen and platelet-platelet binding.

PHARMACOKINETICS

Absorption: Ticlopidine is rapidly and extensively (more than 80%) absorbed after oral administration; plasma levels peak within 2 hours. Food enhances absorption.
Distribution: Drug is 98% bound to serum proteins and lipoproteins.
Metabolism: Drug is extensively metabolized in the liver. More than 20 metabolites have been identified; it's unknown if parent drug or active metabolites are responsible for pharmacologic activity.
Excretion: 60% of drug is excreted in urine and 23% in feces; only trace amounts of intact drug are found in urine. Initially, half-life is 12.6 hours after a single dose; with repeated dosing, half-life increases to 4 to 5 days.

CONTRAINDICATIONS & PRECAUTIONS

Contraindicated in patients with hypersensitivity to ticlopidine, hematopoietic disorders (such as neutropenia, thrombocytopenia, or disorders of hemostasis), active pathological bleeding from peptic ulceration or active intracranial bleeding, or severely impaired hepatic function.

INTERACTIONS

Drug-drug. Use with *antacids* decreases plasma ticlopidine levels; separate administration times by at least 2 hours. Use with *aspirin* potentiates effects of aspirin on platelets; don't use together. *Cimetidine* decreases clearance of ticlopidine and increases risk of toxicity; don't use together. Use with *digoxin* slightly decreases serum digoxin levels; monitor serum digoxin levels. Use with *theophylline* decreases theophylline clearance and increases the risk of toxicity; monitor closely and adjust theophylline dosage as indicated.

ADVERSE REACTIONS

CNS: dizziness, *intracerebral bleeding,* peripheral neuropathy.
CV: vasculitis.
EENT: epistaxis, conjunctival hemorrhage.
GI: *diarrhea, nausea, dyspepsia, abdominal pain,* anorexia, vomiting, flatulence, bleeding, light-colored stools.
GU: hematuria, *nephrotic syndrome,* dark-colored urine.
Hematologic: *neutropenia, pancytopenia, agranulocytosis, immune thrombocytopenia.*
Hepatic: *hepatitis,* cholestatic jaundice, abnormal liver function test results.
Metabolic: *hyponatremia.*
Respiratory: *allergic pneumonitis.*
Skin: *rash,* pruritus, ecchymoses, maculopapular rash, urticaria, *thrombocytopenic purpura.*
Other: arthropathy, myositis, *hypersensitivity reactions,* postoperative bleeding, systemic lupus erythematosus, *serum sickness, increased serum cholesterol levels.*

▣ KEY CONSIDERATIONS

• Clearance of ticlopidine is somewhat less in geriatric patients; however, no difference in safety and efficacy has been observed between geriatric patients and younger patients.
• If drug is being substituted for a fibrinolytic or anticoagulant, discontinue previous drug before starting ticlopidine therapy.
• If necessary, 20 mg of methylprednisolone I.V. has been shown to normalize the bleeding time within 2 hours. Platelet transfusions may also be necessary.
• Monitor CBC and WBC and differential q 2 weeks for the first 3 months of therapy. Drug may cause severe hematologic adverse effects.
• After the first 3 months of therapy, perform CBC and WBC with differential determinations in patients showing signs of infection.
• Perform baseline liver function tests and repeat when liver dysfunction is suspected. Monitor closely, especially during the first 4 months of treatment.
• Drug has been used investigationally for many conditions, including intermittent claudication, chronic arterial occlusion, subarachnoid hemorrhage, primary glomerulonephritis, and sickle cell disease. When used preoperatively, it may decrease incidence of graft occlusion in patients receiving coronary artery bypass grafts and reduce severity of decreased platelet count in patients receiving extracorporeal hemoperfusion during open-heart surgery.
• In rare cases, a positive antinuclear antibody titer has been reported.

Patient education

• Inform patient that an information leaflet that discusses safe use of ticlopidine is available.
• Tell patient to take drug with meals because food substantially increases bioavailability and improves GI tolerance.
• Instruct patient scheduled for elective surgery to notify his health care provider and be prepared to discontinue drug 10 to 14 days before procedure.
• Be sure that patient understands the need to report for regular blood tests. Neutropenia can result in an increased risk of infection. Tell patient to immedi-

---

Reactions may be *common*, uncommon, *life-threatening*, or COMMON AND LIFE-THREATENING.

ately report signs and symptoms of infection, such as fever, chills, or sore throat.
• Tell patient to immediately report yellow skin or sclera, severe or persistent diarrhea, rash, subcutaneous bleeding, light-colored stools, or dark urine.
• Emphasize that drug prolongs bleeding time. Tell patient to report unusual bleeding and to inform dentists and other health care providers that he's taking ticlopidine.
• Warn patient to avoid aspirin and aspirin-containing products, which may also prolong bleeding. Instruct him to call before taking OTC drugs because many contain aspirin.

tiludronate disodium
Skelid

Bisphosphonate analogue, antihypercalcemic

Available by prescription only
Tablets: 200 mg

INDICATIONS & DOSAGE
Paget's disease
Adults: 400 mg P.O. once daily for 3 months, taken with 180 to 240 ml (6 to 8 oz) of water 2 hours before or after meals.

PHARMACODYNAMICS
Antihypercalcemic action: Tiludronate is thought to suppress bone resorption by reducing osteoclastic activity. Drug appears to inhibit osteoclasts by disrupting the cytoskeletal ring structure, possibly by inhibiting protein-tyrosine-phosphatase, thus leading to detachment of osteoclasts from the bone surface, and by inhibiting the osteoclastic proton pump.

PHARMACOKINETICS
Absorption: Bioavailability of tiludronate on an empty stomach is 8%. Food and beverages other than water can reduce bioavailability by up to 90%.
Distribution: Drug is widely distributed in bone and soft tissue; protein-binding is about 90% (mainly albumin).

Metabolism: Drug doesn't appear to be metabolized.
Excretion: Drug is excreted principally in urine; mean plasma half-life, 150 hours.

CONTRAINDICATIONS & PRECAUTIONS
Contraindicated in patients with known hypersensitivity to a component of tiludronate and in patients with creatinine clearance less than 30 ml/minute.
Use cautiously in patients with upper GI disease, such as dysphagia, esophagitis, esophageal ulcer, or gastric ulcer.

INTERACTIONS
Drug-drug. *Aluminum antacids, calcium supplements,* and *magnesium antacids* may dramatically reduce bioavailability of tiludronate by 80%, 60%, and 60%, respectively, when administered 1 hour before tiludronate. *Aspirin* may decrease bioavailability by up to 50% when taken 2 hours after tiludronate. *Indomethacin* may also increase bioavailability of tiludronate.

ADVERSE REACTIONS
CNS: anxiety, dizziness, headache, insomnia, involuntary muscle contractions, paresthesia, somnolence, vertigo.
CV: chest pain, hypertension, edema.
EENT: cataracts, conjunctivitis, glaucoma, pharyngitis, sinusitis, rhinitis.
GI: anorexia, constipation, diarrhea, dry mouth, dyspepsia, flatulence, gastritis, nausea, tooth disorder, vomiting.
Metabolic: vitamin D deficiency.
Musculoskeletal: arthralgia, arthrosis, back pain, *whole-body pain.*
Respiratory: bronchitis, coughing, crackles.
Skin: pruritus, diaphoresis.
Other: hyperparathyroidism.

KEY CONSIDERATIONS
• Plasma levels may be higher in geriatric patients; dosage adjustment unnecessary.
• Tiludronate should be used in patients with Paget's disease who have serum alkaline phosphatase levels at least twice the upper limit of normal or who are symptomatic or at risk for future complications from disease.

• Administer drug for 3 months to assess response.
• Hypocalcemia and other disturbances of mineral metabolism (such as vitamin D deficiency) should be corrected before initiating therapy.

Patient education
• Tell patient to take tiludronate with 180 to 240 ml (6 to 8 oz) of water.
• Instruct patient that drug shouldn't be taken within 2 hours of food.
• Advise patient to maintain adequate vitamin D and calcium intake.
• Inform patient that calcium supplements, aspirin, and indomethacin shouldn't be taken within 2 hours before or after tiludronate.
• Tell patient that aluminum- and magnesium-containing antacids can be taken 2 hours after taking tiludronate.

timolol maleate
Blocadren, Timoptic, Timoptic-XE

Beta blocker, antihypertensive, adjunct therapy for an MI, antiglaucoma drug

Available by prescription only
Tablets: 5 mg, 10 mg, 20 mg
Ophthalmic gel: 0.25%, 0.5%
Ophthalmic solution: 0.25%, 0.5%

INDICATIONS & DOSAGE
Hypertension
Adults: Initially, 10 mg P.O. b.i.d. Usual maintenance dosage is 20 to 40 mg/day. Maximum dosage is 60 mg/day. There should be an interval of at least 7 days between dosage increases.
Reduction of risk for CV mortality and reinfarction after an MI
Adults: 10 mg P.O. b.i.d. initiated within 1 to 4 weeks after an MI.
Migraine headache
Adults: 10 mg P.O. daily b.i.d., then increase up to 20 mg; or 30-mg dose (10 mg P.O. in the morning and 20 mg P.O. in the evening).
◊*Angina*
Adults: 15 to 45 mg P.O. daily given in three divided doses.

Glaucoma
Adults: 1 gtt of 0.25% or 0.5% solution to the conjunctiva once or twice daily; or 1 gtt of 0.25% or 0.5% gel to the conjunctiva once daily.

PHARMACODYNAMICS
Antihypertensive action: Exact mechanism of action is unknown. Timolol may reduce blood pressure by blocking adrenergic receptors (thus decreasing cardiac output), by decreasing sympathetic outflow from the CNS, and by suppressing renin release.
MI prophylactic action: Exact mechanism by which drug decreases mortality after an MI is unknown. Drug produces a negative chronotropic and inotropic activity. This decrease in heart rate and myocardial contractility results in reduced myocardial oxygen consumption.
Antiglaucoma action: Beta-blocking action of drug decreases the production of aqueous humor, thereby decreasing intraocular pressure.

PHARMACOKINETICS
Absorption: About 90% of oral dose is absorbed from the GI tract; plasma levels peak in 1 to 2 hours.
Distribution: After oral administration, timolol is distributed throughout the body; depending on assay method, drug is 10% to 60% protein-bound.
Metabolism: About 80% of a given dose is metabolized in the liver to inactive metabolites.
Excretion: Drug and its metabolites are excreted primarily in urine; half-life is about 4 hours. After topical application to the eye, effects last up to 24 hours.

CONTRAINDICATIONS & PRECAUTIONS
Contraindicated in patients with bronchial asthma, severe COPD, sinus bradycardia and heart block greater than first degree, cardiogenic shock, heart failure, or hypersensitivity to timolol.

Use cautiously in patients with diabetes, hyperthyroidism, or respiratory disease (especially nonallergic bronchospasm or emphysema). Use oral form cautiously in patients with compensated heart failure and hepatic or renal disease. Use ophthalmic form cautiously in patients with cerebrovascular insufficiency.

INTERACTIONS
Drug-drug. Timolol may potentiate antihypertensive effects of *antihypertensives; NSAIDs* may antagonize timolol's antihypertensive effects. Timolol may antagonize the effects of *beta stimulants* or *xanthines.* Use with *calcium channel blockers* or *cardiac glycosides* may cause cardiac arrhythmias. Ophthalmic or oral timolol may cause excessive hypotension when administered *fentanyl* or *general anesthetics.* Timolol may increase the plasma *phenothiazine* levels.

ADVERSE REACTIONS
CNS: fatigue, lethargy, dizziness, depression, hallucinations, confusion (with ophthalmic form).
CV: *arrhythmias, bradycardia,* hypotension, *heart failure,* peripheral vascular disease, *pulmonary edema* (with oral administration); *CVA, cardiac arrest,* heart block, palpitations (with ophthalmic form).
EENT: minor eye irritation, decreased corneal sensitivity with long-term use, conjunctivitis, blepharitis, keratitis, visual disturbances, diplopia, ptosis (with ophthalmic form).
GI: nausea, vomiting, diarrhea (with oral administration).
Hematologic: slightly decreased hemoglobin levels and hematocrit.
Metabolic: slightly increased serum potassium, uric acid, and blood glucose levels.
Respiratory: dyspnea, *bronchospasm,* increased airway resistance (with oral administration); *asthma attacks in patients with history of asthma* (with ophthalmic form).
Skin: pruritus (with oral administration).

▣ KEY CONSIDERATIONS
Besides the recommendations relevant to all beta blockers, consider the following:
• Geriatric patients may require lower oral maintenance dosages of timolol because of increased bioavailability or delayed metabolism; they also may experience enhanced adverse effects. Use cau-

tiously because half-life may be prolonged in geriatric patients.
• Dosage adjustment may be necessary for patient with renal or hepatic impairment.
• Although controversial, drug may need to be discontinued 48 hours before surgery in patients receiving ophthalmic timolol because of systemic absorption.

Patient education
• For ophthalmic form of timolol, teach patient how to properly administer eyedrops. Warn patient not to touch dropper to eye or surrounding tissue, and to lightly press lacrimal sac with finger after administration to decrease systemic absorption.
• Instruct patient to invert ophthalmic gel container once before each use.
• Instruct patient to administer other ophthalmic drugs at least 10 minutes before the ophthalmic gel.

Overdose & treatment
• Signs and symptoms of overdose include severe hypotension, bradycardia, heart failure, and bronchospasm.
• After acute ingestion, induce vomiting or perform gastric lavage and give activated charcoal to reduce absorption. Subsequent treatment is usually symptomatic and supportive.

tioconazole
Vagistat-1

Imidazole derivative, antifungal

Available by prescription only
Vaginal ointment: 6.5%

INDICATIONS & DOSAGE
Treatment of vulvovaginal candidiasis
Adults: Insert 1 applicator (about 4.6 g) intravaginally h.s. as a single dose.

PHARMACODYNAMICS
Antifungal action: Tioconazole is a fungicidal imidazole that alters cell-wall permeability.

PHARMACOKINETICS

Absorption: Only a negligible amount of drug is absorbed.
Distribution: Unknown.
Metabolism: Unknown.
Excretion: Unknown.

CONTRAINDICATIONS & PRECAUTIONS

Contraindicated in patients hypersensitive to tioconazole or other imidazole antifungals (miconazole, ketoconazole).

INTERACTIONS

None reported.

ADVERSE REACTIONS

GU: *burning, pruritus,* discharge, vaginal pain, dysuria, dyspareunia, vulvar edema, irritation.

▣ KEY CONSIDERATIONS

• Because tioconazole is useful only for candidal vulvovaginitis, the diagnosis should be confirmed by potassium hydroxide smears or cultures before treatment with drug.

Patient education

• Review correct use of tioconazole with patient; drug should be inserted high into the vagina. Detailed instructions for the patient come with the product.
• Tell patient to avoid sexual intercourse during therapy or advise partner to use a condom to prevent reinfection.
• Warn patient to open applicator just before using product to avoid contamination.
• Tell patient to watch for and report irritation or sensitivity.
• Emphasize need for patient to continue therapy for the full course, even if symptoms have improved.
• Advise patient to use a sanitary napkin to prevent staining of clothing.

tobramycin

tobramycin ophthalmic
Tobrex

tobramycin sulfate
Nebcin

tobramycin solution for inhalation
TOBI

Aminoglycoside, antibiotic

Available by prescription only
Injection: 40 mg/ml
Ophthalmic solution: 0.3%
Ophthalmic ointment: 0.3%
Nebulizer solution for inhalation: single-use 5-ml (300 mg) ampule

INDICATIONS & DOSAGE

***Serious infections caused by sensitive* Escherichia coli, Proteus, Klebsiella, Enterobacter, Serratia, Staphylococcus aureus, Pseudomonas, Citrobacter, *or* Providencia**
Adults: 3 mg/kg I.M. or I.V. daily, divided q 8 hours. Up to 5 mg/kg I.M. or I.V. daily, divided q 6 to 8 hours for life-threatening infections.

For I.V. use, dilute in 50 to 100 ml normal saline solution or D_5W for adults. Infuse over 20 to 60 minutes.
✦ *Dosage adjustment.* In patients with impaired renal function, initial dosage is same as for those with normal renal function. Subsequent doses and frequency are determined by renal function study results and blood levels; keep peak serum levels between 4 and 10 μg/ml and trough serum levels between 1 and 2 μg/ml. Several methods have been used to calculate dosage in renal failure.

After a 1-mg/kg loading dose, adjust subsequent dosage by reducing doses administered at 8-hour intervals or by prolonging the interval between normal doses. Both of these methods are useful when serum tobramycin levels can't be measured directly. They're based on either creatinine clearance (preferred) or serum creatinine level because these values correlate with drug's half-life.

To calculate reduced dosage for 8-hour intervals, use available nomograms; or, if patient's steady-state serum creatinine values are known, divide the normally recommended dose by patient's serum creatinine value. To determine frequency in hours for normal dosage (if creatinine clearance rate isn't available), divide the normal dose by patient's serum creatinine value. Dosage schedules derived from either method require careful clinical and laboratory observations of patient and should be adjusted as appropriate. These methods of calculation may be misleading in geriatric patients and in those with severe wasting; neither should be used when dialysis is performed.

Hemodialysis removes 50% to 75% of a dose in 6 hours. In anephric patients receiving maintenance dialysis, 1.5 to 2 mg/kg after each dialysis session usually maintains therapeutic, nontoxic serum levels. Patients receiving peritoneal dialysis twice weekly should receive a 1.5- to 2-mg/kg loading dose followed by 1 mg/kg q 3 days. Those receiving dialysis q 2 days should receive a 1.5-mg/kg loading dose after first dialysis and 0.75 mg/kg after each subsequent dialysis.

◊ **Intrathecally or intraventricularly**
Adults: 3 to 8 mg q 18 to 48 hours.
***Management of cystic fibrosis patients with* Pseudomonas aeruginosa**
Adults: 1 single-use ampule (300 mg) administered q 12 hours for 28 days, then off for 28 days, then on for 28 days as advised by health care provider. There's no dosage adjustment for age or renal failure.
Treatment of external ocular infection caused by susceptible gram-negative bacteria
Adults: For mild to moderate infections, instill 1 or 2 gtt into affected eye q 4 to 6 hours. For severe infections, instill 2 gtt into affected eye hourly or apply a small amount of ointment into conjunctival sac t.i.d. or q.i.d.

PHARMACODYNAMICS
Antibiotic action: Tobramycin is bactericidal; it binds directly to the 30S ribosomal subunit, thereby inhibiting bacterial protein synthesis. Its spectrum of activity includes many aerobic gram-negative organisms, including most strains of *P. aeruginosa* and some aerobic gram-positive organisms. Drug may act against some bacterial strains resistant to other aminoglycosides; many strains resistant to drug are susceptible to amikacin, gentamicin, or netilmicin.

PHARMACOKINETICS
Absorption: Tobramycin is absorbed poorly after oral administration and usually is given parenterally; serum levels peak 30 to 90 minutes after I.M. administration. Inhaled drug remains concentrated in the airway, with serum level after 20 weeks of therapy of 1.05 µg/ml 1 hour after dosing.
Distribution: Drug is distributed widely after parenteral administration; intraocular penetration is poor. CSF penetration is low, even in patients with inflamed meninges. Protein-binding is minimal. Inhaled drug remains primarily concentrated in the airway.
Metabolism: Not metabolized.
Excretion: Excreted primarily in urine by glomerular filtration; a small amount may be excreted in bile. Elimination half-life in adults is 2 to 3 hours. In severe renal damage, half-life may extend to 24 to 60 hours. With inhalation use, unabsorbed drug is probably eliminated in the sputum.

CONTRAINDICATIONS & PRECAUTIONS
Contraindicated in patients with hypersensitivity to tobramycin or other aminoglycosides. Use injectable form cautiously in patients with impaired renal function or neuromuscular disorders and in geriatric patients.

INTERACTIONS
Drug-drug. Use with the following drugs may increase the hazard of nephrotoxicity, ototoxicity, and neurotoxicity: *amphotericin B, capreomycin, cephalosporins, cisplatin, methoxyflurane, other aminoglycosides, polymyxin*

B, and *vancomycin;* hazard of ototoxicity is also increased during use with *bumetanide, ethacrynic acid, furosemide, mannitol,* or *urea. Other antiemetics* and *antivertigo drugs* and *dimenhydrinate* may mask tobramycin-induced ototoxicity. Tobramycin may potentiate neuromuscular blockade from *general anesthetics* or *neuromuscular blockers,* such as *succinylcholine* and *tubocurarine.* Use with some *penicillins* results in a synergistic bactericidal effect against *P. aeruginosa, E. coli, Klebsiella, Citrobacter, Enterobacter, Serratia,* and *Proteus mirabilis;* however, drugs are physically and chemically incompatible and are inactivated when mixed or given together. In vivo inactivation has been reported when aminoglycosides and *penicillins* are used together.

ADVERSE REACTIONS

CNS: headache, lethargy, confusion, disorientation (with injectable form).
EENT: *ototoxicity* (with injectable form); blurred vision (with ophthalmic ointment); burning or stinging on instillation, lid itching or swelling, conjunctival erythema (with ophthalmic administration).
GI: vomiting, nausea, diarrhea (with injectable form).
GU: *nephrotoxicity* (with injectable form).
Hematologic: anemia, eosinophilia, *leukopenia, thrombocytopenia, granulocytopenia* (with injectable form).
Metabolic: elevated BUN, nonprotein nitrogen, and serum creatinine levels; increased urine excretion of casts.
Respiratory: *bronchospasm* (with inhalation form).
Skin: rash, urticaria, pruritus (with injectable form).
Other: fever, *hypersensitivity reactions,* overgrowth of nonsusceptible organisms (with ophthalmic administration).

▣ KEY CONSIDERATIONS

Besides the recommendations relevant to all aminoglycosides, consider the following:
• Because tobramycin has nephrotoxic and hematologic adverse effects, use cautiously in geriatric patients.
• For I.V. administration, the usual volume of diluent (normal saline injection or D_5W) for adult doses is 50 to 100 ml; infusion should be over 20 to 60 minutes.
• Don't premix tobramycin with other drugs; administer separately at least 1 hour apart.
• Discontinue ophthalmic preparation if keratitis, erythema, lacrimation, edema, or lid itching occurs.
• Because drug is dialyzable, patients undergoing hemodialysis may need dosage adjustments.
• Inhaled tobramycin is an orphan drug used specifically to manage cystic fibrosis patients with *P. aeruginosa.*

Patient education
• Advise patient that inhaled doses should be taken as close to 12 hours apart as possible and no less than 6 hours apart.
• Teach patient how to correctly use and maintain nebulizer.

Overdose & treatment
• Signs and symptoms of overdose include ototoxicity, nephrotoxicity, and neuromuscular toxicity.
• Remove tobramycin through hemodialysis or peritoneal dialysis. Treatment with calcium salts or anticholinesterases reverses neuromuscular blockade.

---

tocainide hydrochloride
Tonocard

Local anesthetic (amide type), ventricular antiarrhythmic

Available by prescription only
Tablets: 400 mg, 600 mg

INDICATIONS & DOSAGE
Suppression of symptomatic ventricular arrhythmias, including frequent ventricular tachycardia
Dosage must be individualized based on antiarrhythmic response and tolerance.

Adults: Initially, 400 mg P.O. q 8 hours. Usual dosage is between 1,200 and 1,800 mg/day, divided into three doses. Drug may be administered on a b.i.d. regimen with careful monitoring if patient is able to tolerate the t.i.d. regimen.

✦ *Dosage adjustment.* Patients with impaired renal or hepatic function may be adequately treated with less than 1,200 mg/day.

◊ *Myotonic dystrophy*
Adults: 800 to 1,200 mg/day P.O.

◊ *Trigeminal neuralgia*
Adults: 20 mg/kg/day P.O. in three divided doses.

PHARMACODYNAMICS

Antiarrhythmic action: Tocainide is structurally similar to lidocaine and possesses similar electrophysiologic and hemodynamic effects. A class IB antiarrhythmic, it suppresses automaticity and shortens the effective refractory period and action potential duration of His-Purkinje fibers and suppresses spontaneous ventricular depolarization during diastole. Conductive atrial tissue and AV conduction aren't affected significantly at therapeutic levels. Unlike quinidine and procainamide, drug doesn't significantly alter hemodynamics when administered in usual doses. Drug exerts its effects on the conduction system, causing inhibition of reentry mechanisms and cessation of ventricular arrhythmias; these effects may be more pronounced in ischemic tissue. It doesn't cause a significant negative inotropic effect. Its direct cardiac effects are less potent than those of lidocaine.

PHARMACOKINETICS

Absorption: Tocainide is rapidly and completely absorbed from the GI tract; unlike lidocaine, it undergoes negligible first-pass effect in the liver. Serum levels peak in 30 minutes to 2 hours after oral administration. Bioavailability is nearly 100%.
Distribution: Drug's distribution is only partially known. However, it appears to be distributed widely and apparently crosses the blood-brain barrier in animals (however, it's less lipophilic than li-

docaine). Only 10% to 20% binds to plasma protein.
Metabolism: Drug is metabolized apparently in the liver to inactive metabolites.
Excretion: Excreted in urine as unchanged drug and inactive metabolites. Some 30% to 50% of orally administered dose is excreted in urine as metabolites. Elimination half-life is 11 to 23 hours, with an initial biphasic plasma level decline similar to that of lidocaine. Half-life may be prolonged in patients with renal or hepatic insufficiency. Urine alkalization may substantially decrease the amount of unchanged drug excreted in urine.

CONTRAINDICATIONS & PRECAUTIONS

Contraindicated in patients with hypersensitivity to lidocaine or other amide-type local anesthetics and in those with second- or third-degree AV block without an artificial pacemaker.

Use cautiously in patients with heart failure, diminished cardiac reserve, preexisting bone marrow failure, cytopenia, or impaired renal or hepatic function.

INTERACTIONS

Drug-drug. *Allopurinol* increases effects of tocainide. *Cimetidine* and *rifampin* may decrease elimination half-life and bioavailability of tocainide. Use with *lidocaine* may cause CNS toxicity. Use with *metoprolol* may cause additive effects on cardiac index, left ventricular function, and pulmonary artery wedge pressure, necessitating monitoring for decreased myocardial contractility and bradycardia. When used with *other antiarrhythmics,* tocainide may cause additive, synergistic, or antagonistic effects.

ADVERSE REACTIONS

CNS: *light-headedness, tremor,* paresthesia, *dizziness, vertigo,* drowsiness, fatigue, confusion, headache.
CV: hypotension, *new or worsened arrhythmias, heart failure, bradycardia,* palpitations.
EENT: blurred vision, tinnitus.
GI: *nausea, vomiting,* diarrhea, anorexia.
Hematologic: *blood dyscrasia.*

Hepatic: abnormal liver function test results, *hepatitis.*
Respiratory: *respiratory arrest, pulmonary fibrosis, pneumonitis, pulmonary edema.*
Skin: rash, diaphoresis.

◙ KEY CONSIDERATIONS

• Use with caution in geriatric patients; increased serum tocainide levels and toxicity are more likely in these patients. Monitor carefully.
• Geriatric patients are more likely to experience dizziness and should have assistance walking.
• Use cautiously and with lower doses in patients with hepatic or renal impairment.
• Perform chest X-ray if pulmonary symptoms exist.
• Monitor blood levels; therapeutic levels range from 4 to 10 µg/ml.
• Monitor periodic blood counts for the first 3 months of therapy and frequently thereafter. Check CBC promptly if patient develops signs of infection.
• Observe patient for tremors, a possible sign that maximum safe dosage has been reached.
• Adverse effects tend to be frequent and problematic.
• Drug is considered an oral lidocaine and may be used to ease transition from I.V. lidocaine to oral antiarrhythmic therapy.

Patient education

• Instruct patient to report unusual bleeding or bruising, signs or symptoms of infection (such as fever, sore throat, stomatitis, or chills), or pulmonary signs or symptoms (such as cough, wheezing, or exertional dyspnea).
• Tell patient he may take tocainide with food to lessen GI upset.
• Tell patient drug may cause drowsiness or dizziness and to observe caution performing tasks that require alertness.

Overdose & treatment

• Signs and symptoms of overdose include extensions of common adverse reactions, particularly those associated with the CNS or GI tract.

• Treatment generally involves symptomatic and supportive care. For acute overdose, induce vomiting or perform gastric lavage. Respiratory depression necessitates immediate attention and maintenance of a patent airway with ventilatory assistance, if required. Seizures may be treated with small incremental doses of a benzodiazepine, such as diazepam or a short or ultra short–acting barbiturate such as pentobarbital or thiopental.

---

tolazamide
Tolinase

Sulfonylurea, antidiabetic

Available by prescription only
Tablets: 100 mg, 250 mg, 500 mg

INDICATIONS & DOSAGE
Adjunct to diet to reduce blood glucose levels in patients with type 2 diabetes mellitus
Adults: Initially, 100 mg P.O. daily with breakfast if fasting blood glucose level is less than 200 mg/dl; or 250 mg P.O. daily if this level is more than 200 mg/dl. May adjust dosage at weekly intervals in increments of 100 to 250 mg based on blood glucose response. Maximum dosage is 500 mg b.i.d. before meals.
Geriatric patients: 50 to 125 mg P.O. once daily.

PHARMACODYNAMICS
Antidiabetic action: Tolazamide reduces blood glucose levels by stimulating insulin release from functioning beta cells of the pancreas. After prolonged administration, the drug's hypoglycemic effects appear to reflect extrapancreatic effects, possibly including reduction of basal hepatic glucose production and enhanced peripheral sensitivity to insulin.

PHARMACOKINETICS
Absorption: Tolazamide is absorbed well from the GI tract and serum levels peak at 3 to 4 hours. Onset of action occurs within 4 to 6 hours; maximum hypoglycemic effect, within 10 hours.

Distribution: Drug probably is distributed into the extracellular fluid.
Metabolism: Drug is metabolized probably in the liver to several mildly active metabolites.
Excretion: Drug is excreted in urine primarily as metabolites, with a small amount excreted as unchanged drug; half-life, 7 hours.

CONTRAINDICATIONS & PRECAUTIONS

Contraindicated in patients hypersensitive to drug or other sulfonylureas; in patients with type 1 diabetes mellitus; in patients with diabetes that can be adequately controlled by diet; in patients with type 2 diabetes complicated by ketosis, acidosis, coma, or other acute complications such as major surgery, severe infection, or severe trauma; and in patients with uremia.

Use cautiously in geriatric, debilitated, or malnourished patients and in those with impaired renal or hepatic function or in those with adrenal or pituitary insufficiency.

INTERACTIONS

Drug-drug. Use with *beta blockers* (including *ophthalmics*) may increase the risk of hypoglycemia, mask its symptoms (increasing pulse rate and blood pressure), and prolong it by blocking gluconeogenesis. *Calcium channel blockers, corticosteroids, estrogens, isoniazid, oral contraceptives, phenothiazines, phenytoin, sympathomimetics, thiazide diuretics, triamterene,* and *thyroid hormones* may decrease hypoglycemic effect and require dosage adjustments. *Chloramphenicol, insulin, MAO inhibitors, NSAIDs, probenecid, salicylates,* or *sulfonamides* may enhance hypoglycemic effect. Use with *oral anticoagulants* may increase hypoglycemic activity or enhance anticoagulant effect.

Drug-lifestyle. Use with *alcohol* may produce a disulfiram-like reaction consisting of nausea, vomiting, abdominal cramps, and headaches.

ADVERSE REACTIONS

CNS: fatigue, dizziness, vertigo, malaise, headache, weakness.

GI: nausea, vomiting, epigastric distress, heartburn.
Hematologic: *leukopenia,* hemolytic anemia, ***thrombocytopenia,*** aplastic anemia, ***agranulocytosis,*** pancytopenia.
Skin: photosensitivity reactions.

◳ KEY CONSIDERATIONS

Besides the recommendations relevant to all sulfonylureas, consider the following:
• Geriatric patients may be more sensitive to the effects of tolazamide because of reduced metabolism and elimination.
• Hypoglycemia causes more neurologic symptoms in geriatric patients.
• Geriatric patients usually require a lower initial dosage.
• To avoid GI intolerance for those patients receiving dosages of 500 mg/day or more and to improve control of hyperglycemia, divided doses are recommended; these are given before the morning and evening meals.
• Tablets may be crushed to ease administration.
• When substituting tolazamide for chlorpropamide, monitor patient closely for 1 to 2 weeks because of chlorpropamide's prolonged retention in the body which may possibly result in hypoglycemia.
• Oral antidiabetics may increase the risk of CV-related death, compared with diet or diet and insulin therapy.
• To change from insulin to oral therapy with tolazamide take the following steps: If insulin dosage is less than 20 U daily, insulin may be stopped and oral therapy started at 100 mg P.O. daily with breakfast. If insulin dosage is 20 to 40 U daily, insulin may be stopped and oral therapy started at 250 mg P.O. daily with breakfast. If insulin dosage is more than 40 U daily, decrease insulin dosage by 50% and start oral therapy at 250 mg P.O. daily with breakfast. Increase dosages as above.

Patient education

• Emphasize the importance of following prescribed diet, exercise, and drug regimen.
• Advise patient to take tolazamide at the same time each day: A missed dose should be taken immediately unless it's

almost time to take the next dose. Patient shouldn't double-dose.

• Warn patient to avoid alcohol when taking drug. Remind him that many foods and nonprescription drugs contain alcohol. Alcohol in moderate to large amounts will cause a disulfiram-like reaction.

• Encourage patient to wear a medical identification bracelet or necklace.

• Instruct patient to take drug with food if it causes GI upset.

• Teach patient to monitor blood glucose, urine glucose, and ketone levels, as prescribed.

• Teach patient how to recognize the signs and symptoms of hypoglycemia and hyperglycemia and what to do if they occur.

Overdose & treatment

• Signs and symptoms of overdose include low blood glucose levels, tingling of lips and tongue, hunger, nausea, decreased cerebral function (lethargy, yawning, confusion, agitation, nervousness), increased sympathetic activity (tachycardia, sweating, tremor), and ultimately seizures, stupor, and coma.

• Mild hypoglycemia without loss of consciousness or neurologic findings responds to treatment with oral glucose and adjustments in drug dosages and meal patterns. If the patient loses consciousness or develops neurologic findings, he should receive rapid injection of D_5W followed by a continuous infusion of $D_{10}W$ at a rate to maintain blood glucose levels greater than 100 mg/dl. Monitor for 24 to 48 hours.

tolbutamide
Orinase

Sulfonylurea, antidiabetic

Available by prescription only
Tablets: 500 mg

INDICATIONS & DOSAGE
Adjunct to diet to lower blood glucose in patients with type 2 diabetes mellitus
Adults: Initially, 1 to 2 g P.O. daily as single dose or divided b.i.d. or t.i.d. May

adjust dosage to maximum of 3 g P.O. daily.

PHARMACODYNAMICS
Antidiabetic action: Tolbutamide reduces blood glucose levels by stimulating insulin release from functioning beta cells of the pancreas. After prolonged administration, the drug's hypoglycemic effects appear to reflect extrapancreatic effects, possibly including reduction of basal hepatic glucose production and enhanced peripheral sensitivity to insulin.

PHARMACOKINETICS
Absorption: Tolbutamide is absorbed readily from the GI tract. Levels peak in 3 to 4 hours.
Distribution: Drug probably is distributed into the extracellular fluid; 95% is plasma protein-bound.
Metabolism: Drug is metabolized in the liver to inactive metabolites.
Excretion: Drug and metabolites are excreted in urine and feces. Half-life is 4.5 to 6.5 hours.

CONTRAINDICATIONS & PRECAUTIONS
Contraindicated in patients with hypersensitivity to drug or other sulfanylureas; in patients with type 1 diabetes or diabetes that can be adequately controlled by diet; in patients with type 2 diabetes complicated by fever, ketosis, acidosis, coma, or other acute complications such as major surgery, severe infection, or severe trauma, or severe renal insufficiency.

Use cautiously in geriatric, debilitated, or malnourished patients and in those with impaired renal or hepatic function or porphyria.

INTERACTIONS
Drug-drug. Use with *oral anticoagulants* may increase hypoglycemic activity or enhance the anticoagulant effect. Use with *beta blockers (*including *ophthalmics)* may increase the risk of hypoglycemia by masking its developing symptoms, such as increasing pulse rate and blood pressure, and may prolong hypoglycemia by blocking gluconeogenesis. Use with *chloramphenicol, insulin, MAO inhibitors, NSAIDs, probenecid,*

salicylates, or *sulfonamides* may enhance the hypoglycemic effect. *Calcium channel blockers, corticosteroids, estrogens, isoniazid, oral contraceptives, phenothiazines, phenytoin, sympathomimetics, thiazide diuretics, triamterene,* and *thyroid products* decrease hypoglycemic effect.

Drug-lifestyle. Use with *alcohol* may produce a disulfiram-like reaction consisting of nausea, vomiting, abdominal cramps, and headaches.

ADVERSE REACTIONS
CNS: headache.
GI: nausea, heartburn, epigastric distress, altered taste.
Hematologic: *leukopenia,* hemolytic anemia, ***thrombocytopenia, aplastic anemia, agranulocytosis.***
Metabolic: *hypoglycemia, dilutional hyponatremia.*
Skin: rash, pruritus, erythema, urticaria.
Other: *hypersensitivity reactions.*

▣ KEY CONSIDERATIONS
Besides the recommendations relevant to all sulfonylureas, consider the following:
• Geriatric or debilitated patients and those with impaired renal or hepatic function usually require a lower initial dosage.
• Tablets may be crushed for ease of administration.
• Physiological stress (for example, infection) may impair control of blood glucose levels.
• To avoid GI intolerance for those patients on larger doses and to improve control of hyperglycemia, divided doses given before the morning and evening meals are recommended.
• Patients should avoid taking tolbutamide at bedtime because of the potential for nocturnal hypoglycemia.
• To change from insulin to oral therapy with tolbutamide, take the following steps: If insulin dosage is less than 20 U daily, insulin may be stopped and oral therapy started at 1 to 2 g daily. If insulin dosage is 20 to 40 U daily, insulin dosage is reduced 30% to 50% and oral therapy started as above. If insulin dosage is more than 40 U daily, insulin dosage is decreased 20% and oral thera-

py started as above. Further reductions in insulin dosage are based on patient's response to oral therapy.
• Oral antidiabetics may increase the risk of CV-related death, compared with diet or diet and insulin therapy.
• Drug therapy alters cephalin flocculation (thymol turbidity) and ^{131}I thyroid uptake.
• Geriatric patients may be more sensitive to drug's effects because of reduced metabolism and elimination.
• Hypoglycemia causes more neurologic symptoms in geriatric patients.
• When substituting tolbutamide for chlorpropamide therapy, monitor patient closely for the first 2 weeks because chlorpropamide's prolonged retention in the body could result in hypoglycemia.

Patient education
• Emphasize to patient the importance of following prescribed diet, exercise, and drug regimen.
• Instruct patient to take tolbutamide at the same time each day.
• Inform patient that missed dose should be taken immediately unless it's almost time to take the next dose; patient shouldn't double-dose.
• Advise patient to avoid alcohol while taking drug; remind patient many foods and OTC drugs contain alcohol.
• Encourage patient to wear a medical identification bracelet or necklace.
• Suggest that patient take the drug with food if it causes GI upset.
• Teach patient to monitor blood glucose, urine glucose, and ketone levels, as prescribed.
• Teach patient how to recognize the signs and symptoms of hypoglycemia and hyperglycemia and what to do if they occur.

Overdose & treatment
• Signs and symptoms of overdose include low blood glucose levels, tingling of lips and tongue, hunger, nausea, decreased cerebral function (lethargy, yawning, confusion, agitation, nervousness), increased sympathetic activity (tachycardia, sweating, tremor), and ultimately seizures, stupor, and coma.

• Mild hypoglycemia without loss of consciousness or neurologic findings responds to treatment with oral glucose and dosage adjustments. If patient loses consciousness or develops neurologic findings, the patient should receive rapid injection of D_5W, followed by a continuous infusion of $D_{10}W$ at a rate to maintain blood glucose levels greater than 100 mg/dl. Monitor for 24 to 48 hours.

tolcapone
Tasmar

Catechol-O-methyltransferase (COMT) inhibitor, antiparkinsonian

Available by prescription only
Tablets: 100 mg, 200 mg

INDICATIONS & DOSAGE
Adjunct to levodopa and carbidopa for treatment of signs and symptoms of idiopathic Parkinson's disease
Adults: Recommended initial dose is 100 mg (preferred) or 200 mg P.O. t.i.d. If initiating treatment with 200 mg t.i.d. and dyskinesias occur, then a decrease in dosage of levodopa may be necessary. Maximum daily dose is 600 mg. Always give with levodopa/carbidopa. The first tolcapone dose of the day should always be taken with the first levodopa/carbidopa dose of the day.
✦ ***Dosage adjustment:*** Don't use dosages of more than 100 mg t.i.d. in patients with severe hepatic or renal dysfunction.

PHARMACODYNAMICS
Antiparkinsonian action: Exact mechanism of action is unknown. Tolcapone is thought to reversibly inhibit human erythrocyte COMT when given with levodopa/carbidopa, decreasing clearance of levodopa and increasing bioavailability of levodopa twofold. The decrease in clearance of levodopa prolongs the elimination half-life of levodopa from 2 to 3.5 hours.

PHARMACOKINETICS
Absorption: Tolcapone is rapidly absorbed; plasma levels peak within 2 hours. After oral administration, absolute bioavailability is 65%. Onset of effect occurs after administration of first dose. Drug absorption decreases when given within 1 hour before or 2 hours after food; however, drug can be administered without regard to meals.
Distribution: Drug is highly bound to plasma proteins (more than 99.9%), primarily albumin. Steady-state volume of distribution is small.
Metabolism: Drug is completely metabolized before excretion. The main mechanism of metabolism is glucuronidation.
Excretion: Only 0.5% of dose is found unchanged in urine. Drug is a low extraction ratio drug with a systemic clearance of 7 L/hour. Elimination half-life is 2 to 3 hours. Dialysis isn't expected to affect clearance because of significant protein-binding.

CONTRAINDICATIONS & PRECAUTIONS
Contraindicated in patients with known hypersensitivity to tolcapone or its components; in patients with liver disease or ALT or AST levels exceeding the upper limit of normal; in patients withdrawn from therapy due to drug-induced hepatocellular injury; and in patients with history of nontraumatic rhabdomyolysis or hyperpyrexia and confusion, possibly related to drug.

Use cautiously in patients with Parkinson disease because syncope and orthostatic hypotension may worsen.

INTERACTIONS
Drug-drug. Although risk of interactions with *cytochrome substrates 3A4 and 2A6* exists, none have been reported. Use with *desipramine* may increase the risk of adverse effects; use together cautiously. MAO and COMT are two enzyme systems involved in the metabolism of catecholamines; use with *nonselective MAO inhibitors (phenelzine, tranylcypromine)* may inhibit these pathways. Avoid use with *MAO inhibitors* because hypertensive crisis may occur. No interaction is apparent between tolcapone and *selective MAO-B inhibitors* (*selegiline*).

Reactions may be *common*, uncommon, *life-threatening*, or COMMON AND LIFE-THREATENING.

ADVERSE REACTIONS

CNS: *dyskinesia, sleep disorder, dystonia, excessive dreaming, somnolence, dizziness, confusion, headache, hallucinations,* hyperkinesia, fatigue, falling, syncope, balance loss, depression, tremor, speech disorder, paresthesia.
CV: *orthostatic complaints,* chest pain, chest discomfort, palpitation, hypotension.
EENT: pharyngitis, tinnitus.
GI: *nausea, anorexia, diarrhea,* flatulence, *vomiting,* constipation, abdominal pain, dyspepsia, dry mouth.
GU: urinary tract infection, urine discoloration, hematuria, urinary incontinence, impotence.
Musculoskeletal: *muscle cramps,* myalgia, stiffness, arthritis, neck pain.
Respiratory: bronchitis, dyspnea, upper respiratory tract infection.
Skin: increased sweating, rash.

▣ KEY CONSIDERATIONS

• Because of the risk of potentially fatal, acute fulminant liver failure, use tolcapone only in patients taking levodopa and carbidopa who don't respond to or aren't suitable for other adjunctive therapy.
• Don't use drug until the risks have been discussed and the patient has given a written informed consent.
• Diarrhea occurs commonly with drug. It may occur 2 weeks after therapy begins or after 6 to 12 weeks. Although it usually resolves with discontinuation of drug, hospitalization may be required in rare cases.
• Dosage adjustments aren't needed in patients with mild to moderate renal dysfunction; use cautiously in patients with severe renal impairment.
• Withdraw drug in patients who fail to benefit from the drug within 3 weeks of treatment.
• Monitor liver enzyme levels every 2 weeks for the 1st year of therapy, then every 8 weeks. Stop drug if hepatic transaminase levels exceed the upper limits of normal or if patient appears jaundiced.
• Avoid use with a nonselective MAO inhibitor.

Patient education

• Advise patient to take tolcapone exactly as prescribed.
• Warn patient about risk of orthostatic hypotension and to use caution when rising from a seated or recumbent position.
• Caution patient to avoid hazardous activities until CNS effects of drug are known.
• Tell patient that nausea may occur and to report signs of liver injury immediately.
• Advise patient about risk of increased dyskinesia or dystonia.
• Inform patient that he may experience hallucinations.

tolmetin sodium
Tolectin, Tolectin DS

NSAID, nonnarcotic analgesic, antipyretic

Available by prescription only
Tablets: 200 mg, 600 mg
Capsules: 400 mg

INDICATIONS & DOSAGE

Rheumatoid arthritis and osteoarthritis, juvenile rheumatoid arthritis
Adults: Initially 400 mg P.O. t.i.d. Maximum dosage is 1,800 mg/day; usual dosage ranges from 600 to 1,800 mg daily in three divided doses.
◊ ***Ankylosing spondylitis,*** ◊ ***frozen shoulder,*** ◊ ***tennis elbow,*** ◊ ***sprains***
Adults: 600 to 1,600 mg P.O. daily.
◊ ***Nephrogenic diabetes insipidus***
Adults: 100 mg P.O. t.i.d. given with hydrochlorothiazide, 12.5 mg b.i.d.

PHARMACODYNAMICS

Anti-inflammatory, analgesic, and antipyretic actions: Mechanisms of action are unknown; tolmetin is thought to inhibit prostaglandin synthesis.

PHARMACOKINETICS

Absorption: Tolmetin is absorbed rapidly from the GI tract.
Distribution: Drug is highly protein-bound.
Metabolism: Drug is metabolized in the liver.

Excretion: Essentially all of the drug is excreted in urine within 24 hours as an inactive metabolite or conjugates of tolmetin. Elimination is biphasic consisting of a rapid phase with a half-life of 1 to 2 hours followed by a slower phase with a half-life of about 5 hours.

CONTRAINDICATIONS & PRECAUTIONS
Contraindicated in patients with hypersensitivity to tolmetin or in whom acute asthma attack, urticaria, or rhinitis is precipitated by aspirin or NSAIDs.

Use cautiously in patients with renal or cardiac disease, GI bleeding, history of peptic ulcer, hypertension, and conditions predisposing to fluid retention.

INTERACTIONS
Drug-drug. *Antacids* delay and decrease the absorption of tolmetin. The platelet-inhibiting effect of tolmetin may potentiate the effects of *anticoagulants* and *thrombolytics.* Use with *aspirin* may decrease plasma tolmetin levels. Use with *highly protein-bound drugs (phenytoin, salicylates, sulfonamides, sulfonylureas, warfarin)* may cause displacement of either drug and increase adverse effects; monitor therapy closely. NSAIDs decrease renal clearance of *lithium carbonate,* thus increasing serum lithium levels and risk of adverse effects. Use with *other GI irritants* (such as *antibiotics, corticosteroids, NSAIDs*) may potentiate the adverse GI effects of tolmetin; use together with caution. *Methotrexate* may increase methotrexate toxicity.
Drug-food. *Food* delays and decreases the absorption of tolmetin.

ADVERSE REACTIONS
CNS: headache, dizziness, drowsiness, asthenia, depression.
CV: chest pain, hypertension, edema.
EENT: tinnitus, visual disturbances.
GI: epigastric distress, peptic ulceration, occult blood loss, *nausea,* vomiting, abdominal pain, diarrhea, constipation, dyspepsia, flatulence, anorexia.
GU: urinary tract infection.
Hematologic: elevated BUN level, decreased hemoglobin level, decreased hematocrit.
Metabolic: weight gain, weight loss.

Skin: irritation.
Other: *anaphylaxis.*

▣ KEY CONSIDERATIONS
Besides the recommendations relevant to all NSAIDs, consider the following:
• Patients older than age 60 are more sensitive to the adverse effects of tolmetin.
• Because of its effect on renal prostaglandin, drug may cause fluid retention and edema. This may be significant in geriatric patients and in those with heart failure.
• Assess cardiopulmonary status closely; drug may cause sodium retention. Monitor vital signs closely, especially heart rate and blood pressure; schedule routine ophthalmic examinations during prolonged therapy.
• Assess renal function periodically during therapy; monitor intake, output, and daily weight.
• Monitor for presence and amount of edema.
• Therapeutic effect usually occurs within a few days to 1 week of therapy; evaluate patient's response to drug as evidenced by relief of symptoms.
• Administer drug on empty stomach for maximum absorption. However, to lessen GI upset, drug may be taken with meals.

Patient education
• Explain that therapeutic effects may occur in 1 week but could take 2 to 4 weeks. Tell patient to report adverse reactions.
• Advise patient to avoid use of OTC drugs such as NSAIDs unless his health care provider has approved them. Warn patient not to take sodium bicarbonate, which may decrease effectiveness of tolmetin.
• Instruct patient to follow prescribed regimen and recommended schedule of follow-up.
• Advise patient to report signs of edema; encourage routine check of blood pressure.
• Instruct patient to routinely check weight and to report gain or loss of 1.5 kg (3 lb) within 1 week.

Reactions may be *common,* uncommon, *life-threatening,* or COMMON AND LIFE-THREATENING.

Overdose & treatment
• Signs and symptoms of overdose include dizziness, drowsiness, mental confusion, lethargy.
• To treat tolmetin overdose, immediately induce vomiting or perform gastric lavage; then administer activated charcoal. Provide symptomatic and supportive measures (respiratory support and correction of fluid and electrolyte imbalances). Monitor laboratory parameters and vital signs closely. Alkalization of urine by sodium bicarbonate ingestion may enhance renal excretion of drug.

tolterodine tartrate
Detrol

Muscarinic receptor antagonist, anticholinergic

Available by prescription only
Tablets: 1 mg, 2 mg

INDICATIONS & DOSAGE
Treatment of patients with overactive bladder with symptoms of urinary frequency or urgency or urge incontinence
Adults: Initial dosage is 2 mg P.O. b.i.d. May reduce to 1 mg b.i.d. based on response and tolerance.
✦ *Dosage adjustment.* In patients with significantly reduced hepatic function or who are taking a drug that inhibits the cytochrome P-450 3A4 isoenzyme system, recommended dosage is 1 mg b.i.d.

PHARMACODYNAMICS
Anticholinergic action: Tolterodine is a competitive muscarinic receptor antagonist; both urinary bladder contraction and salivation are mediated through cholinergic muscarinic receptors.

PHARMACOKINETICS
Absorption: Tolterodine is well absorbed with about 77% bioavailability; serum levels peak within 1 to 2 hours after administration. Food increases bioavailability by 53%.
Distribution: Volume of distribution is about 113 L. Drug is highly protein-bound (96%).

Metabolism: Drug is metabolized in the liver primarily through oxidation by the cytochrome P-450 2D6 pathway and leads to the formation of a pharmacologically active 5-hydroxymethyl metabolite.
Excretion: Most of drug is recovered in urine; the rest, in feces. Less than 1% of dose is recovered as unchanged drug and 5% to 14% is recovered as the active metabolite. Half-life is 1.9 to 3.7 hours.

CONTRAINDICATIONS & PRECAUTIONS
Contraindicated in patients with urine or gastric retention and uncontrolled angle-closure glaucoma. Also contraindicated in patients hypersensitive to tolterodine or its ingredients.
 Use with caution in patients with significantly reduced hepatic or renal function.

INTERACTIONS
Drug-drug. For patients receiving *antifungals (itraconazole, ketoconazole, miconazole)* or *cytochrome P-450 3A4 inhibitors* such as *macrolide antibiotics (clarithromycin, erythromycin),* the maximum dosage of tolterodine is 1 mg b.i.d. *Fluoxetine,* a selective serotonin reuptake inhibitor and potent inhibitor of cytochrome P-450 2D6, significantly inhibits the metabolism of tolterodine in rapid metabolizers; no dosage adjustment is required.

ADVERSE REACTIONS
CNS: paresthesia, vertigo, dizziness, *headache,* nervousness, somnolence, fatigue.
CV: hypertension, chest pain.
EENT: abnormal vision (including accommodation), xerophthalmia, pharyngitis, rhinitis, sinusitis.
GI: *dry mouth,* abdominal pain, constipation, diarrhea, dyspepsia, flatulence, nausea, vomiting.
GU: dysuria, micturition frequency, urine retention, urinary tract infection.
Metabolic: weight gain.
Musculoskeletal: arthralgia, back pain.
Respiratory: bronchitis, coughing, upper respiratory tract infection.
Skin: pruritus, rash, erythema, dry skin.
Other: flulike syndrome.

▣ KEY CONSIDERATIONS
• Food increases the absorption of tolterodine; no dosage adjustment is needed.
• Dry mouth is the most commonly reported adverse effect.

Patient education
• Inform patient that antimuscarinics such as tolterodine may produce blurred vision.
• Caution patient to avoid hazardous activities until drug's effects are known.

Overdose & treatment
• Overdose can result in severe central anticholinergic effects and should be treated accordingly.
• Perform ECG monitoring if overdose occurs.

topiramate
Topamax

Sulfamate-substituted monosaccharide, antiepileptic

Available by prescription only
Tablets: 25 mg, 100 mg, 200 mg

INDICATIONS & DOSAGE
Adjunctive therapy of partial-onset seizures
Adults: Adjust dosage up to maximum daily dose of 400 mg in two divided doses. Adjust dosage as follows.

Week	a.m. dose	p.m. dose
1	None	50 mg
2	50 mg	50 mg
3	50 mg	100 mg
4	100 mg	100 mg
5	100 mg	150 mg
6	150 mg	150 mg
7	150 mg	200 mg
8	200 mg	200 mg

✦*Dosage adjustment.* For patients with moderate to severe renal impairment, reduce dosage by 50%. A supplemental dose may be required during hemodialysis.

PHARMACODYNAMICS
Antiepileptic action: Topiramate is thought to block action potential, which suggests a state-dependent sodium channel–blocking action. Drug may increase the frequency at which gamma-aminobutyric acid (GABA) activates $GABA_A$ receptors and may enhance GABA's ability to induce a flux of chloride ions into neurons, suggesting drug potentiates the activity of the inhibitory neurotransmitter. Drug may also antagonize kainate's ability to activate the kainate/amino-alpha 3-hydroxy-5-methylisoxazole 4-propionic acid subtype of excitatory amino acid (glutamate) receptor. Drug also has weak carbonic anhydrase inhibitor activity, unrelated to its antiepileptic properties.

PHARMACOKINETICS
Absorption: Topiramate is rapidly absorbed; plasma levels peak about 2 hours after 400-mg oral dose. Relative bioavailability of drug is about 80% compared with solution, and food doesn't affect drug.
Distribution: Plasma levels increase proportionately with dose; mean elimination half-life is 21 hours. Steady state is reached in 4 days in patients with normal renal function. Drug is 13% to 17% bound to plasma proteins.
Metabolism: Drug isn't extensively metabolized.
Excretion: Drug is primarily excreted unchanged in urine (about 70% of administered dose); mean plasma elimination half-life is 21 hours.

CONTRAINDICATIONS & PRECAUTIONS
Contraindicated in patients with history of hypersensitivity to a component of topiramate.
    Use cautiously in patients with hepatic or renal impairment because drug clearance may be decreased.

INTERACTIONS
Drug-drug. Use with *carbamazepine* or *phenytoin* decreases topiramate levels. Use with *carbonic anhydrase inhibitors (acetazolamide, dichlorphenamide)* may increase the risk of renal calculi; avoid using together. Although *CNS depres-*

Reactions may be *common*, uncommon, **life-threatening**, or COMMON AND LIFE-THREATENING.

sants haven't been evaluated, because of the risk of topiramate-induced CNS depression and other adverse cognitive and neuropsychiatric effects, use with caution. *Phenobarbital, primidone,* and *valproic acid* either weren't evaluated or had minimal effects on topiramate levels. Topiramate increased *phenytoin* levels.

ADVERSE REACTIONS
CNS: malaise; *fatigue;* abnormal coordination; agitation; apathy; asthenia; *ataxia; confusion;* depression; difficulty with attention level, language, or memory; *dizziness;* emotional liability; euphoria; **generalized tonic-clonic seizures;** hallucination; hyperkinesia; hypertonia; hypoaesthesia; hypokinesia; insomnia; mood problems; *nervousness; nystagmus; paresthesia;* personality disorder; *psychomotor slowing;* psychosis; *somnolence; speech disorders;* stupor; suicidal attempts; *tremor;* vertigo.
CV: edema, chest pain, palpitations.
EENT: *abnormal vision,* conjunctivitis, *diplopia,* eye pain, hearing or vestibular problems, pharyngitis, sinusitis, epistaxis, taste perversion, tinnitus.
GI: abdominal pain, anorexia, constipation, diarrhea, dry mouth, dyspepsia, flatulence, gastroenteritis, gingivitis, *nausea,* vomiting.
GU: dysuria, hematuria, impotence, micturition frequency, renal calculus, urinary incontinence, urinary tract infection, leukorrhea, vaginitis.
Hematologic: anemia, *leukopenia.*
Metabolic: increased or decreased weight.
Musculoskeletal: back pain, leg pain, myalgia.
Respiratory: bronchitis, coughing, dyspnea, *upper respiratory tract infection.*
Skin: acne, alopecia, aggressive reaction, increased sweating, pruritus, rash.
Other: body odor, fever, flulike syndrome, hot flashes.

▣ KEY CONSIDERATIONS
• Although no age-related differences or adverse effects were seen in geriatric patients, age-related renal abnormalities should be considered.

• Carefully review dosing schedule with patient to avoid underdosing or overdosing.
• If necessary, withdraw antiepileptics (including topiramate) gradually to minimize risk of increased seizure activity.
• Tablets shouldn't be broken because of the bitter taste.

Patient education
• Tell patient to maintain adequate fluid intake during therapy because of potential for renal calculi.
• Advise patient to avoid hazardous activities until topiramate's effects are known.
• Tell patient he may take drug without regard to meals.

topotecan hydrochloride
Hycamtin

Semisynthetic camptothecin derivative, antineoplastic

Available by prescription only
Injection: 4-mg single-dose vial

INDICATIONS & DOSAGE
Metastatic carcinoma of the ovary after failure of initial or subsequent chemotherapy
Adults: 1.5 mg/m²/day as an I.V. infusion given over 30 minutes for 5 consecutive days, starting day 1 of a 21-day cycle. Minimum of four cycles should be given. In the event of severe neutropenia occurring during a course, reduce the dose to 0.25 mg/m² for subsequent courses. Alternatively, administer granulocyte colony-stimulating factor (G-CSF) starting from day 6 of subsequent courses (24 hours after completion of topotecan) before resorting to dosage reduction.
✦ Dosage adjustment. In adults with renal impairment and creatinine clearance of 20 to 39 ml/minute, adjust dosage to 0.75 mg/m². For patients with mild renal impairment (creatinine clearance, 40 to 60 ml/minute), adjustment isn't required. Because of insufficient data, a specific dosage for patients with creatinine clear-

ance less than 20 ml/minute isn't recommended.

If severe neutropenia occurs during therapy, reduce dose to 0.25 mg/m^2 for subsequent therapy. Alternatively, administer G-CSF starting from day 6 of subsequent courses (24 hours after completion of topotecan) before resorting to dosage reduction.

PHARMACODYNAMICS
Antineoplastic action: Topotecan relieves torsional strain in DNA by inducing reversible single-strand breaks. It binds to the topoisomerase I-DNA complex and prevents religation of these single-strand breaks. Double-strand DNA damage produced during DNA synthesis when replication enzymes interact with the ternary complex formed by topotecan, topoisomerase I, and DNA is likely responsible for the cytotoxicity of topotecan.

PHARMACOKINETICS
Absorption: Topotecan is given only I.V.
Distribution: About 35% binds to plasma protein.
Metabolism: Drug undergoes a reversible pH-dependent hydrolysis of its lactone moiety; the lactone form that's pharmacologically active.
Excretion: About 30% of drug is excreted in urine; terminal half-life is 2 to 3 hours.

CONTRAINDICATIONS & PRECAUTIONS
Contraindicated in patients hypersensitive to topotecan or its components and in those with severe bone marrow depression.

INTERACTIONS
Drug-drug. Myelosuppression is more severe when topotecan is given with *cisplatin;* use together with extreme caution. Administration with *G-CSF* can prolong the duration of neutropenia; if G-CSF is to be used, don't initiate until day 6 of the course of therapy, 24 hours after treatment with topotecan is completed.

ADVERSE REACTIONS
CNS: *fatigue, asthenia, headache,* paresthesia.
GI: *nausea, vomiting, diarrhea, constipation, abdominal pain, stomatitis, anorexia.*
Hematologic: NEUTROPENIA, LEUKOPENIA, THROMBOCYTOPENIA, *anemia.*
Hepatic: transient elevations of liver enzyme levels.
Respiratory: *dyspnea.*
Skin: *alopecia.*
Other: fever, *sepsis.*

◉ KEY CONSIDERATIONS
● Before first course, baseline neutrophil count should exceed 1,500 cells/mm^3 and platelet count should exceed 100,000 cells/mm^3.
● Prepare topotecan under a vertical laminar flow hood wearing gloves and protective clothing. If drug solution contacts skin, wash skin immediately and thoroughly with soap and water. If mucous membranes are affected, flush areas thoroughly with water.
● Reconstitute each 4-mg vial with 4 ml sterile water for injection. Then dilute appropriate volume of reconstituted solution in either normal saline solution or D$_5$W before use.
● Because the lyophilized dosage form contains no antibacterial preservative, use reconstituted product immediately.
● Protect unopened vials of drug from light. Reconstituted vials are stable at 68° to 77° F (20° to 25° C) and ambient lighting conditions for 24 hours.
● Bone marrow suppression (primarily neutropenia) is the dose-limiting toxicity of drug. The nadir occurs at about 11 days. If severe neutropenia occurs during therapy, reduce dose by 0.25 mg/m^2 for subsequent therapy. Alternatively, administer G-CSF after subsequent therapy (before dose is reduced) starting from day 6 (24 hours after topotecan is administered). Neutropenia isn't cumulative over time.
● Thrombocytopenia occurred with a median duration of 5 days and platelet nadir at a medium of 15 days; anemia occurred with a median nadir at day 15. Blood or platelet (or both) transfusions may be necessary.

Reactions may be *common,* uncommon, *life-threatening,* or COMMON AND LIFE-THREATENING.

• Frequent monitoring of peripheral-blood cell counts is necessary. Don't give patients subsequent courses of drug until neutrophil counts exceed 1,000 cells/mm³, platelet counts exceed 100,000 cells/mm³, and hemoglobin levels are 9 mg/dl (with transfusion if needed).

• Inadvertent extravasation with drug has been associated with only mild local reactions, such as erythema and bruising.

torsemide
Demadex

Loop diuretic, antihypertensive

Available by prescription only
Tablets: 5 mg, 10 mg, 20 mg, 100 mg
Solution: 2-ml ampule (10 mg/ml), 5-ml ampule (10 mg/ml)

INDICATIONS & DOSAGE
Diuresis in patients with heart failure
Adults: Initially, 10 to 20 mg P.O. or I.V. once daily. If response is inadequate, double the dose until response is obtained. Maximum dosage is 200 mg daily.
Diuresis in patients with chronic renal failure
Adults: Initially, 20 mg P.O. or I.V. once daily. If response is inadequate, double the dose until response is obtained. Maximum dosage is 200 mg daily.
Diuresis in patients with hepatic cirrhosis
Adults: Initially, 5 to 10 mg P.O. or I.V. once daily with an aldosterone antagonist or a potassium sparing diuretic. If response is inadequate, double the dose until response is obtained. Maximum dosage is 40 mg daily.
Hypertension
Adults: Initially, 5 mg P.O. daily. Increase to 10 mg once daily in 4 to 6 weeks if needed and tolerated. If response is still inadequate, add another antihypertensive.
Note: If fluid and electrolyte imbalances occur, torsemide should be discontinued until the imbalances are corrected. Drug may then be restarted at a lower dose.

PHARMACODYNAMICS
Diuretic and antihypertensive actions: Loop diuretics such as torsemide enhance excretion of sodium, chloride, and water by acting on the ascending portion of the loop of Henle. Drug doesn't significantly alter GFR, renal plasma flow, or acid-base balance.

PHARMACOKINETICS
Absorption: Torsemide is absorbed with little first-pass metabolism; serum levels peak within 1 hour after oral administration.
Distribution: Volume of distribution is 12 to 15 L in healthy patients and in those with mild to moderate renal failure or heart failure. In patients with hepatic cirrhosis, volume of distribution is about doubled. Drug binds extensively (97% to 99%) to plasma protein.
Metabolism: Drug is metabolized in the liver to an inactive major metabolite and to two lesser metabolites that have some diuretic activity; for practical purposes, metabolism terminates action of drug. Duration of action is 6 to 8 hours after oral or I.V. use.
Excretion: From 22% to 34% of dose is excreted unchanged in urine by active secretion by the proximal tubules.

CONTRAINDICATIONS & PRECAUTIONS
Contraindicated in patients with anuria or hypersensitivity to torsemide or other sulfonylurea derivatives.
Use cautiously in patients with hepatic disease and associated cirrhosis and ascites.

INTERACTIONS
Drug-drug. *Cholestyramine* may decrease torsemide absorption; administration times should be separated by at least 3 hours. *Digoxin* decreases torsemide clearance, whereas torsemide decreases the renal clearance of *spironolactone;* no dosage adjustments are necessary. Torsemide may increase the risk of *lithium toxicity.* Administration with *NSAIDs* may cause renal dysfunction; use together with caution. Use with *ototoxic drugs* such as *aminoglycosides* increases the risk of auditory toxic reactions. *Probenecid* decreases the diuretic effect of

torsemide, and *indomethacin* decreases the diuretic effect in sodium-restricted patients; avoid using these drugs together. Torsemide reduces the excretion of *salicylates,* possibly leading to salicylate toxicity; avoid using these drugs together.

ADVERSE REACTIONS

CNS: dizziness, headache, asthenia, nervousness, insomnia, syncope.
CV: ECG abnormalities, chest pain, edema.
EENT: rhinitis, cough, sore throat.
GI: diarrhea, constipation, nausea, dyspepsia.
GU: *excessive urination,* altered renal function test results.
Metabolic: altered electrolyte balance.
Musculoskeletal: arthralgia, myalgia.

▣ KEY CONSIDERATIONS

• Geriatric patients are at greater risk for dehydration, blood-volume reduction, and possibly thrombosis and embolism with excessive diuresis; dosage adjustment usually isn't necessary. Monitor fluid intake and output, serum electrolyte levels, blood pressure, weight, and pulse rate during rapid diuresis and routinely with long-term use.
• Tinnitus and hearing loss (usually reversible) have been observed after rapid I.V. injection of other loop diuretics and also have been noted after oral torsemide administration. Inject drug slowly over 2 minutes; single dose shouldn't exceed 200 mg.
• In patients with CV disease, especially those receiving cardiac glycosides, diuretic-induced hypokalemia may be a risk factor for the development of arrhythmias. The risk of hypokalemia is greatest in patients with hepatic cirrhosis, brisk diuresis, or inadequate oral intake of electrolytes and in those taking corticosteroids or corticotropin. Periodically monitor serum potassium and other electrolyte levels.

Patient education

• Encourage patient to follow a high-potassium diet, including citrus fruits, tomatoes, bananas, dates, and apricots.
• Instruct patient to take torsemide in the morning to prevent nocturia.

• Advise patient to change positions slowly to prevent dizziness.
• Inform patient to report ringing in ears immediately because this may indicate toxicity.
• Tell patient to call before taking OTC drugs.
• Advise patient to take protective measures against exposure to sunlight or ultraviolet light.

---

tramadol hydrochloride
Ultram

Synthetic derivative, analgesic

Available by prescription only
Tablets: 50 mg

INDICATIONS & DOSAGE

Moderate to moderately severe pain
Adults: 50 to 100 mg P.O. q 4 to 6 hours, p.r.n. Maximum dosage is 400 mg/day.
✦ *Dosage adjustment.* In patients with creatinine clearance less than 30 ml/minute, increase dosing interval to q 12 hours; maximum daily dose is 200 mg.

In patients with cirrhosis, recommended dosage is 50 mg q 12 hours.

PHARMACODYNAMICS

Analgesic action: Mechanism of action is unknown. Tramadol is a centrally acting synthetic analgesic compound not chemically related to opiates but is thought to bind to opioid receptors and inhibit reuptake of norepinephrine and serotonin.

PHARMACOKINETICS

Absorption: Tramadol is almost completely absorbed; mean absolute bioavailability of 100-mg dose is about 75%. Mean plasma levels peak at about 2 hours.
Distribution: Drug is about 20% bound to plasma protein; may cross the blood-brain barrier.
Metabolism: Drug is extensively metabolized.
Excretion: About 30% of dose is excreted unchanged in urine and 60% as

---

Reactions may be *common,* uncommon, *life-threatening*, or COMMON AND LIFE-THREATENING.

metabolites; half-life of drug is 6 to 7 hours.

CONTRAINDICATIONS & PRECAUTIONS
Contraindicated in patients with hypersensitivity to tramadol or acute intoxication with alcohol, hypnotics, centrally acting analgesics, opioids, or psychotropic drugs.

Use cautiously in patients at risk for seizures or respiratory depression; in those with increased intracranial pressure or head injury, acute abdominal conditions, impaired renal or hepatic function; and in patients physically dependent on opioids.

INTERACTIONS
Drug-drug. *Carbamazepine* increases tramadol metabolism; patients receiving long-term carbamazepine therapy at dosages up to 800 mg daily may require up to twice the recommended dose of tramadol. *CNS depressants* produce additive effects; use together with caution, dosage of tramadol may need to be reduced. *MAO inhibitors* and *neuroleptic drugs* increase the risk of seizures; monitor patient closely.
Drug-lifestyle. *Alcohol* use may cause additive effects.

ADVERSE REACTIONS
CNS: malaise, *dizziness, vertigo, headache, somnolence, CNS stimulation, asthenia,* anxiety, confusion, coordination disturbance, euphoria, nervousness, sleep disorder, *seizures.*
CV: vasodilation.
EENT: visual disturbances.
GI: *nausea, constipation, vomiting,* dyspepsia, dry mouth, diarrhea, abdominal pain, anorexia, flatulence.
GU: urine retention, urinary frequency, proteinuria, increased creatinine clearance, menopausal symptoms.
Hematologic: decreased hemoglobin levels.
Hepatic: increased liver enzyme levels.
Musculoskeletal: hypertonia.
Respiratory: *respiratory depression.*
Skin: *pruritus,* diaphoresis, rash.

▣ KEY CONSIDERATIONS
• Use cautiously in geriatric patients because serum levels are slightly elevated and elimination half-life of drug is prolonged; don't exceed daily dose of 300 mg in patients older than age 75.
• Monitor patient's CV and respiratory status and stop tramadol if respirations decrease, rate is less than 12 breaths/minute, or patient shows signs of respiratory depression.
• Constipation is a common adverse effect and may require laxative therapy.
• For better analgesic effect, give drug before patient has intense pain.
• Monitor patient at risk for seizures closely; drug has been reported to reduce seizure threshold.
• Monitor patient for drug dependence. Because drug dependence similar to codeine or dextropropoxyphene can occur, the potential for abuse exists.

Patient education
• Instruct patient to take tramadol only as prescribed and not to alter dosage or dosage interval without medical approval.
• Caution ambulatory patient about getting out of bed or walking. Warn outpatient to avoid driving and other potentially hazardous activities that require mental alertness until adverse CNS effects of drug are known.
• Advise patient not to take OTC drugs unless instructed because drug interactions can occur.

trandolapril
Mavik

ACE inhibitor, antihypertensive

Available by prescription only
Tablets: 1 mg, 2 mg, 4 mg

INDICATIONS & DOSAGE
Hypertension
Adults: In patient not taking a diuretic, initially 1 mg for the nonblack patient and 2 mg for the black patient P.O. once daily. If control is inadequate, dosage can be increased at intervals of at least 1 week. Maintenance dosage ranges from

2 to 4 mg daily for most patients; there's little experience with doses of more than 8 mg. Patients receiving once-daily dosing at 4 mg may use b.i.d. dosing.

For patient receiving a diuretic, initially 0.5 mg P.O. once daily. Subsequent dosage adjustment is made based on blood pressure response.

Heart failure post-MI or left ventricular dysfunction post-MI
Adults: initially 1 mg P.O. daily, adjusted to 4 mg P.O. daily. If patient can't tolerate 4 mg, continue at highest tolerated dose.

PHARMACODYNAMICS

Antihypertensive action: Unknown. Trandolapril is thought to inhibit circulating and tissue ACE activity, thereby reducing angiotensin II formation, decreasing vasoconstriction, decreasing aldosterone secretion, and increasing plasma renin. Decreased aldosterone secretion leads to diuresis, natriuresis, and a small increase in serum potassium level.

PHARMACOKINETICS

Absorption: Absolute bioavailability after oral administration of trandolapril is about 10% for drug and 70% for its metabolite, trandolaprilat.
Distribution: Drug is about 80% protein-bound.
Metabolism: Drug is metabolized in the liver to the active metabolite, trandolaprilat, and at least seven other metabolites.
Excretion: Drug is about 66% excreted in feces; 33%, in urine. Elimination half-lives of drug and trandolaprilat are about 6 and 10 hours, respectively, but like all ACE inhibitors, trandolaprilat also has a prolonged terminal elimination phase.

CONTRAINDICATIONS & PRECAUTIONS

Contraindicated in patients with hypersensitivity to trandolapril and history of angioedema related to previous treatment with an ACE inhibitor.

Use cautiously in patients with impaired renal function, heart failure, or renal artery stenosis.

INTERACTIONS

Drug-drug. *Diuretics* increase risk of excessive hypotension; stop diuretic or reduce dose of trandolapril. Trandolapril increases serum *lithium* levels and lithium toxicity; don't use together. *Potassium sparing diuretics* and *potassium supplements* increase the risk of hyperkalemia; monitor serum potassium levels closely.
Drug-food. *Sodium substitutes containing potassium* increase the risk of hyperkalemia; monitor serum potassium levels closely.

ADVERSE REACTIONS

CNS: dizziness, headache, fatigue, drowsiness, insomnia, paresthesia, vertigo, anxiety.
CV: chest pain, *AV first-degree block, bradycardia,* edema, flushing, hypotension, palpitations.
EENT: epistaxis, *throat inflammation,* upper respiratory tract infection.
GI: diarrhea, dyspepsia, abdominal distention, abdominal pain or cramps, constipation, vomiting, *pancreatitis.*
GU: urinary frequency, elevated creatinine clearance and BUN level, impotence, decreased libido.
Hematologic: *neutropenia, leukopenia.*
Hepatic: elevated liver enzyme and uric acid levels.
Metabolic: hyperkalemia, hyponatremia.
Respiratory: dry, persistent, tickling, nonproductive cough; dyspnea.
Skin: rash, pruritus, pemphigus.
Other: *anaphylactoid reactions, angioedema.*

▣ KEY CONSIDERATIONS

● Monitor for hypotension. Excessive hypotension can occur when trandolapril is given with diuretics. If possible, diuretic therapy should be discontinued 2 to 3 days before starting trandolapril to decrease potential for excessive hypotensive response. If drug doesn't adequately control blood pressure, diuretic therapy may be reinstituted with care.
● Assess patient's renal function before and periodically throughout therapy. Monitor serum potassium levels.

Reactions may be *common,* uncommon, *life-threatening,* or COMMON AND LIFE-THREATENING.

- Other ACE inhibitors have been associated with agranulocytosis and neutropenia. Monitor CBC with differential counts before therapy, especially in patients who have collagen vascular disease with impaired renal function.
- Angioedema associated with involvement of the tongue, glottis, or larynx may be fatal because of airway obstruction. Appropriate therapy, such as 0.3 to 0.5 ml of S.C. epinephrine 1:1,000 and equipment to ensure a patent airway, should be readily available.
- If jaundice develops, discontinue drug because ACE inhibitors have (in rare cases) been associated with a syndrome of cholestatic jaundice, fulminant hepatic necrosis, and death.

Patient education
- Advise patient to report signs of infection (such as fever and sore throat) and the following signs or symptoms: easy bruising or bleeding; swelling of tongue, lips, face, eyes, mucous membranes, or extremities; difficulty swallowing or breathing; and hoarseness.
- Tell patient to avoid sodium substitutes; these products may contain potassium, which can cause hyperkalemia.
- Light-headedness can occur, especially during the first few days of therapy. Tell patient to rise slowly to minimize this effect and to report symptoms. If syncope occurs, tell patient to stop taking trandolapril and notify the health care provider immediately.
- Instruct patient to use caution in hot weather and during exercise. Inadequate fluid intake, vomiting, diarrhea, and excessive perspiration can lead to light-headedness and syncope.

Overdose & treatment
- Signs and symptoms of overdose are believed to be similar to other ACE inhibitor overdose, with hypotension as the main adverse reaction.
- Because the hypotensive effect of trandolapril is achieved through vasodilation and effective hypovolemia, it's reasonable to treat overdose by infusion of normal saline solution. In addition, renal function and serum potassium levels

should be monitored. Drug is removed by hemodialysis.

tranylcypromine sulfate
Parnate

MAO inhibitor, antidepressant

Available by prescription only
Tablets: 10 mg

INDICATIONS & DOSAGE
Severe depression, ◊***panic disorder***
Adults: 30 mg P.O. daily in divided doses. If patient shows no improvement after 2 weeks, increase dosage in 10-mg/day increments q 1 to 3 weeks; maximum daily dose is 60 mg.

PHARMACODYNAMICS
Antidepressant action: Endogenous depression is thought to result from low CNS levels of neurotransmitters, including norepinephrine and serotonin. Tranylcypromine acts by inhibiting effects of MAO, an enzyme that normally inactivates amine-containing substances, thus increasing level and activity of these drugs.

PHARMACOKINETICS
Absorption: Tranylcypromine is rapidly and completely absorbed from the GI tract. Serum levels peak at 1 to 3 hours; onset of therapeutic activity may not occur for 3 to 4 weeks.
Distribution: Unknown. Dosage adjustments are determined by therapeutic response and adverse reaction profile.
Metabolism: Drug is metabolized in the liver.
Excretion: Drug is excreted primarily in urine within 24 hours; some drug is excreted in feces via the biliary tract. Half-life is 2½ hours; enzyme inhibition is prolonged and unrelated to half-life.

CONTRAINDICATIONS & PRECAUTIONS
Contraindicated in patients receiving antihistamines, antihypertensives, excessive quantities of caffeine, cheese or other foods with a high tyramine or tryptophan content, some CNS depressants (including narcotics and alcohol), bupro-

pion hydrochloride, buspirone hydrochloride, dextromethorphan, diuretics, MAO inhibitors or dibenzazepine derivatives, meperidine, sedatives or anesthetics, selective serotonin reuptake inhibitors, or sympathomimetics (including amphetamines). Also contraindicated in patients with a confirmed or suspected cerebrovascular defect, pheochromocytoma, history of liver disease, severe impairment of renal function, CV disease, hypertension, or history of headache and in those undergoing elective surgery.

Use cautiously in patients with renal disease, diabetes, seizure disorders, Parkinson's disease, or hyperthyroidism; in those at risk for suicide; and in patients receiving antiparkinsonians or spinal anesthetics.

INTERACTIONS
Drug-drug. Use of tranylcypromine with *amphetamines, ephedrine, phenylephrine, phenylpropanolamine,* or *related drugs* may result in serious CV toxicity; most *OTC cold, hay fever,* and *weight-reduction products* contain these drugs. Use cautiously and in reduced dosage with *barbiturates, dextromethorphan, narcotics,* and *other sedatives. Cocaine* or *local anesthetics containing vasoconstrictors* should be avoided. Use with *disulfiram* may cause tachycardia, flushing, or palpitations. Use with *general or spinal anesthetics,* normally metabolized by MAO inhibitors, may cause severe hypotension and excessive CNS depression; tranylcypromine should be discontinued for at least 1 week before using these drugs. Tranylcypromine decreases effectiveness of *local anesthetics* (such as *lidocaine, procaine*), resulting in poor nerve block. Circulatory collapse and death have occurred after administration of *meperidine.* Wait at least 2 weeks before switching to *tricyclic antidepressants.*
Drug-food. *Beverages* and *foods containing tyramine or tryptophan* (such as *wines, beer, cheeses, preserved fruits, meats,* and *vegetables*) or *caffeine* may cause hypertensive crisis; don't use together.

Drug-lifestyle. *Alcohol* use may cause enhanced CNS effects; don't use together.

ADVERSE REACTIONS
CNS: *dizziness,* headache, anxiety, agitation, paresthesia, drowsiness, weakness, numbness, tremor, jitters, confusion.
CV: *orthostatic hypotension, tachycardia,* paradoxical hypertension, edema, palpitations.
EENT: blurred vision, tinnitus.
GI: dry mouth, *anorexia,* nausea, diarrhea, constipation, abdominal pain.
GU: impotence, SIADH, increased urine catecholamine levels, urine retention, impaired ejaculation.
Hematologic: anemia, *leukopenia, agranulocytosis, thrombocytopenia.*
Hepatic: elevated liver function test results, *hepatitis.*
Musculoskeletal: muscle spasm, myoclonic jerks.
Skin: rash.
Other: chills.

▣ KEY CONSIDERATIONS
● Tranylcypromine isn't recommended for patients older than age 60 because geriatric patients have less compensatory reserve to cope with serious adverse effects of drug.
● Consider the inherent risk of suicide until significant improvement of depressive state occurs. Closely supervise high-risk patients during initial drug therapy. To reduce risk of suicidal overdose, prescribe the smallest quantity of tablets consistent with good management.
● Drug may have a more rapid onset of antidepressant effect than other MAO inhibitors (7 to 10 days versus 21 to 30 days). MAO activity also returns rapidly to pretreatment values.

Patient education
● Warn patient to avoid taking alcohol and other CNS depressants or self-prescribed drugs such as cold, hay fever, or diet preparations without medical approval.
● To minimize daytime sedation, tell patient to take tranylcypromine at bedtime.

Reactions may be *common,* uncommon, *life-threatening,* or COMMON AND LIFE-THREATENING.

• Explain that many foods and beverages containing tyramine or tryptophan (such as wines, beer, cheeses, preserved fruits, meats, and vegetables) may interact with drug. A list of foods to avoid can be obtained from the hospital dietary department or pharmacy.

• Tell patient to avoid hazardous activities that require alertness until full CNS effect of drug is known.

• Inform patient to lie down after taking drug and avoid abrupt postural changes, especially when arising to prevent dizziness induced by orthostatic blood pressure changes.

• Tell patient to take drug exactly as prescribed, not to double-dose if a dose is missed, and not to stop taking drug abruptly. Patient should promptly report adverse reactions. Dosage reduction can relieve most adverse reactions.

• Advise patient to store drug safely away from children.

• Tell patient to inform dentist or other health care providers about the use of a MAO inhibitor.

• Tell patient to report severe headache, palpitations, tachycardia, sweating, tightness in throat and chest, dizziness, stiff neck, nausea, vomiting, or other unusual signs or symptoms.

Overdose & treatment

• Signs and symptoms of overdose include exacerbations of adverse reactions or an exaggerated response to normal pharmacologic activity; such signs and symptoms become apparent slowly (24 to 48 hours) and may persist for up to 2 weeks. Agitation, flushing, tachycardia, hypotension, hypertension, palpitations, increased motor activity, twitching, increased deep tendon reflexes, seizures, hyperpyrexia, cardiorespiratory arrest, or coma may occur. Death has occurred with doses of 350 mg.

• Treat symptomatically and supportively. Treat hypertensive crisis with 5 to 10 mg of phentolamine I.V. push; seizures, agitation, or tremors, with I.V. diazepam; tachycardia, with beta blockers; and fever, with cooling blankets. Monitor vital signs and fluid and electrolyte balance. Sympathomimetics (such as norepinephrine and phenyl-

ephrine) are contraindicated in hypotension because of MAO inhibitors.

trazodone hydrochloride
Desyrel

Triazolopyridine derivative, antidepressant

Available by prescription only
Tablets: 50 mg, 100 mg
Tablets (film-coated): 50 mg, 100 mg
Dividose tablets: 150 mg, 300 mg

INDICATIONS & DOSAGE
Depression
Adults: Initial dosage is 150 mg daily in divided doses, which can be increased by 50 mg/day q 3 to 4 days. Average dose ranges from 150 mg to 400 mg/day. Maximum dosage is 400 mg/day in outpatients; 600 mg/day in hospitalized patients.
◊ **Aggressive behavior**
Adults: 50 mg P.O. b.i.d.
◊ **Panic disorder**
Adults: 300 mg P.O. daily.

PHARMACODYNAMICS
Antidepressant action: Trazodone inhibits reuptake of norepinephrine and serotonin in CNS nerve terminals (presynaptic neurons), which results in increased level and enhanced activity of these neurotransmitters in the synaptic cleft. Drug shares some properties with tricyclic antidepressants. It has antihistaminic, alpha-blocking, analgesic, and sedative effects as well as relaxant effects on skeletal muscle. Unlike tricyclic antidepressants, drug counteracts the pressor effects of norepinephrine, has limited effects on the CV system, and in particular, has no direct quinidine-like effects on cardiac tissue; it also causes relatively fewer anticholinergic effects. Drug has been used in patients with alcohol dependence to decrease tremors and alleviate anxiety and depression. Adverse reactions are somewhat dose related; incidence increases with higher dosage levels.

PHARMACOKINETICS

Absorption: Trazodone is well absorbed from the GI tract after oral administration. Effect peaks in 1 hour. Food delays absorption, extends peak effect of drug to 2 hours, and increases amount of drug absorbed by 20%.

Distribution: Widely distributed in the body; drug doesn't concentrate in a particular tissue. About 90% is protein-bound. Proposed therapeutic drug levels haven't been established. Plasma levels reach steady state in 3 to 7 days; onset of therapeutic activity occurs in 7 days.

Metabolism: Drug is metabolized by the liver; more than 75% of metabolites are excreted within 3 days.

Excretion: Drug is mostly excreted in urine; rest is excreted in feces via the biliary tract.

CONTRAINDICATIONS & PRECAUTIONS

Contraindicated during initial recovery phase of an MI or in patients with hypersensitivity to trazodone.

Use cautiously in patients with hear disease and in those at risk for suicide.

INTERACTIONS

Drug-drug. Additive effects are likely after use of trazodone with *antihypertensives,* such as *clonidine, guanabenz, guanadrel, guanethidine, methyldopa,* and *reserpine* (hypotension); and *with CNS depressants,* such as *analgesics, barbiturates, narcotics, tranquilizers,* and *anesthetics* (oversedation). Trazodone may increase serum levels of *digoxin* and *phenytoin. Warfarin* may increase or decrease PT and INR.

Drug-lifestyle. *Alcohol* use may cause additive CNS effects.

ADVERSE REACTIONS

CNS: *drowsiness, dizziness,* nervousness, fatigue, confusion, tremor, weakness, hostility, anger, nightmares, vivid dreams, headache, insomnia, **generalized tonic-clonic seizures.**

CV: orthostatic hypotension, tachycardia, hypertension, syncope, shortness of breath, ECG changes.

EENT: blurred vision, tinnitus, nasal congestion.

GI: dry mouth, dysgeusia, constipation, nausea, vomiting, anorexia.

GU: urine retention; priapism, possibly leading to impotence; decreased libido; hematuria.

Hematologic: anemia, decreased WBC count.

Hepatic: elevated liver function test results.

Metabolic: altered serum glucose levels.

Skin: rash, urticaria, diaphoresis.

◙ KEY CONSIDERATIONS

• Geriatric patients usually require lower initial dosages; they're more likely to develop adverse reactions. However, trazodone may be preferred in geriatric patients because it has fewer adverse cardiac effects.

• Consider the inherent risk of suicide until significant improvement of depressive state occurs. Closely monitor high-risk patients during initial drug therapy. To reduce risk of suicidal overdose, prescribe the smallest quantity of tablets consistent with good management.

• Administering drug with food helps prevent GI upset and increases absorption.

• Adverse effects are more common when dosages exceed 300 mg/day.

• May break 150-mg tablet on the scoring to obtain doses of 50 mg, 75 mg, or 100 mg.

• Tolerance to adverse effects (especially sedative effects) usually develops after 1 to 2 weeks of treatment.

• Drug has been used in alcohol dependence to decrease tremors and relieve anxiety and depression; dosages range from 50 to 75 mg daily.

• Drug has fewer adverse cardiac and anticholinergic effects than tricyclic antidepressants.

• Drug may cause prolonged painful erections that may require surgical correction; consider carefully before prescribing for male patients, especially those who are sexually active.

• Don't withdraw drug abruptly; discontinue drug at least 48 hours before surgical procedures.

• Sugarless chewing gum or hard candy or ice may relieve dry mouth.

Reactions may be *common*, uncommon, *life-threatening*, or COMMON AND LIFE-THREATENING.

- Monitor blood pressure because hypotension may occur.
- Drowsiness may require administration of a major portion of the daily dose at bedtime or, alternatively, a reduced dose.

Patient education
- Tell patient that full effects of trazodone may not become apparent for up to 2 weeks after therapy begins.
- Tell patient to take drug exactly as prescribed and not to double dose for missed doses, not to share drug with others, and not to discontinue drug abruptly.
- Inform patient that drug may cause drowsiness or dizziness; instruct patient not to participate in activities that require mental alertness until full effects of drug are known.
- Tell patient to avoid alcoholic beverages or medicinal elixirs while taking drug.
- Warn patient to store drug safely away from children.
- Suggest taking drug with food or milk if it causes stomach upset.
- To prevent dizziness, tell patient to lie down for about 30 minutes after taking drug and avoid sudden postural changes, especially rising to upright position.
- Tell patient that sugarless chewing gum or sugarless hard candy may relieve dry mouth.
- Advise patient to report unusual effects immediately and to report prolonged, painful erections; sexual dysfunction; dizziness; fainting; or rapid heartbeat. He should regard an involuntary erection lasting more than 1 hour as a medical emergency.

Overdose & treatment
- The most common signs and symptoms of overdose are drowsiness and vomiting; other signs and symptoms include orthostatic hypotension, tachycardia, headache, shortness of breath, dry mouth, and incontinence. Coma may occur.
- Treatment is symptomatic and supportive and includes maintaining airway and stabilizing vital signs and fluid and electrolyte balance. Induce vomiting if gag reflex is intact; follow with gastric lavage (begin with lavage if induced vomiting is unfeasible) and activated charcoal to prevent further absorption.

Forced diuresis may aid elimination. Dialysis is usually ineffective.

triamcinolone (systemic)
Aristocort, Kenacort

triamcinolone acetonide
Kenalog, Triam-A

triamcinolone diacetate
Amcort, Aristocort, Aristocort Forte, Aristocort Intralesional, Articulose-L.A., Cenocort Forte, Kenacort, Triam-Forte, Triamolone 40, Tristoject

triamcinolone hexacetonide
Aristospan Intra-articular, Aristospan Intralesional

Glucocorticoid, anti-inflammatory, immunosuppressant

Available by prescription only
triamcinolone
Tablets: 1 mg, 2 mg, 4 mg, 8 mg
Syrup: 2 mg/ml, 4 mg/ml
triamcinolone acetonide
Injection: 10-mg/ml and 40-mg/ml suspensions
triamcinolone diacetate
Injection: 25-mg/ml and 40-mg/ml suspensions
triamcinolone hexacetonide
Injection: 5-mg/ml and 20-mg/ml suspensions

INDICATIONS & DOSAGE
Adrenal insufficiency
triamcinolone
Adults: 4 to 12 mg P.O. daily in single or divided doses.
Severe inflammation or immunosuppression
triamcinolone
Adults: 8 to 16 mg P.O. daily in single or divided doses.
triamcinolone acetonide
Adults: Initially, 60 mg I.M. Additional doses of 20 to 100 mg may be given p.r.n. at 6-week intervals. Alternatively, administer 2.5 to 15 mg intra-articularly, or up to 1 mg intralesionally p.r.n.

triamcinolone diacetate
Adults: 40 mg I.M. once weekly; or 2 to 40 mg intra-articularly, intrasynovially, or intralesionally q 1 to 8 weeks; or 4 to 48 mg P.O. divided q.i.d.
triamcinolone hexacetonide
Adults: 2 to 20 mg intra-articularly q 3 to 4 weeks p.r.n.; or up to 0.5 mg intralesionally per square inch of skin.
Tuberculosis meningitis
triamcinolone
Adults: 32 to 48 mg P.O. daily.
Edematous states
triamcinolone
Adults: 16 to 48 mg P.O. daily.
Collagen diseases
triamcinolone
Adults: 30 to 48 mg P.O. daily.
Dermatologic disorders
triamcinolone
Adults: 8 to 16 mg P.O. daily.
Allergic states
triamcinolone
Adults: 8 to 12 mg P.O. daily.
Ophthalmic diseases
triamcinolone
Adults: 12 to 40 mg P.O. daily.
Respiratory diseases
triamcinolone
Adults: 16 to 48 mg P.O. daily.
Hematologic diseases
triamcinolone
Adults: 16 to 60 mg P.O. daily.
Neoplastic diseases
triamcinolone
Adults: 16 to 100 mg P.O. daily.

PHARMACODYNAMICS
Anti-inflammatory action: Triamcinolone stimulates the synthesis of enzymes needed to decrease the inflammatory response. It suppresses the immune system by reducing activity and volume of the lymphatic system, thus producing lymphocytopenia (primarily of T lymphocytes), decreases immunoglobulin and complement levels, decreases passage of immune complexes through basement membranes, and possibly depresses reactivity of tissue to antigen-antibody interactions.

Drug is an intermediate-acting glucocorticoid. The addition of a fluorine group in the molecule increases the anti-inflammatory activity, which is five times more potent than an equal weight of hydrocortisone. It has essentially no mineralocorticoid activity.

Drug may be administered orally. The diacetate and acetonide salts may be administered by I.M., intra-articular, intrasynovial, intralesional or sublesional, and soft-tissue injection. The diacetate suspension is slightly soluble, providing a prompt onset of action and a longer duration of effect (1 to 2 weeks). Triamcinolone acetonide is relatively insoluble and slowly absorbed. Its extended duration of action lasts for several weeks. Triamcinolone hexacetonide is relatively insoluble, is absorbed slowly, and has a prolonged action of 3 to 4 weeks. Don't administer the parenteral suspensions I.V.

PHARMACOKINETICS
Absorption: Triamcinolone is absorbed readily after oral administration. After oral and I.V. administration, effects peak in about 1 to 2 hours. The suspensions for injection have variable onset and duration of action, depending on injection site (that is, whether they're injected into an intra-articular space or a muscle) and the blood supply to that area.
Distribution: Drug is removed rapidly from the blood and distributed to muscle, liver, skin, intestines, and kidneys. It binds extensively to plasma proteins (transcortin and albumin); only the unbound portion is active.
Metabolism: Drug is metabolized in the liver to inactive glucuronide and sulfate metabolites.
Excretion: The inactive metabolites and a small amount of unmetabolized drug are excreted by the kidneys; insignificant quantities of drug are also excreted in feces. Biological half-life of triamcinolone is 18 to 36 hours.

CONTRAINDICATIONS & PRECAUTIONS
Contraindicated in patients with hypersensitivity to a component of the formulation or systemic fungal infections.

Use cautiously in patients with GI ulcer, renal disease, hypertension, osteoporosis, diabetes mellitus, hypothyroidism, cirrhosis, diverticulitis, nonspecific ulcerative colitis, recent intestinal

---

Reactions may be *common*, uncommon, *life-threatening*, or COMMON AND LIFE-THREATENING.

anastomosis, thromboembolic disorders, seizures, myasthenia gravis, heart failure, tuberculosis, ocular herpes simplex, emotional instability, or psychotic tendencies.

INTERACTIONS

Drug-drug. Glucocorticoids may enhance hypokalemia from *amphotericin B* or *diuretic* therapy; the hypokalemia may increase the risk of toxicity in patients receiving *cardiac glycosides. Antacids, cholestyramine,* and *colestipol* decrease the effect of triamcinolone by absorbing the corticosteroid, decreasing the amount absorbed. *Barbiturates, phenytoin,* and *rifampin* may cause decreased corticosteroid effects because of increased hepatic metabolism. Use with *estrogens* may reduce the metabolism of triamcinolone by increasing the level of transcortin; the half-life of the corticosteroid is then prolonged because of increased protein-binding. Glucocorticoids increase the metabolism of *isoniazid* and *salicylates* and cause hyperglycemia, requiring dosage adjustment of *insulin* or *oral antidiabetics* in diabetic patients. In rare cases, triamcinolone decreases the effects of *oral anticoagulants.* Administration with *ulcerogenic drugs* such as *NSAIDs* may increase the risk of GI ulceration.

ADVERSE REACTIONS

Most adverse reactions to corticosteroids are dose- or duration-dependent.
CNS: *euphoria, insomnia,* psychotic behavior, pseudotumor cerebri, vertigo, headache, paresthesia, *seizures.*
CV: *heart failure, thromboembolism,* hypertension, edema, *arrhythmias,* thrombophlebitis.
EENT: cataracts, glaucoma.
GI: *peptic ulceration,* GI irritation, increased appetite, *pancreatitis,* nausea, vomiting.
Metabolic: hypokalemia, hyperglycemia, hypocalcemia, and carbohydrate intolerance; decreased T_3 and T_4 levels; increased urine glucose and calcium levels.
Musculoskeletal: muscular weakness, osteoporosis.

Skin: delayed wound healing, acne, various skin eruptions.
Other: cushingoid state (moonface, buffalo hump, central obesity), hirsutism, susceptibility to infection, *acute adrenal insufficiency with increased stress (infection, surgery, or trauma).*
After abrupt withdrawal: rebound inflammation, fatigue, weakness, arthralgia, fever, dizziness, lethargy, depression, fainting, orthostatic hypotension, dyspnea, anorexia, hypoglycemia, *acute adrenal insufficiency. After prolonged use, sudden withdrawal may be fatal.*

▣ KEY CONSIDERATIONS

• Recommendations for use of triamcinolone and for care and teaching of patients during therapy are the same as those for all systemic adrenocorticoids.
• Geriatric patients may be more susceptible to osteoporosis with long-term use.
• Always adjust dosage to the lowest effective one.
• For better results and less toxicity, give a once-daily oral dose in the morning with food.
• Don't use diluents that contain preservatives; flocculation may occur.
• Give I.M. injection deep into gluteal muscle; rotate injection sites to prevent muscle atrophy.
• Monitor patient's weight, blood pressure, and serum electrolyte levels.
• Watch for allergic reaction to the dye, tartrazine, in patients with sensitivity to aspirin.
• Watch for depression or psychotic episodes, especially in high-dose therapy.
• Keep in mind that patients with diabetes may need increased insulin; monitor blood glucose levels.
• Drug may mask or exacerbate infections, including latent amebiasis.
• Unless contraindicated, give low-sodium diet that's high in potassium and protein; administer potassium supplements as needed.
• Drug suppresses reactions to skin tests; causes false-negative results in the nitroblue tetrazolium test for systemic bacterial infections.

• Drug decreases ^{131}I uptake and protein-bound iodine levels in thyroid function tests.

Patient teaching
• Tell patient not to discontinue triamcinolone abruptly or without consent.
• Instruct patient to take drug with food or milk.
• Teach patient signs and symptoms of early adrenal insufficiency: fatigue, muscular weakness, joint pain, fever, anorexia, nausea, dyspnea, dizziness, and fainting.
• Instruct patient to carry a card identifying his need for supplemental systemic glucocorticoids during stress. This card should contain health care provider's name, drug, and dose taken.
• Warn patient on long-term therapy about cushingoid symptoms; instruct him to notify his health care provider of sudden weight gain and swelling.
• Tell patient to report slow healing.
• Instruct patient to avoid exposure to infections and to notify his health care provider if exposure occurs.

triamcinolone acetonide (oral and nasal inhalant)
Azmacort, Nasacort

Glucocorticoid, anti-inflammatory, antasthmatic

Available by prescription only
Oral inhalation aerosol: 100 mcg/metered spray, 240 doses/inhaler
Nasal aerosol: 55 mcg/metered spray

INDICATIONS & DOSAGE
Corticosteroid-dependent asthma
Adults: 2 inhalations t.i.d. or q.i.d. Maximum dosage, 16 inhalations daily.
Rhinitis, allergic disorders, inflammatory conditions, nasal polyps
Adults: 2 sprays in each nostril daily; may increase dosage to maximum of 4 sprays per nostril daily, if needed.

PHARMACODYNAMICS
Anti-inflammatory and antasthmatic actions: Glucocorticoids stimulate the synthesis of enzymes needed to decrease the inflammatory response. Triamcinolone acetonide is used as an oral inhalant to treat bronchial asthma in patients who require corticosteroids to control symptoms.

PHARMACOKINETICS
Absorption: Systemic absorption from the lungs is similar to oral administration; levels peak in 1 to 2 hours.
Distribution: After oral inhalation, 10% to 25% of triamcinolone is distributed to the lungs; rest is swallowed or deposited within the mouth. After nasal use, only a small amount reaches systemic circulation.
Metabolism: Drug is metabolized mainly in the liver; some that reaches the lungs may be metabolized locally.
Excretion: The major portion of dose is eliminated in feces; biologic half-life is 18 to 36 hours.

CONTRAINDICATIONS & PRECAUTIONS
Oral form is contraindicated in patients hypersensitive to a component of the formulation and in those with status asthmaticus. Nasal form is contraindicated in patients with hypersensitivity or untreated localized infections.
  Use oral form cautiously in patients with tuberculosis of the respiratory tract; untreated fungal, bacterial, or systemic viral infections; or ocular herpes simplex and in those receiving corticosteroids.

INTERACTIONS
None reported.

ADVERSE REACTIONS
Most adverse reactions to corticosteroids are dose- or duration-dependent.
EENT: dry or irritated nose or throat, hoarseness, *oral candidiasis,* dry or irritated tongue or mouth.
Respiratory: cough, wheezing (with oral form).
Other: facial edema (with oral form).

▣ KEY CONSIDERATIONS
• Recommendations for use of triamcinolone and for care and teaching of patients during therapy are the same as those for all inhalant adrenocorticoids.

Reactions may be *common*, uncommon, **life-threatening**, or COMMON AND LIFE-THREATENING.

• When excessive doses are used, signs and symptoms of hyperadrenocorticism and adrenal axis suppression may occur; drug should be discontinued slowly.

Patient education

• Urge patient to read the patient instruction sheet contained in each package before using triamcinolone for the first time.

• To instill, instruct patient to shake container before use; blow nose to clear nasal passages; and tilt his head slightly forward and insert nozzle into nostril, pointing away from the septum. Tell him to hold the other nostril closed and then inhale gently and spray. Next, have patient shake container and repeat procedure in other nostril.

• Tell patient to discard the canister after 100 actuations.

• Stress importance of using drug on a regular schedule because its effectiveness depends on regular use. However, caution patient not to exceed the prescribed dosage because serious adverse reactions may occur.

• Tell patient to notify health care provider if symptoms don't diminish within 2 to 3 weeks or if condition worsens.

• Warn patient to avoid exposure to chickenpox or measles and, if exposed to either, to notify his health care provider.

• Instruct patient to watch for signs and symptoms of nasal infection. If they occur, tell him to notify health care provider because drug may need to be discontinued and appropriate local therapy given.

• Instruct patient to rinse mouth or gargle after inhaler use.

triamcinolone acetonide (topical)
Aristocort, Flutex, Kenalog, Kenalog in Orabase, Triacet, Triaderm*

Topical adrenocorticoid, anti-inflammatory

Available by prescription only
Cream, ointment: 0.025%, 0.1%, 0.5%
Lotion: 0.025%, 0.1%
Paste: 0.1%

INDICATIONS & DOSAGE
Inflammation of corticosteroid-responsive dermatoses
Adults: Apply cream, ointment, or lotion sparingly one to four times daily. Apply paste to oral lesions by pressing a small amount into lesion without rubbing until thin film develops. Apply b.i.d. or t.i.d. after meals and h.s.

PHARMACODYNAMICS
Anti-inflammatory action: Glucocorticoids stimulate the synthesis of enzymes needed to decrease the inflammatory response. Triamcinolone is a synthetic fluorinated corticosteroid. The 0.5% cream and ointment are recommended only for dermatoses refractory to treatment with lower levels.

PHARMACOKINETICS
Absorption: Triamcinolone absorption depends on potency of preparation, amount applied, and nature of skin at application site. It ranges from about 1% in areas with a thick stratum corneum (such as the palms, soles, elbows, and knees) to as high as 36% in areas of the thinnest stratum corneum (face, eyelids, and genitals). Absorption increases in areas of skin damage, inflammation, or occlusion. Some systemic absorption of corticosteroids occurs, especially through the oral mucosa.
Distribution: After topical application, drug is distributed throughout the local skin layer. Drug absorbed into circulation is rapidly distributed into muscle, liver, skin, intestines, and kidneys.
Metabolism: After topical administration, drug is metabolized primarily in the skin. The small amount absorbed into systemic circulation is metabolized primarily in the liver to inactive compounds.
Excretion: Inactive metabolites are excreted by the kidneys, primarily as glucuronides and sulfates, but also as unconjugated products. A small amount of metabolites is also excreted in feces.

CONTRAINDICATIONS & PRECAUTIONS
Contraindicated in patients hypersensitive to triamcinolone.

INTERACTIONS
None reported.

ADVERSE REACTIONS
Metabolic: hyperglycemia, glycosuria.
Skin: burning, pruritus, irritation, dryness, erythema, folliculitis, hypertrichosis, hypopigmentation, acneiform eruptions, perioral dermatitis, allergic contact dermatitis, *maceration, secondary infection, atrophy, striae, miliaria* (with occlusive dressings).
Other: *hypothalamic-pituitary-adrenal axis suppression,* Cushing's syndrome.

▣ KEY CONSIDERATIONS
• Recommendations for use of triamcinolone, for care and teaching of patients during therapy, and for use in geriatric patients are the same as those for all topical adrenocorticoids.
• Don't apply near eyes or in ear canal.
• Stop drug if skin infection, striae, or atrophy occurs.
• For patients taking antifungals or antibiotics, stop corticosteroid therapy until infection is controlled.
• Systemic absorption is likely with the use of occlusive dressings, prolonged treatment, or extensive body surface treatment. Watch for symptoms.

Patient teaching
• Teach patient or family member how to apply triamcinolone. Gently wash skin before applying. To avoid skin damage, rub drug in gently, leaving a thin coat. When treating hairy sites, part hair and apply directly to lesions.
• If an occlusive dressing is to be used, advise patient not to leave it in place longer than 12 hours each day and not to use occlusive dressings on infected or exudative lesions.
• Tell patient to stop drug and report signs of systemic absorption, skin irritation or ulceration, hypersensitivity, infection, or no improvement.

triamterene
Dyrenium

Potassium sparing diuretic

Available by prescription only
Capsules: 50 mg, 100 mg

INDICATIONS & DOSAGE
Edema
Adults: Initially, 100 mg P.O. b.i.d. after meals. Total daily dose shouldn't exceed 300 mg.

PHARMACODYNAMICS
Diuretic action: Triamterene acts directly on the distal renal tubules to inhibit sodium reabsorption and potassium excretion, reducing the potassium loss associated with other diuretic therapy.

Triamterene is commonly used with other more effective diuretics to treat edema associated with excessive aldosterone secretion, hepatic cirrhosis, nephrotic syndrome, and heart failure.

PHARMACOKINETICS
Absorption: Triamterene is absorbed rapidly after oral administration, but the extent varies. Diuresis usually begins in 2 to 4 hours. Diuretic effect may be delayed 2 to 3 days if used alone; maximum antihypertensive effect may be delayed 2 to 3 weeks.
Distribution: Drug is about 67% protein-bound.
Metabolism: Drug is metabolized by hydroxylation and sulfation.
Excretion: Drug and its metabolites are excreted in urine; half-life of drug is 100 to 150 minutes.

CONTRAINDICATIONS & PRECAUTIONS
Contraindicated in patients receiving other potassium sparing drugs, such as spirolactone or amiloride hydrochloride, and in those with hypersensitivity to triamterene, anuria, severe or progressive renal disease or dysfunction, severe hepatic disease, or hyperkalemia.

Use cautiously in patients with impaired hepatic function or diabetes mellitus and in geriatric or debilitated patients.

Reactions may be *common*, uncommon, **life-threatening**, or COMMON AND LIFE-THREATENING.

INTERACTIONS

Drug-drug. Triamterene increases the hazard of hyperkalemia when administered with *ACE inhibitors (captopril, enalapril), other potassium sparing diuretics, potassium supplements,* and *potassium-containing drugs (parenteral penicillin G).* Use with *amantadine* has increased risk of amantadine toxicity. *Cimetidine* may increase the bioavailability of triamterene and decrease its renal clearance and hydroxylation. Diuretics may decrease *lithium* clearance. *NSAIDs* such as *ibuprofen* or *indomethacin* may alter renal function and thus affect potassium excretion. Triamterene may potentiate the hypotensive effects of *other antihypertensives;* this may be used to therapeutic advantage.
Drug-food. *Potassium-containing salt substitutes* and *potassium-rich foods* may contribute to an increased risk of hyperkalemia.
Drug-lifestyle. *Sun exposure* may cause photosensitivity reactions to occur.

ADVERSE REACTIONS

CNS: dizziness, weakness, fatigue, headache.
CV: hypotension.
GI: dry mouth, nausea, vomiting, diarrhea.
GU: transient elevation in BUN or creatinine levels, interstitial nephritis.
Hematologic: megaloblastic anemia related to low folic acid levels, ***thrombocytopenia.***
Hepatic: jaundice, abnormal liver enzyme levels.
Metabolic: *hyperkalemia,* acidosis, hypokalemia, azotemia.
Musculoskeletal: muscle cramps.
Skin: photosensitivity, rash.
Other: *anaphylaxis.*

▣ KEY CONSIDERATIONS

• Recommendations for the use of triamterene and for the care and teaching of the patient during therapy are the same as those for all potassium sparing diuretics.
• Geriatric and debilitated patients require close observation because they're more susceptible to drug-induced diuresis and hyperkalemia; reduced dosages may be indicated.
• Drug therapy may interfere with enzyme assays that use fluorometry, such as serum quinidine levels.

Patient education

• Advise patient to avoid prolonged sun exposure, wear protective clothing, and use a sunblock to prevent photosensitivity reactions.
• Tell patient that triamterene may be taken with meals if GI upset occurs.
• Tell patient to notify health care provider if weakness, sore throat, headache, fever, bruising, bleeding, mouth sores, nausea, vomiting, or dry mouth occur or become severe.
• If a single daily dose is prescribed, instruct patient to take it in the morning to prevent nocturia.
• Warn patient to avoid excessive ingestion of potassium-rich foods (such as citrus fruits, tomatoes, bananas, dates, and apricots), potassium-containing salt substitutes, and potassium supplements to prevent serious hyperkalemia.
• Tell patient urine may turn blue.

Overdose & treatment

• Signs and symptoms of overdose include those indicative of dehydration and electrolyte disturbance.
• Treatment is supportive and symptomatic. For recent ingestion (less than 4 hours), induce vomiting or perform gastric lavage. In severe hyperkalemia (more than 6.5 mEq/L), reduce serum potassium levels with I.V. sodium bicarbonate or glucose with insulin. A cation-exchange resin, sodium polystyrene sulfonate, given orally or as a retention enema may also reduce serum potassium levels.

triazolam
Halcion

Benzodiazepine, sedative-hypnotic
Controlled substance schedule IV

Available by prescription only
Tablets: 0.125 mg, 0.25 mg

INDICATIONS & DOSAGE
Insomnia
Adults: 0.125 to 0.25 mg P.O. h.s.
(0.5 mg P.O. h.s. only in exceptional patients; maximum dose, 0.5 mg).
Geriatric patients: 0.125 mg P.O. h.s.
May give up to 0.25 mg.

PHARMACODYNAMICS
Sedative-hypnotic action: Triazolam depresses the CNS at the limbic and subcortical levels of the brain. It produces a sedative-hypnotic effect by potentiating the effect of the neurotransmitter gamma-aminobutyric acid on its receptor in the ascending reticular activating system, which increases inhibition and blocks both cortical and limbic arousal.

PHARMACOKINETICS
Absorption: Triazolam is well absorbed through the GI tract after oral administration; levels peak in 1 to 2 hours, onset of action at 15 to 30 minutes.
Distribution: Drug is distributed widely throughout the body; 90% protein-bound.
Metabolism: Drug is metabolized in the liver primarily to inactive metabolites.
Excretion: Metabolites of triazolam are excreted in urine. Half-life of triazolam ranges from 1½ to 5½ hours.

CONTRAINDICATIONS & PRECAUTIONS
Contraindicated in patients with hypersensitivity to benzodiazepines. Also, contraindicated in patients taking ketoconazole, itraconazole, nefazodone, or other drugs that impair the oxidative metabolism of triazolam by cytochrome P-450 3A.

Use cautiously in patients with impaired renal or hepatic function, chronic pulmonary insufficiency, sleep apnea, mental depression, suicidal tendencies, or history of drug abuse.

INTERACTIONS
Drug-drug. Triazolam potentiates the CNS depressant effects of *antidepressants, antihistamines, barbiturates, general anesthetics, MAO inhibitors, narcotics,* and *phenothiazines.* Use with *cimetidine, isoniazid,* and possibly *disulfiram* causes diminished hepatic metabolism of triazolam, which increases its plasma level. *Erythromycin* decreases clearance of triazolam. Triazolam may decrease serum levels of *haloperidol.* Benzodiazepines may decrease the therapeutic effects of *levodopa.*
Drug-food. *Grapefruit juice* increases triazolam levels.
Drug-lifestyle. *Alcohol* potentiates the CNS depressant effects of triazolam; even a small amount of alcohol will enhance amnestic effects. *Heavy smoking* accelerates triazolam metabolism, thus reducing effectiveness.

ADVERSE REACTIONS
CNS: *drowsiness, dizziness, headache,* rebound insomnia, amnesia, lightheadedness, incoordination, mental confusion, depression, nervousness, ataxia, minor changes in EEG patterns.
GI: nausea, vomiting.
Hepatic: elevated liver function test results.
Other: physical or psychological dependence.

▣ KEY CONSIDERATIONS
Besides the recommendations relevant to all benzodiazepines, consider the following:
• Geriatric patients are more susceptible to CNS depressant effects of triazolam. Use with caution.
• Lower doses are usually effective in geriatric patients because of decreased elimination.
• Geriatric patients who receive drug require supervision with ambulation and activities of daily living during initiation of therapy or after an increase in dose.
• Monitor hepatic function studies to prevent toxicity.
• Onset of sedation or hypnosis is rapid; patient should be in bed when taking drug.
• Store in a cool, dry place away from light.

Patient education
• Instruct patient not to take OTC drugs or to change triazolam regimen without medical approval.

Reactions may be *common,* uncommon, *life-threatening*, or COMMON AND LIFE-THREATENING.

• As necessary, teach safety measures to prevent injury, such as gradual position changes.

• Suggest other measures to promote sleep, such as drinking warm fluids, listening to quiet music, not drinking alcohol near bedtime, exercising regularly, and maintaining a regular sleep pattern.

• Advise patient that rebound insomnia may occur after stopping drug.

• To prevent falls, encourage safety precautions at start of therapy.

• Advise patient of the potential for physical and psychological dependence.

• Advise patient not to take drug when a full night's sleep and clearance of the drug from the body is not possible before normal daily activities resume.

Overdose & treatment

• Signs and symptoms of overdose include somnolence, confusion, hypoactive reflexes, dyspnea, labored breathing, hypotension, bradycardia, slurred speech, unsteady gait or impaired coordination, and ultimately coma.

• Support blood pressure and respirations until drug effects subside; monitor vital signs. Flumazenil, a specific benzodiazepine antagonist, may be useful. Mechanical ventilatory assistance by endotracheal tube may be required to maintain a patent airway and support adequate oxygenation. Use I.V. fluids and vasopressors such as dopamine and phenylephrine to treat hypotension as needed. If patient is conscious, induce vomiting; perform gastric lavage if ingestion was recent, but only if an endotracheal tube is present to prevent aspiration. Then, administer activated charcoal with a cathartic as a single dose. Don't use barbiturates if excitation occurs. Dialysis is of limited value.

trifluoperazine hydrochloride
Apo-Trifluoperazine,* Novo-Flurazine,* Solazine,* Stelazine, Terfluzine*

Phenothiazine (piperazine derivative), antipsychotic drug, antiemetic

Available by prescription only
Tablets (regular and film-coated): 1 mg, 2 mg, 5 mg, 10 mg
Oral concentrate: 10 mg/ml
Injection: 2 mg/ml

INDICATIONS & DOSAGE
Anxiety states
Adults: 1 to 2 mg P.O. b.i.d. Increase dosage p.r.n., but don't exceed 6 mg/day.
Schizophrenia and other psychotic disorders
Adults: For outpatients, 1 to 2 mg P.O. b.i.d., increased p.r.n. For hospitalized patients, 2 to 5 mg P.O. b.i.d., may increase gradually to 40 mg daily. For I.M. injection, 1 to 2 mg q 4 to 6 hours, p.r.n.

PHARMACODYNAMICS
Antipsychotic and antiemetic actions: Trifluoperazine is thought to act by postsynaptic blockade of CNS dopamine receptors, thereby inhibiting dopamine-mediated effects; antiemetic effects are attributed to dopamine receptor blockade in the medullary chemoreceptor trigger zone. Drug has many other central and peripheral effects; it produces alpha and ganglionic blockade and counteracts histamine- and serotonin-mediated activity. Its most common adverse effects are extrapyramidal; it has less sedative and autonomic activity than aliphatic and piperidine phenothiazines.

PHARMACOKINETICS
Absorption: Rate and extent of absorption vary with route of administration: Oral tablet absorption is erratic and variable; onset of action ranges from ½ to 1 hour, oral concentrate absorption is much more predictable. I.M. drug is absorbed rapidly.
Distribution: Trifluoperazine is distributed widely in the body. Drug is 91% to

99% protein-bound. Effect peaks in 2 to 4 hours; serum levels reach steady state within 4 to 7 days.

Metabolism: Drug is metabolized extensively in the liver, but no active metabolites are formed; duration of action is 4 to 6 hours.

Excretion: Drug is mostly excreted in urine from the kidneys; some excreted in feces from the biliary tract.

CONTRAINDICATIONS & PRECAUTIONS
Contraindicated in patients with hypersensitivity to phenothiazines or in patients experiencing coma, CNS depression, bone marrow suppression, or liver damage.

Use cautiously in geriatric or debilitated patients; in those exposed to extreme heat; and in patients with CV disease, seizure disorders, glaucoma, or prostatic hyperplasia.

INTERACTIONS
Drug-drug. Pharmacokinetic alterations and subsequent decreased therapeutic response to trifluoperazine may follow use with *aluminum-* or *magnesium-containing antacids* or *antidiarrheals* (decreased absorption) or *phenobarbital* (enhanced renal excretion).

Additive effects are likely after use with *antiarrhythmics, disopyramide, procainamide,* or *quinidine* (increased incidence of cardiac arrhythmias and conduction defects); *atropine* or *other anticholinergics,* including *antidepressants, antihistamines, antiparkinsonians* (oversedation, paralytic ileus, visual changes, and severe constipation); *MAO inhibitors, meperidine,* and *phenothiazines; CNS depressants,* including *analgesics, barbiturates, narcotics, tranquilizers, anesthetics (epidural, general, and spinal),* and *parenteral magnesium sulfate* (oversedation, respiratory depression, and hypotension); *metrizamide* (increased risk of seizures); and *nitrates* (hypotension).

Use with *appetite suppressants* or *sympathomimetics*—including *ephedrine* (found in many nasal sprays), *epinephrine, phenylephrine,* and *phenylpropanolamine*—may decrease their stimulatory and pressor effects. *Beta blockers* may

inhibit trifluoperazine metabolism, increasing plasma levels and toxic effects. Trifluoperazine may antagonize therapeutic effect of *bromocriptine* on prolactin secretion; it also may decrease the vasoconstrictive effects of *high-dose dopamine* and may decrease effectiveness and increase toxic effects of *levodopa* (by dopamine blockade). Trifluoperazine may inhibit blood pressure response to *centrally acting antihypertensives,* such as *clonidine, guanabenz, guanadrel, guanethidine, methyldopa,* and *reserpine.* Using *epinephrine* as a pressor drug in patients taking trifluoperazine may result in epinephrine reversal or further lowering of blood pressure. Use with *lithium* may result in severe neurologic toxicity with an encephalitis-like syndrome and in decreased therapeutic response to trifluoperazine; use with *propylthiouracil* increases risk of agranulocytosis. Trifluoperazine may inhibit metabolism and increase toxic effects of *phenytoin.*

Drug-food. *Caffeine* increases the metabolism of the drug and therefore decreases therapeutic effects.

Drug-lifestyle. *Alcohol use* causes additive effects when used with trifluoperazine. *Heavy smoking* increases metabolism of drug and therefore decreased therapeutic effects. *Sun exposure* leads to increased photosensitivity reactions.

ADVERSE REACTIONS
CNS: *extrapyramidal reactions, tardive dyskinesia,* pseudoparkinsonism, dizziness, drowsiness, insomnia, fatigue, headache.

CV: *orthostatic hypotension,* tachycardia, ECG changes.

EENT: ocular changes, *blurred vision.*

GI: *dry mouth, constipation,* nausea.

GU: *urine retention,* gynecomastia.

Hematologic: *transient leukopenia, agranulocytosis.*

Hepatic: cholestatic jaundice, elevated liver function test results.

Metabolic: weight gain.

Skin: *photosensitivity,* allergic reactions, sterile abscess, rash.

Other: elevated protein-bound iodine levels, pain at I.M. injection site.

Reactions may be *common*, uncommon, *life-threatening*, or COMMON AND LIFE-THREATENING.

After abrupt withdrawal of long-term therapy: gastritis, nausea, vomiting, dizziness, tremor, feeling of warmth or cold, diaphoresis, tachycardia, headache, insomnia, anorexia, muscle rigidity, altered mental status, and evidence of autonomic instability.

▣ KEY CONSIDERATIONS

Besides the recommendations relevant to all phenothiazines, consider the following:

• Geriatric patients tend to require lower doses, adjusted to effect. Adverse effects, especially tardive dyskinesia and other extrapyramidal effects and hypotension, are more likely to develop in such patients.

• Other drugs, such as benzodiazepines, are preferred for the treatment of anxiety. When drug is given for anxiety, don't exceed 6 mg daily for longer than 12 weeks. Some health care providers recommend using trifluoperazine only for psychosis.

• Administer I.M. injection deep in the outer upper quadrant of the buttock. Massaging the area after administration may prevent formation of abscesses. I.M. injection may cause skin necrosis; don't extravasate.

• Solution for injection may be slightly discolored. Don't use if excessively discolored or a precipitate is evident. Contact pharmacist.

• Monitor blood pressure before and after parenteral administration.

• Shake concentrate before administration.

• Chewing sugarless gum or hard candy or ice may help relieve dry mouth.

• Worsening anginal pain has been reported in patients receiving drug; however, ECG reactions are less common than with other phenothiazines.

• Liquid and injectable formulations may cause a rash after contact with skin.

• Drug may cause pink to brown discoloration of urine or blue-gray discoloration of skin.

• Drug commonly causes extrapyramidal symptoms and photosensitivity reactions; patient should avoid exposure to sunlight or heat lamps.

• Monitor regularly for abnormal body movements (at least every 6 months).

• Oral formulations may upset stomach; administer with food or fluid.

• Concentrate must be diluted in 2 to 4 oz (60 to 120 ml) liquid—preferably water, carbonated drinks, fruit juice, tomato juice, or milk—or pudding.

• Protect liquid formulation from light.

• Drug causes false-positive test results for urine porphyrins, urobilinogen, amylase, and 5-hydroxyindoleacetic acid levels from darkening of urine by metabolites.

Patient education

• Explain risks of dystonic reactions, akathisia, and tardive dyskinesia, and tell patient to report abnormal body movements.

• Explain that many drug interactions are possible. Tell patient to seek medical approval before taking any nonprescribed drug.

• Tell patient that dosage reduction may alleviate adverse reactions. Instruct him to report difficulty urinating, sore throat, dizziness, or fainting; male patients should be warned about inhibited ejaculation.

• Warn patient against hazardous activities that require alertness until the effect of trifluoperazine is established; reassure patient that sedative effects usually subside in several weeks.

• Tell patient to avoid sun exposure and wear sunscreen when going outdoors to prevent photosensitivity reactions. (Explain that heat lamps and tanning beds also may cause burning of the skin or skin discoloration.)

• Warn patient to avoid extremely hot or cold baths and exposure to temperature extremes, sunlamps, and tanning beds; drug may cause thermoregulatory changes.

• Tell patient to take drug exactly as prescribed and to avoid double dosing for missed doses, taking drug abruptly, or sharing drug with others.

• Advise patient to store drug in a safe place, away from children.

• Tell patient to avoid alcohol and other drugs that may cause excessive sedation.

• Inform patient that sugarless candy or gum, ice chips, or artificial saliva may relieve dry mouth.

Overdose & treatment
• CNS depression is characterized by deep sleep (in which the patient can't be aroused) and possible coma, hypotension or hypertension, extrapyramidal symptoms, dystonia, abnormal involuntary muscle movements, agitation, seizures, arrhythmias, ECG changes, hypothermia or hyperthermia, and autonomic nervous system dysfunction.
• Treatment is symptomatic and supportive and includes maintaining vital signs, airway, stable body temperature, and fluid and electrolyte balance. Don't induce vomiting: trifluoperazine inhibits cough reflex, and aspiration may occur. Perform gastric lavage, then administer activated charcoal and sodium chloride cathartics; dialysis is usually ineffective. Regulate body temperature as needed. Treat hypotension with I.V. fluids. Don't give epinephrine. Treat seizures with parenteral diazepam or barbiturates; arrhythmias with 1 mg/kg of parenteral phenytoin, with rate titrated to blood pressure; and extrapyramidal reactions with 1 to 2 mg of benztropine or 10 to 50 mg of parenteral diphenhydramine.

trihexyphenidyl hydrochloride
Apo-Trihex,* Artane, Artane Sequels, Trihexy-2, Trihexy-5

Anticholinergic, antiparkinsonian

Available by prescription only
Tablets: 2 mg, 5 mg
Capsules (sustained-release): 5 mg
Elixir: 2 mg/5 ml

INDICATIONS & DOSAGE
Idiopathic parkinsonism
Adults: 1 mg P.O. on first day, 2 mg on 2nd day, then increase by 2 mg q 3 to 5 days until 6 to 10 mg is given daily. Usually given t.i.d. with meals and, if needed, q.i.d. (last dose should be before bedtime). Postencephalitic parkinsonism may require 12 to 15 mg total daily dose.

Patients receiving levodopa may need 3 to 6 mg daily. Sustained-release capsules shouldn't be used as initial therapy, but after the patient's condition has been stabilized on the conventional dosage forms. Sustained-release capsules can be dosed on a milligram-per-milligram of total daily dose and administered as a single dose after breakfast or in two divided doses 12 hours apart.
Drug-induced parkinsonism
Adults: 5 to 15 mg daily.

PHARMACODYNAMICS
Antiparkinsonian action: Trihexyphenidyl blocks central cholinergic receptors, helping to balance cholinergic activity in the basal ganglia. It may also prolong the effects of dopamine by blocking dopamine reuptake and storage at central receptor sites.

PHARMACOKINETICS
Absorption: Trihexyphenidyl is rapidly absorbed after oral administration; onset of action is within 1 hour.
Distribution: Drug crosses the blood-brain barrier; little else is known about its distribution.
Metabolism: Exact metabolic fate is unknown. Duration of effect is 6 to 12 hours.
Excretion: Excreted in the urine as unchanged drug and metabolites.

CONTRAINDICATIONS & PRECAUTIONS
Contraindicated in patients hypersensitive to trihexyphenidyl.

Use cautiously in patients with impaired renal, cardiac, or hepatic function; glaucoma; obstructive disease of the GI or GU tract; or prostatic hyperplasia.

INTERACTIONS
Drug-drug. Use with *amantadine* may amplify anticholinergic adverse effects of trihexyphenidyl, causing confusion and hallucinations. *Antacids* and *antidiarrheals* may decrease absorption of trihexyphenidyl. Use with *CNS depressants* such as *sedative-hypnotics* and *tranquilizers* increases sedative effects of trihexyphenidyl. Use with *haloperidol* or *phenothiazines* may decrease the an-

tipsychotic effectiveness of these drugs, possibly from direct CNS antagonism; use with *phenothiazines* also increases the risk of anticholinergic adverse effects. When used with *levodopa,* dosage of both drugs may need adjustment because of synergistic anticholinergic effects and possible enhanced GI metabolism of *levodopa* from reduced gastric motility and delayed gastric emptying.
Drug-lifestyle. *Alcohol* use increases sedative effects of trihexyphenidyl.

ADVERSE REACTIONS
CNS: nervousness, dizziness, headache, hallucinations, drowsiness, weakness.
CV: tachycardia.
EENT: blurred vision, mydriasis, increased intraocular pressure.
GI: *dry mouth, nausea,* constipation, vomiting.
GU: urinary hesitancy, urine retention.

▣ KEY CONSIDERATIONS
Besides the recommendations relevant to all anticholinergics, consider the following:
• Use caution when administering trihexyphenidyl to geriatric patients; lower doses are indicated.
• Store drug in tight containers.
• Monitor patient for urinary hesitancy.
• Arrange for gonioscopic evaluation and close intraocular pressure monitoring, especially in patients older than age 40.
• Tolerance may develop to drug, necessitating higher doses.
• Use drug with caution in hot weather because of the increased risk of heat prostration.

Patient education
• Tell patient to avoid activities that require alertness until CNS effects of trihexyphenidyl are known.
• Advise patient to report signs of urinary hesitation or urine retention.
• Tell patient to relieve dry mouth with cool drinks, ice chips, sugarless gum, or hard candy.
• Tell patient to take drug with food if GI upset occurs.

Overdose & treatment
• Signs and symptoms of overdose include central stimulation followed by depression, with such psychotic symptoms as disorientation, confusion, hallucinations, delusions, anxiety, agitation, and restlessness. Peripheral effects may include dilated, nonreactive pupils; blurred vision; flushed, dry, hot skin; dry mucous membranes; dysphagia; decreased or absent bowel sounds; urine retention; hyperthermia; headache; tachycardia; hypertension; and increased respirations.
• Treatment is primarily symptomatic and supportive, as needed. Maintain patent airway. If patient is alert, induce vomiting (or perform gastric lavage) and follow with sodium chloride cathartic and activated charcoal to prevent further drug absorption. In severe cases, physostigmine may be administered to block antimuscarinic effects of trihexyphenidyl. Give fluids, as needed, to treat shock; diazepam to control psychotic symptoms; and pilocarpine (instilled into the eyes) to relieve mydriasis. If urine retention occurs, catheterization may be necessary.

trimethobenzamide hydrochloride
Arrestin, Stemetic, Tebamide, T-Gen, Ticon, Tigan, Tiject-20, Trimazide

Ethanolamine-related antihistamine, antiemetic

Available by prescription only
Capsules: 100 mg, 250 mg
Suppositories: 100 mg, 200 mg
Injection: 100 mg/ml

INDICATIONS & DOSAGE
Nausea and vomiting
Adults: 250 mg P.O. t.i.d. or q.i.d.; or 200 mg I.M. or P.R. t.i.d. or q.i.d.

PHARMACODYNAMICS
Antiemetic action: Trimethobenzamide is a weak antihistamine with limited antiemetic properties. Its exact mechanism of action is unknown. Drug effects may occur in the chemoreceptor trigger

zone of the brain; however, drug apparently doesn't inhibit direct impulses to the vomiting center.

PHARMACOKINETICS
Absorption: About 60% of oral dose is absorbed. After oral administration, action begins in 10 to 40 minutes; after I.M. administration, in 15 to 35 minutes.
Distribution: Unknown.
Metabolism: Some 50% to 70% of dose is metabolized, probably in the liver.
Excretion: Drug is excreted in urine and feces. After oral administration, duration of effect is 3 to 4 hours; after I.M. administration, 2 to 3 hours.

CONTRAINDICATIONS & PRECAUTIONS
Contraindicated in patients with hypersensitivity to trimethobenzamide. Suppositories are contraindicated in patients hypersensitive to benzocaine hydrochloride or similar local anesthetic.

INTERACTIONS
Drug-drug. *CNS depressants*—including *antihypertensives, belladonna alkaloids, phenothiazines,* and *tricyclic antidepressants*—may increase the toxic effects of trimethobenzamide.
Drug-lifestyle. *Alcohol* use may increase drug toxicity.

ADVERSE REACTIONS
CNS: *drowsiness,* dizziness (in large doses), headache, disorientation, depression, parkinsonian-like symptoms, ***coma, seizures.***
CV: hypotension.
EENT: blurred vision.
GI: diarrhea.
Hepatic: jaundice.
Musculoskeletal: muscle cramps.
Other: *hypersensitivity reactions* (pain, stinging, burning, redness, swelling at I.M. injection site).

▣ KEY CONSIDERATIONS
• Use trimethobenzamide with caution in geriatric patients because they may be more susceptible to adverse CNS effects.
• Give I.M. dose by deep injection into outer upper gluteal quadrant to minimize pain and local irritation.

• Record frequency and volume of vomiting; observe patient for signs and symptoms of dehydration.
• Drug may be less effective against severe vomiting than other drugs.
• Drug has little or no value in treating motion sickness.

Patient education
• Warn patient to avoid hazardous activities that require alertness because trimethobenzamide may cause drowsiness, and to avoid consuming alcohol to prevent additive sedation.
• Instruct patient to report persistent vomiting.
• Instruct patient using suppositories to remove foil and, if necessary, moisten suppository with water for 10 to 30 seconds before inserting; tell patient to store suppositories in refrigerator.

Overdose & treatment
• Signs and symptoms of overdose may include severe neurologic reactions, such as opisthotonos, seizures, coma, and extrapyramidal reactions.
• Discontinue trimethobenzamide and provide supportive care.

---

trimethoprim
Proloprim, Trimpex

Synthetic folate antagonist, antibiotic

Available by prescription only
Tablets: 100 mg, 200 mg

INDICATIONS & DOSAGE
Treatment of uncomplicated urinary tract infections
Adults: 100 mg P.O. q 12 hours or 200 mg q 24 hours for 10 days.
◊ ***Prophylaxis of chronic and recurrent urinary tract infections***
Adults: 100 mg P.O. h.s. for 6 weeks to 6 months.
◊ ***Traveler's diarrhea***
Adults: 200 mg P.O. b.i.d. for 3 to 5 days.

◊ **Pneumocystis carinii**
Adults: 20 mg/kg P.O. in four divided doses in conjunction with dapsone, 100 mg daily for 21 days.
✦ *Dosage adjustment.* If creatinine clearance is 15 to 30 ml/minute, give 50 mg q 12 hours. If creatinine clearance is less than 15 ml/minute, the drug manufacturer doesn't recommend using trimethoprim.

PHARMACODYNAMICS
Antibacterial action: Trimethoprim is usually bactericidal. It interferes with the action of dihydrofolate reductase, thus inhibiting bacterial synthesis of folic acid. Drug is effective against many gram-positive and gram-negative organisms, including most Enterobacteriaceae organisms (except *Pseudomonas*), *Proteus mirabilis, Klebsiella,* and *Escherichia coli.*

PHARMACOKINETICS
Absorption: Trimethoprim is absorbed quickly and completely; serum levels peak in 1 to 4 hours.
Distribution: Drug is widely distributed; 42% to 46% of dose binds to plasma protein.
Metabolism: Less than 20% of dose is metabolized in the liver.
Excretion: Most of dose is excreted in urine through filtration and secretion. In patients with normal renal function, elimination half-life is 8 to 11 hours; in patients with impaired renal function, half-life is prolonged.

CONTRAINDICATIONS & PRECAUTIONS
Contraindicated in patients with hypersensitivity to trimethoprim and in those with documented megaloblastic anemia caused by folate deficiency.
Use cautiously in patients with folate deficiency and impaired hepatic or renal function (especially those with creatinine clearance of 15 ml/minute or less).

INTERACTIONS
Drug-drug. Trimethoprim may inhibit *phenytoin* metabolism, causing increased serum phenytoin levels.

ADVERSE REACTIONS
GI: *epigastric distress, nausea, vomiting,* glossitis.
GU: increased BUN and serum creatinine levels.
Hematologic: *thrombocytopenia, leukopenia,* megaloblastic anemia, methemoglobinemia.
Hepatic: elevated liver enzyme levels.
Skin: *rash, pruritus,* exfoliative dermatitis.
Other: fever.

▣ KEY CONSIDERATIONS
• Geriatric patients may be more susceptible to hematologic toxicity.
• Obtain specimen for culture and sensitivity tests before starting therapy.
• Trimethoprim is usually used with other antibiotics (especially sulfamethoxazole) because resistance develops rapidly when used alone.
• If patient is receiving phenytoin, monitor serum phenytoin levels.
• Advanced age, malnourishment, debilitation, renal impairment, and prolonged high-dose therapy increase risk of hematologic toxicity, as does therapy with folate antagonistic drugs (such as phenytoin).
• Sore throat, fever, pallor, and purpura may be early signs and symptoms of serious blood disorders. Monitor blood counts regularly.

Patient education
• Instruct patient to continue taking trimethoprim as directed until it's completed, even if feeling better.
• Advise patient to report signs or symptoms of blood disorders (sore throat, fever, pallor, and purpura) immediately.

Overdose & treatment
• Signs and symptoms of acute overdose include nausea, vomiting, dizziness, headache, confusion, and bone marrow depression. Signs and symptoms of chronic toxicity caused by prolonged high-dose therapy include bone marrow depression, leukopenia, thrombocytopenia, and megaloblastic anemia.
• Treatment of acute overdose includes gastric lavage and supportive measures. Urine may be acidified to enhance drug

elimination. Treatment of chronic toxicity includes discontinuing drug and administering 3 to 6 mg of leucovorin I.M. daily for 3 days or 5 to 15 mg P.O. daily until normal hematopoiesis returns.

trimipramine maleate
Surmontil

Tricyclic antidepressant, anxiolytic

Available by prescription only
Capsules: 25 mg, 50 mg, 100 mg

INDICATIONS & DOSAGE
Depression
Adults: For outpatients, give 75 mg/day in divided doses and increase to 200 mg/day; maintenance dosage, 50 to 150 mg/day. Dosage for inpatients is 100 mg/day in divided doses and increased p.r.n. Maximum daily dose is 300 mg.
Geriatric patients: 50 to 100 mg/day.

PHARMACODYNAMICS
Antidepressant action: Trimipramine is thought to exert its antidepressant effects by equally inhibiting reuptake of norepinephrine and serotonin in CNS nerve terminals (presynaptic neurons), which results in increased level and enhanced activity of these neurotransmitters in the synaptic cleft. Trimipramine also has anxiolytic effects and inhibits gastric acid secretion.

PHARMACOKINETICS
Absorption: Trimipramine is absorbed rapidly from the GI tract after oral administration.
Distribution: Drug is distributed widely in the body; 90% binds to protein. Effect peaks in 2 hours; drug reaches steady state within 7 days.
Metabolism: Drug is metabolized in the liver; a significant first-pass effect may explain variability of serum levels in different patients taking the same dosage.
Excretion: Drug is mostly excreted in urine; some excreted in feces via the biliary tract.

CONTRAINDICATIONS & PRECAUTIONS
Contraindicated during acute recovery phase of an MI, in patients with hypersensitivity to trimipramine, or in those receiving MAO inhibitor therapy within 14 days.
  Use cautiously in geriatric or debilitated patients; in those receiving thyroid drugs; and in those with CV disease, increased intraocular pressure, hyperthyroidism, impaired hepatic function, or history of seizures, urine retention, or angle-closure glaucoma.

INTERACTIONS
Drug-drug. Use with *antiarrhythmics (disopyramide, procainamide, quinidine), pimozide,* or *thyroid drugs* may increase incidence of cardiac arrhythmias and conduction defects. Additive effects are likely after use with *atropine* or *other anticholinergics,* including *antihistamines, antiparkinsonians, meperidine,* or *phenothiazines* (oversedation, paralytic ileus, visual changes, and severe constipation); *CNS depressants,* including *analgesics, anesthetics, barbiturates, narcotics,* or *tranquilizers* (oversedation); or *metrizamide* (increased risk of seizures). *Barbiturates* induce trimipramine metabolism and decrease therapeutic efficacy; *beta blockers, cimetidine, methylphenidate,* and *propoxyphene* may inhibit trimipramine metabolism, increasing plasma levels and toxic effects; and *haloperidol* and *phenothiazines* decrease its metabolism, decreasing therapeutic efficacy. Trimipramine may decrease hypotensive effects of *centrally acting antihypertensives,* such as *clonidine, guanabenz, guanadrel, guanethidine, methyldopa,* and *reserpine.* Use with *disulfiram* or *ethchlorvynol* may cause delirium and tachycardia. *SSRIs (fluoxetine, paroxetine, sertraline)* increase the pharmacologic and toxic effects of trimipramine. Use of trimipramine with *sympathomimetics,* including *ephedrine* (found in many nasal sprays), *epinephrine, phenylephrine,* and *phenylpropanolamine,* may increase blood pressure; use with *warfarin* may increase PT and cause bleeding.

Reactions may be *common,* uncommon, *life-threatening,* OR COMMON AND LIFE-THREATENING.

Drug-lifestyle. Use with *alcohol* is likely to cause additive effects. *Heavy smoking* induces trimipramine metabolism and decreases therapeutic efficacy.

ADVERSE REACTIONS

CNS: *drowsiness, dizziness,* paresthesia, ataxia, hallucinations, delusions, anxiety, agitation, insomnia, tremor, weakness, confusion, headache, EEG changes, *seizures,* extrapyramidal reactions.
CV: *orthostatic hypotension,* tachycardia, hypertension, *ECG changes, arrhythmias, heart block, MI, stroke.*
EENT: *blurred vision,* tinnitus, mydriasis.
Hematologic: decreased WBC counts, altered PT.
Hepatic: elevated liver function test results.
GI: *dry mouth, constipation,* nausea, vomiting, anorexia, paralytic ileus.
GU: *urine retention.*
Metabolic: altered serum glucose levels.
Skin: rash, urticaria, *diaphoresis,* photosensitivity.
Other: *hypersensitivity reaction.*
After abrupt withdrawal of long-term therapy: nausea, headache, malaise (doesn't indicate addiction).

▣ KEY CONSIDERATIONS

Besides the recommendations relevant to all tricyclic antidepressants, consider the following:
● Recommended starting dose for geriatric patients is reduced because geriatric patients may be more vulnerable to adverse cardiac effects.
● Consider the inherent risk of suicide until significant improvement of depressive state occurs. Closely monitor high-risk patients during initial trimipramine therapy. To reduce risk of suicidal overdose, prescribe the smallest quantity of capsules consistent with good management.
● May give the full dosage at bedtime to offset daytime sedation.
● Drug also has been used to decrease gastric acid secretion in peptic ulcer disease. The safety and efficacy of drug in peptic ulcer disease hasn't been established.

● Watch for bleeding because drug may cause alterations in PT.
● Don't withdraw drug abruptly; however, it should be discontinued at least 48 hours before surgical procedures.
● Tolerance generally develops to the sedative effects of drug.
● Manic or hypomanic episodes may occur in some patients, especially those with cyclic-type disorders, when taking drug.

Patient education
● Advise patient to take full dosage at bedtime to minimize daytime sedation.
● Explain that full effects of trimipramine may not become apparent for up to 4 to 6 weeks after therapy begins.
● Tell patient to take drug exactly as prescribed and to avoid double dosing for missed doses, discontinuing the drug suddenly, and sharing drug with others.
● Warn patient that drug may cause drowsiness or dizziness and to avoid activities that require mental alertness until the full effects of drug are known.
● Warn patient not to drink alcoholic beverages or medicinal elixirs while taking drug.
● Tell patient to store drug safely away from children.
● Suggest taking drug with food or milk if it causes stomach upset and to ease dry mouth with sugarless chewing gum, hard candy, or ice.
● To prevent dizziness, advise patient to lie down for about 30 minutes after each dose and to avoid abrupt postural changes, especially when rising to an upright position.
● Tell patient to report adverse reactions promptly, especially confusion, movement disorders, rapid heartbeat, dizziness, fainting, or difficulty urinating.

Overdose & treatment
● The first 12 hours after acute ingestion are a stimulatory phase characterized by excessive anticholinergic activity (agitation, irritation, confusion, hallucinations, parkinsonian symptoms, seizure, urine retention, dry mucous membranes, pupillary dilation, constipation, and ileus). This is followed by CNS depressant effects, including hypothermia, de-

creased or absent reflexes, sedation, hypotension, cyanosis, and cardiac irregularities (including tachycardia, conduction disturbances, and quinidine-like effects on the ECG). Prolongation of QRS interval beyond 100 msec, which usually represents a serum level in excess of 1,000 ng/ml, best indicates severity of overdose; serum levels generally aren't helpful. Metabolic acidosis may follow hypotension, hypoventilation, and seizures.

• Treatment is symptomatic and supportive and includes maintaining airway, stable body temperature, and fluid and electrolyte balance. Induce vomiting with ipecac if patient is conscious; then perform gastric lavage and administer activated charcoal to prevent further absorption. Dialysis is of little use. Physostigmine given I.V. slowly has been used to reverse most of the CV and CNS effects of overdose. Treat seizures with parenteral diazepam or phenytoin; arrhythmias with parenteral phenytoin or lidocaine; and acidosis with sodium bicarbonate. Don't give barbiturates; these may enhance CNS and respiratory depressant effects.

---

troglitazone
Rezulin

Thiazolidinedione, antidiabetic

Available by prescription only
Tablets: 200 mg, 300 mg, 400 mg

INDICATIONS & DOSAGE

As monotherapy for patients with type 2 diabetes mellitus that can't be controlled with diet alone
Adults: Initially, 400 mg P.O. once daily; may increase to 600 mg after 1 month if needed. For patients not responding to 600 mg after 1 month, drug should be discontinued and alternative therapeutic options taken.

Combined with sulfonylureas in patients with type 2 diabetes mellitus
Adults: Initially, 200 mg P.O. once daily; continue current sulfonylurea dose. Increase dosage after 2 to 4 weeks p.r.n. to maximum dosage of 600 mg/day. Sulfonylurea dose may have to be reduced.

Adjunct to diet and insulin therapy in patients with type 2 diabetes mellitus that isn't adequately controlled
Adults: Initially, for patients using insulin, continue with current insulin dose and begin with 200 mg of troglitazone P.O. once daily, taken with a meal. Dosage may be increased after 2 to 4 weeks p.r.n. Usual daily dose is 400 mg; maximum recommended daily dose, 600 mg. Insulin dose may be decreased by 10% to 25% when fasting glucose levels are less than 120 mg/dl in patients receiving both troglitazone and insulin.

PHARMACODYNAMICS

Antidiabetic action: Troglitazone reduces blood glucose levels by improving target cell response to insulin, but action depends on insulin. Drug also decreases hepatic glucose output and increases insulin-dependent glucose disposal in skeletal muscle. Its mechanism of action is thought to involve binding to nuclear receptors that regulate the transcription of a number of insulin responsive genes critical for the control of glucose and lipid metabolism.

PHARMACOKINETICS

Absorption: Troglitazone is rapidly absorbed after oral administration; plasma levels peak within 2 to 3 hours. Food increases absorption from 30% to 85%. Plasma levels reach steady state in 3 to 5 days.
Distribution: Drug extensively binds (more than 99%) to serum albumin. Volume of distribution after multiple doses is 10.5 to 26.5 L/kg of body weight.
Metabolism: Drug is metabolized to three major metabolites.
Excretion: Drug is excreted as metabolites in feces (85%) and urine (3%); plasma elimination half-life is 16 to 34 hours.

CONTRAINDICATIONS & PRECAUTIONS
Contraindicated in patients with known hypersensitivity to troglitazone and in patients with type 1 diabetes mellitus or diabetic ketoacidosis.

Use cautiously in patients with hepatic disease and class III or IV cardiac status. Drug shouldn't be initiated in patients with ALT levels more than 1.5 times the upper limit of normal.

INTERACTIONS

Drug-drug. *Cholestyramine* reduces absorption of troglitazone by 70%; don't administer together. Troglitazone may induce drug metabolism by CYP 3A4 in *drugs metabolized by CYP 3A4 (calcium channel blockers, cisapride, corticosteroids, cyclosporine, 3-hydroxy-3-methylglutaryl coenzyme A reductase inhibitors, tacrolimus, triazolam, and trimetrexate).*

ADVERSE REACTIONS

CNS: asthenia, dizziness, *headache.*
CV: peripheral edema.
GI: diarrhea, nausea.
GU: urinary tract infection.
Hematologic: decreased hemoglobin level, hematocrit, and neutrophil count.
Hepatic: transient elevations in AST and ALT levels, *jaundice, hepatitis.*
Musculoskeletal: back pain.
Respiratory: pharyngitis, rhinitis.
Other: accidental injury, *death, infection, pain.*

▣ KEY CONSIDERATIONS

• Troglitazone doesn't stimulate insulin secretion; don't use to treat patients with type 1 diabetes mellitus or diabetic ketoacidosis.
• When used with insulin, monitor patient for hypoglycemia. Insulin dose may need to be reduced.
• Before starting therapy, investigate and address secondary causes of poor glycemic control (including infection and poor injection technique).
• Monitor glucose levels, especially during increased stress such as infection, fever, surgery, and trauma because insulin requirements may change.
• Monitor serum transaminase levels at baseline and every month for the first 8 months, then q 2 months for the remainder of the 1st year of drug therapy. Continue checking serum transaminase levels periodically thereafter.

• If patient has jaundice or ALT level increases to greater than three times the upper limit of normal, discontinue drug.
• Rare cases of severe idiosyncratic hepatocellular injury have been reported. The injury is usually reversible, but very rare cases of hepatic failure, including death, have been reported. Injury has occurred after both short- and long-term drug therapy.

Patient education

• Advise patient to report such signs or symptoms as nausea, vomiting, abdominal pain, fatigue, anorexia or dark urine that may indicate hepatitis or hepatic failure and require immediate attention.
• Instruct patient about nature of diabetes and the importance of following drug regimen and personal hygiene programs, avoiding infection, adhering to specific diet; reducing weight, and exercising. Explain how and when to self-monitor blood glucose level and teach signs and symptoms of hypoglycemia and hyperglycemia (and explain what to do if he experiences them). Include responsible family members in teaching.
• Tell patient that troglitazone should be taken with a meal. If a dose is missed, take it with the next meal. If a dose is missed, patient shouldn't double-dose on the next day.
• Instruct patient to carry medical identification at all times.

trovafloxacin mesylate
Trovan Tablets

alatrofloxacin mesylate
Trovan I.V.

Fluoroquinolone derivative, antibiotic

Available by prescription only
Tablets: 100 mg, 200 mg
Injection: 5 mg/ml in 40-ml (200 mg) and 60-ml (300 mg) vials

INDICATIONS & DOSAGE

For the treatment of infections caused by susceptible microorganisms, the following dosages are administered once q 24 hours:

Gynecologic and pelvic infections, complicated intra-abdominal and postsurgical infections
Adults: 300 mg I.V. daily followed by 200 mg P.O. daily for 7 to 14 days.

Nosocomial pneumonia
Adults: 300 mg I.V. daily followed by 200 mg P.O. daily for 10 to 14 days.

Community-acquired pneumonia
Adults: 200 mg P.O. or I.V. daily followed by 200 mg P.O. daily for 7 to 14 days.

Complicated skin and diabetic foot infections
Adults: 200 mg P.O. or I.V. daily followed by 200 mg P.O. daily for 10 to 14 days.

Surgical prophylaxis (colorectal, abdominal and vaginal hysterectomy)
Adults: 200 mg P.O. or I.V as a single dose 30 minutes to 4 hours before surgery.

Acute sinusitis, chronic prostatitis, cervicitis, and pelvic inflammatory disease (mild to moderate)
Adults: 200 mg P.O. daily for 5 days (cervicitis), 10 days (acute sinusitis), 14 days (pelvic inflammatory disease), or 28 days (chronic prostatitis).

Uncomplicated urinary tract infections, uncomplicated skin and soft-tissue infections, bacterial bronchitis, uncomplicated gonorrhea
Adults: 100 mg P.O. daily for 7 to 10 days (3 days for urinary tract infection, single dose for gonorrhea).

✦ ***Dosage adjustment.*** Adjustments are unnecessary when switching from I.V. to oral forms. For patients with renal impairment, dosage doesn't need to be adjusted; however, for patients with mild to moderate hepatic disease (cirrhosis), reduce 300 mg I.V. to 200 mg I.V., reduce 200 mg I.V. or P.O. to 100 mg I.V. or P.O.; no reduction needed for 100 mg P.O.

PHARMACODYNAMICS
Antibiotic action: Trovafloxacin is related to the fluoroquinolones with in vitro activity against a wide range of gram-positive and gram-negative aerobic and anaerobic microorganisms. The bactericidal action of trovafloxacin results from inhibition of DNA gyrase and topoisomerase IV, two enzymes involved in bacterial replication.

PHARMACOKINETICS
Absorption: Trovafloxacin is well absorbed after oral administration with an absolute bioavailability of about 88%. Serum levels peak about 1 hour after oral administration, and levels reach steady state by the 3rd day of oral or I.V. administration.
Distribution: Drug is widely and rapidly distributed throughout the body, resulting in significantly higher tissue levels than in plasma or serum. Mean plasma protein-bound fraction is about 76%.
Metabolism: Drug is primarily metabolized through conjugation, although minimal oxidative metabolism occurs with cytochrome P-450. About 13% of a dose appears in the urine as the glucuronide ester and 9% as the N-acetyl metabolite.
Excretion: Primary route of elimination is fecal. About 50% of oral dose (43% in feces and 6% in urine) is excreted as unchanged drug.

CONTRAINDICATIONS & PRECAUTIONS
Contraindicated in patients with hypersensitivity to trovafloxacin, alatrovafloxacin, or other quinolone antimicrobials.

Use cautiously in patients with history of seizures, psychosis, or increased intracranial pressure.

INTERACTIONS
Drug-drug. The bioavailability of trovafloxacin is significantly reduced after administration with *aluminum-, iron-,* or *magnesium-containing preparations* such as *antacids* and *vitamin minerals. I.V. morphine* and *sucralfate* also significantly reduce plasma trovafloxacin levels.

ADVERSE REACTIONS
CNS: *dizziness,* light-headedness, headache, ***seizures.***
GI: diarrhea, nausea, vomiting, abdominal pain, pseudomembranous colitis.
GU: vaginitis.

Reactions may be *common,* uncommon, ***life-threatening,*** or COMMON AND LIFE-THREATENING.

Hematologic: *bone marrow aplasia (anemia, thrombocytopenia, leukopenia).*
Hepatic: elevated hepatic transaminase levels.
Musculoskeletal: arthralgia, arthropathy, myalgia.
Skin: pruritus, rash, injection site reaction, photosensitivity.

▣ KEY CONSIDERATIONS
• At recommended doses, trovafloxacin is as well tolerated and efficacious in patients ages 65 and older as in younger patients.
• Changes in laboratory values during therapy didn't produce clinical abnormalities, and levels generally returned to normal 1 to 2 months after therapy was discontinued.
• Perform periodic assessment of liver function because drug increases ALT, AST, and alkaline phosphatase levels.
• Oral form is more cost-effective and carries less risk; both forms have similar efficacy and pharmacokinetics. Patients started with I.V. therapy may be switched to oral therapy when clinically indicated and at the discretion of the health care provider.
• Drug can be given as a single daily dose without regard for food.
• Administer I.V. morphine at least 2 hours after oral dose in fasting state and at least 4 hours after oral dose taken with food.
• As with other quinolones, neurologic complications such as seizures, psychosis, or increased intracranial pressure may occur; monitor patients with these preexisting conditions closely.
• Safety and efficacy of prolonged treatment (more than 4 weeks) haven't been studied.
• Alatrofloxacin mesylate is supplied in single-use vials which must be further diluted with a compatible I.V. solution, such as D_5W or half-normal saline, before administration. Do not dilute drug with normal saline or lactated Ringer's solution. Follow package insert for specific instructions regarding preparation of desired dosage.
• After dilution, I.V. drug should be administered as a 60-minute infusion.

Patient education
• Inform patient that trovafloxacin may be taken without regard to meals; however, tell him to take sucralfate, antacids containing citric acid buffered with sodium citrate, or products containing iron, aluminum, or magnesium (vitamin minerals, antacids) at least 2 hours before or after a trovafloxacin dose.
• Advise patient who experiences lightheadedness or dizziness to take drug with meals or at bedtime.
• Warn patient to avoid excessive sunlight or artificial ultraviolet light.
• Instruct patient to discontinue treatment, refrain from exercise, and seek medical advice if pain, inflammation, or rupture of tendon occurs.
• Advise patient to discontinue treatment if he experiences rash, hives, difficulty swallowing or breathing, or other signs or symptoms that suggest an allergic reaction and to seek medical help immediately.
• Instruct patient to report severe diarrhea because this could indicate pseudomembranous colitis.

tuberculosis skin test antigens

tuberculin purified protein derivative (PPD)
Aplisol, Tubersol

tuberculin cutaneous multiple-puncture device
Aplitest (PPD), Mono-Vacc Test (Old Tuberculin), Sclavo-Test PPD, TINE TEST (Old Tuberculin), TINE TEST PPD

Mycobacterium tuberculosis *and* Mycobacterium bovis *antigen, diagnostic skin test antigen*

Available by prescription only
tuberculin PPD
Injection (I.D.): 1 tuberculin U/0.1 ml, 5 tuberculin U/0.1 ml, 250 tuberculin U/0.1 ml

tuberculin cutaneous multiple-puncture device
Test: 25 devices/pack

INDICATIONS & DOSAGE
Diagnosis of tuberculosis; evaluation of immunocompetence in patients with cancer or malnutrition
Adults: I.D. injection of 5 tuberculin U/0.1 ml.

A single-use, multiple-puncture device is used for determining tuberculin sensitivity. All multiple-puncture tests are equivalent to or more potent than 5 tuberculin U PPD.
Adults: Apply the unit firmly and without twisting to the upper one-third of the forearm for about 3 seconds, to help stabilize the dried tuberculin B in the tissue lymph. Exert enough pressure to ensure that all four tines have entered the skin of the test area and a circular depression is visible.

PHARMACODYNAMICS
Diagnosis of tuberculosis: Administration to a patient with a natural infection with *M. tuberculosis* usually results in sensitivity to tuberculin and a delayed hypersensitivity reaction (after administration of old tuberculin or PPD). The cell-mediated immune reaction to tuberculin in tuberculin-sensitive individuals, which results mainly from cellular infiltrates of the dermis of the skin, usually causes local edema.
Evaluation of immunocompetence in patients with cancer or malnutrition: PPD is given I.D. with three or more antigens to detect anergy, the absence of an immune response to the test. The reaction may not be evident. Injection into a site subject to excessive exposure to sunlight may cause a false-negative reaction.

PHARMACOKINETICS
Absorption: When PPD is injected I.D. or when a multiple-puncture device is used, a delayed hypersensitivity reaction is evident in 5 to 6 hours and peaks in 48 to 72 hours.
Distribution: Injection must be given I.D. or by skin puncture; an S.C. injection invalidates the test.
Metabolism: None.

Excretion: None.

CONTRAINDICATIONS & PRECAUTIONS
Severe reactions to tuberculin PPD are rare and usually result from extreme sensitivity to the tuberculin. Inadvertent S.C. administration of PPD may result in a febrile reaction in highly sensitized patients. Old tubercular lesions aren't activated by administration of PPD.

INTERACTIONS
Drug-drug. False-negative reactions may also occur if test is used in patients receiving *aminocaproic acid* or *systemic corticosteroids.* When PPD antigen is used 4 to 6 weeks after immunization with *inactivated* or *live viral vaccines,* the reaction to tuberculin may be suppressed. *Topical alcohol* theoretically may inactivate the PPD antigen and invalidate the test.

ADVERSE REACTIONS
Other: local pain, pruritus, vesiculation, ulceration, or necrosis in some tuberculin-sensitive patients; hypersensitivity (immediate reaction may occur at test site in form of wheal or flare that lasts less than a day, which shouldn't interfere with PPD test reading at 48 to 72 hours); *anaphylaxis;* Arthus reaction.

▣ KEY CONSIDERATIONS
● Geriatric patients not having a cell-mediated immune reaction to the test may be anergic or they may test negative.
Tuberculin PPD
● Obtain a history of allergies and previous skin test reactions before administering the test.
● Epinephrine 1:1,000 should be available to treat rare anaphylactic reaction.
● I.D. injection should produce a bleb on the skin that's 6 to 10 mm in diameter; if bleb doesn't appear, retest at a site at least 5 cm from the initial site.
● Read test in 48 to 72 hours. An induration of 10 mm or greater is a significant reaction in patients who aren't suspected to have tuberculosis and who haven't been exposed to active tuberculosis, indicating present or past infection. An induration of 5 mm or more is significant in patients with AIDS or in those sus-

---

Reactions may be *common,* uncommon, *life-threatening,* or COMMON AND LIFE-THREATENING.

pected to have tuberculosis or who have recently been exposed to active tuberculosis. An induration of 5 to 9 mm is inconclusive in patients not suspected of having been exposed or having tuberculosis infection; therefore, test should be repeated if there's more than 10 mm of erythema without induration. The size of the induration, not the erythema, determines the significance of the reaction.

• For either test, keep a record of the administration technique, manufacturer and tuberculin lot number, date and location of administration, date test is read, and the size of the induration in millimeters.

Multiple-puncture device
• Obtain history of allergies, especially to acacia (contained in the TINE TEST as stabilizer), and reactions to skin tests.
• Report all known cases of tuberculosis to appropriate public health agency.
• Reaction may be depressed in patients with malnutrition, immunosuppression, or miliary tuberculosis.
• Read test at 48 to 72 hours. Measure the size of the largest induration in millimeters. A large reaction may cause the area around the puncture site to be indistinguishable.

Positive reaction: If vesiculation is present, the test may be interpreted as positive if induration is larger than 2 mm, but consider further diagnostic procedures.

Negative reaction: An induration smaller than 2 mm signals a negative reaction. There's no reason to retest the patient unless the patient has had contact with a patient with tuberculosis or if the patient has signs or symptoms of the disease.

Diagnosis of tuberculosis: PPD administration to a patient with a natural infection with *M. tuberculosis* usually results in sensitivity to tuberculin and a delayed hypersensitivity reaction after administration of old tuberculin or PPD. The cell-mediated immune reaction to tuberculin in tuberculin-sensitive individuals is seen as erythema and induration, which mainly results from cellular infiltrates of the dermis of the skin, usually causing local edema.

Diagnosis of immunocompetence in patients with such conditions as cancer or malnutrition: PPD is given I.D. with three or more antigens (such as Multitest CMI) to detect anergy.

Patient education
• Advise patient to report unusual adverse effects; explain that induration will disappear in a few days.
• Reinforce the benefits of treatment if test is positive for tuberculosis.

typhoid vaccine
Vivotif Berna

Bacterial vaccine

Available by prescription only
Oral vaccine: enteric-coated capsules of 2 to 6 × 10⁹ colony-forming U of viable *Salmonella typhi* Ty-21a and 5 to 10 × 10⁹ bacterial cells of nonviable *S. typhi* Ty-21a
Injection: suspension of killed Ty-2 strain of *S. typhi;* provides 8 U/ml in 5-ml, 10-ml, and 20-ml vials
Powder for suspension: killed Ty-2 strain of *S. typhi;* provides 8 U/ml in 50-dose vial with 20 ml diluent/dose

INDICATIONS & DOSAGE
Primary immunization (exposure to typhoid carrier or foreign travel planned to area endemic for typhoid fever)
Parenteral
Adults: 0.5 ml S.C.; repeat in 4 or more weeks.
Booster
Adults: 0.5 ml S.C. or 0.1 ml I.D. q 3 years.
Oral
Adults: Primary immunization, 1 capsule on alternate days (for example, days 1, 3, 5, 7) for four doses. Booster, repeat primary immunization regimen q 5 years.

PHARMACODYNAMICS
Typhoid fever prophylaxis action: Vaccine promotes active immunity to typhoid fever in 70% to 90% of patients vaccinated.

PHARMACOKINETICS
Absorption: Duration of vaccine-induced immunity is at least 2 years.
Distribution: Unknown.
Metabolism: Unknown.
Excretion: Unknown.

CONTRAINDICATIONS & PRECAUTIONS
Contraindicated in patients with immunosuppression and in those with hypersensitivity to vaccine. Vaccination should be deferred in patients with acute illness. Also, oral vaccine shouldn't be given to patients with acute GI distress (diarrhea or vomiting).

INTERACTIONS
Drug-drug. Use with *corticosteroids* or *immunosuppressants* may impair the immune response to this vaccine. *Other anti-infectives* and *sulfonamides active against S. typhi* may inhibit multiplication of the bacterial strain from the live attenuated oral vaccine, which may prevent a protective immune response from developing. Use with *phenytoin* may decrease antibody response to S.C. typhoid vaccine.

ADVERSE REACTIONS
CNS: malaise, headache, pain (at injection site).
GI: nausea, abdominal cramps, vomiting.
Musculoskeletal: myalgia.
Skin: rash, urticaria, swelling, inflammation (at injection site).
Other: *fever, anaphylaxis.*

◉ KEY CONSIDERATIONS
● Obtain a thorough history of allergies and reactions to immunizations.
● Have epinephrine solution 1:1,000 available to treat allergic reactions.
● Shake vial thoroughly before withdrawing dose.
● Store injection at 36° to 50° F (2° to 10° C); don't freeze.
● Store oral capsules at 36° to 46° F (2° to 8° C).

Patient education
● Tell patient what to expect after vaccination: pain and inflammation at the injection site, fever, malaise, headache, nausea, or difficulty breathing. These reactions occur in most patients within 24 hours and may persist for 1 to 2 days. Recommend acetaminophen for fever.
● Encourage patient to report adverse reactions.
● Tell patient traveling to an area where typhoid fever is endemic to select food and water carefully. Vaccination isn't a substitute for careful selection of food and water.
● Inform patient that not all recipients of typhoid vaccine are fully protected. Travelers should take all necessary precautions to avoid infection.
● Advise patient that it's essential that all four doses of oral vaccine be taken at the prescribed alternate-day interval to obtain a maximal protective immune response.
● Tell patient to take oral vaccine capsule about 1 hour before a meal with a cold or lukewarm (not exceeding body temperature) drink and to swallow the capsule as soon as possible after placement in the mouth. Remind patient not to chew the capsule.

Reactions may be *common*, uncommon, ***life-threatening**,* or COMMON AND LIFE-THREATENING.

urokinase
Abbokinase, Abbokinase Open-Cath

Thrombolytic enzyme

Available by prescription only
Injection: 5,000-IU/ml U-dose vial;
250,000-IU/vial

INDICATIONS & DOSAGE
Lysis of acute massive pulmonary emboli and of pulmonary emboli accompanied by unstable hemodynamics
Adults: For I.V. infusion only by constant infusion pump; priming dose:
4,400 IU/kg over 10 minutes, followed with 4,400 IU/kg hourly for 12 hours.
Coronary artery thrombosis
Adults: 6,000 IU/minute of urokinase intra-arterially via a coronary artery catheter until artery is maximally opened, usually within 15 to 30 minutes; however, drug has been administered for up to 2 hours. Average total dose is 500,000 IU.
Venous catheter occlusion
Adults: Instill 5,000 IU into occluded line.

PHARMACODYNAMICS
Thrombolytic action: Urokinase promotes thrombolysis by directly activating conversion of plasminogen to plasmin.

PHARMACOKINETICS
Absorption: Urokinase isn't absorbed from GI tract; plasminogen activation begins promptly after infusion or instillation; adequate activation of fibrinolytic system occurs in 3 to 4 hours.
Distribution: Drug is rapidly cleared from circulation; most accumulates in kidney and liver.
Metabolism: Drug is rapidly metabolized by the liver.
Excretion: Small amount is eliminated in urine and bile. Half-life is 10 to 20 minutes; it's longer in patients with hepatic dysfunction. Anticoagulant effect may persist for 12 to 24 hours after infusion is discontinued.

CONTRAINDICATIONS & PRECAUTIONS
Contraindicated in patients with active internal bleeding, history of CVA, aneurysm, arteriovenous malformation, known bleeding diathesis, recent trauma with possible internal injuries, visceral or intracranial malignancy, ulcerative colitis, diverticulitis, severe hypertension, hemostatic defects including those secondary to severe hepatic or renal insufficiency, uncontrolled hypocoagulation, chronic pulmonary disease with cavitation, subacute bacterial endocarditis or rheumatic valvular disease, and recent cerebral embolism, thrombosis, or hemorrhage. Also contraindicated within 10 days after intra-arterial diagnostic procedure or any surgery (liver or kidney biopsy, lumbar puncture, thoracentesis, paracentesis, or extensive or multiple cutdowns) and within 2 months after intracranial or intraspinal surgery. I.M. injections and other invasive procedures are contraindicated during urokinase therapy.

INTERACTIONS
Drug-drug. *Aminocaproic acid* inhibits urokinase-induced activation of plasminogen. Use with *anticoagulants* may cause hemorrhage, so *heparin* must be stopped and its effects allowed to diminish; it may also be necessary to reverse effects of *oral anticoagulants* before beginning therapy. Use with *aspirin, drugs affecting platelet activity, indomethacin,* or *phenylbutazone* increases risk of bleeding; don't use together.

ADVERSE REACTIONS
CV: *reperfusion arrhythmias.*
Hematologic: increased thrombin time, APPT, PT, and INR; decreased hematocrit; *bleeding.*
Respiratory: *bronchospasm,* minor breathing difficulties.
Skin: rash.
Other: phlebitis at injection site, fever, *anaphylaxis.*

▣ KEY CONSIDERATIONS

Besides the recommendations relevant to all thrombolytic enzymes, consider the following:

• Patients ages 75 or older are at greater risk for cerebral hemorrhage because they're more apt to have preexisting cerebrovascular disease.

• To reconstitute I.V. solution, add 5.2 ml sterile water for injection; dilute further with normal saline injection or D_5W injection before infusion; don't use bacteriostatic water, which contains preservatives. A catheter-clearing product is available in a Univial containing 5,000 IU urokinase with the proper diluent. Discard unused portion; product contains no preservatives.

• Urokinase is commonly used in peripheral arterial occlusions; however, the FDA hasn't approved the drug for this use.

Overdose & treatment

• Signs and symptoms of overdose include signs of potentially serious bleeding: bleeding gums, epistaxis, hematoma, spontaneous ecchymoses, oozing at catheter site, increased pulse, and pain from internal bleeding.

• Discontinue urokinase and restart when bleeding stops.

valacyclovir hydrochloride
Valtrex

*Synthetic purine nucleoside,
antiviral*

Available by prescription only
Caplets: 500 mg

INDICATIONS & DOSAGE
***Treatment of herpes zoster in immuno-
competent patients***
Adults: 1 g P.O. t.i.d. daily for 7 days.
***Treatment of initial episode of genital
herpes***
Adults: 1 g P.O. b.i.d. for 10 days.
***Treatment of recurrent genital herpes
in immunocompetent patients***
Adults: 500 mg P.O. b.i.d. for 5 days.
***Long-term suppressive therapy of re-
current genital herpes***
Adults: 1 g P.O. once daily.
✦ *Dosage adjustment.* Base dosage ad-
justments in renally impaired patients on
creatinine clearance levels.

PHARMACODYNAMICS
Antiviral action: Valacyclovir rapidly
converts to acyclovir. Acyclovir incorpo-
rates into viral DNA and inhibits viral
DNA polymerase, thus inhibiting viral
multiplication.

PHARMACOKINETICS
Absorption: Valacyclovir is rapidly absorbed from the GI tract; absolute
bioavailability is about 54.5%.
Distribution: Drug is 13.5% to 17.9%
protein-bound.
Metabolism: Drug is rapidly and nearly
completely converted to acyclovir and L-
valine by first-pass intestinal or hepatic
metabolism.
Excretion: Drug is excreted in urine and
feces. Half-life of drug is 2.5 to 3.3
hours.

CONTRAINDICATIONS & PRECAUTIONS
Contraindicated in patients with hypersensitivity or intolerance to valacyclovir,
acyclovir, or a component of the formulation and in immunocompromised patients.
Use cautiously in patients with impaired renal function and in those receiving other nephrotoxic drugs.

INTERACTIONS
Drug-drug. *Cimetidine* and *probenecid*
reduce the rate, but not the extent, of
valacyclovir conversion to acyclovir and
reduce the renal clearance of acyclovir,
thus increasing acyclovir blood levels;
monitor patient for possible toxicity.

ADVERSE REACTIONS
CNS: *headache,* dizziness, asthenia.
GI: *nausea,* vomiting, diarrhea, consti-
pation, abdominal pain, anorexia.

▣ KEY CONSIDERATIONS
• Dosage adjustment may be necessary
in geriatric patients based on underlying
renal status.
• Initiate therapy at first signs or symptoms of an episode, preferably within 24
hours after onset.
• Thrombotic thrombocytopenic purpura
and hemolytic uremic syndrome have
occurred, resulting in death in some patients with advanced infection with HIV
and also in bone marrow transplant and
renal transplant patients participating in
clinical trials of valacyclovir.

Patient education
• Inform patient that valacyclovir may be
taken without regard to meals.
• Advise patient about signs and symptoms of herpes infection (such as rash,
tingling, itching, and pain), and advise
him to call immediately if they occur.
Treatment should be initiated as soon as
possible after symptoms appear and is
most effective when initiated within 48
hours of the onset of zoster rash.
• Tell patient to avoid contact with lesions and to avoid intercourse when lesions or symptoms are present.

Overdose & treatment
• Although no overdoses have been reported, precipitation of acyclovir in renal

tubules may occur when the solubility (2.5 mg/ml) is exceeded in the intratubular fluid.

• If acute renal failure and anuria occur, hemodialysis may be helpful until renal function is restored.

---

valproic acid
Depakene, Epival*

divalproex sodium
Depakote, Depakote Sprinkle

valproate sodium
Depacon

Carboxylic acid derivative, anticonvulsant

Available by prescription only
valproic acid
Capsules: 250 mg
Syrup: 250 mg/5 ml
divalproex sodium
Tablets (enteric-coated): 125 mg, 250 mg, 500 mg
Capsules (sprinkle): 125 mg
valproate sodium
Injection: 5-ml single-dose vials

INDICATIONS & DOSAGE
Simple and complex absence seizures and mixed seizure types, ◊ tonic-clonic seizures
Adults: P.O.: Initially, 15 mg/kg P.O. daily, divided b.i.d. or t.i.d.; may increase by 5 to 10 mg/kg daily at weekly intervals up to a maximum of 60 mg/kg daily, divided b.i.d. or t.i.d. The b.i.d. dosage is recommended for enteric-coated tablets.

Note: Dosages of divalproex sodium (Depakote) are expressed as valproic acid.

Adults: I.V.: Initially, 10 to 15 mg/kg/day as a 60-minute I.V. infusion (rate, 20 mg/minute or less). May increase dosage by 5 to 10 mg/kg daily at weekly intervals up to a maximum of 60 mg/kg daily. Drug should be diluted in at least 50 ml compatible diluent. Use of valproate sodium injection for periods of more than 14 days hasn't been studied. Patients should be switched to oral products as soon as it's feasible. When switching from I.V. to oral therapy or oral to I.V. therapy, the total daily dose should be equivalent with the same frequency.
Mania
Adults: 750 mg P.O. in divided doses (divalproex sodium).
Migraine prophylaxis
Adults: 250 mg P.O. b.i.d. Some patients may benefit from doses up to 1 g daily.
◊ *Status epilepticus refractory to I.V. diazepam*
Adults: 400 to 600 mg P.R. q 6 hours.

PHARMACODYNAMICS
Anticonvulsant action: Valproic acid's mechanism of action is unknown; effects may be from increased brain levels of gamma-aminobutyric acid (GABA), an inhibitory transmitter. Drug also may decrease GABA's enzymatic catabolism. Onset of therapeutic effects may require a week or more. Drug may be used with other anticonvulsants.

PHARMACOKINETICS
Absorption: Valproate sodium and divalproex sodium quickly convert to valproic acid after administration of oral dose. Plasma levels peak in 1 to 4 hours (with uncoated tablets), 3 to 5 hours (with enteric-coated tablets), 15 minutes to 2 hours (with syrup), and immediately (with I.V. administration); bioavailability of drug is same for all dosage forms.
Distribution: Valproic acid is distributed rapidly throughout the body; 80% to 95% binds to protein.
Metabolism: Valproic acid is metabolized in the liver.
Excretion: Valproic acid is excreted in urine; some drug is excreted in feces and exhaled air.

CONTRAINDICATIONS & PRECAUTIONS
Contraindicated in patients with hypersensitivity to valproic acid.

Use cautiously in patients with history of hepatic dysfunction. Don't administer valproate sodium injection to patients with hepatic disease or significant hepatic dysfunction.

INTERACTIONS
Drug-drug. Use with *clonazepam* may cause absence seizures and should be

---

Reactions may be *common,* uncommon, ***life-threatening,*** or COMMON AND LIFE-THREATENING.

avoided; with *felbamate* and *salicylates,* increased valproate levels; and with *lamotrigine,* increased lamotrigine levels. Valproic acid may potentiate effects of *MAO inhibitors* and *other CNS antidepressants* and of *oral anticoagulants.* Besides additive sedative effects, valproic acid increases serum levels of *phenobarbital, phenytoin,* and *primidone;* such combinations may cause excessive somnolence and require careful monitoring.
Drug-lifestyle. *Alcohol* use causes decreased drug effectiveness and increased CNS adverse effects.

ADVERSE REACTIONS
Because valproic acid usually is used with other anticonvulsants, the drug may not be solely responsible for the adverse reactions reported.
CNS: *sedation,* emotional upset, depression, psychosis, aggressiveness, hyperactivity, behavioral deterioration, tremor, ataxia, headache, dizziness, incoordination.
EENT: nystagmus, diplopia.
GI: *nausea, vomiting, indigestion,* diarrhea, abdominal cramps, constipation, increased appetite and weight gain, anorexia, *pancreatitis.* (*Note:* less GI adverse reactions occur with divalproex sodium.)
Hematologic: *thrombocytopenia,* increased bleeding time, petechiae, bruising, eosinophilia, *hemorrhage, leukopenia, bone marrow suppression.*
Hepatic: *elevated liver enzyme levels, toxic hepatitis.*
Musculoskeletal: muscular weakness.
Skin: rash, alopecia, pruritus, photosensitivity, *erythema multiforme.*

▣ KEY CONSIDERATIONS
• Geriatric patients eliminate valproic acid more slowly; lower dosages are recommended.
• Evaluate liver function, platelet count, and PT at baseline and monthly intervals, especially during first 6 months.
• Therapeutic blood drug level is 50 to 100 mcg/ml.
• Don't withdraw drug abruptly.
• Tremors may indicate need for dosage reduction.

• Administer drug with food to minimize GI irritation; enteric-coated formulation may be better tolerated.
• When switching from oral to I.V. route, total daily dose I.V. should be equivalent to the oral daily dose with the same frequency. Monitor plasma level and make dosage adjustments as needed.
• Administer I.V. as 60-minute infusion with rate not exceeding 20 mg/minute.
• Drug may cause false-positive test results for urine ketones.

Patient education
• Advise patient not to discontinue valproic acid suddenly, not to alter dosage without medical approval, and to call health care provider before changing brand or using generic drug because therapeutic effect may change.
• Tell patient to swallow tablets or capsules whole to avoid local mucosal irritation and if necessary to take with food, but not carbonated beverages, because tablet may dissolve before swallowing, causing irritation and unpleasant taste.
• Warn patient to avoid alcohol while taking drug because it may decrease drug's effectiveness and increase CNS adverse effects.
• Advise patient to avoid tasks that require mental alertness until CNS sedative effects are determined. Drowsiness and dizziness may occur. Bedtime administration of drug may minimize CNS depression.
• Teach patient signs and symptoms of hypersensitivity and adverse effects and the need to report them.
• Encourage patient to wear a medical identification bracelet or necklace, listing drug and seizure disorders, while taking anticonvulsants.

Overdose & treatment
• Signs and symptoms of overdose include somnolence and coma.
• Treat overdose supportively: maintain adequate urine output, and monitor vital signs and fluid and electrolyte balance carefully. Naloxone reverses CNS and respiratory depression but also may reverse anticonvulsant effects of valproic acid. Hemodialysis and hemoperfusion have been used.

---

valsartan
Diovan

Angiotensin II antagonist, anti-hypertensive

Available by prescription only
Capsules: 80 mg, 160 mg

INDICATIONS & DOSAGE
Hypertension, used alone or with other antihypertensives
Adults: Initially, 80 mg P.O. once daily as monotherapy in patients who aren't volume depleted. Blood pressure reduction should occur in 2 to 4 weeks. If additional antihypertensive effect is needed, may increase dosage to 160 or 320 mg daily or add diuretic. (Addition of diuretic has greater effect than dosage increases beyond 80 mg.) Usual dosage range is 80 to 320 mg daily.

PHARMACODYNAMICS
Antihypertensive action: Valsartan blocks the binding of angiotensin II to receptor sites in vascular smooth muscle and the adrenal gland, which inhibits the pressor effects of the renin-angiotensin-aldosterone system.

PHARMACOKINETICS
Absorption: Absolute bioavailability is about 25%; plasma level peaks 2 to 4 hours after dosing.
Distribution: Valsartan doesn't distribute extensively into tissues; it's highly bound to serum proteins (95%), mainly to serum albumin.
Metabolism: Only about 20% is metabolized. The enzyme(s) responsible for metabolism haven't been identified, but don't appear to be cytochrome P-450 enzymes.
Excretion: Drug is excreted primarily through feces (83% of dose) and about 13% in urine. Average elimination half-life is about 6 hours.

CONTRAINDICATIONS & PRECAUTIONS
Contraindicated in patients with known hypersensitivity to valsartan.
Use cautiously in patients with renal or hepatic disease.

INTERACTIONS
Drug-drug. *Diuretics* may increase risk of excessive hypotension; assess fluid status before starting concomitant therapy.

ADVERSE REACTIONS
CNS: fatigue, dizziness, headache.
CV: edema.
EENT: pharyngitis, rhinitis, sinusitis.
GI: abdominal pain, diarrhea, nausea.
Hematologic: *neutropenia.*
Metabolic: hyperkalemia.
Musculoskeletal: arthralgia.
Respiratory: cough, upper respiratory tract infection.
Other: viral infection.

▣ KEY CONSIDERATIONS
• Although no overall difference in efficacy or safety was observed, greater sensitivity of some geriatric patients can't be ruled out.
• Excessive hypotension can occur when valsartan is given with high doses of diuretics; correct volume and salt depletions before initiating therapy.

Patient education
• Tell patient valsartan may be taken without regard to food.

vancomycin hydrochloride
Lyphocin, Vancocin, Vancoled

Glycopeptide, antibiotic

Available by prescription only
Pulvules: 125 mg, 250 mg
Powder for oral solution: 1-g and 10-g bottles
Powder for injection: 500-mg, 1-g, and 5-g vials

INDICATIONS & DOSAGE
Severe staphylococcal infections when other antibiotics are ineffective or contraindicated
Adults: 500 mg I.V. q 6 hours, or 1 g q 12 hours.
Antibiotic-associated pseudomembranous and staphylococcal enterocolitis
Adults: 125 to 500 mg P.O. q 6 hours for 7 to 10 days.

Reactions may be *common*, uncommon, ***life-threatening***, or COMMON AND LIFE-THREATENING.

Endocarditis prophylaxis for dental, GI, biliary, and GU instrumentation procedures; surgical prophylaxis in patients allergic to penicillin
Adults: 1 g I.V. given slowly over 1 hour, starting 1 hour before procedure. In high-risk patients, dose may be repeated in 8 to 12 hours.
✦ *Dosage adjustment.* In patients with renal failure, adjust dosage based on degree of renal impairment, severity of infection, and susceptibility of causative organism. Base dosage on serum drug levels.

Recommended initial dose is 15 mg/kg. Subsequent doses should be adjusted p.r.n. Some health care providers use the following schedule.

Serum creatinine level (mg/dl)	Dosage in adults
< 1.5	1 g q 12 hr
1.5-5	1 g q 3-6 days
> 5	1 g q 10-14 days

PHARMACODYNAMICS
Antibacterial action: Vancomycin is bactericidal by hindering cell-wall synthesis and blocking glycopeptide polymerization. Its spectrum of activity includes many gram-positive organisms, including those resistant to other antibiotics. It's useful for *Staphylococcus epidermidis* and methicillin-resistant *Staphylococcus aureus*. It is also useful for penicillin-resistant *Staphylococcus pneumococcus*.

PHARMACOKINETICS
Absorption: Minimal systemic absorption occurs with oral administration. (However, vancomycin may accumulate in patients with colitis or renal failure.)
Distribution: Drug is distributed widely in body fluids, including pericardial, pleural, ascitic, and synovial. It achieves therapeutic levels in CSF in patients with inflamed meninges. Therapeutic drug levels are 18 to 26 µg/ml for 2-hour postinfusion peaks; 5 to 10 µg/ml for preinfusion troughs (these values may vary depending on laboratory and sampling time).
Metabolism: Unknown.

Excretion: Administered parenterally, drug is excreted renally, mainly by filtration. Administered orally, drug is excreted in feces. In patients with normal renal function, plasma half-life is 6 hours; in those with creatinine clearance of 10 to 30 ml/minute, plasma half-life is about 32 hours; if creatinine clearance is less than 10 ml/minute, plasma half-life is 146 hours.

CONTRAINDICATIONS & PRECAUTIONS
Contraindicated in patients with hypersensitivity to vancomycin.

Use cautiously in patients with impaired renal or hepatic function, preexisting hearing loss, or allergies to other antibiotics; in patients receiving other neurotoxic, nephrotoxic, or ototoxic drugs; and in patients older than age 60.

INTERACTIONS
Drug-drug. Vancomycin may have additive nephrotoxic effects when used with *other nephrotoxic drugs*, such as *aminoglycosides, amphotericin B, capreomycin, cisplatin, colistin, methoxyflurane,* and *polymyxin B*.

ADVERSE REACTIONS
CNS: pain at injection site.
CV: hypotension, thrombophlebitis at injection site.
EENT: tinnitus, ototoxicity.
GI: nausea.
GU: increased BUN and serum creatinine levels, *nephrotoxicity*.
Hematologic: *neutropenia*, eosinophilia.
Respiratory: wheezing, dyspnea.
Skin: red-neck syndrome with rapid I.V. infusion (maculopapular rash on face, neck, trunk, and extremities).
Other: chills, fever, *anaphylaxis*, superinfection.

🔲 KEY CONSIDERATIONS
• Geriatric patients may be more susceptible to vancomycin's ototoxic effects. Monitor serum levels closely and adjust dosage as needed.
• Obtain culture and sensitivity tests before starting therapy (unless drug is used for prophylaxis).

• To prepare drug for oral administration, reconstitute as directed in manufacturer's instructions. Reconstituted solution remains stable for 2 weeks when refrigerated.

• To prepare drug for I.V. injection, reconstitute 500 mg with 10 ml, or 1 g with 20 ml, sterile water for injection to yield 50 mg/ml. Withdraw desired dose and further dilute to 100 to 250 ml with normal saline solution or D_5W; 1 g should be diluted with at least 200 ml diluent. Infuse over at least 60 minutes to avoid adverse effects related to rapid infusion rate. Initial reconstituted solution remains stable for 14 days when refrigerated.

• Don't give I.M. because drug is highly irritating.

• Monitor CBC and BUN, serum creatinine, and drug levels.

• If patient develops maculopapular rash on face, neck, trunk, or upper extremities, slow infusion rate.

• If patient has preexisting auditory dysfunction or requires prolonged therapy, auditory function tests may be indicated before and during therapy.

• Hemodialysis and peritoneal dialysis remove only minimal drug amounts. Patients receiving these treatments require usual dose only once q 5 to 7 days; however, dosage is based on the serum drug level. Some high-flux dialysis systems are capable of removing up to 50% of the drug, creating the need for supplemental doses postdialysis.

Patient education
• If patient is receiving vancomycin orally, remind him to continue taking it as directed, even if he feels better.

• Advise patient not to take antidiarrheals with the drug except as prescribed.

• Instruct patient to call promptly if he develops ringing in the ears.

varicella-zoster immune globulin (VZIG)

Immune serum, varicella-zoster prophylaxis

Available by prescription only
Injection: 10% to 18% solution of the globulin fraction of human plasma containing 125 U varicella-zoster virus antibody in 2.5 ml or less

INDICATIONS & DOSAGE
Passive immunization of susceptible patients, primarily immunocompromised patients after exposure to varicella (chickenpox or herpes zoster)
Adults: 125 U/10 kg of body weight I.M., to a maximum of 625 U. Higher doses may be needed in immunocompromised adults.

PHARMACODYNAMICS
Postexposure prophylaxis: VZIG provides passive immunity to varicella-zoster virus.

PHARMACOKINETICS
Absorption: After I.M. absorption, the persistence of antibodies is unknown, but protection should last at least 3 weeks. Protection is sufficient to prevent or lessen the severity of varicella infections.
Distribution: Unknown.
Metabolism: Unknown.
Excretion: Unknown.

CONTRAINDICATIONS & PRECAUTIONS
Contraindicated in patients with thrombocytopenia, coagulation disorders, immunoglobulin A deficiency, or history of severe reaction to human immune serum globulin or thimerosal.

INTERACTIONS
Drug-drug. Use with *corticosteroids* or *immunosuppressants* may interfere with the immune response to this immune globulin; when possible, avoid using these drugs during the postexposure immunization period. VZIG may interfere with the immune response to *live virus vaccines* (for example, those for

measles, mumps, and *rubella*); don't administer live virus vaccines within 3 months after or 2 weeks before administering VZIG. If it's necessary to administer VZIG with a live virus vaccine, confirm seroconversion with follow-up serologic testing.

ADVERSE REACTIONS

CNS: malaise, headache.
CV: chest tightness.
GI: GI distress.
GU: *nephrotic syndrome.*
Musculoskeletal: myalgia.
Respiratory: respiratory distress.
Skin: rash.
Other: *anaphylaxis,* discomfort at injection site, *angioedema, angioneurotic edema,* fever.

▣ KEY CONSIDERATIONS

• Obtain a thorough history of allergies and reactions to immunizations.
• Have epinephrine solution 1:1,000 available to treat allergic reactions.
• VZIG use, especially in immunocompromised patients of any age and normal adults, should be considered on a case-by-case basis. VZIG isn't for use in immunodeficient patients with history of varicella, unless immunosuppression results from bone marrow transplantation.
• Administer only by deep I.M. injection. Never administer I.V. Use the deltoid or anterolateral thigh in adults. Give no more than 2.5 ml at a single injection site.
• For maximum benefit, administer VZIG within 96 hours of presumed exposure.
• Store unopened vials between 36° and 46° F (2° and 8° C); don't freeze.

Patient education

• Explain that patient's chances of contracting AIDS or hepatitis from VZIG are very small.
• Tell patient some local pain, swelling, and tenderness may occur at the injection site; recommend acetaminophen to alleviate these minor effects.
• Encourage patient to immediately report severe reactions.

vasopressin (antidiuretic hormone [ADH])
Pitressin Synthetic

Posterior pituitary hormone, ADH, peristaltic stimulant, hemostatic

Available by prescription only
Injection: 0.5-ml and 1-ml ampules and vials, 20 U/ml

INDICATIONS & DOSAGE

Nonnephrogenic, nonpsychogenic diabetes insipidus
Adults: 5 to 10 U I.M. or S.C. b.i.d. to q.i.d., p.r.n.
Postoperative abdominal distention
Adults: 5 U I.M. initially, then q 3 to 4 hours, increasing dosage to 10 U, if needed.
To expel gas before abdominal X-ray
Adults: Inject 5 to 15 U S.C. at 2 hours, then again at 30 minutes before X-ray. Enema before first dose may also help to eliminate gas.
Upper GI tract hemorrhage
Adults: 0.2 to 0.4 U/minute I.V. or 0.1 to 0.5 U/minute intra-arterially.

PHARMACODYNAMICS

Antidiuretic action: Vasopressin is used as an antidiuretic to control or prevent signs and complications of neurogenic diabetes insipidus. Acting primarily at the renal tubular level, vasopressin increases cAMP, which increases water permeability at the renal tubule and collecting duct, resulting in increased urine osmolality and decreased urine flow rate.
Peristaltic stimulant action: Used to treat postoperative abdominal distention and to facilitate abdominal radiographic procedures, vasopressin induces peristalsis by directly stimulating contraction of smooth muscle in the GI tract.
Hemostatic action: In patients with GI hemorrhage, vasopressin administered I.V. or intra-arterially into the superior mesenteric artery controls bleeding of esophageal varices by directly stimulating vasoconstriction of capillaries and small arterioles.

PHARMACOKINETICS

Absorption: Vasopressin is destroyed by trypsin in the GI tract and must be administered intranasally or parenterally.
Distribution: Drug is distributed throughout the extracellular fluid, with no evidence of protein-binding.
Metabolism: Most of dose is destroyed rapidly in the liver and kidneys.
Excretion: About 5% of S.C. dose is excreted unchanged in urine after 4 hours. Duration of action after I.M. or S.C. administration is 2 to 8 hours; half-life, 10 to 20 minutes.

CONTRAINDICATIONS & PRECAUTIONS

Contraindicated in patients with known anaphylaxis or hypersensitivity to vasopressin or its components and in patients with chronic nephritis accompanied by nitrogen retention.

Use cautiously in geriatric patients or those with seizure disorders, migraine headache, asthma, CV or renal disease, heart failure, goiter with cardiac complications, arteriosclerosis, or fluid overload; or in preoperative or postoperative patients who are polyuric.

INTERACTIONS

Drug-drug. Use with *carbamazepine, chlorpropamide,* or *clofibrate* may potentiate vasopressin's antidiuretic effect; use with *demeclocycline, epinephrine, heparin, lithium,* or *norepinephrine* may decrease its antidiuretic effect.
Drug-lifestyle. Use with *alcohol* may decrease vasopressin's antidiuretic effect.

ADVERSE REACTIONS

CNS: tremor, headache, vertigo.
CV: angina in patients with vascular disease, vasoconstriction, *arrhythmias, cardiac arrest,* myocardial ischemia, circumoral pallor, decreased cardiac output.
GI: abdominal cramps, nausea, vomiting, flatulence.
Skin: diaphoresis.
Other: *water intoxication* (drowsiness, listlessness, headache, confusion, weight gain, *seizures, coma*), hypersensitivity reactions (urticaria, *angioedema, bronchoconstriction, anaphylaxis*), cutaneous gangrene.

▣ KEY CONSIDERATIONS

Besides the recommendations relevant to all posterior pituitary hormones, consider the following:
• Geriatric patients show increased sensitivity to the effects of vasopressin. Use with caution.
• Establish baseline vital signs and intake and output ratio at the initiation of therapy.
• Monitor patient's blood pressure twice daily. Watch for excessively elevated blood pressure or lack of response to drug, which may be indicated by hypotension. Also, monitor fluid intake and output and daily weight.
• Question patient with abdominal distention about passage of flatus and stool.
• A rectal tube facilitates gas expulsion after vasopressin injection.
• To prevent seizures, coma, and death, observe for signs and symptoms of early water intoxication (drowsiness, listlessness, headache, confusion, and weight gain).
• Use extreme caution to avoid extravasation because of risk of necrosis and gangrene.

Patient education

• Tell patient to drink one or two glasses of water with each dose of vasopressin to reduce certain adverse reactions, including unusual paleness, nausea, abdominal cramps, and vomiting.
• Teach patient how to maintain a fluid intake and output record.
• Show patient how to check the expiration date.
• Tell patient to call health care provider immediately if he experiences chest pain, confusion, fever, hives, rash, headache, problems with urination, seizures, weight gain, unusual drowsiness, wheezing, difficulty breathing, or swelling of face, hands, feet, or mouth.
• Encourage patient to rotate injection sites.

Overdose & treatment

• Signs and symptoms of overdose include drowsiness, listlessness, headache, confusion, anuria, and weight gain (water intoxication).

Reactions may be *common*, uncommon, *life-threatening*, or COMMON AND LIFE-THREATENING.

• Treatment requires water restriction and temporary withdrawal of vasopressin until polyuria occurs. Severe water intoxication may require osmotic diuresis with mannitol, hypertonic dextrose, or urea, either alone or with furosemide.

---

venlafaxine hydrochloride
Effexor, Effexor XR

Neuronal serotonin, norepinephrine, and dopamine reuptake inhibitor, antidepressant

---

Available by prescription only
Capsules (extended-release): 37.5 mg, 75 mg, 150 mg
Tablets: 25 mg, 37.5 mg, 50 mg, 75 mg, 100 mg

INDICATIONS & DOSAGE
Depression
Adults: Initially, 75 mg P.O. daily, in two or three divided doses with food. Increase dosage as tolerated and needed in increments of 75 mg/day at intervals of no less than 4 days. For moderately depressed outpatients, usual maximum dosage is 225 mg/day; in certain severely depressed patients, dosage may be as high as 375 mg/day (divided into three doses). For extended-release capsules, 75 mg/day P.O. in a single dose. For some patients, it may be desirable to start at 37.5 mg/day P.O. for 4 to 7 days before increasing to 75 mg/day. Dosage may be increased at increments of 75 mg/day q 4 days to a maximum of 225 mg/day.
✦ *Dosage adjustment.* Reduce dosage by 50% in patients with impaired hepatic function and by 25% in patients with moderate renal impairment (GFR, 10 to 70 ml/minute). In hemodialysis patients, reduce dose by 50% and withhold drug until after dialysis treatment.
Note: Discontinue drug if patient develops seizures.

PHARMACODYNAMICS
Antidepressant action: Venlafaxine is thought to potentiate neurotransmitter activity in the CNS. Preclinical studies have shown that venlafaxine and its active metabolite, o-desmethylvenlafaxine (ODV), are potent inhibitors of neuronal serotonin and norepinephrine reuptake and weak inhibitors of dopamine reuptake.

PHARMACOKINETICS
Absorption: Venlafaxine is about 92% absorbed after oral administration.
Distribution: Drug is about 25% to 29% protein-bound in plasma.
Metabolism: Drug is extensively metabolized in the liver; ODV is the only major active metabolite.
Excretion: About 87% of dose is recovered in urine within 48 hours (5% as unchanged venlafaxine, 29% as unconjugated ODV, 26% as conjugated ODV, and 27% as minor inactive metabolites).

CONTRAINDICATIONS & PRECAUTIONS
Contraindicated in patients hypersensitive to venlafaxine and within 14 days of MAO inhibitor therapy.
Use cautiously in patients with impaired renal or hepatic function, diseases or conditions that could affect hemodynamic responses or metabolism, or history of seizures or mania.

INTERACTIONS
Drug-drug. Use with *cimetidine* or *CNS-active drugs* may increase venlafaxine level; use together cautiously.
MAO inhibitors may precipitate a syndrome similar to neuroleptic malignant syndrome when used with venlafaxine, so don't start venlafaxine within 14 days of stopping a MAO inhibitor and don't start a MAO inhibitor within 7 days of stopping venlafaxine.

ADVERSE REACTIONS
CNS: *headache, somnolence, dizziness, nervousness, insomnia,* anxiety, tremor, abnormal dreams, paresthesia, agitation, *asthenia.*
CV: hypertension, vasodilation.
EENT: blurred vision.
GI: *nausea, constipation,* vomiting, *dry mouth, anorexia,* diarrhea, dyspepsia, flatulence.
GU: *abnormal ejaculation,* impotence, urinary frequency, impaired urination.

Metabolic: weight loss.
Skin: *diaphoresis,* rash.
Other: yawning, chills, infection.

▣ KEY CONSIDERATIONS

• No overall difference in effectiveness or safety has been observed between geriatric and younger patients, but greater sensitivity to venlafaxine in geriatric patients can't be excluded.
• Because drug may cause sustained increases in blood pressure, monitor blood pressure regularly. For patients who experience a sustained increase in blood pressure while receiving drug, consider reducing the dosage or discontinuing the drug.
• Monitor patients with major affective disorders because drug may activate mania or hypomania.
• When discontinuing drug therapy after more than 1 week, taper dosage. If patient has received drug for at least 6 weeks, gradually taper dosage over 2 weeks.

Patient education

• Caution patient not to operate hazardous machinery until the effects of the drug are known.
• Instruct patient to call primary health care provider before taking other drugs, including OTC preparations, because of potential interactions.
• Tell patient to avoid alcohol while taking drug.
• Instruct patient to report rash, hives, or a related allergic reaction.

---

verapamil hydrochloride
Calan, Calan SR, Covera-HS, Isoptin, Isoptin SR, Verelan

Calcium channel blocker, antianginal, antihypertensive, antiarrhythmic

---

Available by prescription only
Tablets: 40 mg, 80 mg, 120 mg
Tablets (sustained-release): 120 mg, 180 mg, 240 mg
Capsules (sustained-release): 120 mg, 180 mg, 240 mg, 360 mg
Injection: 2.5 mg/ml

INDICATIONS & DOSAGE

Management of Prinzmetal's or variant angina or unstable or chronic, stable angina pectoris
Adults: Initial dose of 80 to 120 mg P.O. t.i.d. Dose may be increased at weekly intervals. Some patients may require up to 480 mg/day.
Supraventricular tachyarrhythmias
Adults: 0.075 to 0.15 mg/kg (5 to 10 mg) I.V. push over 2 minutes. If patient doesn't respond, give a second dose of 10 mg (0.15 mg/kg) 15 to 30 minutes after the initial dose.
Control of ventricular rate in patients receiving digoxin with chronic atrial flutter or fibrillation Adults: 240 to 320 mg/day P.O. in three or four divided doses.
Prophylaxis of repetitive paroxysmal supraventricular tachycardia
Adults: 240 to 480 mg/day P.O. given in three or four divided doses.
Hypertension
Adults: Usual starting dose is 80 mg P.O. t.i.d. Daily dose may be increased to 360 to 480 mg.

Initiate therapy with sustained-release capsules at 180 mg (240 mg for Verelan) daily in the morning. A starting dose of 120 mg may be indicated in patients who have an increased response to verapamil. Adjust dosage based on effectiveness 24 hours after dosing. Increase by 120 mg/day to a maximum dosage of 480 mg/day. Sustained-release capsules should be given only once daily. Antihypertensive effects are usually seen within the 1st week of therapy. Most patients respond to 240 mg/day.

PHARMACODYNAMICS

Antianginal action: Verapamil manages unstable and chronic stable angina by reducing afterload both at rest and with exercise, thereby decreasing oxygen consumption. It also decreases myocardial oxygen demand and cardiac work by exerting a negative inotropic effect, reducing heart rate, relieving coronary artery spasm (via coronary artery vasodilation), and dilating peripheral vessels. The result of these effects is relief of angina-related ischemia and pain. In patients with Prinzmetal's variant angina,

---

Reactions may be *common,* uncommon, *life-threatening,* or COMMON AND LIFE-THREATENING.

drug inhibits coronary artery spasm, resulting in increased myocardial oxygen delivery.

Antihypertensive action: Drug reduces blood pressure mainly by dilating peripheral vessels. Its negative inotropic effect blocks reflex mechanisms that lead to increased blood pressure.

Antiarrhythmic action: Drug's combined effects on the SA and AV nodes help manage arrhythmias. Drug's primary effect is on the AV node; slowed conduction reduces the ventricular rate in atrial tachyarrhythmias and blocks reentry paths in paroxysmal supraventricular arrhythmias.

PHARMACOKINETICS

Absorption: Verapamil is absorbed rapidly and completely from the GI tract after oral administration; however, only 20% to 35% of drug reaches systemic circulation because of first-pass effect. When administered orally, effects peak within 1 to 2 hours with conventional tablets and within 4 to 8 hours with sustained-release preparations. When administered I.V., effects occur within minutes after injection and usually persist for 30 to 60 minutes (although they may last up to 6 hours). Therapeutic serum levels are 80 to 300 ng/ml.

Distribution: Steady-state distribution volume in healthy adults ranges from 4.5 to 7 L/kg but may increase to 12 L/kg in patients with hepatic cirrhosis. About 90% of circulating drug binds to plasma proteins.

Metabolism: Drug is metabolized in the liver.

Excretion: Excreted in urine as unchanged drug and active metabolites. Elimination half-life is normally 6 to 12 hours and increases up 16 hours in patients with hepatic cirrhosis.

CONTRAINDICATIONS & PRECAUTIONS

Contraindicated in patients with hypersensitivity to verapamil, severe left ventricular dysfunction, cardiogenic shock, second- or third-degree AV block or sick sinus syndrome except if the patient has a functioning pacemaker, atrial flutter or fibrillation and accessory bypass tract syndrome, severe heart failure (unless secondary to verapamil therapy), or severe hypotension. I.V. verapamil is also contraindicated in patients receiving I.V. beta blockers and in those with ventricular tachycardia.

Use cautiously in geriatric patients and in those with impaired renal or hepatic function or increased intracranial pressure.

INTERACTIONS

Drug-drug. Use with *antihypertensives* may lead to combined antihypertensive effects, resulting in significant hypotension. Use with *beta blockers* may cause additive effects leading to heart failure, conduction disturbances, arrhythmias, and hypotension, especially if high doses of beta blockers are used, if drugs are administered I.V., or if patient has moderately severe to severe heart failure, severe cardiomyopathy, or a recent MI. Use with *carbamazepine* may cause increased serum carbamazepine levels and subsequent toxicity; with *disopyramide,* combined negative inotropic effects; with *flecainide,* added negative inotropic effect and prolonged AV conduction; and with *quinidine* to treat hypertrophic cardiomyopathy, excessive hypotension. Use of oral verapamil with *digoxin* may increase serum digoxin level by 50% to 75% during the first week of therapy. Use with *drugs that attenuate alpha-adrenergic response* (such as *methyldopa* and *prazosin*) may excessively reduce blood pressure. Verapamil may potentiate the action of *neuromuscular blockers. Rifampin* may substantially reduce oral bioavailability of verapamil. Verapamil may inhibit the clearance and increase the plasma *theophylline* levels.

Drug-lifestyle. Use with *alcohol* may prolong the intoxicating effects of alcohol.

ADVERSE REACTIONS

CNS: dizziness, headache, asthenia.
CV: *transient hypotension,* **heart failure,** pulmonary edema, **bradycardia,** AV block, **ventricular asystole, ventricular fibrillation,** peripheral edema.
GI: *constipation,* nausea.
Hepatic: elevated liver enzyme levels.
Skin: rash.

▣ KEY CONSIDERATIONS

• Geriatric patients may require lower doses. In geriatric patients, administer I.V. doses over at least 3 minutes to minimize risk of adverse reactions.

• If verapamil is initiated in patient receiving carbamazepine, carbamazepine dosage may need to be reduced by 40% to 50%; monitor patient closely for signs of toxic reaction.

• Reduce dosage in patients with renal or hepatic impairment.

• If patient is receiving I.V. verapamil, monitor ECG and blood pressure continuously.

• If patient is also receiving digoxin, reduce digoxin dosage by half and monitor serum drug levels.

• During long-term therapy with verapamil and digoxin, monitor ECG periodically to observe for AV block and bradycardia.

• Obtain periodic liver function tests.

• Use reduced dosage in patients with severely compromised cardiac function and those receiving beta blockers. Monitor closely.

• Discontinue disopyramide 48 hours before starting verapamil, and don't reinstitute until 24 hours after verapamil has been discontinued.

• Generic sustained-release verapamil tablets can be substituted for Isoptin SR or Calan SR, not Verelan capsules. The capsule formulation should be given only once daily. When using sustained-release tablets, doses exceeding 240 mg should be given twice daily.

Patient education

• Instruct patient to report signs and symptoms of heart failure, such as swelling of hands and feet or shortness of breath.

• Urge patient receiving a nitrate while verapamil dose is being adjusted to comply with prescribed therapy.

Overdose & treatment

• Signs and symptoms of overdose are primarily extensions of adverse reactions. Heart block, asystole, and hypotension are the most serious reactions and require immediate attention.

• Treatment may include administering I.V. isoproterenol, norepinephrine, epinephrine, atropine, or calcium gluconate in usual doses. Ensure adequate hydration. In patients with hypertrophic cardiomyopathy, use alpha-adrenergics—including methoxamine, phenylephrine, and metaraminol—to maintain blood pressure. (Avoid using isoproterenol and norepinephrine.) Use inotropic drugs, including dobutamine and dopamine, if necessary. If severe conduction disturbances, such as heart block and asystole, occur with hypotension that doesn't respond to drug therapy, initiate cardiac pacing immediately, with cardiopulmonary resuscitation measures as indicated. In patients with Wolff-Parkinson-White or Lown-Ganong-Levine syndrome and a rapid ventricular rate caused by hemodynamically significant antegrade conduction, use synchronized cardioversion, with lidocaine and procainamide as adjuncts.

---

vinblastine sulfate (VLB)
Velban, Velbe

Vinca alkaloid (cell cycle–phase specific, M phase), antineoplastic

---

Available by prescription only
Injection: 10-mg vials (lyophilized powder), 10 mg/10-ml vials

INDICATIONS & DOSAGE

Dosage and indications vary. Check current literature for recommended protocol.

Breast or testicular cancer, Hodgkin's and malignant lymphomas, choriocarcinoma, lymphosarcoma, neuroblastoma, lung cancer, mycosis fungoides, histiocytosis, Kaposi's sarcoma
Adults: 0.1 mg/kg or 3.7 mg/m² I.V. weekly or q 2 weeks. May be increased in weekly increments of 50 mcg/kg or 1.8 to 1.9 mg/m² to maximum dosage of 0.5 mg/kg or 18.5 mg/m² I.V. weekly, based on response. Dose shouldn't be repeated if WBC count is less than 4,000/mm³.

PHARMACODYNAMICS

Antineoplastic action: Vinblastine arrests the cell cycle in the metaphase portion of cell division, thus blocking mitosis. Drug also inhibits DNA-dependent RNA synthesis and interferes with amino acid metabolism, inhibiting purine synthesis.

PHARMACOKINETICS

Absorption: Vinblastine is absorbed unpredictably across the GI tract after oral administration; drug must be given I.V.
Distribution: Drug is distributed widely into body tissues, crosses the blood-brain barrier, but doesn't achieve therapeutic levels in CSF.
Metabolism: Drug is metabolized partially in the liver to an active metabolite.
Excretion: Excreted primarily in bile as unchanged drug; smaller portion is excreted in urine. Plasma elimination of drug is described as triphasic, with half-lives of 3.7 minutes, 1.6 hours, and 24.8 hours for the alpha, beta, and terminal phases, respectively.

CONTRAINDICATIONS & PRECAUTIONS

Contraindicated in patients with severe leukopenia, granulocytopenia (unless result of disease being treated), or bacterial infection.

Use cautiously in patients with hepatic dysfunction.

INTERACTIONS

Drug-drug. Use with *erythromycin* may cause vinblastine to have a toxic affect on the patient. Use with *mitomycin* has produced acute shortness of breath and severe bronchospasm. Use with *phenytoin* may result in lower plasma phenytoin levels, requiring increased dosage of phenytoin.

ADVERSE REACTIONS

CNS: depression, *paresthesia, peripheral neuropathy and neuritis, numbness, loss of deep tendon reflexes, muscle pain and weakness, seizures, CVA,* headache.
CV: hypertension, *MI.*
EENT: pharyngitis.
GI: *nausea, vomiting,* ulcer, bleeding, *constipation, ileus, anorexia,* diarrhea, *weight loss,* abdominal pain, *stomatitis.*

Hematologic: *anemia, leukopenia* (nadir occurs days 4 to 10 and lasts another 7 to 14 days), *thrombocytopenia.*
Metabolic: increased blood and urine uric acid levels.
Respiratory: *acute bronchospasm,* shortness of breath.
Skin: reversible alopecia, vesiculation.
Other: *irritation, phlebitis,* cellulitis, necrosis with extravasation.

▣ KEY CONSIDERATIONS

● Patients with cachexia or ulceration of the skin (more common in geriatric patients) may be more susceptible to leukopenic effect of vinblastine.
● To reduce nausea, give an antiemetic before administering drug.
● To reconstitute drug, use 10 ml preserved normal saline injection to yield 1 mg/ml.
● Don't dilute drug into larger volume for infusion into peripheral veins. This method increases risk of extravasation. Drug may be administered as an I.V. infusion through a central venous catheter.
● Drug may be administered by I.V. push injection over 1 minute into the tubing of a freely flowing I.V. infusion.
● After administering drug, monitor for life-threatening acute bronchospasm. This reaction is most likely to occur in patient also receiving mitomycin.
● Don't administer more frequently than every 7 days. Before administering the next dose, review effect of drug on leukocyte count. Leukopenia may develop.
● Reduced dosage may be required in patients with liver disease.
● Prevent uric acid nephropathy by giving patient generous amounts of oral fluids and administering allopurinol.
● Treat extravasation with liberal injection of hyaluronidase into the site, followed by warm compresses to minimize the spread of the reaction. (Some health care providers treat extravasation with cold compresses.) Prepare hyaluronidase by adding 3 ml normal saline solution to 150-U vial.
● Give laxatives as needed. Stool softeners may be used as prophylactics.

• Don't confuse vinblastine with vincristine or the investigational drug vindesine.

• Drug is less neurotoxic than vincristine.

Patient education

• Encourage adequate fluid intake to increase urine output and facilitate excretion of uric acid.

• Reassure patient that therapeutic response isn't immediate; adequate trial is 12 weeks.

• Advise patient to avoid exposure to people with infections and to report signs of infection or unusual bleeding immediately.

• Reassure patient that hair should grow back after treatment has ended.

Overdose & treatment

• Signs and symptoms of overdose include stomatitis, ileus, mental depression, paresthesia, loss of deep reflexes, permanent CNS damage, and myelosuppression.

• Treatment is usually supportive and includes transfusion of blood components and appropriate symptomatic therapy.

vincristine sulfate
Oncovin, Vincasar PFS, Vincrex

Vinca alkaloid (cell cycle–phase specific, M phase), antineoplastic

Available by prescription only
Injection: 1 mg/1-ml, 2 mg/2-ml, and 5 mg/5-ml multiple-dose vials; 1 mg/1-ml and 2 mg/2-ml preservative-free vials

INDICATIONS & DOSAGE
Dosage and indications vary. Check current literature for recommended protocol.

Acute lymphoblastic and other leukemias; Hodgkin's disease; lymphosarcoma; reticulum cell, osteogenic, and other sarcomas; neuroblastoma; rhabdomyosarcoma; Wilms' tumor; lung and ◊ breast cancer
Adults: 10 to 30 mcg/kg I.V. or 0.4 to 1.4 mg/m^2 I.V. weekly.

✦ *Dosage adjustment.* Reduce dose by 50% in patients with direct serum bilirubin level exceeding 3 ml/dl or other evidence of significant hepatic impairment.

PHARMACODYNAMICS
Antineoplastic action: Vincristine arrests the cell cycle in the metaphase portion of cell division, thus blocking mitosis. Drug also inhibits DNA-dependent RNA synthesis and interferes with amino acid metabolites, inhibiting purine synthesis.

PHARMACOKINETICS
Absorption: Vincristine is absorbed unpredictably across the GI tract after oral administration; drug must be given I.V.
Distribution: Drug is rapidly and widely distributed into body tissues; binds to erythrocytes and platelets. Drug crosses the blood-brain barrier but doesn't achieve therapeutic levels in CSF.
Metabolism: Drug is extensively metabolized in the liver.
Excretion: Drug and its metabolites are primarily excreted into bile; smaller portion is eliminated from the kidneys. Plasma elimination is described as triphasic, with half-lives of about 4 minutes, 2¼ hours, and 85 hours for the distribution, second, and terminal phases, respectively.

CONTRAINDICATIONS & PRECAUTIONS
Contraindicated in patients hypersensitive to vincristine or those with the demyelinating form of Charcot-Marie-Tooth syndrome. Don't give to patients who are receiving radiation therapy through ports that include the liver.

Use cautiously in patients with hepatic dysfunction, neuromuscular disease, or infection.

INTERACTIONS
Drug-drug. *Asparaginase* decreases the hepatic clearance of vincristine. *Calcium channel blockers* enhance vincristine accumulation in cells. Use with *digoxin* decreases digoxin levels; monitor serum digoxin levels. Use with *methotrexate* increases the therapeutic effect of methotrexate; this interaction may be used to therapeutic advantage because it allows a lower dose of methotrexate, re-

---

Reactions may be *common*, uncommon, *life-threatening*, or COMMON AND LIFE-THREATENING.

ducing the risk of a toxic reaction to methotrexate. Use with *mitomycin* may increase the frequency of bronchospasm and acute pulmonary reactions. Use with other *neurotoxic drugs* increases neurotoxicity through an additive effect. Use with *phenytoin* may decrease plasma phenytoin levels; dosage adjustments may be needed.

ADVERSE REACTIONS

CNS: *peripheral neuropathy,* sensory loss, *loss of deep tendon reflexes, paresthesia, wristdrop and footdrop, seizures, coma,* headache, ataxia, cranial nerve palsies, *jaw pain,* hoarseness, vocal cord paralysis, *muscle weakness and cramps*—some neurotoxicities may be permanent.
CV: hypotension, hypertension.
EENT: diplopia, optic and extraocular neuropathy, ptosis, photophobia, transient cortical blindness, optical atrophy.
GI: diarrhea, *constipation, cramps,* ileus that mimics surgical abdomen, paralytic ileus, *nausea, vomiting,* anorexia, weight loss, dysphagia, *intestinal necrosis, stomatitis.*
GU: urine retention, SIADH, dysuria, acute uric acid neuropathy, polyuria.
Hematologic: anemia, *leukopenia, thrombocytopenia.*
Metabolic: increased blood and urine uric acid levels, hyponatremia.
Respiratory: *acute bronchospasm,* dyspnea.
Skin: *reversible alopecia.*
Other: fever, severe local reaction with extravasation, *phlebitis,* cellulitis at injection site.

▣ KEY CONSIDERATIONS

• Weak or bedridden patients may be more susceptible to neurotoxic effects; use cautiously.
• Vincristine may be administered by I.V. push injection over 1 minute into the tubing of a freely flowing I.V. infusion.
• Don't dilute drug into larger volumes for infusion into peripheral veins; this method increases risk of extravasation. Drug may be administered as an I.V. infusion through a central venous catheter.
• Necrosis may result from extravasation. Manufacturer recommends treat-

ment with cold compresses and prompt administration of 150 U I.D. hyaluronidase, sodium bicarbonate, and local injection of hydrocortisone, or a combination of these treatments. However, some health care providers prefer to treat extravasation only with warm compresses.
• After administering drug, monitor for life-threatening bronchospasm; it's most likely to occur in patients also receiving mitomycin.
• Because of potential for neurotoxicity, don't give drug more than once weekly. Neurotoxicity is dose related and usually reversible; reduce dosage if symptoms of neurotoxicity develop.
• Monitor for neurotoxicity by checking for depression of Achilles tendon reflex, numbness, tingling, footdrop or wristdrop, difficulty walking, ataxia, and slapping gait. Also, check ability to walk on heels. Patient should have support while walking.
• Prevent uric acid nephropathy by giving patient generous amounts of oral fluids and administering allopurinol. Urine may need to be alkalized if serum uric acid level is increased.
• Monitor patient's bowel function. Patient should have stool softener, laxative, or water before dosing. Constipation may be an early indication of neurotoxicity.
• Reduced dosage may be required in patients with obstructive jaundice or liver disease.
• Don't confuse vincristine with vinblastine or the investigational drug vindesine.
• Vials of 5 mg are for multiple-dose use only. Don't administer entire vial to patient as single dose.
• Drug may cause SIADH. Treatment requires fluid restriction and a loop diuretic.
• Treatment of patients mistakenly receiving intrathecal vincristine is a medical emergency. Prognosis is generally poor.

Patient education

• Encourage adequate fluid intake to increase urine output and facilitate excretion of uric acid.

• Tell patient to call regarding use of laxatives if constipation or stomach pain occurs.
• Reassure patient that hair growth should resume after treatment is discontinued.

Overdose & treatment

• Signs and symptoms of overdose include alopecia, myelosuppression, paresthesia, neuritic pain, motor difficulties, loss of deep tendon reflexes, nausea, vomiting, and ileus.
• Treatment is usually supportive and includes blood transfusions, antiemetics, enemas for ileus, phenobarbital for seizures, and other appropriate symptomatic therapy. Administration of 15 mg of calcium leucovorin I.V. q 3 hours for 24 hours, then q 6 hours for 48 hours, may help protect cells from the toxic effects of vincristine.

---

vitamin A (retinol)
Aquasol A, Del-Vi-A, Palmitate-A 5000

Fat-soluble vitamin

Available by prescription only
Tablets: 10,000 IU
Capsules: 10,000 IU, 25,000 IU, 50,000 IU
Injection: 2-ml vials (50,000 IU/ml with 0.5% chlorobutanol, polysorbate 80, butylated hydroxyanisole, and butylated hydroxytoluene)
Available without prescription, as appropriate
Drops: 30 ml with dropper (5,000 IU/0.1 ml)
Capsules: 10,000 IU
Tablets: 5,000 IU

INDICATIONS & DOSAGE
Severe vitamin A deficiency with xerophthalmia
Adults: 500,000 IU P.O. daily for 3 days, then 50,000 IU P.O. daily for 14 days, then maintenance dosage of 10,000 to 20,000 IU P.O. daily for 2 months, followed by adequate dietary nutrition and RDA vitamin A supplements.

Severe vitamin A deficiency
Adults: 100,000 IU P.O. or I.M. daily for 3 days, then 50,000 IU P.O. or I.M. daily for 14 days, then maintenance dosage of 10,000 to 20,000 IU P.O. daily for 2 months, followed by adequate dietary nutrition and vitamin A supplements.

PHARMACODYNAMICS
Metabolic action: 1 IU vitamin A is equivalent to 0.3 mcg retinol or 0.6 mcg beta-carotene. Beta-carotene, or provitamin A, yields retinol after absorption from the intestinal tract. Retinol's use with opsin, the red pigment in the retina, helps form rhodopsin, which is needed for visual adaptation to darkness. Vitamin A prevents growth retardation and preserves the integrity of the epithelial cells. Vitamin A deficiency is characterized by nyctalopia (night blindness), keratomalacia (necrosis of the cornea), keratinization and drying of the skin, low resistance to infection, bone thickening, and diminished cortical steroid production.

PHARMACOKINETICS
Absorption: In normal doses, vitamin A is absorbed readily and completely if fat absorption is normal. Larger doses, or regular doses in patients with fat malabsorption, low protein intake, or hepatic or pancreatic disease, may be absorbed incompletely. Because vitamin A is fat soluble, absorption requires bile salts, pancreatic lipase, and dietary fat.
Distribution: Vitamin A is stored (primarily as palmitate) in Kupffer's cells in the liver. Normal adult liver stores are sufficient to provide vitamin A requirements for 2 years. Lesser amounts of retinyl palmitate are stored in the kidneys, lungs, adrenal glands, retinas, and intraperitoneal fat. Vitamin A circulates bound to a specific alpha$_1$ protein, retinol binding protein (RBP). Blood level assays may not reflect liver storage of vitamin A because serum levels depend partly on circulating RBP. Liver storage should be adequate before discontinuing therapy.
Metabolism: Drug is metabolized in the liver.

Reactions may be *common*, uncommon, *life-threatening*, or COMMON AND LIFE-THREATENING.

Excretion: Retinol, which is fat soluble, is conjugated with glucuronic acid and then further metabolized to retinal and retinoic acid. Retinoic acid is excreted in feces via biliary elimination. Retinal, retinoic acid, and other water-soluble metabolites are excreted in urine and feces. Normally, no unchanged retinol is excreted in urine, except in patients with pneumonia or chronic nephritis.

CONTRAINDICATIONS & PRECAUTIONS

Oral form contraindicated in patients with malabsorption syndrome; if malabsorption is from inadequate bile secretion, oral route may be used with administration of bile salts (dehydrocholic acid). Also contraindicated in those with hypervitaminosis A and hypersensitivity to an ingredient in product. I.V. route contraindicated except for special water-miscible forms intended for infusion with large parenteral volumes. I.V. push of vitamin A of any type is contraindicated (anaphylaxis or anaphylactoid reactions and death have resulted).

INTERACTIONS

Drug-drug. Use with *cholestyramine* may decrease the absorption of vitamin A by decreasing bile acids and preventing the micellar phase in the GI lumen; daily vitamin A supplements may be necessary during long-term cholestyramine therapy. Prolonged use of *mineral oil* may interfere with the intestinal absorption of vitamin A. Use with *neomycin* may decrease vitamin A absorption. Because of potential for additive adverse effects, patients receiving *retinoids* (such as *etretinate* or *isotretinoin*) should avoid use with vitamin A. Large doses of vitamin A may interfere with the hypoprothrombinemic effect of *warfarin*.

ADVERSE REACTIONS

CNS: irritability, headache, *increased intracranial pressure,* fatigue, lethargy, malaise.
EENT: papilledema, exophthalmos.
GI: anorexia, epigastric pain, vomiting, polydipsia.
GU: polyuria.

Hepatic: jaundice, hepatomegaly, *cirrhosis,* elevated liver enzyme levels.
Metabolic: decalcification, hypercalcemia.
Musculoskeletal: migratory arthralgia, periostitis, cortical thickening over the radius and tibia.
Skin: alopecia; dry, cracked, scaly skin; pruritus; lip fissures; erythema; inflamed tongue, lips, and gums; massive desquamation; increased pigmentation; night sweats.
Other: splenomegaly; *death, anaphylactic shock (with I.V. use).*

▣ KEY CONSIDERATIONS

• The RDA for vitamin A in men is 1,000 retinol equivalents (RE) or 5,000 IU, which combines retinol and beta-carotene. The RDA in women is 800 RE or 4,000 IU, which combines retinol and beta-carotene.
• Liquid preparations are available to administer via an NG tube.
• In dietary deficiency, suspect multivitamin deficiency.
• For patients with malabsorption caused by inadequate bile secretion, give vitamin A with bile salts.
• Vitamin A given by I.V. push can cause anaphylaxis and death and is thus contraindicated.
• Use special water-miscible form of vitamin A when adding to large parenteral volumes.
• Vitamin A therapy may falsely increase serum cholesterol level readings by interfering with the Zlatkis-Zak reaction. Vitamin A has also been reported to falsely elevate bilirubin levels.

Patient education

• Explain that patient must avoid prolonged use of mineral oil while taking drug because mineral oil reduces vitamin A absorption in the intestine.
• Tell patient not to exceed recommended dosage.
• Instruct patient to report promptly signs and symptoms of overdose and to discontinue drug immediately if they occur.
• Teach patient to consume adequate protein, vitamin E, and zinc, which,

along with bile, are necessary for vitamin A absorption.

• Tell patient to store vitamin A in a tight, light-resistant container.

Overdose & treatment

• Signs and symptoms of overdose include nausea, vomiting, anorexia, malaise, drying or cracking of skin or lips, irritability, headache, and loss of hair.

• In cases of acute toxicity, increased intracranial pressure develops within 8 to 12 hours; cutaneous desquamation follows in a few days. A toxic reaction can follow a single dose of 25,000 IU/kg, which in adults is more than 2 million IU. Chronic toxic reaction results when the patient takes 4,000 IU/kg for 6 to 15 months, which in adults is 1 million IU/day for 3 days, 50,000 IU/day for more than 18 months, or 500,000 IU/day for 2 months.

• Treat, if hypercalcemia persists, by discontinuing vitamin A; administer I.V. sodium chloride solution, prednisone, and calcitonin, if indicated. Perform liver function tests to detect possible liver damage.

---

vitamin E (alpha tocopherol)
Amino-Opti-E, Aquasol E, E-200 IU Softgels, E-400 IU in a Water-Soluble Base, E-1000 IU Softgels, E-Complex-600, E-Vitamin Succinate, Vita Plus E

Fat-soluble vitamin

Available without prescription, as appropriate
Capsules: 100 IU, 200 IU, 400 IU, 500 IU, 600 IU, 1,000 IU
Tablets: 100 IU, 200 IU, 400 IU, 500 IU, 600 IU, 1,000 IU
Oral solution: 50 IU/ml

INDICATIONS & DOSAGE

Vitamin E deficiency in patients with impaired fat absorption (including patients with cystic fibrosis); biliary atresia
Adults: 60 to 75 IU P.O. daily, depending on severity. Maximum dose is 300 IU/day.

PHARMACODYNAMICS

Nutritional action: As a dietary supplement, the exact biochemical mechanism is unclear, although it's believed to act as an antioxidant. Vitamin E protects cell membranes, vitamin A, vitamin C (ascorbic acid), and polyunsaturated fatty acids from oxidation. It also may act as a cofactor in enzyme systems, and some evidence exists that it decreases platelet aggregation.

PHARMACOKINETICS

Absorption: GI absorption depends on the presence of bile. Only 20% to 60% of the vitamin obtained from dietary sources is absorbed. As dosage increases, the fraction of vitamin E absorbed decreases.
Distribution: Distributed to all tissues and is stored in adipose tissue.
Metabolism: Vitamin E is metabolized in the liver through glucuronidation.
Excretion: Excreted primarily in bile; some enterohepatic circulation may occur. Some metabolites are excreted in urine.

CONTRAINDICATIONS & PRECAUTIONS

No known contraindications. Use cautiously in patients with liver or gallbladder disease.

INTERACTIONS

Drug-drug. Use with *cholestyramine, colestipol, mineral oil,* or *sucralfate* may increase vitamin E requirements. Vitamin E may have anti–*vitamin K* effects; patients receiving *oral anticoagulants* may be at risk for hemorrhage after large doses of vitamin E.

ADVERSE REACTIONS

None reported with recommended dosages. Hypervitaminosis E signs and symptoms include fatigue, weakness, nausea, headache, blurred vision, flatulence, diarrhea.

▣ KEY CONSIDERATIONS

• The RDA for vitamin E in men is 15 alpha tocopherol equivalent (TE), which is equal to 1 mg d-alpha-tocopherol or 1.49 IU; in women, 12 TE.

• Give with bile salts if patient has malabsorption caused by lack of bile.

Patient education
• Inform patient about dietary sources of vitamin E.
• Tell patient to store vitamin E in a tight, light-resistant container.
• Instruct patient to swallow capsules whole and not to crush or chew them.

Overdose & treatment
• Signs and symptoms of overdose include an increase in blood pressure.
• Treatment is generally supportive.

vitamin K derivatives

phytonadione
AquaMEPHYTON, Konakion

Vitamin K, blood coagulation modifier

Available by prescription only
Tablets: 5 mg
Injection (aqueous colloidal solution): 2 mg/ml
Injection (aqueous dispersion): 10 mg/ml

INDICATIONS & DOSAGE
Hypoprothrombinemia secondary to vitamin K malabsorption or drug therapy, or when oral administration is desired and bile secretion is inadequate
Adults: 5 to 10 mg P.O. daily, or titrated to patient's requirements.
Hypoprothrombinemia secondary to vitamin K malabsorption, drug therapy, or excess vitamin A
Adults: 2 to 25 mg P.O. or parenterally, repeated and increased up to 50 mg, if necessary.
Hypoprothrombinemia secondary to effect of oral anticoagulants
Adults: 2.5 to 10 mg P.O., S.C., or I.M., based on PT and INR and repeated, if necessary, 12 to 48 hours after oral dose or 6 to 8 hours after parenteral dose. In emergency, give 10 to 50 mg slow I.V., rate not to exceed 1 mg/minute, repeated q 6 to 8 hours, p.r.n.

Prevention of hypoprothrombinemia related to vitamin K deficiency in long-term parenteral nutrition
Adults: 5 to 10 mg I.M. weekly.

PHARMACODYNAMICS
Coagulation modifying action: Vitamin K is a lipid-soluble vitamin that promotes hepatic formation of active prothrombin and several other coagulation factors (specifically factors II, VII, IX, and X).
Phytonadione (vitamin K_1) is a synthetic form of vitamin K and is also lipid soluble. Vitamin K doesn't counteract the action of heparin.

PHARMACOKINETICS
Absorption: Phytonadione requires the presence of bile salts for GI tract absorption. Once absorbed, vitamin K enters the blood directly. Onset of action after I.V. injection is more rapid but of shorter duration than that occurring after S.C. or I.M. injection.
Distribution: Vitamin K concentrates in the liver for a short time. Action of parenteral phytonadione begins in 1 to 2 hours; hemorrhage is usually controlled within 3 to 6 hours, and normal prothrombin levels are achieved in 12 to 14 hours. Oral phytonadione begins to act within 6 to 10 hours.
Metabolism: Metabolized rapidly in the liver; little tissue accumulation occurs.
Excretion: Data are limited. High levels occur in feces; however, intestinal bacteria can synthesize vitamin K.

CONTRAINDICATIONS & PRECAUTIONS
Contraindicated in patients with hypersensitivity to vitamin K.

INTERACTIONS
Drug-drug. *Broad-spectrum antibiotics* (especially *cefamandole, cefoperazone,* and *cefotetan*) may interfere with the actions of vitamin K, producing hypoprothrombinemia. *Mineral oil* inhibits absorption of oral vitamin K; give drugs at well-spaced intervals, and monitor result. Vitamin K antagonizes the effects of *oral anticoagulants;* patients receiving these drugs should take vitamin K only for severe hypoprothrombinemia.

ADVERSE REACTIONS

CNS: headache, pain, dizziness, convulsive movements.
CV: transient hypotension after I.V. administration, rapid and weak pulse, *arrhythmias.*
GI: nausea, vomiting.
Respiratory: *bronchospasm,* dyspnea.
Skin: diaphoresis, flushing, erythema, urticaria, pruritus, allergic rash.
Other: cramp-like pain, *anaphylaxis and anaphylactoid reactions* (usually after too-rapid I.V. administration), swelling, hematoma at injection site.

▣ KEY CONSIDERATIONS

• The RDA for vitamin K in men is 80 mcg; in women, 65 mcg.
• Check particular product for approved routes of administration.
• If severity of condition warrants I.V. infusion, mix with preservative-free normal saline solution, D_5W, or dextrose 5% in normal saline solution. Monitor for flushing, weakness, tachycardia, and hypotension; shock may follow. Deaths have occurred.
• Discontinue drug if allergic or severe CNS reactions appear.
• Monitor PT and INR to determine effectiveness.
• Monitor patient response, and watch for adverse effects; failure to respond to vitamin K may indicate coagulation defects or irreversible hepatic damage.
• Excessive use of vitamin K may temporarily defeat oral anticoagulant therapy; higher doses of oral anticoagulant or interim use of heparin may be required.
• Phytonadione is the vitamin K analogue of choice to treat an oral anticoagulant overdose.
• Patients receiving phytonadione who have bile deficiency require bile salts to ensure adequate absorption.
• Phytonadione can falsely elevate urine steroid levels.
• When I.V. administration is considered unavoidable, the drug should be injected very slowly, not exceeding 1 mg/minute.

Patient education

• For patients receiving oral form, explain rationale for drug therapy; stress importance of complying with medical regimen and keeping follow-up appointments.
• Tell patient to take a missed dose as soon as possible, but not if it's almost time for next dose, and to report missed doses.

Reactions may be *common*, uncommon, *life-threatening*, or COMMON AND LIFE-THREATENING.

warfarin sodium
Coumadin, Panwarfin

coumarin derivative, anticoagulant

Available by prescription only
Tablets: 1 mg, 2 mg, 2.5 mg, 3 mg,
4 mg, 5 mg, 6 mg, 7.5 mg, 10 mg
Injection: 5 mg/vial

INDICATIONS & DOSAGE
Pulmonary emboli, deep vein thrombosis, MI, rheumatic heart disease with heart valve damage, atrial arrhythmias
Adults: Initially, 2 to 5 mg P.O. or I.V.,
then daily PT and INR are used to establish optimal dose. Usual maintenance
dosage is 2 to 10 mg P.O. daily.

PHARMACODYNAMICS
Anticoagulant action: Warfarin inhibits
vitamin K–dependent activation of clotting factors II, VII, IX, and X, which are
formed in the liver; it has no direct effect
on established thrombi and can't reverse
ischemic tissue damage. However, warfarin may prevent additional clot formation, extension of formed clots, and secondary complications of thrombosis.

PHARMACOKINETICS
Absorption: Warfarin is rapidly and
completely absorbed from the GI tract.
Distribution: Drug is highly bound to
plasma protein, especially albumin.
Metabolism: Drug is hydroxylated in liver into inactive metabolites.
Excretion: Metabolites are reabsorbed
from bile and excreted in urine. Half-life
of parent drug is 1 to 3 days, but is highly variable. Because therapeutic effect is
relatively more dependent on clotting
factor depletion (factor X has half-life of
40 hours), PT won't peak for 1½ to 3
days despite use of a loading dose. Duration of action is 2 to 5 days, more closely
reflecting drug's half-life.

CONTRAINDICATIONS & PRECAUTIONS
Contraindicated in patients with bleeding or hemorrhagic tendencies, GI ulcerations, severe hepatic or renal disease,
severe uncontrolled hypertension, subacute bacterial endocarditis, aneurysm,
ascorbic acid deficiency, history of
warfarin-induced necrosis, regional or
lumbar block anesthesia, polycythemia
vera, and vitamin K deficiency; in those
in whom diagnostic tests or therapeutic
procedures have potential for uncontrolled bleeding; in unsupervised patients with senility, alcoholism, psychosis, or lack of cooperation; and after recent eye, brain, or spinal cord surgery.

Use cautiously in patients with diverticulitis, colitis, hypertension, hepatic or
renal disease, drainage tubes in orifice,
infectious disease or disturbance of intestinal flora, trauma, a large exposed
surface resulting from surgery, indwelling catheters, known or suspected
deficiency in protein C or S, heart failure, severe diabetes, vasculitis, or polycythemia vera; in patients also taking an
NSAID; and in patients at risk for hemorrhage.

INTERACTIONS
Drug-drug. Oral anticoagulants interact
with many drugs; changes in drug regimen, including use of *OTC compounds,*
require careful monitoring. The most
significant interactions follow. Use with
*allopurinol, cefamandole, cefoperazone,
cefotetan, danazol, diflunisal, erythromycin, glucagon, heparin, miconazole, quinidine, sulindac,* or *vitamin E*
increases warfarin's anticoagulant effects; monitor carefully. Use with *amiodarone, anabolic steroids, chloramphenicol, cimetidine, clofibrate, dextrothyroxine, disulfiram, metronidazole,
other thyroid preparations, salicylates,
streptokinase, urokinase,* or *sulfonamides* markedly increases warfarin's
anticoagulant effects; don't use together.
Barbiturates may inhibit anticoagulant
effect for several weeks after barbiturate
withdrawal, and fatal hemorrhage can
occur after cessation of barbiturate effect; if barbiturates are withdrawn, reduce anticoagulant dose. Use with *carbamazepine, corticosteroids, ethchlor-*

vynol, griseofulvin, or *vitamin K* may decrease anticoagulant effect; monitor carefully. *Cholestyramine* decreases warfarin's anticoagulant effect when used close together; administer 6 hours after warfarin. Use with *chloral hydrate* may increase or decrease warfarin's anticoagulant effect; monitor therapy carefully and avoid using together when possible. Use with *ethacrynic acid, indomethacin, mefenamic acid, phenylbutazone,* or *sulfinpyrazone* increases warfarin's anticoagulant effect and causes severe GI irritation (may be ulcerogenic); avoid using together when possible. Use with *glutethimide* or *rifampin* causes decreased anticoagulant effect of major significance and should be avoided.

Drug-lifestyle. *Acute alcohol intoxication* increases warfarin's anticoagulant effect. *Alcohol abuse* decreases anticoagulant effect but may predispose patient to bleeding problems.

ADVERSE REACTIONS

GI: anorexia, nausea, vomiting, cramps, *diarrhea,* mouth ulcerations, sore mouth.
GU: hematuria.
Hematologic: prolonged PT, INR, and PTT; *hemorrhage* (with excessive dosage).
Hepatic: *hepatitis,* elevated liver function test results, jaundice.
Skin: dermatitis, urticaria, necrosis, gangrene, alopecia, *rash.*
Other: *fever,* enhanced uric acid excretion.

▣ KEY CONSIDERATIONS

• Geriatric patients are more susceptible to effects of anticoagulants and are at increased risk for hemorrhage; this may be caused by altered hemostatic mechanisms or age-related deterioration of liver and kidneys.
• I.V. warfarin provides an alternative for patients who can't tolerate or receive an oral drug. The I.V. dose is the same as the oral dose. Administer over 1 to 2 minutes into peripheral vein.
• To reconstitute, add 2.7 ml sterile water for injection to vial labeled as containing 5 mg warfarin. Inject appropriate dose slowly over 1 to 2 minutes.

• Store drug in light-resistant containers at controlled room temperature (59° to 86° F [15° to 30° C]). After reconstitution, warfarin injection is stable for 4 hours at controlled room temperature.
• Discard solution that contains a precipitate.
• Drug may interfere with the Schack and Waxler ultraviolet method for serum theophylline determinations, resulting in falsely decreased theophylline levels.

Patient education

• Warn patient to avoid taking OTC products containing aspirin, other salicylates, or drugs that may interact with the anticoagulant, causing an increase or decrease in action of drug, and to seek medical approval before stopping or starting drug.
• Advise patient not to substantially alter daily intake of leafy green vegetables (asparagus, broccoli, cabbage, lettuce, turnip greens, spinach, or watercress) or of fish, pork or beef liver, green tea, or tomatoes. These foods contain vitamin K and widely varying daily intake may alter anticoagulant effect of warfarin.
• Instruct patient to inform all health care providers (including dentists) about use of warfarin.
• Instruct patient to inform health care provider if unusual bleeding or bruising occurs.

Overdose & treatment

• Signs and symptoms of overdose vary with severity and may include internal or external bleeding or skin necrosis of fat-rich areas, but most common sign is hematuria. Excessive prolongation of PT or minor bleeding mandates withdrawal of therapy; withholding one or two doses may be adequate in some cases.
• Treatment to control bleeding may include oral or I.V. phytonadione and, in severe hemorrhage, fresh frozen plasma or whole blood. Use of phytonadione may interfere with subsequent oral anticoagulant therapy.

Reactions may be *common,* uncommon, *life-threatening,* or COMMON AND LIFE-THREATENING.

X

xylometazoline hydrochloride
Otrivin

Sympathomimetic, decongestant, vasoconstrictor

Available without prescription
Nasal drops: 0.05%
Nasal spray: 0.1%

INDICATIONS & DOSAGE
Nasal congestion
Adults: Apply 2 or 3 gtt or sprays of 0.1% solution to nasal mucosa q 8 to 10 hours, not to exceed three times in 24 hours.

PHARMACODYNAMICS
Decongestant action: Xylometazoline acts on alpha-adrenergic receptors in the nasal mucosa to produce constriction, thereby decreasing blood flow and nasal congestion.

PHARMACOKINETICS
Absorption: Unknown.
Distribution: Unknown.
Metabolism: Unknown.
Excretion: Unknown.

CONTRAINDICATIONS & PRECAUTIONS
Contraindicated in patients with acute angle-closure glaucoma or hypersensitivity to xylometazoline.

Use cautiously in patients with hyperthyroidism, cardiac disease, hypertension, diabetes mellitus, and advanced arteriosclerosis.

INTERACTIONS
Drug-drug. Xylometazoline may potentiate the pressor effects of *tricyclic antidepressants* if significant systemic absorption occurs.

ADVERSE REACTIONS
EENT: transient burning, stinging; dryness or ulceration of nasal mucosa; sneezing; rebound nasal congestion, irritation (with excessive or long-term use).

▣ KEY CONSIDERATIONS
● Use with caution in geriatric patients with cardiac disease, diabetes mellitus, or poorly controlled hypertension.
● Monitor carefully for adverse effects in patients with CV disease, diabetes mellitus, or hyperthyroidism.
● Nasal spray is less likely to cause systemic absorption and is more effective if 3 to 5 minutes elapse between sprays and nose is cleared before next spray.

Patient education
● Tell patient that xylometazoline should only be used for short-term relief of symptoms, no longer than 3 to 5 days.
● Teach patient how to use correctly. Have patient hold head upright and sniff spray briskly. To correctly administer drops, tell patient to recline on a bed and hang head over the edge as able. Patient should remain in that position for several minutes, turning head side to side. Only one person should use dropper bottle or nasal spray.
● Caution patient not to exceed recommended dosage to avoid rebound congestion.
● Tell patient to report insomnia, dizziness, weakness, tremor, or irregular heartbeat.

Overdose & treatment
● Signs and symptoms of overdose include somnolence, sedation, sweating, CNS depression with hypertension, bradycardia, decreased cardiac output, rebound hypotension, CV collapse, depressed respirations, coma.
● Because of rapid onset of sedation, emesis isn't recommended in therapy unless given early. Activated charcoal or gastric lavage may be used initially. Monitor vital signs and ECG. Treat seizures with I.V. diazepam.

Z

zafirlukast
Accolate

Leukotriene receptor antagonist, antasthmatic

Available by prescription only
Tablets: 20 mg

INDICATIONS & DOSAGE
Prophylaxis and long-term treatment of asthma
Adults: 20 mg P.O. b.i.d. taken 1 hour before or 2 hours after meals.

PHARMACODYNAMICS
Antasthmatic action: Zafirlukast selectively competes for leukotriene receptor (LTD_4 and LTE_4) sites, blocking inflammatory action.

PHARMACOKINETICS
Absorption: Zafirlukast is rapidly absorbed after oral administration; plasma levels peak 3 hours after dosing.
Distribution: More than 99% binds to plasma proteins, predominantly albumin.
Metabolism: Drug is extensively metabolized through the cytochrome P-450 2C9 (CYP 2C9) system; also inhibits the CYP 3A4 and CYP 2C9 isoenzymes.
Excretion: Drug is primarily excreted in feces; mean terminal half-life is about 10 hours.

CONTRAINDICATIONS & PRECAUTIONS
Contraindicated in patients with known hypersensitivity to zafirlukast or its components.

Use cautiously in geriatric patients and those with hepatic impairment.

INTERACTIONS
Drug-drug. *Aspirin* increases plasma levels of zafirlukast. Although no formal drug interactions have been found, administer *calcium channel blockers, carbamazepine, cisapride, cyclosporine, dihydropyridine, phenytoin,* and *tolbutamide* with caution because these drugs are metabolized by CYP 2C9 and CYP 3A4 isoenzymes. Use with *erythromycin* and *theophylline* decreases plasma levels of zafirlukast. Use with *warfarin* causes increased PT; monitor PT and INR levels, and adjust dosage of anticoagulant.
Drug-food. *Food* decreases bioavailability of drug; give 1 hour before or 2 hours after a meal.

ADVERSE REACTIONS
CNS: asthenia, dizziness, *headache.*
GI: abdominal pain, diarrhea, dyspepsia, nausea, vomiting.
Hepatic: elevated liver enzyme levels.
Musculoskeletal: back pain, myalgia.
Other: accidental injury, fever, infection.

▣ KEY CONSIDERATIONS
• Zafirlukast clearance is reduced in geriatric patients; use with caution.
• Drug isn't indicated for the reversal of bronchospasm in acute asthma attacks.
• Drug is known to inhibit CYP 3A4 and CYP 2C9 in vitro; it's reasonable to use appropriate clinical monitoring when drugs metabolized by this isoenzyme system are administered together.

Patient education
• Tell patient that zafirlukast is used for long-term treatment of asthma and that he should keep taking drug even if symptoms disappear.
• Advise patient to continue taking other antiasthma drugs as prescribed.
• Instruct patient not to take drug with food; take 1 hour before or 2 hours after meals.

zalcitabine (dideoxycytidine, ddC)
HIVID

Nucleoside analogue, antiviral

Available by prescription only
Tablets (film-coated): 0.375 mg, 0.75 mg

INDICATIONS & DOSAGE
Patients with advanced HIV infection (CD4 count less than 300/mm³) who have shown significant clinical or immunologic deterioration
Adults weighing 30 kg (66 lb) or more: 0.75 mg P.O. q 8 hours. Can be taken with zidovudine (200 mg P.O. q 8 hours).
✦ *Dosage adjustment.* For patients with impaired renal function, use this table.

Creatinine clearance (ml/min)	Dosage
> 40	0.75 mg P.O. q 8 hr
10-40	0.75 mg P.O. q 12 hr
< 10	0.75 mg P.O. q 24 hr

PHARMACODYNAMICS
Antiviral action: Zalcitabine is active against HIV. Within cells, it's converted by cellular enzymes into its active metabolite, dideoxycytidine 5′-triphosphate. It inhibits the replication of HIV by blocking viral DNA synthesis. The drug inhibits reverse transcriptase by acting as an alternative for the enzyme's substrate, deoxycytidine triphosphate.

PHARMACOKINETICS
Absorption: Mean absolute bioavailability is more than 80%; administering zalcitabine with food decreases rate and extent of absorption.
Distribution: Steady-state volume of distribution is 0.534 ± 0.127 L/kg. Drug enters the CNS.
Metabolism: Drug doesn't appear to undergo significant hepatic metabolism; phosphorylation to the active form occurs within cells.
Excretion: Drug is excreted primarily from the kidneys; about 70% of dose appears in urine within 24 hours. Mean elimination half-life, 2 hours.

CONTRAINDICATIONS & PRECAUTIONS
Contraindicated in patients with hypersensitivity to zalcitabine or component of the formulation.
   Use cautiously in patients with preexisting peripheral neuropathy, impaired renal function, hepatic failure, and history of pancreatitis, heart failure, or cardiomyopathy.

INTERACTIONS
Drug-drug. *Cimetidine* and *probenecid* decrease elimination of zalcitabine. Use with *drugs that cause peripheral neuropathy* (such as *chloramphenicol, cisplatin, dapsone, didanosine, disulfiram, ethionamide, glutethimide, gold salts, hydralazine, iodoquinol, isoniazid, metronidazole, nitrofurantoin, phenytoin, ribavirin, vincristine*) may increase risk for peripheral neuropathy. *Drugs that may impair renal function* (such as *aminoglycosides, amphotericin B,* and *foscarnet*) may also increase risk for zalcitabine-induced adverse effects. Use with *pentamidine* isn't recommended because of the risk of pancreatitis.

ADVERSE REACTIONS
CNS: *peripheral neuropathy, headache, fatigue,* dizziness, confusion, **seizures,** impaired concentration, amnesia, insomnia, mental depression, tremor, hypertonia, anxiety.
EENT: pharyngitis, ocular pain, abnormal vision, ototoxicity, nasal discharge.
GI: nausea, vomiting, diarrhea, abdominal pain, **pancreatitis,** anorexia, constipation, stomatitis, esophageal ulcer, glossitis.
Respiratory: cough.

▣ KEY CONSIDERATIONS
● If zalcitabine is discontinued because of toxicity, resume recommended dosage for zidovudine alone, which is 100 mg every 4 hours.
● If symptoms indicating peripheral neuropathy occur, discontinue drug if symptoms are bilateral and persist beyond 72 hours. If these symptoms persist or worsen beyond 1 week, permanently withdraw drug. However, if all findings relevant to peripheral neuropathy have resolved to minor symptoms, drug may be reintroduced at 0.375 mg P.O. every 8 hours.
● The peripheral neuropathy seen with drug therapy is a sensorimotor neuropathy, initially characterized by numbness and burning in the extremities. If drug isn't withdrawn, patient may experience sharp, shooting pain or severe, continuous burning pain requiring narcotic anal-

gesics, both of which may not be reversible.

• Toxic effects of drug may cause abnormalities in several blood test results, including CBC; leukocyte, reticulocyte, granulocyte, and platelet counts; and hemoglobin, AST, ALT, and alkaline phosphatase levels.

Patient education

• Make sure patient understands that zalcitabine doesn't cure HIV infection and that he can still transmit HIV. Opportunistic infections may continue to occur despite use of drug. Review safe sex practices with patient.

• Tell patient that drug may cause peripheral neuropathy and life-threatening pancreatitis. Review signs and symptoms of these reactions, and instruct patient to report them immediately.

zidovudine (AZT)
Retrovir

Thymidine analogue, antiviral

Capsules: 100 mg
Syrup: 50 mg/5 ml
Injection: 10 mg/ml

INDICATIONS & DOSAGE
Symptomatic HIV, AIDS, or advanced AIDS-related complex
Adults: 100 mg P.O. q 4 hours (600-mg daily dose). Or administer by I.V. infusion, 1 mg/kg (at a constant rate over 1 hour) q 4 hours for total of 6 mg/kg/day.
Asymptomatic HIV infection (CD4 count less than 500/mm³)
Adults: 100 mg P.O. q 4 hours while awake (for total of five doses or 500 mg daily). Alternatively, administer 1 mg/kg I.V. over 1 hour q 4 hours while awake (5 mg/kg daily).
✦ *Dosage adjustment.* Dosage may need to be adjusted in patients undergoing dialysis because the drug is partially removed. Dosage may also need to be adjusted in patients with decreased liver function.

PHARMACODYNAMICS
Antiviral action: Zidovudine is converted intracellularly to an active triphosphate compound that inhibits reverse transcriptase (an enzyme essential for retroviral DNA synthesis), thereby inhibiting viral replication. When used in vitro, drug inhibits certain other viruses and bacteria, but the significance of this effect is unknown.

PHARMACOKINETICS
Absorption: Zidovudine is absorbed rapidly from the GI tract. Average systemic bioavailability is 65% of dose (drug undergoes first-pass metabolism).
Distribution: Preliminary data reveal good CSF penetration. About 36% of dose is plasma protein-bound.
Metabolism: Drug is metabolized rapidly to an inactive compound.
Excretion: Parent drug and metabolite are excreted through glomerular filtration and tubular secretion in the kidneys. Urine recovery of parent drug and metabolite is 14% and 74%, respectively. Elimination half-lives of these compounds is 1 hour.

CONTRAINDICATIONS & PRECAUTIONS
Contraindicated in patients with hypersensitivity to zidovudine.
Use cautiously in patients in advanced stages of HIV and in those with severe bone marrow suppression, renal insufficiency, or hepatomegaly, hepatitis, or other risk factors for hepatic disease.

INTERACTIONS
Drug-drug. When used with *drugs that are nephrotoxic or that affect bone marrow function or formation of bone marrow elements (such as amphotericin B, dapsone, doxorubicin, flucytosine, ganciclovir, interferon, pentamidine, vinblastine, vincristine)*, zidovudine may increase the risk of drug toxicity. Use with *probenecid* may impair elimination of zidovudine.

ADVERSE REACTIONS
CNS: *headache,* **seizures,** paresthesia, *asthenia, malaise,* insomnia, *dizziness,* somnolence.
EENT: taste perversion.

Reactions may be *common,* uncommon, **life-threatening,** or COMMON AND LIFE-THREATENING.

GI: *nausea, anorexia, abdominal pain, vomiting,* constipation, *diarrhea,* dyspepsia.
Hematologic: *severe bone marrow suppression (resulting in anemia), agranulocytosis, thrombocytopenia.*
Musculoskeletal: myalgia.
Skin: diaphoresis, *rash.*
Other: *fever.*

⊡ KEY CONSIDERATIONS

• Optimum duration of treatment as well as dosage for optimum effectiveness and minimum toxicity is unknown.
• Monitor CBC and platelet count at least every 2 weeks. Significant anemia (hemoglobin level less than 7.5 g/dl or reduction of more than 25% of baseline) or significant neutropenia (granulocyte count less than 750 cells/mm^3 or reduction of more than 50% from baseline) may require interruption of zidovudine therapy until evidence of bone marrow recovery occurs. In patients with less severe anemia or neutropenia, a reduction in dosage may be adequate.
• I.V. dosage equivalent to 100 mg P.O. every 4 hours is about 1 mg/kg I.V. every 4 hours.
• Observe patient for signs and symptoms of opportunistic infection (including pneumonia, meningitis, and sepsis).
• Store undiluted injection, capsules, and syrup at room temperature (77° F [25° C]); protect from light. Dilute I.V. form to less than 4 mg/ml with D$_5$W before administering. Don't mix with protein-containing solutions. To minimize potential for microbial contamination, administer within 8 hours of mixing if left at room temperature or within 24 hours if refrigerated (36° to 46° F [2° to 8° C]).
• Drug doesn't cure HIV infection or AIDS but may reduce morbidity resulting from opportunistic infections and thus prolong the patient's life.

Patient education

• Because zidovudine commonly causes a low RBC count, advise patient that he may need blood transfusions or epoetin alfa therapy during treatment.
• Teach patient about the disease, ways to prevent disease transmission, rationale for drug therapy, and limitations of the drug.
• Teach patient about proper drug administration. When drug must be taken every 4 hours around the clock, explain the importance of maintaining an adequate blood level and suggest ways to avoid missing doses, such as using an alarm clock.
• Inform patient about importance of follow-up medical visits to evaluate for adverse effects and to monitor status.
• Instruct patient how to recognize adverse drug effects and to report them immediately.
• Warn patient not to take other drugs for AIDS (especially from the street) without medical approval.
• Make sure patient understands that he can still transmit HIV infection while taking the drug.

zileuton
Zyflo Filmtab

5-lipoxygenase inhibitor, antasthmatic

Available by prescription only
Tablets: 600 mg

INDICATIONS & DOSAGE
Prophylaxis and chronic treatment of asthma
Adults: 600 mg P.O. q.i.d.

PHARMACODYNAMICS
Antasthmatic action: Inhibits enzyme responsible for the formation of leukotrienes, thus reducing inflammatory response.

PHARMACOKINETICS
Absorption: Zileuton is rapidly absorbed with oral administration (mean time to peak level, 1.7 hours).
Distribution: Apparent volume of distribution is 1.2 L/kg. Drug is 93% bound to plasma proteins, primarily albumin.
Metabolism: Drug is metabolized by the cytochrome P-450 system via oxidation. Several active and inactive metabolites of zileuton have been identified.

Excretion: Elimination of drug is predominantly by metabolism, with a mean terminal half-life of 2½ hours.

CONTRAINDICATIONS & PRECAUTIONS

Contraindicated in patients with known hypersensitivity to zileuton or its components and in those with active hepatic disease or a transaminase level that's at least three times the normal upper limit.

Use with caution in patients with hepatic impairment or history of heavy alcohol use.

INTERACTIONS

Drug-drug. Use cautiously when administered with *drugs metabolized by the cytochrome P-450 3A4 isoenzyme (calcium channel blockers, cisapride, cyclosporine, dihydropyridine, estradiol, ethinyl, prednisone).* Administration with *propranolol* and *other beta blockers* may increase beta-blocker effect; monitor patient and reduce dosage of beta blocker. Administration with *theophylline* decreases theophylline clearance (on average, serum theophylline levels double); reduce theophylline dose and monitor serum levels. Administration with *warfarin* increases PT; monitor PT and INR and adjust dosage of anticoagulant.

ADVERSE REACTIONS

CNS: malaise, asthenia, dizziness, *headache,* insomnia, nervousness, somnolence.
CV: chest pain.
EENT: conjunctivitis.
GI: abdominal pain, constipation, dyspepsia, flatulence, nausea.
GU: urinary tract infection, vaginitis.
Hematologic: *leukopenia.*
Hepatic: elevated liver enzyme levels.
Musculoskeletal: arthralgia, hypertonia, myalgia, neck pain and rigidity.
Skin: pruritus.
Other: accidental injury, fever, lymphadenopathy, pain.

🔲 KEY CONSIDERATIONS

• Zileuton isn't indicated for use in the reversal of bronchospasm in acute asthma attacks.

• Obtain liver enzyme levels at baseline, then once a month for the first 3 months, every 2 to 3 months for the remainder of the 1st year, and periodically thereafter.

Patient education

• Tell patient that zileuton is used for long-term treatment of asthma and to continue taking drug even if his symptoms disappear.
• Caution patient that drug isn't a bronchodilator and shouldn't be used to treat acute asthma attack.
• Advise patient to continue taking other antasthmatics.
• Instruct patient to call if the short-acting bronchodilator is not effective in relieving symptoms.
• Tell patient to call immediately if signs and symptoms of hepatic dysfunction develop (right upper quadrant pain, nausea, fatigue, pruritus, jaundice, malaise).
• Advise patient to avoid alcohol and to seek approval before taking OTC or newly prescribed drugs.

---

zinc

Orazinc, Verazinc, Zinc 15, Zinc-220, Zincate

zinc sulfate (ophthalmic)

Eye-Sed

Trace element, anti-infective, nutritional supplement

Available by prescription only
Injection: 10 ml (1 mg/ml), 30 ml (1 mg/ml with 0.9% benzyl alcohol), 5 ml (5 mg/ml); 10 ml (5 mg/ml), 50 ml (1 mg/ml)
Capsules: 220 mg (50 mg zinc)
Available without prescription, as appropriate
Tablets: 66 mg (15 mg zinc), 110 mg (25 mg zinc), 200 mg (47 mg zinc)
Capsules: 110 mg (25 mg zinc), 220 mg (50 mg zinc)
Solution: 15 ml (0.25%)

INDICATIONS & DOSAGE

Metabolically stable zinc deficiency
Adults: 2.5 to 4 mg/day I.V.; add 2 mg/day for acute catabolic states.

Reactions may be *common,* uncommon, **life-threatening,** or COMMON AND LIFE-THREATENING.

Stable zinc deficiency with fluid loss from the small bowel
Adults: Add 12.2 mg/L total parenteral nutrition solution or 17.1 mg/kg stool output.
Dietary supplement
Adults: 25 to 50 mg P.O. daily.
For relief of minor eye irritation
Adults: 1 or 2 gtt ophthalmic solution into the eye b.i.d. or q.i.d.

PHARMACODYNAMICS

Metabolic action: Zinc serves as a co-factor for more than 70 different enzymes. It facilitates wound healing, normal growth rates, and normal skin hydration and helps maintain the senses of taste and smell.

Adequate zinc provides normal growth and tissue repair. In patients receiving total parenteral nutrition with low plasma zinc levels, alopecia has followed dermatitis. Zinc is an integral part of many enzymes important to carbohydrate and protein mobilization of retinal-binding protein.

Zinc sulfate ophthalmic solution shows astringent and weak antiseptic activity, which may result from precipitation of protein by the zinc ion and by clearing mucus from the outer surface of the eye. Drug has no decongestant action and produces mild vasodilation.

PHARMACOKINETICS

Absorption: Zinc sulfate is absorbed poorly from the GI tract; only 20% to 30% of dietary zinc is absorbed. After administration, zinc resides in muscle, bone, skin, kidney, liver, pancreas, retina, prostate, and particularly RBCs and WBCs. Zinc binds to plasma albumin, alpha-2 macroglobulin, and some plasma amino acids, including histidine, cysteine, threonine, glycine, and asparagine.
Distribution: Major zinc stores are in the skeletal muscle, skin, bone, and pancreas.
Metabolism: Zinc is a cofactor in many enzymatic reactions. It's required for the synthesis and mobilization of retinal-binding protein.
Excretion: After parenteral administration, 90% of zinc is excreted in stool, urine, and sweat. After oral use, the major route of excretion is secretion into the duodenum and jejunum. A small amount is also excreted in urine (0.3 to 0.5 mg/day) and sweat (1.5 mg/day).

CONTRAINDICATIONS & PRECAUTIONS

Parenteral use of zinc sulfate is contraindicated for patients with renal failure or biliary obstruction (and requires caution in all patients); monitor plasma zinc levels frequently. Don't exceed prescribed doses. In patients with renal dysfunction or GI malfunction, trace metal supplements may need to be reduced, adjusted, or omitted. Hypersensitivity may result.

Administering copper in the absence of zinc or administering zinc in the absence of copper may result in decreased serum levels of either element. When only one trace element is needed, it should be added separately and serum levels monitored closely. To avoid overdose, administer multiple trace elements only when clearly needed. In patients with extreme vomiting or diarrhea, extreme amounts of trace element may be needed. Excessive intake in healthy persons may be deleterious.

INTERACTIONS

Drug-drug. Zinc sulfate ophthalmic solution may precipitate *acacia* and certain proteins. Use of oral zinc sulfate with *fluoroquinolones* or *tetracycline* impairs antibiotic absorption. Zinc sulfate ophthalmic solution has a dehydrating effect on *methylcellulose suspensions,* causing precipitation of *methylcellulose.* When zinc sulfate ophthalmic solution is used with *sodium borate,* precipitation of zinc borate may occur; glycerin may prevent this interaction.
Drug-food. Use with *dairy products* reduces zinc absorption.

ADVERSE REACTIONS

CNS: restlessness.
GI: distress and irritation, nausea, vomiting with high doses, gastric ulceration, diarrhea.
Skin: rash.
Other: dehydration.

▣ KEY CONSIDERATIONS

• The RDA for zinc is 15 mg/day P.O. for adults.
• Results may not appear for 6 to 8 weeks for patients with zinc deficiency.
• Zinc decreases the absorption of tetracyclines and fluoroquinolones.
• Monitor for severe vomiting and dehydration, which may indicate overdose.
• Calcium supplements may confer a protective effect against the toxic effects of zinc.
• Because of potential for infusion phlebitis and tissue irritation, don't administer an undiluted direct injection into a peripheral vein.
• Don't exceed prescribed dosage of oral zinc; if oral zinc is administered in single 2-g doses, patient will vomit.
• If ophthalmic use causes increasing irritation, discontinue use.

Patient education

• Tell patient not to take zinc with dairy products, which can reduce zinc absorption.
• Teach patient how to instill ophthalmic solution and to prevent contamination. Tell him to avoid contacting the tip of the container with other surfaces and to tightly close the container after use.
• Warn patient not to take zinc sulfate ophthalmic solution for more than 3 days. Patient should report increased irritation or redness.
• Warn patient that GI upset may occur after oral administration but may be diminished if zinc is taken with food. Patients must avoid foods high in calcium, phosphorus, or phytate during zinc therapy.

Overdose & treatment

• Signs and symptoms of severe toxic reaction include hypotension, pulmonary edema, diarrhea, vomiting, jaundice, and oliguria.
• Dosage must be discontinued and supportive measures begun.

zolmitriptan
Zomig

Selective 5-hydroxytryptamine receptor agonist, antimigraine drug

Available by prescription only
Tablets: 2.5 mg, 5 mg

INDICATIONS & DOSAGE
Treatment of acute migraines with or without aura
Adults: Initially, 2.5 mg P.O. or less; for a smaller dose, break a 2.5-mg tablet in half. If migraine returns after initial dose, a second dose may be given after 2 hours. Maximum dose is 10 mg/day.
✦ *Dosage adjustment.* In patients with liver disease, use doses less than 2.5 mg.

PHARMACODYNAMICS
Antimigraine action: Zolmitriptan binds with high affinity to human recombinant 5-HT_{1D} and 5-HT_{1B} receptors, causing constriction of cranial blood vessels and inhibition of proinflammatory neuropeptide release—thus relieving migraine.

PHARMACOKINETICS
Absorption: Zolmitriptan is well absorbed after oral administration; plasma levels peak in 2 hours. Mean absolute bioavailability is about 40%.
Distribution: Apparent volume of distribution is 7 L/kg; drug is 25% plasma protein-bound.
Metabolism: Drug is converted to an active N-desmthyl metabolite. Metabolite level peaks in 2 to 3 hours. Mean elimination half-life of drug and active N-desmethyl metabolite is 3 hours.
Excretion: Mean total clearance is 31.5 ml/minute/kg, of which one-sixth is renal clearance. The renal clearance is greater than the GFR, suggesting renal tubular secretion. About 65% of dose is excreted in urine and 30% in feces.

CONTRAINDICATIONS & PRECAUTIONS
Contraindicated in patients with hypersensitivity to zolmitriptan or its components; in those with uncontrolled hypertension, ischemic heart disease (angina pectoris, a history of MI, or documented

silent ischemia), or other significant heart disease such as Wolff-Parkinson-White syndrome.

Avoid use within 24 hours of other 5-HT$_1$ agonists or ergot-containing drugs or within 2 weeks of discontinuing MAO inhibitor therapy. Also avoid use in patients with hemiplegic or basilar migraine.

Use cautiously in patients with liver disease.

INTERACTIONS
Drug-drug. *Cimetidine* doubles the half-life of zolmitriptan. *Ergot-containing drugs* may cause additive vasospastic reactions. *Fluoxetine, fluvoxamine, paroxetine,* and *sertraline* may cause weakness, hyperreflexia, and incoordination. *MAO inhibitors* increase plasma zolmitriptan levels.

ADVERSE REACTIONS
CNS: somnolence, vertigo, *dizziness,* hyperesthesias, paresthesia, asthenia.
CV: palpitations; pain or heaviness in chest; *pain, tightness, or pressure in the neck, throat, or jaw.*
GI: dry mouth, dyspepsia, dysphagia, nausea.
Musculoskeletal: myalgia.
Skin: sweating.
Other: warm or cold sensations.

▣ KEY CONSIDERATIONS
• The pharmacokinetic disposition is similar in younger and older patients. However, because geriatric patients were excluded from clinical trials, these patients should be observed.
• Monitor blood pressure in patients with liver disease.
• Zolmitriptan isn't intended as prophylaxis for migraines or for use in hemiplegic or basilar migraines.
• Safety hasn't been established for cluster headaches.
• Serious cardiac events, including some that have been fatal, have occurred rarely after use of 5-HT$_1$ agonists. Events reported have included coronary artery vasospasm, transient myocardial ischemia, MI, ventricular tachycardia, and ventricular fibrillation.

Patient education
• Tell patient that zolmitriptan is intended to relieve the symptoms of migraines, not prevent them.
• Advise patient to take drug only as prescribed and not to take a second dose unless instructed. If a second dose is indicated and approved by the health care provider, take it 2 hours after initial dose.
• Advise patient to report pain or tightness in the chest or throat, heart throbbing, rash, skin lumps, or swelling of the face, lips, or eyelids at once.
• Remind patient that drug shouldn't be taken with other antimigraine drugs.

zolpidem tartrate
Ambien

Imidazopyridine, hypnotic
Controlled substance schedule IV

Available by prescription only
Tablets: 5 mg, 10 mg

INDICATIONS & DOSAGE
Short-term management of insomnia
Adults: 10 mg P.O. immediately before bedtime.
Geriatric patients: 5 mg P.O. immediately before bedtime. Maximum daily dose is 10 mg.
✦ *Dosage adjustment.* In debilitated patients or patients with hepatic insufficiency, 5 mg P.O. immediately before bedtime. Maximum daily dose is 10 mg.

PHARMACODYNAMICS
Hypnotic action: Zolpidem is a hypnotic with a chemical structure unrelated to benzodiazepines, barbiturates, or other drugs with known hypnotic properties; it interacts with a gamma-aminobutyric acid (GABA)–benzodiazepine or omega-receptor complex and shares some of the pharmacologic properties of the benzodiazepines. It exhibits no muscle relaxant or anticonvulsant properties.

PHARMACOKINETICS
Absorption: Zolpidem is absorbed rapidly from the GI tract; mean level peaks at 1.6 hours. Food delays drug absorption.

Distribution: Drug is about 92.5% protein-bound.

Metabolism: Drug is converted to inactive metabolites in the liver.

Excretion: Drug is primarily eliminated in urine; elimination half-life is about 2.6 hours.

CONTRAINDICATIONS & PRECAUTIONS

No known contraindications.

Use cautiously in patients with conditions that could affect metabolism or hemodynamic response and in those with decreased respiratory drive, depression, or history of alcohol or drug abuse.

INTERACTIONS

Drug-drug. Other *CNS depressants* enhance the CNS depression of zolpidem; don't use together.

Drug-lifestyle. *Alcohol* enhances the CNS depressant effects of zolpidem; don't use together.

ADVERSE REACTIONS

CNS: daytime drowsiness, abnormal dreams, light-headedness, amnesia, dizziness, *headache,* hangover, sleep disorder, lethargy, depression.

CV: palpitations.

EENT: sinusitis, pharyngitis, dry mouth.

GI: nausea, vomiting, diarrhea, dyspepsia, constipation, abdominal pain.

Musculoskeletal: myalgia, arthralgia, back or chest pain.

Skin: rash.

Other: flulike syndrome, *hypersensitivity reactions.*

◉ KEY CONSIDERATIONS

• Geriatric patients may experience impaired motor or cognitive performance after repeated exposure or unusual sensitivity to sedative-hypnotics.

• Observe patients with history of addiction to or abuse of drugs or alcohol because they're at risk for habituation and dependence.

• Limit zolpidem therapy to 7 to 10 days; reevaluate patient if drug is to be taken for more than 2 weeks.

• Because sleep disturbance may be the only sign of physical or psychiatric disorder, initiate symptomatic treatment of insomnia only after carefully evaluating the patient.

• Drug has CNS depressant effects similar to other sedative-hypnotics. Because of its rapid onset of action, drug should be given immediately before going to bed.

• Dosage may need to be adjusted if drug is given with other CNS depressants because of the potentially additive effects.

• Hospitalized patients who are depressed, suicidal, or known to abuse drugs may try to hoard or overdose on zolpidem.

Patient education

• Tell patient not to take zolpidem with or immediately after a meal.

• Stress importance of taking drug only as prescribed; inform patient of potential drug dependency from long-term therapy with hypnotics.

• Inform patient that tolerance may occur if drug is taken for more than a few weeks.

• Warn patient against use of alcohol or other drugs used to treat insomnia during therapy to avoid serious adverse effects.

• Caution patient to avoid activities that require alertness, such as driving a car, until adverse CNS effects of drug are known.

• Tell patient not to increase dosage and to call if he feels drug is no longer effective.

Overdose & treatment

• Signs and symptoms may range from somnolence to light coma. CV and respiratory compromise also may occur.

• General symptomatic and supportive measures should be used and gastric lavage performed immediately when appropriate. I.V. fluids should be administered as needed. Flumazenil may be useful. Hypotension and CNS depression should be monitored and treated. Sedatives should be withheld after zolpidem overdose, even if excitation occurs.

Reactions may be *common*, uncommon, *life-threatening*, or COMMON AND LIFE-THREATENING.

Components of analgesic combination products

Many common analgesics are combinations of two or more generic drugs. This table lists the generic components of common analgesic combination products.

NONNARCOTIC ANALGESICS	
Trade name	**Generic drugs**
Allerest No-Drowsiness Tablets, Coldrine, Ornex No Drowsiness Caplets, Sinus-Relief Tablets, Sinutab Without Drowsiness	• acetaminophen 325 mg • pseudoephedrine hydrochloride 30 mg
Amaphen, Anoquan, Butace, Endolor, Esgic, Femcet, Fioricet, Fiorpap, Isocet, Medigesic, Repan	• acetaminophen 325 mg • caffeine 40 mg • butalbital 50 mg
Anacin, Gensan	• aspirin 400 mg • caffeine 32 mg
Arthritis Foundation Nighttime, Extra Strength Tylenol PM, Midol PM	• acetaminophen 500 mg • diphenhydramine 25 mg
Ascriptin	• aspirin 325 mg • magnesium hydroxide 50 mg • aluminum hydroxide 50 mg • calcium carbonate 50 mg
Ascriptin A/D	• aspirin 325 mg • magnesium hydroxide 75 mg • aluminum hydroxide 75 mg • calcium carbonate 75 mg
Doan's P.M. Extra Strength	• magnesium salicylate 500 mg • diphenhydramine 25 mg
Esgic Plus	• acetaminophen 500 mg • caffeine 40 mg • butalbital 50 mg
Excedrin Extra Strength	• aspirin 250 mg • acetaminophen 250 mg • caffeine 65 mg
Excedrin P.M. Caplets	• acetaminophen 500 mg • diphenhydramine citrate 38 mg
Fiorinal, Fiortal, Lanorinal	• aspirin 325 mg • caffeine 40 mg • butalbital 50 mg
Phrenilin	• acetaminophen 325 mg • butalbital 50 mg
Phrenilin Forte, Sedapap	• acetaminophen 650 mg • butalbital 50 mg
Sinus Excedrin Extra Strength	• acetaminophen 500 mg • pseudoephedrine hydrochloride 30 mg
Sinutab Maximum Strength	• acetaminophen 500 mg • pseudoephedrine hydrochloride 30 mg • chlorpheniramine maleate 2 mg

(continued)

NARCOTIC AND OPIOID ANALGESICS

Trade name	Controlled substance schedule	Generic drugs
Aceta with Codeine	III	• acetaminophen 300 mg • codeine phosphate 30 mg
Anexsia 7.5/650, Lorcet Plus	III	• acetaminophen 650 mg • hydrocodone bitartrate 7.5 mg
Azdone, Damason-P	III	• acetaminophen 500 mg • hydrocodone bitartrate 5 mg
Capital with Codeine, Tylenol with Codeine Elixir	V	• acetaminophen 120 mg • codeine phosphate 12 mg/5 ml
Darvocet-N 50	IV	• acetaminophen 325 mg • propoxyphene napsylate 50 mg
Darvocet-N 100, Propacet 100	IV	• acetaminophen 650 mg • propoxyphene napsylate 100 mg
E-Lor, Genagesic, Wygesic	IV	• acetaminophen 650 mg • propoxyphene hydrochloride 65 mg
Empirin With Codeine No. 3	III	• aspirin 325 mg • codeine phosphate 30 mg
Empirin With Codeine No. 4	III	• aspirin 325 mg • codeine phosphate 60 mg
Fioricet with Codeine	III	• acetaminophen 325 mg • butalbital 50 mg • caffeine 40 mg • codeine phosphate 30 mg
Fiorinal With Codeine	III	• aspirin 325 mg • butalbital 50 mg • caffeine 40 mg • codeine phosphate 30 mg
Innovar Injection	II	• droperidol 2.5 mg • fentanyl citrate 0.05 mg/ml
Lorcet 10/650	III	• acetaminophen 650 mg • hydrocodone bitartrate 10 mg
Lortab 2.5/500	III	• acetaminophen 500 mg • hydrocodone bitartrate 2.5 mg
Lortab 5/500	III	• acetaminophen 500 mg • hydrocodone bitartrate 5 mg
Lortab 7.5/500	III	• acetaminophen 500 mg • hydrocodone bitartrate 7.5 mg
Percocet	II	• acetaminophen 325 mg • oxycodone hydrochloride 5 mg
Percodan-Demi	II	• aspirin 325 mg • oxycodone hydrochloride 2.25 mg • oxycodone terephthalate 0.19 mg

NARCOTIC AND OPIOID ANALGESICS *(continued)*

Trade name	Controlled substance schedule	Generic drugs
Percodan, Roxiprin	II	• aspirin 325 mg • oxycodone hydrochloride 4.5 mg • oxycodone terephthalate 0.38 mg
Phenaphen/Codeine No. 3	III	• acetaminophen 325 mg • codeine phosphate 30 mg
Phenaphen/Codeine No. 4	III	• acetaminophen 325 mg • codeine phosphate 60 mg
Propoxyphene Napsylate/ Acetaminophen	IV	• propoxyphene napsylate 100 mg • acetaminophen 650 mg
Roxicet	II	• acetaminophen 325 mg • oxycodone hydrochloride 5 mg
Roxicet 5/500	II	• acetaminophen 500 mg • oxycodone hydrochloride 5 mg
Roxicet Oral Solution	II	• acetaminophen 325 mg • oxycodone hydrochloride 5 mg/5 ml
Talacen	IV	• acetaminophen 650 mg • pentazocine hydrochloride 25 mg
Talwin Compound	IV	• aspirin 325 mg • pentazocine hydrochloride 12.5 mg
Tylenol With Codeine No. 2	III	• acetaminophen 300 mg • codeine phosphate 15 mg
Tylenol With Codeine No. 3	III	• acetaminophen 300 mg • codeine phosphate 30 mg
Tylenol With Codeine No. 4	III	• acetaminophen 300 mg • codeine phosphate 60 mg
Tylox	II	• acetaminophen 500 mg • oxycodone hydrochloride 5 mg
Vicodin, Zydone	III	• acetaminophen 500 mg • hydrocodone bitartrate 5 mg
Vicodin ES	III	• acetaminophen 750 mg • hydrocodone bitartrate 7.5 mg

Appendix 2

Adverse reactions misinterpreted as age-related changes

Some conditions result from aging, others from drug therapy. However, some can result from aging and drug therapy. The chart below indicates drug classes and their associated adverse reactions.

DRUG CLASSIFICATIONS	Agitation	Anxiety	Arrhythmias	Ataxia	Changes in appetite	Confusion	Constipation	Depression	
Alpha₁ adrenergic blockers		●					●	●	
ACE inhibitors						●	●	●	
Antianginals	●	●	●			●			
Antiarrhythmics			●				●		
Anticholinergics	●	●	●			●	●	●	
Anticonvulsants	●		●	●	●	●	●	●	
Antidepressants, tricyclic	●	●	●	●	●	●	●		
Antidiabetics, oral									
Antihistamines						●	●	●	
Antilipemics							●		
Antiparkinsonians	●	●		●	●	●	●	●	
Antipsychotics	●	●	●	●	●	●	●	●	
Barbiturates	●	●	●			●			
Benzodiazepines	●			●		●	●	●	
Beta blockers		●	●					●	
Calcium channel blockers		●	●				●		
Corticosteroids	●					●		●	
Diuretics						●			
NSAIDs		●				●	●	●	
Opioids	●	●				●	●	●	
Skeletal muscle relaxants	●	●		●		●		●	
Thyroid hormones			●		●				

	Difficulty breathing	Disorientation	Dizziness	Drowsiness	Edema	Fatigue	Hypotension	Insomnia	Memory loss	Muscle weakness	Restlessness	Sexual dysfunction	Tremors	Urinary dysfunction	Visual changes
			●	●	●	●	●	●				●		●	●
			●			●	●	●				●			●
			●		●	●	●	●			●	●		●	●
	●		●		●	●	●								
		●	●	●		●	●		●	●	●			●	●
	●		●			●	●						●	●	●
	●	●	●			●	●	●			●	●	●	●	●
			●			●									
		●	●	●		●							●	●	●
			●			●	●	●		●		●		●	●
		●	●	●		●	●	●		●				●	●
			●	●		●	●	●			●	●	●	●	●
	●	●		●		●	●				●				
	●	●	●	●		●			●	●			●	●	●
	●		●			●	●		●			●	●	●	●
	●		●		●	●	●					●		●	●
					●	●		●		●					●
			●			●	●				●			●	
			●	●		●	●				●				●
	●	●	●	●		●	●	●	●			●	●	●	●
			●	●		●	●	●					●		
								●					●		

Creatinine clearance calculations

In patients with stable renal function, these formulas provide a reliable estimate of creatinine clearance (Cl_{cr}). In patients with falsely low serum creatinine (such as paraplegic patients with muscle wasting), the calculations will give an artificially high creatinine clearance. In patients with rapidly increasing serum creatinine (over 0.5 to 0.7 mg/dl/day), the calculations will give an unreliable estimate of creatinine clearance.

Method 1: Estimated creatinine clearance (ml/minute)*

$$\text{Male } Cl_{cr} = \frac{(140 - \text{age in years}) (IBW)}{(72) (S_{cr})}$$

Female Cl_{cr} = (Estimated male Cl_{cr}) (0.85)

IBW = ideal body weight in kilograms:
    IBW (Male) = 50 + [(2.3) (height in inches over 5 feet)]
    IBW (Female) = 45.5 + [(2.3) (height in inches over 5 feet)]
    Note: The use of the patient's IBW is recommended except when patient's actual body weight is less than IBW.
S_{cr} = Serum creatinine in mg/dl

Method 2: Estimated creatinine clearance (ml/minute/1.73 m²)†

$$\text{Male } Cl_{cr} = \frac{98 - [(0.8) (\text{age in years} - 20)]}{S_{cr}}$$

Female Cl_{cr} = (Estimated male Cl_{cr}) (0.90)

S_{cr} = serum creatinine in mg/dl.

*Cockroft, D.W., and Gault, M.H. "Prediction of Creatinine Clearance From Serum Creatinine," Nephron 16:31, 1976.
†Jelliffe, R.W. "Creatinine Clearance: Bedside Estimate," Ann Intern Med 79:604, 1973.

Using antipsychotics in long-term care facilities

The Health Care Financing Administration (HCFA) has updated its guidelines for using antipsychotics in long-term care facilities. These updates became effective July 1, 1999.

Guidelines for use

Before initiating antipsychotic therapy in any patient, take nonpharmacologic steps to modify his behavior and environment. If such measures are unsuccessful, you may use an antipsychotic provided that your patient has one of the following conditions:

1. schizophrenia
2. schizoaffective disorder
3. delusional disorder, which may include characteristics of other disorders
4. psychotic mood disorders, including mania or depression with psychotic features
5. acute psychotic episodes
6. brief reactive psychosis (related to an event and lasting less than 1 month)
7. schizophreniform disorder
8. atypical psychosis (covers psychotic disorders not otherwise specifically diagnosed)
9. Tourette syndrome
10. Huntington's disease
11. symptomatic 7-day treatment of hiccups, nausea, vomiting, or pruritus. Residents with nausea and vomiting secondary to cancer or cancer chemotherapy can be treated longer.
12. organic mental syndromes—including dementia, delirium, and amnestic and other cognitive disorders—accompanied by psychotic or agitated behaviors.

However, behaviors must be quantitatively (number of episodes) and objectively (for example, hitting, kicking, scratching) documented and mustn't be caused by preventable reasons. Behaviors must present a danger to the resident or others or involve continuous crying, screaming, yelling, or pacing if these behaviors impair functional capacity. And, psychotic symptoms (hallucinations, paranoia, delusions) mustn't otherwise be related to the above behaviors, which cause distress to the resident or impair functional capacity.

If a patient has a history of recurring psychotic symptoms and has 1 of the first 10 conditions—and if that condition has been stabilized with an antipsychotic with no significant adverse effects—dosage doesn't need to be reduced for a finding that dosage reduction is contraindicated. If the patient has an organic mental syndrome such as Alzheimer's, attempt gradual dosage reductions twice a year. If attempts are unsuccessful, a finding that further attempts at dosage reduction are contraindicated must be established and documented.

Don't use an antipsychotic if one of the following is the only indication: agitated behaviors that don't pose a danger to resident or others, anxiety, depression (without psychotic features), fidgeting, indifference to surroundings, insomnia, memory impairment, nervousness, poor self care, restlessness, uncooperativeness, unsociability, or wandering.

Guidelines for dosing

The table of daily doses on the next page is only for patients with organic mental syndromes. Avoid exceeding the total daily dose, unless higher doses are necessary to maintain or improve the patient's functional status—and unless evidence of that need is documented. Reduce dosage for a patient taking an antipsychotic, unless doing so is contraindicated. Monitor any patient taking an antipsychotic for adverse effects such as tardive dyskinesia, orthostatic hypotension, cognitive or behavioral impairment, akathisia, and parkinsonism.

Generic name (brand name)	Daily dose (mg/day)
chlorpromazine (Thorazine)	75
clozapine (Clozaril)	50
fluphenazine (Prolixin, Permitil)	4
haloperidol (Haldol)	4
loxapine (Loxitane)	10
mesoridazine (Serentil)	25
molindone (Moban)	10
olanzapine (Zyprexa)	10
perphenazine (Trilafon)	8
prochlorperazine* (Compazine)	10
quetiapine (Seroquel)	200
risperidone (Risperdal)	2
thioridazine (Mellaril)	75
thiothixene (Navane)	7
trifluoperazine (Stelazine)	8

*May exceed dose for up to 7 days when treating nausea and vomiting.

Adapted from American Society of Consultant Pharmacists, *Nursing Home Survey Procedures and Interpretive Guidelines*, 2nd edition, 1999.

Appendix 5

Using anxiolytics and sedatives in long-term care facilities

According to the Health Care Financing Administration (HCFA), a health care provider must consider, rule out, and document other reasons for distress before treating a patient in a long-term care facility with an anxiolytic or sedative. If used, the drug must maintain or improve the patient's functional status—and documentation must support its use.

Short-acting benzodiazepines and other anxiolytics and sedatives

These drugs may only be used for sleep disorders and the following indications:
• generalized anxiety disorder
• organic mental syndromes, including dementia, accompanied by a quantitatively and objectively documented agitated state that's a source of distress or dysfunction to the patient or that poses a danger to the patient or others
• panic disorder
• symptomatic anxiety that's accompanied by another diagnosed psychiatric disorder, such as depression or adjustment disorder.

Limit daily use of the drugs in the table below to less than 4 consecutive months, unless one or more dosage reductions are unsuccessful. If two attempts at dosage reduction in 1 year are unsuccessful, reduction is contraindicated. Don't exceed the total daily dose, unless doing so is necessary to maintain or improve functional status.

Generic name (brand name)	Daily dose (mg/day)
alprazolam (Xanax)	0.75
chloral hydrate (Noctec)	750
diphenhydramine (Benadryl)	50
hydroxyzine (Atarax, Vistaril)	50
lorazepam (Ativan)	2
oxazepam (Serax)	30

Long-acting benzodiazepines

Avoid using long-acting benzodiazepines, unless short-acting benzodiazepines have failed. Limit daily use of drugs listed in the table below to less than 4 consecutive months, unless gradual dosage reductions are unsuccessful. If two attempts at dosage reduction in 1 year are unsuccessful, dosage reduction is contraindicated. For patients receiving duplicate therapy—that is, more than one drug with the same effect—monitor for adverse reactions.

Don't exceed the total daily dose, unless doing so is necessary to maintain or improve functional status. Exceptions include diazepam (Valium) for neuromuscular syndromes (such as cerebral palsy, tardive dyskinesia, and seizure disorders); clonazepam (Klonopin) for bipolar disorders, tardive dyskinesia, nocturnal myoclonus, and seizure disorders; and any long-acting benzodiazepines if used to withdraw patients from short-acting benzodiazepines.

Generic name (brand name)	Daily dose (mg/day)
chlordiazepoxide (Librium)	20
clonazepam (Klonopin)	1.5
clorazepate (Tranxene)	15
diazepam (Valium)	5
flurazepam (Dalmane)	15

Drugs to induce sleep

Before considering drug therapy to treat insomnia, first eliminate the external causes of the condition—for example, noise, light, caffeine, pain, and depression. Then, initiate hypnotic drug therapy as appropriate to induce sleep with lower doses, and increase doses only gradually when necessary. Avoid exceeding the total daily dose, unless it can be shown that higher doses are necessary to maintain or improve the patient's functional status. Limit daily use of the drugs listed in the table below to less than 10 continuous days, unless gradual dosage reduction is unsuccessful. If three attempts at dosage reduction in 6 months are unsuccessful, dosage reduction is contraindicated.

Generic name (brand name)	Daily dose (mg/day)
alprazolam (Xanax)	0.25
chloral hydrate* (Noctec)	500
diphenhydramine* (Benadryl)	25
estazolam (ProSom)	0.5
hydroxyzine* (Atarax, Vistaril)	50
lorazepam (Ativan)	1
oxazepam (Serax)	15
temazepam (Restoril)	7.5
triazolam (Halcion)	0.125
zolpidem (Ambien)	5

*Not a drug of choice for sleep disorders, but it may be used.

Anxiolytics and sedatives to avoid

Certain anxiolytics and sedatives shouldn't be used for patients in long-term care facilities, including amobarbital (Amytal), amobarbital-secobarbital (Tuinal), butabarbital (Butisol and others), ethchlorvynol (Placidyl), glutethimide (Doriden), meprobamate (Equanil, Miltown), methyprylon (Noludar), paraldehyde (many brands), pentobarbital (Nembutal), phenobarbital (many brands), and secobarbital (Seconal).

To help eliminate or modify the symptoms for which such a drug is prescribed, reduce the patient's dosage; however, a newly admitted patient may have an adjustment period before his dosage is reduced. If two attempts at dosage reduction in 1 year are unsuccessful, reduction is contraindicated. Because rapid withdrawal of such drug may result in severe physiological symptoms, reduce all dosages gradually.

Adapted from American Society of Consultant Pharmacists, *Nursing Home Survey Procedures and Interpretive Guidelines,* 2nd edition, 1999.

Unnecessary drugs in long-term care facilities

The Health Care Financing Administration (HCFA) has updated its guidelines for using unnecessary drugs in long-term care facilities. Such drugs are characterized as either high severity or low severity, with *severity* being defined as "a combination of both the likelihood that an adverse outcome would occur and the clinical significance of that outcome should it occur."

High severity

The following drugs are inappropriate for geriatric patients and are characterized as high severity:

● anticholinergics for patients with BPH, including anticholinergic antidepressants; anticholinergic antihistamines and GI antispasmodics that are used more frequently than every 3 months for 7 days (a surveyor must review drug use that's more frequent); and antiparkinsonians.

● aspirin, dipyridamole (Persantine), NSAIDs, or ticlopidine (Ticlid) for residents taking anticoagulants.

● hypnotics or sedatives for residents with COPD. Short-acting benzodiazepines are acceptable for patients with mild COPD.

● metoclopramide (Reglan) for patients with seizures or epilepsy.

● NSAIDs for patients with active or recurrent gastritis, peptic ulcer disease, or gastroesophageal reflux disease. COX-2 inhibitors such as celecoxib [Celebrex] aren't included on the HCFA list of NSAIDs.

● tricyclic antidepressants in patients with arrhythmias, if started within past month.

The following drugs may be inappropriate for geriatric patients because of the high potential for severe adverse reactions:

● amitriptyline (Elavil). May be used for neurogenic pain if another tricyclic antidepressant, such as desipramine (Norpramin), failed.

● chlorpropamide (Diabinese).

● digoxin (Lanoxin). Unless an atrial arrhythmia is being treated, dosages greater than 0.125mg/day increase the risk of adverse reaction without improving outcomes. High severity is considered if started within the past month.

● disopyramide (Norpace).

● doxepin (Sinequan).

● GI antispasmodics (belladonna alkaloids, clidinium, dicyclomine, hyoscyamine, propantheline) that are used more frequently than every 3 months for 7 days (a surveyor must review drug use that's more frequent).

● meperidine (Demerol), oral. High severity is considered if started within the past month.

● meprobamate (Equanil, Miltown).

● methyldopa (Aldomet). High severity is considered if started within the past month.

● pentazocine (Talwin).

● ticlopidine (Ticlid). May be used for patients who are intolerant of aspirin or who have had a previous stroke or evidence of stroke precursors (for example, transient ischemic attacks).

Low severity

The following drugs are inappropriate for geriatric patients and are characterized as low severity:

● antipsychotics in patients with seizures or epilepsy. Treatment of acute psychosis for 72 hours or less is permissible.

● corticosteroids in patients with diabetes, if started within past month.

● narcotics and bladder relaxants such as oxybutynin (Ditropan) and bethanechol (Urecholine) in patients with BPH. A surveyor doesn't need to review drug use if drug is used for 7 days or less once every 3 months for symptoms of an acute self-limiting condition.

• potassium supplements or aspirin (dosages exceeding 325 mg/day) in patients with active or recurrent gastritis, peptic ulcer disease, or gastroesophageal reflux disease. Use of potassium supplements to treat low potassium levels until they return to normal range is permissible in these patients if the health care provider determines that using fresh fruits and vegetables or other dietary supplementation is inadequate or impossible.

The following drugs may worsen constipation:
• anticholinergic antidepressants
• anticholinergic antihistamines. A surveyor doesn't need to review drug use if drug is used for 7 days or less once every 3 months for symptoms of an acute self-limiting condition.
• antiparkinsonians
• GI antispasmodics
• narcotics. A surveyor doesn't need to review drug use if drug is used for 7 days or less once every 3 months for symptoms of an acute self-limiting condition.

The following drugs may worsen insomnia:
• beta agonists
• decongestants
• MAO inhibitors
• selective serotonin reuptake inhibitors and desipramine (Norpramin)
• theophylline.

The following drugs may be inappropriate for geriatric patients because of the high potential for less severe adverse outcomes:
• antihistamines with anticholinergic properties.
• digoxin (Lanoxin). Unless an atrial arrhythmia is being treated, dosages exceeding 0.125mg/day increase the risk of adverse reaction without improving outcomes. Low severity is considered if therapy exceeds 1 month.
• diphenhydramine (Benadryl). A surveyor doesn't need to review drug use if drug is used for 7 days or less once every 3 months for treatment of allergies.
• dipyridamole (Persantine).

• indomethacin (Indocin). Drug may be used for 1 week to treat acute gouty arthritis.
• meperidine (Demerol), oral. Low severity is considered if therapy is exceeds 1 month.
• methyldopa (Aldomet). Low severity is considered if therapy is longer than 1 month.
• muscle relaxants, such as carisoprodol (Soma), chlorzoxazone (Paraflex), cyclobenzaprine (Flexeril), dantrolene (Dantrium), methocarbamol (Robaxin). A surveyor doesn't need to review drug use if drug is used for 7 days or less once every 3 months for acute self-limiting condition.
• trimethobenzamide (Tigan).

Adapted from American Society of Consultant Pharmacists, *Nursing Home Survey Procedures and Interpretive Guidelines,* 2nd edition, 1999.

Appendix 7

Age-related changes in laboratory values

Standard normal laboratory values reflect the physiology of 20 to 40 year olds. Many normal values for geriatric patients differ because of age-related physiologic changes.

Certain tests, though, remain unaffected by age. These include PTT, PT, serum acid phosphatase, serum carbon dioxide, serum chloride, AST, and total serum protein levels. This table lists tests that are affected and provides important considerations.

TEST VALUES AT 20 TO 40 YEARS OLD	AGE-RELATED CHANGES	CONSIDERATIONS
Blood tests		
Albumin level 33.5 to 5.0 g/dl	Younger than 65; Higher in males Older than 65; Levels equalize then decrease at same rate	Increased dietary protein intake needed if liver function is normal; edema is a sign of low albumin level. May affect highly proteinbound drugs
Alkaline phosphatase level 13 to 39 IU/L	Increases 8 to 10 IU/L	May reflect liver function decline or vitamin D malabsorption and bone demineralization
µ-globulin level 2.3 to 3.5 g/dl	Increases slightly	Increases in response to decrease in albumin if liver function is normal; Increased dietary protein intake needed
Blood urea nitrogen (BUN) level Men: 10 to 25 mg/dl Women: 8 to 20 mg/dl	Increases, possibly to 69 mg/dl	Slight increase acceptable in absence of stressors, such as infection or surgery
Cholesterol level 120 to 220 mg/dl	Men: Increases to age 50; then decreases Women: Lower then men until age 50, increases to age 70, then decreases	Rise in cholesterol level (and increased cardiovascular risk) in women as a result of postmenopausal estrogen decline; dietary changes; weight loss, and exercise needed
Creatinine kinase (CK) level 17 to 148 U/L	Increases slightly	May reflect decreasing muscle mass and liver function
Creatinine level 0.6 to 1.5 mg/dl	Increases, possibly to 1.9 mg/dl in men	May remain in the normal range due to a decrease in muscle mass yet the patient may be severely renally impaired Important factor to prevent toxicity when giving drugs that are excreted in urine
Creatinine clearance 104 to 125 ml/min	Men: Decreases; formula: $(140 - age \times kg$ body weight$)/72 \times$ serum creatinine Women: 85% of men's rate	Reflects reduced GFR, important factor to prevent toxicity when giving drugs that are excreted in urine.
Glucose tolerance (fasting plasma glucose level) 1 hr: 160 to 170 mg/dl 2 hr: 115 to 125 mg/dl	Rises faster in first 2 hr, then drops to baseline more slowly	Reflects declining pancreatic insulin supply and release and diminishing body mass for glucose uptake. Rapid *rise* can quickly trigger hyperosmolar hyperglycemic nonketotic syndrome.

(continued)

TEST VALUES AT 20 TO 40 YEARS OLD	AGE-RELATED CHANGES	CONSIDERATIONS
Blood tests (continued)		
Glucose tolerance (continued) 3 hr: 80 to 110 mg/dl		Rapid *decline* can result from alcohol, certain drugs, such as beta blockers, and MAO inhibitors
High-density lipoproteins (HDL) level 80 to 310 mg/100 ml	Levels higher in women than men; levels equalized with age	Compliance with dietary restrictions required for accurate interpretation of test results
Leukocyte count 4,300 to 10,800/mm^3 B: 50 to 200/mm^3	Drop to 3,100 to 9000/mm^3	Decreases proportionate to lymphocytes
Lymphocyte count T: 500 to 2,400/mm^3 B: 50 to 200 /mm^3	Decrease	Decreases proportionate to leukocytes
Platelet count 150,00 to 350,000/mm^3	Change in characteristics; decreased granular constituents, increased platelet-release factors	May reflect diminished bone marrow, increased fibrinogen levels
Potassium level 3.5 to 5.5 mEq/L	Increases slightly	Requires food-label vigilance, knowledge of hyperkalemia's signs and symptoms, and avoidance of potassium-containing salt substitutes.
Thyroid-stimulating hormone (TSH) level 0.3 to 5.0 micron IU/L	Increases slightly	Suggests primary hypothyroidism or endemic goiter at much higher levels
T$_4$ level 4.5 to 13.5 µg/100 ml	Decreases 25%	Reflects declining thyroid function
Triglyceride level 40 to 150 mg/100 ml	Range widens: 20 to 200 mg/100 ml	Suggests abnormalities at any other levels, requiring additional tests such as serum cholesterol level
T$_3$ level 90 to 220 ng/100 ml	Decreases 25%	Reflects declining thyroid function
Urine tests		
Glucose level 0 to 15 mg/100 ml	Decreases slightly	May reflect renal disease or UTI; unreliable check for geriatric diabetic patients, as glycosuria may not occur until plasma glucose level exceeds 300 mg/100 ml
Protein level 0 to 5 mg/100 ml	Increases slightly	May reflect renal disease or UTI
Specific gravity 1.032	Decreases to 1.024 by age 80	Reflects 30% to 50% decrease in number of nephrons available to concentrate urine

Resources for geriatric care

Administration on Aging
330 Independence Ave., S.W.
Washington, DC 20201
Phone: (202) 619-7501
Fax: (202) 260-1012
E-mail: aoainfo@aoa.gov
Website: www.aoa.gov

Alliance for Aging Research
2021 K St., N.W., Suite 305
Washington, DC 20006
Phone: (202) 293 2856
1-800-639-2421
Fax: (202) 785-8574
E-mail: info@agingresearch.org
Website: www.agingresearch.org

Alzheimer's Association
National Headquarters
919 N. Michigan Ave., Suite 1000
Chicago, IL 60611-1676
Phone: 1-800-272-3900
Fax: (312) 335-1110
Website: www.alz.org

American Academy of Orthopaedic Surgeons
6300 North River Rd.
Rosemont, IL 60018-4262
Phone: (847) 823-7186
1-800-346-AAOS
Fax: (847) 823-8125
Website: www.aaos.org

American Association for Geriatric Psychiatry
7910 Woodmont Ave., Suite 1050
Bethesda, MD 20814-3004
Phone: (301) 654-7850
Fax: (301) 654-4137
Website: www.aagpgpa.org

American Association of Retired Persons (AARP)
601 E St., N.W.
Washington, DC 20049
Phone: 1-800-424-3410
Website: www.aarp.org

American Diabetes Association
ATTN: Customer Service
1701 N. Beauregard St.
Alexandria, VA 22311
Phone: (703) 549-1500
1-800-DIABETES
Website: www.diabetes.org

American Geriatrics Society
The Empire State Bldg.
350 5th Ave., Suite 801
New York, NY 10118
Phone: (212) 308-1414
Fax: (212) 832-8646
E-mail: info.amger@
americangeriatrics.org
Website: www.americangeriatrics.org

American Heart Association
National Center
7272 Greenville Ave.
Dallas, TX 75231-4596
Phone: 1-800-AHA-USA1
Website: www.Americanheart.org

American Society on Aging
833 Market St., Suite 511
San Francisco, CA 94103
Phone: (415) 974-9600
Fax: (415) 974-0300
Website: www.asaging.org

Arthritis Foundation
1330 W. Peachtree St.
Atlanta, GA 30309
Phone: (404) 872-7100
1-800-283-7800 (Arthritis Answers)
Fax: (404) 872-0457
Website: www.arthritis.org

Gerontological Society of America
1030 15th St., N.W., Suite 250
Washington, DC 20005
Phone: (202) 842-1275
Fax: (202) 842-1150
Website: www.geron.org

Health Care Financing Administration
7500 Security Blvd.
Baltimore, MD 21244
Phone: (410) 786-3000
Website: www.hcfa.gov

Institute for Safe Medication Practices
1800 Byberry Rd., Suite 810
Huntingdon Valley, PA 19006
Phone: (215) 947-7797
Fax: (215) 914-1492
E-mail: ismpinfo@ismp.org
Website: www.ismp.org

John A. Hartford Foundation Institute for Geriatric Nursing
New York University
Division of Nursing
50 W. 4th St., 429 Shimkin Hall
New York, NY 10012
Phone: (212) 998-5355
Fax: (212) 995-4770
Website: www.nyu.edu/education/nursing/hartford.institute/

Leonard Davis School of Gerontology
Ethel Percy Andrus Gerontology Center
University of Southern California
Los Angeles, CA 90089-0191
Phone: (213) 740-5156
Fax: (213) 740-0792
Website: www.usc.edu/dept/gero

National Association for Home Care
228 Seventh St., S.E.
Washington, DC 20003
Phone: (202) 547-7424
Fax: (202) 547-3540
Website: www.nahc.org

National Council on the Aging—MaturityWorks
409 Third St., S.W.
Washington, DC 20024
Phone: (202) 479-1200
Fax: (202) 479-0735
Website: www.maturityworks.org

National Gerontological Nurses Association
7250 Parkway Dr., Suite 510
Hanover, MD 21076
Phone: 1-800-723-0560
Fax: (850) 484-8762
Website: www.nursingcenter.com/people/nrsorgs/ngna

National Hospice Organization
1700 Diagonal Rd., Suite 300
Alexandria, VA 22314
Phone: (703) 243-5900
Fax: (703) 525-5762
Website: www.nho.org

National Institute on Aging
Public Information Office
Bldg. 31, Room 5C27
31 Center Drive, MSC 2292
Bethesda, MD 20892
Phone: 1-800-222-2225
Fax: (301) 496-1072
Website: www.nih.gov/nia

National Library of Medicine
8600 Rockville Pike
Bethesda, MD 20894
Website: www.nlm.nih.gov

National Osteoporosis Foundation
1232 22nd St., N.W.
Washington, DC 20037-1292
Phone: (202) 223-2226
Website: www.nof.org

National Stroke Association
96 Inverness Dr. E., Suite I
Englewood, CO 80112-5112
Phone: 1-800-787-6537
Website: www.stroke.org

Acknowledgments

We would like to thank the following companies for granting us permission to include their drugs in the full-color photoguide.

Abbott Laboratories
Biaxin®
Depakote®
Depakote® Sprinkle
E.E.S.®
Ery-Tab®
Erythrocin Stearate
Filmtab®
Erythromycin Base
Filmtab®
Hytrin®
PCE®

AstraZeneca LP
Nolvadex®
Prilosec®
Tenormin®
Toprol XL®
Zestril®

Bayer Corporation
Adalat® CC
Cipro®

Bristol-Myers Squibb Company
BuSpar®
Capoten®
Cefzil®
cephalexin
Duricef®
Estrace®
Glucophage®
Pravachol®
Sumycin®
Trimox®
VeetidsÇ

DuPont Pharmaceuticals Company
Coumadin®

Endo Pharmaceuticals, Inc.
Percocet®

ESI Lederle Division of American Home Products Corporation
atenolol

Ethex Corporation
potassium chloride

Forest Pharmaceuticals, Inc.
Lorcet® 10/650

Glaxo Wellcome, Inc.
Ceftin®
Lanoxin®
Zantac®
Zantac® EFFERdose®
Zovirax®

Hoechst Marion Roussel
Allegra®
Altace®
Carafate®
Cardizem®
Cardizem® CD
DiaBeta®
Lasix®
Trental®

Janssen Pharmaceutica, Inc.
Propulsid®
Risperdal®

Jones Pharma
Levoxyl®

KV Pharmaceutical Company
Micro-K Extencaps

Eli Lilly and Company
Axid®
Ceclor®
Darvocet-N® 100
Lorabid®
Prozac®

McNeil-PPC, Inc.
Motrin®

Medeva Pharmaceuticals
methylphenidate hydrochloride

Merck & Co., Inc.
Cozaar®
Fosamax®
Mevacor®
Pepcid®
Prinivil®
Sinemet®
Sinemet® CR
Vasotec®
Zocor®

Mylan Pharmaceuticals, Inc.
amitriptyline hydrochloride
cimetidine
cyclobenzaprine hydrochloride
doxepin hydrochloride
furosemide
glipizide
naproxen
propoxyphene napsylate with acetaminophen

Novartis Corporation
Fiorinal® with Codeine
Lotensin®
Pamelor®

Novopharm USA, Inc., Division of Novopharm Limited
amoxicillin trihydrate

Ortho-McNeil Pharmaceutical
Floxin®
Tylenol® with Codeine No. 3
Ultram®

971

Pfizer, Inc.
Cardura®
Diflucan®
Glucotrol®
Glucotrol XL®
Norvasc®
Procardia XL®
Zithromax®
Zoloft®
Zyrtec®

Pharmacia & Upjohn
Deltasone®
Glynase®
Micronase®
Provera®
Xanax®

**Proctor and Gamble
Pharmaceuticals, Inc.**
Macrobid®

**Rhône-Poulenc Rorer
Pharmaceuticals, Inc.**
Dilacor XR®
Slo-bid™ Gyrocaps®

**Roche Laboratories,
Inc.**
Bumex®
Klonopin®
Naprosyn®
Ticlid®
Toradol®
Valium®

**Roxane Laboratories,
Inc.**
Roxicet™

**Schein Pharmaceutical,
Inc.**
nortriptyline
hydrochloride

**Schering Corporation
and Key
Pharmaceuticals, Inc.**
Claritin®
K-Dur®
Theo-Dur®

Schwarz Pharma
Verelan®

G.D. Searle & Company
Ambien®
Calan®
Daypro®

**SmithKline Beecham
Pharmaceuticals**
Amoxil®
Augmentin®
Compazine®
Coreg®
Dyazide®
Paxil®
Relafen®
Tagamet®

**Tap Pharmaceuticals,
Inc.**
Prevacid®

**Warner-Lambert
Company**
Accupril®
Dilantin® Infatabs®
Dilantin® Kapseals®
Lipitor®
Lopid®
Nitrostat®

**Watson Laboratories,
Inc.**
hydrocodone bitartrate
and acetaminophen

**Wyeth-Ayerst
Laboratories**
Ativan®
Cordarone®
Effexor®
Inderal®
Lodine®
Oruvail®
Premarin®

**Zenith Goldline
Pharmaceuticals**
verapamil hydrochloride

Index

---

t refers to table; **boldface** indicates full-color photographs.

---

t refers to table; **boldface** indicates full-color photographs.

t refers to table; **boldface** indicates full-color photographs.

t refers to table; **boldface** indicates full-color photographs.

---

t refers to table; **boldface** indicates full-color photographs.

THE COMPLETE
RUGBY
JOKES
OMNIBUS

Also available

MORE RUGBY JOKES
EVEN MORE RUGBY JOKES
RUGBY JOKES IN THE LOCKER ROOM
RUGBY SONGS

THE COMPLETE
RUGBY
JOKES
OMNIBUS

COMPRISING
RUGBY JOKES
SON OF RUGBY JOKES
WHAT RUGBY JOKES DID NEXT

WARNER BOOKS

A *Warner* Book

This edition first published in Great Britain in 1995 by Warner Books

The Complete Rugby Jokes Omnibus Copyright © Sphere Books 1995

Previously published separately:
Rugby Jokes first published in Great Britain in 1968 by Sphere Books
Copyright © Sphere Books 1968
Reprinted by Warner Books in 1995
Son of Rugby Jokes first published in Great Britain in 1970 by Sphere Books
Copyright © Sphere Books 1970
What Rugby Jokes Did Next first published in Great Britain in 1970
Copyright © Sphere Books 1970

The moral right of the authors has been asserted.

A CIP catalogue record for this book
is available from the British Library.

ISBN 0 7515 1703 8

Printed and bound in Great Britain by Clays Ltd, St Ives plc

Warner Books
A Division of
Little, Brown and Company (UK)
Brettenham House
Lancaster Place
London WC2E 7EN

RUGBY JOKES

RUGBY JOKES
AND COARSE LIMERICKS

Table of Contents

In Bed with the Doctor

A spinster suffered more and more from "nerves". She was not the doctor's best customer, so when the National Health came in he grew wearier than ever of her "nerves" and told her frankly that there was only one thing the matter with her.

"Doctor," she said, "I've left it too late, no face, no figure, who would take me to bed and perform, now?"

The doctor scratched his head.

"Doctor, would YOU do it, for twenty pounds?"

The Doc thought "Well, she's not as bad as all that, and it will work out at over a pound a minute" and said: "Yes, I'll call after surgery."

* * *

As she reached for her handbag to pay him, she said: "How about a repeat performance?"

"But Miss Rustyfan, you're a poor woman."

"Yes doctor, but I've saved up enough though to make sure of a respectable funeral; there's another twenty under the mattress, the Parish can bury me!"

BENDING OVER BACKWARDS

There was a sprightly old maid who lived to be a hundred, and all the Press men went after the story. One asked about her health. . . .

"I've never been to a doctor in my life!"

"Really Miss, in a hundred years do you mean to say that you were never bedridden, even for a short time?"

"Of course I was, young man, and table-ended, but there's no need to put that in the paper."

9

ILLUMINATING

A man went to his doctor, complaining of a pain in his member. The doctor examined him, and said:

"You can't be healthy without sex, what are you getting?"

The patient explained that he had a young lady, and went to the woods with her, twice a week.

"Yes, and does your member burn after intercourse?"

"I don't know doctor, I've never put a match to it."

INDEED I DO

There was an old specialist in the Diseases of Women, who simply could not stand the fat middle aged matron who ate and drank too much, and "never enjoyed good health". He could spot them a mile away.

One day he sat in his Consultant's chair at the hospital with students and nurses in attendance, when one such woman waddled up, and plonked her carcass in a chair without being asked. He went on writing, then suddenly looked up and said:

"Well, what's the matter with you!"

She sighed, rocked like a jelly, and said:

"Ooh doctor, you do feel terrible when you're on the change, don't you?"

"I do, I do, indeed I do!"

IT'S ALL MY EYE!

A hospital secretary moved to a new post, and decided immediately to tighten up on "security". He set up a man in the gatehouse with very strict instructions to challenge all comers. Those not on business were to be turned firmly away.

Quite soon a young woman marched up, seeking to enter.

"Hi, wait a bit, what's your business?" shouted the gatekeeper.

"I'm a maternity patient," said the girl.

"Can you prove it? are you pregnant?"

"Don't be daft, I haven't seen anything for six months."

"Ah, I thought so, you've come to the wrong place, the Eye Hospital's further down the road."

CONCRETE PROOF

A man went to the doctor and complained that he could not get an erection. The doctor gave him every treatment in the book, but none of them worked. After weeks of this, the doctor said:

"There's an old fashioned remedy which involves an injection in a very delicate place, but we'll try it."

It worked so well that the man had a permanent erection so that he asked for it to be reduced, if only for a time.

"Sorry my man, that's impossible."

"Surely doctor, to every known drug there is an antidote?"

"Yes, but this wasn't a drug."

"What did you inject it with then?"

"Just three of sand and one of cement."

YOU CAN KISS MY ARM

A man with a beautiful wife was in a car accident, and his wife's face was badly scarred. He went to the best plastic surgeon in the business to seek help.

"It will cost you three hundred pounds, but I can do it, if you will allow me to take the skin off your behind for grafting."

"Gladly!" said the husband, and so the operation was carried out, and it was a brilliant success; the wife was more lovely than ever.

The surgeon got a cheque for £400 and rang up to say: "Hey, you sent me a hundred quid too much."

"Oh no I didn't, the extra hundred is for the sheer pleasure I get from watching my mother-in-law kiss my arse!"

RIDING FOR A FALL

The doctor told the working chap that he could not complete his examination without a sample of urine. The small boy who was sent with the "specimen" spilled most of it while messing about. Fearing a good hiding, he topped it up from a cow in a field.

The doctor hastily sent for the man, who returned home to his wife in a furious temper, and said: "That's you and your fancy positions! You would be on top wouldn't you, and now I'm going to have a baby."

STICKING OUT

A man was told by his doctor: "You are going to make medical history, you are the only male ever recorded who has become pregnant."

The man replied: "This is terrible, whatever will the neighbours say, I'm not even married."

SITTING IT OUT

An old lady went to the doctor because she was constipated.
"Well, d'you do anything about it?" he enquired.
"Of course I do, doctor, I sit there for hours."
"No, no, Mrs Bloggs, I mean, do you take anything?"
"Oh yes, doctor, I takes me knitting."

ITHN'T IT NITH

The school doctor was examining a girl of goodly proportions, and, taking up his stethoscope, said:
"Big breaths."
"Yeth," said the girl, "and I'm not thirteen yet."

SHORT AND CURLY

There was a chap lay in hospital all too long, and he got very bored. One day out of devilment he said to a very straightlaced nurse: "Hey nurse, where does a woman's hair grow thickest and blackest and curliest?"
The nurse coloured up, walked away, and came back with Matron. Said that dragon:
"Young man, before I have you thrown out, tell me what you said, because nurse is too upset to repeat it."
"Certainly Matron, I simply asked her where does a girl's hair grow thickest and blackest and curliest."
"And where DOES it?" she said, outfacing him.
"Why Matron, in Central Africa, of course!"

THE BALD TRUTH

An old Alderman found himself getting balder and balder. He couldn't bear the idea of taking his turn as Mayor, with a bald head, so he consulted his doctor. Said the quack:

"In the first place, nothing can be done, in the second place it's a sign of passion and you ought to be pleased."

The Alderman resigned from the Council, and spent the rest of his years and the rest of his fortune, searching for a bald woman.

A BLOODY MOUTHFUL

A woman went to the doctor and complained she could not get passionate. The doctor examined her, and told her that if she would follow his special diet she would get very randy. This was agreed, but after a few weeks she was back, and said:

"There's something gone wrong! Last night I got so passionate I chewed my boyfriend's ear off."

"Oh, don't worry about that trifle, it's only protein, no carbohydrates."

A BAREFACED LIE

Two Harley Street men were talking of professional difficulties. Said one who was a specialist in beauty treatment for rich women:

"You can't win, I warned Lady Mucke against having so many facelifts, but she would go on, and now she's suing me!"

"Really, what's the matter?"

"She's got a beard."

A LEAP IN THE DARK

A man came to the surgery covered with blood and bruises.
. . . "What's the matter?" said the doctor.

"It's my wife – another of her nightmares!"

"Don't talk daft man! She might have kicked you, but
not these injuries. . . ."

"Listen doc, she had one of her nightmares, she shouted
out: 'Get out quick, my husband's coming home' and me
being only half awake, naturally, I jumped straight out of
the window."

FOR WHEEL OR FOR WOE

A man was off work without a medical note, and the foreman wanted an explanation . . .

"Where've you been, you lousy ignorant lazy B?"

"It was my wife Sir, she was giving birth to a wheel-
barrow."

The foreman knew the man was stupid, but this was too
much. . . . "If you can't do better than that, you'll get your
cards, come on, what was the real trouble?"

The man pondered, and said: "I got it wrong, my wife
was in bed having a pushchair."

"Go and get your cards! You're too dim even for this
firm, you're fired!"

The labourer went home, and said: "Hes missus, what
was wrong with you when you was poorly?"

"Jack, I told you, I had a miscarriage!"

"Ah, I knowed it was something with wheels on."

UNIDENTIFIED FLYING OBJECT

There was a young woman who did not seem very well, so her mother took her to the doctor. Mother did all the talking, she was that sort.

"She's pregnant," said the doc.

"Doctor, I must call you a fool, my daughter has never so much as kissed a man, have you darling?"

"No momma, I haven't even held a man's hand."

The doctor left his chair, walked to the window and gazed at the sky. There was a long silence, then mother asked –

"Is there anything wrong out there doctor?"

"Not at all, not at all! Only the last time this happened a star appeared in the east, and I don't want to miss it this time."

VIRGIN ON THE RIDICULOUS

An innocent young woman told her doctor she was not feeling at all well lately.

After examination, the doctor told her she was pregnant. . . .

"But that's impossible, I've never been with a man!"

The doctor patiently explained the facts of life to her in some detail.

"Well!" she said, "and that lousy First Aid Instructor told me it was artificial respiration."

ALL BALLS AND FESTIVITIES

A man went to the doctor with a pain in his loins.

After examination the doctor said: "You're a big man, doing a navvy's job, you need to wear a suspensory bandage."

"I'm on'y a hignorant navvy, wot's one o' them doctor?"

"Why man, it's a band for your balls, now good day, I'm busy."

The poor old navvy wandered around until by chance he came to a music shop, which was also an agency. There was a card in the window: BANDS FOR BALLS:

He went in, and said: "Is that right, bands for balls?"

"Yes indeed' said the bright and shapely girl behind the desk, "We have brass bands for large balls, and string bands for small balls, and . . .

"And," said the navvy, undoing his trouserflies, "what have you got for these?"

The modern miss did not bat an eyelid: "I'm afraid," she said, "You'll have to go to a sports shop and buy a hammock!"

STRETCHING IT A BIT

Said the plain nurse to the pretty nurse: "Hey, you know that big commando in the third bed?"

"Oh, you mean the one who's tattooed all over?"

"Yes, that's him, have you ever bathed him?"

"Yes, why?"

"Well, when I bathed him yesterday I noticed he had 'Ludo' tattooed on his er, thing."

"That's not 'Ludo', that's 'Llandudno'."

There was a young man of Kings Lynn
Who was so exceedingly thin
That when he essayed
Making love to a maid
He slipped on the mat, and fell in!

There were two young ladies of Grimsby
Who wondered, what use could their quims be?
The bit in the middle
Was, clearly, for piddle,
But what could those hair-covered rims be?

There was a young curate named Batt
In the Lord Bishop's seat he was sat,
He was thinking of Venus
While pulling his penis,
And catching the drops in his hat

There was a young WAAF in the Ritz
Wearing officers' pips on her tits
A bit further down
Was an RSM's crown
Which gave further scope for the wits

There was young lady named Anna
Who thought she would like a pianner,
Her Mother said "No!"
And bought her a po
Saying "Now you can have a pee, Anna"

Pump! You Beggars Pump!

A certain tough old sea captain bought a young parrot at a foreign port (being assured it was a marvellous learner) and hung it on the bridge. Coming back through the Bay of Biscay, a fearful black cloud came over, and the skipper remarked: "It's gone bloody dark all at once." Soon after, the cloud burst in dreadful torrent, and the captain said to the mate: "It's bloody hissing down!" The storm got worse, the ship lurched and developed a leak, so that one of the men called up:

"What shall we do to be saved?" He got the reply: "Pump! you lousy shower! Pump you poxed-up beggars, pump!"

The ship, and all, were lost; a wet, swearing, washed-up parrot alone survived, and after some adventures, finished up with a dear spinster, who was just expecting the vicar. As a precaution she threw a cloth over the cage, so that the vicar was greeted with:

"It's gone bloody dark all at once."

The lady was livid, and put the parrot immediately under the cold water tap, at which he shrieked:

"It's bloody hissing down!"

"No, no, Miss Fantight! You mustn't be so cruel to God's creatures, rather bring him to church on the Sabbath, and expose him to good influences." This was done, and the parrot behaved like an angel, even joining in the hymns. The vicar, beaming at his own success, rose to announce his text: "Brethren today we ask What shall we do to be saved?" and down the aisles rang the parrot's clear tones. . . .

THE ARM OF THE LAW

There was a policeman with a dog on night duty, and he met up with a pretty young policewoman, also on night duty. It was a very cold night, and the policewoman was shivering. . . .

"What's the matter, can I do anything?"

The policewoman explained that she had come on duty late, and in a hurry, and had forgotten to put on her black woollen issue knickers. Being late already, she dare not go back and fetch them.

The dog handler said not to worry. He explained that the dog was superbly trained: "Let the dog sniff you between the legs, then we'll send him back to the station, and you can bet he'll return with your passion-killers."

This was agreed upon, and the dog trotted off, while they resumed their beat.

Half an hour later the dog returned, bearing part of the sergeant's hand!

SUCK IT AND SEE

A man went into his club leading a snake on a string.

The barman took a poor view of this, and fetched the Secretary, who said:

"Hey, is that snake poisonous?"

"Yes."

"Then what happens if he bites one of the members?"

"Oh that's no trouble, he just gets a friend to suck the wound."

"Suppose he gets bitten up the backside?"

"That's when he finds out who his friends are!"

IN DEATH AS IN LIFE

There was a spinster who kept a lady parrot and a gentleman parrot, which were her pride and joy. Then the lady parrot took cold and died, and, alas, the gentleman parrot died of a broken heart soon afterwards.

The spinster, very distressed, took the two dead birds to the taxidermist, so that they might be stuffed and preserved in the house as a memento.

"I'll send you a card in a week or so," said the man.

A month went by, with no news, so the spinster drove into town to enquire. "I forgot to ask you," said the taxidermist, "but do you want them mounted?"

"It's a nice thought," she said, "but the Vicar would never approve, so we'd better have them just holding hands."

TEARING A STRIP OFF

The costermonger had a donkey, and one day the animal said:

"Hey, it's twenty years today I've worked for you, in all weathers."

"So you have," said the cockney, "what can I get you for a special treat?" – "A night with a female," said the ass. So the cockney scoured London, but he could not find a female donkey on hire. When he had given up hope, he came to a circus, where the boss said that for £5 he'd loan out a female zebra.

The cockney took the zebra, shoved it in the stable, and went home for a late supper. Next day, he asked the moke: "How'd you get on – alright?"

"Bloody awful, I couldn't get her pyjamas off."

The spinster had a parrot who kept repeating:

"I want to poke, I want to poke."

She found this slightly irritating, until a married friend explained what it meant, then she became very alarmed. . . .

"I love that bird, but I'll have to get rid of him, or the vicar will never call again," she said. But her more experienced friend said:

"Well, if you really love him, you'll get him what he longs for, which is a female, then he won't keep on about it all the time." Off went the spinster to the bird shop, but the man said: "No can do, no lady parrots coming in at all this season Miss, but I can do you a lady owl at a reasonable price."

Anything was better than nothing, so she popped the owl into the parrot's cage, and waited with thrilled anticipation. . . .

"I want to poke, I want to poke," said the parrot.

"Oooh, Ooh," said the lady owl.

"Not you, you goggle eyed freak," said the parrot, "I can't stand women who wear glasses."

A LOT OF BULL

A city visitor, a ventriloquist, was being shown round a farm. For a joke he made the bull appear to say: "How d'ye do". The attendant yokel did not seem impressed, until the hen said: "Hodge has been stealing my eggs," when he became very flustered, and the farmer said:

"Hodge, what have you to say to that, hey?"

"What I says to that master's this, when you gets to that young sow across the yard, don't you believe a word her tells ye, because it ain't true."

SERVED HER RIGHT!

The new young farmer was all for modernisation. The first thing he did was to put radio on in the cowsheds, and the effect of the music was greatly to increase milk output. He was so pleased that he went over to TV, and although the farm-hands scoffed, he scored once more, with a higher yield.

Then he achieved his greatest ambition, sold the bull, and went in for A.I.D. Much to his distress, milk output dropped to an all-time low.

One day a labourer rushed in and said: "Master, I don't know why 'tis, but they cows are giving double milk today, I've never know'd anything like it."

The farmer ran down to the cowsheds, and the first thing which caught his eyes was the TV, which was reading:

"Normal service will shortly be resumed."

HORSE SENSE

There was a Vicar who was always being approached by young people in his flock as to whether it was or was not better to have sexual experience before marriage.

As he knew little of these matters he wrote to an old college friend who was now a Consultant Psychologist, and he finished: "When you write back, phrase it tactfully, as my wife reads all my letters."

The Psychologist wrote back:

"Dear Revd. John,

There was once a recruit who joined the cavalry. The sergeant said: 'Have you ever ridden a horse before?' and the young man said 'No', so the sergeant said: 'Here's a horse that's never been ridden, you can start together'."

23

There was a man whose wife had a pet parrot, but it died, and she was very upset. Her good natured husband went off to the shop to get another bird, but nothing the man had on offer would do. One was too dear, one was too dull, another too big, until the Pet Shop man was fed up, and the customer made for the exit.

In the doorway he saw a parrot he really fancied:

"How much for this chap," he asked.

"That's a very special parrot; I don't really want to part with it, but if I do, it's £200."

"What's so very special about it?"

"Well, you see Sir, she's the only parrot in Great Britain that lays square eggs!"

The caller was not disposed to believe this, but the vendor took him into the back room, and showed him a dish of eggs, each a perfect cube.

"It's a deal, I'll take the bird with me," he said.

While the shopkeeper was making out the bill, an uneasy thought struck the man (thinking of his wife) and he said:

"I suppose the parrot can talk, as well?"

"Well, Sir, she can, but so far she only seems to have one expression."

"Oh indeed, what's that?"

"Ooooo Ooooo Ker – rist!"

NUTS TO YOU TOO

There was a workingclass Cockney who had given his young son a big build-up about the monkeys at the Zoo. If only the lad would be good, Dad would take him on Saturday to the Monkey House at Regents Park.

The kid was good, Saturday came, and off went the two of them to the Zoo. Alas! there was not a monkey in sight. This made Father very angry, and he fetched a Head Keeper. . . .

"Well, of course," said the Keeper, this happens to be the breeding season – they're all inside the hut."

"Do you think they'd come out for a nut?"

"Well, would you?"

SORRY FRED

A man had a buck rabbit at stud, and one day the buck complained of overwork. . . . "I want an assistant," he said.

"How could I get another as gentlemanly as yourself?"

"You buy a healthy young buck, I'll teach him good manners," said the rabbit, "if you pop him in with me."

This was done, and the man stood back to listen. . . . "Tomorrow there will be a row of does lined up; I'll start at one end, you at the other, and just remember your manners. "You will say, 'darling that was divine' or 'thanks a million' or something, but don't forget manners manners."

Next day early, the owner dropped the bucks, one at each end of the row of does, and was astonished to hear: "Ta duck, ta duck, ta duck, ta duck, SORRY FRED, ta duck, ta duck. . . ."

LIMERICKS II

There was a young lady of York
Seducing herself with a cork,
It stuck in her vagina
And can you imagine 'er
Probing it out with a fork!

There was a young girl of Kinsale
Who offered her body for sale,
To be kind to the blind
She engraved her behind
With detailed instruction in Braille.

There was a young lady named Starkie
Who had a night out with a darkie
The result of her sins
Was quads and not twins,
One black, one white, and two khaki!

There was a young lady at sea
Who said: "It is so hard to pee"
"Oh indeed?" said the Mate,
"That accounts for the state
Of the Captain, the Purser, and me."

There was a young girl of Dumfries
Who said to her boyfriend "Oh, please,
It will give me great bliss
If you play more with THIS,
And give less attention to THESE."

Nicer than Pork, isn't it

A priest and a rabbi happened to find themselves sharing a first class carriage on a long rail journey. They argued without rancour about the truths of religion, until the priest, feeling he was getting the worst of it, said rather sharply:

"Look here rabbi, on your oath as a man of religion, can you swear you never enjoyed the taste of pork?"

The rabbi coloured up, wrestled with his conscience a moment, and said:

"Very well Father, I'll admit it, I have eaten pork."

"And it's very nice, isn't it!" exclaimed the triumphant man of Rome. The rabbi retired behind his Jewish Times in a long and thoughtful silence. Suddenly re-emerging he said:

"I say Father. . . ."

"Yes brother, what is it?"

"Can you swear as a Christian priest that you have never enjoyed sex with a girl out of the flock?"

The priest tried to beg off, but the rabbi insisted:

"The truth, come on, the truth?!"

"Well rabbi, I confess it, I have."

"Nicer than pork, isn't it?!"

MATERNAL CARE

The Curate reading the Church Notices: "Next Sunday is Easter, will those ladies who have eggs please lay them in the church porch: The Young Mothers meet each Wednesday, will those who wish to become young mothers, please meet me in the vestry any Tuesday evening."

A DELIGHTFUL SPOT

A curate went on his honeymoon to a Lakeland hotel. As he was a natural early riser, he came down before breakfast after his bridal night, and found the lounge deserted, except for a regular resident, an old retired Army Officer. The officer looked across at the vista of lakes and mountains in the clear air, and remarked:

"A delightful spot Sir!"

"Yes indeed," said the curate, "and so cunningly concealed."

THE WORM TURNED

A woman died and went up to the Pearly Gates. Saint Peter came out, and said: "Come in."

"I want you to find my husband," said the woman, "I can't be happy unless we are reunited."

"What was his name?" said the Gate Keeper.

"Why, Smith," she said.

"Upon my everlasting soul! we've millions of Smiths in Heaven. Had he any distinguishing peculiarity?"

"He was a most peculiar man, his last words were, 'Missus, if you're ever unfaithful, I shall turn in me grave."

Peter said: "Oh, you mean *revolving* Smith."

A GOOD MAN AT BOTTOM

The Vicar had been prominent in local affairs for many years, so when he retired a dinner was given in his honour, by the Council he had so ably chaired.

The Distinguished Guest was no Churchman, but he thought that in thanking the Vicar he must work in a religious reference. Unfortunately the wine had gone round too often, and he said:

"Ladies and gentlemen, when a child is born its Guardian Angel gives it a kiss; if it is kissed on the head it will be brainy, if on the mouth, a good singer, if on the hands a clever craftsman. I don't know where our Vicar was kissed, but he certainly makes a damn good Chairman!"

USUAL PERFORMANCE

An earnest spinster wanted to work on a newspaper. She had no experience, but as her father was a Bishop and very influential in the district, they took her on.

Her first assignment was to write up the wedding of a young actor and actress who were prominent in the local Repertory Company. Said the Editor:

"Your angle on this is: 'The Show Must Go On' – write it up from that point of view."

She wrote: "Sally Promptside married Arthur Script at Mugsborough Register Office this afternoon. The usual performance will take place tonight."

ALL BULL

A girl about eleven was walking down the village street leading a cow on a rope. She met the Vicar, who said: "Little girl, little girl, what are you doing with that cow?"

"Please sir," said the child, "it's my father's cow, and I'm taking it to the bull."

"Disgusting, disgusting," said the parson, "can't your father do it?"

"No indeed Vicar, it has to be the bull."

OLD AGE WENCHIONER

There was a very old parson who married an innocent girl of eighteen. He took her off on honeymoon, and soon had her to bed.

She said: "Ooh dear, I do feel something strange coming over me," and he said: "Yes, it's old age creeping on."

VICE – VERSA!

There was a girl married a curate and when he got her to bed he seemed to know his way around with a great deal of expertise. She said:

"Darling, have you ever done anything like this before?"

The question took him by surprise, and he coloured up.

The girl, pressing home her advantage said: "Come on, come on, own up, own up, we must start with a clean sheet, who WAS it?"

After a deal of stammering and stuttering he said it was with one of the choir boys.

Writing to her mother the next day, the bride said: "Do you know, I didn't know which way to turn."

COCKSURE

A young woman was alone in a railway carriage until a clergyman got in. Seeking to be sociable, he said:

"That's a fine baby you've got there."

The woman replied that it was indeed a lovely child, conceived after six years of marriage, when hope had almost gone.

"Yes," said the parson, "persistence, persistence, is always blessed in the end; take my case, I breed pigeons; for years I never won a race, but lately I'm winning silver cups all the time."

"Indeed," said the young married woman, "what made the break-through?"

"Oh, I changed the cock."

"Yes, that's what I did."

TIME FLIES

It was the Rugby Club dinner, and the main speaker, a Bishop, was drivelling on and on. . . . On the right of the chairman sat the Mayor.

"I wish to cripes I knew how to stop the beggar," said the first to the second. "That's easy," said the experienced old Mayor, "pass that paper serviette," upon which, he scribbled a few words and passed the note to the speaker.

The speaker, in full flow, glanced, suddenly mumbled a conclusion, and sat down. Said the chairman to his friend: "You're a genius, what did you write?"

"Only four little words – 'Your flies are undone.'"

SHE HAD GOOD PULL

The Mothers Union were on their annual coach outing, and unfortunately Mrs Bloggs began to tipple. Indeed, after the last stop, which was at a truly rural pub, they couldn't find Mrs Bloggs at all.

The Vicar said he would go and look for her, and, wandering round the back of the "Farmers Arms" he found a cowshed in which was a cow. Hanging onto the cow's teat was Mrs Bloggs.

"Come along now dear," he said, "come and get in your seat like a good woman."

"Shan't move," said Mrs Bloggs in a very slurred voice. "Shert'nly not. I sat by the driver coming along, I shall sit by the driver goin' back."

TENORS – AND BASS

The new doctor was making his first-ever round of the Maternity Ward. Seeking to be friendly, he asked the woman in the first bed when her baby was due.

"March 11th," she said. The next woman he came to said her event would be March 11th, and so it went on.

"Extraordinary!" said the doctor to the Matron, "extraordinary coincidence." However, the last patient he spoke to said her due date would be March 17th.

"That's more extraordinary still, that nineteen women should be on the same date and just the twentieth should be different."

"Ah well, you see doctor, I wasn't on the Choir Outing."

HE WAS A BAR – STEWARD

There was a man went to his Club on a weekday to play golf, and the only person available was a parson, a stranger who had called in while on holiday.

Off they went, and the man said: "Ah, reverend, I hope you don't mind, but we always play for a pound in this club."

The parson was put out, not approving of gambling, but he thought "only a pound", and teed up. His opponent played dirty, sneezed at the wrong moment, used filthy language, cheated when he could, and finished up thrashing the poor old parson. . . ."In this Club, the loser buys the drinks" he told him, adding: "And may I trouble you for six quid."

"I thought we agreed a pound?"

"A hole!" said the villain.

Over the drinks, the cad said: "If you're ever this way again vicar, drop in and I'll always gladly give you a game."

"Yes," was the reply, and here's my card, come to my church, and it would be a good idea if you brought your parents, too."

"Brought my father and mother? Why?"

"Well, I could marry them."

SOME'S SPEED!

The Mothers' Meeting were on their annual coach outing, and unfortunately the driver was a reckless sort, and drove faster and faster.

Down one narrow winding lane in Wales he was getting up to sixty mp.h. when the Dear Vicar observed that old Mrs Moggs had gone white in the face with fear. He went up, put his arm on her shoulders and said, with a great show of jocularity: "Some speed, eh Mrs Moggs, some speed!"

"I don't know about the others, Vicar, but I certainly have."

A HARD PROPOSITION

A parson was anxious that the church social and dance should be a success. An actress famous for her voluptuous figure was doing a local show, and he got her to support it. The lady was wearing a tight sheath dress with a daring corsage, and as she and the vicar led off in the first dance he remarked:

"You know, Miss Tartly, you're a wonderful actress."

"Thank you vicar."

"And you are also very beautiful."

"That's nice of you vicar," and they danced on. "But I ought to tell you," he went on, blushing, "that I've got just one thing against you."

She said: "Yes, I can feel it."

A MAN OF POSITION

This same vicar thought he ought to do something to "save" this actress, and he innocently suggested to her that he should visit her in her room, to "get down to fundamentals".

She readily agreed, and when the vicar arrived she was stark naked on the bed with her legs wide open.

"I prayed for you all last night . . ." he began.

"Well, I'm on the phone, but anyway, you can have me now for five pounds."

"No no Miss Tartly, you misunderstand, I expected to find you on your knees, and I think that even now we should begin by kneeling down."

"Of course vicar, if that's how you want it, but it hurts a bit, and anyway if you want it kinky it's ten pounds."

JIMMY'S RIDDLE

A curate went to his first parish, and was met by the vicar, who said: "Ah James, you've just come at the right moment, the Parish Mothers are having their weekly meeting in the Hall, you must go down and introduce yourself to them."

When the curate entered the Parish Mothers' meeting the cackle suddenly stopped, and there was an embarrassed silence. The curate beamed round the room, and said:

"Well well, I can see we're all knitting or sewing, but can't someone tell a story or ask a riddle to enliven the proceedings?"

"Yes," said old Mrs Bloggs in the corner, "you've been to college, what is it a man stands up to do, a woman sits down to do, and a dog holds out his leg to do?"

Scarlet and stammering, the curate blurted out that he had not the least idea. . . .

"Why!" said the old gossip, "to shake hands, of course!"

COMING WITH A LETTER

The wealthy widow of a Rural Dean was explaining her duties to the new housemaid. The widow would be lying in bed late each morning, the maid would bring her up a cup of tea, and should then go back down and fetch the post, for she was a massive correspondent.

The girl listened carefully, and followed her instructions, except that she didn't come back up again:

"Mary, Mary! Hasn't the postman come yet?"

"Not yet Mum, but he's breathing hard."

TAKING THE MICKY

There was a young nun who went to the Mother Superior in some distress, and after a great deal of beating about the bush, admitted she was pregnant.

"Who was it? Who was this wicked wicked man?" said the Mother Superior.

"Oh Reverent Mother, I wouldn't commit a carnal offence with a man!" exclaimed the nun.

"Well it wasn't fathered by a woman, was it!" said the M.S., beginning to lose her temper.

"No indeed blessed mother, but it was fathered by one of the Holy Angels" (simper, simper).

"Holy Angels – what is this nonsense?"

"Yes Blessed Mother, he came down to me in the middle of the night in my sleep, and when I asked him who he was he said "Saint Michael" and showed me his name on his vest, to prove it."

WHITE FRIARS

There was a man went to a laundry for a job, and the Manager said: "Trade's terribly slack, but if you can fetch in any fresh business, I'll give you 5% on the take."

"That's me!" said the man, "the best order-getter in the business," and off he set, whistling. He was back in half an hour with a black eye.

"Hallo," said the Manager, "what's going on?"

"Well Sir, I thought I'd try that monastery down the road. I asked to see the Father Superior, and when I was admitted I said I felt sure the monks must have some dirty habits."

PUNCTURED

The parson was a worried man, "Listen," he said to his verger, "somebody's stolen my bicycle."

"Where've you been on it rector," enquired that worthy.

"Only round the parish on my calls."

The verger suggested that the best plan would be for the rector to direct his Sunday sermon to the ten commandments. . . . "When you get to 'Thou Shalt Not Steal', you and I'll watch their faces, we'll soon see."

Sunday came, the rector started in fine flow about the Commandments, then lost his thread, changed the subject, and tailed off lamely.

"Sir," said the verger, "I thought you was going to. . . ."

"I know Giles, I know, but you see, when I got to 'Thou Shalt Not Commit Adultery' I suddenly remembered where I'd left my bicycle."

FISHY STORY

The Trappists needed something for supper, and the Father Abbot made signs to two of the monks to go out early and fish.

They fished silently all day without a single bite, and were thoroughly fed up, when, at the end of the day, the younger monk caught a mermaid. He looked at this naked and beautiful catch, fondled it all over, then hurled it back into the lake.

The other Trappist could keep his fearful vow of silence no longer, he exploded:

"Why?"

"How?"

THE BEST OF THE RUBBER

To a highly select parish in Cheltenham came a new curate who, within a short time married a sexy young woman. In ten months they had a child, and eleven months after that, another. At the end of five years they had five children and were expecting a sixth. The worthies of the parish were deeply shocked, and wrote to the Bishop about it.

The Bishop sent the curate a strong letter.

HE WAS STONED

When the new curate arrived, the vicar said:

"I'm giving you a break, the Bishop's coming next Sunday, I'll stand down for you; this will be your great chance to get marked for preferment."

By Sunday the curate was a nervous wreck, but the vicar he'd been through it all and knew the answer, with which he took the curate into the vestry.

"As you preach and your mouth goes dry, take a sip of this", and he gave him a glass of water well laced with gin. But his hand slipped and he overdid the gin.

The curate preached like a fireball, then, lurching down, staggered to the Bishop, slapped his back and said: "Not a bad shermon, eh m'Lord, hey? hic!"

"Ah, a fair start my son, but you know, there were ten commandments not twelve, twelve apostles not ten, and David slew Goliath with a stone, he did *not* do up the stupid bleeder with the jawbone of a bloody ass."

THE LONG AND THE SHORT OF IT

A young hardworking and devout farmer in the Irish village shocked the priest by marrying a girl from away, and a Protestant at that. However, much to his relief, the girl became a Catholic.

In his middle age the farmer lost his wife; again he married a stranger and a Protestant and shocked the priest, but she too was converted.

In his old age the same thing happened, but the priest did not worry, until several months passed, and the new bride did not come to mass. He then went and gave Patrick a piece of his mind . . .

"Jabers father, the old converter isn't what it was!"

THE SEX MANIAC

The newly appointed priest thought he'd walk this vast parish and meet the flock. One day he followed a dusty track for miles to find a devout family with fourteen children.

"Good day Connelly, you're a credit to Ireland, the biggest family in the parish."

"Good day father, but this is not the biggest family in the parish – that's Doylan, over the hill."

It was a tired priest who greeted Doylan and his sixteen children, but . . . "God bless all these eighteen little Catholics" he said.

"Sorry father, but this is a Protestant family!"

"Then I'll go at once," said the priest, "for it's nothing but a dirty sex maniac that ye are!"

CIRCUMSCRIBED

A rabbi and a priest were neighbours, and there was a certain amount of "needle" between them. If the Cohens had their drive done up, Father O'Flynn had his relaid, and so it went on.

One day the priest had a new Jaguar, so the rabbi bought a Bentley. When the rabbi looked out of his window it was to see the priest pouring water over the top of the car bonnet. He opened the window and shouted:

"That's not the way to fill the radiator, you know."

"Aha," said the priest, I'm christening it with holy water, that's more than you can do to yours."

A little while later the priest was taken aback to see the rabbi lying in the road, hacksaw in hand, sawing the last inch of his car's exhaust pipe.

THE LITTLE MOTHER

A sincere clergyman was out walking when he saw three Salvation Army girls sitting on a bench crying their eyes out. He lifted his hat, saying: "Pardon me, but this is a wretched sight, can I help?"

There was no reply, only more sobs.

He tried again: "Over there in the pavillion we can have a nice cup of tea, that always improves things."

When the tea and cream cakes arrived the girls cheered up. As the waitress put the tray down, the parson beamed and said:

"Who's going to be the 'little mother'?"

They all burst into tears again.

A FOUR-LETTER WORD!

A curate and a bishop were in opposite corners of a railway carriage on a long journey. As the bishop entered, the curate put away his copy of "Playboy" and was reading the "Church Times". The bishop ignored him, and went on doing the "Times" crossword. Silence prevailed.

After a while the curate tried to make conversation, and when the bishop began to do a lot of head scratching and "tut-tut-tut-ing" he tried again. . . .

"Can I help you Sir?"

"Perhaps; I'm only beaten by one word; what is it that has four letters, the last three are U, N, T, and the clue is: 'Essentially feminine'?"

"Why Sir," said the curate after a slight pause: "that'll be 'Aunt'."

"Of course, of course!" said the bishop, "I say young man, can you lend me a rubber?"

T-T-T-T-TEE TOTALLER!

A shy young curate went to a strange golf club while on holiday, and asked the Secretary to find him a game. The Sec. was very busy, and said:

"Look here, there's a pretty girl just gone out, she's a stranger like you, catch her up and introduce yourself."

So the shy young man went after the girl and said:

"M-my name's P-peter, b-but I'm n-no s-saint."

The girl replied with a flashing smile:

"M-my name's M-mary, b-but I'm n-not a v-v-v-very g-good player!"

SHOTGUN WEDDING?

A pretty young married woman went to her vicar and asked for some advice. She did not wish to start a family yet, and (putting the matter delicately) asked the parson if he knew how to prevent the stork from settling on the roof.

The vicar said that as an old bachelor he could not answer the question, but his sister had a very wise parrot, Oxford educated, and they had best ask the bird.

The parrot, duly put in humour by sugar, cocked his head when the vicar said:

"Polly, tell the young lady how to prevent the stork from landing" and shouted:

"Shoot it in the air!"

CONVENT-IONAL

The nuns ran an orphanage, and one day the Mother Superior summoned to her office three buxom girls who were leaving, and said:

"Now, you're all going out into the big sinful world, and I must warn you against certain men. There are men who will buy you drinks, take you to a room, undress you, and do unspeakable things to you. Then they give you two or three pounds, and you're sent away, ruined!"

"Excuse me Reverend Mother," said the boldest one, "did you say these wicked men do this to us and give us three pounds?"

"Yes, dear child, why do you ask?"

"Well, the priests only give us apples."

There were two young ladies of Birmingham
There is a good story concerning 'em,
They lifted the frock
And played with the cock
Of the Bishop engaged in confirming 'em;
Now, the worthy old Bish was no fool
(He'd been to a Sec. Modern school)
He took off the britches
Of those dirty bitches
And used his episcopal tool!

There once was a wicked old actor
Who waylaid a young girl and attacked 'er,
In reply to this trick,
She bit off his wick
And thus remained virgo intacta!

There was a young man of Cape Horn
Who wished he had never been born,
He wouldn't have been
If his father had seen
That the end of the letter was torn

There was a young plumber named Lee
Who was plumbing his girl by the sea,
When she said: "Stop your plumbing!
"There's somebody coming!"
Said the plumber (still plumbing) "It's me!"

Nuts Screws Washers and Bolts

A certain rich man had a wastrel son who was the family's despair. Finally, the old man, whose name was Nuts, bought his son a laundry business in a remote country town, also appointing a reliable manager. All was peace for a time; then came an urgent call from the manager to go down at once. Sure enough, the manager was at the station:

"It's terrible Sir, your son has put half the laundry girls in the family way."

"That's bad, but could be worse."

"Worse than that Sir, he's scarpered, gone away!"

"That's bad, is that the lot?"

"Much worse Sir, the local paper's on to the story, and they're going to splash it. . . ."

The old man was sure there was nothing money could not do, so he called on the local editor, and offered a good bribe to suppress the scandal, "for the sake, not of my worthless son, but his ailing mother."

The editor said too much was known already, he dare not kill the story, but for a hundred quid he could print it in a form well understood in the town, but not likely to be picked up by the National press.

This being agreed, an anxious father awaited the week-end and read: "Special Ironmongery Announcement – NUTS SCREWS WASHERS AND BOLTS".

GOOD FOR NOTHING

In a first-class carriage rode an icy Deb, very "top drawer". Opposite was a middle aged business man. Suddenly he lowered his Financial Times and said:

"Would you sleep with me just one night for a thousand pounds?"

The snooty girl said any more of this talk and she would pull the alarm cord! The man smiled patiently and said: "Money is nothing to me if I fancy anything, and I fancy you . . . TEN thousand pounds?"

The girl was beginning to waver, and he pressed:

"At the Hilton, in pound notes, cash in advance?"

After a little more hesitation the young lady said yes, the deal was on.

"Right, will you get down on the seat now, for thirty bob?"

"My dear Sir, how dare you! What sort of person do you think I am?!" she blazed.

"Now now, that's already settled, we're merely haggling on price."

GONE TO POT

A man narrowly reared by a widowed mother, got married. He telephoned back to his mother from the honeymoon hotel, to say that he knew there was something he had to do in bed, but he didn't know what it was.

"Why," said his mother, "you put your . . . er, that is, you put the hardest part of yourself in the place where your wife wee-wees."

At midnight the hotel rang the Fire Brigade for help. . . .

"We've got a young man with his head jammed in a chamber-pot."

FAST AND LOOSE

A noble lord whose wife had died, was making all arrangements for his daughter's "coming out". At the last moment he was sent for on urgent government work, so he asked the butler – a faithful old family retainer – to see that the Coming Out Ball details were finalised and keep on eye on the daughter.

The Deb daughter went to her Ball, and she did not come back until 3 a.m. When she awoke, very late, she was in bed, and the faithful retainer was standing by with black coffee. . . .

"James, how did I come to be in this bed?"

"You came home very late and very tired, my lady."

"But James, I'm undressed and in my nightdress!"

"I could not let you spoil that dress, my lady."

"Good lord James, do you mean you undressed me and put me to bed without my knowing it?"

"Yes Madam."

"James, tell the truth, was I tight?"

"Not after the first time, my lady."

IT'S A WISE CHILD

A certain little girl, when asked her name, would reply:

"I'm Mr Smithbrown's daughter."

Her mother told her this was wrong, she must say:

"I'm Jane Smithbrown."

Then the Vicar spoke to her in Sunday School, and said: "Aren't you Mr Smithbrown's daughter?"

She replied:

"I thought I was, but mother says I'm not."

THE STUPID COUNT

A sweep's son was his mother's only darling, and when they won the pools, mother insisted the boy must go to college, although father protested.

The son sent home for rowing togs, cricket togs, tennis togs, and no matter what father said, Willy was refused nothing. Finally, he wrote and said the college ball was coming due, could he have a suit of tails. Father went mad, but mother sent the money.

The boy wrote to say that he had been a great success at the Ball. . . . "Everybody said I looked like a proper Count," he wrote.

"He never could spell," said his father.

WIRE PULLING

A pompous self-made grocer named Bates got his son into a posh college. Of course, the whole family had to go up with Johnny, to see him start his first term, and to meet the Principal.

"I'm Sir Snortweight Bates," announced the rich grocer, "this is my good lady, Lady Bates, my daughter, Miss Bates, and my son Master Bates."

"Oh does he? Well, we'll soon get him out of that."

IN PRAISE OF VICE

It was a Tory convention, and the President introduced a smashing matron, "and I must tell you that Lady Goodbody is also chairman of the Northern Federation."

"No no," said the speaker, "Sir Bragge Bloodworthy is our chairman, I am his vice. . . ."

TOWN AND GOWN

The Oxford student was walking out late at night with a sleazy blonde on his arm, when he ran straight into the proctor: "Sir!" said the proctor, "are you a member of this University?"

"Yes, Sir, I am."

"Then introduce me to the young gentlewoman."

(The undergrad was a quick thinker . . .). "Certainly Sir," he said, "this is my elder sister. . . ."

"Gosh dammit," said the proctor, beginning to lose his temper, "everybody knows this is the most notorious old bag in Oxford!"

"Oh Sir, how unkind of you to throw the family misfortunes into my face in such a manner."

PROCTOR-COL

The proctor was prowling along the river bank at night, seeking whom he could catch, and he came to a punt tied up in some bushes. He could just make out a scholastic gown and a pair of silken legs.

The proctor turned to his bulldogs (strong-arm men) and said: "Fetch him here!" The unfortunate fellow was lifted off and placed in a dishevelled state before the proctor. In accordance with ancient protocol he asked the time-honoured question: "Sir, are you a member of this University?"

"Gore dammiy and suck yourself!" stormed the angry victim, "I am chairman of the governing body of this university!"

The proctor turned calmly to the bulldogs and said:
"Replace the gentleman."

"EXCEEDINGLY SMALL...."

The Proctors of Cambridge were watching a house of ill
repute to see if they could catch any undergrads using it.
They hid in a doorway and saw three young men enter;
after an hour one came out. . . .

"Your name and college sir?"

"Smith of Jesus," he said.

Two hours went by before the second victim came out,
and it was getting dark and cold when he admitted to being
"Jones of Trinity."

It was two in the morning, and snowing before the last
one was caught: "You needn't tell us," they said, "you're
Mills of God."

VIVE LA DIFFERENCE!

A stodgy professor, in Paris on business, was approached at
night by a girl offering her charms for cash. The prof
stuttered:

"I don't understand you, and I've left my dictionary at
the hotel." The girl lifted her skirt and said: "Voici le
dictionaire universel, qui les savants de tout pays ont
ouvert" (Behold the universal dictionary, which the learned
of all nations have opened.)

VIVE LE SPORT!

An English gentleman of breeding was standing face to
wall in a dark corner of Paris one night, when a gendarme
tapped him smartly on the shoulder, and said:

"Defense de pisser!"

The gentleman replied: "Pardonnez moi M'sieur, je
n'pisse pas, je m'abuse.'

"Ah, pardonnez *moi*, vive le sport!"

HE BOOBED!

It was a select Society dinner, and the old waiter was training the young waiter. The great art of the job, he told him, was to be quick in any emergency. . . . "For instance I was on a job at the Palace when a lady with a low blouse and a big chest laughed, and they both popped out. Did I use my bare hands to put them back? no, I. . . ." Here they were interrupted.

The dinner went on, and the young waiter noticed a Peeress with a large chest, a low dress and a hearty laugh. He hung around expecting the worst, and sure enough it happened! Quick as a flash he seized a large serving spoon, and popped them back.

When he rejoined his boss round the back, he said:

"How about that eh? Not bad for a learner?"

"Young man, when you really know the trade you will use a *warm* spoon."

ON THE JOB

A pukka sahib was entertaining the Governor's party; and his wife, in spite of warnings, wore a low dress. Sure enough, in the middle of dinner, there was a calamity when the lady's large bubs flopped out. The husband, quick as a flash, caused a diversion by pointing out of the big window to the lawn, on which was a newly installed fountain:

"I say, look at that splendid sight will you."

They all looked.

A pair of monkeys were coupling on the fountain.

FAMILY TRADITION

A middle-aged colonel left the Indian army and in accordance with his family's tradition, married a young woman. Nine months later he engaged the best Harley Street obstetrician. . . . "See about my son."

"How do you know it'll be a son?"

"It will, family tradition."

When the doctor rang through, it was a son.

"Circumcise him," said the father, against all the doctor's protests, "it's family tradition."

Later the doctor rang and said the child seemed ill. . . .

"Give him a stiff brandy, I'm paying, don't argue."

The doctor rang yet again, and said the child was no better: "Then put him to the breast; I'll come over."

Sure enough, when the father arrived the child was feeding well, and was obviously a very fit baby indeed.

"Splendid," shouted the colonel "there's a real father's son for you, belly full of brandy, mouth full of tit and a sore cock!"

APING HIS BETTERS?

Two old cavalry colonels were talking about a third. . . .

"I say, Smithers old chap, did you hear about Jenkins?"

"No, what's that devil up to now?"

"You'll never believe this old boy, but Jenk has started living in sin with a monkey!"

"By jove! I say what! Male monkey or female monkey?"

"Dammit Smithers, don't say that. Female monkey of course, nothing unnatural about old Jenkins."

PINCHED

The Deb gave a snooty party, and hired a maid, just to show off. Alas, the maid was not really experienced. A second party was organised, and when the Agency sent the same girl along, the Deb said:

"Look here Mary, don't forget the sugar tongs this time: it's not very nice when the men go in the loo, and they take themselves out, and they put themselves back, and then they have to pick up the sugar lumps with their fingers."

The girl swore she would remember this time, but, after the guests had gone, the Deb said: "Mary I thought I told you about the sugar tongs!"

"I put them out My Lady, I swear I did!"

"Well, *I* didn't see them on the table!"

"On the table? My Lady, I should think not, I put them in the toilet."

WHO WOULDN'T?

The Master of an Oxford College invited a well-known public figure to dine at High Table with him, and laid on the best old port for the occasion. Now the visitor was a "temperance" bigot, and when the Master said:

"Will you have some port Sir?" gave the reply:

"By the lord harry! I'd rather commit adultery than drink a single glass of port."

"Who wouldn't?!" said the Master.

SAILOR'S HORNPIPE

An Admiral of the Fleet was a widower, so he sent his daughter to an exclusive and rather narrow boarding school. To his horror, when her education was finished she began courting a common sailor. She waited until she was of age, and then announced that she would marry the Jack Tar. The day before the wedding, the Admiral took his daughter aside, and said:

"This is very difficult for me, in fact I'd rather face the enemy in battle than talk to you about the Facts of Life, but the truth is, well, you see, it's like this, sailors spend months at sea, and they sometimes get peculiar habits, or, er, let me put it this way, if he ever demands sex in a funny way, you tell me and I'll speak to him."

"A funny way father, what exactly d'you mean?"

"Well er, if he er, ever wants it the other way round."

The girl left it at that, and was soon married and on honeymoon. For months she bloomed, then one night going to bed, she said to her sailor husband:

"Jack, have you ever thought you'd like to try sex 'the other way round' whatever that means?"

"What! and fill the bloody house with kids!"

THROUGH THE HOOP

The circus came, and as a treat the nuns were given a block of seats. Most of all they enjoyed the clown. Alas, a great fire broke out in the "big top" and everybody fled for their lives, except one young nun who was a cripple. The clown, with great courage, went into the smoke, and brought her out on his back, which was virgin on the ridiculous!

THE BITER BIT

The Noble Lord and the Noble Lady were middle aged and not on good terms. In fact Her Ladyship was convinced that he was carrying on with the pretty housemaid, so she laid a trap: she suddenly sent Mary home for the weekend.

That night when they went to bed, His Lordship came the Old Story: "Excuse me my dear, my stomach," and promptly disappeared. Her Ladyship promptly dashed along the corridor, up the back stairs, into the maid's bed. She just had time to switch the light off, when in he came. . . .

. . . He wasted no time or words, but quickly took his will. He was still panting when Her Ladyship switched on the light and said: "You didn't expect to find me in this bed, did you?"

"No indeed, Madam," said James, the Butler.

CAME TOO SOON

Mrs Kaysor-Bondor was dressing for a very Grand Occasion, but as she put on her expensive nylons, one laddered. She put on a fresh pair, but they laddered leaving the house; yet another pair went as she entered the car. Her husband was furious. . . . "You're not going back AGAIN! We're late already!"

She replied: "It would never do for Mrs Kaysor-Bondor to appear in laddered stockings, what *would* people think?"

He replied: "Listen, the last big 'do' I went to, that charming Mrs Rendels was there, *and* her four children!"

WITHOUT A.I.D.

The Squire and his Lady were Chief Patrons of the Agricultural Show, and after the opening ceremony they dutifully walked round, mixing with the tenants and peasantry, and looking at the exhibits.

But his Lordship spent so much time in the beer tent that her Ladyship wandered off to admire the prize bull. Never was a male animal so splendidly equipped.

"My, but that's a fine beast you have there Giles," she said to the yokel in charge.

"Yes my Lady, he be champion, and father o' champions."

"Go on, tell me all about him."

"Well Mam, this here bull went to stud three hundred times last year."

"Indeed? Well, go over to his Lordship will you, my good fellow, and tell him that there's a bull here went to stud three hundred times in one year, will you."

Giles dutifully trotted up to Squire and gave the message. . . .

"Very interesting indeed," was his comment, "always the same cow, I presume?"

"Oh, no indeed Sir, three hundred different cows."

"Aha, go and tell her Ladyship that, will you."

There was a young lady of Barking Creek
Who had her monthlies twice a week,
Said a man from Working:
"How provoking"
"You'd get no poking so to speak!"

There was an old man of Pagoda
Would not pay a whore what he owed'er,
"I'll show you!" she said,
And she jumped out of bed,
And peed in his whisky and soda.

There was a young girl of Malacca
Who played with her boyfriend's left knacker,
One night they were tight
And she played with his right –
The b*gger went off like a cracker!

There was an old fellow of Cosham
Who took out his ballocks to wash'em,
His wife said: "Now Jack,
If you don't put'em back
I shall jump on the beggars and squash'em."

From a tart, a young man of Cape Anchor
Caught syph, gonnorrhea, clap and canker,
In addition to crabs
And scabs on the tabs,
So he sent her a postcard, to thank'er.

Feather Pluckers

Three louts were brought before the Beak for "loitering with intent". The first convinced the Court that he had a steady occupation as a "Car Dealer" and got off. The second said he was a "Street Trader" and after his Pedlars License had been produced, he too was dismissed. The third had to do some quick thinking, and recalled that he had sometimes helped the Market people to get their Christmas poultry ready. . . .

"Your occupation or employment?" said the Beak.

"Sir, I'm one of those what they call, you know, er, feather pluckers. . . ."

"Clever WHAT?"

JUST A MINT

A Banker went up the West End for a night, picked up a tart and asked the price. She told him not to worry, it would be reasonable. After a good night out, she asked for fifty pounds.

"Fifty pounds! far too much!"

"Surely you've heard of me, Polly, the dearest in the game."

"What did you say your name was – Polo?"

"No, silly, Polly. Why Polo?"

"Well you've certainly got a hole with a mint in it!"

THE TACTFUL PLUMBER

The plumber impressed on his new apprentice that tact was essential on the job. "For instance" he said, "I was once following a pipe through a house and I walked into an unlocked bathroom, and there was a woman stark naked. Quick as a flash, I said: "Excuse me, Sir," and went away – "that's tact see."

The next job they went on, the plumber started in the kitchen and sent the kid upstairs to look for the tank. There was a disturbance, and the boy re-appeared with a black eye and a bleeding nose.

"What the hell have you been up to?"

"It's all your fault, you and your bloody tact. There was a courting couple stark naked on a bed upstairs, doing things, and I said: "Excuse me, gentlemen.""

HIGHLAND FLING

There was an elocution master went to a ball, and seemed to be getting on famously with a young woman he had picked up.

After a while he said: "You're Scottish, aren't you?"

"How did ye knaw that?" she said.

He replied: "I could tell by the way you roll your R's."

"Nae, nae" she said, "that's just th'effect o' my high heels!"

A man went to his solicitor and said: "I am very rich, so money is no object, but I want to be rid of my wife, who is a bitch, without being had for murder, so tell me what to do."

"Buy her a strong horse and it may throw her."

A month later the man came back and said his wife was now the best horsewoman in the district. . . .

"Try" said the lawyer, "buying her a mini and send her up the M 1 in it."

The man did this, but she drove like Stirling Moss, putting in danger everybody but herself. The husband told the solicitor he was desperate. . . .

"Buy her a big Jaguar."

The man was back in a week delighted. "Name your fee," he said, "it worked!"

"What happened then?"

"Well, when she opened the cage door to feed the jaguar, it bit her bloody head off!"

ON THE MARK

Two old friends went on honeymoon together, and had a bet who would perform the most times first night. It was a point of honour to tell the truth, and each would chalk up his score outside the bedroom door. Jack performed three times altogether, and chalked them up thus: 1 1 1 .

Bill staggered along at breakfast time to see the state of the parties, observed the marks, and said:

"Cor blimey, one hundred and eleven, beat me by two!"

AS YE RAPE, YE SHALL SEW

A man had just done five years in prison for a double rape, and was being discharged. Said the warder: "Here's your civvies, here's the £50 you came in with, sign for them and be off."

As the man departed the warder added: "I suppose you'll be up the West End tonight, looking for a woman."

"A woman? Me? Don't be daft, I've been impotent all my life."

"Impotent? Don't talk like a bloody fool, how can you be impotent when you've just done time for raping two women?"

"I know, I know," said the convict, sadly, "I think I didn't have a very good solicitor."

REDUCIO AD ABSURDAM

A woman complained to her solicitor that every time she had intercourse with her husband it hurt her past all bearing, "He's enormous, simply enormous," she added.

The solicitor said: "In that case madam, the best thing you can do is to file your petition."

"Oh, certainly not! Let him sandpaper his. . . ."

NO CHANGE OUT OF HIM

A man in full morning dress was descending the steps of the Strand Law Courts when a blowsy made-up blonde asked him if he felt like a bit.

"Madam," he replied very haughtily, "permit me to inform you that I am the Crown Solicitor."

"That's quite alright me old cock! I'm the half-crown solicitor!"

PERILS OF POLYGAMY

A Chief in darkest Africa sent his son and heir to London to be educated. The boy divided happy days between classrooms and the West End, until he got a sudden call to go home and take over – his father had suddenly died. Of one thing he was quite certain, he was going to take home an English, king-sized double bed (the like of which he had not previously seen), to accommodate a King Size harem.

All the tribe turned out to see their new ruler, as he arrived accompanied by massive packing cases. As soon as formalities were concluded he ordered the bed to be erected in the Royal Kraal, but here arose trouble. Much of the space was occupied by an enormous ancestral throne made of logs:

"Take that thing outside" said the youth, but at this point a terrible wail arose from the Witch Doctor, who pointed out that for time out of mind it had been known that should the throne leave the Kraal, the Royal Line must die out. After a good deal of argument the boy agreed to leave it in, but to make room for the King Size royal bed, he had the throne lashed to the rafters with primitive ropes.

For a time all went very well, but alas, the insects which lived in the straw roof came out and nibbled at the ropes. One night, when the young Chief was in bed with four of his favourite wives, the throne came crashing down, and killed the lot of them.

PEOPLE WHO LIVE IN GRASS HOUSES SHOULDN'T STOW THRONES!

LOOPING THE LOOP

There was a certain lass who had more bust than brains and she was what is known as a P.T. or "teaser".

It was her custom to go out with men, get her drinks and entertainment paid for, and then "cry off" when the chap claimed his reward.

One day she met her match; he was a sportsman who had a big old saloon car with a useful-sized back seat, and here he was up before the Court charged with rape.

The Chairman of the Bench looked over his glasses at the peroxide blonde in the witness box and said: "But my dear, there wasn't a mark on you – why didn't you struggle in the car?"

"I couldn't!" said the girl, "you know those loops in the corners? Well, he stuck one of my legs through one loop, and the other through the other loop, and there. I was, fixed."

"Remarkable, remarkable" said the Beak, "now I know what those loops are for, I often wondered."

"Yes, yes," put in his fellow magistrate, another ancient man, "and what a sign of progress too!"

"Progress? What the blazes are you on about, progress?"

"Why yes, progress my dear Chairman, when I was a young feller there was nothing like that, we had to make do with winding down each window, shoving her foot out and winding it up again."

PENNIES FROM HEAVEN

To the Council of a country town was elected an old farmer, determined to "reduce the rates". When the Surveyor's report was read, it included a scheme to bridge the local stream. "Disgraceful!" shouted the old man, "bridge that! Why I could piss across it."

"You're out of order, completely out of order," bellowed the Mayor.

"Aye, I knows I am, or I could piss twice as far as that."

Later on came a proposal to have a urinal in the market place. "I'm dead agen that," said the farmer, "I move rejection!"

"Shut up you fool" whispered his companion, "we've got to have somewhere to have a run-out."

"Oh, is that what it is? Sorry, Mr Mayor, I withdraw my objection, in fact I move we have an arsenal as well."

A SHINING LIGHT

There was a policeman on night duty who thought he heard something up an entry. He shone his torch up, and observed a young woman with her blouse undone and her knickers round her ankles, calmly eating from a bag of crisps. . . .

"Hey, what's going on there?"

The girl looked up, chewing, and said:

"Blimey! Has he gorn?"

DESIGNING WOMEN

Two men in a London Professional Men's club got into a heated argument as to who had originally designed woman. The architect said only an architect could have designed such beauty, the sweeping curves leading the eye to the essentials, all in perfect proportion . . . etc."

"That's all piffle, not to say balls and codswallop," said the engineer: "Woman is functional from first to last, ideally designed to reproduce the race, clearly the work of a skilled engineer."

Finally they referred the matter to the arbitration of a fellow clubman, a retired judge. He thought for a while, then he said:

"You are both wrong, woman was designed by a 'planner' without any doubt."

"How do you make that out?" they both wanted to know.

"Why because only a planner would have placed the pleasure gardens between the Waterworks on one side, and the Sewage Disposal Plant on the other.

STIFF WORK

A young man owned a small and ancient open tourer with a tired engine. One day he took a hefty girl out for a ride in the country, and when they arrived at a remote and steep hill, the car spluttered and finally stopped.

"Shall we get out and push it up?" said the man to the girl.

"A good idea that, but will it be alright to leave the car here?"

NIGHT "MARE"

Twins had been told of the coming of a new baby. As it was due near their birthday, mother, along with the Facts of Life, had also built it up as her additional birthday present to them. And, great joy, the baby did arrive on their birthday and was much loved. Came the next year, and the mother asked the twins what they wanted for a present. They didn't know, so she gave them time to think it over. They came back and said:

"If it wouldn't blow you up too much, do you think you could manage a pony this year?"

HIAWAFFLE

A certain young man was articled as a Civil Engineer, but he could not pass his exams because the Theorem of Pythagorus beat him time after time. In despair he ran away to sea. He deserted ship in the USA, and wandered across the continent. Months later, ragged and hungry, he drifted into an Indian reservation, where they took him in and nursed him back to health. One day he told the Chief the whole story, and the Chief said:

"Our Medicine Man, heap wise, him solve this one."

The Medicine Man listened gravely, and said:

"Paleface, a Brave takes three squaws, one sleeps on a buffalo's skin and has papoose, another sleeps on sheep's skin and has papoose, the third sleeps on hippopotamus's skin, and has twins, what does that prove?"

"Why" said the youth, "it proves the squaw on the hippopotamus's equals the sum of the squaws on the other two's hides."

"Precisely!" said the Medicine Man.

DIRTY WEEKEND

The chemist impressed upon the new boy that in business, politeness was everything. "It doesn't matter if they only come in to ask what time it is, courtesy costs nothing, always be friendly and polite."

With which the chemist departed to have his lunch. When he came back the boy was in a shocking state, with two black eyes and his clothes torn. "It's all your fault, you and your daft advice, look what it's done for me."

"Why, what happened?" said the boss.

"Well, a courting couple came in, arm in arm, and the girl bought a packet of S.T.'s. I remembered what you said, and while I was wrapping them up I politely remarked:

"It looks like being a dull weekend, Sir."

"MISS" UNDERSTOOD

An Oxford student off for a weekend at a country house party arrived at this rustic town realising he had left part of his luggage behind. He went into the only chemists shop in the place, a real old-fashioned pharmacy, and rapped boldly on the counter. The chemist's wife, a right battleaxe, appeared from the back and said: "Yes?"

"Three french letters, Miss," said the young man in loud clear tones.

"Don't you dare 'Miss' me," said the old matron.

"Oh, sorry, four french letters, please."

YOU'RE ALL WRONG, JACK

Two broken-down unemployed actors thought they were certain of a job in the pantomime season, but all the Agent could offer was the cow, in Jack and the Beanstalk. They were hungry, so swore they'd done the part before. "You'd better be good" said the Agent as he threw the skin at them, "we open next week."

To get some practice they went into the country at dawn, and wore the cow's skin up and down in a field. Then the one at the front, who could see, said: "Jack can you run fast?"

"I'll be b*ggered if I can run at all!"

"You'll be b*ggered if you can't, there's a bull coming up behind us."

SHE HAD A CLUE!

A sweep's wife used to bath him every Saturday, but one time when he came in late she set about him with the bathbrush and half killed him.

"What's all this in aid of?" he groaned.

"Always before you've been home at 12 a hundred percent black, now you're home at two, one percent white."

UNREELED HIS HOSEPIPE

A ladder was placed against the bedroom window of a burning house, and a young fireman rushed up. Inside was a curvy brunette in a see-through nightie.

"Aha," said he, "you're the second pregnant girl I've rescued this year!"

"But I'm not pregnant."

"You're not rescued yet."

MANHOLE COVERS

An old railway driver went into a chemists shop and said he had some heavy parcels, would they give him a hand. The chemist went out, read the label, picked up the box, and said:

"I'm an old man, like you, but dammit I can carry a box of ST's without yelling for assistance."

"Blimey!" said the old van driver, "they said at the depot they was manhole covers."

". . . HOW MUCH IT IS"

Two Frenchmen landed in England on a pleasure trip, were told that English girls required a sheath to be used. Not knowing English, the first entered a chemists, put his member on the counter, and a shilling beside it. The other thought that was not enough, so he placed his member on the counter with a florin beside it.

The chemist came out, looked, placed his own member on the counter, picked up the money and walked away.

OF MICE AND MEN

A women entered the chemists and shyly asked for some condoms. The chemist showed her several sizes, but she said they were all too big. Finally he found some dwarf-sized – they were still too big.

"Pardon me Madam," he said, "but your husband seems to be rather, er, ill blessed."

"*My Husband!* Oh you insolent man, we're over-run with mice!"

GROUNDSHEETS, TROOPS, FOR THE USE OF

An ATS driver, after a long journey across Salisbury Plain, arrived at her destination, a remote camp, at midnight.

The Sergeant of the Guard showed her where to leave the lorry, and then said: "Where will you sleep tonight?"

The girl explained that the only thing she could do was to kip down in the cab. It was a cold night, and the Sergeant thought for a moment and said:

"If you like you can have my bunk, I'll sleep on the floor." The offer was accepted with thanks.

After the girl had turned in, she felt very sorry for the Sergeant lying down there on the hard cold floor, and, leaning out, said:

"This isn't right, why don't you get up here and squeeze in alongside of me?" This being done, the "sarge" said: "Well how's it to be? Do you want to sleep 'single' or 'married'?"

The girl giggled and said: "I think it would be nice if we slept 'married', don't you?"

"Right, I'm not fussy, we'll sleep 'married' then," he said, turning his back on her and going off to sleep.

MILITARY MANŒUVRES

There were three ATS girls . . .
The first gave her discharge to an Officer,
The second jumped over a campfire and got deferred,
The third (a driver) swerved to avoid a child,
(and fell out of bed!)

DAUGHTER OF THE REGIMENT

There was an old Colonel who in his middle age suddenly married a young and beautiful girl, in the hope, as he told people, of starting a family.

However, some time went by and nothing happened. Then one day he suddenly paraded the whole regiment:

"Officers, non-commissioned officers, and men of the Thirtyninth Royal Loamshires, I have called you together to make a special announcement: This morning my wife gave birth to a fine girl weighing eight pounds; Officers, non-commissioned officers, and men, of the Thirtyninth Royal Loamshire Regiment, I thank you, one and all."

YOU'LL CARRY THE BANNER

There was once a young woman joined the A.T.S. and went for her "medical". The doctor had her stripped off, and then called over his assistant. "Look at that, the biggest navel I've ever seen in all my career!"

The young doctor looked, and said: "By George girl, that's a huge navel, can I take a photograph of it for the medical press?"

The girl was fed up, and could not understand what all this was in aid of: "You'd have a big navel if you'd been in the Salvation Army for as many years as I have."

This only heightened the mystery: "The Salvation Army, what's that got to do with it?"

"I carried the banner for ten years."

WHORTICULTURE

A Parks Director from the West Country was up in London for a big conference. He went up town at night and picked up a girl. He told this girl that if she would look after him for a week, entertain him, and show him all the hot spots, she should be well rewarded.

At the end of the week this Parks Director told the girl that never in all his life has he had such a wonderful time. Her reward, he said, should be exceptional, for he had succeeded in growing a perfect black rose, which, as soon as he announced the news, would become an international sensation. He would name the rose after her.

She said she'd rather have fifty pounds in cash, thank you.

Which only goes to show, that you may take a horse to water but you can't take a horticulture.

SWEET VIOLETS

An old navvy went into a chemists shop and said: "I want some arse paper" to the sweet young woman behind the counter. The chemist was furious, and he followed the chap into the street: "Look here you!" he said, "we don't mind your custom, but we won't have that language to young lady shop assistants, see."

"I'm on'y an ignorant navvy, what should I a' said?"

"Why 'toilet paper' of course, and remember!"

A week later he came back and said: "I want some soap."

"Yes sir," said the girl with a sweet smile, "toilet soap?"

"Don't be daft miss, I on'y want to wash my hands and face."

LIMERICKS V

There was a young sailor named Guest
Who was struggling to get on the nest,
Said his young Chinese wanton
Don't forget you're in Canton
The tram lines all run East to West!

There was a young man of Devizes
Whose balls were of two different sizes,
One was so small
It was no use at all
While the other took several prizes!

There was an old farmer named Pitt
Whose cart a large boulder did hit
The load of manure
Was so insecure
He was up to his neck in the sh*t!

There was a gym mistress of Munich
Whose muscular action was unique
She wrestled with men
Again and again
And burst all the seams of her tunic!

There was a young lady named Gluck
Who suffered some terrible luck,
Stripping off in a punt
She fell off the front
And was pecked in the dunt by a cuck!

All trains to Aldershot

An old railway servant had spent his whole life at one station on the (former) Great Western line. One of his main jobs was to call out:

"Next train for Oxshott, Aldershot and Bagshot."

"Change for Uppingham, Woking, and Buckingham," not for Hants, Dorset and the West."

One day the District Manager came, and explained that under the Beeching reforms he would be replaced by a Tannoy system, and was now redundant.

On the old man's last day at work, startled commuters heard:

"Next train for Ox sh*t, pig sh*t and all the sh*t."

"Change for tupping'em, poking and *uckingham, not your pants, corsets and vest."

"Furthermore, rollocks, pollocks and asholes to the fornicating railway, I've had me cards!"

A SOFT ANSWER – ON TOILET PAPER

An old miner suddenly won £20,000 on the pools, and told his wife he would never again go down the pit. She insisted he ought to send in a proper letter of resignation, and after much argument he took pen and paper, and wrote:

"Dear Coal Board, – you can keep your lousy, poxy, clapped-up mucking job, and put it where the monkey put the nut. Tell the Overman to stuff my tools up his dirt-box while you're at it.

Yours Truly,

Wm. Bloggs."

"PS: Insulting letter to follow – W.B."

AFTER MANY EXERTIONS

There was a man rushed into a small-town newspaper office in a great state of excitement, and said to the counter clerk:

"Quick, I want to put something in the paper, marvellous! what d'you think, after ten years my wife's had a baby, a fine son, fabulous...."

"Yes, Sir," said the clerk, calmly, when the caller stopped for breath – "How many insertions?"

"Oh, we lost count – bloody hundreds!"

A SITTING TARGET

In the Black Country it is common for the cottage gardens to run down to the canal, with a privy sitting on the edge. Young Albert pushed the privy into the water one night, for devilment....

"Albert, did you push that closet in the cut last night?"

"No, Dad, I didn't do it."

Father tried the friendly approach, and told the boy about George Washington, who cut down the cherry tree, and then owned up, thus escaping dire punishment.

"Now you young beggar, own up, did you push that closet in the cut last night?"

"Father, I cannot tell a lie, I did it."

At which the old man gave his son the hiding of a lifetime.

"Here!" said the kid, sobbing, "you said as how when young George owned up, his dad let him off for telling the truth."

"Listen here you young beggar, when young Washington cut that tree down, his father wasn't sitting in the branches!"

COME TO THE FAIR

During the last war, a farmer was sent a young and pretty Land Girl. He lived with his two sons, his wife being dead, so he thought it wiser to fix the girl up in a small empty cottage on the other side of the farm.

After supper on the day she arrived, he told his younger son, who he thought he could trust, to take the girl home, and come straight back. But the boy returned after midnight, which upset the old man. Next time, he told the older son to see the girl home, and behave himself, but he came home at two a.m.

By now the farmer was worried, and feeling he owed a duty to the girl, although his legs were bad, he decided that he personally would take her home that night. He didn't get back until breakfast time!

The sons teased him unmercifully. . . .

"But father, you'll admit she's pretty?"

"Aye indeed."

"And father, isn't she passionate?"

"Aye, pretty she be, passionate she be, but above all, she's patient!"

PUBLIC RIGHT OF WAY?

There was a Squire's daughter who went to a country Solicitor and complained that a man had put his hand on her leg, and she wanted a prosecution.

This put the lawyer in a spot, because this girl was notorious for scandalous conduct at hunt balls and the like, and the local Bench would react accordingly. The old man stroked his beard, and said:

"Look here, are you sure it was his hand, and not his foot?"

"Hell no, don't be bloody stupid, of course it was his hand."

"What a pity, what a pity, if it had been his foot, we could have run him for trespass."

BLACK SHEEP IN THE FAMILY WAY

A farmer said to his man, "Hodge go down and plough up the old pasture behind the hill, and don't waste any time."

At the end of the day the farmer went to inspect progress, and was pleased to see the pasture all nicely ploughed save for one bit about six by three. . . .

"Hey Hodge, why've you missed this bit?"

"Sorry Master, I can't possibly plough yon, for sentimental reasons, never ask me gaffer, I can't do it."

"Sentimental reasons, what are you on about you girt lout?"

"Well Master, that bit o' grass there was where I had my first experience o' sex."

"Oh, I see Hodge, that's where you first had sex."

"Yes Gaffer, and her mother were looking at us, though that hole in the hedge there."

"Good Lord! Her mother saw you! What did she say?"

"Oh, nothing only just, baa baa ba-a-aa."

UP AND COMING

A farmer complained to the Vet that his stock were not breeding, so the Vet said: "Don't worry, I'll make up a sack of stuff that'll get them going, send your man for it." So the man was sent, but returning, he carelessly ripped the sack on some wire; the stuff was trailed across the fields, and a month's supply instantly consumed.

That evening, Hodge rushed in, shouting: "Master, Master, the goat's doing the sow, the cock's doing the ducks, the bull's doing the mare. . . ."

"Don't stand there like a fool – get out and throw some cold water over them!"

"I can't the donkey's doing the pump."

SUCK IT AND SEE

There was a farmer whose best sow was not at all well, so he consulted the Vet.

Said the Vet: "No real trouble, I'll give you a pessary to put up its backside, that'll put things right."

"And how the heck do I get it up its backside," said the farmer.

"Not to worry, there's a little plastic tube comes with the outfit, you simply insert and blow it up."

When the farmer got home he was late for dinner, so he said to his man: "Take this tube, and blow this pessary up Bluebell's backside."

Half an hour later Hodge was still puffing and blowing, but with no success. The farmer came out and said: "Here! give it to me" with which he reversed the tube, re-insterted it, and blew the pessary up first time.

"Master, master," said Hodge, "why did you turn the tube round?"

"Why did I turn the tube round? Well, I wasn't going to suck the end that had been in your dirty mouth!"

SHE LET THE BOROUGH SURVEY'ER?

A Deb who had a sudden yen to work with sweaty animals applied for a job on a farm, and got herself an interview.

The old farmer showed her the sheep and she said: "What nice pigs." He showed her the hens and she said: "What nice ducks," and this went on all over, so great was her ignorance.

Finally he showed her his prize bull, who was wonderfully equipped, and she said: "What a sweet mare."

"Gore dammee wench! When didst see a mare wi' a pair o' barls loike to yon? Ther never was such!"

"Oh yes indeed" said she, with a sweet smile: "The Mayor of Nuneaton."

GOING TO FOCUS

Two Black Country girls on holiday at Blackpool were walking along the front when one of these beach photographers stepped forward. . . .

"Stand still a minute, Mary, he's going to focus."

"What, both on we?"

NIGHT WORK IF YOU CAN GET IT

It was Friday afternoon, and the foreman told Enoch he'd have to work overtime, so Enoch asked his mate to call home and tell the missus.

Accordingly, Ziah called at the cottage and said:

"Your old man aint coming home until late, how about a bit o' love upstairs?"

The shocked young wife became less shocked when he offered her five pounds, but she still would not.

"Ten pounds then?"

"Er, no."

"Fifteen pounds then."

"Er, well no, it wouldn't hardly be right, would it."

"Come on my wench, fifteen pounds just for half an hour on the bed, and Enoch'll never find out!'

She needed no more persuading, but took him in the bedroom, giving due value for money.

When the husband came home late, he said:

"Did my mate tell you I'd be working over?"

"Yes, duck, he called in for a minute."

"Oh, and I suppose he handed you my wages like I asked him."

A SHAGGY DOG

A countryman went into a London pub with a dog. The man ordered a pint, the dog ordered a whisky.

"What the hell!" said the barman.

"Yes," said the owner, "he's the most intelligent dog in the West Country; I brought him to see the sights of town."

"If I give him fivepence, will he get me a paper?" said the barman, "because I forgot to get one."

"Of course I will," piped up the dog, then, receiving the money, "back soon, tat ta."

The dog did not return, so, after an hour, the worried owner went in search. He finally found his dog in a back alley, nicely on the job with a bitch.

"Well I'm damned!" said the owner, "you've never done that before."

"No," said the dog "I've never had the money before."

UP AND DOWN ALONG

A yokel married the curviest girl in the village, and she was also the dimmest.

He took her to a little cottage after the wedding, and soon after dusk he had her upstairs, in bed, and on the job.

After a repeat performance he excused himself, left the bedroom, but returned in five minutes to perform again.

This happened about six times more, after which the girl protested:

"George, you be going to the lavatory a terrible lot o' times tonight!"

To which she got the reply:

"I ain't George. George is downstairs taking the half-crowns."

THE SODS HAVE GONE

In a council house lived a man who went to much trouble growing a front lawn from seed. The day came when he had got a better job in another town, and in putting his notice in, he told the rent collector he was going to take the lawn with him.

When this was reported to the Council, they took a poor view of it, holding that as the soil in the garden was theirs, the lawn must be theirs. The row became public, and the Town Clerk told the rent collector to watch the position very closely.

One day the Clerk found a note on his desk which read:
"The sods have gone."
He sent one back:
"Yes, but what's become of the lawn?"

MUCKING ABOUT WITH LANGUAGE

A woman had a daughter who began to bring home a "superior" bank clerk. Father insisted on showing the superior young man his garden, which was a very fine one. . . .

"Sir, how d'you get such lovely roses?"
"Muck, young man, muck."
"And that superb rhubarb?"
"I does it wi' muck. Lots and lots on it. Muck on the taters, muck on the cabbages, muck on everything."

Afterwards the daughter took her mother on one side and said: "Can't you please get father to use a more respectable word than 'muck' when somebody decent comes to the house?"

"My dear girl! It's taken me 25 years to get him to say 'muck'."

A RATTLING GOOD STORY

Two Portsmouth prostitutes picked up two sailors, and each took one home for the night.

They met the next day and compared notes:

"How'd yer get on, Mabel?"

"Nicely thank you, Mary, he had it three times, gave me fifteen pounds, and helped wash up after breakfast. How about you?"

"Terrible, terrible! Never gave me a moment's rest all night, stuck an old-fashioned pop bottle up my fanny, and cleared off without paying!"

"You were a bit slow, why didn't you take out the pop bottle and hit him on the head with it?"

"I didn't know it was there until I heard the marble rattling as I was coming down the stairs this morning."

WORSE THAN DEATH?

There was a Irish village girl left home for the great lights, and returned home loaded with money and finery.

"Is it indade a great good job yez have in London thin?" enquired her mother. The girl wouldn't say what the job was, but after much badgering she whispered in her mother's ear. The old lady shrieked, groaned and fainted right off.

When they'd brought her round she asked: "Whit's that ye said ye wuz agin?"

The girl told her.

"Arrahh, praise be to arl the saints! Oi thought at first ye said ye'd become a *protestant*."

ONE OF OURS

The Irish navvies were digging the road outside a house full of made-up floozies. A parson came along, pulled down his hat and went in. Says Pat to Mike:

"Did you see that! Just what you'd expect with one of them parsons!" Soon after a rabbi arrived, turned up his collar, and in he went. Says Mike to Pat: "Is it not a terrible thing that the priest of God's Own People should go in there!"

Lastly a Catholic priest arrived, wrapped his cloak round his head, and dived quickly into the bawdy house.

"Pat, isn't that dreadful now, to think that one o' the girls must have been taken ill."

LITTLE BY LITTLE

A much married man who had been repressed, won a free holiday, a week in Paris. He asked the porter at the hotel how to get to a brothel. He was told not to worry, just go down Montmatre, and he would find English visitors catered for. Sure enough, he soon found a chap in uniform who said: "You want a sexy girl? Pay at the desk, and follow the signs."

He paid up, and followed an arrow "British this way" leading to doors: "Under ten stone" and "Over ten stone". Thus to: "Under 5 ft 6" and "Over 5 ft 6". Still following directions he came to "Under 50" and "Over 50", and finally: "Under four inches" and "Over four inches".

Opening the appropriate door, the would-be roué found himself back in the street!

THREE-DIMENTIONAL

A six foot, 16-stone, 25-year-old Australian came in from the outback when gold was discovered on his land, and took a plane to London, where he sought the pleasures of the West End, and its well known "ladies".

Unfortunately, although he got many girls as far as the bedroom, one sight of his monstrous member caused one and all to faint, or feign illness. Not even for a hundred pounds would any girl risk damaging her ration book. One night, disconsolate, he was stopped by a girl on the game, who said: "What about it? I've got the smallest, tightest. . . ."

"Listen Marm, that's what I'm *not* looking for," and he explained his difficulty. The little tart said she had many friends in the game, and among them one who could satisfy even this over-endowed cowboy.

The Aussie had his doubts, but the tart said her friend was trained by the USA Army from the age of 12, so off they went in a taxi to Big Fanny's. It was to be £100 for the fee, and £10 for the agent, and in went the agent to tell Big Fanny all about it. The latter came out, and said:

"I fear no man born, come on Aussie, tell me how big it is?"

The Colonial flustered, and finally said:

"Four inches!"

"Four inches! Cripes, you don't call that a man's size do you? Cor what a fuss over nothing!"

"Thick, Marm, thick."

THE LAST OF WAILS

A man who wished to walk in the Welsh mountains made his headquarters at a pub in a country town. He found his evenings dull, for nothing happened and pub conversation was mostly about sheep, mostly in Welsh. He asked the landlord how to set about finding the Ladies of the Town, and that worthy was shocked:

"Look man, this is Wales man, we couldn't have prostitutes, the Chapel would never allow it." The visitor looked sad, and the man continued: "Of course we have human nature the same as anywhere, but the thing you mention is kept out of sight."

He went on to explain that up the mountain at the back were caves, well furnished and with all mod con. What the stranger must do was go up the mountain at dusk and shout "Yoo-oo-hoo" and if the lady yoo-hoo'd back, terms could be negotiated. If she was already engaged, there would be no answer.

That evening the Englishman yoo-hoo'd his way from cave to cave, but with no luck at all. He finally decided to go back and get drunk, but at the foot of the mountain he found a fresh cave.

"Yoo-hoo, yoo-hoo," he shouted.

"Yoo-hoo yoo-hoo-oo-oo-oo," came back so clearly.

He rushed into the cave and was killed by a train.

BOTTOMS UP

This man married the curviest girl in the office, and all his mates envied him. In particular an unmarried young Scot, who said one day: "You ken, I'd give a hundred pounds to smack the pretty bottom of yon wee wife o' yours."

Smith was furious, and went home raging to his wife about it. But the wife had Scots blood too, and she said: "You know the furniture isn't paid for, and I could do with a fur coat, what's a few smacks on the bottom?"

Finally she wore her husband down, and he was forced to tell Jock that it was on for him to smack the wife's bare bottom for a hundred pounds, but only on terms. The husband was to be there, and no funny business.

So the three were in a suburban bedroom, the blushing wife removed her panties and bent over. . . . Jock threw her skirt up and gently stroked her, saying "What beautiful curves, what pinkness, what dimples, what firmness, . . ." and all the time rubbing and stroking, while the husband was nearly in hysterics. When Jock suddenly produced a flash camera and took a photo, the husband yelled, "Get on, get on and smack it, or else the deal's off."

"Och no!" said Jock, "I could not bring myself to smack such a beautiful bottom as this one, and besides, it would cost me a hundred pounds if I did!"

INTENT

Mac was courting a wee girl, and this wee girl had a wee flat, but Mac could never get further than the doorstep. Always he would take her home and say: "Can I come in for a whiles, Mary?"

And always she would reply:

"Nae, nae, Mac, I can see the glint in your eye!"

Mac saw that this glint-in-his-eye business was his undoing, so one night as he took the girl towards her flat, he craftily put on a pair of sun-glasses:

"Can I come in the flat a wee whiles, Mary?"

"Nae, nae, Mac."

"But Mary, you cannot see any glint in my eye!"

"Nae, nae, Mac, but I can see the tilt in your kilt!"

HIS YARDSTICK

Jock's young lady mentioned that her birthday was coming up, and Jock could not think of an inexpensive present. His mother had just finished making him a pair of breeks for wearing under his Sunday kilt, and she remarked that there was a yard of the material left, no-doubt clever Jeannie could make something of it.

Jock thought that was a splendid plan, and when he had taken the girl a walk on the heath, he stopped, spun round fast on his heels until his kilt flew up:

"Jean, did ye see anything?"

She blushed, and said that she had not, so Jock then spun round until his kilt was horizontal, blissfully unaware that he had in fact forgotten to put his breeks on. . . . "Surely Jeannie, ye saw it that time?"

"Aye Jock, I did."

"Well, you're having a yard of it for your birthday."

ODD STORY

An Insurance Agent went into a pub and remarked as he stood at the bar:

"I've just taken over London Road, and do you know, every housewife along there is an easy pushover!"

"Every one?" enquired a bystander who was listening.

"Well, to be exact, all but one."

Now, this bystander lived in London Road and he went home deep in thought, and repeated to his wife what he had just heard.

". . . all but one?" echoed his wife.

"All but one!"

"Dear me, I wonder who that can be."

A LONG RIDE

A chap in a sports car picked up a girl and drove into the country. The car began to cough and splutter, and they just managed to get into a lay-by before it conked out.

"Excuse me," said the driver, with which he got out and crawled underneath. He was there some time when the girl called out:

"Can I do anything for you?" to which he replied:

"Yes, come under here, and hold this."

An hour later a lorry driver tapped the young man on the shoulder, and said:

"Excuse me, but your car's been gone a long time."

LIMERICKS VI

There was a young lady named Dodd
Who thought that her child came from God
It was not the almighty
Who lifted her nightie
But Roger, the lodger, the sod!

There was a young lady named May
Who purchased a new whirling spray
She said: "Ah, that's better!"
As she washed out a letter,
"It's been there since Victory Day."

Said a young homo twin to his brother:
(When told of the death of their mother)
"Now don't look so sad
"For it isn't that bad –
"After all, we can still have each other."

There once was a Bey of Algiers
Who said to his harem: "My Dears,
"Though you may think it odd o' me,
"I've given up sodomy,
"Tonight we start breeding" – LOUD CHEERS!

There was a young lady named Wallace
Used monkeys and snakes for her solace,
The children had scales
And prehensile tales
And voted for Governor Wallace

Too late my love, Too late my love

A famous old violinist was proud of just two things, his Stradivarius and his virtuous young wife. They went on a long sea voyage on one of these cargo boats, and the captain with whom they dined daily, was much attracted to the wife. One day he said: "You know, I'd give a hundred pounds to have your wife in my cabin for an hour." The violinist replied:

"It wouldn't do you any good, her virtue is proof against all temptation."

The end of the argument was, that the captain bet his ship against the "Strad" that if he could have the young girl in his cabin for an hour, he would conquer. When everything was signed and sealed, the captain took the lady to his cabin and quickly pulled the curtains.

The fiddler, very confident up to now, began to panic, and after ten minutes, crept round and listened at the ventilator. What he heard alarmed him, and he shouted down:

Be true my love, be true my love,
Be true for one short hour
Just close your legs, your husband begs
And then this ship is ours!

*　　*　　*

Too late my love, too late my love,
He's got me round the middle,
He's locked the door, I'm on the floor . . . (Ooh–ow!)
You've lost your bleeding fiddle!

The Bishop was lacking in golf practice, and going out on a strange course he removed a fearful divot.

The Professional had warned the caddy, that, going out with a Bishop, he must mind his language most carefully, so when the latter said:

"Where did that little sod go to?" the boy said:

"Over the bleeding hedge, and don't forget, you started it."

NOT CAUGHT BY THE SHORTS

There was a man went to a new district, and being a keen golfer, joined the local club.

"Go in the Club House," said the Secretary, "and get yourself a drink, two if you like, we don't charge new members, first day."

The man had several drinks, and thought perhaps he'd take a lunch before playing. As he'd had the drinks for free, he ordered a blowout, but when he called for the bill, the waiter said: "That's all right, new member, first day."

Off went the man to play, but found he'd not brought any balls, so he went to see the Professional, who gave him six. "By the way," said the Professional, "those balls are £5 each cash down, if you don't mind, Sir."

The man said: "There's one thing about this Club, they don't catch you by the food and drink."

ALL FOR ONE, AND ONE FOR ALL

There was a young married man who was very keen on trade union work, so he was given the job of going to a country town to get a new branch going. About a dozen new members turned up, but, the business taking much longer than was expected, he missed the last train back.

"Never mind," said one chap who had taken him to the station, "come and kip at my place, we'll get you some early breakfast, you can whip off in the morning straight to your office, and no harm done."

All went as agreed, but when the chap got home at night, his wife, who was a jealous bitch, gave him a fearful doing. It was worse when she asked him who he'd stayed with, because he couldn't remember, as they were all equally strangers. She was convinced he'd been with a woman.

She would not rest, but at the first opportunity searched his drawers, and discovered the list of names and addresses of those who had attended the meeting. Then she wrote to each and every one, demanding: "Did my husband sleep at your house on the night of the 31st?"

All twelve wrote back and said: "Yes".

NOT STANDING?

There was a man who was a keen political worker, and when the General Election came along, they asked him to be the Party Agent.

The Vicar met him one day and said: "Moggs, you look terribly depressed, is anything the matter?"

"Yes, indeed, Vicar, I'm having great difficulty in getting my member in."

"Dear me, dear me, have you tried vaseline?"

SWEET VIOLETS

There was a fellow went to a dance, and he was going round the floor with a pretty girl, to whom he said:

"Your name's Rose, isn't it?"

"How did you know?"

"I could tell by the scent you are wearing."

The same thing happened later on with a girl named Violet, again he could tell by the scent she was wearing.

The bystanders however were somewhat startled towards the end of the evening to hear a girl saying to him sharply:

"But how did you know my name was Fanny?"

HIS OLD CHINA

A young chap had to go to London on his firm's business, and he said to his older and more experienced colleague:

"What's the best chance for a bit of fun?"

His mate told him of a private hotel where the special feature was early morning tea brought up by a very voluptuous chambermaid, who could be made agreeable at a reasonable price.

"The hotel's a bit dear, but it's good value, if you see what I mean."

The man made a special point of staying at this place and ordered early morning tea very firmly.

The early morning tea was brought up by an old, scruffy, and unfriendly porter. . . .

"Hey," said the guest, "where's the chambermaid?"

"I've no idea, but the teapot's made in Stoke-on-Trent."

FUNNY BONE

A stranger got into a suburban railway carriage in which two men were already sitting. One of them had a peculiar mannerism, he scratched his elbow again and again.

This elbow-scratching was nearly driving the stranger mad, by the time the victim got out at his station.

"Gravely afflicted, your friend," he said to the other man.

"Yes, indeed, he's got a terrible dose of piles."

"I'm not talking about piles, I'm talking about all that scratching just now."

"Yes, that's right, piles, you see, he's a civil servant, can't tell his arse from his elbow."

SHE'D HAD HER CHIPS

There was a woman went to go on a coach trip, and she had a baby in her arms. The driver said:

"Hey there, missus, no babies allowed on long-distance coaches."

The woman went away, but she was determined to travel, so she wrapped the baby up in a bundle and boarded the next coach.

The driver enquired: "What've you got in that bundle, missus?"

"Just fish and chips," she said.

"Well, you'd better hurry up and eat them, the vinegar's running out."

NINETY-NINE, BONK!

Two gentlemen centipedes were in the King's Road, Chelsea, when they spied a lady centipede.

Says one to the other: "Look, George, there's a nice pair o' legs, pair o' legs, pair o' legs. . . ."

BALLADS TO YOU, TOO!

A man who worked as a humble clerk went along to a Hilton Hotel, and asked if they could use an evening pianist.

"As a matter of fact," said the manager, "I've just heard my regular pianist is ill this week, I can find you a job provided you are a good pianist."

"Anything you can hum, I can play," said the applicant.

"O.K.," said the manager, "there's one other thing, you must wear a dinner suit."

The man explained that his dinner suit was very tatty, owing to lack of engagements lately, but it would be all right if the manager agreed to lower the lights on the stage.

All went according to plan, in fact the pianist played brilliantly, but when the man stood up to receive the applause, the manager was horrified. He dashed on the stage and hissed:

"For cripes sake! Do you know your balls are hanging out?"

"You hum it, I'll play it," was the reply.

OUT IF IN, IN IF OUT

The rent collector told the woman she'd be thrown out if she didn't pay the rent. She explained that she was always in debt through having so many children. . . .

"Whose fault's that?" snapped he, "it must be either you or your husband to blame!"

"Well, I suppose you could say it's 'Sex of one and half a dozen of the other'."

WHAT BRASS!

A dashing man went to a dance where he was unknown, and looked around for a prospect. Across the room he saw what he thought was a very curvaceous piece, so he waved and began to walk over.

As he approached he could see she was by no means pretty, and as he got near he could see she was an elderly gargoyle.

It was too late, she had risen to accept his offer. . . .

Suddenly he saw his escape route: "Pardon me," he said, "but I mistook you for my mother."

"But," she said, "you couldn't possibly have mistaken me for your mother: don't you see, I'm wearing a wedding ring."

ALL FOR THE UNION

The Director of a large motor manufacturing company was walking through his factory when he saw a man and a woman having intercourse on a bench during working hours.

He turned to the manager at his side and said:

"Sack that man at once!"

"We can't do that," said the manager, "he's the shop steward for this section."

"Then sack the woman!"

"You can't do that either, Sir, she's the Convenor's secretary."

"Damn and blast it! I'll show you who gives the orders in this place, take that bench outside!"

THE KEYHOLE IN THE DOOR

A certain mayor and some councillors were leaving the town hall late one night after a function. Somebody noticed a light on in the Medical Officer's room, and they all went over to have a peep.

The mayor's pretty secretary was naked on the floor, and the MoH was on top of her, indulging in social intercourse.

They looked at each other aghast, and one councillor said:

"We must sack the mayor's secretary at once!"

"Certainly not!" said the mayor, "we must sack the doctor."

Somebody protested that the secretary would be a loss, the Medical Officer of Health would be a greater loss ... and was interrupted by a Scots councillor:

"Could we not," he said, "could we not just buy a wee curtain?"

HOW UNFEELING

There was a medical student went on honeymoon, and a telegram was received and opened by the manager: COME HOME AND GET MARRIED ALL IS FORGIVEN. He made up his mind to have revenge on the man he thought had played this trick, a man by the name of Smith.

Smith was too clever, when he got married he gave a false address, and even hid his car so that it could not be interfered with.

On returning from his honeymoon he met his old tutor, who said: "Smith, you are walking round in a thoughtful and rather grim manner, are you looking for something?"

"Yes, Sir, I'm looking for the gentleman who put local anaesthetic in the vaseline."

THE NAKED TRUTH

A New Zealand city, founded in 1868, was presented by the founder with a pair of statues to stand in the Market square. They were life size, naked, very obviously male and female, and they faced each other a few feet apart for a hundred years.

One night Venus, Goddess of Love, appeared to them and said: "For a hundred years you have faced each other with arms outstretched, I will reward your patience with any one wish, if you ask."

The man replied: "We have only ever had one thought, will you make us human for just 24 hours, so that we may do what we have in mind?"

"At dawn you shall come alive," said Venus.

Accordingly they came alive and rushed into each others arms. . . . "How shall we begin?" said the woman.

"I know!" said the man, "I'll catch the beggars in those cabbage nets, and you pull their necks."

OUTSTANDING DIFFICULTY

A young typist complained that her machine was faulty; it was always making extra spaces in her typing copy. The makers sent mechanic after mechanic, but the defect remained. Finally the boss said: "This is our best customer," and sent the Sales Manager in person.

The Sales Manager sent a wire almost at once: "Solved it" and was back the same day. A delighted Director asked him, how?

"Easy, I simply raised her seat three inches."

BEGGAR YOU JACK

A certain civil servant had a cold wife, three howling kids, and when his mother-in-law came to live with them it was the last straw.

The man fled to Tibet and took refuge in a monastery.

The Head Llama said: "You cannot stay unless you work hard, speak little, and eat less."

The man looked downcast, but he said he would try it.

"Mind you," went on the Llama, "we understand the weakness of men, and when you feel that you can remain celibate no longer, you can have a one-night pass to go up the mountain at the back."

"And what good will that do me, O Blessed Llama?"

"You see my son, on top of the mountain is a yak, and you can spend the night with it. It isn't much, but it makes a break in the long round."

When it was the civil servant's turn, he went up the mountain and had his session with the yak. On returning the Llama said:

"Did you enjoy yourself?"

"Yes, O Blessed One, I took full advantage of the opportunity."

"Good! and of course, you fed and watered the yak, and cleaned out the hut afterwards?"

"No, I certainly did not!"

"Ah just as I thought – the English civil servant – 'b*gger you yak, I'm alright!' "

A LITTLE OF WHAT YOU FANCY

A man who had felt unwell for some time went to his doctor and asked for a check-up. The doctor gave him a going over and said:

"Either you pack up smoking, drinking and sex, or you'll be dead in twelve months."

After a while the man went back and said "Look, I'm so bloody miserable I might just as well be dead, *please* can I smoke just a little."

"Very well, just five filter-tips a day," said the medico, who was a very abrupt man.

Some weeks later the man was back again: "Look here, I do miss my pint, please . . . ?"

"All right, two halves a day then, and no spirits."

Time went by, and the patient approached the doctor for the third time –

"Yes, yes, but only with your wife – no excitement!"

SHE THOUGHT HE WAS A CLOSET

A newly-made Lord Mayor found himself at a big dinner, seated opposite a very well-upholstered dowager; her generous charms were generously exposed, and stuck in the vee-line of her more-than-ample was a rose.

The Lord Mayor found the scenery most distracting, he could not take his eyes off it, and finally, catching the lady's questioning glare, blurted out:

"Madam, I was wondering if you would blush if I plucked your rose?"

In clear ringing tones she replied: "Sir, would you flush if I pulled your chain?"

"A HAND IN THE BIRD'S WORTH . . ."

There was a young chap taking a girl out, and doing pretty well. The girl thought an engagement ring was on the way, but the man left London for a better job in Newcastle. He wrote regularly at first, but then tailed off, and his girl wrote and demanded to know the reason. The reply was:

"Sorry, but I've found a regular girl up here."

To the further question: "What has she got that I haven't got?" came a final note:

"Nothing, but she's got it here."

CORNY JOKE

A young lady mouse lived in a cornfield. One day, just as she was all dressed up to go out and meet her boyfriend, a gigantic machine came along, and mouse nest and all were swept up, bashed, and thrown out again, inside a tight bale.

The mouse, much damaged, managed at last to nibble her way out, and fell at the feet of her boyfriend. She was scratched all over, an ear and part of her tail were missing. . . .

"What on earth's happened to you,?' he asked.

"I've been reaped!"

LOVING CUPS

Two fleas got locked up in a ladies dress shop, and went to sleep in a brassiere.

That's how they became bosom friends.

FED UP, FOULED UP, AND FAR FROM HOME

There was a man in a railway carriage who was joined by another man who had with him a crowd of dirty and ill-behaved kids: before they had gone very far he gave one of his kids a fearful belting.

"Look here," said the other man, "you stop beating that child, or I'll get you into trouble."

"You'll do what?"

"I said: 'I'll get you into trouble.'"

"Listen, my friend . . . my wife has run off with a black man taking every penny I've got; I am on my way to leave these kids with a relative who drinks; the girl in the corner is fifteen, and eight months pregnant, that kid over there has messed his pants, the baby has thrown the flask out of the window, and the one I've just beaten has swallowed our tickets. For being off my work I've had the sack, did you say you were going to get me into trouble?"

BLESS YOU!

A young lady suffering from a cold went to a dance with two handkerchiefs, one in her evening bag and a reserve tucked down the front of her dress. During the course of the evening she finished using the one in her bag and tried to retrieve the second, but she couldn't find it. A gentleman at a nearby table who had been watching with interest was amazed to hear her remark.

"I could have sworn I had two when I came!"

ROCK BOTTOM

A certain man was head of a firm of Industrial Consultants. One night at his Club a member came up whom he knew slightly and said:

"Look here old man, you're an efficiency expert, I wonder if you could help me."

"What's the problem?"

The man explained that he owned a factory making seaside lettered rock, and it was losing money.

The expert went round to the rock factory, cut out overtime, tightened up the piecework system, and installed new time clocks. "In a few months time you'll be rolling in the money," he told the owner.

Not many weeks later the owner was back, looking depressed . . . he was still losing money. So the expert went along, cut out the tea breaks, speeded up the conveyor belts, and again departed.

Two weeks later the owner told him he was calling a meeting of his creditors. . . .

"What's gone wrong old boy?"

"Well, you tell me how I can sell ten thousand sticks of rock with ROTTEN BLEEDER lettered in them."

THE ELASTIC LIMIT

A girl from the factory floor was giving evidence against a youth who had stolen her purse. The Beak listened and said: "But my dear girl, if it was in the top of your stocking, how is it you didn't realise?"

"Oh, Sir, I didn't think it was that he was after."

There was a young lady of Wantage
Of whom the Town Clerk took advantage
Said the Borough Surveyor:
"You'll now have to pay 'er
"You've altered the line of her frontage!"
It was really a female of Thame
Who fled there to cover her shame,
She was heavy with child
And it makes them so wild
That their shortsighted Clerk took the blame

A policeman of Paddington Junction
Whose organ had long ceased to function
All the days of her life
Deceived his poor wife
By the dexterous use of his truncheon

There was a young girl of Malay
Who got put in the family way
By the mate of a lugger,
An ignorant b*gger
Who even spelled quim with a K!

A young man of Aberdeen
Invented a screwing machine
Concave or convex
To suit either sex
And a bucket below for the cream

I am the Vicar

You'll carry the banner tonight!
I don't wanna carry the banner tonight
You'll carry the beggar tonight, TONIGHT!
I'll not carry the banner any night
Then you'll come away to the woods, TO THE WOODS!
I don't wanna go to the woods
You're going to come away to the woods!
But I'm in the family way
You're in every beggar's way!
But I'm only thirteen
I'm not superstitious!
I'll tell the Vicar
I AM the Vicar!

AND THE LITTLE PIECES OVER THERE

It was in the days of unemployment that the little labourer walked into the yard and asked for a job. "You're in luck," said the ganger, "see that great big pile of scrap timber, well, the gaffer wants the little pieces over there and the big pieces over there." For two hours he toiled, and had just finished when the ganger said: "He made a mistake, he wants the little pieces over *there*, and the big pieces over *there*." The little man had just finished, and was going for his dinner when a further message came, to move them all back again. Said the man to the ganger:

"I'll tell you what he wants, he wants them up . . .' (The foreman, a huge hairy fellow, had just walked up behind, and said:) "Yes, go on, what do I want then?"

"Why, Sir, you want the little pieces over *there* and the big pieces over *there*."

HIS PENCIL

A girl married a chap, a quiet unpushing sort, a humble clerk. When they had been married a week the man came home rather out of temper and said:

"When I got to work this morning, I found a pencil tied on John Thomas!"

"Yes," she said, "I thought if you couldn't come you could write."

SPREAD THE BLESSINGS

A man took his little lad to the pantomime. They secured seats in the front row of the gods, and as they entered, father said: "Do you want a wee-wee before we settle down?"

The kid swore he did not.

No sooner were they well hemmed in than the lad started off that he must have a wee-wee. Father was furious, and told the boy to shut up until the lights went out. The kid fidgeted no end, but at last the lights went out, and father said: "Go quietly over the front edge."

Quite soon an extremely toffee-nosed voice from the stalls shouted up: "I say you cads, play the White Man, wave it about a bit."

A SHOT IN THE DARK

In the old days of the silent film, every decent cinema had its own orchestra. Then, as now, they were the haunt of courting couples, and this pair were sitting in the dark near the front, having a right good maul.

"Mary," whispered the man, "keep on playing with it and making it bigger."

"All right," said the girl, "if you promise to control yourself, and not make a mess."

The man solemnly promised, but what with the heat, and the X-certificate picture, and one thing and another, he broke his word.

"There!" hissed the girl, "now you've done it, you've come in my hand, whatever shall I do with it?"

"Raise your hand and flip it away."

The girl did as she was bid, and flipped it away.

Down at the front there was another whispered argument, between the conductor and the first fiddle:

"Hey, for cripes sake, you're about three bars late!"

"Well, somebody's come in my eye!"

"I'm not surprised, you've been playing like a twat all night."

NELL'S DILEMMA

Nellie Wallace would rush breathless on to an empty stage and say: "Sorry I'm late folks, but the manager blocked my passage."

A variant was: "I got to the theatre late, I was on one of those cliff walks when I met a man, and I didn't know whether to toss him off or let him block my passage."

A TICKLISH JOB!

An army unit crossing the Western Desert, complete with camel transport. Bombardier Smith had a particularly difficult stubborn camel, which finally stopped altogether. The others pressed on regardless.

Smith was stuck there for hours, trying every trick in the book to make the camel go, but in vain.

An ATS driver came along, and asked what the trouble was, so he told her. "That's easy, leave it to me," she said, and proceeded to put her hands beneath the camel's belly. The camel jumped up, and disappeared at the rate of knots after its long-departed companions.

"What on earth did you do Miss, what's the trick?"

"Quite simple, Bombardier, I simply tickled its balls!"

"By cripes then, you'd better tickle mine quick, I've got to catch the b*gger!"

AND KISS HER BETWEEN THE DRAWS?

There was a clippie on a bus late in the evening, who noticed a boy sitting downstairs and calmly smoking. She thought he was out late anyway, and she said to him: "How old are you?"

"Twelve."

"Twelve, and smoking!"

"Yes."

"What if the Inspector gets on?"

"Well, what if he does?"

"Do you want to get me into trouble?"

"Yes thanks, what time do you finish work?"

SHACKED OUT

A sultan had thirty wives, and they made so much racket he built a special suite for them half a mile from his palace. He kept a strong youth, and whenever he felt like it he would press a bell, and when the youth appeared would say: "Fetch me number 15" or "Fetch me number 37" or whatever the case might be.

The youth would have to run all the way with the message, and such was the sultan's nature that he was kept pretty busy. One day he trotted off with the usual message, but he didn't come back.

The sultan sent out servants to search, and they found the young man dead, from heart failure.

The moral of this story is: It isn't sex that kills a man, but the running about after it.

NOT UP AND COMING

There was a gormless young man going out with a well shaped and sexy girl, but she could make no progress with him. She got him alone in the woods and put his hand in her blouse. He took it out again. She lifted up her skirts to show her knickers, and he talked about the weather.

Finally she stepped out of her pants, thrust her thighs towards him, and said:

"Don't you know what this is?"

"No, I don't, what is it?"

"Why you fool, it's a twat!"

"Oh, how interesting, that's what they call me at work."

CROSS EYED

A man went to his local Health Executive, and asked for a new pair of glasses. The man looked up the record and said: "You only had the last pair a month ago."

"I know," said the man, "but I got them broken in an accident."

The clerk looked up the Book of Words—"Domestic Accident, Road Accident, Accident at Work, . . ." no, it wasn't any of those.

"What was it then?" said the clerk.

"I – I don't like to tell you," stammered the applicant.

"No satisfactory explanation, no new glasses," snapped the clerk, getting fed up.

"Very well then," said the man, "I was kissing my girl."

"How the hell could you break your glasses kissing a girl?"

"You see, she crossed her legs."

WASHED HIS HANDS OF IT

A Frenchman was staying in England, and a friend asked him how he was getting on. He said he was doing very well, except for one thing: "When I go to a party, the hostess, she does not tell me where is the *pissoir*. . . ."

"Ah, Georges, you mean she does not tell you where the toilet is? That's just our English prudery; actually, she will say, 'Do you want to wash your hands?' and that means the same thing."

The Frenchman made a mental note of this, and the next time he went to a party, with the hostess waiting for him, the guests standing around heard: "Good evening Mr Du Pont, do you want to wash your hands?"

"No tank you Madame, I have just washed them up against de tree in de front garden."

IN GLAMORGAN

"Dai, did you hear the news? Megan Evans is getting married."

"Indeed now, I did not even know she was pregnant!"

"Steady there Dai, Megan Evans is not pregnant."

"What! Getting married and not even pregnant, bloody middle-class snobbery, that's what that is!"

UP AND DOWN

A courting couple were out walking and could not find a privy place to start petting in. At last they came to a gentleman's park with a high wall all round it; just the job, only the girl couldn't climb the wall.

"Here, stand on this," said the man, producing from his trousers a splendid specimen of manhood.

"No fear! How will I be able to get back?"

V.G. OR V.D.?

There was a courting couple out in the country and they entered a wood and lay down under some bushes. Very shortly afterwards they heard the tramp tramp of marching feet; a squad of troops just back from the Near East was coming along the nearby road: "Company, halt! Fall out for five minutes," at which dozens of soldiers entered the woods and began to relieve themselves all over the place.

The girl watched fascinated through the leaves, and after the soldiers had fallen into their ranks again, and departed, she said:

"George, I suppose those were the officers, those who had theirs wrapped in cotton wool?"

An Arabian Oil Magnate sent for a famous dance band from England, to go and play before his courtiers, harem, etc, and this was arranged.

The band played their best, the Magnate was delighted. He clapped his hands and said:

"Let their instruments be stuffed with gold pieces."

All were delighted except the poor old flautist, whose instrument was too small in diameter to take even one gold piece.

Next night they played again, but the Magnate had got indigestion, and he shouted: "Seize them, and let their instruments be stuffed up their. . . ."

Again the flautist was the unlucky one.

CURTAINS!

Says Mum to Dad: "Those two are very quiet in the front room, go and see what's going on." Dad went through, came back, said nothing, and resumed his paper.

Next night, Mum left it rather longer before she made Dad visit the parlour, and again he made no comment. The third night he went unprompted after waiting two hours, and then there was a commotion, the sound of a youth being thrown out, and a girl crying. Mum wanted an explanation. . . .

"Well," said Dad, "I said nothing about him stripping our Mary, I said nothing when I found him doing our Mary, that's what they call 'progress' I thought, but I do draw the line when I find him wiping his filthy wick on our best curtains."

ALL BALLS

An old couple had promised themselves a seaside holiday when the husband retired. Foolishly, they did not book, and every hotel in Seaville was full. Worn out, they went to the Police Station, where a kind Inspector took pity. "There's just one manager who'll fix you up as a favour to me," he said, "take this note to the Majestic."

The manager said that as a favour he would open up the bridal suite, but the old man was not grateful:

"Her and me's 65, what would we want with a bridal suite!" The annoyed manager said: "Look you old sod, I've slept people in the billiard room before now, but they didn't have to play billiards all night!"

CLOSED SHOP

One day old Maggie asked her husband, as they were going to bed, what would become of them when he could no longer work. Old Jack said: "Look out of the window, I own those two cottages, and the shop on the corner."

The wife wanted to know how he had done this on a modest wage. . . .

"From the day we were wed, I put a half-crown under the mattress every time you let me."

"Well I never!"

"Yes, and if you hadn't been such a cold mean frigid old sod we'd have had two hotels and a pub!"

IN AND OUT THE WINDOW'S

Two men were on a walking tour of the New Forest when they got caught in a black storm and lost their way. After wandering around until dark they became very tired, but happened to see a light in the distance. Struggling across, they found it was the abode of a presentable widow, who made them welcome with supper and wine.

As the evening drew to a close she said: "You are both decent respectable looking men, so I suggest that you toss up; the loser sleeps in the spare room, the winner sleeps with me."

Jack won the toss, and had a marvellous night of it.

Next morning, well fortified with breakfast, they set off in bright sunshine to resume their travels. There was a long pregnant silence before Bill said:

"How d'yer get on?"

"Marvellous! but in the morning she began to get worried, and pressed for my name and address, so I gave her yours."

This led to a bitter quarrel, and the break-up of the friendship, until some nine months later Bill called on Jack:

"Hey," he said, "you remember that widow? Well, I've had a solicitor's letter and . . ."

"Look," said Jack, "I'm very sorry, old pal, I know I let you down, but what could I do, you know what my wife is, she'd have . . ."

"I was saying," said Bill icily, "before you interrupted me, I was saying, she's died and left me five thousand pounds."

THE ELASTIC LIMIT

A boy of twelve was sent to the psychologist because he was such a complete pest. He made catapults all the time, and broke everything in sight.

The Head Shrinker was convinced that "sex" lay behind everything, and he asked the kid what he would do if he found himself alone for the afternoon in the house with a girl his own age.

"I'd kiss and fondle her to get her in a nice mood."

(Here we go, thought the psychologist).

"What next?"

"I'd get her in the mood and take her knickers off."

"What would you do after that?"

"Next," said the kid "I'd get out my pocket knife and threaten her with it to make her give way to my wishes."

"Which would be what . . . ?"

"Why mister, I'd want to cut her knickers up to get the elastic out and make some more catapults."

THEN THE BALLOON WENT UP

A small boy wandered into his mother's bathroom when she forgot to lock the door, and said:

"Mother, what nice balloons you've got!"

"Balloons, Jimmy, why do you call them balloons?"

"Well, I saw father blowing the maid's up when you were out yesterday."

There was a man who lived a righteous and upright life, while his neighbour loved drinking and fornicating, which were his two main hobbies.

In course of time the wicked man died as the result of his excesses, whilst still a young man, and the good respectable neighbour continued to flourish, and be a pillar of the church.

At last, however, the second man died, and, naturally, went straight to Heaven. Imagine his surprise however, when he got inside, to see his old neighbour apparently doing more than well. The wicked man was sitting at the side of a large barrel of beer, and in his arms was a naked lady angel with obvious and luscious attractions.

The pillar of the church hastened off to Saint Peter and complained bitterly:

"Look," he said, "I denied myself all the good things of life, on earth, so that I could come to Heaven, and have the consolation of knowing that Smith was in hell; now look at him . . . . unlimited beer and a naked girl to. . . ."

"Stop!" said Saint Peter, "the man is in hell, as he deserves to be."

"In hell?" said the other, "in hell? I can't say that's my idea of hell!"

"Ah," said Peter, "that's because you don't know the facts."

"What facts?"

"Well, you see, the barrel's got a hole in it, but the woman hasn't."

FEATHERBEDDED

A man was crossing a wild heath late on a filthy night, when his car broke down. He staggered on for some miles, and at last came to a lonely cottage, where an old couple were just going to bed. The old man looked at the wet and shivering stranger and said:

"We've only got two bedrooms and our spinster daughter sleeps in the other one, but you can lie downstairs on the sofa.

The chap was well pleased, but such a bitter wind got up in the night that Mother woke Father and said:

"Go down and see how he is."

So Father went down to the unhappy stranger and said:

"We're poor folk, but seeing it's so cold, would you like our eiderdown?"

"Good lord no! She's been down twice already."

STORY WITH WHISKERS ON

It was a family re-union, and everybody had to double up. Young Willy, who was 13, and of an enquiring turn of mind, was put to sleep with a young and attractive "Auntie".

No sooner was the light out, than Willy's hands began to wander. Auntie wriggled about to avoid his clutch, and bade him behave himself.

Finally his hand went under her armpit, and he said:

"Oh, you crafty madam, you've shifted it."

THE BLIND

There was a couple went on honeymoon and retired to bed early, in their hired bungalow.

It was late when they finally got up, the sun shining outside.

"Charles, get out of bed please, and let the blind up, I haven't got the strength," said the bride.

Charles got out of bed to do as he was asked, but when the blind went up, he went up with it!

When he had somewhat recovered, the man opened the window, and said to a passing policeman: "Excuse me officer, what time do the Sunday papers arrive around here?"

"Sunday papers!" said the policeman, "today's Wednesday."

NO FLIES ON HIM

There was a spinster sitting knitting in the corner of a railway carriage on a long journey. The only other person in the carriage was a student type who lolled back in the opposite corner.

The old maid observed that the young man's flies were undone. He didn't seem to know or care, and began to doze off. The rolling of the train was producing an effect which made bad worse, and the spinster was getting very concerned. Finally she reached over, nudged him, and said:

"Excuse me young man, excuse me."

"Yes, what is it, Miss?"

"Well, er, well, it really is very wicked of you, but you've got your thing sticking out."

"Miss, you flatter yourself, it's hanging out."

PUTTING ONE AND ONE TOGETHER

There was a couple got married, and the reception was at her home. Half way through the reception, Father called for order, and said: "The bride will now cut the cake."

At this there was confusion, the bride and groom had disappeared!

"Hey mother, where's John and Mary?" roared father.

"Don't panic and take on so, Father," said mother, "they've only gone upstairs a minute, to put their things together."

FROLICS

There was a couple on honeymoon who went to bed in an expensive hotel. Having had a very tiring day, and then having exhausted themselves in the jousts of Venus, the couple tried to go to sleep. However, there was a great deal of noise coming from downstairs, and the longer they lay there trying to doze off, the more the noise increased. Finally the groom rang the bell for the night porter. . . .

"What the hell's going on in this place?" he roared.

"Sorry, Sir, but they're holding the Oddfellow's Ball."

"Oh, are they, well for cripes sake tell them to let go of it."

COCKSURE

A mother was dressing her daughter for the wedding. "Darling, aren't you the weeniest bit nervous?" enquired Momma.

"Certainly not mother! I was never so cocksure in my life."

Titian was mixing rose madder
To paint a lewd nude on a ladder
The condition of Titian,
Indicated coition
So he rushed up the ladder and 'ad 'er!

There was a young lady of Hitchin
Who was scratching her quim in the kitchen
Her mother said: "Rose
"It's the pox I suppose?"
She snapped: "Rollocks get on with your stitchin'."

There once was a spinster named Perkins
Whose gardener gave her some gherkins,
And times out of number
She tried his cucumber
Which swelled up her internal workings.

There was a young Scottie named Coates
Who wearied of living on groats,
For a change, in the end
He married a Friend
And nightly enjoys Quaker oats!

There was a young lady named Hyde
Who tried a banana and cried
And stormed, and lamented
That the fruit had fermented
Inside her, inside her inside

You have to stand on a chair

A very wealthy spinster rang the Grande Hotel to book a suite. The Manager laid on everything of the best, but no sooner were her trunks carried up than she sent for him, and said:

"This is a *dreadful* room! I look out of the window across the courtyard, and what do I see but men undressing, and running about naked."

The Manager leapt to the window, and he looked right and he looked left, but no naked men could he see. . . .

"What men do you refer to, Madam? I can't see any."

"Oh, well of course, you have to stand on a chair."

DEAD EASY

A certain prominent business man lost his wife, and the funeral became a public occasion. All the dignitaries of the town attended, and almost all were known to the bereaved. There was however a stranger, and he seemed more upset than anyone, and before the funeral was over he broke down completely.

The widower-husband asked who was this weeping stranger. . . .

"Ooh!" whispered someone, "didn't you know? He was your late wife's lover!"

The bereaved moved across to the sobbing man, patted him on the back, and said:

"Cheer up old boy, cheer up, I shall probably marry again."

GETTING THE MESSAGE THROUGH

A man went up to the West End looking for tarts. To each girl in turn he said: "Have you got the pox?" and when each indignantly said "No" he turned and walked away.

Finally one girl said: "In all London I only know one girl on the game who's got a dose. . . ."

"Take me to her," said the man, "and I'll pay her double, and give you a present as well."

"Listen, chap, are you barmy, or what?"

"I'll explain: If I can catch the pox I can go home and give it the maid, who'll give it my father, who'll give it my mother, who'll give it the vicar, who'll give it his daughter; she'll give it to her headmaster, and that's the old devil I'm after."

CHIPS OFF THE OLD JOCK?

There was a mean old Scot who suddenly surprised his three sons by saying he would buy them each a present, provided it was something tartan.

"I want a tartan bonnet," cried the first, quickly.

"I want a tartan kilt," cried the second, more bold.

"I want fifty pounds," said the youngest.

"Fifty pounds!! what are you thinking o' getting?"

"I'm not, father, I've got it already!"

"Got what?"

"I've got a tart 'n trouble!"

ALL FOR LOVE

Three sisters fell on hard times when their factory closed down. When they were very hungry and behind with the rent, they held a council, and decided that one of them would have to go on the streets. The first said she was too old, the second said she was too plain, and it came down to the youngest to go out and find a customer. For all she protested her virtue they removed her knickers and left her standing outside a pub. She was instructed to ask for at least £3.

It was very late when she got in. "Hurry up!" they said, "before the fish and chip shop shuts."

"I haven't got any money!"

"Why, what happened?"

The young sister explained that a man had picked her up, taken her to a room, stripped her bare, had his will twice, and given her three pounds. . . .

"Come on then, what did you do with it?"

"Well, you see, I liked it so much, I gave it him back to do it again."

BUS OR PRAM?

Two women, strangers had been waiting at the bus stop for ages. Finally one spoke:

"When's it due?"

"March!"

"Cripes, the ruddy service gets worse don't it."

CHEAP AT HALF THE PRICE

An Alderman had to go to London, and his wife tagged along. While he was at the Ministry she went shopping, and they arranged to meet for tea. The Alderman's business being soon finished, he went looking for a tart. In the West End he met a Real High Class, and it was all arranged when the girl mentioned that it would be ten pounds.

"Struth! I've only got thirty shillings."

So she left him flat, and the man collected his wife and took her to a restaurant. At the next table sat the "model" he had picked up an hour before. She leaned over and said very loudly:

"Serves you right, that's what you get for thirty shillings."

LOVE FROM A STRANGER

A man swore that if his Premium Bond came up, he'd do a good deed. He won a good prize, so he told the Warden of an Old Peoples Home to choose a deserving couple and he would send them to Blackpool for a weekend.

"No, you go in and pick your own."

The man picked his couple, gave them money, vouchers and everything needed for a luxury hotel visit. After they were back the donor met the woman one day in the street. She thanked him very much, and went on. . . .

"By the way, who was that gay old kipper you sent with me?"

A BLOCK OFF THE OLD CHIPPY

A frustrated spinster was a pest to the police, she kept ringing up saying there was a man under her bed. She was sent to a Mental Hospital, but she still told the doctors there was a man under her bed. They gave her the latest drugs, and she suddenly declared she was cured.

"You mean, Miss Rustyfan, you can't see a man under the bed now?"

"No I can't. I can see two."

One doctor told the other that there was only really one sort of injection that would cure her complaint, which he called "Malignant virginity" – why did they not shut her up in her bedroom with Big Dan, the hospital carpenter?

Big Dan was fetched, told what her complaint was, and told he would be locked in with her for an hour. He said it wouldn't take that long, and an anxious group gathered on the landing . . . they heard:

"No, stop it, Dan, mother would never forgive."

"Shut up yelling, it's got to be done some time, it should have been done years ago."

"Have your way by force then, you brute!"

"It's only what your husband would have done, had you had one."

The medics could not wait, they burst in.

"I've cured her," said the carpenter.

"He's cured me," said Miss Rustyfan.

He had sawn the legs off the bed.

BOARD AND LODGINGS

The old Pioneer and the young Pioneer were off on the Yukon trail. They slogged on and on, pulling a sledge, until they came to the last outpost, which was simply a place in the snow where two tracks crossed, and there was a hutted store.

The old Pioneer entered the Store and said:

"Howde, pard – got my gunpowder?"

"Yes, Jake."

"Got my traps, got my pemmican?"

"Yes, sure thing, here y'are."

"Got my board all ready?"

"Yep, all wrapped up and ready."

* * *

So they loaded stores and resumed their treck. Soon the young Pioneer said: "Hey, what's this about a board, what the heck do we wanna board for?"

The old Pioneer explained that in the Yukon it was possible to go six months without seeing a woman, therefore the old and experienced traveller arranged to have a board with a hole in it, and a naked woman painted on it.

* * *

Only a short time later Jake returned to the Store, alone.

"Gees, Jake, youze back early, didya strike gold or what?"

"Nope, just a bit o' bad luck I had, had to shoot me pardner."

"Hadta shoot yer pardner, that's bad. For Pete's sake, why?"

"Caught that guy sleeping with ma board."

FOR BEDDER OR WORSE

A Cambridge student rushed into his friend's study un-announced. His friend was not there, so he went on into the bedroom, and there was his friend lying face down on the bed, on top of a life-size cinema poster.

"I say Charles, old boy, what the bloody h—"

His friend looked up rather breathless and panted:

"It's all right, Mortiboys, I've got the charwoman under-neath."

HOLE IN NONE

Four middle-aged men were on a Irish golf course. The little quiet feller was just teeing off when a leprechaun appeared to him, and asked if he would like to hole in one.

"Where's the catch in it?"

"Not a catch. You have to give up five years of your sex life, but think of the glory."

The man thought of that, agreed, and holed in one, to the astonishment of the onlookers.

At the next hole, the leprechaun offered another hole-in-one in exchange for ten years of the man's lovelife. The result was sensational, it had only been done four times in history.

The fairy said: "Bet all you've got you can do it three times, the odds will be fantastic, but no relations with any women for the rest of your life, remember!"

And that is how Father O'Flynn got his name in all the record books.

A TRIPLE EVENT

A father approached his child of ten and said: "I think I'd better tell you, your mother's going to have another baby; it's in her tummy now, waiting to be born."

"Are you sure, daddy?"

"Of course I'm sure, what are you looking so worried about?"

"Well, daddy, auntie says the stork's bringing me a brother or a sister, and will drop it down the bedroom chimney; Mrs Smith says the doctor will be bringing one in a little black bag, so it looks as if the bloody place'll soon be overrun with kids."

THE PRIMROSE PATH

There was a mother of two boys who said to her oldest: "Look you're eighteen now, your father's dead, I think you should tell your younger brother the facts of life."

The youth sought out his kid brother of sixteen, and said: "Here you, listen, what did we do last night?"

"Why, we went up the boozer, had a couple, and picked up Poppy Tinne and Lucy Tupper the bar-room floozies."

"Yes, go on."

"Well, we bought them some gins, and then we gave them five bob each and took them round the back of the boozer."

"Yes, what next?"

"Well, we took one each, pushed them up against the wall and . . . look, what's all this in aid of?"

"Nothing. It's just that mother says I've got to tell you it's just the same with birds and the bees and the flowers."

NO USA ANY MORE

In the village was an old widower of 80, whose family had long since grown up. He suddenly married a girl of 20, and shortly afterwards astonished the vicar with:

"I shall want you soon parson, there be a christening on the way."

When the vicar had recovered he managed to stammer:

"Congratulations you old rascal; a child eh? Your wife's young yet; is this the first of several?"

"Nay, vicar, no more after this. You see, my big son's left for Americky."

At this a black thought entered the vicar's mind, but he put it away, and said: "I don't follow you Dad, what's your son going to America got to do with it?

"Well, you see, vicar, he used to lift me on and off."

FISHY

A certain youth had a party piece in which he could insert two fingers in his mouth and give a whistle audible a quarter of a mile away.

This man started courting, and one evening he took his girl right out into the countryside. They dallied long, and, as they approached the terminus, the last bus was moving off.

"Stop him – whistle!" cried the girl.

The man put his two fingers to his mouth, paused, and said: "It's a lovely evening, the walk won't hurt us."

PREGNANT WITH POSSIBILITIES

There was an old man in the village who had been a widower many years; he was known to have money. He went to the doctor and asked for a check over. The doctor said, "For a man of 87 you're doing well, why a check up?" The old rascal explained that he was going to marry a girl of twenty.

He would not be dissuaded, so the doctor's final advice was: "Then, if you hope for a peaceful, not to say a fruitful marriage, take a lodger in as well."

They did not meet for eight months, when the old man said: "Congratulate me doctor, the wife's pregnant."

The doctor collected his thoughts, and said: "Ah yes yes, so you took my advice, and had a lodger as well?"

"Of course, grinned the old devil through his toothless gums, she's pregnant as well!"

THREE TIMES A DAY AFTER MEALS

A courting couple went into a chemists shop, and after some shy whispering the girl said:

"What's that stuff they advertise – 'Makes bonny babies'?"

"Ah," said the pharmacist, "you mean Glaxo, do you want a medium or a large size?"

"Just a minute," said the girl, "who has to take it, me, or my young man?"

FUN WITH DUCKS

A young man married and took his girl to one of these farms where they did holiday accommodation, for their honeymoon.

Half way through the week, over breakfast, the farmer hummed and ha'd a bit and then said:

"Look here, are you two getting enough?"

"I don't know what you mean!" stammered the man.

"I mean, enough to eat?"

"Oh, yes, plenty thanks, why?"

"I only thought," said the farmer, "that if you must keep eating sausages in the bedroom, I wish you wouldn't throw the skins out of the window, they be choking my ducks."

STRETCHING IT A BIT

A man consulted his doctor because his wife was having far too many children. The doctor gave him a sheath and said follow the instructions and all would be well.

A month later the man was back saying his wife was pregnant again. . . .

"Did you follow the instructions?"

"Well doctor, it said: 'Stretch over the organ before intercourse', but as we hadn't got an organ I stretched it over the piano. . . ."

JUST A PRECAUTION

Twins were waiting to be born; said one:

"Don't let's go out yet."

Said the other: "Why not?"

"It's raining outside."

"How d'you know?"

"There's a man just come up the entry with his mac on!"

GETTING HIS MEMBER IN

A Socialist girl and a Tory man were very much in love, and finally married. On the first night of their wedding, instead of love and passion, they finished up in a double bed with their backs turned on each other, all because of a silly quarrel about politics.

After twenty minutes a timid girl's voice said:

"Darling."

"Yes, what is it?"

"There's a split in the Labour Party, and if the Conservative member stood now, he'd get in easily."

"Too bloody late! He's stood as an independent, and lost his deposit."

ICE-HOLES TO YOU

A hunter tried to catch a polar bear for a zoo, but had no luck, until an Eskimo, in exchange for whisky, told him what to do . . .

"They love dried peas. You make a neat hole in the ice, three feet across, and each night you put dried peas round the edge. After a few days he gets over-confident, then, you creep up behind him quietly and . . ."

"And what?"

"Kick him in the ice-hole!"

MISTAKEN IDENTITY

The husband gets drunk, and insists on taking a friend home from pub to show him posh home. They get in the hall, and:

"Shee that chandelier, thash mine!"

They progress through the house. . . . "Shee that gran' pianer, thash mine."

"Shee that colour tel'vision shet, thash mine."

Then upstairs: "Shee that king-shise double bed, thash mine."

"Shee that lovely woman naked in bed, thash my wife."

"Shee that feller lyin' on top of her. Thash me."

DO OR DIE

Dai was popular in the Welsh village, and easily won at the Rural District Election. "Congratulations Dai!" said the barman in the local.

"Councillor Jones, now, if you please."

The landlord came in – "Congratulations Dai!"

"Councillor Jones from now, IF you don't mind."

The Minister popped in for a lemonade – "Well done Dai!"

"Councillor Jones now, Minister, please."

He went home late and rather sloshed, and the house was dark but for a light upstairs. As he entered, a voice from above said:

"Is that you, Dai?"

"Shertainly not!" was the very slurred response, "Ish Counshellor Jones."

"Oh good, but come on up quick, we've only got a few minutes and Dai'll be coming home."

TICKED OFF

A young couple with single beds had been married a month when they realised someone had stolen their alarm clock. They sat down and thought and thought, and working it out backwards, they remembered that on the day of the wedding, Uncle Geroge had been seen much admiring the clock. Taking a chance, they wrote and asked him if by any chance he could say what had happened to it – had he by accident walked off with it?

A telegram came back: "In the other bed you fools."

HARD AND SOFT

A "Modern" couple started off their married life with single beds. One night soon after they had turned in, a little voice was heard:

"Ooh, dahling." – – – – – – "Yes dahling?"

"Would poppa's likkle iggy-wiggy lovvy-duvvy cuddle-some girl like to come over into this ikkle warm beddy?"

She replied: "Of course poppas ikkle sugar-bunch wants to come into dahlin's beddy-weddy," but alas on the way over she tripped on the mat, and he said: "Oh honey, oh likkle dewdrop, diddums hurtums ikkle self?"

But, she had't hurt herself, and was soon locked with him in the jousts of Venus. Fifteen minutes later, when returning to her own bed, she fell over the mat again. . . .

"Why don't you look where you're putting your great big ugly feet you stupid little fool!!!!"

NO TREAD!

A very shapely girl got married to a young man who was mad about motor cars and everything to do with them. After they had been married a week the girl's father happened to meet her, and asked her how she was getting on.

"It's terrible," she said, "he gets into bed and goes straight to sleep, he doesn't *do* anything!"

Father thought for a moment and said: "Listen, when you go to bed tonight, lie flat on your back, and as he begins to doze off, take hold of his hand and stroke it straight down the middle of your belly: nature will do the rest."

The girl carefully remembered her instructions, and when they were in bed, took hold of her sleepy husband's hand and stroked the palm of it down her tummy. Her husband suddenly cried out: "Scandalous, I've been swindled! Only five hundred miles and not a bit of tread left on it."

SHORT TRIPS

A girl was courting a sailor, and he used to send her all his money to get a home together ready for the wedding day. When at last he came home to make her his bride, she showed him with pride the house she had got, and the furniture in it. All went well until he saw the bridal bedroom, in which were twin beds.

"Twin beds, by cripes what's this, a joke?"

"Darling, darling think of the money we shall save."

"Rubbish, think of the carpets we shall wear out!"

EXPENSIVE BOARD!

A man's wife died, and he decided to get right away on a long-distance cargo boat. After a while he began to regret it, and said: "Captain, what do we do for sex?" Said the Captain: "You know damn well Australia is three months away; there's nothing doing."

A week later the man returned to the old subject:

"What do the crew do for sex?"

"I'll tell you, they have a board with a naked female painted on it, and a hole in it; the cook bends down on the other side. I daresay they'll give you a turn if you'll pay."

So the man had a go, and the Captain said:

"That'll be six pounds two and six."

"What?! How can it be that much?."

"Half a crown for the cook, and two pounds each for the men who hold him; you see, he don't like it very much."

BLACK AND WHITE

A negro boy came home painted white, and said:

"The kids at school painted me white all over," so his mother beat him for getting messed up. Father came home, and said: "What's going on?" so Mother told him: "The kids at school painted our Sam white." So father gave him another thrashing for not standing up for himself. Shortly afterwards a small voice was heard:

"I've only been a white boy for two hours but already I hate you black b*ggers."

There was a young fellow of Poole
Who found a red ring round his tool,
He ran to the clinic,
But the doctor, a cynic,
Said: "That's only lipstick, you fool!"

A Magdalen Dean of Divinity
Had a daughter who kept her virginity,
The Fellows of Magdalen
They must have been dawdlin'
'Twould never have happened at Trinity

There was a young fellow of Trinity
Who ruined his sister's virginity
He rogered his brother
Had twins by his mother –
And now he's a Dean of Divinity!

There was a good Bishop of Birmingham
Who did all young girls whilst confirming 'em,
Amidst screams of applause
He dragged off their drawers,
And slipped the episcopal worm in 'em!

Two school-kids around Aberystwyth
Made love with the lips that they kissed with
But as they grew older
They also grew bolder
Making love with the things that they pissed with

Repairs to gun

A man went for a job as a Commercial Traveller, and told the Sales Manager he was the best in the business provided his expenses were met without dispute.

"No bother at all," said the latter, "you sell the stuff, we pay up without question."

In the first few months the man doubled the sales, but sent in a bill for £45. He was told that on those sort of figures he must set out the details.

Accordingly, next time, the bill showed such items as:

Intercourse with Molly	=	£5
Laying Big Mabel	=	£4
Knee-trembler, Mrs Loveit	=	£3
		and so on ...

The Sales Manager was aghast because these matters were dealt with by young girls in the Accounts Section, and the Traveller was ordered to disguise his goings-on in diplomatic terms. So, month after month there appeared:

"Shooting = £3" or "Game Birds = £10" and so on, and all went well.

However, after a wonderful year the accounts stopped coming in, and so did the orders. The firm wrote anxiously to enquire progress, and received no reply except:

Repairs to gun = £150

HOT STUFF

A man got married, and when he returned to work after his honeymoon, all his mates "ribbed" him.

"Come on Jack," said one, "how's your wife now?"

"I left her smoking in bed this morning," he replied.

"Cripes, what lovemaking," said an envious forewoman.

BOOT ON THE OTHER FOOT?

A commercial traveller, staying at a hotel, fancied the chambermaid. He offered her £5 for an hour upstairs, but the girl replied indignantly that she was not like that. She added that when she did it was for love, not money, and just now she had "gone off" and could not get passionate if she tried.

The traveller played his trump card, he was selling shoes, and here was an extremely fine sample pair. . . .

The girl's vanity conquered, and she took the traveller upstairs, stripped naked, and lay back on the bed. The traveller got going, and to his delight found the girl very responsive. She wrapped her right arm round him, then her left leg, then her left arm, then her right leg, and he found these wriggles and embraces delicious.

"I thought you said you couldn't get worked up?"

"I'm not," she replied, "I'm simply trying the shoes on."

FRENCH LEAVE

A Frenchman staying at an English country house for the weekend was attracted to a Debutante type, and without much difficulty, seduced her. Several months later they met by chance at a very select Society ball. He stepped forward with outstretched hand, but she walked straight past him without acknowledgement. As soon as he could, the Frenchman cornered her and said: "Surely you remember me?"

Of course I do young man, but you are not to assume that in England a one-night frolic constitutes an introduction."

A well-built navvy was signing on at the "Labour" when when one day the clerk said: "Would you like to have a go at this job? It's a middle-aged spinster lady, very wealthy. Her butler's died, and she must have a big lusty man in the livery, even if he can't buttle."

So off went the navvy to the Great House, again assured by the Labour Exchange that his ignorance was no bar.

He returned, crestfallen.

"How did you get on?"

"I got on lovely at first; she said stand up straight, turn round, yes, yes, try the coat on, and I did perfect. She smiled and said: I'm sure you'll do, now show me your testimonials."

"Believe me mister, I lorst that job through sheer bloody ignorance."

WHO'RE YOU SPEAKING OF?

The small urchins playing in a back street. Rolls Royce arrives, befurred and bejewelled young woman gets out and cries: "Willy!"

The snottier of the two raggamuffins goes over and the girl says: "Here's five pounds, take it straight to mother. Here's five shillings, that's for you, now be a good boy!"

With which she re-entered the chauffeur-driven Phantom, and disappeared in a cloud of perfume.

"Hey, 'oo's that?" said the other kid.

"That's my sister wot's bin ruined."

COLD LOVER

There was a man had a most attractive wife, but he began to be suspicious of her. At last he could stand it no longer. Being on "nights" he asked the foreman for a "pass-out" and went home at two in the morning to find his best friend's car outside, just as he had feared.

He let himself in, crept up the stairs, and rushed into his wife's bedroom. There she lay, on top of the bed, stark naked, but smoking a cigarette and reading a book.

He went wild and searched under the bed, in the wardrobe, even in the airing cupboard, but he could find no man. He went berserk, wrecked the bedroom, then he started on the living room, threw the TV out of the window, slashed the armchairs, overturned the table and sideboard, then turned his attention to the kitchen, where he smashed all the crocks and threw the fridge out of the window. Then he shot himself.

When he got up to Heaven's gates, who should he see waiting for admission, but his late best friend, who said:

"What are you doing up here?"

So the wronged husband explained how he had lost his temper, and all about it, and added: "But how does it come about that you are up here too?"

"Oh me? I was in the fridge."

A FUNNEL FOR THE MISSUS

There was an old farmer who all his life had wanted to stay at an expensive hotel. At last he achieved his aim, but, as he and the old woman went to bed, he observed something lacking. He asked the night porter, where was the chamber pot?

The man explained that they didn't have them, but there was a bathroom at the end of the corridor. The farmer said he didn't want a bath, and the end of the matter was, the night porter, in exchange for half a crown, fetched an empty quart bottle.

"Well Sir, how did you get on?" he enquired next morning.

"I was all right," said the old farmer, "myself, but I was up half the night trying to make a funnel for the missus."

HE FLUSHED

A man who had been living in the slums was granted a council house.

"How's it going?" asked a mate at work, a few days later. Jack explained that it was a bit of all right, except for that mysterious chain and tank arrangement in the bathroom.

"Why! You bloody fool, you pull down the chain, and that makes the water flow."

The next day, Jack said he'd tried it out, but it was no good.

"What went wrong?"

"Well, I pulled the chain, and the water came, like you said, but before I could grab the soap and towel, it had all gone again."

THE RESULT OF PRAYER

Two girl friends married on the same day, and took their new husbands to the same honeymoon hotel. The four of them sat in the lounge thinking how obvious it would look if they all went to bed at the same early hour, but after a while it was decided that the girls should go out in the direction of the "Ladies" and then slip up to their rooms, and the men would have a last drink at the bar. After about ten or fifteen minutes the men would leave casually in the same manner, and join their brides.

However, just as they were about to follow the girls, every light in the place failed, which was disconcerting in a strange building. Nevertheless, each was convinced he could find his room, and so they set off.

Harry groped up stairs and along passages, counting doors in his careful way (for he was a very careful man) and found the room. Just to make sure he struck a match and saw bits of confetti on the landing. Then, quietly entering he carefully took off his clothes, put on his pyjamas, kneeled down and said his prayers, climbed into bed, and began to make love.

At that very moment all the lights came on, and he saw that he was in the "right room" as it were, but on the wrong floor, and this was the other man's bride! He grabbed his clothes and hurried off to his own proper room, only to find that the other man was an atheist!

Two business girls shared a flat. One night one of them was out on a date, and her friend went to bed. She had not been in bed long when the other one returned, and, not wishing to disturb her mate, got undressed in the dark. As she did so, there was a curious tinkling noise. As neither of them could make sense of this, they went to sleep.

In the morning Jane said: "Hey Mary, what was that rattling last night when you were going to bed?"

"I don't know Jane, let's look round."

They scrabbled on the floor, and found an American dime.

"Oh the swine!" said Mary, "he told me it would melt in three minutes."

PERIODS

Two friends got married about the same time. After five years Pat, the Roman Catholic had one child, Jack, the Protestant, had four. One Saturday they were drinking, and Jack asked Pat how it was that he, an RC had fathered only one child, while he Jack, was fathering one a year.

"It's the 'safe period'," said Pat.

"Garn! The doctors say it doesn't work."

"It works if you know exactly when it is, it's different for each individual. In my case, I have sex every third week, late at night, weekdays only."

"Well Pat, why is that the safe period for you?"

"You see Jack, that's when you're on nights."

A certain fishing club ran an annual outing. One year, when they were preparing the outing, the Chairman said:

"Look, just for once we'd better take the ladies; my wife is for ever on at me that we clear off fishing every weekend, and we never take them anywhere."

After discussions this was agreed on, and the day of the outing came round. It turned out to be nothing but a long booze-up, and only after the last pub was closed did they make for home. It was a long way, and after a while the Chairman told the driver he must make a comfort stop.

"Impossible!" said the driver, "this is a 'No stopping highway'."

The coach went on and on and on, and the men were bursting. Finally the Chairman said: "Never mind the law, stop soon for cripes sake."

"O.K.," said the driver, "if you're that desperate I'll stay in the next lay-by, but it's got a street lamp in it, you'll have to put up with that.'

He stopped by the lamp, while drunk and desperate men got out and relieved themselves, neither knowing nor caring what the wives, sitting in the bus, could see.

Late that night, going to bed, the Chairman's wife said:

"You are nothing but a lot of disgusting beasts. First you get stupid drunk, then you flash yourselves without shame in front of a whole bus full of wives . . ." she stopped for breath, and then continued:

"Mind you Jack, I was very proud of ours!"

BISHOP'S BAD BACK

Three Business men were off to a conference. They sat in the train with a parson. One buried his head in the Times, the other two conversed – What will you do with your spare time at Brighton? asked the first. Replied the second: Pubs! they've got wonderful pubs there, not one will remain unvisited – what will you do?

Girls! replied the other. Brighton's full of girls, all sorts of girls, I'm off on the tiles every night!

The parson was shocked, and was about to make some remark when the Delegate who was reading the Times looked up, and said: Does anybody know what sciatica is?

Yes! said the parson quickly, it is a painful disease caused by alcoholic indulgence, and promiscuity.

Ah, that's very odd, said the questioner, for I see that your Bishop has got a bad attack of it!

TAKING A CHANCE

There was a fireman who was horribly mean both to his wife and his lodger. One night he brought home a splendid pork pie and ate half of it for his supper. His wife and the lodger had to make do with dry bread and cheese.

He carefully put the rest of the pie away, and they all went to their beds.

In the middle of the night the fire bells rang, and off the landlord had to run. The wife, stark naked, entered the lodger's room, shook him awake and said: "He's gone out, quick, now's your chance."

"Are you sure it's all right?" enquired the lodger.

"Of course! Hurry up, lose no time!"

So the lodger went downstairs and finished the pork pie.

LOOK LIVELY!

A chap went to bed with his wife, and he was just dozing off when she shook him hard. . . .

"John, don't go to sleep darling! Listen, I've made a mistake and instead of my sleeping tablets I've taken my pep pills. . . ."

"Aha! Whacko!, and you want me to . . . ?"

"Yes, of course, I want you to teach me the Gay Gordons."

DOWN WITH THE PILL

Two farmers drinking, and one says to the other:

"How is it your stock breed so well, and mine are hardly breeding at all?"

The other explained that he was getting some special sex-pills from the Vet to give the animals.

"Sex pills, what be they? What's in them?"

"Oh, I don't know what's in 'em, but they taste like peppermints."

BAG AND BAGGAGE

A man was going to a distant town on business, and not taking his wife. He asked his pal if he'd got any addresses. His pal said; "any house in Blanco Street will produce women who've got everything a man could wish for."

The stranger knocked on many doors, and each produced a slut more odious than the last. He had nearly given up hope, when, at the last house the door was answered by a woman with everything a man might wish for . . . beard, moustache, muscles. . . .

THE BOSS, THE TYPIST, AND THE LINGERIE

On the staff of Beatherfed UDC was a young woman of excellent figure who was considered "fast". She was, however, popular with her male colleagues, all of whom claimed at some time or other to have had her favours. All, that is, except the Head Clerk, who was oldish, and somewhat crabby. He dropped her several hints, but all in vain.

Suddenly, last year just before Christmas, she said to him: "It's my birthday to-morrow – I thought perhaps you'd like to come down in the evening, bring a bottle of wine and cut yourself a slice of cake."

Overjoyed, he arrived on time, bottles bulging from his pockets, and knocked the outer door. She admitted him to the lobby, and said: "Wait a minute darling, I'm not quite ready," with which she disappeared within. He waited about fifteen minutes, and was getting properly cheesed off, when the inner door opened, and she stood there in ravishing black nylon lingerie.

I'll not keep you long now," she said, "I'm nearly ready – why don't you strip off while you're waiting."

Sure enough, in a few minutes a sweet voice called: "Coo-ee, come i-in darli-i-ing."

He needed no second bidding! He stepped boldly in, his clothes (neatly folded) over his left arm, his shoes held in his right hand. There she sat, lit by soft candles, more desirable than ever. Her table was loaded with food and wine. Round it, in festive attire, sat fourteen men and women – the whole office staff – wearing paper hats.

A HAND IN THINGS

A mother and her seventeen-year-old daughter sat on a bus. Outside the hospital a man got on who had been in an accident, and he had both his arms in slings.

When the conductor came round for the money the man said:

"Excuse me Miss, will you put your hand in my trousers pocket and get out a shilling for my fare."

The girl did this, but she was so embarrassed that she dropped the money, and it rolled under the seats, causing quite a kerfuffle.

When they got off the bus, the woman said:

"Really Mary, you did make a lot of fuss and bother over nothing, you could see the poor man could not help himself, and yet you go all goofy, just over putting your hand in his pocket."

She said: "Oh mother, I did feel a big soft thing."

A PILL IN THE EAR

"Oh yes," said this working-class woman. "Nye Bevan was the greatest man who ever lived."

"Why's that Mrs Moggs?"

"Well luv, he started this here National Health and saved me from having about fourteen kids."

"But don't be silly Mrs Moggs, you don't get birth control on the National Health!"

"Course yer do, I get me deaf aid on it. Saved me having a string o' kids it did."

"I don't foller yer Mrs Moggs, how could a deaf aid stop yer having kids?"

"I'll tell yer, Mrs Bloggs: every night when we went to bed me and my old man, he'd say: 'Are we going to go to sleep or what?' and me being so deaf I'd say 'what'.

PUT HIS FOOT IN IT

A man stayed out late, drinking, and crept into bed in the dark. When he awoke at daybreak he saw three pairs of feet sticking out at the bottom of the bed, and one was a black pair. He woke his wife up, and said:

"Hey Mary, look at that, three pairs!"

She said: "Don't talk bloody daft, you're drinking yourself stupid, go down and count them." So the husband got out, carefully counted and examined the objects, and said:

"You're quite right, only two pairs, and aint mine dirty!"

IT'S THE KNACK AS DOES IT

A young bull, newly on the farm, was put in with the old bull.

"What would you like to do?" enquired the old bull.

"Well, I hear there's a hundred cows right across the far side of the farm; I suggest we run over and do two or three each?"

"Certainly not! We'll WALK there, and do them all."

SQUATTERS RIGHTS

An Indian Chief came into big money when oil was discovered on his reservation, so he booked a room in a London hotel for himself and his favourite squaw. In the night he woke her up with:

"Big Chief, him want water, plenty water."

She fetched him some, but from then on, about every hour he made the same demand. Finally he got a refusal:

"Big Chief, him no can have water! White woman sitting on well."

LOST AND FOUND

"Is that the Salvation Army?"
  "Yes, speaking."
  "Do you save lost girls?"
  "Indeed we do!"
  "Save one for Saturday night for me, will you please?"

MAIDEN'S DREAM

A "difficult" schoolgirl of fifteen was sent to the Psychologist, who asked her a number of very personal questions. He was sure that "sex" lay at the bottom of the trouble, and asked her:
  "Do you suffer from sexy or erotic dreams?"
  "Certainly not!"
  "Are you sure?"
  "Quite sure, in fact, I enjoy them."

IN A JAM

Two strawberries were cooking in a pot, and it got hotter and more uncomfortable every moment. Said one to the other:
  "You know, if us two hadn't been found in the same bed, we wouldn't be in this jam now."

SHOWED HER PINK FORM

A working girl who applied for a job at a big factory was told to fill in the usual form calling for name, address, age, etc., etc.
  She brought it back and under the heading "Sex" had entered: "Four times a week."

WHAT THE BUTLER DIDN'T SEE

The London fog was swirling over the Thames as a young tramp settled himself on the embankment for the night.

Suddenly he was roused by a gentle voice and, looking up, saw a beautiful brunette alighting from her chauffeur-driven Rolls-Royce.

"My poor man," she said, "you must be terribly cold and wet. Let me drive you to my home and put you up for the night."

Of course, the tramp didn't refuse this invitation and climbed into the car beside her.

After a short drive the car stopped before a large Victorian mansion and the brunette stepped out, beckoning the tramp to follow her. The door was opened by the butler, into whose charge the lady gave the tramp, with instructions that he should be given a meal, a bath and a comfortable bed in the servants' quarters.

Some while later, as the brunette was preparing to retire, it occurred to her that her guest might be in need of something, so, slipping on her negligee, she hurried along to the servants' wing.

As she rounded the corner a chink of light met her eye, indicating that the young man was awake.

Knocking softly on the door she entered the room and enquired of the young man why he was not sleeping.

"Surely you are not hungry?"

"Oh no, your butler fed me royally."

"Then perhaps your bed is not comfortable?"

"But it is – soft and warm."

"Then you must need company. Move over a little. . . ." The young man, overjoyed, moved over. . . .

(and fell into the Thames. . . .)

There was a young girl of Madrid
Who wouldn't be done for a quid,
There came an Italian
With a stalk like a stallion
Who swore that he would, and he did!
Now, this clever young girl of Madrid
When she found she was having a kid,
She stopped up her water
For a month and a quarter,
And drownéd the b*gger, she did!

There was a young lady of Durbar
Who swore that no man could curb 'er,
But a man from Khartoum
Knocked the top off her womb
With a fifteen inch kidney disturber!

There was a young lady of Tottenham
Her manners? She'd simply forgotten 'em,
During tea at the Vicar's
She whipped off her knickers,
Because she was feeling too hot in 'em!

There was a young lady of Twickenham
Of candles she never grew sick on 'em,
She prayed in the nude
And Venus she sued –
To-lengthen, and strengthen, and thicken 'em

A Tribute to Mr. Wilson

Dear Secretary – We have the honour to be members of a Committee set up to raise £50,000 for the purpose of erecting a statue to H. Wilson Esq. at Westminster. The Committee is in somewhat of a quandary as to where to place it, it could not go next to that of George Washington who never told a lie, nor Lloyd George who never told the truth, since Harold Wilson could not tell the difference.

After careful consideration we have decided to put it next to Christopher Columbus, the greatest Socialist of them all, in that he started out not knowing where he was going, arriving did not know where he was, and returning, did not know where he had been, and he did all this on borrowed money. The inscription will read: "Five thousand years ago, Moses said to the Children of Israel, 'Pick up your shovels, mount your asses and camels, and I will lead you to the Promised Land'." Nearly 5,000 years later, George Brown said: "Lay down your shovels, sit on your asses, light up a camel, this IS the promised land." Now Wilson is stealing your shovels, kicking your asses, increasing the tax on camels, and taking over the Promised Land.

Therefore, naturally, we expect a generous contribution from you towards our noble project.

Yours,

Wm Muggins

THE DIRECTOR'S LARK

A meeting of the Education Committee was recently called for the purpose of presenting Miss Lark, the Director's Secretary with a testimonial on the occasion of her leaving to take up another sphere of labour.

In making the presentation the Director, Dr Heluva B. Lyar, in a few well-chosen words, referred to Miss Lark's extraordinary capabilities. The Dr remarked that for quickness of conception, easy delivery, and faithful reproduction of all matters imparted to her, Miss Lark surpassed any secretary he had ever had under him, and which, the Director facetiously remarked, had not been few. He further remarked that he had never known his efforts with Miss Lark to miscarry.

Miss Lark, in thanking the Director for his great kindness, felt bound to refer to his gentleness, firmness and strength in his treatment of her when she had the pleasure of working under him. Miss Lark spoke feelingly of his energy and force of action, his powers of duration, his dexterity in grasping his subjects, and above all, his precision in driving home his point. Concluding, Miss Lark trusted that the germ so skilfully imparted to her by Dr Heluva B. Lyar would fructify, and if, as she hoped, the Doctor would find time to visit her in her new home, he would find that his labours had not been in vain.

LOVE LETTER

To –

My Dear Ever-Loving Wife

During the past year I have tried to make love to you 365 times, an average of once per day, and the following is a list of the reasons you gave for rejecting me:

Wrong week	11
It will wake the children	7
It is too hot	15
It is too cold	3
Too tired	19
Too late	16
Too early	9
Pretending to sleep	33
Window is open, neighbours might hear	3
Backache	16
Toothache	2
Headache	6
Not in the mood	31
Baby restless, might cry	18
Watched late show	15
Mud-pack	8
Grease on face	4
Too drunk	7
Forgot to visit chemists	10
Visitors sleeping in next room	7
Just had hair done	28
Is that all you think about?	62

Dearest, do you think we can improve on our record during the forthcoming year?

Your ever-loving Husband,

Jack.

Late one evening two gentlemen were walking down the avenue when they passed a very respectable-looking girl. As she passed one says to the other: "I'd give fifty pounds to spend a night with her." The girl overheard, turned, and said: "It's a bargain"! The man immediately said Goodnight to his friend and took the lady to her flat.

The next morning the man got up, put £25 on the dresser, and prepared to go. She asked for the rest of the money, adding "If you don't pay up I'll sue you for it." The man laughed, and departed.

A few days later, he got a Summons. He rushed off to his Solicitor, who said: "She can't possibly recover from you for *that*, but it will be interesting to see what her lawyer makes of it.

After the usual preliminaries, the lady's Counsel rose and said "Your Honour, my client, this lady, is the owner of a delightful piece of property, a garden spot, surrounded by shrubbery, which she agreed to rent to the defendant for a special length of time for fifty pounds. The defendant took possession, used it repeatedly for the purpose for which he had rented it, but upon leaving the premises he paid only one half the agreed rent. The rent was not excessive since this was restricted property, and we ask for judgement for the balance."

Defendant's lawyer was amused by this, but he thought it would save his client embarrassment if he replied in the same terms. "Your Honour," he said, "my client agrees that this young lady has a very attractive piece of property, that he did rent it, and derived great pleasure from the transaction. However, my client found a well on the property, around which he placed his own stones, opened a shaft, and erected a pump, supplying all his own materials, and personally using his own labour. These improvements to the property were more than enough to offset the unpaid amount, and we submit that plaintiff was adequately compensated."

The modest maiden's lawyer replied: "My client agrees that the defendant did find a well on the property, and that he did carry out the work and make the improvements described. However, had defendant not known the well was there, he would not have rented the shrubbery in the first place. Also, on giving up the lease, defendant removed his stones, pulled up the shaft, and took the pump away with him. Moreover, your Honour, in doing so he not only dragged his equipment through the shrubbery, but he left the hole much larger than it was prior to his occupancy, making it easily accessible to small boys. I ask for Judgement for the lady."

The Judge said that in view of her actions, it was only right that the young lady should be covered, and he found accordingly.

WHAT A LOVELY DEATH!

Dear Friend – this chain letter was started by a man like yourself, to bring happiness to tired business men. It costs no money! Simply send a copy to five of your business friends who are tired. Then bundle up your wife, send her to the man whose name heads the list, and add your own name.

When your name reaches the top you will receive 16,487 women, and some of them will be smashers. Have faith! One man broke the chain, and got his own wife back.

Yours sincerely, ————

PS: At today's date a friend of mine had received 18 women. They bury him tomorrow with a smile on his face not seen there for seven years.

THE SAILORS DICTIONARY

By: Rollicking William, the Mariner.

Engineering

Naval Cutter	– Knicker elastic
Grub Screw	– Lunchtime intercourse
Endless Belt	– Night out with a sailor
Ball Race	– Tom cat 3 yds in front of Vet
Insulated Screw	– Barmaid in gumboots
Breeze Block	– Sex in the entry
Blunderbuss	– Perambulator

Love Sex and Marriage

Mothers Day	– Nine months after Fathers Day
Brassiere	– Device for making mountains out of molehills
Divorce	– When a couple can't stomach each other
Kiss	– Application at H.Q. for a position at base

Mistress	– Between a Mister and a Mattress
Prostitute	– A busybody
Salesmanship	– Difference between rape and seduction
Twins	– Womb mates who become bosom pals
Kept Woman	– One who wears mink by day and fox by night
Perfect Secretary	– One who never misses a period
Pyjamas	– Articles placed under the pillow in case of fire
Board of Trade	– A bench in Hyde Park
Love	– A fellow feeling
Jealousy	– Another fellow feeling
Taxidermist	– A man who stuffs animals
Insomnia	– When a bridegroom can't get OFF to sleep
Pansy	– One who likes vice versa
Welsh rarebit	– A Cardiff virgin
Wife	– A device which you screw on the bed and it does all the housework
Sob Sister	– A girl who sits on your knee and bawls, and makes it hard for you
Adolescence	– The time between infancy and adultery
Dancing	– Vertical expression of horizontal intention
Lady	– A woman who never smokes or drinks, and only swears when it slips out
Music Lover	– A man who hears a lady singing in the bath and puts his EAR to the keyhole
Cad	– A man who, when his girls asks for the loan of a penny, gives her two halfpennies

My wife said to me: "George, it's about time you learned to play golf – you know, that game where you chase a little ball all over the place when you're too old to chase women."

So I went to see Jones, and asked him if he would teach me to play golf. "Sure," he said "you've got balls haven't you?" I said: "Yes, but sometimes on cold mornings they're kinda hard to find."

Bring them to the Club House tomorrow, he said, and we will tee off. What's tee off? I said. He said, it's a golf term and we have to tee off in front of the Club House. Not for me, I said, you can tee off there if you want to, but I'll tee off behind a barn somewhere. No, he said, a tee is a little thing about the size of your little finger that you carry with you. Yes, I said, I've got one of those. Well, he said you stick it in the ground and put your balls on top of it. Do you play sitting down? I asked him, I always thought you walked around. He said, you stand up when you put a ball on the tee.

Well, folks, I thought that would be stretching things a bit too far, and said so. Then he asked me if I knew how to hold my club; well, after fifty years I should have some sort of an idea, so when he said you take hold of your club in both hands I knew right then he didn't know what he was talking about.

Then he said, you swing your club over your right shoulder – no! that's not me, that's my brother you're talking about. So he said, well how do you hold your club? and I said in two fingers. He said that wasn't right, and he told me to bend over and he would put two arms round me and show me how to do it. He couldn't catch me there folks! – I didn't put four years naval service in for nothing. He said, you hit your balls with your club, and they will soar and soar, and I said I could well believe that. Then he said, and when you're on the green. . . . What's the green? I asked. That's where the hole is, surely you're not colour-blind? he asked. No? then you take your putter, and you put the ball in the hole . . . you mean the putter, I corrected. He said no, the hole isn't big enough for the ball and the putter. Well – I've seen holes big enough for a horse and wagon.

Then, he said, after making the first hole, you go on and do the next seventeen. He wasn't talking to me! After two holes I'm shot to hell. You mean, he said, you can't make 18 holes in one day? Hell no, I said, it takes me 18 days to make one hole, besides I said, how will I know when I'm in the 18th hole?

He said, you'll know, because then the flag will go up. That would be just my luck.

A MAN'S LIFE

Years	Times
20 – 30	Tri-weekly
30 – 40	Try weekly
40 – 50	Try weakly
Over 50	Beer is Best

WOMEN – AND THE FIVE CONTINENTS

At 14–18 she is like Africa, partly virgin and partly explored.

At 18–24 she is like Australia, highly developed in the built up areas.

At 24–30 she is like America, highly technical, and always seeking new methods.

At 30–35 she is like Asia, sultry, hot and mysterious.

At 35–45 she is like Europe, devastated, but still interesting in places.

(At 45–65 she is like Antarctica, everybody knows where it is, but nobody wants to go there!)

INSTRUCTIONS FOR USING THE NEW
DIAL TELEPHONES

On the telephone there is a dial with letters to indicate the Exchange required. For instance, S for south, P for pussy if using the phonetic code, and O for the operator.

If south is required, put your finger in the S hole or in the P hole for pussy, according to requirements. If the operator is wanted, put your finger in the Operator's hole and work your finger until she comes, then she will give you the required connection.

If you have fingered the P hole correctly, you will hear a purring sound, but if you have inserted your finger in the wrong hole, the R's hole for instance, you will hear a high-pitched scream. In this event, remove your finger, and put the end of your pencil in pussy. When you have finished the operator may have lost her ring.

Where satisfactory connection proves difficult, this may be due to more than one person fingering the operator's hole at the same time, or the cable engineers may have slipped a length in the operator's socket. You must then wait for service until he removes his tool.

To remedy faults

Hold your instrument tightly round the middle, and feel underneath until the operator responds. Remove your finger from either the P hole or the R's hole, grasp the flex and pull your wire until you hear a buzzing in the ears.

Foreign connections

These involve the use of small French letters or else Dutch caps.

There was a young man of Bavaria
Who peed in a clergyman's area
Said the maid to the cook,
"Cook, do come and look,
"It's longer than master's, and hairier!"

There was a young fellow of Kent
Whose wick was exceedingly bent,
To save himself trouble
He had it bent double
And instead of coming, he went!

There was a young Scottie named Dave
Who kept a dead whore in a cave
And when he was told
"You'll find her too cold!"
Said: "Think o' the siller I save!"

There was a young lady named Grace
Whose corset no longer would lace,
Her mother said: "Nelly!"
"There's more in your belly,
"Than ever went in through your face!"

There was a young lady of Rye
Who said to a gent passing by:
"I've looked in my bag
And I haven't a rag...."
So he gave her his Old School Tie.

Up Spake a Brave old Pauper

It was Christmas Day in the Workhouse
The one day of the year
When paupers' hearts were full of joy,
Their bellies full of beer.

Then rose the Workhouse Master
He was a wicked sod:
"You'll do your tasks this afternoon,
"Or else you get no pud."

Up spake a brave old pauper,
His face as bold as brass:
"You can keep your Christmas pudding mate
"And stuff it up your ass!"

They seized the Workhouse Master
He fought with might and main
They cut his bloody privates off
And pulled the bloody chain

BROKEN DOWN BY AGE AND SEX

In days of old, when knights were bold,
And paper not invented,
They wiped the ass, with tufts of grass
And they were quite contented

In days of old, when knights were bold,
And women not invented
They drilled great holes in telegraph poles
And they were quite contented.

MINI-POME

'Tis God who sends the roaring winds
To blow the skirts on high
But God is just and sends the dust
To blind the bad man's eye.

NURSERY RHYME

There was a little girl
And she had a little curl
Right in the middle of her forehead
And when she was good she was very very good
And when she was bad she was marvellous!

EPITAPH

Here lie the remains of Schultz's Charlotte
Who died a highly respected harlet,
For fourteen years she kept her virginity
A very long time for this vicinity.

TRIBUTE

Mae loved for profit, not for fun
And she was scorned by everyone.
Dee loved for fun, and not for profit
And made a very good thing off it!

ANOTHER MINI-POME

If skirts get any shorter,
Said the typist, with a blush,
There'll be two more cheeks to powder
And a lot more hair to brush!

LITTLE MARY'S LITTLE MARY

Little Mary pinned her hopes
On a book by Mary Stopes
Judging by the girl's condition
It must have been an old edition.

Mary had a little lamb
Its fleece was white as snow
And everywhere that Mary went
A ram was sure to go.

Mary had a little lamb. . . .
And the midwife was treated for shock!

BLACK OUTLOOK

A Labourite rose in the House for to speak
"We support the new Vice Act, the best thing this week,
Experience teaches, if life's to be sweet,
"We must shift all these floozies away from the street.
"Life will be better, I swear I'll be bound
"If we put prostitution right under the ground!"

Then up rose a Tory, a man from the Shires
He called them all spoilsports, and twisters, and liars,
"For backing this Act now, your reason is plain —
"To pamper the miners, yet once more again."

THE RADCLIFFE CAMERA

(Oxford University Reading Room)

Whenever I work in the Radder
I wish it could truly be said
That my head was as full as my bladder
My bladder as void as my head!

GODIVA PROCESSION

Early this century there was controversy whether Coventry
Corporation were right to erect only one row of stands. . . .

It was worth more than a fiva
To watch Lady Godiva –
When the wind blew off the wig
Of Miss Nan Gigg,
She continued her ride
With stands on either side

EXPENSES ACCOUNT!

In Warwick she was Winnie, she was Margaret in Perth
In Stratford she was Maisy, the sweetest thing on earth
In Brighton she was Betty, the cutest of the bunch
But down in his expenses, she was Petrol, Oil, and Lunch!

EFFLUENCE

He was our Sewage Manager, was Mr Moses Mudge
And he never thought of anything, but activated sludge,
He never heard us laughing but he gazed with great regret at us,
For his mind was just as murky as his own discoloured detritus;
Promotion had come soon to him (hard work combined with piety)
And thus he was outstanding in the Effluent Society!

FOOTPRINTS ON THE DASHBOARD, UPSIDE DOWN

My wife bought me a lighter
And I'm such a clever blighter
That when it stuck, it didn't mean a thing —
For I'd also had a knife, from my jealous little wife
Which screws the screw that screws the little spring.

I was sitting in my car
When I got a nasty jar
While I fiddled and I twiddled at that spring. . . .
As I poked away, I cursed, for there came a sudden burst
Of metal objects, flying with a "ping!"

My search was microscopic
And I nearly went myopic
My limbs were twisted all ways and my breath was nearly stopped,
As I stretched round nooks and crannies finding peppermints of
*   grannies,*
But not the little lighter parts that popped.

When I found them, it was late
She was waiting at the gate,
With black suspicion written in her frown
"I've been a fool my dear. . ." but all she did was leer
At my footprints on the dashboard upside down!"

LEAVE, COMPASSIONATE, CHILDREN, FOR THE PRODUCTION OF

In 1945 troops serving abroad were offered home leave subject to certain conditions:

In distant lands the stalwart bands of would-be fathers wait,
Certificates to join their mates, upon affairs of state.
For para (3), Appendix (b), will authorise a chap
To reproduce (for scheduled use) the species Homo Sap.

When Good Sir James takes down their names, in files, to procreate
This caveat the unborn must circumnavigate:
"All who have wives past thirtyfive, and children unbegot,
And certified that they have tried, are able, and have not,
May stake a claim. But if they have not, or succeeded,
We can't allow that here and now their services are needed.
All who apply must certify, that they can understand
What lies behind the subtle mind of Middle East Command."

The Middle East has now released a gallant group of men,
Of future Dads, like Galahads, who have the strength of ten,
And every dame must be the same, for it is infra dig
That they should dare a child to bear, uncertified by Grigg.

THOUGHTS ON A.I.D.
By A COW

Though I've just given birth to a heifer
And of pride and of milk I am full
It is sad to relate that my lacteal state
Was NOT brought about by a bull.

I have never been rogered, I swear it,
In spite of the calves I have borne
I swear by that tractor, I'm virgo intacta
I never took bull by the horn!

How dreary this farmyard and meadow
This cowshed seems gloomy and grey
For the one bit of fun in the year's dreary run
By science is taken away.

I know that the farm is a business,
In which we must all pull our weight,
And I'd pull and I'd pull, for a strongly built bull,
But this phoney business I hate.

It mustn't be thought that I'm jealous
There are things a mere cow shouldn't say,
But the Land Army tarts who handle our parts
Still get it the oldfashioned way.

THE 1951 BUDGET

Big Ben it is chiming the hour is now late
The Commons are sitting in deepest debate,
Discussing the gravest of National matters,
Concerning the conduct of tarts queers and hatters.

The Chancellor rose, and said: "Striking at vice?"
"Then the easiest way is by raising the price"
"I feel certain Hon Members will never revoke"
"A Bill I'm presenting called 'Pay as you Poke'."

"The Customs and Excise will find it a cinch"
"To collect these new duties – one shilling an inch"
[Amid shouts from the House, of 'Get out!' and 'Resign']
"And I'll pay my quota each time I have mine –."

"There's the Member for Mudsport, a cuddlesome lass"
"Who performs anytime for a bottle of Bass"
"There's the Member for Ticklam, who says in a daze"
"For a packet of Woodbines she'll take it both ways."

Clem Attlee was up, on his feet in a flash
Denouncing this tariff on crumpet for cash,
And then, in a slashing attack on the Tories –
"You've stuffed benches and wenches you randy old whorers."

The Labourites raved against privilege and wealth,
Demanding free crumpet upon National Health,
While Bevin created an odour of haddocks
By pulling the pants down off Dame Molly Maddox.

Herbert Morrison tossed all the Clerks at the table
While Bevin was stroking and pulling his cable.
And the member for Tamworth enjoyed several jerks
With Postmaster General and Minister of Works.

The member for Bannock, a big buxom wench
Was waving her tits at the Government bench
And the Member for Bilston, tho' three times a grannie
Induced Ebby Edwards to tickle her fanny.

Sir Winston came in, and with V-sign and topper
Induced Lady Astor to play with his chopper
Whilst poor Hughie Gaitskell then left the front rank
And walked round the lobbies in search of a wank.

The Closure was moved then, to end the debate
Just as Black Rod was tickling the balls of his mate
Whilst Megan Lloyd George let go a right squeaker
When having it off with the Rt Hon, the Speaker.

So voters take heed, if you have an erection
There's no need to wait for a General Election
For married or widowed, bachelor or spinster
There's plenty of Crumpet and Cock at Westminster.

TENDER LOVE

Boy meets girl, holds her hand, visions of a promised land
Tender words, cling and kiss, crafty feel, heavenly bliss
Nibbles nipples, squeezes thighs, gets a beat, feels a rise,
Flies agape, drawers well down, really starts to go to town,
Legs outspread, virgin lass, fanny froths like bottled bass.
Love is great, a Cupid stunt, soon he'll feel a stupid. . . .

Love's a jewel, pearls he's won, shoots his load – what's he done?
Comes the pay-off, here's the rub, now she's in the Pudding Club!
Shotgun wedding, bridesmaids flap, Love and Cherish, all that crap.
A tubby tummy, weight she gains, prams and nappies, lubour pains,
Realises what he did, nagging missus, shrieking kid.

Sweats his balls off, works his stint, all the same he's always skint,
Only pleasure, evenings when, mattress creaks she's off again.
Can't forsake those sexy habits, breeding kids like bleeding rabbits,
Curses marriage, starts to bicker, swears he'll choke the bleeding vicar.
Work and worry take their toll, gets cheesed off with same old hole.

Bit of fluff, quite a kick, auburn hair, likes her dick,
Gets it in, lovely fit, durex bursts, he's in the shit.
Up in Court, nowt to say, ten at home, one away,
That silky hole with hair all round has dug his grave in stony ground.
As he draws his final breath, knows he's shagged himself to death,
On his tombstone, plainly lacquered, his epitaph, just
   *f***ing knackered!*

LIMERICKS XII

There was a young lady named Joan
Who went to the dentist's alone
In a fit of depravity
He filled the wrong cavity
She nurses the filling at home.

There was a young fellow named Hyde
Who fell down a closet and died;
He had a brother
Who fell down another,
And now they're interred side by side.

There was a young man of Cawnpore
Whose dick was one inch and no more,
It was lovely for keyholes
And little girls' peeholes
But lost in a bloody great whore!

There was a young lady of Exeter
And all the young men craned their necks at 'er,
Save one dirty sod
Who did six months in quod
Far waving his organ of sex at 'er.

There was a young lady of Gloucester
Whose parents thought they had lost her,
But they found in the grass
The marks of her ass,
And the knees of the man who had crossed her!

SON OF RUGBY JOKES

"Rugby is a game played by men with peculiarly shaped balls"   William Webb Ellis

One With Whiskers On

An army officer who had been abroad for a long time, returned home to his wife. He had become used to high-class floozies in Japan, and was discontented because his wife would not shave her bush. She made all sorts of excuses, it was too cold in winter, it was shocking to her modesty, etc., and neither threats nor bribes would change her mind.

Her husband got fed up, and one night when he had been out with the Rugger Club boys for a drink, he decided to settle the matter. He carried his wife upstairs, threw her on the bed, and tied her hands and feet to the four corners with neckties.

She cried, she begged and she pleaded, but in vain. He plugged in his electric razor and was away. She told him he would regret it all the days of his life, but he scoffed at her suggestion.

As he finished and blew away the whiskers he found neatly tattooed underneath—KILROY WAS HERE.

TOOK THE STUFFING OUT OF HER

A shapely girl was being forced to marry for money, a man she did not love. On the night before her wedding she decided to have one last wild fling with her former lover. He was not expecting her, and had not got a sheath.

In desperation they decided to use the skin of a saveloy, but owing to their passionate exertions, it came adrift, and could not be recovered.

On the wedding night she put up a very good show of violated innocence, but her rich middle-aged husband took his lust in five minutes and withdrew. He was amazed to find himself decorated with what looked like a sausage skin.

"I told you," she sobbed, "it's my maidenhead, and you've half killed me."

"Mary," he said, "I've seen a good many, but I never saw one with 'Marsh & Baxters' printed on it before."

THAT SHOOK HIM!

There was a rich man's daughter who was rather plain, and in addition she had an unfortunate affliction—every time she got emotionally worked up, she developed a fearful fit of shuddering. Thus in spite of her money, she remained a virgin.

Along came a dashing young man who could charm the pants off any girl, and to the surprise of everyone, he married the rich man's daughter. Even more to the surprise of everyone, he seemed well content with his bargain, and as for the girl she purred like a pussy full of cream.

A famous doctor who had rather lost face by failing to cure the girl of her shakes, sent for the young husband, and said: "I've got one or two cases like this, a thousand quid if you'll tell me how you cured her?"

"Sorry, Doctor, but I haven't cured her."

"Then how do you account for your own satisfaction and the girl's manifest good health?"

"Hand over the money and I'll tell you."

The young man then explained that all he used was four neckties and a sharp penknife. "Good Lord! Go on."

"I take her to bed, and undress her. I kiss and fondle her, and she starts to shake. I lay her down and she begins to thrash about like a harpooned whale. Then I tie her hands and feet to the corners of the bed."

"Yes, and after that?"

"I get well in, then I cut the neckties, doctor, it's absolutely bloody fantastic!"

MADE A MEAL OUT OF IT

A man married a slut. She would neither keep the house clean nor get him a decent meal. She never took a bath, and he took to sleeping alone.

He got so fed up he asked an old friend what he could do, and the friend advised that the best plan would be to kill her with sex, which was not a capital offence. So the man went home one Friday, took a little food and wine into the bedroom, dragged his wife up and locked the door. On Monday morning he could hardly crawl to work.

He came home to find his wife in a spotless kitchen. She was stark naked, her quim shaved, her breasts reeked of eau de cologne, and she was cooking a splendid meal. . . . "You treat me right, darling, and I'll treat you right."

THEN HER DRAWS CAME UP

There was a small boy who was caught by his father indulging in betting. This greatly upset father, who consulted the boy's teacher. She said the best thing would be for him to lose one really heavy bet, and get hurt, and that would cure him, and she promised father every cooperation.

That evening, when the class dismissed she told Johnnie to stay behind.

"I want to talk to you about wicked habits," she said.

"Ah," he replied, "and I want to talk to you Miss too, you're a cheat!"

This took her breath away, and Johnnie went on: "You pretend to be natural blonde, but you've got black hair between your legs—yah!"

"Indeed I haven't," she replied instinctively, before she fully grasped the enormity of what he'd said.

"I bet you ten shillings, two weeks' pocket money, you have," said the kid.

She'd landed herself in a trap, and anyway, she'd promised to help, there was no one around, so she took the bet. She dropped her knickers, lifted her skirt, and picked up the money.

She could hardly wait to dismiss the boy before phoning his father with the good news.

"Hell and damnation!" he said, "only this morning he bet me five pounds he'd see your quim before the day was out!"

MEAT SAFE

The farmer was old, and his wife was young. To keep up with the work they set on a strong youth.

One day the farmer's wife went round the back of the barn and found the strong youth about to masturbate between two pieces of bullocks liver.

"Don't do that," she said, "there's a much better way, come with me and I'll show you."

"What about Maister?"

"Master's gone to market, come on upstairs." At which she got on the bed, took off her pants, and said: "Now put it in here."

"Both pieces Missus?"

GOT HIS TEETH INTO IT

There was a strapping young fellow who was on holiday alone in a strange town, and he thought he would go and watch some Club rugger on the Saturday.

The Secretary recognised him at once as a chap who had played scrum half for Northampton Town. "Look man," he said, "we've turned out a man short, the situation's desperate. PLEASE play for us."

The visitor explained that he hung up his boots when he had to have false teeth. The Secretary said this was only local Club stuff, several players wore dentures . . . the visitor looked, and it seemed to him that several of them wore crutches as well, and he allowed himself to be persuaded.

It turned out to be a hell of a rough match, and half way through the young man got a fearful kick in the mouth which broke his dentures to fragments.

He told the Club President that he had to return home that evening and lecture to Rotary, was there a chance of getting his teeth repaired, on a Saturday afternoon?

"Not a cat in hell's chance, but come home with me, I'll fix you."

* * *

An hour later he was drinking whisky in a very handsome lounge while his host kept trotting in with various sets of false teeth. . . . "Try these . . . now try these. . . ."

Some were too large, some too small, but at about the seventh go, they found a set of teeth that were near enough a perfect fit.

The young man shook hands and departed.

"It was vile luck to get my teeth shattered," he said, "but by the Lord Harry I could not have had a better break than to fall in with a dental surgeon, could I?"

"Dental Surgeon? Me? Not me, I'm a Funeral Undertaker."

THICK SKINNED

The Royal Engineers were on a jungle exercise. They had to cross a raging river by means of a rope. The difficulty was to get the rope across, for the stream was wide and deep, and full of crocodiles.

The first volunteer to swim got eaten alive.

The crocodiles also got the second volunteer.

"Sapper Jones," yelled the Sergeant, "strip and swim with the line."

The Captain was aghast: "You can't send him to his death, he isn't even a volunteer!"

"Leave this to me, he's a Brummy football supporter, Sir."

By now, Sapper Jones was across, the crocodiles just sniffed and went away.

"Brummy football supporter! What the hell are you on about?"

The Sergeant said that if the Officer would go and look at the tattooing on the soldier's backside, he would understand everything.

On the left cheek he had: "Villa for the Cup," and on the right cheek: "Birmingham City League champions."

"Oh, I see what you mean, Sergeant, not even a crocodile could swallow that, hey?"

ALL TASTES CATERED FOR

There was an oil rig in a vast and inhospitable desert. A visitor asked the Manager what on earth they did with themselves other than working. "Oh, we have lots of fun, let me see, today's Monday, when they fly the booze in. Would you like to stay for a blind-up?" The man said he was tee-total.

"Never mind," said the Manager, "hang on until Wednesday, that's when they fetch in the birds, lovely, young, coffee coloured. . . ." The visitor said he didn't like women.

"What are you then, are you a Queer?"

"No indeed I am not!"

"No, well in that case you'd better not be here on Saturday then."

WHAT HAD SHE PRAYED FOR?

The Mother Superior had just concluded a prayer meeting in chapel to celebrate the forgiving of Sister Theresa who had been found in bed with a man. She went straight up to her cell and started to pack.

"What's the matter blessed mother?" asked the novice who was her personal maid.

"Matter!" she said, "I've been here fifteen years and three months. During all that time it's been penis and penance, fornicating and forgiving, well it's time for me to stop doing the forgiving and do some of the fornicating."

A LITTLE FRICTION

Two old maids were getting neurotic, and consulted a doctor. He said, far better than cucumbers was a real man. He knew two students who were hard up, so had started a bull shop where frustrated women could go for treatment at a fee.

He gave the address, and off they trotted; on the way they passed a barber-shop, where the hairdresser was giving a customer a singe. There was a smell of burned hair in the air.

"Steady Mabel, I think we're walking too fast."

THE RUB-OUT

A business man going to Japan was asked by a friend to bring back a parcel which could not be trusted to a shipping agent. When the man got back he was intrigued to know what could be in the large box, so he took it in the bedroom and carefully unwrapped it. It turned out to be a rubber woman, and he decided to give it a trial run. He inserted himself and touched a knob, which fell off, at which the thing went mad and began to suck him dry. He shouted to his wife, and gasped that he could not stop it.

She was a woman of resource, and cabled Japan: RUBBER WOMAN WEARING OUT MY HUSBAND HOW DO YOU STOP IT QUESTION MARK.
The reply came back: ORDER FUNERAL LADY WOUND UP ONE MONTH FOR WEST END BROTHEL.

THE NAKED TRUTH

The local paper had been dropping some pretty hot hints about the conduct of the Lord Mayor and his sexy secretary.

Finally, a lawyer's letter was sent, and the paper promised to print a bold statement, clearing the matter up. There followed a headline:

THERE IS NOTHING BETWEEN THE LORD MAYOR AND HIS SECRETARY.

The Lord Mayor's lawyer rang up the Editor and said this wouldn't do, it could be taken two ways, next week's edition would have to put the matter clear beyond doubt.

All this time the Editor had been playing for time; he wanted to get enough on the Lord Mayor to be able to defend a libel action, and now he had got it. Therefore he gladly promised to put his meaning beyond doubt. The next edition came out with:

NOT EVEN A SHEET.

FED UP

A machine operator in a newspaper printing office was getting married. The mechanics worked evenings in their own time to build him a splendid double bed with spring mattress.

After a few days he brought it back.

"What's the matter?" enquired the foreman, "aint it good enough?"

"No, just a question of adjustment gaffer, it feeds too fast!"

THE GROANGREASER AND THE VIRGINS

Two old maids went out shopping, and, entering the greengrocers, enquired the price of cucumbers. The shopkeeper said: "Tenpence each, but you can have three for two shillings, it's a better bargain."

They looked at each other?

"Come on, Veronica, we can always eat the other one."

188

IN THE PINK

A snobbish young woman did a great deal of hunting and horse riding, for her family kept a high-class hiring stable, with provision for little children as well. However, after a row with her parents she went off to London, determined to get work as a model.

She finished up with a top photographer who told her to strip off, and then, gazing with interest, said:

"You've certainly got rosy cheeks."

"Yes," she said. "I get those from horse-riding."

"So I see. You've certainly got the tits for modelling, but what about your ass?"

"Oh daddy will take care of that, it only needs stuffing with hay and a going over occasionally with a good stiff brush."

NO BOTTLE

A woman went to a doctor with a bottle of urine, and said:

"My husband wants you to prescribe some medicine for his stomach pains, and he's too busy to come himself, so he's sent this."

The doctor emptied out the bottle, peed into it himself, and said:

"I believe your husband is a tailor. Take this and tell him to cut a suit to fit me, if he succeeds just by looking at it, I will do the same for him."

SILLY ASS

A grumpy customer was playing up the waitress. "Would he like some oxtail?" "Don't be disgusting, Miss, I know where it comes from."

"Would he like some tongue?"

"I don't want anything that's been in an animal's mouth!"

"Yes, Sir, can I get you an egg."

TWO FAST WOMEN

Two girls were driving through the pouring rain, and they were late for a date.

"Go on Mary," says the passenger, "put your foot down!"

"No fear," said the other girl, "we couldn't hope to buy off any speed-cops with the grass this wet."

WHERE HAVE ALL THE YOUNG GIRLS GONE

There was a fourteen-year-old girl who developed a splendid figure, and she began to take a real interest in the lads.

Mother said to father: "You know, Dad, I'm getting very worried about our Mary, she spends too much time in the churchyard with the boys."

"Girls will be girls," said the old man, "you did at her age."

"Yes, but I didn't come home with my knickers starched and a shilling's worth of coppers!"

"Is that all? It could be worse."

"It is. Yesterday I found 'In Loving Memory' imprinted on the back of her best school coat."

STANDING INSTRUCTION

There was a respectable businessman and Sunday-school teacher who liked to fill the house with "improving" texts.

One day the maid said to the mistress of the house: "I want to put my notice in."

"Why, Mary, you've always had a good place here, and been treated well."

"Yes, madam, but you don't know what the master's been up to in my bedroom."

The woman paled, steeled herself, and said: "What has he done?"

"He's stuck up one of them cards!"

The mistress rushed upstairs and read: "Be Ye Prepared, For Ye Know Not At What Hour The Master Cometh."

SUBJECT NORMAL

Two hotel chambermaids were talking when the bell rang, and one had to go up to the room of a commercial traveller. He laid her straight down on the bed, took his will and in less than five minutes she was back downstairs.

"What did he want?" said her mate.

"Do you know, I honestly don't know, I think he must have forgotten, himself."

POETIC INJUSTICE

Three daughters were getting ready to go out after tea.

Mother: "Where are you off to?"

First daughter: "I'm going off with Neal for a ride and a meal."

Second daughter: "I'm meeting Mick to visit a flick."

Third daughter: "I'm off with Hugh for a . . ."

Mother: "Oh no you're not!"

ONE TRACK MIND

Three women with young children went to a psychiatrist for advice.

To the first he said: "You've got a fixation on drinking, you even called your child 'Sherry'."

To the second he said: "All you think about is your stomach, you even called your little girl 'Candy'."

The third woman said: "I must go, I'm not staying to listen to this."

"I know where you're going too, you're going to meet your son Dick out from school."

LONG TIME COMING

A girl was asked by her mother: "When you got home last night you stayed a long time downstairs with your boyfriend, I want an explanation."

"Oh Mother, if a boy takes you to the cinema you've got to kiss him goodnight for it afterwards, haven't you?"

"The pictures! I thought he was taking you to a very expensive night club?"

"Yes, Mother, he did."

SINGLE MINDED

A newly married couple were in the back of a taxi on the way to the station. The groom interfered with her blouse, but she fought him off. He tried again up her leg. She turned to him angrily and said:

"Hey, lay off that stuff will you, don't forget, I'm a respectable married woman now."

DUSTY ANSWER

A little girl came home, and asked her mother:

"Mummy, are dustmen religious?"

"I never thought so, why do you ask dear?"

"Well, this man emptied a full bin into the cart and he didn't see the other man, and he tipped it all over him and he just stood up and told God all about it."

The same little girl was too much under her mother's feet, so she was given the money to go to the pictures, a treat she had never previously enjoyed. When she came home, mother said: "How did you get on dear?"

"Well mummy, it was a bit like Sunday School."

"Like Sunday School, what do you mean?"

"Well, at Sunday School they sing 'Stand Up Stand Up For Jesus' and in the pictures they shout 'For Christ's Sake Sit Down'."

192

PANNED

There was a girl had her eye on this chap, and she wangled it for her parents to be out when he called. She took him in the front room, turned up the gas fire, turned out the light, poured him a drink, and sat with him on the sofa.

She thought he would be slow, but he proceeded with every confidence. He stroked her hair, kissed her neck, then her lips. He crushed her to him, he pressed her back, he laid her down, he lay on top of her . . . then he stopped.

"Go on, go on," she moaned, "don't stop now or I shall die."

"But dearest, I don't know what to do next."

"You don't know what to do next you nit, what DO you mean?"

"Well darling, the pictures always fade out at this point."

A BRUSH WITH THE FOREMAN

A young and innocent schoolgirl left and went to work in a broom factory. She worked well, and the foreman was annoyed when she gave her notice in.

"What's the matter, you're on good bonus, and doing well?"

"Oh no gaffer, I'm not stopping in this place, I'm catching a horrible complaint, it's all the stuff you use here, it's not nice."

After a lot of questioning he got her to say what the trouble was, since handling all these bristles, a lot of black hairs had grown between her legs, where all was bare before. The foreman explained that this happened to everybody, as they grew up, but she would not believe it.

Finally he took her into the Rest Room, dropped his trousers, and said: "Look here then what did I tell you?"

"Oh dear, it's worse than I thought," said the girl, "you've grown the broom handle as well."

EXPANDING TRADE

In the old days, in East London, of a Saturday night, the butchers' and fishmongers' stocks would be laid out next the pavement on open slabs. The poorer women would come along looking for "bargains" and the tradespeople had a line of sales patter, and patience, up to a point.

But this woman hovered around, buying nothing. She picked up one bit of meat, put it down, poked it, picked it up again. . . .

Finally the butcher shouted: "Nah then Missus, taint like yer old man's yer know, gets bigger as yer play wiv it!"

NOT LEGITIMATE

There was a certain boy, who, every Friday night of his life, had to go across town to his father. The father would hand the boy the affiliation money, which the boy took back to his mother. This had been going since sixteen years before, when the mother had obtained a Bastardy Order against the man.

One day the father said to the boy: "You're 16 today, is that right?"

"Yes, Dad, I am."

"Right, here's the last payment, here's a quid for yourself, now go back and tell your mother, I'm not your father any more."

"Yes, Dad, she told me to tell you, you never were."

FOXS OFF!

A retired Ironmonger wanted to join the gentry, and he sent such large contributions to the hunt, that they felt they must let him join.

After the first "Meet" the MoF took the man on one side, and said:

"Look here, Bloggs old boy, d'you mind if I give you a hint?"

"I ain't bleedin' fussy, say what yer likes."

"Well old man, it is customary, when the fox is sighted, to shout 'Tally Ho!', not 'Get cracking you lousy buggers, there the little bleeder goes!'"

TRUNK CALL

An optimist and a pessimist were in Trafalgar Square, watching a political demonstration.

Said the pessimist: "I bet I get crapped on by a pigeon."

Said the optimist: "Nonsense, there are ten thousand other people here."

The man WAS bombed by a pigeon, and he said: "Go on, you daft sod, tell me just one thing to be optimistic about, go on, just tell me, while I ruin my best handkerchief by wiping my hat with it."

"Indeed," said his friend, "let us be grateful that elephants can't fly."

A BRUSH WITH THE LAW

A man went to the Health Insurance Offices and said he wanted a new National Health wig.

"What have you done with your old one?"

"I lost it."

"When?"

"Three months ago."

When they asked him why he had not reported the loss sooner, he said it was because he had been in jail.

They then asked whether he searched for it when he first lost it. . . . "Because unless you can prove you searched diligently, you don't get a replacement."

"Diligently! Listen! I was sitting in the cinema next to a girl in a mini-skirt when I lost it. Cor, diligently! I was groping around in the dark, and I could swear I had my hand on it twice. That's how I finished up in jail."

HE WAS ON THE BOX

There was a notable rugby player who was about to get married. The boys advised him to lay off the game and save his strength, but he was too keen. The afternoon before his wedding he turned out for the Club, and, alas, got a fearful kick in the groin, and was taken to hospital where his member was put in splints.

After the wedding, when he and his new bride got to their hotel, and retired to bed, she was coyly undressing. . . .

"Look," she said, showing her breasts and quim, "untouched by man, these goods have never been unwrapped before."

"Don't you worry," said he, "mine's still in the box, as well."

HE BOPPED A DROLLOCK!

Doctor Spooner, Warden of New College, used to live at famous Boar's Hill, Oxford. But he moved to the Marston Ferry Road, and when asked why, said:

"Ah well you know, I got tired of running up the whore's bill, I thought it would be cheaper to move to the fast and merry road."

Doctor Spooner got into serious trouble in Blackwell's bookshop whilst trying to purchase copies of *A Tale of Two Cities* and *Friar Tuck*. Until the dust settled, he moved to Cambridge, and greatly shocked a Dean's wife when he told her that his favourite inn was the "Fish and Duck".

ALL BULL

There was a rough workingman who had been "signing on" at the Labour Exchange for all too long. One day the clerk asked him if he'd like a job abroad.

"What sort of a job?"

The man said it was rather a "blind date". All he knew was, it was for one of those rich oil magnates in Arabia. There was a book of travel vouchers, £50 in advance of wages. . . .

The labourer said, "Oh alright, he'd try anything once."

When he got there he was met by a Sultan's private physician, who said:

"My master wishes fifty maidens to be impregnated by an Englishman at five pounds apiece."

"Bloody hell!" said the man, "isn't that like Wolverhampton Labour Exchange to send a man all this way for two days' work?"

A FELLOW FROM EALING?

Mae West was in her flat when three sailors arrived one after the other. Mae poured out drinks and said: "Only one of you can stay the night, we'll have to have a competition: I shall strip naked, the first man to pee on the floor can stay, the others must go."

Only one sailor could manage it, and he was disqualified for standing on his head.

SOCIAL INTERCOURSE

There was a Debutante who married a Naval Officer, and he certainly knew his way about. He took her to Naples for their honeymoon.

When they awoke late on the first morning, they started again. . . .

"Dahlingest."

"Yes, Dahling?"

"Do the poo-ah do this, the proles?"

"Yes, Dahling."

"That should nevvah be allowed, it's much too good for them."

* * *

After a week he said they'd better move on, he had heard that an earthquake was imminent.

"Yes, Dahling, but surely, those things are always confined to the poorah quarters of the town?"

* * *

The Deb's sister wrote to her from America, where she had gone to try and improve the family fortunes. She said that already she had bought a new fur coat, and it only cost her a hundred bucks.

"She never could spell," said her sister.

DEATH AND BENEFIT SOCIETY

Two Brummies met.

"Eh, Albert, is that right, you've joined the Conservative Club?"

"Ar, joined it last week!"

"But yo've allus bin a Labour man, all yower life."

"I know, but the doctor said I'd only got six months to live!"

"On'y got six months to live, wot the 'ells that got to you joining the Conservatives?"

"Well, I thought as how if any body'd got to lose a member it had better be them buggers."

BLOODY IMPUDENCE

A Black Country chap said to his daughter: "I don't like that young chap as you're courtin', rough, and common, he is, and bloody stupid with it!"

"No, Dad, no!" replied the girl, "Albert's the cleverest chap I know."

"How d'yer mek that out?"

"Well, Dad, we've only bin courting nine weeks and already he's cured that little illness as I used to have every month."

LIMERICKS I

There was a young lady named Muir
Perversion she would not endure
But opened her dimple
For sex pure and simple,
Saying: "Only the simple are pure."

As I went for my train to the station
My watch stopped, Oh Hell and damnation!
So I said to this dame:
"Have you got the time?"
She said: "Yes, and a strong inclination."

There was an old spinster named Flowers
Who watched the TV at all hours
She dreamed that "Night Rider"
Was in bed beside 'er
And stayed there for "Twenty-four Hours."

There were two young ladies named Feather
Who were feeling quite under the weather,
The Vicar, named Morgan,
Said: "Purchase an organ
And then you can play 'hims' together."

As this couple came out of a clutch
The kiss that she gave him was such
That he said to her: "Right
Are you free tonight?"
She said: "No, but I never charge much."

Nudist "Camp"

There was a woman whose husband was a devil for the women. One day she told her best friend that the pair of them had joined a Nudist Club.

"Oh my dear, no! You don't mean to say you let him loose in that summer park, with all those woods and shrubberies; that you let him mix with big-breasted dollies, all starkers. You're asking for trouble."

"Not at all, we both love going there."

"But how can you take such risks? They say the wife is always last to learn, but surely you know what he is?"

"Of course, but you see, I always take jolly good care to decant him, immediately before we set out from home."

LITTLE BIG HORN?

A rancher's daughter went for a long ride across the prairie, her horse fell and broke his leg, and she was very late back. Her anxious father looked out, and saw an Indian "whoo-oo-ing" towards the ranch with the girl mounted up behind him. He gave the Indian a dollar, and said: "How did you manage to stay on, my dear?"

"Father, I nearly fell off, but he told me to reach round him and hang on to the saddle horn."

"Dern it! Don't you know Indians always ride bareback."

THE SILLY ASS

It was a poor roadside cottage. The widow told her daughter who was doing the washing out at the front, that she must on no account take her hands out of the washtub as a regiment of soldiers were coming by. Moreover, she was not on any account to look round.

A number of soldiers, finding the girl's underclothes in rags, were able to take advantage of the opportunity presented. The girl said nothing for fear her mother should hear. The regimental mascot, a donkey, also saw his chance.

The girl said: "Will the last gentleman please leave his name and address?"

OLD MARRIAGE CUSTOMS

A peasant youth from a mountain village in the Apennines went into the big city to work in hotels, and became educated by the chambermaids, who liked his rustic muscles and lack of inhibition.

He made enough money to go home and marry a virgin in the village.

On the wedding night he shaved off her pubic hair, took her in all three directions, smacked her behind with a hair brush, and finished up playing 69's. She started off objecting, but was very disconcerted to find that the longer it went on, the more she enjoyed it. She felt that this could not be right, and consulted the village priest, who, deeply shocked, immediately excommunicated the young man.

He took his new bride to New York, and a job at the Hotel Metropole. The local priest enquired why a good Italian boy was not coming to church. "It's a long story father, perhaps you could spare half an hour?"

"Tonight, at the presbytery," said the priest, "bring some whisky."

When the whisky, and the story were poured out, the New York priest laughed, and said: "That's all right my son, you're in again, don't worry."

"What father, no penances, nothing to pay?"

"Not a dime."

"But our village priest way back home said. . . ."

"Listen Alfonso, I don't want to denigrate my brothers, but really, what would a hick priest from the mountains be expected to know about normal modern western marriage customs."

RUCKING THE DUCK

A society woman had a son of eighteen, and she was very worried about him, and went to consult a psychiatrist. "Tell me all about it," said he. The lady explained that the son had gone downstairs in the night, and eaten a duck out of the fridge. Then she had caught him masturbating . . .

"No harm so far," said the doctor.

". . . in the knickers of my thirteen-year-old niece!" She added that she thought the boy would have to be put in the looney-bin.

"Not at all," said the doctor, "had he masturbated in the duck, and eaten the young lady's knickers there would have been cause for concern, but up to now it's all been natural and normal."

CAT CREPT IN CROFT

There was a clergyman in a tough district who was not satisfied with the behaviour of his congregation. The trouble was, they didn't believe in Hell Fire any more, so he decided to teach them a lesson.

He said to the Verger: "Listen, next Sunday morning I'm going to preach Hell Fire and damnation at this shower, I'm really going to get stuck into them and frighten the wit out of them."

He went on to explain that the Verger was to hide up in the rafters of the roof, armed with lots of bits of scrap paper. The parson would preach, and when he got to the line: "And fire rained down upon them" the Verger was to light the pieces of paper and float them down on the heads of the congregation.

Afterwards the parson would explain it was only a trick, but . . . "You never know."

The parson preached his heart out, he got them really worked up, and when he got to the payoff line: "And flames of fire rained down out the heavens upon them . . ." nothing happened.

This was appalling! He tried again: "And flames of fire rained. . . ."

There was a silence penetrated only by:

"It's no bloody use, Vicar, the cat's pissed on the matches."

PART OF HIS EDUCATION

There was a new young priest went to his first parish, a mining village, and the old priest arranged to be in the back of the confessional, to see if the young beginner did it right. The young man tried hard, and afterwards said:

"I didn't do too badly, did I father?"

"Well, not too badly for the first time, but next time can we have a little less: 'Whew oo-oo-ew!' and a lot more 'Tut-tut-tut'?"

WORTH PRAYING FOR

There was an Irishman visiting a strange town along with his English friend, and they were pretty bored in the evening. The Irishman decided to go to confession, and told the priest he'd been having sex with a girl.

The priest cross-examined him at length, but he wouldn't say who it was, so he got thrown out.

Waiting outside the church, his pal said: "Did you get absolution?"

"I damn well didn't, but I got some useful names and addresses."

PUT HER FOOT IN IT

The Mother Superior of the Convent awoke in a particularly happy mood, dressed, and set off to visit her flock at their labours. The first nun she came to was Sister Theresa:

"Good morning, Sister, God bless you! Are you happy at your work?"

"Yes indeed, Reverend Mother, but I'm sorry to see that you got out of bed on the wrong side this morning."

The remark distressed the Reverend Mother, but she decided to ignore it, and passed on to where another nun was busy at her task. . . .

"Good morning, Sister Bridgid, you look pleased with yourself this lovely day."

"Indeed I am Reverend Mother, everything's all right with me, but it's a pity you got out of bed on the wrong side today!"

The Mother Superior, greatly puzzled, moved on to where a little novice was working:

"Before I wish you God's blessing and a happy day, little Sister, tell me something – do you get the impression I must have got out of bed on the wrong side?"

The nun blushed, hesitated, and said: "I'm afraid so, Reverend Mother!"

"And in the name of the holy Church, why do you all say that – am I not as happy as a songbird, and pleasant to you all?"

"Yes indeed Mother, but you see, er, but you see, you're wearing Father O'Connor's house slippers."

TO THE POINT

There was a businessman who was middle-aged and not very prepossessing. He set on a typist of 18, and soon began to take her out to dine. However, he saw he was making no progress, so he started to buy her presents.

Asked what she wanted for her birthday, she said, "A real leopard-skin coat." This cost the earth, but he got her one.

One day in the office he said: "Joan, your knickers are coming down."

She blushed, hastily explored under her very short skirt, and said: "Oh no they're not."

"Yes they are, or else that coat goes back to the shop."

SUPPLY AND DEMAND

A little boy and a little girl playing alone in a shed. They decide to take their clothes off, and little girl is very upset to see that little boy has got something she hasn't got. Little boy torments her about his superiority, and she runs home to Mammy, crying.

"What's the matter dear?" said Mother, "has Johnny been hitting you?"

"No," says little girl, pointing to her fanny, "but he's got something there that I haven't got."

"Don't worry my dear," says Mother, very relieved, "believe me darling, as long as you've got one of *these*, you'll always be able to get one of *those*."

OLD CHINESE CUSTOM

Three Chinese girls discussing marriage. One said she hoped to marry a man of good birth, with two dragons on his shirt.

The next said she hoped to marry a man of good birth and great wealth, with three dragons on his shirt.

The third said she had no ambition for birth or wealth, she simply hoped to marry a man with one dragon on the floor.

WHERE DID THAT SOD GO?

There was a peppery old Colonel went to play golf. The only other man waiting for a game was the newly appointed Bishop, so they introduced themselves and set off.

The Colonel drove a mighty drive, and removed a large divot, the ball remaining stationary.

"Bugger it, missed!" said he.

The Bishop was put out, and said so.

A bit further on the Colonel again foozled a shot, and hissed: "Bugger it, missed!"

At this point the Bishop really told him off about his language, and finished up: "I warn you, the Almighty is not mocked, if you come out with any more swearing, something dreadful will happen to you."

The Colonel kept himself under control, and, needing the last hole for the match, was left with a six-inch putt.

He took careful aim and . . . missed!

His flow of blasphemies was interrupted by a terrible clap of thunder, a flash of lightning came out of the sky, and struck the Bishop dead.

From behind a black cloud was heard a deep-throated rumble: "Bugger it, missed!"

BALLS TO YOU, MISS

It was during the London air-raids, when many town children were evacuated to the country for the first time. A party of cockney kids were entering the hallway of a great manor. On the table was a brass dish, in which by chance there happened to be a couple of old golf balls.

"Wot's them rahnd things?" said a girl of twelve to the Squire's wife.

"They're golf balls my dear."

As everybody knows, the children drifted back, until the coming of the V-2 rockets, when there was another mass evacuation. . . .

The same child entered the same hallway, and this time there were four golf balls in the dish.

"Ah, missis, I see your old man's shot another golf."

A REAL GENTLEMAN

There was a parson noted for good works amongst the poor. One day he was visited by a woman in distress. She was the most unpleasing female he had ever set eyes on, dirty, bedraggled and foul of breath. Her ragged blouse had no buttons, exposing shrivelled dugs beneath. He thought she was sixty, but it turned out she was forty-five.

She told a long tale of how her husband had run away and left her with ten children, and all the time she spoke the parson was hypnotised by her one tooth, a long black fang.

She wanted the Vicar to help her get the kids in an orphanage. He was kind, he was patient, and he explained that there were various funds which would help to keep the family together, rather than break it up. After a great deal of work he got her afloat again.

*　　*　　*

Twelve months later the Vicar was in his study when his wife came in and said: "There's a fearful drab on the doorstep, and she must see you."

"Really," he said, "you know I'm writing my sermon, tell her to come back some other time."

"You're quite right dear," said his wife, "really, she's got one black tooth that. . . ."

"Oh her, she's a friend of mine, send her in at once."

The drab had come to explain that she was in trouble again – there was a new baby. The Vicar, who was a slow thinker, counted on his fingers, and said: "Here, your husband has been missing for 12 months!"

"I know," she said.

"Well, who is this man, the father? Is he going to pay you?"

"I don't know his name, Vicar, he was an Irish lodger I had, he only stayed two weeks."

cont'd over

"Good Lord in Heaven woman, you had all the troubles in the world already, what in the name of all that's holy possessed you to do a daft thing like this?"

"Well, Vicar, I thought it was very nice of him to ask me."

OLD COUNTRY CUSTOM

An elderly landed gentlewoman was riding round her estates, with an old manservant in attendance. Away on a grassy bank she thought she saw something unusual.

"Heathers," she said, "What do you see over there?"

"A blanket, Madam."

"What is it doing over there, hey?"

"Moving up and down, Madam."

"Do you see anything else Heathers?"

"A pair of lady's legs wide apart, my lady."

"What else do you see?"

"A pair of gentleman's legs between them."

"And what do they think they're doing, hey?"

"Having intercourse, Madam."

"Good Lord, does that still go on?"

DROPPED A CLANGER

There was a man went for a Government job, and when he was given a start the Labour Officer wanted his full name.

"What, just for a dockyard sweeper, my full name?"

"Yes my man, that is the strict rule."

The new sweeper was very shy about giving his full name, but at last said:

"All right then John Blast And Bugger It Smith."

Trying to keep a straight face, the Labour Officer said:

"How did you come by that name?"

"Well, Sir, it was like this, just as the parson was christening me, some silly clot knocked the lid of the font on his foot."

THOUGHT HE WAS NICKED

There was a youth in Ireland lived in the priest's house as his servant. As the boy grew towards 16 he began to feel certain urges, and asked if he could go to a dance. The priest explained that dancing meant moving around with young women in tight blouses, short skirts, etc. . . . in short, he was agen it.

The boy kept on so, that finally he was allowed to go to a dance at a town about six miles away, provided he got home by midnight. The dance finished very late, at two in the morning the frightened lad was creeping across the wild and lonely bog that led to his home. When he came to the "haunted rock" just as he feared, a dreadful creature jumped out. It had horns, and a tail, and flames were roaring out of its arse.

"Who are ye?" said the kid.

"I'm Old Nick, I'm the Devil himself," said the apparition.

"Och thank God for that, I was afraid you might be the priest!"

THE HAYCOCK

It was the church outing, and they all picnicked on a farm. After the meal one young man climbed up a bank and lay down on his back on some hay, to rest. His girl came along, and said: "Let's make love." He said he was too tired, but she said, never mind, she'd do all the work. With which she slipped her pants off, undid his trousers, and squatted across him. She heard someone scrambling up the bank, so quick as a flash, she covered him up with hay.

The Minister appeared, and said: "Oh Miss Molly, why are you sitting there like that?" She explained that her grandfather owned the farm, and when it came to her she would build a new barn over *there* (wriggling round). She would also chop down that spinney over *there* (wriggling round the other way). And when she married, she would build a little cottage over *there* (swinging round again) with a track running back to the main road over *there* (wriggle, wriggle). "Indeed, Minister, you won't recognise the place when I've finished with it."

"Perhaps not," said the Minister, but I'm sure I recognise that pair of boots sticking out of the hay, they belong to my son." "Yes, Father," said a muffled voice, "and thanks to your bloody interference she'll need to build a nursery and a pram shed."

THE SPIRIT MOVED HIM

There was a parson, full of good works, who used to do much jail visiting. One day he called in the cell of an "old lag" and said could he do anything for the man.

The man said yes, he would like to be read to, from the bible, of course.

"What would you like me to read?"

"The 119th Psalm please parson."

"My goodness brother, that's the longest psalm in the whole bible."

"Nemmind parson, I likes it."

So the good man read it over to him, and when he had finished, the old rascal said please could he have the psalm read to him all over again.

The parson said: "Yes, of course, I take it you have found true religion at last brother?"

"Well, it's not exactly that, but you see, I haven't had a drink for three years, and the smell of your breath's doing me a power o' good."

NOT IN COLDSTREAMS!

There was a strict wartime rule that water, especially hot water, was not to be wasted.

A sergeant of the Guards was taking a bath, and two ATS girls were caught peeping through a crack in the bath hut.

Put on a charge, they said it was in the course of duty.

"And what the hell d'you mean by that?"

"Sir, we wanted to see if he had more than five inches."

AT COVENT GARDEN?

A lady of the town was up before the Bench, and was asked to declare her occupation, she said she was a "dealer".

"Hey, what's that?" said the Beak, unbelieving.

"Sir, I am an old-established street trader."

"I'm not having that either," said the Beak.

The Learned Clerk, who wanted to press on, said: "Leave it to me, Sir, we'll just put down that she's in the 'wholesale' business."

"MISS" UNDERSTANDING

Some troops were stationed in a remote part of the Western Desert. One day a Brigadier flew in on inspection. They tried to keep him away from a thorn thicket that lay on the edge of the camp, but he would not have it so, and forced his way into the small enclosure. In the middle was a scruffy female camel.

Very suspiciously he bawled: "What the hell's all this?"

The young Lieutenant in charge explained that the place was a terrible long way from any women, and this camel was kept for the use of the men when they got desperate. The C.O. said it was disgusting: "Get rid of the wretched animal at once."

It so happened that some time later the Brigadier was actually posted to that camp, and after a few weeks he sent for the Lieutenant and asked what had become of the camel.

"After you'd gone, Sir, we put it back in the thicket."

That night when all was still the sentry saw the Brigadier enter the thicket carrying a stool, on which he stood and began to have intercourse with the beast.

"Hi, Sir! You're making a terrible mistake, the camel is only for the troops to ride to the nearest town on."

DOGGED DOES IT

A cowed little much-married man thought he would give his wife a birthday surprise by buying her a bra. He entered a ladies shop all flurried, but the girls took him in charge . . . what colour? . . . He settled for white. The price . . . forty shillings . . . very good.

All that remained was the size. He hadn't the faintest idea. "Now, Sir, can we say, a pair of melons? Coconuts? Grape fruit? Oranges?"

"No," he said, worried, "nothing like that."

"Come on, Sir, think! There must be something your wife's bust resembles." He thought long and earnestly, then looked up, and said:

"Have you ever seen a spaniel's ears?"

A Stockbrokers Clerk of Ostend
Whose wife caught him bulling *her friend*
(And cried: "I can't bear *it*
Why shouldn't we share *it?*")
Said: "I never withdraw *till I* spend."

There was an old spinster named Mead
Who was prudish in thought word and deed,
Yet held it no scandal
To press on the handle
Of the vessel in which she wee-weed.

There was a young Scottie named Brown
Who offered a tart half a crown,
"We Campbells," she cried,
"Have still got our pride,
I'll never take that *lying down.*"

There was a Director named Mitty
Whose blonde was all bottom and titty,
To his wife, he said: "Dear
I'll be latish, I fear,
I've a fair bit to do in the city."

A dropout and wastrel named Humming,
Did nothing but scrounging and bumming,
When his mother one day
Caught him having a lay,
He said: "I am now up and coming."

As the Bishop said to the Actress

As the Bishop said to the Actress:
I'll try and come more often. . . .

        *   *   *

"Do it Now" is a good motto. . . .

        *   *   *

We take off in half an hour. . . .

        *   *   *

It sticks out a mile. . . .

        *   *   *

Isn't it nearly opening time?

        *   *   *

HE WAS KNACKERED

There was a very uneducated man who by drive, and ruthless methods amassed a large fortune. The older he got, the richer he got, the richer he got the more women he kept, the more women he kept the less use he was to them.

One day he went to the foremost surgeon in the business, and said:

"I want to be castrated."

"You want to be WHAT?"

"I said castrated, my sexual powers are failing."

The surgeon was a bit dubious, but in view of this last statement, and for a consideration of five hundred guineas, he carried out the operation.

A few weeks later the rich illiterate man was in his club, listening to the conversation at the bar, which was "subject normal". "I say Smithers," says one Clubman to his drinking partner, "do you think there's anything in this yarn that if a man gets himself circumcised it improves his sexual performance?"

The rich illiterate retired muttering to himself . . . "*Circumcised*, that was the word I've been trying to think of."

217

NOT TOP HOLE

A certain farm labourer was down the bottom meadow when he carelessly cut his thumb in the mowing machine. It bled badly, and they had no first-aid box.

"There's on'y one remedy for that there," said the boss, a sage old farmer – "Ye must goo and put ee in a virgin's bottom, that'll stop the bleeding right away."

The labourer said where would he find such an object, and the farmer replied that a new dairymaid had started that day, he had better go up to the farm house and ask a favour.

The new dairymaid was a good-natured girl, and when Giles explained his difficulty, and showed her his thumb, she without more ado, dropped her bloomers, and bent down.

After a few moments she cried out: "Hey, Garge, that baint my bottom!"

"Baint my thumb, noither."

WAXING HOT

Some nuns were getting very restless. The weather was very hot, and quarrelling was breaking out.

The Mother Superior called them together and demanded that cards be put on the table – what exactly was the matter.

Nobody would speak until at last a Novice who had not long been in, said: "What this place needs is some healthy males."

The Reverend Mother was shocked, but another, emboldened, said: "Well, she's right, it's only human nature, isn't it?" Mother Superior had met this one before: "Very well then, as it's such hot weather I will issue you all with candles, and you have my dispensation to comfort yourselves with them."

"They're no good, we've tried them," cried several voices.

"Well indeed! when I was young they were all right, what's the objection?"

"Well, Reverend Mother, you get tired of the same thing wick in and wick out!"

LUCY LOCKET'S POCKET

One morning bright and early an old farmer set off to market to do some shopping and sell two piglets. He and his youngest daughter put the horse in the cart, but Mother decided not to come.

They sold the pigs, bought a few necessities, and set off back. Passing through a lonely wood they were set on by robbers, who took everything, including the farmer's watch. The farmer was broken-hearted, "We're ruined, we're ruined," he kept on saying.

"No Father, we're not," said the girl, "We've still got the pig money, I hid it." "You hid it? But they stripped you!"

"I know, but I stuffed the fivers up my you-know-what."

"Oh, what a pity, what a pity we didn't bring your mother, we'd have saved the sack of flour as well."

ELASTIC LIMIT

A rather fat bride would wear the latest thing in "foundation garments" and she was indeed strapped in.

The honeymoon was at her mother's house, and her mother was waiting for the floor to start rocking, but nothing much happened. Worried, the old lady crept upstairs and listened at the door. . . .

The trouble had been that the bride's zipper was firmly jammed, and she could not get undressed. Mother arrived just in time to hear:

"It's no use, Darling, we'll never make any progress unless I cut it."

"No no!" shouted mother, "don't be such a fool, just put two fingers in and gradually stretch it!"

I'LL DO IT TO "SUTURE"!

There was a well-built but rather tom-boyish schoolgirl who was always sliding down the bannisters. One day she lost control, and collided with the knob at the bottom. She was taken to a plastic surgeon, who said of course it would have to be sewn up. He was a kindly old boy, and with a merry twinkle said: "What size shall I make it?"

"Can I have it the same as my mother's?"

"Oh, all right, go back and slide down twice more."

The members of the Women's Institute in this particular country parish, fell into a series of quarrels as to whose husband had the biggest phallus.

Feeling ran really high because the Chairwoman said her husband, the Squire, had one so big that there could be no argument, and the matter was not worth discussion.

The women then challenged her to prove this. If her husband would display his weapon, they could judge whether any of their husbands could make a bigger show.

Her Ladyship was now in a right predicament, and she went home and told her husband. He said: "You know I'm small, you've lost your bets." She was so upset that in the end the Squire went to a good friend and said:

"Look here, you've got a huge one. The reputation of the gentry will be tarnished for ever through that damnfool wife of mine, if you won't cooperate."

"What do you want me to do?" said his good friend.

* * *

The upshot was that it was agreed for the judging to take place in a barn, and the great phallus was to be pushed through a knothole in a screen, so that the owner should not be embarrassed. The Committee of the Institute stood round expectantly, and when the monster was pushed through the knot hole, her Ladyship felt she had won. Alas, one of the women instantly cried:

"Hey, that's the Vicar's, I recognise the wart on the end."

WITH FUR ROUND IT

A wealthy young man had the chance to take a girl home to her flat. On the way they passed a small furriers shop, and the man said: "If you play ball with me, you can have the best fur coat in that window."

Now the girl was greedy, and she knew a shop where the coats were of a much higher quality. After the rich young man had had his lust on her, she took him round to "Superior Modes", but all he bought her was a rabbit-skin wrap for three pounds.

Home at the weekend she was crying her eyes out, and her father asked her why, so she told him.

"Good God! Didn't your poor mother teach you anything at all about men? Rule number one: When they're hard they're soft: Rule number two: when they're soft they're hard."

THE LITTLE LESS, HOW MUCH IT IS

A wealthy Bishop had three daughters. He went to his lawyer and said that as their mother was dead he wished to leave a small share of his fortune to two of the girls, but the bulk of it to the third – whichever was the most virtuous.

The lawyer said: "We can't get any further with this my lord, unless you find out definitely which is the most virtuous, you'd better devise a sure test."

The Bishop went away and thought about it, and one summer day he took his oldest daughter, who was twenty, into the shrubbery, and dropped his trousers:

"Forgive me my dear," he said, "but it's only a little test, I want to know if you know what this is?"

"Why, it's a prick," said the girl.

The Bishop thought that wasn't a very good sign of innocence, so he carried out the test with the eighteen-year-old. "It's a prick," she said.

The Bishop hoped things might be a little better with the sixteen-year-old, so he dropped his trousers and said: "My dear, can you tell me what this is?"

"To tell the truth, dear Father, I don't know what to call it."

"Ah my sweet virtuous child, I'm delighted with you, you shall be rewarded. I thought you might say it was a prick."

"My goodness! you don't call that thing a prick, do you?"

LONGED FOR OLD TIMES

A refugee from Europe had brought his mother to England with him. He prospered, but his widowed mother, who was not really old, began to pine and go into a decline. He decided to send her to a psychiatrist, but to put him in the picture, first. "Don't worry," said the head-shrinker, "I haven't forgotten my Yiddish, I'll be sympathetic."

When the old lady came in he called her "Mudder" and made her feel right at home. Then he held up a spoon, and said: "What's this?"

"Doss iss a leffel." "Fine" (showing fork). "What's this?"

"Doss iss a gappel." "Lovely, what's this?" (holding up a banana).

The widow burst into tears: "Doss iss a phallic symbol."

SMALL THINGS PLEASE SMALL MINDS

A man was urinating in one of those old-fashioned green iron pee-corners when he heard a lot of giggling, and beheld an eye glued to a crack in the plating.

He was pretty angry, and rushed outside to find a married woman and a girl about fifteen.

"Dammit, you really are vulgar," he shouted, as the girl still giggled.

The mother said: "Oh Sir, take no notice of her, she's only a child, she laughs at any little thing."

WATERING THE MILK

A little boy had never seen a horse and cart until his family moved to a country town. One day there appeared outside his home a milk float pulled by a horse. He stared in disbelief for some minutes.

When the milkman returned, the little boy said: "You won't get very far!"

"Why not?" enquired the milkman, puzzled.

"All the petrol's just run out and gone down the drain."

WHO LAVS LAST LAUGHS LAST

There was a fearful row in the nunnery, and in the end the parish priest had to be sent for.

"Sisters, sisters," he said, "what is all this storm about?"

"It's the Reverend Mother," said a bold young nun, "she keeps making the most terrible insinuations about us."

"Indeed," said the priest, "out with it, what's the charge?"

"I haven't charged anybody, and I haven't insinuated anything; I merely demanded to know how it was I found one of the lavatory seats tipped up."

PIPED

On the Sunday School outing a great deal of lemonade was drunk, and several little girls retired behind a bush to pee, and there was a certain amount of trouble with nettles and thistles.

A small boy who was with them simply pulled out his wee-wee and stood there performing.

"My," said one little girl, "that's a real handy thing to bring on a picnic."

SONG OF SOLOMON

There was a middle-class suburb of stockbrokers, young businessmen and the like, which was noted for orgies. Wife-swapping was normal, high-class floozies haunted its pubs, while actresses and models kept open house.

The Vicar of the parish, having a rich and generous congregation, was on a good thing. Everybody used to say: "Our Vicar's got a really modern outlook" as they dropped the pound notes on the plate.

However, word got round to the Bishop, who ordered the Vicar to preach strongly against these goings-on. Accordingly, the Vicar got up before the congregation, and said:

"The sins of Sodom are with us, fornication and adultery flourish, and I must, in a fashion warn you, that unless you, as it were, repent, and, so to say, change your ways, you may be, after a manner of speaking, damned."

HE SAW THE RED LIGHT

The Colonel retired from the Indian army in middle age, and settled in a London flat with his faithful black servant.

After some time he married, and brought his beautiful and toffee-nosed bride home. After the first night he rose at six, as was his custom, to take his constitutional in the park.

The black servant entered the bedroom, pulled all the sheets off the naked bride, and gave her a resounding smack on the backside. . . .

"Dawn him come. Dolly-girl now go back to naughty house."

BLACK MAGIC

A Missionary came to live with a tribe of Pygmies, and by his gifts of clothing, and superior pills, soon put the Witch Doctor out of business.

However, when the rainy season came the Pygmies developed a peculiar rash behind the knees, and the Missionary failed to cure it. The Pygmies drifted back to the Witch Doctor, who was having great success. The Missionary was beaten, he had to eat humble pie. He went to the Witch Doctor, and said: "Oh father of wisdom, tell me the secret of your cure, and I will reward thee. Blankets? Beads? Mirrors? name thy price and tell me how you get rid of the rash."

The Witch Doctor said that this was most difficult magic, and the only price he was interested in, was a night with the Missionary's daughter in western lingerie, and in the presence of his other wives. The Missionary went home and cried. His daughter (who was as plain as a stick) asked him why, and he told her. Now this girl, ever since she had come to live among these naked savages, had had a craving for black pudding. So, weeping all the while, she said she would reluctantly sacrifice her virginity to save her father's reputation.

Thus the daughter spent a long and busy night in the Witch Doctor's kraal, and returned home late next morning, pale but placid.

Father couldn't wait to hear of her sufferings. . . . "The secret?" he said, "what is this rare medicine, so valuable that only my dear girl's honour could purchase it?"

She yawned, and replied absently, "Oh, that. All he does is cut the tops off their wellingtons."

BAPTISED BY IMMERSION

Three men went out in a boat to fish in a lake. The protestants were friends – a parson and a minister, but the third, a priest, was a newcomer.

It was a beautiful sunny day, and as they weren't catching much they amused themselves looking at the scenery.

Now it happened that a very shapely young woman came down the strand, stripped off her clothes, and began paddling and bathing in the water. When she saw that she was observed, far from being coy she stood up naked on a rock, exposing her nubile charms, and waved to indicate that she wouldn't mind company.

The men were silent, but after a time the parson said:

"You know, I am a fool, I've left my prayer book on the shore, I hope you will excuse me," with which he upped and walked on top of the water to the shore. He then disappeared into the bushes with the girl, and an hour later he walked back, still dry-shod.

The minister looked thoughtful, then brightened up, and said:

"Dear me, nearly lunch time, and I've left my sandwiches in the car, pray pardon me while I fetch them." With this he stepped out of the boat, walked briskly on the water, and the nude girl was again conducted to a suitable area of green sward.

When the minister at last came back the priest was in a tidy state. He could hardly wait before he leapt overboard, and with no apologies, simply said: "I really must go and get my whisky."

As the priest went down for the third time, and only bubbles came up, the minister turned to the parson and said: "Brother, I know you and I have no time for Popish practices, yet I cannot help feel, before God and the Church, that it would have been an act of Christian charity to have told Father Brown where the stepping-stones were."

THOSE WHO'RE SAVED

A couple of London whores who had had a very busy season were feeling exhausted, and decided to "Get away from it all". They asked a travel agent, who advised a small town in rural Scotland, where all was peace and quiet.

Off they went, and terrified of being recognised for what they were, dressed very quietly, and behaved in a discreet manner. All was well until the Sabbath, when to keep up the deception, they went off to kirk with the rest of the township.

Now a new minister had arrived, and he was determined that the whole congregation should take part in the hymn singing; this was a fetish of his. It so happened that neither of these whores could sing a note, but to avoid notice, they opened and shut their mouths in time.

But in the middle of the second hymn the minister lost his patience, and shouted in "braid Scots":

"Stop, will ye, stop! It's nae guid enough! There's those that are singin' weel, but there's those who're singin' tae saft."

"Let's get out quick Mary, we're damn-well discovered again."

MADE IN CAPE HORN?

A man up in Scotland called on a garage where they did a big business in tyres and tyre repairs. Somewhat sheepishly he asked if the Manager would see him in his private office. He then produced from his wallet a somewhat tatty rubber sheath, and said:

"How much wull ye charge tae vulcanise a patch on yon?"

The Manager looked somewhat surprised, but saying nothing examined the article carefully. "About half a crown, and as you can buy a new one for three shillings, I don't see any point in it."

"Verra weel," said the caller, "Ah wull let ye know in a day or so. Ah'll have tae ask them."

"Them, them? Who the hell's them?"

"The Aberdeen Golf Club."

UN "CONVENT" IONAL!

There was a Catholic priest who had been overworking for years. He finally went to a sympathetic doctor who said: "You're worn out, father, you must go away for a really long holiday." The doctor then wrote to the Bishop, who put up the money for Father Reilly to have three months' paid vacation.

Father Reilly tried everything. He fished, he sailed boats, he walked in the mountains, and soon was again a man in the prime of health.

He had often heard about life in the West End, and as he must soon return to duty, thought he would like to see a strip club. Thus he turned up one night amid the smoke and dim lights, with a double whisky in his hand, enjoying the cabaret. Then the stripper came on, and as she did her act his bulging eyes met hers, and she gave him a wondrous smile.

After her show, the stripper came to the priest's table, placed her bare breasts under his nose, and said: "Can I fetch you another drink, Father Reilly?"

He blenched. "Now by the Holy Church, I'm discovered! I'm utterly ruined! I'll be unfrocked!"

"Don't worry, Father," said the girl, "I'm Sister Theresa, I think we must have the same doctor."

RAISING COCKS?

On Monday morning teacher asked three boys in the class:

"What was your mother doing when you left the house?"

The first said: "Doing the washing."

The second said: "Vaccing the bedrooms."

The third said: "Getting ready to go out and shoot pheasants."

"What ARE you on about" said teacher.

"Well Miss, me dad's left home and she threw her knickers on the fire and said she was going back to the game."

230

TOOK HIMSELF IN HAND

The Jones' were social climbers, and when they moved into a "select" district they decided to ask some of the more superior neighbours in to play bridge one evening. Everything was laid out perfectly, and they packed Junior, who was twelve off to bed, and settled down for a nice evening. Unfortunately, Junior misbehaved. He kept coming back downstairs . . . he couldn't sleep . . . his leg hurt . . . he wanted water. There was interruption after interruption.

Finally a distinguished old gentleman who was a church-warden and a much respected schoolmaster was appealed to.

"Yes," he said, "I can quieten him, somebody take my hand for ten minutes and leave the rest to me," with which he took Jimmy upstairs.

The rest of the evening was perfect, and not a sound was heard from Junior. As the guests departed, Mrs Jones thanked the old gentleman profusely, and asked him what the secret was.

"Quite easy, Madam, quite easy. I simply taught him to masturbate."

EXTRA SENSORY PERCEPTION

An old gentleman went into a public convenience and found a grammar school boy about sixteen masturbating himself.

"And what do you think you're doing?" he asked angrily.

"Never mind what I'm doing – duck off," said the boy.

"You think I don't know what you're doing, but I do know what you're doing," went on the old gent.

"You think you know what I'm doing, but you don't," said the boy.

"Well, what are you doing then?" said the man.

"I'm a Christian Scientist, and I'm doing my girl in Edinburgh."

SHORTCOMING

Two men went behind a hedge to pee. Says one: "I wish I had a big one like my brother's. His is so big he has to hold it with four fingers."

His friend paused, looked, and said:

"But you're holding yours with four fingers!"

"Yes, but I'm wetting on three of them."

RELIGIOUS PRINCIPLES

There was a young woman who was naturally kind hearted, and she used to go round to her Granny's every Saturday to do the old lady's bedrooms for her. Quite by chance she opened an old box in the wardrobe, and found about five hundred pounds in loose money. She rushed down to Granny, who explained: "It's very simple my dear, next year your Granddad retires, and I've saved and scraped a bit together over the years, so's we can have just a few comforts when we go on pension."

The girl said it was absolutely daft not to put the money into the Post Office to avoid theft, and she kept on about it until Granny agreed to let her take it there and then. It was a fine warm day, so the young woman took a short cut through the woods, to reach the village post office. In the very darkest part, a rough youth jumped out flourishing a knife, and said: "Give me your handbag or I'll cut your throat."

The girl was desperate to distract him. She opened her dress, exposed a very fine pair of bubs, and said: "I'm sure you'd rather play with these."

"No, I must have the money!"

She stepped out of her knickers, lay down on her back, opened her very nice thighs, and said: "Surely a fully blooded male would rather have a virgin than thirty bob out of a handbag?"

He said: "I'd just love to, but I can't."

"Do you mean to say, you snivelling wretch, that you're impotent?"

"No, not at all, but I've given it up for Lent."

AS IN LIFE SO IN DEATH

Something had gone wrong at the Crematorium. The Manager looked out of his window, and saw a queue of hearses all up the drive. He rushed out and said to his foreman: "What the blazes is the hold up?"

"Sorry boss, but we've got a coffin stuck, it won't go in the oven."

The Manager rushed to have a look, and to his amazement, he saw that it was a Y-shaped coffin. He ran back to the office, rang up the undertaker, and said: "What the hell d'you mean by sending me a Y-shaped coffin?"

"I couldn't help it, I had no choice," said the Undertaker.

"What do you mean – you couldn't help it."

"She was a very sexy young woman."

THE HEIGHT OF OPTIMISM

Mary: What's the meaning of the saying "The height of optimism?"

Jane: When you're six months gone and rub it with vanishing cream.

* * *

CHILD'S ESSAY

Sir Francis Drake circumcised the globe with a forty-foot cutter.

* * *

ALL BULL

The Papal Bull is kept at the Vatican to provide milk for the Pope's children.

* * *

ASS OVER PIP?

A man came out of a pub, trod on some orange peel, and fell arse over tip. Little girl: Mummy, how did that man know it was a blood orange?

* * *

233

THE FIRST TRADE UNIONIST

Teacher: Who invented the Five Day week?

Johnny: Please Miss, it was Robinson Crusoe.

Teacher: What makes you say that?

Johnny: My Dad says Robinson Crusoe had to work hard all the week and he was always buggered by Friday.

* * *

DEAD A LONG TIME

Letter from a Coroner to a Town Clerk: I must have a Deputy, I never get a holiday, I haven't slept outside my own bed for twenty years, and my wife badly needs a change.

* * *

PILLS TO THAT GAME

Mary: What do they call a man whose wife refuses to take the Pill?

Jane: "Daddy" I should think.

* * *

WHO'S ZOO

Biology Teacher: How do hedgehogs make love?

Bright Student: With the utmost caution, I suspect!

* * *

LIMERICKS III

There was a young laundress named Gert
Who couldn't get into her skirt,
Her dildo she'd smothered
With starch which had covered
The front of a clergyman's shirt.

A reckless young sculler named Box
Forced the Oxford crew on to the rocks,
The Eight shouted: "Rowlocks!
You've ripped off our bowlocks
And terribly injured our cox."

There was a young lady named Lee
Whose quim was as small as could be
When needing a lay
A search fee she'd pay
And loan the binoculars, free.

A pious young widow named Dove
Was wearing black garters, for love,
"They remind me," she'd say,
As she stripped for a lay
"Of many who've gone up above."

A sexy young lady named Hall
Whose tits were exceedingly small
Made up for the lack
With a very large crack,
Her love life was "having a ball".

The Crusader and the Chastity Belt

There was a Baron who had a most beautiful young wife, and he wished to ride forth on the Crusades. Knowing his wife's passionate nature, and that he would be gone at least a year, he consulted his Magician, who advised fitting the lady with a chastity belt. So the Baron went to the best man in the business, and duly the lady, although protesting a great deal, was locked up in it.

"But my Lord," she cried: "If by any mischance you are killed, I shall be encased in it to my grave." Her husband took the point, and consulted with his Magician again, following which, he announced to all the Court that he would leave the key with the most trustworthy man in England, namely, the Archbishop of Canterbury.

* * *

Thus it came to pass a few days later, a ship loaded with Crusaders was just casting off from Dover when a very dusty Archbishop arrived on the quayside on a very exhausted horse. . . .

"Hey!" he shouted, "this is the wrong key!"

"You're telling me!" said the Baron.

THE BITER BIT

There was a King who wanted to go on the Crusades, but he was very worried about his wife, who was a bit too oolalla to be left alone for a long time. The King consulted his Bishop, who had a bright idea. He explained that he knew a smith so cunning that he could make a suitable device to fix on the lady and keep the men off.

Thus it came to pass that the Bishop produced a man-trap device with fearful teeth, so set that if any male approached it, it would snap shut, with devastating results.

When the King returned from his travels he lined all the Courtiers up, and demanded from each in turn, whether he had behaved like a true gentleman to the King's wife. Each swore that he had, and the King noted with grim satisfaction that each had a high-pitched voice. Only the Court Jester acted awkward, he wouldn't answer any questions at all.

"He seems to have lost his tongue!" said the King.

"Indeed he has," said the Bishop.

DIRTY DOG FASHION

There was a miner who went off to the pit for the afternoon shift, but when he got there it was to find that there was a breakdown in the plant, and they were all sent home again.

The miner returned to find his plump wife bending down over the sink, washing up. Without a word he upped her skirts, dragged her drawers down and quickly had his will on her.

Having finished he gave her bare behind two or three vicious blows.

"You nasty rotten bleeder!" she said, "I stood there and let you have your will on me, and all the thanks I got for it was a good 'idin'."

"That was for not looking round to see who it was," he said.

WAAL BRUSH MA NUTS!

There was an American gentleman of the Deep South who was proud of his family and traditions. One day there called a distant cousin, an Englishman. A splendid meal was laid on, followed by genuine old Scotch, and ceegars worth five dollars apiece. Just "Southern hospitality".

"Now, Sir," said the host, "As Ah wuz naat a-ware of yo' arrival, Ah arranged to go to Rotary right now, but my wife, wa-al, I guess she'll entertain ya, an' show y' th' garden an' ma prerry lawns." With which he departed.

The wife showed the guest the house and garden, and then, in a shady corner of the lawn, began to undress. "I say!" said the Englishman, "I'm not an utter cad you know."

She explained that this was just part of famous "Southern hospitality" – what else did her husband mean by "show him the lawns"? They couldn't do it in the house with the children in bed, now, could they?

She lay on her back, the Englishman stripped and got on with it. Quite soon the husband returned however, but the first the guest knew about it was when he heard the husband's voice from the porch of the house:

"Sadie, Sadie, aint y'shure ashamed! Is this what you call Southern hospitality. Arch up you' back at once, an' raise the ge'man's boils off of the demp grass!"

SPIRITUAL NEEDS

There was an Irishman hastening up and down a train, putting his head in every compartment and asking for a priest. He was clearly distressed, and when he came back a second time, a Methodist Minister looked up from the Church Herald and said: "We are all brothers in the Lord, although I am only a humble Methodist minister, if you will take me to your friend who is ill or distressed, I will comfort him as well as I may."

"It's meself that's after bein' distressed!" said the Irishman, "and noone else besides."

"What can I do for you brother?"

"Nothing! I must have a priest, I'm stuck for a bottle opener."

COFFEE IN BED

There was a soldier who had been abroad for some years, and his turn came round for home leave. He gave his wife the date, but by getting a lucky air-lift he arrived a week early. His wife, who had had a black baby in his absence, was startled to see the husband coming up the garden path, and she hastily hid the baby in the wardrobe.

Husband came in, brown from the African sun, ordered his wife upstairs immediately, and followed her. While she was undressing he casually looked in the wardrobe, and saw the coloured child.. . . .

"I – I'm sorry about that," stammered the wife.

"So am I," said the husband, "how did the little devil manage to follow me all this way?"

COULDN'T LOVE FOR TOFFEE

A married couple began to have rows, and the upshot of it was she locked him out of her bedroom for three weeks. He slept in the spare room, and seemed so little bothered that she greatly regretted her rashness.

One night she was just retiring when there came a knocking on the door.

"It's me knocking," he said.

"Of course I know it's you knocking."

"But I bet you don't know what I'm knocking with, or you'd open the door."

"Will you let me have it darling, if I let you in?"

"Of course I will, it's here, ready in my hand, I'm dying to give it you."

She threw her nightie off and slid back the bolts.

He entered and gave her a tin of caramels.

HOLEY SMOKE?

Two Irishmen were approached by the priest, and asked what they would give up for Lent.

After discussion Kelly said he would pack in smoking. Reilly said he would renounce sex.

Two weeks later Reilly was asleep and having a marvellous dream in which he lay in a bath full of beer watching a TV horserace in which his 20–1 fancy was leading the field. . . . His wife shook him awake.

"Pat," she said, "Pat wake up, I want to tell yez somethink."

"What is it now woman?" said her husband irritably.

"Pat, today I saw Mike Kelly smoking back o' the bike shed."

HOPE FOR THE FUTURE GENERATION

An earnest spinster schoolteacher got herself seduced by a preacher.

As she rose from her bed and began to get dressed, she said: "Oh, I can't get up in front of those children next week and tell them to be good, now I'm nothing but a regular sinner!"

"Regular sinner, Gwendoline, you've only done it once!"

"Yes, but we've got the whole weekend in front of us haven't we?"

HACKING

There was an English working man who won some money on the "pools" and decided that he and his wife should "see the world". However, by the time they got as far as Texas they had spent much more than they bargained for.

There was a rodeo advertised, with many cash prizes on offer, so in they went. The star event was for a "greenhorn" to ride the bucking broncho.

Over the loudspeakers came the message, that if any amateur could stay on the unbroken bronc for fifteen seconds he should have a thousand dollars. Many brave young men had a go, but they all got hurt, for he was indeed a vicious animal.

Suddenly, Dad got up and said he'd have a go. Mother clutched his jacket, but he slipped out of it, and entered the ring. Everybody laughed, but he stayed on, and collected the thousand dollars.

When he got back to his seat, his wife said: "But you've never been on a horse in your life, how DID you do it?"

"I know Mother, but don't you recall how when we went on honeymoon you had the whooping cough?"

DOING IT THE HARD WAY

There was a man whose wife led him a hell of a life. He went to consult an old friend on his problems, and the friend says: "Do you ever have sex with her?"

"What! That skinny old stringbag, why it would kill her."

"There you are then," said the friend, "get on a diet of oysters and raw egg, get in training, then do her three times every night. She can't refuse you, that's grounds for a divorce, but at the end of a month she'll be dead."

The man went into training, and did as he was bid. Three weeks later his old friend met him in the street. His back was bowed, his hands trembled, his head shook, his eyes rolled about, and he could scarcely walk.

"Ha," said his friend, "how's your wife?"

"Well, Jack, outwardly she looks very plump and well, but I'm laughing, because, although she doesn't know it, she's only got a week to live!"

STORY WITH NO WHISKERS ON IT

A businessman had a shapely young wife and he rather neglected her in favour of the Stock Exchange. When she suggested a holiday he said: "You go off my dear, I've got a lot to do at the office."

She fixed herself up for a fortnight away, and the husband was very pleased, until he found out it was at a Nudist Camp, when he began to be very suspicious. In the end, when she swore to be modest in her conduct, he let her go.

When the wife came home and went to bed with her husband, she tried to get undressed in the dark, which was unusual. He switched the light on again, and observed that she was bare at the fork, her dark brown curly thatch was missing.

His worst fears were aroused. He demanded an instant explanation: "And it had better be good, or you're divorced, and without a penny!"

The girl said it was that long spell of wet weather.

"Wet weather?"

"Yes, it rained three days running, there was nothing to do but sit in the Social Hut and play cards."

"And now you're going to say you lost your Ace of Spades – come on, the truth girl, the truth?"

"I'm telling you, we played Strip Poker."

"How could you play Strip Poker in a Nudist Camp?"

"We used pairs of tweezers. Oh darling, I had a most terrible bad run of cards, and you wouldn't want your little wife to come home without any eyebrows now, would you?"

PUSHING THE BOAT OUT

An innocent girl got a date with a man and they went for a long walk in the country. Coming to a pond, the young man boldly flashed himself out and urinated into the water.

The girl was in need too, and thought if he could make a splash, she could, so she dropped her drawers and did the same.

"Oh dear," she said, "I think I wee-weed into a canoe!"

"No dear, that was just your own reflection."

SOLD HIM THE DUMMY

An ignorant man was left some money in a will, provided he had an heir. As he had been married several years with no offspring, he consulted the doctor. The doctor said, after tests, that this man could never become a father. "Doctor, I could afford to pay you a hundred pounds if you could solve this one for me." "Easy," said the doctor, "have you never heard of A.I.D.?"

The man said he hadn't. The doctor explained that the woman was made pregnant by another man's seed. The patient said that under no circumstances would he have another man doing his wife.

"Don't be silly, there's no intercourse involved, leave this to me." He went on to say that the wife must come to his surgery next evening, to see if she approved of the Donor. A suspicious husband followed behind. He peeped through the curtains, he saw his wife introduced to a handsome young man, he saw the doctor called to the telephone, and he saw the doctor leave to answer an urgent call.

When he resumed his vigil at the window he saw his naked wife thrashing about under the Donor, who was giving her the belting of a lifetime. When the doctor returned up the garden path he was met by the husband, who said:

"Come and look doctor"—the doctor peeped—"you know doctor, you said there would be no intercourse, and it's a good job I trust you, or else I would have swore he was doing her."

244

SEDUCTION NO RAPE

There was a convent bred girl who went out with a man who used to kiss her goodnight against a dark wall. She began to get slightly worried, and she went back to the convent to ask for advice.

"Tell me all about it from the beginning my child," said the Mother Superior. The girl explained that at first this young man got out a hard thing and pressed it against her. After a few weeks he was pushing an inch, and then two inches up her wee-wee. Lately it had been five inches, and last night it was six.

"And what is it you want to ask me, my child?"

"Well, Reverend Mother, I want to know if I'm taking too much risk, I mean, do you think that if I let him go on like this, one night he might rape me?"

CAVES OF DELIGHT

A widow married for the second time, and she was greatly disappointed with her new husband's equipment. One evening she was in such a bad temper he asked what was the matter.

"I had a bad dream last night."

"Tell me about it?"

"I dreamed I was at a big auction sale, and men were bidding for phalluses. The long ones made up to five pounds, the thick ones were fetching six pounds, and the long thick ones over ten pounds."

"I see, and what about those like mine?"

"Those like yours were withdrawn, not reaching the reserve."

The husband said that was a strange coincidence, for he too had had a similar dream. . . .

"I dreamed they were auctioning quims, the tight muscular ones fetched really high bids, and the unbroken ones over twenty quid each."

"And now I suppose you are going to make out that one like mine was considered useless?"

"Not at all dear, that's where they held the auction."

HE BELTED HER WELL

A young bride was very ill-educated. When she found herself pregnant she rushed off to the doctor for advice. He told her a number of things. Then she asked: "What is the best position for actually having the baby?"

The doctor said the nurse would see to all that. The young woman explained that her husband was just taking her out to Arabia where he'd got a good job, there would only be native help: "What's the best English position for delivering it?"

"Exactly the same as when you conceived it."

"Great heavens doctor, do you mean I've got to give birth in the back of a car parked in a field with my ankles lashed up in the safety belts?"

SINGULAR

A young woman went to the doctor and said she wanted an operation or some drugs or something, as, try as she might, she could not conceive a baby, and her husband was nearly worn out.

"How long have you been married my dear?"

"Two years doctor."

"Two years! Good lord, give Nature a chance girl, go away and keep trying. If in another four years, nothing has happened, come back and we will see if intervention is indicated."

The woman said: "But doctor, I was brought up in total innocence, ignorance would be a better word, but the one thing I've known since I was at school, was this, that if you wanted a baby, all you had to do was have one night in bed with a man."

"Ah yes," said the old doctor, *"but only when you're single."*

CHALKING IT UP

A man lived an average sort of life, and he died, and went up to meet Saint Peter, and said: "Can I come into Heaven?"

"Heaven," said Peter, "this isn't Heaven." He went on to explain that the Pearly Gates were much higher up, and could only be reached by very long ladders, which varied according to circumstances. . . .

"You take this chalk and start climbing. For each sin of adultery, fornication, lechery, or whatever, you chalk off one rung."

The man kept going for ages, his legs ached, his arms ached, and he met no one. All at once he saw a fellow in a curious garb descending the neighbouring ladder.

"Excuse me, Sir," he said, "are you by any chance an angel going back for more candidates?"

"No indeed, I'm the Archbishop of Canterbury going back for more chalk."

A LOAD OF TRIP-LETS

There was a young parson whose wife was expecting, and he was pacing up and down outside a Maternity Ward.

At last the midwife came out and said: "Congratulations, you've got a bonny pair of twins!"

"Oh dear, oh dear," said the parson, "I'm afraid that's the end of our marriage, I never thought she would be unfaithful."

"Unfaithful, don't talk daft."

"But you see nurse, I was only wicked once, the other one isn't mine."

WHIRLED AROUND

There was a man in a strange town, and he thought he might as well go to a dance. He entered the local "Palais", but before long he was taken short, and not knowing the place, he could not find the toilets. He asked an attendant, who replied in an unfamiliar dialect that it was: "Up thur, and rahnd thur, and up them stairs."

More and more desperate he wandered through store rooms and attics, and in the end did the job in a cleaners' cupboard (as he thought).

When the young man got back down to the big ballroom, the place was empty, except for the commissionaire.

"Where have they all gone?"

"Where have they all gone? They've all gone to look for the rotten bleeder that used the fan room as a lavatory."

GROUP SEX

A young woman rushed into a police station, and said:
"I've been graped!"

"Beg pardon, Miss, do you mean you've been raped?"

"No Sergeant, there was a bunch of them."

THE LONG AND THE SHORT OF IT

There was a strongminded woman married to a meek little man, though all his pals at work kept telling him to assert himself.

One day she told him: "We're going up town this afternoon to buy you a new pair of trousers." Off they went to the shop, and she chose the trousers for him. The shop assistant said: "Now these come in several styles, do you want button flies or zipper flies?"

"Zipper," replied the man, quickly.

"Very good, Sir, and do you want a five-inch zip or a ten-inch?"

"Ten inch," said the man, before his wife could intervene.

* * *

When they got outside, she was furious. "You!" she said, "You and your ten-inch zip! Why you remind me of the man who lives next door to my father. Every morning he goes down his garden and unlocks his garage, then he opens the eight-foot double doors, then he wheels his bike out."

TOOK HIS GIRL FOR A SPIN

There was a girl went home and told her mother she must break her engagement. Her mother asked why, and she said: "He's too tall, and too fond of practical jokes." Mother explained that tall men were to be preferred, and a sense of humour was vital in marriage. . . . "Tell me more about the trouble – confide frankly in your mother," she said.

"Well, Mother, when he says goodnight to me in the back porch he puts his hand in my blouse." "That's no harm," says mother, "go on."

"Then he lifts my skirt, pulls down my knickers, and puts it in."

"After all," said mother, "this is the age we live in, and you ARE engaged."

"But Mother, next he straightens his legs, lifts me clear of the ground, and applies his famous sense of humour."

"A little uncomfortable perhaps," said mother, "but hardly grounds for a broken engagement."

"Ho, alright Mother! How would YOU like to be spun round like an aeroplane propellor?"

STRIPPING THE OLD GEYSER

Workmen's Time Sheets received by Borough Surveyor
4 hours stripping old geyser in bathroom (would not get hot).

* * *

Trimming the virgins on either side of the highway, 8 hours.

* * *

4 hours mating on sewers.

* * *

8 hours mating with tractor (horse not available).

* * *

Half day, stripping young Ivy at rear of Park Pavilion.

* * *

HE MUST HAVE BEEN A LITTLE WET

There was a woman with a large family of small children. As she was married to a jockey they were quite well off, and set on an Au Pair girl. The first evening the Au Pair arrived the woman was called away to a sick relative. She said to her: "I want you to bath all the children, littlest first, and put them to bed. I warn you, some of the boys are little devils."

"I am peasant daughter, ver' sthrong, und I hab brudders, I vill conquer, Madame, you vill see."

So the woman went out, and when she came back she asked how the bathing time had gone. The girl explained that with only one exception she had washed and bedded the kids with no trouble. . . .

"Only dat big boy mit der red 'air, 'e stroggle und fight sometink terrible. I am mit der blows smitten, but I overcomen him at last."

"With red hair?" said the mother, "my God, that was my husband!"

LIMERICKS IV

Here lieth an innocent maid
By a medical student betrayed
Caesarian section
Came after injection,
She thought he was teaching First Aid.

A lesbian just out of jail
Was asked how she managed for tail
Said: "Up inside 'holloway'
Putting dildol away,
A Miss is as good as a Male."

There was a young baker named Hall
Whose wife had a child every Fall,
His partner, an oaf
Said: "I use my loaf
My Missus has no kids at all."

A jungle explorer named Bunce
Took photos of native-girls' fronts
In no beads enveloped,
But they're not developed,
He's going again in twelve months.

There was a young sailor named Viner
Who failed to get in a vagina
When visualised frontal
It ran horizontal
He forgot he was stationed in China.

Cock and Bull Story

A farmer kept the parish bull, and made a good thing out of the stud fees. However, during a busy harvest season he and his older son had to be down in the fields a great deal.

The farmer said to his young son, who was twelve, "Sam, stay in the yard, if anybody brings a cow, turn the bull out, and take three pounds off them."

The boy had several customers, then things went quiet, and he was just about to lock the bull up when a big angry-looking man came up carrying a shotgun and a whip.

"I'm farmer Giles," he said, "where's your father?"

"He's out, Sir, and my brother's out. There's only me in, can I help you?"

"No you can't, your brother has put my daughter in the family way!"

"That's right, Sir, you'll have to see father, I don't know how much he charges for Harry."

LOOKING FOR A WIRE

There was a young working man whose wife was expecting their first baby. Mother-in-law, who was as thrilled as the rest of them, lived a long way off. Mother-in-law insisted that she should be sent a telegram immediately the child arrived, giving full details. Son-in-law said he was much too shy to write such things out in front of a Post Office girl.

After a deal of argument, Mother-in-law said it would do if the telegram was in code.

The great day arrived, and Mother-in-law was somewhat surprised to receive a telegram reading: BICYCLE ARRIVED SAFELY PUNCTURED BACK AND FRONT PUMP AND TOOLBAG MISSING.

SHE'D HAD A NIBBLE

There was a small boy who kept biting his nails. His mother warned him that if he didn't stop he'd get like *that* (pointing to a pregnant woman sitting opposite in the bus).

From then on, the boy never took his gaze off the woman's belly, until in the end she angrily said: "Little boy why are you staring at me?"

Down the crowded bus rang his reply: "Because I know how you got like that."

CIRCUMSTANTIAL EVIDENCE

There was a commercial traveller called on a farmer to sell him a new tractor. The farmer didn't want a new tractor. "In fact, I'm thinking of packing in farming," he said.

The traveller was persistent. The farmer was obdurate.

Finally the farmer said: "Look here, I'm in real trouble, and if you can get me out of it, I'll buy a tractor." He went on to explain his problem. The previous afternoon he had brought home a new cow. . . .

"When I went to milk her she turned out a devil. She brought round her right leg and kicked the bucket over, so I tied her leg to the stall. Then she brought round her left leg, and kicked ME, so I lashed it to the other post. Next she swung her tail and knocked my hat off, so I tied her tail to the rafters.

"By this time I was sweating, so I took my coat off. Then I needed a piss, so I undid my trousers and stood behind the cow to relieve myself.

"At that moment my wife walked in, and if you can convince HER. . . ."

GETTING DOWN TO IT

There was a widow who had one son, and when he got married she was envious. Her son and his wife had the front parlour, and every evening she used to go and listen outside the door.

Every evening after tea she would hear her son say: "Come on Mary, let's have half an hour on the rug." Sometimes it would be the girl who would say: "Don't bother about the telly Jack, let's have a bit of time on the rug together."

Mother's suspicions got worse when she once heard:

"Whatever else happens, Mother mustn't find out about this."

Christmas came, and imagine mother's surprise when the couple presented her with a lovely rug, assuring her they had made it themselves!

PRAYING FOR IT

A woman was being treated by a doctor for sore knees. She made no improvement so he said: "Look, something's rubbing the skin off your knees as fast as it heals – is it prayer?"

"No Doctor, it's my husband, he will have his sex dogfashion on the floor, and in no other way."

The doctor sent for the man, and gave him a telling-off: "There's plenty of other positions for sex," he told him.

"No Doctor, no there aint, not if we're going to watch the telly as well."

HAND REARED

A man went to his doctor because he was so run down.

"Do you get a regular sex life?" asked the doctor.

"Oh yes," said the man, "with my wife, twice a day."

"I see, anyone else?"

"Yes, Doctor, with my secretary, twice a day."

"Now you look here young man, you'll have to take yourself in hand."

"But I do Doctor, twice a day."

THE PEDLAR CALLED

A busy Registrar of Births Deaths and Marriages noticed that on four birth notifications for the same day, the father was the same Joe Bloggs, though the mothers lived far apart.

He made it his business to visit the father on pretext of checking the facts: he turned out to be a little runt of a middle-aged plumber.

"Look here," said the Registrar, "North Side, South Park, East End, and Western Boulevard, all miles apart. And four in one day, how DO you manage it?"

"It's quite easy, Sir, you see, I've got a bicycle."

THE PEEHOLE

There was a most virtuous spinster, who boasted that no man had ever been near her. When she was forty-five a wide boy married her for her considerable fortune. When he went along to draw a couple of thousand to put on the gee-gees, her solicitor said:

"She tells me the marriage is not consummated, therefore it's not a marriage. If you don't give her what she got married for, not only do you draw nothing, but she can divorce you, and make you pay the costs."

"But listen mister, I can't, I can't, her quim's too small!"

"What do you mean, too small? You ought to be damn pleased."

"I tell you it's too small ever to operate."

The solicitor sent for a doctor neighbour of his to come over and hear the tale.

"What do you MEAN by small?" said the latter. "Is it like a banana split?"

"Smaller than that."

"Is it like the cleft of my chin?" – "Smaller than that!"

"Like a cowrie shell?" – "No."

"Well, for cripes sake, what is it like?"

"Listen, Doctor, have you ever seen a mouse's earhole?"

LOVE'S ENTANGLEMENT

There was a rich old devil who married a young shapely piece, and really fancied himself in bed.

On the first night he began to grind away, and soon she was squeaking and squawking. "Am I stretching you honey?" he chortled through his toothless gums.

"No dammit, but your truss is tangled with my whiskers."

PUTTING UP THE MAINMAST

There was a low-class whore who swore she could take any man. A Portsmouth sailor took her round the back of a pub and put her against the wall. She began to get really frightened: "Here," she said, "steady up past my heart."

"Never mind your heart, hold your hat on."

UPS AND DOWNS OF MARRIAGE

A man went home and told his wife he had received a great honour – he had been asked to lecture to the Rotary Club.

"What will you lecture on dear?"

"Flying," he said.

"Why you silly fool, you've had no experience of flying since you left the Royal Flying Corps in 1918, and then you got grounded!"

They had quite an argument, and the man knew his wife was right, but he wasn't going to admit it. Privately he decided to lecture on sex instead, but he didn't tell her.

* * *

A day or two later the wife met another Rotary wife. "Did you hear how my husband's talk went?" she enquired.

"Yes, they said it was very good indeed."

"Was it, you amaze me!"

"Why do you say that, dear?"

"Well, my husband has only been up three times in his life; the first time he was sick, the second time, he blacked out, and the third time, his hat blew off."

257

HIGH OCTANE

A man had the bonnet of his car up, and his head inside.

A drunk came by, and became a nuisance. . . .

"Wash marrer ol' man, gorrer sphot o' trouble. What ish it, eh?"

The motorist was abrupt. . . . "Piston broke."

"Ah, thash bad luck, pishton broke, sho am I, sho am I."

WRONG ORGAN

There was a girl sitting on the settee in the front room with her new young man. After speaking about the weather he fell into a long silence.

"Look here," she said, "when you have a girl all by herself, can't you do something?"

"Oh, ar," he said, with which he produced a mouth-organ and began to play it.

VERY INDUSTRIOUS

The famous Climax engines and fork-lift trucks are made in Coventry. A group of students from the University of Warwick were given a "project" namely, to research into the habits of young married couples who both went to work, to see if it affected their sex life. They went from door to door with their questionnaires, and one student was greeted by a smashing young housewife, who said, Yes, she was willing to give information.

"How old are you?"

"I'm 22, he's 25."

"I see, and how often do you have sex?"

"Every night, and twice on Saturdays and Sundays."

"Now, Madam, this is rather personal, and if you feel you do not want to answer it, it's up to you, but, er, how long does it generally take you to get to orgasm?"

"I beg your pardon, I don't follow?"

"How long does it take you to reach the climax?"

"Well, ten minutes if I catch the bus, but half an hour if I have to walk."

RATTLING IDEA

Some Secondary School girls were having an intimate conversation about what they did when they went out with boyfriends.

"I always carry a sheath in my handbag," said the first.

"I get some pills off my mother's dressing table," said the next.

There was silence. "Come on, Theresa, what do you do?"

"You know Catholics aren't allowed to use those things, they're artificial."

"Yes, but you're not frustrated, what do you DO?"

"I carry a biscuit tin with a few stones in it."

(Both together): "A biscuit tin! How does that work?"

"Easy, I make him stand on it, and when it starts to rattle I kick it from under him."

DUCKING THE ISSUE

Three girls in distress went to a centre of Religious Healing. The Reverend Master in charge asked what could he do for them? One had got tiny breasts and wanted them bigger, one had got legs like beansticks and she wanted plump sexy thighs, the third was doubled up in a wheelchair.

It was explained to them that this was much too tall an order for a provincial healing centre, but if they were to go to the River Jordan and totally immerse themselves, they would stand a good chance, provided they had *faith* as well. The Reverend Master, who had questioned them closely, was satisfied that Mary and Jean had faith, but about Agnes in the wheelchair he was very doubtful. However she swore she had faith too, and he sent them off to the Jordan with the necessary documents and introductions.

When the great day arrived, Mary went first, totally immersed herself in the icy stream, and came out with a superb pair of breasts.

Jean went next, bravely ducked, and walked up with splendid thighs and a round bottom to match.

It was necessary to get local assistance to get the wheelchair out, and when it was pulled up the bank the anxious watchers noticed that it now had a brand new pair of tyres.

IT DEPENDS WHAT YOU MEAN

A young married man was thrilled when his wife was expecting their first child. As soon as she was in labour he took her off to the Maternity Hospital.

The same night he rushed up to the hospital enquiry desk to enquire.

"Ward 3B," they said, "and she's had triplets."

He ran up the stairs and was barging into the ward when a frosty Sister promptly threw him out again.

"How dare you come in here, you're not sterile!" she said.

"Sterile! Me? I should bloody well think I'm not sterile, I've just fathered triplets!"

ACTIONS SPEAK LOUDER THAN WORDS

There was a Professor of English in the University of Oxford, who was a very great stickler for the correct use of words. Unfortunately he had a termagant wife who led him a hell of a life.

One day this nagging bitch announced that she would go and have a holiday with her mother. She packed her bags, summoned a taxi, and departed.

The Professor couldn't wait. He took the very sexy housemaid into his study, pressed a five pound note into her hand, and found her only too willing.

Unfortunately the wife had forgotten her handbag, and ten minutes after departure, she returned. Finding no one downstairs, and hearing some unusual noises she rushed aloft and opened the study door. The maid's knickers and bra were on a chair, and the maid was not inside them. The Professor was far too busy to notice her entry until she shouted:

"John, John, I AM surprised!"

Occupied as he was, yet this gross abuse of English pulled him up short:

"No no, my dear, it is WE who are surprised, YOU are amazed."

THE BLACK PUDDING CLUB?

There was an old Professor of Anthropology at Oxford who had a hatred of women, and especially of women students. One day he noticed half a dozen of them sitting in the front row, legs and busts in full view.

The Professor addressed the class: "Gentlemen, this morning we are going to talk about the Trobriand Islanders. This race of naked barbarous savages never wash, and they smell. They live upon herbs which give their breath a foul odour. Their male members are twice normal size, and they place on a ring of thorns before intercourse. In these wretched islands there are four men to every woman, so even the ladies of Lady Margaret Hall might find a husband there."

The girls were so disgusted they rose in a body and walked out.

As they got to the door he shouted: "Don't hurry, the steamers only go every six months."

APPRECIATIVE AUDIENCE

There was a young married woman who went to her doctor for some help. She explained that her husband never made love to her, was she lacking in something, she was certainly frustrated. The doctor examined her all over, one excuse was as good as another, for she had a really shapely body.

"It's not you, it's him," he said, "but put one of these pills in his tea at breakfast time, and I think by bedtime he'll be a bit randy." He added: "Come back and let me know, because they're experimental."

Two days later the woman was back, and she was furious.

"Didn't it work then?"

"Work! Work! We were just sitting down to tea when he glared at me with lust in his eyes. Then he swept all the crocks on the floor, dragged the cloth off, dragged my knickers off, and did me violently straight across the table. I was never so angry in my life."

"Angry, madam? I thought that was just what you wanted."

"I said angry, Doctor. Why, I shall never dare go in that branch of Lyons again."

BUCKED UP

There was a man whose wife was frigid and a shrew. He had a rotten life with her. Yet, when he died she gave him a posh funeral, and even went to the Spiritualists to see how he was getting on.

The Spiritualist said that for a suitable fee he thought he could get in touch with the dear departed, and after a little effort, with the widow and her relations sitting in the dark round a table, a signal came through.

"Hush," hissed the Spiritualist, "I am in tune with our Brother, speak to him Mrs Faggott."

"Hallo Harry, are you very happy dear?"

"Yes my dear, I am more happy than words can speak."

"Oh, I'm glad of that Harry, what's it like being an angel in heaven?"

"Angel in heaven! I'm a buck rabbit on Salisbury Plain!"

263

CAUGHT IN A NET

A woman went to a solicitor and said she must have a divorce.

Was her husband unfaithful? – No, nothing like that, she wanted a divorce for "cruelty".

She went on to explain that her husband was peculiar, he had a twisted mind. He never played billiards but with crooked cues, he liked to shave standing on his head . . . whatever he did, he did the hard way.

The solicitor said this was eccentricity but not cruelty, it was not enough. "But," said the wife, "he wants to make love in the garden."

"Good lord woman!" said the solicitor, losing patience, "that's a compliment. . . ."

"All right," said the woman, "then YOU try having intercourse standing up in a hammock."

The following are actual reports from a Northern Matrimonial Court:

(a) Young woman: My husband's a sexual monster, I must leave him.

Magistrate: What do you mean "sexual monster"?

Y.W.: He wants it nearly every night!

M.: Of course he does, that's what he married you for.

Y.W.: But he wants it in a most unnatural way!

M.: Aha, that's different. Tell us about his bestial practices.

Y.W.: Well, he wants it with the light on!

(b) Wife: I demand a divorce, I can't stay with him.

Magistrate: On what grounds, Madam?

Wife: Unreasonable demands! He's wrecking my health with his lusts.

Mag.: I see, well what "unreasonable demands" – how often?

Wife: I can't bear to talk about it, it's disgusting!

Mag.: Come, Madam, we can't help you if you won't help us. How often?

Wife: Twice a week!

Mag.: Good God almighty! Women have stood where you're standing now, and called twice a week desertion!

Enoch and Eli had been going to see Wolverhampton Wanderers for years. Every home game they would meet behind the Molineux end goal, and cheer their team. Then, one season early, Enoch failed to turn up. Three times he missed. Eli sought him out:

"I ay seen yo down the Wanderers lately, where've y'been?"

Enoch explained that he had married a plump and passionate wife. Every time he was getting ready to go to the match, she would grab him and pull him down on to the hearthrug. . . .

Eli explained that it was quite unmanly to be ruled by a woman in this manner: "Next Satday, if her does that, yo must pull her bloomers down and put her acrost yer knee, and slap her backside good and hard. If her cries, do it harder, then come to the match."

Enoch swore that he would, but he didn't turn up at the game.

Eli was furious, and quickly sought his mate for an explanation.

"Did y'do what I told yer?"

"Ar, well, I caught hold of her and put her over me knee. I dragged her drawers down, I raised me 'ond, but well, the Wolves haven't been playing very well lately, have they?"

A WILLING STAND-IN

Two working men were leaning on a bar discussing marriage.

"My wife's cold, dead cold," complained one, "I'm only too anxious any time, but she always says she don't feel like it."

"Ah that's it," said the other, "you lack technique."

"What the hell's that when it's out?"

"Now listen, you nit. When you go home Friday, give her a box of chocolates. After tea, fetch a bottle of her favourite tipple. Then take her on your knee, open her dress and play with her tits for an hour. . . ."

"Yes," said the husband, "then what?"

"Take her pants off, lay her on her back, stroke her thighs, play with her clit. . . ."

"Then what?"

"Send for me."

There was a small boy who was always a chatterbox.

One morning, after Daddy had gone to work, he said:

"Mamma, you know you went out to Grannie's all day yesterday."

"Yes, my son. What about it?"

"Well, Daddy came home after lunch, and do you know what him and the maid were doing in your bedroom. . . ."

"Be quiet! How dare you talk like that!" she said. Then, after a moments reflection: "Jimmy, when Mamma wants you to speak about it she will ask you."

That same evening, when Daddy came home for his evening meal, and they were all seated at the table, Mother said: "Now Jimmy, what was it you were telling me this morning about Daddy and the maid yesterday?"

"Well, Mamma, I was playing at hiding in the wardrobe when Daddy brought Mary in, and I peeped out and they were taking their clothes off. . . ."

"Really, my dear," said Father, "this is most unfair. . . ."

"You shut up!" said Mother, "I'm off to my solicitor in the morning; go on Jimmy, there's a good boy."

"Well she lay on the bed, and he got on top of her."

"Yes, go on."

"Then they started to do what you and Uncle John did last summer when Daddy was away on his business trip."

GREEK COMEDY

A labourer who lived in a very small cottage went to the Marriage Guidance Council and said that his sex life was unsatisfactory, his wife said she didn't enjoy it.

He was instructed that variation might make it more interesting. For instance, why not try the Greek position? He went away, thoughtful.

Three months later he was back, still in trouble. . . .

"Did you try the Greek position?" – "Yes."

"And your wife didn't like it?" "No guvnor, she loved it."

"Then why are you back here?" – "We had to give it up."

"Why, for goodness' sake?" "Well guv, doing it like that, the kids kept laughing at us."

LIMERICKS V

A land-hungry farmer named Jakers
Was stealing a yard off some Quakers
An Elder named Halls
Just jumped on his balls
And gave him a couple of acres.

There was a young man from Llandinging
Who long kept the bed-springs a-pinging
The girl said: "Ooh Bevan
You said it was Heaven,
And now I can hear the harps ringing."

A girl engineer named Miss Holt
Had a foreman as spry as a colt
When she asked for a screw
What did the man do
But offer two nuts and a bolt.

There was a young lady loved salmon
She said to her boy: "Though I am on,
And I can't, as we wish
Have your fish in my dish
We can do just as well with some gammon."

Don was chokkers, to speak in vernacular
To find that Flo's flow was spectacular
She tried to be kind:
"Have a drink, never mind —"
"Flo! My name is Donald, not Dracula."

You for Coffee?

The London–Manchester express train was crowded with business men.

In a first-class carriage a Chinaman was sitting reading quietly, when a white-coated waiter came down the corridor, put his head in the door and said:

"You for coffee?"

"No, you ferk offee, I got first-class ticket."

HONEYMOON SALAD – LETTUCE ALONE

There was a waitress who went up to the Head Waiter and said:

"I'm not going to serve that cheeky devil over there!"

"Why not?"

"Well, he asked me for 'French Salad', and when I said, 'What's that?' the devil said, 'It's the same as any other salad, only you serve it without dressing'."

TO FILL A GAP?

The Bishop came down to breakfast and said to his wife: "Any post?"

"Yes," she said, "there's a letter from the Rector of Little Crumpet, and you'd better read it, because it's upset me, it's disgusting!"

The Bishop unfolded the Rector's letter, and read:

My Lord, my wife died suddenly yesterday and it is most urgent and important that you send a substitute for the week-end.

271

FINGERED HER ORGAN

There was a piano in the front room, where Mary did her courting.

One evening the young man called, and soon afterwards Mother thought she heard funny noises emanating. She put her head in, and said:

"Is everything all right?"

"It's nothing," said the young man, "only that she started to laugh and giggle when I began to play. . . ."

"Ah, yes," said her mother, "she always was ticklish."

SPLITTING THE DIFFERENCE

There was a Chorus Master whose job in life was to train young girls for dancing acts in night clubs. He set on a new leading girl, who turned out to be stubborn and self-willed as well.

They were rehearsing a new show, and she wanted to dance topless, he wanted her in a see-through blouse, and a row was brewing up. Suddenly she stopped, and said: "Life's too short to quarrel, let's have a little contest – if I win, topless, if you win, see-through."

"Very well then, what's the competition?"

"Simple," said she, "we'll just see who can do the splits the best!"

"What, and you've got a start!"

BAD AUSPICES?

There were two men in a bar having a fearful row about whether Burton beer was better than London beer. They were nearly coming to blows, so the landlord said: "Gentlemen, do not fight, simply lay your bets with me, and I'll send two samples to the County Analyst."

This was agreed upon, but unfortunately the covering letter went astray.

A crowded bar heard the landlord read the report: "I beg to assure you that neither of these women is pregnant."

THE LAST TRUMP

There was an old maid went to the doctor, and complained that she was passing wind all day. The doctor, who was busy, said: "A lot of people do."

"Yes, Doctor, but mine is entirely odourless!"

He took notice, "Can you do it now?"

"Yes, indeed, I never stop."

The doctor looked concerned, and said an immediate operation was indicated.

"Oh dear, Doctor, on my backside?"

"No indeed Miss, on your nose."

PERMISSIVE SOCIETY

Hodge and Giles were old friends who ran neighbouring farms. Hodge had a daughter, Giles a son. One fine evening Hodge walked over to Giles' place and after a long conversation about weather and crops, said:

"By the way, Garge, I ought to tell 'ee, I caught your lad lyin' on top o' Mary in th'ay loft larst night."

"Well, dammit, Tom! – there's a young devil, he'll be smokin' next!"

Nine months went by.

Again Hodge called on Giles. They discussed farm prices and the rotten government. As he turned to go, Hodge added:

"Oh, Garge, that there lad o' yourn, he have put my Mary in the pod."

"Oh, Tom, I dunno what to do wi' 'im 'e be gettin' so careless, only last week 'e broke a teacup."

BACK TO THE LAND

Two London girls wanted badly to get work on a farm, and when the farmer asked them if they were experienced they rather misunderstood the question, and swore that they were.

"Very well," he said, "you can start. The cow's due for service, and the bull is being driven up in half an hour, so just get Bluebell ready for him, will you?"

With that, he went indoors for his dinner. Shortly there was a good deal of disturbance, which he ignored until the girls rushed in, with their clothes nearly torn off them.

"What be the matter then, for the lord's sake?"

"Oh farmer, it's Bluebell, we can't get her to lie on her back."

A SORE POINT

There was a shapely farmer's daughter, sixteen, who had to drive her father's cow to another farm where the bull was kept. She put the cow in the yard, and the young labourer drove the bull in and shut the gate. The bull wasted no time, and as the labourer stood watching, beads of sweat came to his forehead: "By golly, I wish I was doing that," he said.

"Go on then," said the girl, "I'm not stopping you."

"No miss, but perhaps the cow wouldn't like it."

ALL A LOT OF BULL

There was an old farmer, very set in his ways. When the bull died he tried to buy another, but everywhere he went he met with same response:

"No bulls for sale now, it's all this artificial insemination."

He didn't like to admit he didn't know what it was about, but finally, in desperation he rang up the A.I. centre and enquired about the drill.

When the Vet realised the farmer was a novice with A.I. he gave him some pretty strict instructions:

"I'll come next Monday and do it, and remember: I shall expect the cowshed well whitewashed and the floor scrubbed: I shall want hot water, soap and clean towels. . . ."

"Yes, Sir," said the farmer, "is that all?"

"And I shall not go near the animal unless she's spotlessly clean, understand?"

The farmer said he did understand. When the day came the farmer said to the Vet: "I've done arl ye said, I've got ye arl ye want, and I've put ye an 'ook, as well."

"A hook, a hook! What the hell would I want a hook for?"

"Well, Sir, I didn't think you'd want to throw your trousers down on the floor, even if it is clean."

COULDN'T FATHOM IT OUT

An old sportsman had supported his local rugger club loyally for many years, but alas the Old Borstalians had a series of bad seasons, and became somewhat of a joke. As the old sportsman lay on his deathbed he sent for the Club Secretary.

"Jenkins," he said, "I've supported the club loyally, always coughed up the shekels when the hat came round, what!"

"Yes you have, Sir," said the Sec., "we'll miss you very much."

"Will you do me one last favour Jenkins, will you and the club come and stand for a few moments on my grave, in remembrance like?"

"Why of course, of course – where are you going to be buried?"

"At sea old boy, at sea!"

HE PUT HIS FOOT IN IT!

The captain of a rugby club was much concerned because his best player was losing form, he asked what the trouble was?

The player explained that he was depressed because he was getting no sex life. The captain knew that this splendid athlete was very attractive to women, so he asked him why he didn't just go out and get it.

The player, after a great deal of humming and haa-ing, explained that he was a fetishist, and when it came to the point the girls cried off, because they would not let him put his number-ten-size foot in it.

The captain was a man of resource; he must get this man back into form, so he gave him ten pounds out of the kitty, and told him to go up the West End, where services, however kinky, were available for money.

* * *

It had been a hard day at the hospital, and as the doctor sat down wearily to his tea, he said to his colleague: "You know Smithers, you never stop learning on this job, do you. Who would have thought that in one day I would have to treat a prossy with athletes foot in her fanny, and a big hulking footballer with syph in his great toe."

SEX WITH KNOBS ON

A woman went to a solicitor and said she must have a divorce, owing to her husband's sexual demands. "Tell me?" said the man of law.

The wife explained that her husband wanted sex every night and twice on Sundays. "That's not unreasonable," said the solicitor.

"That's not all," she went on. "He takes me in the day time. I can't enter any room that he's in, but he rushes across for a stand-up job."

"My dear lady," said the lawyer, losing patience, "you are lucky to have a virile husband, and sexual intercourse up against a door is not grounds for a divorce."

"Oh, indeed!" said the woman, "then how would you like it if you had to keep going to hospital to have a brass doorknob removed from your backside?"

THAT WAS THE WHOLE IDEA

It was a family wedding, the house was crowded with people, and at bedtime everybody had to "double up". A bridesmaid of sixteen, made randy by the occasion, was put to bed with a cousin a year older.

There was a deal of fidgetting, and the girl said: "Let's change sides, you roll over me, and I'll roll over you."

"Don't bother," said the lad, "I can just as easily get out and walk round."

This happened several times more, and the frustrated girl said:

"You know, I don't think you really understand what I want!"

"Oh yes, I do," he said, "you want the whole bloody bed, but you're not going to get it."

HOT STUFF

Outside a West End cinema which was showing a film called "The Facts of Life" was a young man kicking an older man. A policeman came along to make an arrest, but the younger man explained that the older man had asked him to do it.

The older man then explained: twenty years ago he had been taken to the flat of a young woman who removed her jumper and skirt because she was too hot, and he had got up and turned off the gas fire. Then she took off her knickers and bra, upon which the man got up to go. As he left, she had said to him: "One day you will think about this, and you will ask the first man you meet to kick you."

"I've just found out what she meant," said the man.

"Kick him again," said the policeman.

THE OAF AND THE LOAF

There was a country chap in London during the war stopped a passing girl and said he could not get a lodging.

"My husband's abroad," she said, "come home with me, a slice off a cut loaf is never missed."

"Sorry madam, you misunderstand me, it's a bed I'm looking for, not a meal."

BACKS TO THE LAND

A man went to Russia to study the system. One day he was out in a peasant district, and he saw that the women toiled from morning to night in the fields. He spoke to one of the women and asked her if that was her idea of the "Communist paradise".

By this time a little group of interested bystanders had gathered, and the woman asked the man to explain what happened in Capitalist England. The man spoke good Russian, and he gave quite a fluent account: the men got up early, took their wives a cup of tea, and went off to work all day. At night they helped put the children to bed, and did any odd jobs about the house.

"There comrades," said the woman, "the Capitalist system is hell for the women, just as we were taught; it is a society in which all the men go to bed tired."

ADJUSTABLE SCREW

A man was in the top bunk, of a cross-Channel steamer, and a young woman was in the lower bunk. The man peered over, and saw the girl remove her wig, false teeth, and glass eye. Then she unscrewed her artificial leg.

At that moment she realised the man was watching her, looked up angrily, and said:

"What are you waiting for?"

"Miss, you know damn well what I'm waiting for, hurry up and unscrew it, and throw it up here."

DOWN MEMORY LANE

There was a dear old lady, who had been a widow for many many years.

One day a young married woman came visiting, bringing her baby. When she undressed the infant to bath it, she held it up for Grandma's inspection, and said:

"Isn't that a lovely baby?"

"Heh, heh, yes indeed it is, and, if my memory serves me rightly, a boy."

OLD AGE WENCHIN?

A certain student was told to do research on "Problems of the Aged" so he went and consulted an expert on the subject.

The expert said: "Let us take the women first, over 70 they really don't need it for health, yet they often have a desire for it, and wish they could do it more often. Subject to their physical limitations, such as stiff legs, they may still be enthusiastic. Unfortunately, in most cases their husbands will by then have lost all interest.

"Although women lose their looks early, they often retain more physical vigour than men. Men, even men who have enjoyed it all their lives, men who have spent time and money on it, men who have given a lot of thought to looking after their equipment, don't seem to bother in old age, they would rather watch the telly."

CONCLUSION: "I conclude then," wrote the student, "that men and women over 70 tend to give up gardening."

DOGGED DOES IT

An American entered a crowded railway carriage, but the only spare seat was occupied by a nasty alsatian, owned by a big red-faced woman in hunting tweeds. He asked if the dog might be put on the floor, and got the reply: "You leave the bloody dog alone!"

The Yank searched the train in vain for a seat, came back, and threw the dog out of the window.

"Are you going to stand by and let this wretched American do that to a gentlewoman?" she said to the carriage at large.

A man in a bowler hat lowered his *Times* and said: "The Yanks are always wrong, Miss; they eat with the fork in the wrong hand, they drive on the wrong side of the road, and now this fool's thrown the wrong bitch out of the window."

NOT TRUSTWORTHY

There was a very keen businessman who met a friend in his club.

"How's trade?" said the friend.

"Trade's excellent, since I have set on a brilliant young accountant. Unfortunately he has seduced my daughter, put my cashier in the family way, and sexually assaulted my wife."

"That's bad Jock, that's bad, what are you going to do?"

"Going to do! I'm going to watch that bleeder like a hawk, and if I catch him fiddling the petty cash, I shan't hesitate, I shall sack him."

WOULD NOT PLAY "POKER"

There were four passengers in the railway carriage, a young gentleman, a red-faced tycoon, a parson and the parson's wife.

The tycoon took out whisky and offered it the boy. "I don't drink, thank you," was the reply.

He took out cigars. . . . "I don't smoke," said the boy.

He took out a pack of cards. . . . "I never gamble," the young man replied.

As they left the train, the parson overtook the young man, and said:

"What a pleasure it is to meet a young man today, so entirely pure and free from sin. My wife here, and I, would like you to come down to our place for the weekend, and meet our charming daughter."

"Thank you," said the young man, "I'm a homo, on the run from the police."

OATS AND BREAKFAST

A man lost in the country begged a lodging with a small-time farmer.

In the morning, he asked what he owed.

"I don't rightly know," said the farmer, "I aint never took anyone in afore. Let me see, there's your supper, and your bed, and your breakfast; then you screwed my wife once, and my daughter twice, do you think thirty bob would be asking too much?"

LET US SPRAY

It was a crowded men's hairdressers. In one seat sat a retired Colonel, and the barber was saying: "Shall I spray a little scent on it Sir?"

"How dare you!" said the Colonel, "If I went home with that muck on my hair, my wife would say I smelled like a brothel."

Just then a private in the Pioneer Corps was asked the same question, by the barber at the next chair.

"Yes, a'course, spray me with all of 'em, my wife don't know what a brothel smells like."

FOR SALE AND WANTED

A certain Bishop had heard that one of his city parishes was a nest of sin, so he went down one day to have a look round. The Vicar was away, but the Curate undertook to show him round, and off they went through the streets.

They had not gone very far when a girl passed by: high heels, short skirt, big white handbag, and loaded with make-up.

"Upon my soul!" said the Bishop, "what an eyesore."

A little further on two more tarts went by.

"Look my lord," said the Curate, "there are two more nice whores."

CHEESED OFF

A man was getting very fresh with his girl in a railway carriage.

The only other occupant was an old shopkeeper who was sound asleep. Having wrecked the top-hamper the young man investigated the lower end. The girl protested that the old boy opposite might only be pretending to be asleep.

The bold young man said he would soon put the matter to the test, and stuck his fingers under the grocer's nose.

The old man shuffled in his sleep, and murmured, "Gorgonzola".

HE DID NOT RISE TO THE OCCASION

A man and a woman were alone in a railway carriage on a long journey.

The train passed through farmland, and at one point they observed a boar mounting a sow. A bit further on they observed a stallion mounting a mare. Next it was a bull serving a cow.

The woman, who was getting more and more restless, told the man she was unmarried, and wanted to know more about it.

The man, who was a professor, said it would be a pleasure to educate her in the facts of life. He then spoke at great length about the female heat cycle, and how it led to certain odours, and these olfactory indications produced libido in the male, etc., etc.

When they parted as the train reached Euston, he said, he hoped he would meet such a charming lady again.

"Only when your cold in the head is better," she said.

WRESTLING WITH SIN?

A young man boasted to his friend that he was courting a smashing bit of crumpet. The next time they met the young man had a black eye.

"How come you got that black eye?"

"Well," explained the other, "I was harmlessly dancing in the parlour with my girl to music from the radio. Her father walked in, and it turned out he was absolutely stone deaf."

TOPPED AND TAILED

Two factory girls, friends, were talking.

"What's become of that nice fellow you started going out with Mary?"

"Oh, I gave him the push, he was no gentleman."

"What happened?"

"No sooner were we alone on the settee in the front room when he put his hand up my thighs."

"Well, that shows interest, anyway."

"Oh no, I was brought up proper, I'm not having that, every lady knows that with a real gentleman it's always tits first."

THREW THE TOWEL IN

A man was in an upper bunk on a cross-Channel steamer. In the bunk below were a honeymoon couple. Every time the steward passed by, the groom said: "Steward, bring two towels."

After this had happened six times the man in the upper bunk shouted:

"Steward, bring me one towel, and some sleeping tablets."

FRIGHTENING EXPERIENCE

A girl asked her mother what would happen on her wedding night. The mother was old-fashioned and prudish. She said: "Well, he'll take you to bed, and strip all the clothes off you. Then he'll undress, and lie on you, and . . . er, scare you, but you'll have to put up with it."

After the first time the bride looked up coyly, and said: "Darling, scare me again." This was repeated several times more.

When they woke up in the morning the bride at once said: "Darling, scare me again."

The groom opened his bleary eyes, slowly drew in a breath, and said: "Boo!"

ARTIFICIAL INSEMINATION

There was a woman and a little boy sharing the top bunk in a steamer.

No sooner were they in bed than Willy told his mother he must get down and have a wee-wee. It was a long way down, and while mother was wondering how the kid would get back, he reappeared.

"How did you get up so easily, Willy?"

"Mother I put my foot on the bare bum of the man in the bottom bunk."

"Did you indeed, and what did he say?"

"He didn't say anything, but a lady's voice called out 'thankyou'."

WASTE OF POLLEN

A girl student was alone in a train with a boy student. He persuaded her to fondle him, but in case the guard should come by, she did it under a piece of fancy wrapping paper. They both fell asleep. The paper blew down on to the floor.

The guard came along, woke the girl up, and said: "Excuse me, Miss, your bouquet has wilted."

A hospital Sister named Dabbitts
Was noted for slap-happy habits,
Mixing pills for sterility
With those for fertility
Had ten at a birth, plus some rabbits.

He made such a hullaballoo
At finding no "roll" in the loo
That his mother said: "Ted
You've a tongue in your head!"
"Ma! I'm not a giraffe at the Zoo."

A champion swimmer named Last
Was noted for making love fast,
He'd start at the rude end
By grabbing the pudend
And leave the breast-stroking 'till last.

A snob Tory filly at Kew
Wore Union Jack briefs in full view,
Some Communist shirkers
Cried: "Up with the workers
And down with the red white and blue!"

There was a young lady of Eton
Whose figure had plenty of meat on
She said: "Marry me, Neal
And have a good meal,
I can't cook, but I'll get you a 'Beat-on'."

Right Upper Entrance

An old broken-down actor was signing-on for months at the Labour Exchange, and they were sick of him. One day the clerk said: "I'm sending you for a job, and you'd better keep it, or we'll cancel your benefits."

"What's the job?" enquired the old stager.

The clerk explained it was dead easy, it was to be prompter and assistant stage manager for a West End show that was being rehearsed.

The next day the man was back.

"What's your story? and it had better be bloody good, or you've had it," said the clerk sharply.

The actor explained that it was all on account of the Leading Lady being a prude, and the chorus girls having low blouses and low minds.

"Cut the cackle," said the clerk sharply, "and get on with it."

"Well," said the failed prompter, "I called out during rehearsal: *Enter the Duchess with a candle right up her entrance,*' the girls giggled, and the Director said: 'That can't be right, try again' so I started again, and read out, *Enter the Duchess with a candle left upper entrance*. At that point the Duchess swore, the chorus girls laughed until their tits fell out, and I got me bleeding cards."

SHE WOULD BE TORPEDOED

The troopship was crossing the Indian Ocean, and the Major was as randy as hell. He had his eye on the ship's nurse, who was as shapely as she was prudish. However he was a bold warrior, and although it took him a week to get the top button undone, he persisted. With only two more weeks to go, he thought seriously of taking the last bastion by storm, and planting his standard between the ramparts, but his nerve failed.

Alas, the ship got torpedoed, and while the captain was giving emergency orders, the Major appeared on the bridge, and said:

"Is the ship sinking?"

"Oh suck off, I'm busy, what's the matter, are you scared?"

"Not at all, Sir, but if we're going to sink I propose to use the last five minutes making up that bitch's mind for her!"

PAYMENT IN KIND

A theatrical Director was casting a play, and was interviewing a string of "starlets". When one came in whose breasts and backside were pleasing to him, he said she could have a small part if she took off her clothes and got down on the carpet. He had not finished the sentence before she was ready.

Not having wasted any time on finesse, he soon refastened his trousers and said: "Right, rehearsals three months tomorrow."

"Good God!" she said, "three months, I'm starving, can't you advance me a couple of quid to buy food?"

"Miss, do not be offensive, I am not a shop-keeper, and I do not buy sex either, I am a Director, I give free passes."

SAFETY IN NUMBERS

A young man was desperately in need of sex, but he soon found that although respectable girls would never sell sex, they expected expensive presents.

He had little money, but plenty of brains, and he told this typist he would buy her an expensive fur coat if she cared to be cooperative.

In no time at all she was naked on the bed, and so was he.

Afterwards he gave her his card, and told her to go to the furriers and take her choice. "If there's any question," he said, "tell them to phone me at this number."

"Is it your home or your office?" she enquired.

"Actually, it's the sweet shop on the corner, but they'll call me."

STOP IT I LIKE IT

Girl and boyfriend, having a row:

He: "I'll come up tonight and I'll tear the clothes off your back."

She: "Oh no you won't!"

He: "Then I'll do you and do you till you can't get up off the floor."

She: "Oh no you won't!"

He: "And I won't even wear a french letter."

She: "Oh yes you will!"

HOLE FULL OF SOAP

There was a beautiful and shapely young girl married to an actor, who was mostly "resting". One day she told him that if he didn't get a job and bring some money in, she would leave him for a rich sugar daddy.

The upshot was, she had to sleep with a Director to get her spouse a part, and she told him he'd better be good at it, or else. . . .

It was one of those romantic plays which opened with a beautiful young girl lying on a bank in summer, in a frail dress, wafted by a gentle breeze.

He had to come on as a love-lorn prince, and say:

> *Ah, she sleeps, and dreams of peace*
> *Her soul is full of hope.*
> *So shall I quickly snatch a kiss,*
> *And fly off in the air.*

Now, being very nervous he had taken several snifters before going on, and by bad luck the "gentle breeze" had blown up the dress, revealing nothing underneath except perhaps a little barber's rash. He declaimed:

> *Ah, she sleeps and dreams of a piece*
> *Her hole is full of soap.*
> *So shall I quickly kiss her snatch*
> *And shoot off in the air.*

PULLING THE BELLE

There was a college chap and a college girl, returning from a football game. They were rather excited as their team had won, and the girl suggested they stop the car in the woods, and get against a tree for a little smooching.

The man didn't like to admit that he'd never done it before, and when he'd finished he said: "Darling, I suppose you must have enjoyed it a lot, as you kept nodding your head?"

"As a matter of fact Charles, you'd got my scarf tucked in as well."

FAST AND LOOSE

A woman went to Court and demanded a divorce. After a lot of beating about the bush it came out that her husband's member was so big that it really hurt. The divorce was granted.

A year later she was back. She had remarried, and this time she wanted a divorce because her husband's was so tiny it could not satisfy her.

"Case dismissed!" roared the Judge. "Madam, the Court has better things to do than fitting dicks to your vagina."

PUDDING WITH SAUCE

Father was talking to Mother: "You know, I'm not altogether happy about our Mary getting engaged, I hear the chap's a vegetarian."

Mother: "Well if the chap's a vegetarian, it's just not on, we don't want any cranks and weirdies in our family."

Little sister Jane, who was seven, had been listening quietly, and now asked: "What's a vegetarian?"

"A man who will never eat meat."

"Oh, that's all right then."

"What do you mean dear 'that's all right'?"

"Well, yesterday, when I peeped into the front room through the keyhole he was making a good meal off our Mary's tits."

SHE SAW THE DRAWBACK

A respectable high-class Jewish family were at dinner, and Father said to Mother: "By the way, I hear Emmanuel wants to join that Nudist Club down the road."

"I can't really think of any objection," said Mother.

"Mother!" said the thirteen-year-old daughter of the house, "our Manny can't possibly join that Club?"

"Why on earth not, my dear?"

"They're all gentiles!"

"How can you possibly know that, my child?"

"Daddy. Mummy, of course I know. I peeped through a crack in the fence."

AN UPRIGHT OLD MAN

Little Jimmy was playing in the garden, and he pulled a worm out of its hole. Grandad was watching, and to tease little Jimmy, he said:

"I bet you half a crown you can't put it back!"

Little Jimmy said: "Oh yes I can, Grandad, you come back here in half an hour, and I'll show you!"

So, half an hour later, Jimmy reappeared with the worm, which was now as stiff as a pencil, and he threaded it back into its hole without much difficulty.

Grandad was amazed, and asked how it was done.

"Pay up the half crown you owe me, and I'll tell you," said the child.

Grandad handed over the money, and then Jimmy explained the trick. He had gone to his big sister's dressing-table, sprayed the worm with her hair varnish, and after a few minutes it was stiff and hard.

* * *

The following day, Jimmy was again playing in the garden when his Grandfather came along and gave him half a crown. The boy was honest, and said:

"Grandad, you paid me yesterday."

"Yes, I know I did son, this one's from your Grandmother."

CAUTIONARY TALE

Two young farm labourers were mowing the hay when they came across two girl cyclists from the city, picnicking in the grass. They told the girls they would have to pay damages for flattening the hay, but, after a bit of talk, the girls suggested paying on their backs. The boys were only too ready, but the girls produced condoms, saying: "You must wear these to prevent disease."

Two weeks later Herbert said to George: "You got any disease Garge?" – "No, Bert."

"Noither 'ave Oi, let's take these darn things off."

294

COME BACK TO ERRING!

Pat grew up in a remote parish in Ireland, and he came to an understanding with a local colleen. But first he must go to America to establish himself, and he was gone ten years.

Pat returned, city-suited, pockets jingling, to the one-roomed sheiling where his girl's family lived. Naturally he had to stay the night, so he and Father went up to the "bedroom", which was no more than a sort of loft reached by a ladder, while the two women stayed below.

The men were not comfortable, and they lay awake listening to the mother and daughter whispering below:

"Well me darlin', ye'll soon be married now."

"Muther, you know I can't marry him. Have I not had a child, and it put out to adoption whiles he's away!"

Mother pooh-poohed all this, she said he'd never know, shut up about it.

"But mother, I must tell him, it's not honest."

"My child, my dear daughter, did I not myself have a child before I met your father, and him none the worse for not knowing on't?"

* * *

Up aloft there was some shuffling; "Move over will ye," says Pat to father, "and let me get out of the ventilation hole, for am I not off back to Americky this minnit."

"Steady Pat, steady, whin ye get down, bring over the ladder from the hayrick, for it's meself that's coming wid ye."

NO "R" IN THE MONTHLY

There was a shapely young woman went to the doctor because she was not too well. He took a sample of her water and told her to return later.

When the lady came back, he said: "Congratulations Mrs Brown, I have some good news for you. . . ."

"But Doctor, I'm MISS Brown."

"Then Miss Brown, I have some bad news for you."

PENETRATED

A well set up widow of 38 had a daughter of 18. Mother considered herself of superior class, and had a very icy manner. She was quite pleased when her daughter started to go out regularly with the curate.

After some months she said to the daughter: "When are you getting engaged?"

"I'm not getting engaged Mother. We had a row and broke it off a fortnight ago."

"Oh indeed, and did you give him his ring back?"

"Yes I did, the horrible beast, and I secretly made pinholes in those french letters he was proposing to use on me . . . oh Mother, you've fainted!"

UP WITH THE WORKERS

A young porter in an hotel was brought up in Court for raping the chambermaid. She alleged that while she was leaning out of the hotel window to watch a May Day parade, the youth lowered the sash, trapped her, and took his will of her.

"But Miss," said the Judge, "why didn't you start yelling?"

"What, and have everybody thinking I was supporting the Labour Party!"

HANDS UP EVERYBODY

Bandits held up a holiday coach at gun point on a wild and lonely moor. The chief bandit cried: "Right, stand fast, we're going to rob all the men and do all the women."

"Boss," said his assistant, "wouldn't it be safer to rob all the men and then get to hell out of it?"

An old maid at the back: "Who's in charge of this robbery I should like to know."

THAT WON'T WASH

A young man was courting for the first time, and it wasn't long before he got the girl undressed. But she wouldn't let him without a sheath, and he didn't know what they were. "Any chemist will explain," she told him.

So off he went, and the chemist said they were half a crown each, but it was much better to buy ten-shilling ones, because these could be washed and used again.

Some time later he met the chemist in the street, who asked him if he was having any luck with the lady. "That part was OK," he said, "but I got a hell of a stinking note from the manager of the laundry."

THUMBS UP

A chap was making pretty good progress with a girl. She agreed to go away for the weekend, provided he brought a sheath with him.

When they went upstairs to bed, he admitted he didn't know how to wear it, so she rolled it down his thumb to show him. Then they put the light out and got on with it.

After a while the girl said: "You know I'm terribly sticky, I do believe you've broken that thing."

"Oh no I haven't," he said, and (switching the light on) "here it is, still on my thumb."

BLINDED WITH SCIENCE

A man was determined to fail his army "medical" on the grounds of semi-blindness. When the doctor said: "Read that card," he said: "What card?" "The card on the wall, man!" – "What wall doctor?"

The doctor indicated to the shapely nurse to strip naked. "Now, what do you see?" – "The figure 8," said the man, so he was discharged. He was so pleased he rushed up town and went to a Strip Club. When the lights came up at an interval, who should be sitting in the next seat but the doctor who had just failed him. Quick as a flash, he said:

"This is the bus for Charing Cross, isn't it Miss?"

NOBLESSE OBLIGE, BUT NOT TONIGHT

There was a dashing young man, the son of a Peer, who went to a Deb's coming-out ball. The band played, the champers went round, and all was merry. Young Fitznakkers was smitten by a bird whose dress was open down to her navel, and after turning on the old charm he had little difficulty in getting her on a couch in the conservatory, well hidden behind some shrubbery.

Such was his progress that pretty soon her pants and bra were decorating the branches. He was nearly there, when she cried off:

"No no, Charles, that's enough, stop now."

He was in no condition to put the brakes on: "Darling, darling, don't be frightened, this is real love, darling: will you marry me?" (At that moment he really meant it.)

"No darling, I won't. I love you, but I must say No now."

He was obliged to make love to his best silk handkerchief, after which, feeling a little calmer, he fetched some drinks and said:

"Darling, I offered honourable marriage; you love me and I love you, yet you said No."

"You see, Charles," she explained, "it's an old family superstition."

"Old family superstition, what the hell are you on about?"

"Well, you see, my father proposed to my mother in the conservatory, and he died the same night."

THE BRIDE WANTED COVERING

There was a charming and beautiful young girl went on honeymoon with her dashing husband. She went up to bed first to get ready, and he followed soon afterwards. He found her starkers in the bedroom, except for a small beret on her head.

"Darlingest pet," he said, "have you gone crackers?"

"No, Harry darling, I'm just following my mother's good advice; I don't know what she meant, but I'm sure she must have had good reason."

"Why duckiest, what did she say?"

"She said, if I wanted to keep my husband's interest I must never let him see me totally naked."

A DIFFERENT SORT OF RIDE

A chap was up before the Bench for stealing a young woman's bicycle. He pleaded "Not guilty".

"Well, what happened?" said the Beak.

"Well, Sir, I was walking through the woods and this girl came by on her bike and stopped, and she got me to sit down although I wasn't tired, then she took her blouse off, although it wasn't that hot, and then she said 'Kiss me'."

"Yes, go on."

"Well, Sir, I kissed her and she took her jeans off, then she took her panties off, then she said: 'Kiss me again and you can have what you like'."

"And then?"

"Well, Sir, panties is girls clothes, and her jeans wouldn't fit me, so I had her bicycle."

PUT IT DELICATELY

There was a rough navvy up for burglary, but he seemed to have a reasonable alibi. Said the Judge: "Now tell us *everything* you did that night, in detail."

"Well, Sir, I comes 'ome for me *ing tea, and then I 'as a *ing wash and puts my *ing best shoes on. Then I goes up the *ing pub and I 'as several *ing pints, and in comes *ing Nelly. So I buys *ing Nelly a couple of *ing drinks, and takes her round the *ing back and across the *ing fields and into the *ing woods. Then I takes her *ing knickers off and lays her on the *ing ground, and. . . . Sir, I don't like to say any more, it ain't decent."

"Go on, go on," said the Judge, "if you want to stay out of jail, finish the story."

"Well, then we 'as sexual intercourse."

HOLE IN ONE

There was a man went into a bar looking very cheerful, and he instantly called for "drinks on the House".

A stranger enquired what was the source of his joy, and the man said: "This mor..ng my wife gave birth to a fine son, our eleventh, think of that, what a bit of luck!"

"I can't see it old boy, nothing but damned expense, surely?"

"Money doesn't worry me," said the happy father, "but I am a soccer fan, and now I can have a football team . . . more drinks! landlord."

There was a long pause, and the stranger, who had been melancholy, looked up suddenly with a smile, and said:

"No, these are on me, I've just thought of something."

The others enquired as to the source of his inspiration and were told:

"Well gentlemen, you know I've got seventeen daughters, if we have one more I'll have a golf course!"

"HELP! HELP!" SHE WHISPERED

A rather shy man was courting a passionate girl, and each time he visited her home she would make a point of going on the back porch with him as he departed. Little by little she was leading him on, and one night during an embrace he discovered there was nothing else under her dress.

His emotions began to stir, his breath was getting shorter, and finally he said:

"If I were to go all the way, would you yell for your mother?"

"Why!" said the girl, "do you want to do it to her as well?"

NICER THAN PORK?

A factory Welfare Officer was visited by a weeping girl.

"Usual trouble, I suppose?"

"Yes, Miss."

"Married man, I suppose?"

"Yes Miss."

"Here! Aren't you Fanny Hitches who came to me in the same pickle just a year ago?"

"Yes, Miss."

"You stupid little fool, what did you go and do it again for?"

"Well, Miss, if God made anything nicer, you tell me what it is."

CLOSED SHOP

There was a man who was his mother's pet. He didn't get married until he was thirty. "I've brought him up to be choosey," his mother would say.

When he did get married he returned to his mother the next day.

"Why have you left her, Dear?" said Mam.

"I found out she was a virgin, Mother."

"What's the objection to that, son?"

"Well, Mother, if she's not good enough for the lads of the village, she's not good enough for me."

IT GOT UP HER PIPE

Prewar Council houses were not well built. A woman went to her neighbour on the "estate" and said:

"Hey, Mrs Bloggs, have you got the sweep in?"

"What if I has then," replied the other, cautiously.

"This is what, Mrs Bloggs, you just tell him to be a damn sight more careful what he's a-doin'. He's pushed our Johnny off the lavatory twice with his brush."

A honeymoon pair from Nantucket
Went to bed, and by heck, did they ruck it!
Next morning, said he:
"Do you feel like some tea?"
"No! I feel like a billposter's bucket."

A lockkeeper's daughter named Baines
Sobbed: "Loss of virginity pains,
An artist," she said:
"Came through Maidenhead
Whose brushwork left nothing but Staines."

An Ordnance Surveyor of guile
His ranging rod used in such style
That in taxis the sod
Put virgins in pod
On the scale of one inch to one mile.

A certain blonde rider named Hatch
Withdrew from the Hunt with despatch
When she fell at some ditches
And ruptured her britches
The hairs on her brush didn't match.

There was a girl student named Grubb
Too young to be served in a pub,
Said a Yorkshire churchwarden:
"Just come in the garden,
Ah'll serve thee, and put thee in Club."

Custer's Last Stand

In the prairie where Custer made his famous last stand against the Sioux there now stands a prosperous town, and the City Fathers held a meeting. They had to decide what they would do to celebrate the hundredth anniversary of this great piece of American history.

After due debate it was decided to put up ten thousand dollars and engage the best painter they could find to paint a huge mural for the Town Hall, depicting the event.

Picasso was suggested.

"Mister May-yor, ain't he just a bit . . . wal, he's French I guess," said one. "That guy sure paints hot noods," said another. "Wid square boobs!" added a third.

"Sure, sure," said the Mayor, "but fer ten grand we can tie him down like to a prarper picture."

It was agreed that Picasso should have the contract if he would undertake to do a lifelike historical record with no abstract stuff. It was to demonstrate the drama of the scene so that simple cowboys could grasp it.

Picasso had this drummed into him, and at the same time he insisted that the great work should remain under cover until finished.

* * *

When the great day came, hundreds were packed into the hall, including all the big-wigs of the city, county and state. The President sent a message.

A Senator's wife pulled a silk cord, and the drapes fell off, revealing a giant canvas covered all over with naked Indians. The crowd gasped to see that each Indian brave was coupled frankly with a squaw wearing only a head-dress. The detail was marvellous! In the top corner was a fish with a halo over it.

The Mayor turned to Picasso and heaped abuse on him. Picasso mumbled in French. . . . "How in heck does he allow this to hev anny rellervance to Ammurican history?" demanded the Mayor of the interpreter.

cont'd over 305

The interpreter questioned Picasso, and then said: "He makes it out like this Mister May-yor – he says how he's checked up on Custer's very last words on earth. . . . HOLY MACKEREL! LOOK AT ALL THEM ****ING INDIANS!"

HOSPICE

The Women's Institute had a "Men's Night" and all the ladies had to bring their husbands, willing or unwilling.

To liven the proceedings, a "spelling bee" was laid on, and to everyone's surprise, Old Farmer Haycock was out in front of the field.

Indeed, as he said in the Barley Mow afterwards: "Ar, and I'd a-won it an arl, if the last word hadn't been 'Auspices'."

NOT YET WRITTEN OFF

There was an Army P.T. instructor who finished his time out in the Far East. To the disappointment of his family he did not come back to England but took a job out there.

His Dad wrote several times to ask him what the job was, but he always evaded the question. At last he came home on a long vacation, and his Dad took him out for a few drinks. "Now Jack," he said, "out with it, what's this job you're doing?"

The son explained he had a really well-paid number at the court of one of these wealthy oil sheiks.

"Yes, but WHAT?"

"Well, Dad, it's a kind of educational job."

"Educational! Why you bloody ignoramus you were always bottom of the class. Come on, out with it, trust your old Dad."

Jack said: "Well, it's like this here, I has a wall painted black, and I gets sent a lot of well-made fourteen-year-old virgins from the villages, see, and I has to teach them arithmetic, see."

"Do you mean to say you get a fancy salary for that?"

"Well hang on a minnit, Dad, it ain't that easy, it takes perseverance see, but when they pass out trained the Boss is very satisfied."

"What do they have to do to pass out?"

"When they can hold a stick of chalk in the cheeks of their arse, and write one and seventeen-thirtyseconds plus three and twentynine-sixtyfourths equals four and sixtythree-sixtyfourths on the wall, they're ready for the Sultan's harem, see."

A POPULAR GIRL

There was a man who had got on only by his own efforts and made some money. He crowned his success by marrying a debutante of snooty extraction. On the wedding night she told him that she was too modest to undress in front of him, would he stay down, smoke a cigar, and have a final drink, then she would be ready. Actually he did not wait very long, but soon went after her.

When he entered his bedroom his wife was naked on the bed. Two bellboys were sucking her breasts, the night porter was on top, and she was gamming the boots.

"Oh, Delia," he said, "I am surprised!"

"But dahrling, why? I told you I was a bit of a flirt."

SLIPPING THEM IN

A young woman was about to get married, and she was quite innocent. Her mother said: "Before you go to bed the first night, be sure and give him some oysters for supper."

Next day, mother asked daughter how she got on.

"Not very successful mother, I suppose it's because I lack your catering experience. I fed him a dozen, but only nine worked."

BEST OF BOTH WORLDS

Two experienced women were talking. One said she had been in the East where male organs were short and thick, and she preferred them that way.

The other said she had always lived in the West where the male equipment was long and thin.

The daughter of one of them, who was not supposed to be listening, told her mother afterwards that she hoped to marry a man who had been in the Diplomatic Service.

"But why, my dear?"

"Then I might hope to find a man born in the West who had lived in the East a long time."

YOU OUI-OUI OFF!

A working chap won the pools, so he and his wife set out for a holiday in Paris. They went out for a drink, and by chance wandered into Charrington's famous "English Pub".

The working man took out his phrase book and said:

"Voulay vouz donner moi a pint of beer, silver plate."

The waiter said: "Sorry, Sir, no French spoken here."

"Ho, you don't speak bloody French hey, well clear off and come back with the bugger that does."

OVER TO METRIC

On the first day of each month a young man went into a chemist's shop, as regularly as clockwork, and ordered one gross of french letters. Recently the chemist said to him:

"Our industry's gone over to Metric, they come in packets of fifty now, not in dozens, actually it comes out slightly cheaper."

Customer: "Three packets of fifty?"

Chemist: "That's what I said, instead of a gross."

"What do you think I am, a sex maniac?"

OLD RUGBY CUSTOMS

A parson went to his first rugby match. Shortly an excited scrum-half hacked an opponent's leg.

The parson turned to his friend, and said: "Excuse me, but how did that one player know the other player was a Bar steward?"

There was a girl, daughter of a noble house, who had breeding, but no money to go with it. At last she picked up with the son of a Duke, and an engagement was announced.

However, there was trouble, the girl went to her mother, and said:

"Charles says that if he finds I'm not a virgin on our wedding night, he'll make no settlement on me, and we'll all be ruined."

"You should have kept your virginity dear, shouldn't you."

"Dammit, I did keep it until I was eighteen, *you* sent me to Roedean!"

"That's no help now, we'll go and see Doctor Duguid."

The old family doctor shook his head. "When I was a student we weren't taught how to re-fabricate maidenheads. Anyway, it isn't necessary . . . (turning to the girl) this is the oldest trick in the world: go in the bathroom on your wedding night, and dry your orifice out with cotton wool. When your husband, half drunk anyway, gets going, scream the place down." (The girl shook her head.) "I tell you Miss de Hardwick, thousands of men have been taken in like that."

"Doctor, in the first place I'm a rotten actress, in the second, as soon as a man puts his hand on it, it runs like a tap. You'll have to think again."

"Well," said the doctor, "there's a Harley Street chap who was at college with me. . . ." ". . . We haven't got Harley Street money," said Mother.

"Then I'll do a local job for £25, it may work, Miss de Hardwick, come to me the day before."

❋   ❋   ❋

cont'd over

The wedding was not only a great social success, but the screams of the virgin bride disturbed the whole hotel. Mother went to pay the doctor his £25, and said, "It was good value for money, what did you actually do?"

"Well, Mrs De Hardwick, I sat up all night with the old books, but it was no good. Then I suddenly remembered I'd been in the Sea Scouts as a lad."

"And what, may I ask, have the Sea Scouts to do with restored maidenheads?"

"Why, I simply knotted the hairs together."

DELAYED ACTION

Two elderly men met in a bar. They had been soldiers together, and got talking: "How are you getting on?" says one.

"Not very well," says the other, "you know that dope the medical officer used to put in the troops' tea to quieten us down?"

"Yes, what about it?"

"It's just beginning to catch up on me."

DOUBLE MEANING

There was an irritable businessman used to play golf, with his wife. One day a visiting niece of fifteen went round with them. The golfer misses a six-inch putt for the match, and shouts: "Oh f**k!"

The wife is shocked, and soundly rebukes her husband. The man looks at the girl, her full bust, her round bottom, her red lips, and says:

"Surely you must have heard that expression before?"

"Yes, Uncle, but not spoken in anger."

IN A SHROUD

A policeman shone his torch into a graveyard late at night, and saw a courting couple making love. He brought them before the Judge:

"And what were you doing in the churchyard at midnight?" said the Judge to the young man.

"Nothing wrong, Your Honour, just burying a stiff."

"What about you?" he said to the girl.

"Your Honour, I was the undertaker."

MISUNDERSTANDING

A middle-aged motorist and his wife could not find the country pub at which they were booked, and their petrol was running low.

"We can't go much farther," said the wife, when they were in the middle of nowhere, "there's a car in that spinney, go and see if you can get any directions."

The man went across, and came back with a black eye.

"All I did," he said, "was walk across to this couple, and call through the quarter-light: 'How far is the Cock Inn?' "

313

THE MISCARRIAGE TRADE

A farmer had a plain thin daughter, and one day it turned out she was pregnant. The farmer loaded his shotgun and said: "He'll marry you or else. . . ."

"He's married already," said the girl. "It was the Squire."

Father said he'd shoot him just the same, and sallied off to the Hall in a frenzy.

"Here! hold on a minute Hodge old chap," said the Squire, "I mean to do right by the girl. If she has a boy, I'll settle a thousand quid on him, and if it should be a girl, five hundred quid."

"And if it's twins, Squire."

"Fifteen hundred. Now sod off you old blackmailer."

"Excuse me, Squire, just a final word: if it's a miscarriage, can she have another go?"

SHE HAD EXPECTATION

A man of good family had gone abroad to complete his education, but unfortunately squandered all his money in brothels and casinos. He came home broke, and his father said: "Don't look at me, you'll just have to buy a business, if you can raise the dough. Try your Uncle George, he's rich."

The young man went to see Uncle George and said any chance of a loan of ten thousand? "No," said uncle, "I want my cash to marry my daughter off, hey, you'll do. Listen, she's got nice hair, a fine pair of tits, a well-shaped bottom, good teeth, a generous nature, a dowry of ten thousand, and all my expectations."

"And I'm penniless and unemployed!" said the cousin, "where's the catch, Uncle, out with it?"

"Well, my boy, I must confess that she is just the weeniest, teeniest bit pregnant."

314

SHE PUT HER FEET IN IT

An Irish country woman went to the doctor and asked for some birth control pills. The doctor told her that it would be illegal in Ireland, and she said, with ten kids in ten years, and still only thirty years old, what should she do.

The doctor suggested she go back to the farm and cut the top off a two-gallon paraffin tin. If she slept with both feet in that every night, she would not become pregnant.

Six months later she was back, filled out in front. . . .

"I thought I told you. . . ."

"I know you did, Doctor, but you see, Pat buys his paraffin in one-gallon tins, so I put one on each foot."

MEN OF CAPE HORN

A man went from town to town as a traveller in contraceptive goods.

He arrived at his regular hotel, and the reception girl said:

"Your regular room eh, Mr Smith?"

"No dammit, I want two rooms, one with three cots, and a bathroom, I've got three infants in the back of the car."

"Oh dear, has your wife suddenly run away?"

"Not at all, just going back to the factory with customers' complaints."

UNLETTERED OAF

Two attractive girls moved down from college into a country town to open a chemists shop. A bold young man went in and asked for a packet of french letters. "What size, Sir?" – "I don't know."

"Well, go round the back for a fitting."

Round the back the other girl is waiting with her pants down: she slips it in, and shouts, "Size 6 Mary."

The man rushed round to tell his best friend, who at once set off on the same errand. When it came to trying for size however, the rotten hound left it in and came off.

"It's all right, Miss," he said to the furious girl, "I didn't come along to buy any, I just wanted a fitting."

HAND IN GLOVE

A widow had a daughter who was rather innocent. The girl started courting, but one day out in the country the young man went over a hedge for a run out, and the girl peeped through to look, out of curiosity. Terrified by what she had seen, she ran home to mother and swore she could never marry.

Mother pooh-poohed this, and, after discussing it with the young man, it was agreed that they should have a trial run, so that the engagement could be broken off rather than a disastrous marriage be entered into.

Accordingly, the three of them retired upstairs on Saturday afternoon, and the sight of the girl's plump body roused the man to supreme heights. This in turn frightened the girl out of her wits, and she firmly closed her legs. Mother said: "Open them wide dear, and I will grasp him round the base of the stem, one hand above the other. Only if you can bear it will I remove one or both hands."

Operations commenced, and the mother very carefully removed one hand, and after a minute, the other. After five minutes the girl cried out:

"Mother, for cripes sake hurry up and take both hands away."

VIRGIN BIRTH

A young and smarmy lawyer was up before the judge in a paternity case.

He had been actually seen swiving the girl at the relevant date, blood group tests were positive, and the judge could not wait to hear what sort of a case he would make in support of his plea of "Not Guilty".

"Well, my Lord, it's like this. This girl is nothing but a prickteaser. She would take me upstairs when her mother was out, lie naked on the bed, and then not let me put it in. At last she agreed that I could put the first inch in, if I stopped at the maidenhead. I kept my word like a true English gentleman; but on this occasion her mother came in unexpectedly, gave me a series of belts across the bare arse, and I went straight through and came off.

"My Lord, I submit that the father of the child is that girl's mother."

THE OLD BAG

The daughter of a Welsh hill-farmer's family was being courted by a city fellow. One Saturday night there was a fearful storm, and then after that his motorbike wouldn't start, so there was no choice but for him to stay the night. This meant him sleeping in the daughter's bed, and mother was greatly troubled.

"Mother," whispered father, "look now is not the old bundling bag somewhere in grandad's trunk, go and look."

"Indeed to goodness yes," cried mother from the depths of the trunk, but alas, the upper half had been used for something else. So mother put Megan's feet and legs in the bag, tied it round her waist, and made her swear that she would in no circumstances get out of it.

*　　*　　*

Several months later, Megan was pregnant. "Is it not a little liar that you are! Were you not swearing to me that you wouldn't get out of the bag?"

"But Mother, I didn't get out of the bag, at least, shall I put it this way Mother, only one leg."

FIVE TIMES A VIRGIN

A young man was courting a Welsh girl who shared her family's narrow views. He tried drink, he tried gifts, he tried the top end and got encouragement, but when he tried the bottom end he found stout linen bloomers with elasticated legs.

She told him that never mind if the frustration was killing him, her mother would never let them share a bed unless a formal engagement was announced.

Buoyed with hope he bought a most expensive ring, and her parents put the pair of them to bed, but only in bundling bags with knots tied tight behind the neck.

He saw there was nothing to it but he would have to marry her. On the wedding night he said: "You know Olwen my dear, I'm just the same as other men, if you had let me have your virginity before, I wouldn't have been in a hurry to get married."

"I know," she said, "that's how I lost the other four."

EMBARRASSING

A man in a pub was asked by a stranger if he'd got a light.

He said: "I'm a non-smoker, but I've got a match somewhere." With which he turned out all his pockets and produced six packets of aspirins and a quarter of cough lozenges.

"What's the matter mate, you got flu or something?"

"Not at all, it's every time I go into a chemists shop lately, they only seem to have women behind the counter."

RED LETTER DAY

A man was cycling past a house in a narrow street when a used french letter was thrown out of an upper window, and hit him smack in the eye.

As this caused him to take a nasty tumble from the bike, he was very angry, and knocked at the front door of the house. Father came to the door, paper in hand, feet in slippers, and said: "Are you trying to break my door knocker?"

"Never mind that, who's upstairs where that light is?"

"My daughter, as a matter of fact."

"And who is with her?"

"My intended son-in-law, and what business is it of yours?"

"None at all my dear Sir, none at all, but I thought you would like to know that your intended grandson has just been thrown out of the window."

HE WAS FABRIC-ATED

A man at work was very little, and although he had spent a long lifetime there, he was still teased because of his small size.

The day came when he had to put away his broom, and the directors gave a dinner, and Tich drank far more than he was used to. When it came to the speeches the Chairman said: "Now, before I ask my younger daughter to present our retiring labourer with this splendid gold watch, I am going to ask him if he cares to tell us how it is that he is so small."

"As to that," replied Tich, "I was born before french letters was invented." This produced such a shocked silence that he took it for encouragement. ". . . my mother made my father use his handkerchief, and you'd be little if you'd been strained through fine silk."

SHE WAS ONLY AN ADMIRAL'S DAUGHTER . . .

She was only an Admiral's daughter, but she loved a navel encounter, with a great loss of semen.

* * *

She was only the Mayor of Birmingham's daughter, but she knew Five Ways.

* * *

She was only a cardsharper's daughter, but she covered my jack with her deuce.

* * *

She was only a Huntsman's daughter, but all the horse-manure.

* * *

She was only a doctor's daughter, but she liked being bad in bed.

* * *

ENLARGEMENTS WANTED?

There were some explorers pushing up through the jungle where no white man had ever been before. At last they broke through to the bank of a river where some native girls were bathing, together with a naked black man who had the largest chopper ever seen. This massive zeppelin was unique, and they asked through the interpreter if they could photograph it for the Science publications.

There was some mumbling, and then the interpreter returned and said:

"He wants to know what all the fuss is about. Does not the member of the white man shrink in cold water?"

There was a coloured man in Britain whose wife was having so many children that the District Nurse persuaded him to visit a doctor. The doctor, not without difficulty, got through to him that he must wear a sheath. So long as he wore it, his wife could not conceive.

However, she soon conceived again, and the doctor was furious. He had the man in, and this time he laid on an interpreter, through whom he questioned the man.

"He swears he did wear it, he never took it off," said the interpreter.

"Then how the hell did his wife conceive, ask him that?"

"He says that after a week he was dying for a pee, so he cut the end off."

LIMERICKS VIII

There was a great swimmer named Hidges
Whose bottom got bitten by midges
To avoid the attack
He swam on his back
But his hampton got bashed on the bridges.

There was an old whore of Madras.
Who was bushed with a liner of brass
She would tinkle like hell
When they clappered the bell
And play the bass notes with her ass.

There was a young lady named Myrtle
Who would have it straight up or turned turtle
She littered a child
By the late Oscar Wilde
To prove to the world she was fertile.

There was a young lady named Laws
Who worked in a furniture stores
If rich clients pressed
On her very fine chest
She would readily open her drawers.

There was a shy virgin named Grace
Who said: "If the whole human race
Depends upon what
The boys call a twat,
Then it's put in a damned awkward place!"

There was a rugby captain who became so weak they dropped him, and the trainer sent him to the psychiatrist, who asked him all about his dreams. "I have the same dreadful dream every night," said the patient. "I dream I am in the Strand with a barrow full of bricks, and I have to wheel them to Bethnal Green; I wake up completely beggared."

Said the Head Shrinker: "I know I can help you, take one of these pills each night when you go to bed, and that'll be ten guineas please."

The rugby captain took a pill at bed-time, and he had exactly the same dream as before, except that when he got as far as the Mile End Road the psychiatrist met him, took the barrow of bricks from him, and pushed them to Bethnal Green. Thus the man woke up much less exhausted, recovered his strength, and his place in the XV.

The good news went round the club, so that when the full back began to lose form they sent him at once to the same man.

"Explain your dreams," said he.

"Well, Doctor, I dream every night I am in a Sultan's harem. Ten fantastic girls come in, with breasts like melons, big thighs, pink round bottoms. . . ." "Yes-yes," said the quack, "never mind that, what do YOU do?"

"That's just it! One after another they demand my services, I get so I can't refuse, and I wake up shattered and shugged out."

After paying the fee, and taking the pills, he got worse instead of better.

"What's gone wrong?" said the trainer.

"Well, now, when I dream about the ten luscious girls the psychiatrist always arrives to take five of them off me. A rugger man of my age can manage five a night without bother, but, oh dear, when I finish and go outside, I find I am in the Mile End Road with a barrow full of bricks which I have to wheel to Bethnal Green!"

MY KINGDOM FOR A HORSE'S

An enterprising young journalist was always on the lookout for "stories" and one day he read under "Legal Notices" that a Vet and a surgeon had formed a business partnership.

He thought there must be something unusual behind this, and he went round to the address given. Nobody answered the bell, but the door was open, so he pushed through to the back. Looking through a glass door he beheld a remarkable sight. There was a wealthy middle-aged man stretched out naked on an operating table, and he had a very shrivelled-up member. Nearby, on a huge slab, was a stallion under anaesthetic. The young journalist listened at the door, and he heard the surgeon say to the vet:

"You know, Jones, if we can only pull off this particular transplant, we shall both make our bloody fortunes."

NEEDED FRESH HAIR?

There was a boastful young man, who thought he knew all the answers.

He married a girl who knew she knew all the answers.

They went on a Winter honeymoon in Oslo, when the nights were fourteen hours long.

After the bridal night the groom got up, stretched himself and boasted:

"Well, I feel like a new man now."

"So do I," said the bride.

THE PRIMROSE PATH

There was a little girl whose parents brought her up "modern".

One day she was at a wedding, and when the bride and groom came out of the church and stood ready to be photographed, there was a bit of a hush.

Then a little girl's voice piped up: "Mummy dear, will he give her his pollen now, or wait 'til they get home?"

LONG TIME PASSING

There was a methodical German, a passionate Frenchman, and a cold Englishman staying with their new brides at a famous honeymoon hotel. As they retired to bed they agreed that they would get together the next day and exchange experiences over some drinks. Thus it came to pass next day that the German was asked:

"How did you get on last night?"

"Acht, vunce to begin wid, then vunce von hour later, und every time der clock strucken, vunce again, vich vass eight times in eight hour."

"And what did your wife say?"

"Wunderbar, Wunderbar!!"

The Frenchman told them:

"I am straightway on the work. Den I am on the work again when I receive back my breath. Den I sleep and start again, and sleep and start again. Vingt fois, tventy time, them I am halted, finis."

"What did your wife say?"

"Ah, elle dit, Magnifique, encore, magnifique!!"

The Englishman had been very quiet: "Come tell us, how many?"

"Once," he said.

"Once! – what did your wife say at dawn?"

"Get off, we need some sleep."

KEEPING ABREAST OF THINGS

There was a new African State set up and they wished to set up a legal system as good as that in Great Britain. Accordingly they studied the law reports in various papers and went ahead accordingly. When this new system was in full swing they invited the Lord Chancellor to go and give it the O.K. Accordingly the Lord Chancellor paid a visit, and was much impressed with what he saw. Counsel and Judges wore wigs, English fashion, they had a Jury System, and all was according to the Book. However, he was astonished when he attended his first big case. Before the proceedings opened a Pigmy entered the Court, and proceeded to feel the breasts of the policewomen, the lady shorthand writers, and those of the girls who happened to be in the public gallery. "What's all this about?" he gasped.

"Ah, my Lord, we read the papers from your country, and from time to time we know that 'A little titter runs round the Court', well, that's him."

THAT'S MY STORY

A male ballet dancer, having Sunday as his day off, went for a walk in the woods. He met a large and ugly toad, who startled him by saying:

"Hey, don't pass me by!"

"What's going on?" enquired the young man.

"I'm a bewitched human being," said the toad, "and if I can find a man who was born on February 29th, which is less than one chance in a thousand, as you know, I can bring him great good luck."

The young man said he was born on February 29th, what did he have to do to acquire the good luck?

"Take me to your bed, let me sleep all night with you, and in the morning you will have a wonderful surprise."

So the young man took the great ugly toad back, smuggled him into his theatrical digs, and took him to bed. Just as the landlady brought in the morning cup of tea, the toad turned into a handsome prince.

* * *

"Is that the story?" enquired the learned Judge.

"Yes, my Lord, that concludes the case for the defence," replied Counsel.

LIKE FATHER LIKE . . .

Council houses have thin walls. When this couple got married they stayed the night with his parents, who retired to bed, only to be disturbed by the bumping about in the next room.

"Tell you what," whispered father, "every time they do it, we'll do it?"

This was agreed, and after an hour the honeymooners were off again. Father and mother fell into an exhausted sleep, only to be re-awakened at four in the morning. At six father awoke, listened, and said:

"Stop it, Albert, you're killing your mother."

HANDLE WITH CARE

A new bride was getting in the taxi to go to the station. Suddenly she cried: "Wait! Mother, I've left my gloves somewhere in the reception, go and find them please."

"Oh my child, you don't need your gloves, take it in your bare hand, the same as I did with your father."

DIZZY HEIGHTS

A man went to join the army, and was sent before the Medical Board. The doctor examined him in the buff, and then instantly sent out for his students: "Look gentlemen," he said, "the biggest one I've ever seen, and I've been an army doctor twenty years." The students looked with awe, and one said: "Sir, can I ask this recruit a question?"

"By all means, go ahead."

"Right, now pardon me Smith, but you appear to have the biggest one of any army recruit, tell me, what is it like when it's down?"

"It's down now," was the reply.

"Good lord! Then tell us, what is it like when it's up?"

"I'm sorry, I don't know, I've never seen it erect, doctor."

"Do you mean to say that a man as well blessed as you is actually impotent? Bad luck that."

"I didn't say that," protested the soldier, "I said I'd never SEEN it up. You see, I've only got enough blood for one of us, and every time he rises, I faint."

PLEASE LIFT ONLY BY THE HANDLE

By a strange coincidence, two more recruits came in that day with oversize members. They were brothers, and the doctors, unable to believe their eyes, decided to write the matter up in the medical press. Says the head medico, getting out his writing pad: "How do you account for this?"

"It's hereditary, Sir," said the older one.

"Aha" (writing it down) "your father is the cause of these, hey?"

"No, Sir, our mother. It's because of our mother that my brothers and I have such big dicks."

"Your mother! Why you idiot, women don't have them!"

"No, Sir, but she only had one arm, and when it came to getting us in and out of the bath, she had to manage as best she could."

SATAN REBUKING SIN

A man went to a solicitor and said he must have a divorce.

"Why?" said the man of law.

"Because of my wife's filthy habits."

"What filthy habits?"

"Ooh, I couldn't tell you."

The solicitor explained that if the man wouldn't detail the dirty habits of his wife, there could be no possibility of a divorce.

At last the man blurted it out:

"The fact is," he said, "that every time I go to piss in the sink, I always find it full of dirty washing-up."

A SCABBY TRICK

There was a girl who went to a priest to confess that she had been "naughty" with a man. She said it was her first experience, and she was certainly a bit vague about it.

"Look here, daughter," said the priest, undoing her blouse, "did he do this?" – "Yes Father." (Having a right good maul.) "Did he do this?"

"Yes, Father."

The priest took her knickers off. . . . "Did he do this?" – "Yes he did."

Shortly she was on her back and the priest's trousers open. . . . "Did he do this?" "Yes, indeed Father."

After the job was fully completed and they were both doing up their clothes, the priest says: "Well, you've told me everything, you can have absolution."

"But, Father, he did something else."

"Something else?" (His mind visualised several unpleasant ideas.)

"Yes, he gave me the pox!"

SECOND CHILDHOOD

A little girl was in the park crying when a respectable old gentleman asked her why. She said: "I want one of those things like my brother's got, that sticks out, and then lays down, and then sticks out again."

The respectable old gentleman began to cry too.

DESERT ISLAND DISHED

There was a man who was overweight, and this worried him, so he went to his doctor. The doctor said: "I can put you right, but it's rather pricey; take these pills, one each night, and come back in two weeks."

The man returned in a fortnight looking fine. "Tell me?" said the doctor.

"Well, Sir, every night when I went to bed, I dreamed that I was in a harem with twenty of the most voluptuous randy girls, and I had to lay all of them. It was marvellous, and I've lost a stone in weight!"

"That'll be twenty quid," said the doctor.

"And well worth it," said the patient.

Now this patient had an acquaintance, a mean miserable beggar, who was also too fat, so he sent him for the same treatment.

When this miser reported back to the doctor, he too had lost a stone, but he wasn't in the least grateful.

"Look here," he said, "I dreamed I was on a desert island, and every night a huge Blackamoor came out with a long sharp knife; he chased me round and round 'til dawn, swearing he would castrate me. I used to wake up sweating and half dead. . . ."

"But you lost a stone!"

"Yes, but my mate had girls with big. . . ."

"That's your fault. You *would* have yours on the National Health."

AN ODD ONE

An Irishwoman went to the Marriage Guidance clinic to ask about a divorce:

"Does your husband ill-treat you?" – "No, he's a kind, gentle, man."

"Does he drink and gamble?" – "No, he gives me all his money."

"Then of course, unfaithfulness must be the trouble?"

"Yes, I suppose it must be, one of the kids isn't his."

UNITED WE STAND

There had been some massive take-over bids in the Insurance world, and four of Britain's largest companies had amalgamated. They built a new headquarters in the Strand which was truly marvellous. The Planning Authority had insisted that it be finished off with a giant piece of sculpture, as is the modern custom, and this was the problem.

The Directors met, and as money was no object, they decided to engage Einstein. It was written into the contract that the sculpture was not to be "modern", but it was to be a true representation of the amalgamation of four great Insurance companies, no more, no less. In return, Einstein asked that the plinth be close-boarded and the thing kept under drapes until finished, which was readily agreed.

*　　*　　*

When the day of unveiling came, all were there in their toppers, Directors, MPs, and distinguished men as well. The ladies included some of the noblest in the land, with their daughters.

When the Lord Mayor of London pulled the string, a shocking sight was disclosed. The thing was no more than a huge shield divided into four quarters, and in each quarter a naked couple, larger than life, manifestly having intercourse. The Chairman was livid! "We demand an explanation," he shouted, "and it had better be a good one, or you'll never see a penny of that twenty thousand quid!"

Einstein remained calm: "Gentlemen," he said, "I have fulfilled my instructions. Observe in the first quarter an Actuary in a whore's parlour – that is *Commercial Union*. In the second quarter a Director is having his typist across the desk, which is surely *Employers' Liability*. Next we have a Banker's son with his fiancée in an hotel, that's *Mutual Trust*. The last couple are clearly married to each other, which is *Wesleyan and General*." (*They had to pay him the money.*)

RISING TO THE OCCASION

There was a young man who considered himself sex starved. He was randy all the time. He was dying to join a nudist camp, and finally, after a good deal of wangling, got himself invited to a Club, "on probation".

His friend told him what to do. You prove your identity at the gate, then they let you into the hut, and you strip off. Then you walk down a glade, and the Secretary will meet you and introduce you.

"Remember!" he said, "behave yourself, it's all very respectable."

The man swore to be good, and all went according to plan. He left the hut, walked down the path, and spotted a young woman with splendid breasts, a round full bottom, a shaved quim, in fact, the lot.

"Excuse me," he said, "but I'm looking for the Secretary."

"I'm the Secretary."

"Oh indeed, then I'm very glad to meet you."

"Yes, I can see that you are."

HE WASN'T A LABOUR MAN

A midwife on her day off called in the hospital for her wages. At that moment the phone rang, and there was a mild panic. It seemed that yet another emergency case had arisen, and no one to take it. The off-duty midwife must go.

"But I'm in civvies."

"That doesn't matter."

"My car's in dock."

"We'll get you a taxi."

All this took time, and as soon as the taxi arrived, the nurse flung herself into it, and said: "For Pete's sake hurry up, the baby's due in ten minutes."

The taxi driver stopped, opened the door, and said: "Oh no yer don't Missus, not in my cab yer don't."

WISSED IN THE POTTLE

A working-class woman was up before the Beak for assaulting her neighbour on the bus.

"I don't understand it," he said, "you and Mrs Maggs have been neighbours and friends for years, how did this fight start?"

"It was like this, your Worship. I'm on the bus going with me sample to the doctor's see, and Mrs Bloggs gets on, see. . . ."

"Yes yes, get on with it, what happened?"

"Well she asts me 'What have yer got in that bottle?' and I replies 'Piss' and she says, 'Oh it's piss to me is it?' in that case, 'Shit to you too', and that's how it all started."

LOOKING GLASS

A working-class woman was very jealous because all her neighbours were getting things free off the National Health. One had new teeth, another had new glasses, and when the woman next door got a free hearing aid, it was the last straw.

She went to the doctor and said: "I want something free on the National Health as well."

"Oh indeed," said the doctor, humouring her, "and what do you fancy, eh?"

"Well, Doctor, I fancy I'd like you to cut a hole in my stomach."

The doctor thought he could see what was coming, "Ah, I see, your husband is not satisfied with the one you've got, and you want me to make you a new one?"

"Oh no, certainly not, I want you to make the hole and fit a piece of glass in it."

"Look here, Mrs Shufflebottam, I'm a busy man, I'll prescribe some tranquillisers, and please send the next patient in."

"I don't fancy tranquillisers!"

"Well, what do you fancy then?"

"I've just told you – a womb with a view!"

CHEESED OFF

Two rough types were employed as Night Soil men, and one very hot summer day they were approaching their cart, each with a full bucket, when a local factory hooter blew for dinner-hour. They put down their burdens, and each produced a packet of sandwiches, which they proceeded to eat at the roadside. The stench was noisesome, blowflies filled the air, and passers-by crossed the road.

"Hey Dan," said Bill, "it stinks enough now, without you stirring it round with your arm!"

"Stirring it up? Don't be bloody silly, I've dropped me bread and cheese."

MOVING STORY

A Chinaman went to the doctor because he was very constipated, and the doctor gave him a prescription for a good stiff dose of "number nines".

"Come back in three days, and tell me how you get on."

Three days later the Chinaman was back.

"Have you moved yet?"

"No, Slir, me no moovee not at all."

The doctor gave him a double dose, and awaited results.

Three days later, still no results, so the quack gave him the stiffest possible dose of the very strongest purgative, and said: "Come back in three days, without fail."

When the man came back:

"Have you moved yet?"

"No, Slir, me no moovee yet, me moovee tomorrow, house full of slit."

BELLY LIKELY

Sherlock Holmes went up to Heaven. Saint Peter said: "What's your claim?"

"I claim to be the world's greatest detective," said Holmes.

"Pass a test, and you can stay in Heaven," said Peter.

"What test?"

"There are millions of people in here. If you can pick out Adam and Eve, you win."

(Holmes had no difficulty, they were the only two without navels!)

APPEASEMENT

There was a doctor who had a working-class National Health practice, and, just before going on holiday he was explaining the business to a young locum.

"There is one man," he said, "an Irishman, and a proper pest – never satisfied." At this moment the doctor looked out of the window, and added: "Ah, he is coming in now."

The trouble-maker came into the surgery, and started shouting that his wife was having too many kids, why didn't the doctor do something about it?

"Ah yes, I could put your wife on the Pill."

The man protested that Father O'Flynn would never allow it.

"Then why don't *you* do something about it, wear a sheath."

"Damn that for a game – like eating a toffee with the paper on."

After a lot more argument the man shouted that the doctor must put matters right, or he would write to the Medical Council about it.

"Oh very well, very well," said the doctor, "I'll write a prescription; now clear off, I'm busy."

The man set off and found a chemists shop. The chemist broke the seal, read the prescription, and said: "I want none of your funny jokes here, take it to a greengrocer."

As surgery was finishing the Irishman came back. "What the blazes is the meaning of this!" he yelled, flourishing the piece of paper under the doctor's nose. . . . "Half a pound of dried peas, one to be placed in the left shoe each morning."

"It will make you limp all the time," said the doctor.

BACK TO *SKOLL*!

A stranger at a nudist camp had drunk too much tea. He was having a real good pee behind a bush before he saw a nice girl doing the same. Neither could stop, and to cover her embarrassment the girl said:

"Good health, here's to you, and PLEASE don't tell anybody about this."

"That's a bargain," said he, "provided we touch glasses!"

"Agreed," she said, "kiss my quim."

"That's not at all what you promised," he protested.

"Oh yes it is, you will be putting your old mug against my little cup."

WET BLANKET

A well brought up girl went to a dance, missed the last bus, and had to walk home. She lost her way, and finished up sleeping on the porch of a synagogue.

Her mother, when she heard the story, was a little bit upset. "It was such a damp night, I only hope you're going to be all right after the experience."

The girl said she was quite all right. A few months later she was obviously pregnant.

Her mother said: "You didn't tell the truth did you, about where you slept that night?"

"Oh yes I did, Mother, but I forgot to mention that when I woke up in the morning I found a little *dew* on me."

TO HER CREDIT

A man got in touch with a girl through a Marriage Bureau. He rather liked her, but he told the Bureau Manager that he wouldn't consider marriage without a trial of her sexual abilities. "We businessmen never purchase in bulk without a sample," he added.

The girl, when she heard about this, sent back the answer: "I too am business trained, and I don't have to give free samples, but I can, and will give bankers' and solicitors' references."

ANSWER TO PRAYER

A Minister heard that in his rather superior parish the harmless little parties that went on were really orgies. He wangled himself an invite to such a party, and it started off with harmless games and background music.

However, after the drinks had gone round a few times, more and more people began to undress, and everybody was mauling everybody else. The Minister retired to a bedroom to pray furiously.

He had not been there very long when a smashing girl walked in, stark naked. "Do you want me?" he said.

"Not particularly, but I drew you in the raffle."

NUTS TO THAT

A Women's Army Corps officer during the war thought that her girls were getting frustrated. When a Yankee Division straight from the line moved into the next town she saw her chance, and rang up the Commanding Officer.

"Would you like to come and take dinner with me and escort me to the dance afterwards?"

"Deelighted, Marm."

"Could you bring along some enlisted men for the girls?"

"I should tell you, Marm, my privates are black."

"That's all right I can give you a bath before dinner, but can you bring along some enlisted men?"

WHAT A WET

Some toffee-nosed WRENS ran a dance, and, for want of better, sent along some tickets to the Naval barracks. The WREN C.O. was a bit worried about things, and decided to station herself at the ticket desk to see who came in.

The first to arrive was a rough Portsmouth petty officer, he said:

"Before I go in, where's the piss-corner?"

"My good man, proceed right down the corridor until you see a door on your left marked 'Gentlemen Only'. Take no notice of that, just walk right in."

ENLARGEMENT

A young married man took his wife to an overworked National Health doctor to be examined, because he thought she might be pregnant, as she had missed one month.

The doctor took up a rubber stamp, made a tiny imprint on the woman's belly, and dismissed them, calling for the next patient.

The husband, overcome with curiosity undressed the wife as soon as they got home, and got a powerful magnifying glass to work. He read:

"As soon as you can read this in ordinary daylight, without glasses, it's time to bring her back."

There was a young curate named Borrow
Who eloped with two nuns, to his sorrow,
They lived on an isthmus
And one he called Christmas
The other he christened Tomorrow.

"You need exercise man, and fresh air!"
Said the doctor, to Sinjohn Sinclair.
To her joy and surprise
He forced his wife's thighs –
The "exercise" brought a fresh heir!

The learned Lord Chancellor Veres
Suspended a shocked House of Peers
And to Coventry hied
For Godiva's great ride,
As he'd not seen a white horse for years.

There was a yachtswoman of Hale
Who had a leak under the rail,
A caulker named Goat
Put a plug in her boat,
And now she's a ship in full sail.

"My bride was no virgin," said Braining,
"I've never received such a draining!
Mere up and down thrust
Could be natural lust,
But side-to-side action, that's training!"

WHAT RUGBY JOKES DID NEXT

You should be ashamed of yourself, picking up a book like this.

THIS IS A CHAIN LETTER

Dear Friend :
This chain was started in the hope of bringing happiness to all tired business men. Unlike most chains, it doesn't require money. Simply send a copy of this to five male friends, then bundle up your wife and send her to the fellow whose name heads the list. When your name reaches the top of the list, you will receive 15,186 women and some should be corkers. Have faith. Don't break the chain. One man broke it and got his wife back.

Your friend,
Homebreakers, Ltd.

FLAT OUT

A young lady was permitted by her parents to take employment in a large city and live in her own apartment. The one condition was that she would not allow gentlemen friends to her flat as it would worry her mother.

During a long distance phone conversation, the daughter described her date of the previous evening to her mother.

"You didn't permit that man in your flat, did you?" queried the nervous mother.

"Oh, no !" replied the daughter, "we went to his flat. Let his mother worry."

CARRY ON FIREMAN

John, a 6ft. 2in. fireman from Yorkshire, thought he had every reason to be pleased with the results of his first evening out in London. After a few pints at the pub, here he was bedded down with a delightful redhead whom he hadn't known for longer than an hour.

Unfortunately those pints at the pub (not to mention the chasers in between) had a rather softening effect on his otherwise passionate advances. Hoping that his customary vigour would return to him later in the evening, John tried to make conversation :

"I'm a big fireman from Bradford," he told her.

"Well," replied the redhead, "either start paying out more hose, or get closer to the fire !"

FAT WOMAN TO FAT MAN

"Thanks for the tip."

A ROSE BY ANY OTHER NAME

Harold and Mabel were admiring the view from the window of their honeymoon hotel. Slightly flushed with embarrassment Mabel turned to her newly acquired husband and asked:

"Harold, darling, now that we're married at last, please tell me: what is a penis?"

Delighted by her innocence, Harold led her back into the bedroom, took off his trousers and showed her.

"Oh!" she exclaimed, "It's just like a prick, only smaller."

THE ULTIMATE INSULT

"Is it in?"

THE WAGES OF SIN

Three young boys were playing in the street of a London slum. A Rolls Royce stopped and a beautiful, expensively dressed blonde stepped out. She crossed over to the boys, picked up the youngest, hugged him and left a box of candies, and filled his hands with money. Waving goodbye, she re-entered the car and departed. The other boys were goggle-eyed.

One said, "Blimey, Jackie, was that yer fairy godmother?"

Jackie looked at him with scorn and replied, "Naw, that wuz my sister wot was ruined."

AFTERTHOUGHT

Bellhop at the 'Hit and Run' Hotel. "Anything else, sir . . . ?"

Man : "No, that's all. Thank you."

Bellhop : "Anything for your wife . . . ?"

Man : "Why, yes. Come to think of it. Bring me a postcard."

AN APPLE A DAY

Harry's sore throat was bothering him so much that he went along to the doctor's house at lunchtime, even though it was outside normal surgery hours.

The doorbell was answered by the doctor's pretty young wife.

"Is the doctor in?" Harry whispered hoarsely.

"He won't be back till three," she whispered back, "come on in."

THE HORSE'S MOUTH

Sally, a buxom young deb, had been out riding all morning and when she brought the horse back to the stable, it was tired out and lathered with sweat. As she dismounted the groom remarked:

" 'E looks just about done in."

"You'd be tired too," replied Sally, "if you'd been between my legs for as long as that horse has."

TIT FOR TEAT

Despite his good looks and his rich 6oo acre farm, Fred had never managed to have his way with the buxom farmgirl who milked his cows. So he took her away to watch his prize bull servicing a cow, in the hope that the spectacle would set the juices churning in her ripe young body.

"Believe me," he told her as they watched, "I'd like to be doing what that bull is doing right now !"

"Why don't you?" she answered, "it's your cow."

A HARD DECISION

The party was in full flow when George set out on a tour of inspection round the house. In one of the bedrooms he came upon a naked girl fast asleep under an eiderdown. Unable to resist the temptation, he stripped off his own clothes, clambered aboard and began making love to her. She soon woke up and asked him what on earth he thought he was doing.

"Shall I take it out?" asked George.

"Take it out," she replied, "and then put it in again a few times so that I can make up my mind."

THE MARKET PRICE

Everyone looked up as the couple walked through the restaurant to their table. She was young, beautiful and voluptuous while he was old, haggard and stooped. The waiter came over to take their order and the young woman proceeded to order the most expensive dishes in the house. Her escort was somewhat staggered and asked, "Do you eat this well at home?"

"No," she replied, "but then, no one there wants to sleep with me!"

PLAYBACK

A bra manufacturer who sells his product under the slogan "Every Girl Wants EMBARGO" was asked why he picked "EMBARGO" for a trade name. "At first glance you may think it's foolish," he explained, "but spelled backwards, it has tremendous sales appeal."

A DISAPPOINTING SWEET

Mrs Jones was on trial for beating up her husband so badly that he had to spend two weeks in hospital.

On the night of the incident, her lawyer explained, Mrs Jones had locked her husband out of the bedroom because he was disgustingly drunk. But Mr Jones kept hammering on the door, saying :

"I bet you'd let me in if you knew what I was knocking with."

When she got up at once to unlock the door, he came in and gave her a box of chocolates.

FANCY UNDRESS

Fanny ransacked her wardrobe for something to wear at the Fancy Dress Ball. Finding nothing suitable she simply took off all her clothes and went along stark naked as Eve.

But the Doorman turned her away on the grounds that nudity didn't represent anybody in particular.

Twenty minutes later she was back, still naked except for a pair of black gloves and black shoes.

"Who are you supposed to be now?" asked the doorman, preparing to turn her away a second time.

"Can't you see?' answered Fanny, "I'm the five of spades."

BIRD TALK

Aunt Mildred decided to buy a parrot to keep her company. The local pet shop had a good selection, but one bird with bright green and blue feathers immediately caught her attention as the pick of the bunch. Curiously enough the shopkeeper seemed reluctant to sell it.

"I don't think he's really Madame's sort of parrot," he explained evasively.

"Why on earth not?"

"He doesn't come from a very nice home. Now, if madame would care to step this way, I think I have just the bird . . .'

"But I don't *like* any of those. I want this one," Mildred insisted.

"Very well, madam." Noting the glint of determination in Mildred's eye, the shopkeeper sold her the bird and an expensive wrought iron cage to go with it.

Mildred installed the parrot in her sitting room and waited breathlessly for his first words. The parrot flapped his wings, looked around the house and said:

"New house. Very nice."

Mildred was delighted.

At half past four Mildred's two teenage daughters came back from school. The parrot cocked an eye at them and said:

"New girls. Very nice."

Mildred clapped her hands with joy. Not only was the parrot such a magnificent specimen, but he had perfect manners. No wonder the man at the pet store hadn't wanted to part with him!

At half past five her husband Henry returned from the office. The parrot skittered to the front of his cage and said:

"New house. New girls. Same old customer. How are you Henry?"

A SNATCH OF CONVERSATION

Finding himself next to a rather striking mini-skirted blonde in the bus queue on a windy day, George decided to strike up a conversation with her.

"Airy, isn't it?" he remarked.

"Wot did yer hexpect," she answered haughtily, "hostrich feathers?"

CINEMATIC TECHNIQUE

On Saturday nights Tom and Hilda usually went to the pictures to pet in the back row. One night, when they were showing Dracula's Grave, Hilda's squeals and giggles of excitement attracted the attention of the Manager.

"What's the matter young lady?" he asked, "Are you feeling hysterical?"

"No, he's feeling mine."

QUESTIONS AND ANSWERS

Q. What do you call an uncircumcised Jewish baby?
A. A girl.

Q. What is a lesbian?
A. A mannish depressive with delusions of gender.

Q. What is a gynaecologist?
A. A spreader of old wives' tales.

Q. What's the difference between a vitamin and a hormone?
A. You can't hear a vitamin.

Q. What do you call an abortion in Prague?
A. A cancelled cheque.

Q. Why don't prostitutes vote?
A. Because they don't care who gets in.

Q. How do porcupines make love?
A. Very carefully.

HORSE SENSE

Said the worried patient to the psychiatrist: "I'm in love with my horse."

"But that's nothing," replied the psychiatrist. "A lot of people love animals. My wife and I have a dog that we love very much."

"Ah, but doctor, it's a physical attraction that I feel toward my horse!"

"Ummmm!" said the psychiatrist. "What kind of horse is it? male or female?"

"Female of course!" the gent shot back angrily. "What do you think I am, queer?"

UNDERSTATEMENT

A man called the undertaker and cried, "Come over and bury my wife."

"But," said the mortician, "I buried your wife ten years ago."

"I got married again," sobbed the man.

"Congratulations," said the undertaker.

A HEAVENLY REUNION

Elsie died at the age of ninety-two, having outlived a remarkable total of eight husbands. At the funeral one of her neighbours remarked : "At last they're together again."

"Which husband are you talking about?" asked another of the neighbours.

"I'm not talking about her husbands," came the reply, "I'm talking about her legs."

PASS THE BUCK

At dinner Daisy told her stodgy old husband about her visit to the doctor :

"When he examined me, he admired my breasts and said they were very beautiful."

"Did he," asked her husband, "say anything about your great fat arse?"

"No," answered Daisy. "I don't think he mentioned you at all."

A MATTER OF PRINCIPLE

A man was travelling to Manchester with his family by train. Since their compartment was a non-smoker, he went next door to smoke a cigar. The only other occupant was a rather dejected young man, gazing moodily out of the window. Harry offered him a cigar.

"No thank you," said the young man, "I don't smoke."

When Harry had finished with his newspaper, he asked the young man whether he'd like to read it.

"No thank you," he replied, "I don't read."

Still hoping to cheer up his travelling companion, Harry offered to buy him a drink.

"No thank you," came the refrain, "I don't drink."

Refusing to admit defeat, Harry tried again :

"Young man, I admire your principles. I'd like you to come and meet my wife and daughter in the next compartment."

"No thank you. I don't screw either."

LIKE FATHER, LIKE SON

George ran the business in partnership with his son. When his son showed signs of worry and strain, George asked him what the matter was, reminding him that, as partners, they must share their responsibilities.

"Well, Dad, since you put it that way, the typist is pregnant, and she wants *us* to marry her."

NIGHTRIDE

Making love on the backseat of the car, a young couple were interrupted by the arrival of a policeman.

"What are you doing in there?" asked the policeman.

"Just necking officer," replied the young man.

"Well put your neck back in your trousers, and drive on."

A NEW DEAL FOR YOUNG LOVERS

An Irish priest was disturbed by the number of women in his flock who confessed to him that they had been seduced by the grocer's new delivery boy. As a penance he asked them all to put ten shillings in the poor box. When the delivery boy came to make his confession, the priest asked angrily:

"Well, boy, what have you got to say for yourself?"

"Just this father," he replied, "either you give me a fair share of those ten shilling fees, or I take my business to the next parish."

MANSLAUGHTER

A couple, married for thirty years, had never missed a night of connubial bliss. Not feeling well one day, the wife consulted her doctor and was informed that she must have complete rest and quiet for six months or she would not live.

The wife and husband decided that they must stay completely apart during this period. She moved into an upstairs bedroom and he remained downstairs.

After three months of complete abstinence and solitude, his will power collapsed and he started for her bedroom. Just as he was about to ascend the stairs, he saw her coming down. Their eyes met and she said, "Dear, I was just coming down to die." To which he quickly replied, "I'm glad, darling, because I was just going up to kill you."

SAVED BY THE BELLE

A son comes to tell his father that he has got his girlfriend pregnant.

"How much do you need?" asks the father.

"A hundred and twenty pounds."

A few days later the second son arrives with the same story.

"How much?"

"A hundred and fifty pounds, Dad."

The next day the daughter comes and confesses that she is pregnant.

"Thank God," says the father, "business is looking up at last."

A SINNER PRAYS

Oh, Blessed Virgin we believe
That without sin thou didst conceive.
Teach us then how thus believing
We can sin without conceiving.

A LONELY DIET

The young bride asked her doctor for a simple and effective method of birthcontrol.

"Orange juice." he replied.

"Do you take it before or after?" asked the bride.

"Neither—instead."

DIVINE INTERVENTION

There was no doubt about it, Gloria was pregnant.

"Please feel free to use my telephone if you'd like to tell your husband," said the doctor.

"But doctor, I'm not married."

"Well, then, you'd better tell your lover."

"But I've never had a lover!"

"All right. Then I must ask you to go home and tell your mother to get ready for the second coming of Christ."

FAIL SAFE

After lights-out at an exclusive girls' school the conversation turned to the best method of avoiding pregnancy.

"My boy friend takes it out before he comes off," said the first girl, "but I know that's not very safe, so I'm going to get some pills during the holidays."

"I've been using the rhythm method," said the second, "but that means I can't have it very often. I think I'll go on the pill too."

"I wouldn't advise it," said the third, "I've tried and it keeps dropping out."

A SLIPPERY CUSTOMER

The chemist was trying to explain why this particular brand of contraceptive was so much more expensive than the rest.

"These ones," he said, "are guaranteed by the makers."

"But what if they break?"

"Then the guarantee runs out."

A SELLER'S MARKET

A man went into a chemists to find a cure for his persistent erection. He was embarrassed to find that there was only a female assistant, but she did her best to assure him that he could speak freely.

"Well, I've had this erection for two weeks, and I can't get it to go down. What can you give me for it?"

"Just a minute, please sir, I'd like to consult my partner."

The woman disappeared into the back of the shop and came back three minutes later.

"I've talked it over with my partner, and the best we can offer you is the shop and fifty pounds in cash."

GUESS AGAIN

It was at the office Christmas party. As they lay on the office reception couch in the darkened room, their breath came hot and fast.

"Oh, Melvin, Melvin," she said passionately, "you've never made love to me like this before. Is it because of the holiday spirit?"

"No" he panted. "It's probably because I'm not Melvin!"

PHOTO-PLAY

The husband finally cornered the Casanova who had been seducing his wife. "Look," he said, flourishing photos taken by a private detective he had employed. "Here's a shot of you and my wife in the living room of my apartment. Here's another of you drinking together, half undressed. And here's a picture of you two in bed together. Now, what are you going to do about it?"

The adulterer studied the photos carefully, nodding over each one. After a moment he picked up the third one and handed it to the husband. "All right," he said. "I'll take a dozen of this one."

HUMP-TY DUMP-TY

A man was walking down the street one afternoon when he was hit on the head by a used contraceptive thrown out of a second story window. Outraged, he pounded at the door of the offending house until the owner appeared.

"Whose window is that?" he asked, pointing to the second storey.

"My daughter's," replied the owner.

"Is she alone?"

"She's with my intended son-in-law, not that it's any of your business."

"Well in that case you might like to know that your intended grandson has just had a very bad fall."

.

CAUGHT IN THE ACT

Sally's mother, determined on a good marriage for her daughter, instructed her to let her rich boy friend have his way with her, and then, when he lit a cigarette afterwards, to say : "And what shall we call the baby?" He will then be forced to propose to her.

Sally did as she'd been told.

"If he gets out of that," said her boyfriend, throwing the contraceptive into the waste-paperbasket, "we'll call him Houdini."

A SALESMAN'S PITCH

A father of twins was pestered in the station waiting room by a nosey old lady who kept asking questions about his children. Every time she asked him a question, he would simply answer, "I don't know, Madam."

"How is it that you don't even know your own children's names, or whether they're boys or girls," the old lady asked.

"I'm not the father of these children, Ma'am," he answered, "I'm a contraceptive salesman, and these are two complaints I'm taking back to the factory."

CARNAL KNOWLEDGE

After a particularly enjoyable evening out, Susan asked Roger in for a cup of coffee in her parents' house.

Half an hour later her mother came down to find them having intercourse on the sofa. "Well I never . . ." she exclaimed.

"Don't be silly, mother," replied Susan, "of course you did."

THE NAME OF THE GAME

Three sisters were preparing to go out for the evening. All three went to say good-bye to their mother before they left.

"I'm going out with Pete to eat," said the first.

"That's nice, darling," said the mother, "try not to be late."

"I'm going out with Lance to dance," said the second.

"How lovely!" said the mother, "but do keep an eye on the time."

"I'm going out with Chuck," said the third.

"Oh, no you're not," said the mother, 'you're staying right here."

ACROBATICS

The bride and groom realised from the sounds next door that the parents were listening through the wall. So they decided to pack up their belongings and move out to an hotel. Unaware of what was going on, the parents on the other side of the wall mistook the sounds of packing for the sounds of intercourse.

The hastily packed suitcase would not shut properly; "Let me sit on it," said the bride.

"No, I'll sit on it," whispered the groom.

"All right, let's both sit on it," said the bride.

At which point the father burst into the room, saying, "I'm sorry to interrupt, but this I've got to see!"

GENERATION GASP

The elderly gentleman was nearing eighty but refused to accept his loss of sexual desire and stamina. He consulted with his doctor.

The doctor was amused and asked "Why should you be so concerned? It's expected at your age."

"But," pursued the oldster, "a friend of mine who is eighty-five says he makes love to his wife every night."

The doctor smiled. "Well, can't you say the same thing?"

HAND OUT

Girl in theatre : "The man next to me is masturbating !"
Girl-friend : "Ignore him."
"I can't; he's using my hand !"

LISTEN WITH MOTHER

When their son brought his newlywed wife home for their first night together, Mr and Mrs Jones, eavesdropping from the next door bedroom, decided to do everything that the young couple did.

After the newlyweds had made love three times and were starting on number four, the father banged desperately on the wall and shouted:

"Tony, stop! You're killing your mother!"

A NOTE ON THE BRIDAL BED

The cold cream's on the mantle
The shoe-horn's on the shelf;
I saw that great big thing of yours
And I chloroformed myself.

HANDY PANKY

A young couple travelled by train to their honeymoon hotel. During the journey the woman fondled her man under the cover of a newspaper spread across his lap. Later they both dozed off and a breeze blew the newspaper onto the floor. Then the conductor came by.

"Wake up, Madam," he said, shaking her awake. "Your bouquet has wilted."

WELL PRAYED!

The young vicar and his bride had just undressed and were ready to taste the fruits of love. But before the bride could clamber into the marital bed, he suggested they should kneel down together to pray for strength and guidance.

"Just pray for strength," said the bride. "I'll do the rest."

SHAFTED

Sally's girl-friend asked her to describe the first night of the honeymoon:

"All night it was up and down, in and out, up and down, in and out—our room was next to the lift."

ANIMAL INSTINCTS

Coming down to breakfast on the morning after the wedding night, the groom was surprised to find a fresh lettuce on his plate, and nothing else.

"What's this?" he asked.

"I just wanted to see whether you eat like a rabbit too," explained the bride.

TOO MANY COOKS...

A newly married couple were in Paris for their honeymoon. The groom went down to the lobby while his wife undressed upstairs, as she was still too shy to undress in his presence. Imagine his surprise when he came back to the suite ten minutes later to find her lying stark naked on the bed, copulating with one bellboy clutching the ardent members of two others in her hands and ministering to a fourth with her lips.

"Penelope!" cried the groom, "how *could* you?"

"Oh darling," she replied, releasing the fourth bellboy with an audible plop, "you know I've always been something of a flirt."

PUSH OVER

It was sundown, and the young athlete was doing push-ups on the beach when a drunk appeared. The drunk weaved his way to within a few yards of the perspiring young man, sat down on the sand and laughed and laughed. "What in the devil are you laughing about?" asked the annoyed young man. The drunk laughed and laughed, and then spluttered, "Don't look now, but shumbuddy sthole yur girl."

EYE WITNESS

Arriving home unexpectedly from a business trip, the husband found his wife in bed with his best friend, in what may be described as a compromising position.

"See here," shouted the husband, "just what do you two think you're doing?"

"See!" said the wife to the man beside her. "Didn't I tell you he was stupid?"

THE CROWN JEWELS

The groom stood naked in front of the mirror admiring his physique :

"Two inches more and I'd be a king."

"Yes," said the bride, "and two inches less and you'd be a queen."

SIZING OFF

The judge granted them a decree nisi.

As she left the courtroom, the wife turned to her ex-husband, waggled her little finger at him and called out : "Goodbye, Shorty.'

The man stretched the corners of his mouth with two fingers and replied : "Goodbye, Lucy."

THE THEORY OF RELATIVITY

Despite George's reputation as the office Romeo, the new secretary was not impressed by his performance.

"I don't think much of your organ," she said as she retrieved her panties from the IN tray.

"No?" replied George, "well I didn't expect to play in an auditorium."

DRIVING LICENCE

Three weeks before the birth of her firstborn, Lady Caroline paid a visit to her gynaecologist in Harley Street.

"What position," she inquired, "will I have to lie in to give birth to my baby?"

"The same position you were in when you started it," replied the specialist.

"My God," exclaimed Lady Caroline, "do you mean I shall have to drive around Hyde Park in the Rolls for two hours with my feet hanging out of the window?"

A TASTE OF HONEY

Three daughters were all married on the same day, and that night their parents listened at the bedroom doors. They heard the first daughter laughing, the second crying and the third silent. The next morning their mother took them aside and asked them to explain.

"Well," said the first, "you always told me to laugh when something tickled me."

"Well," said the second, "you always told me to cry when something hurt me."

"Well," said the third, "you always told me not to speak when I had my mouth full."

VIVE LA DIFFERENCE 1

What's the difference between a circus and a high class whore house?
A circus is an array of cunning stunts.

VIVE LA DIFFERENCE 2

What's the difference between a donkey, an egg and sex?
You can beat a donkey, you can beat an egg, but you can't beat sex.

VIVE LA DIFFERENCE 3

What's the difference between a fat woman and an old maid?
The fat woman is trying to diet, the old maid is dying to try it.

THE SHORT CUT

HE : (pouring a drink) "Say when."
SHE : "After this drink."

THE PERFECT LOVER

A Frenchman with a nine inch tongue who can breath through his ears.

WILL POWER

She was complaining to the doctor that her husband was too old for her and couldn't consummate the marriage. The doctor gave her some pills for her husband and she left, promising him that she would let him know how things worked out. A week later, she came back and said, "Doctor, the pills were fine. For four days in a row, he did it morning and night."

"That certainly was an improvement," said the doctor.

She replied, "Oh yes! And just yesterday, he did it three times before he died."

FRICTION

A pretty young miss walked up to the bowlegged druggist and asked, "May I have some talcum powder, please."

He said, "Yes M'am, walk right this way."

She replied, "If I could walk that way, I wouldn't need any talcum powder."

ONE GOOD TURN...

Harry, a big powerful man, just didn't seem to hit it off with his fragile little wife after they got married. The house was filthy, the bed unmade, the dishes unwashed and her cooking was awful. After six months of this Harry made up his mind to kill her, using the huge weapon with which nature had endowed him. That night he made love to her for three hours. The next morning he staggered off to work, leaving his wife exhausted on the bed.

When he came home in the evening, he found the house spotlessly clean. Harry decided that the neighbours must have found the body and tidied up the house before the undertaker arrived. But in the kitchen he found his wife stark naked except for a little apron, preparing a six course dinner.

"But, darling..." he began.

"Say no more," she broke in, "you look after me properly, and I'll look after you."

His young wife had recently been displaying herself in various rather expensive new dresses, but he didn't want to ask her how she got the money out of their housekeeping allowance in case they had another row about how mean he was. But when his wife came in wearing a brand new silver mink jacket he was moved to ask her how she came by it.

"Oh, the most exciting thing dear, I won it in a raffle at the tennis club."

The next week he noticed that she was wearing a brand new pair of diamond earrings, and casually enquired how she came by them. The same answer :

"I won them in a raffle at the golf club." Then she went on : "Actually dear, I want to dash out again in a few minutes to get to another raffle reception—would you mind awfully running me a bath?"

"Well, my love," he replied, "I'm not sure that you ought to take a bath just now."

"Now why on earth not, dearest," she asked.

"Well darling I don't want you to get your raffle ticket wet."

FLUSHED OUT

A young English teacher was rather nervously giving her new class of eight year olds a grammar lesson. All was going well and she had explained the use of the word 'perhaps' to them without any interruptions.

"Now, Billy, will you make up a sentence to show that you understand how to use 'perhaps'?"

Billy stood up and after some thought said :

"If we are all very good perhaps teacher will let us go home early."

"Excellent," beamed the teacher, and, encouraged, turned to one of her more difficult pupils : "Now, I'm sure that you can give us another example, Jimmy."

Jimmy shambled sullenly to his feet and said : "Does it have to be made up, Miss ?"

"No, it can be true, Jimmy, as long as the word 'perhaps' is used well."

Immediately, Jimmy started on his sentence : "When I saw Miss and the music teacher taking their pants off in the music room I thought perhaps they are going to shit in the piano."

STAND-IN

A big Yorkshire farmer found it necessary to go to London for several months and decided to leave one of his best workers in charge. "I want you to take care of things, Harry, as if I were here myself. Understand?" Harry nodded.

Four months later the boss farmer returned to find everything in shape. Said Harry, pointing things out, "the chicks have been laying plenty of eggs, the wheat has grown double strong, the vegetables are better than they've ever been, and as for those monthly spells your daughter used to have, I've even got those stopped."

YOU KNOW WHO...

The chorus girl was exuberant over receiving a role in a forthcoming play.

"I was made for the part!" she crowed happily.

"Shhh," cautioned her friend, "you don't have to tell everybody."

TURNING A TRICK

Manny Briggs thought that at last he had found a girl with an act that would put his theatrical agency on the map. He telephoned a big night club owner and launched into his selling line:

"No, but Al, I really have got one for you this time. She's stupendous, eighteen years old with long blonde hair, and . . . wow, Al, her figure is outa this world. Just get this: 66-22-36!"

The big night club owner was interested, and said he thought he could give the girl a dance routine right away: "What sort of a dance act does she have, Manny?"

"Well, she doesn't actually dance," came Manny's reply. "She just sorta crawls out there onto the stage and tries to stand up."

WHAM BAM

A zippy sports car had piled into a lamp post, and the driver sat swearing horribly at the safety belt which was still firmly holding him into his seat.

The local constable who arrived on the scene of the accident tried to calm the young man down by saying :

"Well sir, the safety belt did a lot for you. You ought to be thankful. If you hadn't been wearing it you would have gone straight through the windscreen like your lady."

"Good grief !" screamed the man. "You're joking ! Just look what she's got in her hand."

THANK YOU MA'AM

A man is hit by a tennis ball two days before he is to be married. He is hurt in a vulnerable spot, so he goes to the doctor who says, "Sorry, old man, all I can do is put it in splints."

The wedding night, the bride takes off her dress, drops down her bra and says, "Look at these, aren't they beautiful? Virgin, never been touched by a human hand."

The bridegroom drops his pants and says, "Look at this, it hasn't even been uncrated."

SHEEPISH

A couple of farmers were walking back across the fields after a boozy lunch at the local when they spotted a lamb caught fast in a fence.

"Ahrr, Jem, I could wish that was Ursula Andress stuck in that fence like that," chortled one.

Jem replied: "Well, I'm just after wishing that it was dark."

A SHARP REJOINDER

A doctor performs an operation on a young woman. When she is ready to leave the hospital he tells her, "I've made a terrible mistake. I sewed the scissors up inside of you. However, it won't bother you. Go home and forget about it."

Two weeks later the young woman comes rushing into the doctor's office.

"Doctor, doctor," she cries, "you'll have to do something about those scissors. You must remove them at once. Two of my friends have been circumcised and a casual acquaintance has had his finger cut."

EXCOMMUNICATION

The husband wired home that he had been able to wind up his business trip a day early and would be home on Wednesday. When he walked into his apartment, however, he found his wife in bed with another man. Furious, he picked up his bag and stormed out; he met his mother-in-law on the street, told her what had happened and announced that he was filing suit for divorce in the morning.

"Give my daughter a chance to explain before you do anything," the older woman pleaded. Reluctantly, he agreed.

An hour later, his mother-in-law phoned the husband at his club.

"I knew my daughter would have an explanation," she said, a note of triumph in her voice. "She didn't receive your telegram!"

VIRGIN TERRITORY

He held her close against him, a warm glow of satisfaction covering them both.

"Am I the first man you've ever made love to?" he asked.

She studied him reflectively. "You might be," she said, "Your face looks very familiar."

RING MY CHIMES

The sweet seventeen year old girl had only been married for six weeks when her seventy-year-old husband died.

Talking about her brief marriage to her mother she said :

"We were so terribly happy, and, mama, he was a wonderfully romantic lover. We used to make love all the time, and on Sunday mornings I remember he would make love to the rhythm of the church bells." She wept a little, and then went on : "I feel sure, mama, that if the fire engine hadn't dashed past clanging away on that last Sunday, he would still be alive now."

THE ACE OF HEARTS

A man was playing bridge with three women. He was bidding so badly that his partner was greatly annoyed.

After a few hours, he excused himself to go to the washroom. His partner exclaimed, "This is the first time all night that I know what he has in his hand."

Did you hear about the French bridegroom who was so exhausted by the ceremony and the riotous wedding reception afterwards, that he fell asleep the minute his feet hit the pillow?

DEBUNKING

A honeymoon couple start off on a train. All they can get are two upper bunks opposite each other. During the night the bridegroom wakes up and calls to the bride, "Darling, come over into my bed."

"I can't," she answers. "I've no way of getting over."

"Look," says the bridegroom, "I have something long and hard. I'll turn it in your direction, use it to climb over."

"Oh, yes," came a voice from the lower bunk, "and how in hell do you think she'll get back?"

ALMS FOR THE POOR

A husband comes home and finds his wife in bed with a man. He is furious and wants to leave at once. The wife pleads, "Give me a moment to explain. This man came to my door an hour ago and asked for something to eat. I gave him a sandwich. I noticed that his shoes were worn out, so I looked in your closet and found a pair that you haven't had on your feet for five years, and I gave him the shoes to put on. Then I saw that his jacket was very torn, so I went back to your closet and found a jacket that you haven't worn for eight years. When he took his old jacket off to put yours on, I saw that his shirt was falling to pieces, so I opened your bureau drawer and gave him a shirt that you haven't worn for the past twelve years. Then as this man was going out of the door he turned to me and asked, "Is there anything else around here that your husband doesn't use?"

THE FAMILY WAY

They were crushed together in a passionate embrace when John decided that the psychological moment had arrived to tell Marsha.

"Darling," he murmured, "I think you're a marvellous person and I want you to know that I certainly appreciate your-ah-company, but as far as I'm concerned, marriage is for squares."

Marsha replied with a small sigh of pleasure.

"What I mean," John continued doggedly, "is you're more like a sister to me."

At that Marsha's eyes opened in surprise and she exclaimed, "Good Lord, what a home life you must have!"

MARITAL PROBLEM

". . . I'm in love with him, he loves me, we both enjoy the same things, he earns plenty of money, we're real happy together. . . . My problem is; what shall I tell my husband?"

THIS SPORTING LIFE

A married man, the father of three children, came to London. He met a beautiful girl. They spent the next five days together in a hotel room.

He then had to return to his home town, so he bid her a fond farewell.

As she said goodbye, she remarked, "I've been a good sport, haven't I? I haven't asked for a fur coat or diamond bracelet?"

Five months later she called him up at his factory in Manchester. He couldn't seem to place her. "This is the good sport," she reminded him. "I'm pregnant. I'm desperate. I'm going to have to commit suicide!" she wailed.

"You really are a Damned Good Sport," he commented.

A TASTY MORSEL

What is there in common between a passionate kiss and a spider?

Both lead to the undoing of the fly.

THE TRUANT

Every weekday for several months six commuters found that they invariably managed to travel in the same compartment. Breaking the ice one day, one of them suggested that they might pass the time with a few hands of poker. They started to introduce themselves: "My name's Hitchcock," beamed the man who had suggested the poker school. "I'm Hancock," announced the man on his right. And so it went round the compartment: "Alcock." "Woodcock." "Moorcock." Until they came to the last man, who shifted slightly and cleared his throat before muttering: "Vell, my name's Kuntz, an I don' think I better play with you boys."

ENGAGED

A woman walked into the ladies and saw a man standing up using the toilet.

Shocked, she exclaimed, "This is just for women!"

"So's this," he replied.

A rich American widow had for some years had a fantasy about finding a man who had never ever had any sexual experience with women.

The idea obsessed her completely, and she hired the services of an international detective agency who, after extensive and expensive investigations came up with a strapping young Australian who fitted the requirements. The negotiations were all completed, and the couple were married in New York.

On the wedding night the widow could hardly contain her excitement and she slipped her clothes off quickly in the bathroom and, clad in the flimsiest of negligees, drifted into the bedroom to greet her husband. She was absolutely flabbergasted to find that he had moved all the furniture, including the bed, onto the landing outside. "What on earth have you done with the furniture?" she shrieked in amazement.

"Well," drawled her husband, "I've never slept with a woman before, but I can tell you if it's anything like those there kangaroos, I'll need all the space I can get!"

THRICYCLE

The newlyweds were suffering from exhaustion and after an examination, their doctor advised, "It's not unusual for young people to overdo things during the first weeks of marriage. What you both need is rest. For the next month I want you to limit your sex to those days of the week with an 'r' in them. That is, Thursday, Friday Saturday."

Since the end of the week was approaching, the newlyweds had no immediate difficulty following the doctor's orders. But on the first night of scheduled rest the young bride found herself eager as a beaver. Hubby fell asleep, but she tossed and turned and finally nudged her spouse into partial wakefulness.

Expecting daylight, and confused with the darkness, he asked, "What day is it?"

"Mondray," said his bride, cuddling against him.

PSYCHO-THERAPY

The college psychology class was studying human reaction to sexual stimulus and of special interest was the frequency of amorous relations.

"How many students here," said the professor, "engage more than once a week?"

Five people raised their hands.

"And how many engage once a week?"

Ten hands went up.

"How many twice a month?"

Eight hands went up.

"Once a month?"

Four hands were raised.

"And how many once a year?"

A little guy in the back waved his hand frantically and giggled hysterically.

"If you engage only once a year," said the professor, "I don't see what you're so overjoyed about."

Flushed with excitement, the little guy said, "Yeah, but tonight's the night!"

PARLAY VOO...?

One evening, on an isolated part of the beach near Cannes, a beautiful young French girl tried to drown herself. Seeing this from a distance a man dashed down to the beach and into the water to try and save her. He was too late, but he brought her half naked body back to the beach and laid it on the sand while he went to call the police.

When he came back he was shocked to see another man making love to her, and he ran across the beach shouting: "Eh, monsieur, monsieur!" Out of breath, he reached the spot: "What are you doing, monsieur? That woman is dead!"

"Sacre bleu!!" shrieked the other man, leaping to his feet, "I thought she was an American."

FAIR EXCHANGE

Two couples go away on a two-week holiday together. After a week they are thoroughly bored. The men decide that if they exchange partners maybe life will take on new meaning. They all agree that it's an experiment worth trying. The morning after the exchange, one fellow says,

"I'm glad we tried this. It was exhilarating. Come on, let's go in the other room and see how the girls got on."

PHOTO FINISH

A young hippie bookseller was arrested by a member of the Vice Squad for peddling pornographic photographs.

"But you're making a big mistake," said the hippie. "These aren't dirty pictures!"

The officer selected a particularly intricate study of several naked men and women:

"Now you can't tell me that this isn't a dirty picture!"

"Aw, c'mon, man!" shrugged the hippie. "Haven't you ever seen five people in love before?"

THE EASY WAY IN

"How could you go to dinner with that wolf?" Alice asked her friend.

"Why not?" questioned the friend.

"Didn't you have trouble with him?" persisted Alice.

"No," her friend replied.

"How come?" Alice persevered.

"I said yes."

OVERTIME

"Oh I am so tired today," yawned a pretty young secretary to her girl friend. "Last night I couldn't go to sleep until after three."

"Well, goodness, no wonder you are tired," sympathised the friend. "Twice is usually quite enough for me!"

KISS AND MAKE UP

A man comes home very tired and despondent and tells his wife, "I was late for work today."

"I know," she says.

"I quarrelled with the boss," he adds.

"I know," she answers.

"He fired me," he says glumly.

"I know," she replies.

"How in the hell do you know?" he asks angrily.

"He told me," she replied.

"Screw the boss," said the irate husband.

"I did," said the wife. "You go back to work on Monday."

MAN ERRS

A smart London career girl had married a young farmer from Devon, and was far from pleased with his social manner. She determined to start improving him immediately and throughout the wedding reception she was continuously correcting his mistakes, telling him how to speak, which knife to use at table, and when to pass the salt. Finally the celebrations were all over, and they were in bed at last.

The flustered bridegroom fidgeted about between the sheets, unsure of himself and turning this way and that. Eventually half turning towards his new wife he stuttered :

"Could you pass the pussy, please?"

AIR CONDITIONED

A husband brings home a monkey and two rabbits to the one room in which he and his wife live. She looks dismayed. "What will they eat?"

"The same food as we do," says the husband.

"Where will they sleep?"

"At the foot of the bed."

"What about the smell?" she protests.

"They'll get used to it," he answered. "I did."

S.O.B. STORY

When an attractive young girl returned from her honeymoon she was in a state bordering on desperation, and decided to write to the "Aunt Marge" page of her weekly magazine:

"I am at my wit's end since it seems that the nice boy I married is really a sex-maniac. He never leaves me alone—he makes love to me all night without stopping, and then while I'm cooking breakfast, cleaning the house, while I'm in the bath, while I'm watching television, and so on. He just never stops! Can you please tell me what to do?
Signed,
　　'Exhausted'.
P.S.
Please excuse the jerky handwriting."

Air-hostess: "Would you care for some of our TWA coffee?"

Male Passenger: "No, but I'd love some of your TWA Tea!"

BEASTLY APPETITES

A beautiful girl applied to the circus for a job as a lion tamer. "I already have a lion tamer," said the owner. "But I can take you on as an equestrian or as a trapeze artist."

"No," she protested, "I want to work as a lion tamer."

Just then the lion tamer walked in on them with blood oozing from his arm. "A lion mauled me," he moaned. "I won't go on tonight."

"Okay," said the owner to the girl, "the job is yours." The girl entered the lions' cage, took off her shoes and her stockings, then her dress, her bra and her petticoat. She folded her apparel neatly. Then, naked, she lay down on the floor of the cage using her clothes as a pillow.

Two lions walked over to her and started licking her face, her neck, her breasts.

The owner turned to his lion tamer still nursing his wounded arm and asked, "Why can't you do that?"

"I can," the man answered, "if you'll just remove the lions."

A CLOSE SHAVE

A man is in a barber's shop getting a shave and a manicure. He says to the manicurist, "How about going out to dinner with me tonight?"

"I can't," she answers, "I'm married."

"Tell your husband," says the customer, "that you have to work tonight."

"You tell him," says the manicurist. "He's shaving you!"

IDENTIKIT

Three men were in court before the judge on various charges. Asked to state their occupations, one said he was a cork soaker, the second man said that he was a coke sacker, and the third man said that he was the real thing.

MEASURE FOR MEASURE

A man is sitting in his living room reading the newspaper when his wife comes over and slaps him.

"What was that for?' asks the indignant husband.

"That's for being a lousy lover."

A little while later, the husband goes over to where the wife is sitting watching TV and he gives her a resounding smack.

"What was that for?" she yells at him.

To which he answers, "For knowing the difference."

SAVOIR FAIRE

Two Frenchmen are standing on the platform of the train that is pulling out of Paris. One of them waves to a friend at the station and calls :

"Thanks loads; had a marvellous time; your wife was a wonderful lay!" Then he turns to the man standing next to him and says, "It's not true. She's no good at all. I just wanted the husband to feel good."

TRAFFIC JAM

A Frenchman and his girl were driving past the outskirts of Paris when the man stopped his car and persuaded his girl to climb under the car with him where he could make love to her.

Half an hour later, a gendarme tapped him on the feet and asked him what he was doing.

"Repairing my car," replied the Frenchman.

"Monsieur," replied the policeman, "I'm afraid I cannot accept your explanation. Do you know that behind you is a long line of cars? You are holding up the President of France, the Commissioner of Paris, and the Abbey of Notre Dame—and furthermore Monsieur, someone has stolen your car."

OVER OPTIMISTIC

The professor asked a girl in his physiology class, "What part of the body expands to ten times its natural size under an emotional impact?"

Blushing, the girl said, "I'd rather not answer that."

The professor called on the boy sitting next to her, who promptly replied, "The pupil of the eye."

The professor turned back to the girl and said, "Your confusion shows : one, that you didn't study your lesson; two, that you have a dirty mind; and three, that you will be sadly disappointed."

HOLY WATER

Over drinks, one man asks another, "Ever see an ice cube with a hole in it?"

The other responds, "Yes, I was married to one for twenty years."

STALE MATE

A couple, who were married for years, were making love. He asked, "Dear, am I hurting you?"

"No," she replied, "but why do you ask?"

"You moved," he replied.

EAGER TO PLEASE

A boy meets a girl at a discotheque and she asks him to take her back to her flat. After a lot of kissing the girl refuses to let him make it with her, telling him :

"Look, boyo, anybody that makes me has to have two things—a brand new sports car and a cock at least twelve inches long."

The boy said he would be back, and left it at that.

Two days later he drew up outside her flat in a brand new Aston Martin. The girl gasped in disbelief, but he went on :

"As for that other thing, well my doctor says he can cut it down to any size you like."

COCKSURE

At four o'clock one morning the Madame was most surprised to hear the doorbell ring long and loud. Yawning, she opened the door and stared tiredly at a man who had both arms and both legs in plaster.

"I want a woman," he stated.

"Oh, why don't you go home and go to sleep instead : my girls have all turned in for the night anyway."

"Look, lady, when I say I want a woman, I mean I want a woman and now !"

The Madame began to get cross : "Well, let's be realistic. What on earth do you think you could do with a woman in your condition?"

"Listen, lady," replied the man, "I rang the bell, didn't I?"

THROUGH A GLASS DARKLY

The housemaster found two of his school-boys masturbating and reprimanded :

"If you keep that up you will go blind !"

Only slightly abashed the two boys glanced at each other and the first boy said to the second :

"Well, let's just do it until we need glasses."

WIFEMANSHIP

A travelling salesman was just on the point of checking into a hotel when he caught sight of a stunning piece of skirt who was without doubt giving him the full 'come-hither' treatment. He strolled over to her, and nonchalantly exchanged a few words with her, behaving as though he had known her all his life. Then they both walked back to the reception desk and booked in as man and wife.

After a one-night stay, the salesman went to collect his bill and check out. He was appalled to be presented with a bill for £100.

"Look here, this is out of the question. I've only been here one day!"

"Yes, sir," replied the receptionist, "but your wife has been here a month."

DISCOUNTING SHEEP

A ventriloquist, driving across country from one engagement to another, put up for the night at a farm miles off the beaten track. In the morning he amazed the farmhands by practising his voice-throwing in the farm yard and, apparently, making various animals talk.

One of the yokels grabbed his arm and asked: "Here, can youse make all them animals talk?"

"Why, of course," replied the ventriloquist.

"Ar, well," muttered the yokel, drawing him to one side and lowering his voice, "if that there sheep on the end there says anythin' about me, I tell 'ee now it's all a dirty lie!"

SOUL MATES

A man presented his wife with a tombstone while she was still living. On it he had had carved, "Here lies my wife, cold as usual."

The wife went out and bought her husband a tombstone. She presented it to him with the inscription: "Here lies my husband, stiff at last."

FOREIGN PARTS

A French woman dies. At the funeral the husband is calm and composed, but the lover is beside himself with anguish. He throws himself on the coffin, moaning and groaning. Finally the husband goes over to him and says, "Console yourself; I plan to marry again."

SILLY QUESTION

A man asked a prostitute, "What's your ceiling price?"
She answered, "Same as on the floor."

PUSSY CAT

A pert and rather debbie young actress, just out of drama school, was chatting loudly at a theatre party: "I must say that I'm twenty-eight years old and I still have my cherry."

The leading lady, who certainly didn't have hers and hadn't had it for years, purred at the prissy little angel, "So, you still have your cherry, do you? Fascinating, do tell me just one thing . . . does it get in your way when you screw?"

SELLERS MARKET

A man goes on a business trip to buy up some metal. He is to be gone a week. After the week he wires his wife: "Busy, still buying."

Each week for three or four more weeks he sends his wife the same wire.

At the end of six weeks she telegraphs to him: "Come home at once, darling, before I start selling what I think you're buying."

There was a young man of Kildare
Who was having a girl in a chair.
  At the sixtieth stroke
  The bloody thing broke
And his rifle went off in the air.

There was a young man of Cape Horn
Who wished he had never been born.
  And he wouldn't have been
  If his father had seen?
That the tip of the rubber was torn.

There was a young student of John's,
Who was keen to bugger the swans.
  Said the faithful hall-porter :
  "Pray take my daughter,
But the birds are reserved for the dons!"

The typists at Wheesly and Beasly
All fornicate steadily and easily.
    In this pleasant way
    They add to their pay,
Which at Wheesly and Beasly is measley.

There was an old girl from Kilkenny
Whose usual charge was a penny.
    For half of that sum
    You could roger her bum
—A source of amusement to many.

That naughty old lady of Greece
Said : "What I prefer to a piece
    Is to have my pudenda
    Rubbed hard by the enda
The little pink nose of my niece."

Three suitors called on a girl, and they had to sleep together in the spare bed. Mother and daughter listened outside the door to their conversation.

The first was heard to say that his aunt might leave him ten thousand pounds.

"That's the man for you," says mother.

The next was heard to say that his father was just going to make him a director in the family firm.

"No, that's the man for you," says mother.

The third man was heard to say: "Bill you're lying on the end of my cock, move off it, will you?"

"No, I am not lying on it," said Bill.

"Then it's lying on top of you, and Jack is on the end of it!"

"That's the man for me," said the daughter.

IN A FLAP

Two young girls who were close friends used to exchange confidences.

One day, Mary said : "I've got some smashing news Jane, listen to this, I'm getting engaged to a chap who has promised me a Rolls Royce for a wedding present, and then he's going to give me a Fashion Shop to run, after we're married."

"Congratulations, darling," said the other, a little bleakly.

The next time they met, Jane said :

"Oh, by the way Mary, I'm putting the Banns up for me and a chap at the office."

"Has he any money?" enquired her friend.

"No, I must confess, but he says his phallus is so long that six pigeons can perch on it at once. You must admit that would help a marriage to go."

*   *   *

Several months later they met again. "How's the Rolls Royce?" said Jane.

"Listen, dear, we were always truthful with each other, I'll admit it, the Rolls turned out to be a Ford Popular, and the Fashion House turned out to be assisting in a little tobacconists run by his father."

"Mine was a terrible disappointment, too," said the other girl. "The honest truth is, that only four pigeons can perch on it, and even then the end one has to keep flapping."

TO(I)LET

A Rent Collector got a job in the Black Country. His Chief told him :

"It's different here, the houses are rough, the people are rough, you've got to be persistent." Armed with this information the Collector made his first call—a small boy answered the door :

"Is your mother in?"

"No, she went out when me dad came in."

"Fetch your dad then, will you?"

"Can't, he went out when me brother came in."

"Where is your brother then?"

"He cleared off when me big sister came in."

"Can your sister give me the rent?"

"No, she went out when I came in."

"Look here son, someone's got to pay—No rent, no house, see? You'll all be turned out of this place, see?"

"But look here, mister, this isn't the house, it's the W.C."

FACTS OF LIFE

Johnny came home from school and said : "Oh we had a very extra special film at school this afternoon." "Did you?" said dad.

"Yes," said Johnny, "and all the girls were sent out of the room."

Pa looked at Ma, and changed the subject. When Johnny had gone, Pa looked at Ma again, and she said : "Well, you've got to discuss it with him sometime, even if he is only ten."

Just before bed, father said : "Er, hum, er, Johnny, I want to have a little talk with you. What was that film about, the one where the girls were sent outside?"

"Football," said Johnny.

OLD CHINESE CUSTOM?

A lady Professor was lecturing the Women's Institute. "Do you know," she said, "that somewhere in the world a woman is giving birth to a child every minute of the day and night—What are we going to do about it?"

"I know," said an old countrywoman, "find her, and stop her at it."

I COVER THE WATERFRONT

Or : *It's the knack as does it!*

I really love the BLACK COUNTRY, I come from
Wolverhampton
But BUSHEY PARK I did prefer, and there took out my
HAMPTON
I said : Sweet girl just be a pearl, give me your TAPLOW
do
She said : You may enjoy a lay, if you lay MARLOW too.

I found the way to EGHAM on, to TICKLEHAM and
fookham,
And when I sought to BURNHAM up, by gad I'd really
COOKHAM!
Now, listen Gents, to these events, you don't get sex for
gins, or
Gifts of chocs, or frocks, or clocks, it is the knack as
WINDSOR

I said : My Queen, here's COCKPOLE GREEN, with that
she was most smitten;
Please don't be SLOUGH, but quickly go, oh how I have
LONG DITTON
My HAMPTON COURT, but stopped at naught, and
broke, in spite of pains,
Her MAIDENHEAD, and left the bed a lovely view of
STAINES

*SPLITTING THE DIFFERENCE

Mary had a little blouse, twas busted all to bits,
And everywhere that Mary went, it showed her little tits.
Mary had a little skirt, twas split right down the front,
And everywhere that Mary went, she had to sit down all the
time

*BAWDY GEORDIE

There was a young man of Newcastle
Who did a peculiar trick,
He opened the vent of his astle
And deftly inserted his wick

He didn't do this for honour
He didn't do this for pelf,
He did it to please an old comrade
Who'd told him to roger himself

An oversexed lady named Bright
Insists on two dozen a night.
A fellow named Chedder
Had the brashness to wed her—
His chance of survival is slight.

SHOOTING PRACTICE

A captain of artillery, a sergeant and a bombardier were arguing about the act of love. The captain declared it was ninety percent pleasure and ten percent work; the sergeant said it was ten percent pleasure and ninety percent work. The bombardier, who was scared of both, said it was fifty percent work, fifty percent pleasure.

They decided to ask the first person who came along, and it happened to be a humble gunner. In answer to the question, he said :

"Of course it's a hundred percent pleasure. If it wasn't you lot would make us gunners do it for you."

GEORGE AND THE DRAGON?

A man in a country hotel, a commercial traveller, rang down to the reception desk and said : "Send up a nice whore." The proprietor's wife was very angry, and told her husband to go up and throw the man out. He refused, because he didn't want to lose a good customer, and he said the request was natural and harmless.

The wife said. "If you won't, I will," and off she went upstairs.

There was a fearful racket for about twenty minutes, after which the traveller came down and said : "I suppose that's all you can get in country towns, but she was a tough old bitch. I damn near had to rape her."

STRETCHING IT A BIT

A woman complained to the doctor that her breasts hurt her. He asked a few questions, and she said she was sure it was because her husband would insist on an unnatural practice.

"What sort of unnatural practice?"

"Well, doctor, he will insist on sleeping with my nipple in his mouth!"

"Nothing unusual in that madam," says the medico.

"What, when we're sleeping in separate beds!"

WHORE YOU KIDDIN'?

It was during the war that a Polish officer who did not fully understand the language, picked up a high class prostitute in London, and was taken to her flat. After a remarkable supper with wine, she took him to bed for a series of repeat performances.

After a very good breakfast she helped him into his overcoat, handed him his hat, and said: "What about some money?"

"Oh, but Madame, a Polish officer and a gentleman could never accept money from a woman, it would be a dishonour."

A country chap went up to London during the war, and he could not find a lodging. He by chance met a village maiden who had gone up to town some years before to look for work, and who remembered him.

Rationing was very strict, and the man was very pleased to get a big meal, with food unlimited.

"Go on" she said, "eat, I'm well in with the grocer. Have some wine, I'm well in with the vintner. Have a cigar, I'm well in with the tobacconist."

The visitor was overwhelmed. He rose to make up the fire. "Put plenty on" she said, "I'm well in with the coal-man."

Then she tucked up to the blaze, pulled her skirts well up to warm her thighs, and the young man said : "Mary, be careful !"

"Be careful—why?"

"I should hate you to burn your ration book."

BY THEIR WORDS SHALL YE KNOW THEM

During the war a German spy was dropped behind the British lines with orders to report on what regiments were moving up to the front. The spy sent back such perfect reports that he was afterwards taken before General Rommell to receive the Iron Cross.

"Tell me, Feldwebel Shmit," said the General, "what is the secret of your success?"

The spy explained that he had concealed himself by a Sewage Works, and as the first regiment marched past he heard:

"I thay, Thecil old darling, do you notith a dweadful pongo?"

"Yeth Basil, ithent it fwiteful?" so he knew that must be the Artists Rifles. As the next lot came past he heard: "Jock, d'ye reckon we could dree oot some o' yon stuff, an' smoke it in oor wee pipes" so that must be the Aberdeen Light Infantry.

Finally, he heard men saying: "By cripes Jack, can you smell a mucking smell of mucking grit that stinks like a navvy's piss-corner?"

These, Mein Herr, could only be the South Staffords.

SWEET AND LOW

The old Squire had an estate, and during the war he woke up one morning to find the Americans camped all over it. Honour demanded that he ask the Colonel to dine.

After dinner the dignified old family butler said:

"How do you like your coffee Sir?"

The Colonel was rather an abrupt man, lost in these surroundings, and he replied:

"Lissen, Ah likes ma corfee like Ah likes ma wimmen— hot and sweet, d'you gerrit?"

"Yes Sir," said the butler, unflappable, "black, or white Sir?"

THE SENTIMENTAL COURTESAN

Belle de l'Amour was the most beautiful and exotic courtesan in France under the Empire. When the king had finished with her she set up shop in a fashionable boulevard, and charged one thousand francs a night.

The Cadets of Saint Cyr had heard many stories of her voluptuous charms and passionate nature, and the conversations in the barrack rooms often ended on the note of what any one of them would do if he won the national lottery.

"Lottery!" cried a bright recruit, "that gives me an idea." It was there and then agreed among them that every Cadet should pay one franc, and as there were a thousand of them that would just be the courtesan's fee. Then they would hold a raffle, and the lucky winner should spend a night with the lady.

Thus it was that young Du Pont, the son of a noble house, appeared before the lady. When she saw a boy of 19 she went to send him away, but when she saw the thousand francs, she changed her mind.

The following morning, pulling a transparent silk slip over her voluptuous body, she sat up and asked how such a youth came by so much money, and he told her the whole story.

Her romantic French heart was deeply moved: "Ah, mon petit cheri, quel sentiment!" she cried, and said in the circumstances she felt she ought to give him his money back. The idea thrilled the youth, and as he departed he kissed her and held out his hand. She reached for her jewelled purse and—gave him a franc.

LOCKSMITH LAUGHS AT LOVE

A certain firm set on a commercial traveller. His only qualification was that he was the son of a Director, and had failed at several other jobs. They sent him out after a good "spec" and told him to report next day.

Next day he came in looking very washed up, and without the order. He explained that while driving across the New Forest his car broke down, and when he knocked on a cottage door to ask for help, the place was occupied by a young widow, who asked him to stay the night.

"Go on, go on," said the Sales Manager . . . "and you spent the night screwing? I didn't think you'd got that much sense!"

"You bet I did!" said the young man, "You see, when we went to bed she told me the lock on her bedroom door was broken."

"I see, and you didn't get much sleep?"

"That's what I keep trying to tell you, I felt in honour bound to try and mend it, and it took longer than I thought."

YES SIR, THAT'S MY BABY

A traveller was crossing a wild and lonely moor late at night when his car broke down, and he walked to an isolated farm for help. The farmer had no phone, and anyway it was late and a rough night, so the farmer offered a bed.

"You can either share a single bed with the baby," he said, "or kip down on the hay in the barn."

The traveller thought he wouldn't want to be wet on by any babies, so he chose the barn, and had a pretty rotten night of it.

In the morning he awoke to see a big-breasted rosy-cheeked girl of sixteen entering with a pail: "Who are you?" he said.

"I'm the baby of the family, who are you?"

"I'm the stupid prat that chose to sleep in the barn."

ON THE CARPET

A man was up in London for a Conservative conference, and having a free day was exploring the streets when he got lost.

After a time he suffered an urgent need to ease his bowels, and nowhere could he see. The situation was desperate, so he stopped a stranger and explained the difficulty. The stranger said : "I see from your badge you are a Tory, follow me, it's not far." With which he took him around a few quick corners, entered a Georgian portal, and took him down a long carpeted passage.

"Are you sure this is all right?"

"Quite all right, old boy, just follow."

Thus they went through a gilded lobby into a vast room lit with candelabra, and hung with old masters.

"Here."

"What here, on this posh carpet?"

"Yes, here, on this posh carpet."

The man felt very much better. "Where now?" he said.

"The next," said his new friend, "is to run the hundred yards in eleven seconds, you're in the Russian Embassy."

ONE AND ONE MAKE THREE

A boy of 12 went to his father with a little girl of 10, a neighbour's daughter.

"Dad," he said, "we want to get married."

"Yes, son, in ten years."

"No dad, now !"

"What are you going to live on?"

"We can manage on her pocket money and mine."

Said father (playing the joke along) : "Oh, I see, and what if she has a baby?"

"Well dad, nothing's happened so far."

CALF LOVE

There was a young man went to the doctor and said he wanted to get married but he was worried about the small size of his member. The doctor advised him to go and stay on a farm, dip his wick in milk several times a day, and have it sucked by a calf.

Some months later when they met in the street, the doctor said :

"How's your marriage?"

"Oh, I didn't get married doctor, I bought a calf instead."

BITCH IN SHEEP'S CLOTHING

It was way out in the wild west, and women were very scarce. The tenderfoot went into the saloon, and asked the barman where he could go to get sex. The barman said : "Back o' Jake's place down the track, there's a nice young sheep in a barn. Give Jake a dollar, and you're fixed."

When the tenderfoot arrived at the barn he found a nice young sheep, very clean and decked with ribbons. But Jake came out and told him to clear off. "Listen, Jake, I got my dollar."

"Listen, I said scram t'hell outa it. Sheriff's keepin' her now."

WOOL OVER HIS EYES

The African Chief was very suspicious. His youngest and curviest wife had given birth to a near-white child. He pointedly called the Missionary's attention to it, and at the same time fondled his spear in a thoughtful manner.

The Missionary was calm: "Listen, O chief," he said, "look at all those sheep over there on the mountain (the Chief looked), well, one of those white sheep has just had a black lamb."

"Fair enough, O man of God, you no tell, me no tell."

SWEET CONVERSATION

A woman went into a chemist's shop and said: "Do you fit ladies with dutch caps?" "Certainly madam, certainly," beamed the chemist.

"Well go and wash your dirty filthy hands and serve me with a quarter of cough drops."

BIRDS OF A FEATHER

There was a certain respectable suburb in which there was a high class brothel, which had everything, even a high class parrot. When the Madam had made her pile, and the girls were going off a bit, she decided to sell up. On the day of the sale most of the local worthies were present, bidding for luxury carpets, curtains, etc.

When the parrot was auctioned the auctioneer called: "What am I bid for this beautiful bird . . . five pounds . . . six pounds . . . seven pounds ten." There was a silence, and the parrot shouted out: "Aw, come on daddy, don't be a mean scrooge, make it ten and I'll give you a gam as well."

The bird was finally bought by the Mayor, but he was a bit wary of it, and kept it covered up with a cloth whenever there was an official reception. One day the Mayor was receiving a religious convention when the Bishop's wife, overcome by curiosity, pulled the cloth from the cage. The parrot shouted:

"Oh, hallo! New house, new girls, new lighting, same old customers, howdy Charlie!"

ACTING THE GOAT

A city visitor drove up to a farm, just as the farmer's son was walking up the road wearing wellington boots. It was a fine hot summer day, so the stranger enquired: "Why are you wearing gumboots on a day like this?"

"I allus wears these when I goes courting," replied the yokel.

The visitor could not see why gumboots were essential for courting, so the young man explains: "You've got to have some way of keeping that nanny-goat's back legs still."

MADE A COCK-UP OF IT

There was a poultry farmer who was having no luck at all. His birds just refused to lay or breed. He was telling his troubles one day in a pub to another poultry farmer . . .

"You've come to the right man," said the other, "I've got the randiest cockerel in the business. He's wearing my birds out, you can have him for a quid. If he doesn't liven up every bird you've got, you can have your money back."

The man took the bird home, and really he had a devilish look in his eye. When he was let loose the next morning he not only covered all the pullets within the hour, but he'd done his stuff with a large flock of ducks as well.

After lunch every goose in the place was heard squawking, and by teatime even the turkey-hens were looking placid, and had begun to lay. When the new owner went out in the evening to give the bird a splendid meal, he couldn't find him. He looked everywhere, and at last, peering over a bank, he saw his cockerel stiff and motionless on his back, his legs in the air.

The poultry farmer was broken-hearted . . . the bird had worked himself to death . . . what a tragedy. "Never mind, old son," he said, as he approached, "you had a lovely death, and I'll never eat you, but give you a decent funeral."

"Go away you bloody stupid fool," hissed the cock, "I'm trying to fox down that damn vulture hovering up there."

RETORT COURTEOUS

There was a really curvy girl at a dance, and all the smart men were after her. A spotty youth was much attracted, but he couldn't get a look in. However, during a "Gentleman's Excuse-me" he rushed up and grabbed her.

"Go away!" she glared, "I'm not going to dance with a child."

"Oh, sorry Miss, I didn't know you were pregnant."

A spinster of 40 had a brother at sea, and he sent her a pair of parrots in a double cage. The spinster was intrigued to know which was the cock and which was the hen, as they were exactly alike, so she consulted a Vet.

"Watch them," said the vet, "the one that gets on top is the male."

"I DO watch them," said the lady, "but they never do anything!"

"Then creep down at dawn and have a peep, and when you know which is the cock, be sure and mark it."

The spinster obeyed instructions, and caught the birds in the very act of mating. Thrilled to bits, she tied a white tape round the cock's neck.

The following Sunday the Vicar came to tea. As he removed his coat the cock parrot shouted:

"Hallo, so you've been caught doing a woman as well, have you?"

SAGA OF PASSION

There was a spinster schoolteacher who was plain, skinny and with an impediment in her speech.

She longed for a man, and used to comfort herself by reading 'respectable' erotic stories, namely the adventures of the great classical gods. This only made her worse, but one night a strange thing happened . . . she dreamed that a big blond naked man came to her bed, ripped off her long nightgown, and raped her again and again.

In the morning as he was about to depart through the window, she begged him to stay.

"I must return to Valhalla," he said, "I'm Thor."

"Tho am I, but wathenth it marvellouth!"

STANDING OVATION

There was an elderly Peer who woke up one morning and rang for his valet : "Jenkins, I find I have an erection."

"Congratulations, Sir !—shall I fetch Her Ladyship."

"Certainly not ! Fetch the car, this is a West End job !"

ANSWER TO A MAIDEN'S PRAYER

There was a spinster who had a parrot, and it swore and used some terrible expressions. When the Vicar called she covered it up for shame, and the Vicar enquired the reason.

"I couldn't repeat it," she said, but the Vicar pulled the cover off, and that wicked bird let out a mouthful.

"I'll have to have his neck pulled, the villain," said the spinster.

"Certainly not, Miss Tavvinitt," he said, "I have a lady parrot, a parrot of the utmost virtue, who prays by day and night. I'm sure that if we put them together she will reform him."

This was agreed upon, and the following day Miss Tavvinitt took her bird round to the Vicarage, and he was put in the cage with the devout lady parrot.

Immediately he misbehaved, shouting : "Lift your tail up, come on, I want sex, what are we waiting for !"

Before the Vicar and the spinster could do a thing about it, the lady parrot replied : "What the bloody hell d'you think I've been praying for all these years?"

OLD AGE CREEPING ON

There was a blooming young girl who asked her old grannie how often married people had sex. Grannie explained, it wasn't as simple as that.

Newly married people might have it every night, people in their thirties, three times a week. In the forties and fifties, it might slow up to once a week.

"But grannie, what about people over say, 65?"

"Well then I reckon it's once a quarter."

"Grannie, you're 75, and grandad's 85, how often . . ."

"Once a year," croaked the old dame . . . "Heh, heh . . . TONIGHT ! !"

TWISTED PERSONALITY

> Here lies the body of poor old Mick
> Who went through life with a corkscrew wick
> He spent his days on a fruitless whim
> To find a girl with a corkscrew quim.
> He found one at last, but fell down dead,
> When he found it had a left-hand thread.

WRINGING WET

It was a hard-fought rugger match, and the lads staggered to an inn for some throat oil. After a few pints two players, they were opponents and strangers, went round the back to pump ship. Suddenly one burst out laughing, and said :

"Pardon me old chap, but ho ho! your John Thomas—I hope I'm not being rude—is all twisted. Did you get mangled in the scrum or sumpin?"

"No old feller," replied the other, "it's always been corkscrew-shape, I must admit it bothers me a bit."

"Tell you what," said the first, "my Guvnor's a doctor, come round on Monday, I'll get the old man to have a look at it for you."

Monday came, and the young man kept the appointment. His new friend was waiting, and said :

"Howdyer get on old chap?"

"Oh, it's nothing that plastic surgery won't put right."

"Yes, but how did it get like that?"

"That was through my mother being a widow, and prudish as well."

"I'm not with you old boy, elaborate a little."

"Well, your father has just explained to me for the first time, that when you have a pee, you shake it, you don't wring it out."

A plump stewardess named Byote
Took too many rolls when afloat,
Said her Ma : Tons of grub
Couldn't fill out *that* tub,
You've been messing about in a boat !

She was reared in a bleak institution
And grew up in great destitution,
She married, the bitch,
A man old and rich
And always condemns prostitution

There were three young maidens of Twickenham
Who wanted Tom, Harry, and Dick in 'em,
They prayed hard to Venus
Saying : Surely, between us,
We can lengthen, and strengthen, and thicken 'em

The foxhunting Countess of Mourne
Was hunting her spouse in the corn,
By God did she swear
When she saw the Au Pair
Go to ground as he flourished his horn

Said a Printing House man to his bird :
To wait for the Chapel's absurd
And tho' it would fret 'er
He'd slip in a letter
And act out a four-letter word

THE MODEST MINI MAIDEN

Tune: The Red Flag (Tannenbaum)

Some pad their chests and dye their curls
 That's just to nark the other girls,
And tho' they are like walking-sticks
 I show my legs to get my kicks

Chorus

> Then raise the mini skirts on high
> And bare another piece of thigh
> Tho' young men pinch and old men leer
> I'll keep my hemline right up here !

My mother says I'm in disgrace
Disclosing pants all edged with lace,
I'll leave them off, what do I care
If only MEN will stop and stare

Chorus

> Then raise the mini skirts on high, etc.

And now, dear girls, advice to you,
When men do what you drove them to,
You call a policeman on the spot,
To deal with such a dirty lot

Chorus

> Then raise the mini skirts on high, etc.

For you can raise your skirts on high
Yet pose a virgin modesty,
Stoke up the fire, but never quench
Until he's firmly hooked, my wench.

Chorus

> Then raise the mini skirts on high
> And show another piece of thigh
> Tho' young men pinch and old men leer
> I'll keep my hemline right up here !

BY THEIR FRUITS SHALL YE KNOW THEM

When reading the wafflings of great men of old
Eve fell for the serpent, or so we are told
She must have this reptile so long strong and firm
That even the thought of it caused her to squirm.
But Adam had got it ! The problem to grapple—
When would he uncoil it ? "She offered an *apple*"
And thus there began the erroneous libel—
No *apple* is mentioned in anyone's bible

As everyone knows, without going to College,
She gave him *the fruit of the banned Tree of Knowledge*
And the fruit Eve thrust forth with lascivious zest
The vulgar call *tit* and the learned call *breast*
So that's why the Savants in High Schools and Halls
(Who say *nuts* or else *taters* when speaking of balls)
Have classified breasts, and the way women show them
In various grades : *By their fruits shall ye know them!*

By Their Fruits Shall Ye Know Them (*cont.*)

Some girls have nothing but two little puce-berries
In size and appearance like rather small *gooseberries*,
And others again, without sexy shapes
Can present to their sweethearts mere *cherries* or *grapes*
There's small hope of marriage for those would-be Mums
Who've nothing to offer but *lemons* or *plums*
The fruits that men fall for are bulgy and swell-uns
Like *coconuts, grape-fruit,* or well-rounded *melons*

Girls hardly get any man's serpent to rise
Unless they are blessed with a bust of good size,
But don't overdo it. They only get bumpkins
Whose bra's are just sackfuls of bloody great *pumpkins.*
Last : Ladies ! Take comfort if your tits are small
Far better have small ones than no bust at all,
Grown women I've seen—on their chests not a thing !
Save two tiny spots where a bee left a sting

*CHEESED OFF

Under the spreading chestnut bough
There sat a young milk-maid, a-milking a cow
Along came the farmer, and gave her the sack,
So she turned the cow over, and poured the milk back

*ROMANTIC LOVE

The love of a beautiful maiden
The love of a strong young man
The love of romantic sweethearts
Existed since time began.
But the greatest love of all loves
Greater than that of a mother,
Is the tender, delicate, intimate—lust
Of one randy sod for another !

*THE EXCEPTION

With vain regret I oft remember
Those happy days of youth and fun
When all my limbs were soft and tender
Did I say all? Well, all but one.
Gone are those happy days for ever
Those halycon days of lust and fun,
Now, all my joints, and limbs, are stiffer
Did I say all? Well, all but one.

BOSOM FRIENDS?

When I look at Janet and Jessie and Julia
It seems Nature's plan is very peculia
For some girls are carrying more than a plenitude
While others are moaning they-haven't-got-any-tude.

Thus girls with full hip lines and very good legs
Are filled full of envy by two skinny pegs,
And lassies whose sweaters are tenanted houses
Stare jealous of others with loose flapping blouses

In other men's pastures the grass is much greener
Say Aggie the Scraggy and plump Wilhelmina.

* DOUBLE COVER

When the Censor saw the Dancer
He became a flaming red
First he stuttered, then he stammered
Then he caught his breath and said :

"I am shocked beyond description
At the length to which you've gone
I can't allow this exhibition
Twice as much, you must put on."

When the Dancer heard the Censor
She was very quick to heed
To her dressing-room she hastened
And put on another bead !

* OLD FIDDLES, BEST TUNES

I told my friend one Summer's day
My husband's safe and will not stray
I'll not believe a tale that's told,
He's decent, fine, — and very old

*   *   *

My dear ! How true it is to say
He strayed with me the other day !
Old fiddles play the very best
And play as often as the rest !

LOVELY ENGLISH MAIDEN

See that beauty standing there
Bootblack eyes and Woolworth's hair,
Plastic coat and kinky boots
Blonde (but very dark at roots)
Moth gashed big and quim gashed bigger
All she lacks is face and figure

*   *   *

Those tatty nylons full of holes
Those tatty shoes with cardboard soles
Those skinny legs : a skirt on high
Betrays a piece of skinny thigh,
Skinny bottom, skinny mind,
Behold, this piece of womankind—
This Work of God, this painted face,
Behold ! the Mother of the Race.

*TIME OFF IN LOO?

We see it every morning, it happens every day
A double file of female staff meanders on its way,
The thing that puzzles all the men, and gives the boss
    grey hairs
Is why, when serving Nature's calls, they have to go in
    PAIRS?
Perhaps the trip's demanding, and the toilet dark and lonely?
But two by two they reach the loo by the door marked
    Ladies Only.

The poor Boss stands, and tears his hair, he's simply mad
    with grief,
The day's production goes to pot, while girls go on relief,
At two o'clock each afternoon, the match begins once more,
But what on earth goes on all day, behind that toilet door?
The only way that I can see to make production boom,
Is to move the whole damn Typing Pool inside the Ladies
    Room!

*OVER THE HILL

It's not the grey hair that makes a man old
Or the faraway look in his eye, so I'm told :
But when the mind seeks a contract the body can't fill,
You're over the hill brother, over the hill.

You can fool the dear wife with the cleverest lies,
You can tell her the tale and pull wool on her eyes,
But when she wants an encore, and you say you're ill,
You're over the hill brother, over the hill

When you gaze on a stripper, and just heave a sigh
When you hear a bum joke, and you laugh till you cry,
When sex is plain duty, and never a thrill
You're over the hill brother, over the hill

Love is a conflict the battle is keen,
There are so many rounds in the old magazine
When you've fired your last shell and you cannot refill
You're over the hill brother, over the hill

Repair the old howitzer, boy, if you can,
But oyster and eggs cannot make you a man,
No vigour can last got from powder or pill,
You're over the hill brother, over the hill

This is my story, alas and alack,
When you've squeezed out the toothpaste you can't put it
        back,
If "Whoopee" you're needing, well don't wait until
You're over the hill brother, over the hill

An Optician's clerk named Mollasses
Had a wick far too small for the lassies,
Much pleasure he'd missed
Till his boss made a list
Of spinsters who needed thick glasses

A Pools-winning woman of Fife
Said : Marriage is nothing but strife,
(Her husband asked : Gwen
Do we enter again?)
With my draws up?—Why not on your life !

A Canon of very high station
Wed a woman of no reputation
They'd a child in ten weeks
And whenever she speaks,
It's only to knock fornication

A French woman Maquis named Blérot
Who took Winston C. for her hero
Said : He told the *Entente*
It was hard, tough and long,
And the chance of withdrawal was zero

A skinny young woman of Broom
Took a candle alone in the gloom,
Now and then she would curse
When her lord, and his nurse
Made the bed in the neighbouring room

THE JAPANESE EROTIC

There was a rugby captain, a young man of upright life and modest bearing, an accountant by profession. He found the camp-followers flighty, over made-up and stupid, so he remained a bachelor.

One day in a bar he met a shapely girl who was cultured and intelligent, so he started dating her. One night she asked him to go back to her place, but when they entered the taxi, she gave a Park Lane address. The young man asked how a secretary could pay that sort of rent, and she told him that secretaries in London always took money from men, although seldom admitting it honestly.

He gave her all the money he had, begged her to reform, and fled the scene. When they later met by chance, she said : "Take me out to dinner, I've something to discuss." Over dinner she said :

"When I was 15, and home from school I found in my father's study a rare book he had smuggled in called 'Eastern Sexology'. I lay reading it, with my crotch drilling holes in the carpet, but father caught me, thrashed my bare bottom, and burned the book. I had read only one chapter, but I have never forgotten it, it was called the *Japanese Erotic*, and I have practised it to perfection, but never, I swear, with a man. I love you, take me home and I will do it for you." He eagerly agreed, but alas, the waiter handed him a telegram, his father was dying, he must go at once.

He asked around, but though the club knew lots about sex, they didn't know the *Japanese Erotic*, and told him to find out and report. But the girl had disappeared, and he searched in vain.

Months later she met him from work, and said she was washed up and repentant. If he would marry her she would reform, and make him a perfect wife. "And can I have the *Japanese Erotic* ?" he asked. "Of course, darling, anything you like."

For various reasons the marriage was delayed, and she forgot the promise. On the wedding night he found her waiting naked on the bed, her full pink curves presenting a sexier sight than most men would ever witness.

"Rape me John, make me pregnant," and she opened her glorious thighs.

But he wanted *Japanese Erotic*.

She pressed up her splendid breasts : "Let me crush it between them."

He wanted *Japanese Erotic*.

She pointed to her blood-red mouth : "Put it in here as far as you like."

He wanted *Japanese Erotic*.

The girl smiled, slid gently off the bed, and bent down low over a chair, presenting to him a full round bottom of outstanding beauty.

"Darling," she said, "violate me any way you like, take your savage lust on me."

He wanted *Japanese Erotic*.

She straightened up, turned her liquid eyes to his, and still smiling, said :

"As my master commands; I am his slave. Go into the bathroom and cover yourself with lather, that's an essential part. As soon as I have got everything ready I will call you to come and slay me with your spear."

He could hardly contain himself. As soon as she "Cooeed" he rushed for the bathroom door, fell over the mat, hit his head on the pan, and died of concussion.

Shortly afterwards the girl died of a broken heart, and to this day not a living soul knows what *Japanese Erotic* is.

What is the difference between a Eunuch and an Eskimo?
    A Eunuch is a massive vassal with a passive tassel.
    An Eskimo is a rigid midget with a frigid digit.

*   *   *

What is the difference between an Opera Director and a baby?
    A baby sucks his fingers.

*   *   *

What is the difference between a constipated owl and a bad marksman?
    A bad marksman shoots and can't hit.

*   *   *

What is the difference between frustration and utter frustration?
    Frustration is the first time you find you can't do it the second time.
    Utter frustration is the second time you find you can't do it the first time.

Two into one won't go—true or false?
   Yes, but only one at a time.

* * *

What is the definition of the true music lover?
   A man who hears a lady singing in the bath and puts his *ear* to the keyhole.

* * *

What is the definition of old age?
   When it takes all night to do what you used to do all night.

* * *

What is it that six men can do that three women can't?
   Pee simultaneously in the same bucket.

* * *

HOW TO TELL CHARACTER FROM METHOD OF URINATION

Study this carefully, and determine your friend's character —and your own!

TYPE

Excitable: Pants twisted, can't find hole, rips in a rage.

Sociable: Joins friends in a pee whether he wants to or not, figures it costs nothing anyway.

Cross-eyed: Looks in stall on left, pees in one on right.

Timid: Can't go if anyone is looking. Pretends to, sneaks back later.

Aggressive: Whistles loudly, looks over to see how others are doing.

Indifferent: All stalls being occupied, calmly pisses in basin.

Clever sod: No hands. Adjusts tie. Gazes round for admiration.

Worried: Ex-serviceman, makes furtive but close examination.

Frivolous: Shoots a stream up and down and around. Has never really grown up.

Absentminded: Unbuttons waistcoat, takes out tie, pees in pants.

Disgruntled: Stands for a while, grunts, tries to fart, fails, walks out.

Sneaky: Lets strong silent farts whilst leaking.

Flashy: Tells loud jokes while leaking, shakes drops off with great flourish.

Sloppy: Tell-tale drops on flies. Never misses shoes. Walks out with flies undone. Adjusts balls 30 minutes later.

Childish: Pees directly into pool at bottom of stall. Enjoys the noise and splashing, interrupts to aim at a fly.

Patient: Stands there for hours on end.

Anxious: Leaves it late, wants to go so badly he can't start. Puts it back too soon, wetting leg. Adjusts flies in door-way.

Boastful: Stands back four feet and aims high up the wall. This type are invariably among the world's failures.

CERTIFICATION

THIS IS TO CERTIFY THAT I, the undersigned, being a Female, about to enjoy sexual intercourse with ...... am above the age of Consent. I am in my right mind, and not under the influence of any drink, drug or narcotic, neither does he have to use any kind of force, threat or promise, in order to influence me.

I FURTHER DECLARE that I am in no fear of him of whatsoever kind, that I do not expect him or want him to marry me, nor I to marry him. I do not know whether he is married or not, nor do I care. I am not asleep, or drunk and I enter into this relationship with him because I love it, and want it as much as he does.

UNDERTAKING I hereby undertake, provided I receive the satisfaction I have a right to expect, to play an early return engagement. Furthermore, I agree never to appear as a witness against him under the Bastardy Act, nor do I expect him to wear a contraceptive.

Signed, gladly of my own free will, and at the moment of slipping off my panties

....

This .... day of ...... 19 ....

Address. ....

....

NUTS ON THE BALLS IN THE HALLS

There was an account in a Sunday paper about Friggington; which was said to be a place where bored housewives earned a bit on the side, or more improperly, on the back, and evening parties were held for "social sex". The disclosures were made by Councillor "Ginger" Nutt, a very prominent Liberal.

Alderman Sir John Stonehurst ("Stoney") Balls, leader of the Conservatives on the Council, disagreed : "These lies are all Nutt's," he said, "he's a singular fellow, no-one really knows where he hangs out."

"Nuts," said Nutt, "I am going to expose Balls, he wants to extend Tory spheres of influence, but the Conservative balls at the Town Hall are flopping, as anyone can see."

"I still say nothing is swinging in Friggington," replied Stoney Balls, and I am going to ask my brother, Canon Balls, to preach against the Liberals next Sunday. Everyone knows he bawls like a bull."

The last word was with Ginger Nutt : "The Canon is always shooting off in the pulpit, it doesn't produce any results; as for Stoney Balls, I'm going to keep tabs on him. Excuse me now though, I'm off to see the Rolling Stones."

RELATIVELY SPEAKING

Letter to the Woman's Monthly

Dear Aunt Fanny, Please can I have your advice as I am worried. I have started going serious with a nice young man of good family and with a good job. My mother is an actress and my father is always unemployed as well. My older sister is a model and my younger sister is also on the game. One of my uncles is a garage proprietor and he has a brother also a crook; my cousin is a male ballet dancer and several of his friends have also been convicted. I have a nephew and niece in jail for incest, and my Socialist brother-in-law is attending a VD Clinic.

Do you think I ought to confess to my fiancee that I am related to a Socialist?

Yours, Worried Winnie

TWO INTO ONE WON'T GO (EXCEPT ONE AT A TIME

There are about 25,000,000 females in this country
Of whom at least 12,000,000 are nubile
6,000,000 of them are married
The other 6,000,000 are single or widowed
Of these last, 4,000,000 like sex.
Add 6,000,000 to 4,000,000, that gives 10,000,000 taking sex
Assume 30% out of commission on any one evening
Gives 7,000,000 functioning fannies per night.

*　　*　　*

The average male, ignoring boasting and exaggeration
Is just over five inches when erect
Which, multiplied by 7,000,000 = 360,000,000 inches
Or ten million yards of sex per night!
This is between five and six hundred miles,
Multiplied by seven it is nearly 4,000 miles,
And four thousand miles a week, say 2,000,000 miles a year
Sure is a whole lot of sex.

ARE YOU GETTING YOUR SHARE?

COMMERCIAL UNION

Dear Sirs,

I took out what your agent called a "Comprehensive Policy" and he said if I ever suffered fire flood or theft or got struck by lightning I had only got to claim on you. I am a spinster living on my own, and I feel the cold so I had a man in to fix a wall heater. Yesterday, when I was adjusting a picture, the electric heater melted a big hole in the middle of my nylon dress, and I want to know if I am properly covered.

Yours tryly,
Virginia N. Rustyfann

Dear Miss Rustyfann,

We are sorry to hear about the hole in the front of your dress, and although it does not sound to us as if you are properly covered, we are sending our man at once to look into it. In any case, before he makes you an offer we have instructed him to find out what other cover you may have, and I should warn you that failure to disclose can lead to a breach, so we trust you will hide nothing.

Yours truly,
Commercial Union

Dear Sirs,

Reference the hole in the front of my dress, your man has looked into it, and is quite satisfied that I had no other cover. I must say, he came very quickly, and as he didn't want to offer much money he suggested that I let a piece in the front of the dress. After his expert attentions I shall need to let a piece into the front of my dress anyway. I must say he was very efficient, and offered to come again as often as I wanted.

However, I do not think I shall need this service again for some time, not unless I have the misfortune to sit on a hot stove that is!

Your satisfied customer
V. Nomora Rustyfann

HOW SOON ARE YOU GOING TO FOCUS?

SCENE : *The house of a childless couple, married five years.*

Husband : Well dear, I must be off to work, but don't forget, the "Artificial Insemination" expert is coming this morning.

Wife : Darling, do you think we did the right thing?

H : Of course my dear. You want a child, I want a child, we don't want to adopt, so this is the only way.

W. I hope he doesn't want to do anything to me, I'm not a bit in the mood.

H : Oh you great big silly! He only wants to talk; the action's weeks away. (*He kisses her and departs.*)

There is a loud knock on the door

W : Ooh, good morning, are you the gentleman from . . .?

MAN: Yes, that's right, I've come about the baby. (*Thinks to himself, so this IS the right house. Why the hell can't they bring their babies to the studio to be photographed?*)

W : Won't you take your coat off and put your bag down Mr . . . ?

M : Jones. I hope this is a convenient time. Your husband's at work I presume?

W : Naturally. He wouldn't want to be around as he's not going to do it himself, even though he is mad keen on babies.

M : Quite quite. Takes a professional touch to get results. I suggest two on the settee, two on the mat, and one or two naked on the bed. That'll need a fairly long exposure.

W : (*Alarmed*) You're not going to do it *now?* I thought this was to discuss it !

M : Madam your husband placed a firm order and paid. I don't want to come more than is necessary. Half a dozen shots now, and one is sure to produce an attractive baby. I'm a busy man, I've got two more to do this morning.

W : Two more to do this morning !

M : Yes, a model wants to try various positions in a topless dress. She wants an enlargement for advertising purposes. Afterwards some nuns want me to take them in a group on their knees, part of a religious festival, I gather.

W : You do get around, don't you.

M : Yes indeed, variety is the spice of my job. Want to see some samples (*produces photos of babies*), here's a good one, I got it on top of a moving bus. Mother a film actress, divorced, but wanted one for publicity. I only had the chance of one shot too.

W : Only one shot?

M : Every time the bus turned a corner she rolled off the seat. Here's a good one, I did that in Hyde Park when the snow was on the ground, the ducks kept pecking my equipment.

W : Ooh goodness, there's twins !

M : Ah yes, that was sensational. On the front at Brighton, crowds gathered round, the mother was so pleased and excited she paid me double.

W : I think perhaps we'd better get on with it.

M : Of course, I'm ready when you are, just let me get my tackle ready.

W : But, isn't it?

M : Yes, I mean, I just have to get it out, you see I always reckon to get the best results with a three foot stand . . . my gord, she's fainted !

IT GIVES ME GREAT PLEASURE

Dancing is the vertical expression of horizontal intention.

* * *

Virtue is insufficient temptation.

* * *

A camel is a horse designed by a committee.

* * *

Wife : If you really loved me, you would have married someone else.

* * *

Rear view of any girl in jeans=Two ferrets fighting in a sack.

* * *

A wife=A woman who can turn an old rake into a lawn mower.

* * *

It is easy for a girl to stay on the straight and narrow, if she's built that way.

* * *

Big Ben, to the Leaning Tower : I've got the time if you've got the inclination.

* * *

A doctor was asked to address a crowded meeting on sex. He rose, said : "It gives me great pleasure" and sat down.

* * *

Mummy, Mummy, why can't we give our Alice's baby a proper funeral? Oh, shut up child, and keep pulling the chain.

* * *

Driving Instructor to Vicar (who has just felled a lamp-post) : "Here endeth the first lesson !"

* * *

Report of Camera Club : Our President has produced remarkable results from a 16 year old Brownie.

* * *

There is now on offer a gadget you can screw on the bed and it does all the housework. It is called a wife.

* * *

A clever typist = One who never misses a period.

* * *

A smart secretary : She wears mink by day and fox by night.

* * *

Granddaughter (16) Tell me about the men in your life? Grandma (75) My dear, it isn't the men in your life it's the life in your men that's important.

A schoolgirl who reached adolescence
Asked : What did they mean by pubescence?
Said the Vicar : A dame
And a man, aren't the same,
And he widened the split with the difference !

Said a crafty old doctor named Hammon
Im*pote*nce is getting too common.
Pills, oysters, and honey
Are sheer waste of money,
What works, is to bed a fresh woman.

There was a young lady named Bickers
Whose cousin came off in her knickers,
A tadpole in cream
Found a split through a seam
And they had to rush round to the Vicar's.

There was a young lady named Lees
Whose titties resembled two peas,
Yet she had such technique
She could stiffen the weak,
And leave all the strong on their knees

A "teaser" in spite of all rumours
Would only have sex in her bloomers,
A rigger named Hussett
Drilled right through the gusset
And tapped her for future consumers.

DAMAGED GOODS

He had been a most eligible bachelor, but now he was on his way to get married. As luck would have it, his car was involved in an accident, and a thorough examination revealed only a ligament laceration in a most intimate place. Despite his protestations, the doctor insisted on putting a splint on it, consisting mainly of four small strips of narrow wood bound together.

When the groom and his bride were alone in their boudoir that night she proceeded to disrobe in a most provocative manner. When she unveiled her shoulders she said, "Look, Dear, never been touched by any man."

Then she stripped to the waist and said, "Look, darling, no other man's eyes have ever gazed upon these." She continued this routine until finally the groom could contain himself no longer. Indicating his damaged organ, he said, "That's nothing. Look at this ... still in the original crate!"

NIFTY THINKING

A woman walked into a very busy butcher's shop. Looking at the meats and poultry on display, she suddenly grabbed hold of a dressed chicken. She picked up one wing, sniffed it; picked up the other wing, sniffed it; picked up one leg, sniffed it; picked up the other leg, sniffed it. Just as she finished sniffing the second leg, the butcher walked up to her and said, "Madam, could *you* pass such a test?"

I SPY

There was once a playboy who had the reputation of winding up under the table every time he went to a night club with a pretty girl. Not drunk, you understand . . . just an insatiable curiosity.

And today's story has a vicar alone on the first tee. He sees a fellow standing there and suggests they play together. After a couple of holes, the stranger tells the minister what he's doing wrong. As they play along, the vicar gets more advice, all of it good. The man of the cloth finishes the round six strokes under his usual score. He thanks his golf partner and the fellow says : "That will be £25. I'm the pro here." The vicar argues but to no avail. So he tells the pro to drop over to the rectory that evening to collect his fee. "And when you come," suggests the vicar, "bring your mother and father. I'll marry them at the same time !"

BUTTONS UP

The teacher took her class of little boys and girls on an outing, near a race track. As the children left the bus, several of them had to answer the call of nature.

Naturally, the teacher helped them.

She was helping one very cute little fellow when he said: "Please miss, would you mind letting me button my own pants? I'm in a terrible hurry ... I have to get to the track in time to ride in the third race."

FULL MARKS

Diana lay sprawled in sweet exhaustion on the bed, her attire consisting of one earring. Beside her, Bob wore nothing at all. He slowly lit two cigarettes and passed one to Diana. For a long moment, smoke and silence hung in the air, then: "My mother always told me to be good," Diana said with a little smile. "Was I?"

THE HARD STUFF

The most notorious tippler in an Irish village, making his way unsteadily homeward, encountered the parish priest who inquired about the suspicious bulge in his coat pocket.

"It's holy water, Father," the culprit protested piously.

The priest removed the bottle, sniffed at it and announced that it contained whiskey.

"Glory be," cried the drunk. "A miracle!"

MARITAL BLISS

Marriage is the process of finding out what kind of man your wife would have preferred.

SMELLBOUND

A spirited session of poker was in progress as a new arrival, a practical joker, proceeded to spray the nearest player with the contents of a perfume atomizer.

"Hey, don't spray that on me," the player shouted, "my wife will think I spent the evening in a brothel!"

The player sitting next to him said, "You can squirt me if you like. My wife was never in a brothel and she won't recognize the smell."

SMALL TALK

The wife was understandably furious when she came
home unexpectedly and found her husband in bed with a
lady midget.

"You promised me two weeks ago that you would never
cheat on me again," she stormed.

Her husband shrugged nonchalantly. "Take it easy,
dear," he said airily. "Can't you see I'm tapering off?!"

MIXED EMOTIONS

Watching your mother-in-law drive over a cliff in your
brand new Jaguar.

COLD SHOULDER

The husband leaned over to his wife and asked, "Come on, darling, let's make love."

His wife replied, "George, I wish you wouldn't talk that way; the children might hear you. Whenever you're in the mood, why don't you say to me, 'Honey, I'd like to use your washing machine'."

A few nights later, the wife felt in a romantic mood and leaning over to her husband, asked, "George, would you like to use my washing machine?" George replied, "To tell you the truth, dear, it was just a small bundle. I did it by hand."

WHICH WITCH?

Once upon a time there was a beautiful young girl taking a stroll through the woods. All at once she saw an extremely ugly bull frog seated on a log and to her amazement the bull frog spoke to her.

"Maiden," croaked the frog, "would you do me a big favour? This will be hard for you to believe, but I was once a handsome, charming prince and then a mean, ugly old witch cast a spell over me and turned me into a frog."

"Oh, what a pity!" exclaimed the pretty girl. "I'll do anything I can to help you break such a spell."

"Well, Miss," replied the frog, "the only way that this spell can be taken off and I can be returned to a handsome young man again is for some lovely and pretty young girl to take me home and let me spend the night under her pillow."

The young girl took the ugly frog home and placed him beneath her pillow that night when she retired. When she awoke the next morning, sure enough, there beside her in the bed was a very young, handsome man, and plainly of royal blood.

And so they lived happily ever after, except that until this day her father and mother still do not believe her story.

BUSINESS AS USUAL

A doctor in London for a medical convention was conversing with a gorgeous blonde in the lobby of the Ritz when his wife suddenly emerged from the lift. Eyeing the departing figure, the wife snapped, "How do you happen to know her?"

"Oh, just professionally," the doctor replied.

The wife raised a sarcastic eyebrow. "Yours, or hers?" she asked.

TIDYING UP

The shapely young nurse was walking down the hospital corridor with her uniform askew and part of her bosom showing when she encountered the matron. The matron bawled her out for improper dress and shameful display of her body.

Straightening her clothes in confusion, the young nurse blurted the excuse, "I'm terribly sorry but you know those damned interns never put anything away!"

CORRESPONDENT

Blonde : "I've been receiving threatening letters in the mail—isn't that against the law?"

Lawyer : "Why yes, who has been writing them?"

Blonde : "My lover's wife."

She had her suspicions for a long time, but when he arrived home late one night with signs of lipstick on his cheek, she decided it was time to speak.

"Now look here, Reggie," she complained, "I'll have you know once and for all that I will not play second fiddle!"

"Sec'n fiddle!" he shrieked, "Sec'n fiddle! You can take it from me, Evelyn, you're damn lucky to be in the ruddy band at all!"

MONKEY GLANDS

Two old men meet on a corner.

First old man : "Where have you been for the past eight weeks?"

Second old man : "In jail."

First old man : "You in jail? How come?"

Second old man : "Well, about eight weeks ago I was standing on a corner, and this beautiful young girl rushes up with a policeman and says, 'He's the man, officer. He's the one who attacked me.' I tell you, I felt so flattered, I admitted it."

THE RED LIGHT

Two sailors were walking down the street in a strange town when a girl stuck her head out of a doorway and shouted : "Come in, fellows, and I'll give you something you've never had before." One sailor looked at the other and said : "Run like hell. She's got leprosy."

"Send me the bookkeeper," roared the senior partner.

"Listen you," he bellowed when the bookkeeper appeared. "I can't stand for too much more of this. Last year you forged three cheques in my name, six months ago you stole thousands of pounds. I discovered you were disclosing our business secrets and several nights ago you took advantage of my daughter. Now, I'm warning you—the next least little thing you do, out you go!"

The young girl had not been feeling well and went to her family doctor. "Young lady," said the doctor, "you're pregnant." "But that can't be. The only men I've been with are nudists and in our colony we practise sex only with our eyes." "Well, my dear," said the doctor, "someone in that colony is cockeyed."

MORE RUGBY JOKES

More, More!!

You thought it was all over, didn't you? You thought that the team that brought you dozens of RUGBY SONGS and RUGBY JOKES had packed their sweaty bags and gone away. Well, you were *wrong* – that was just the beginning!

Here's a whole locker-room full of jokes featuring the virgin sturgeon, a mother-in-law, the peasant and his cow, a 3-parent family, and the terrible deeds of Abdul the Bulbul Emir.

Yes, it's MORE RUGBY JOKES!

<u>RUGBY JOKES IN</u>
<u>THE LOCKER ROOM</u>

Lewd, rude and laughing all the way to the locker room
. . .

. . . another instalment of the superselling series of raunchy
rugby rib-ticklers. It's enough to make a cricket team – but
what they get up to between these pages is definitely not
cricket . . .

<u>RUGBY SONGS</u>

Unknown, but certainly not unsung, the anonymous
composers of the bawdy ditties enjoyed by rugby players –
and plenty more besides – deserve a place of honour in
rugby clubs throughout the world.

This comprehensively rude collection of more than 140
songs ranges from such classics as 'Eskimo Nell' and 'The
Good Ship Venus' to lesser known but equally worthy
gems of lewd lyricism.

☐	More Rugby Jokes	£3.50
☐	Rugby Jokes in the Locker Room	£3.50
☐	Rugby Songs	£4.50

Warner Books now offers an exciting range of quality titles by both established and new authors which can be ordered from the following address:

Little, Brown and Company (UK),
P.O. Box 11,
Falmouth,
Cornwall TR10 9EN.

Alternatively you may fax your order to the above address. Fax No. 01326 317444.

Payments can be made as follows: cheque, postal order (payable to Little, Brown and Company) or by credit cards, Visa/Access. Do not send cash or currency. UK customers and B.F.P.O. please allow £1:00 for postage and packing for the first book, plus 50p for the second book, plus 30p for each additional book up to a maximum charge of £3.00 (7 books plus).

Overseas customers including Ireland, please allow £2.00 for the first book plus £1.00 for the second book, plus 50p for each additional book.

NAME (Block Letters) ....

....

ADDRESS ....

....

....

☐ I enclose my remittance for ....

☐ I wish to pay by Access/Visa Card

Number ☐☐☐☐☐☐☐☐☐☐☐☐☐☐☐☐

Card Expiry Date ☐☐☐☐